D0470802

Musculoskeletal Ultrasound

Second Edition

Marnix T. van Holsbeeck, M.D.
Director of Musculoskeletal Radiology and Emergency Radiology in the Department of Diagnostic Imaging and Director of Orthopedic Radiology in the Bone and Joint Center at the Henry Ford Health System, Detroit, Michigan
Associate Professor of Radiology at Case Western Reserve Medical School, Cleveland, Ohio

Joseph H. Introcaso, M.D., D.M.D.
Interim Chairman, Department of Radiology, Director of Interventional and Therapeutic Neuroradiology, Lutheran General Hospital, Park Ridge, Illinois

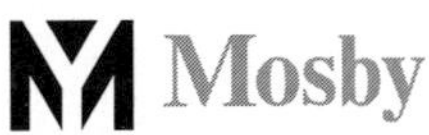

A Division of Harcourt Health Sciences
St. Louis London Philadelphia Sydney Toronto

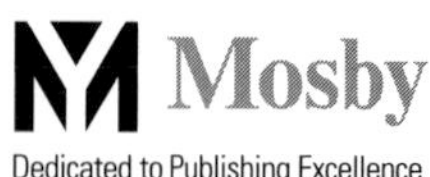

Dedicated to Publishing Excellence

Mosby, Inc.
A Harcourt Health Sciences Company
11830 Westline Industrial Drive
St. Louis, Missouri 63146

Printed in the United States of America

Library of Congress Cataloging-in-Publication Data

van Holsbeeck, Marnix T.
Musculoskeletal ultrasound/Marnix T. van Holsbeeck, Joseph H. Introcaso—2nd ed.
p. ; cm.
Includes bibliographical references and index.
ISBN 0-323-00018-5
1. Musculoskeletal system—Magnetic resonance imaging. 2. Musculoskeletal system—Diseases—Diagnosis. I. Introcaso, Joseph H. II. Title.
[DNLM: 1. Muscular Diseases—ultrasonography. 2. Bone Diseases—ultrasonography. 3. Musculoskeletal System—pathology. WE 141 V256m 2001]
RC925.7.V36 2001
616.7'07543—dc21 00-058417

00 01 02 03 04 / 9 8 7 6 5 4 3 2 1

To Beatrice, Lodewijk, Elise, Annabel, Hendrik, Mona, and Louis

MvH

To Susan, Marian, Joseph, William, and Mary

JHI

Contributors

Ruth Y. Ceulemans, M.D.
Department of Radiology
Leiden University Medical Center
Leiden, The Netherlands

Rethy K. Chhem, M.D., Ph.D., FRCPC
Associate Professor of Radiology
Chief, Musculoskeletal Imaging Section
Diagnostic Radiology Department
National University Hospital
National University of Singapore
Singapore

Michael DiPietro, M.D.
Professor of Radiology
University of Michigan
School of Medicine
Pediatric Radiologist
C. S. Mott Children's Hospital
Ann Arbor, Michigan

David P. Fessell, M.D.
Clinical Assistant Professor
Department of Radiology
University of Michigan
Ann Arbor, Michigan

H. Theodore Harcke, M.D.
Chief of Imaging Research
A. I. duPont Hospital for Children
Wilmington, Delaware
Professor of Radiology and Pediatrics
Jefferson Medical College
Philadelphia, Pennsylvania

Ronnie Ptasznik, MBBS, FRANZCR
Director of Radiology
Latrobe University Medical Centre
Visiting Radiologist
Epworth Hospital
Melbourne, Australia

Foreword

I am pleased to have been asked to contribute a foreword to Drs. van Holsbeeck and Introcaso's book on *Musculoskeletal Ultrasound.* In the present atmosphere of rapidly advancing techniques in imaging, as well as the increasing pressure for cost containment, this is an extremely timely work.

Vast areas of investigation have been opened as a result of the development of ultrasound as an imaging tool. In the past 15 years, there have been dramatic advances in imaging in the form of computerized tomography and magnetic resonance. These have developed, however, as highly expensive procedures with fixed facilities. By contrast, ultrasound provides economic, noninvasive imaging of tissues in static or dynamic states, and in serial studies where indicated. Its capacity to be easily transported adds to its value.

These unique aspects of imaging have made ultrasound especially valuable in the field of sports medicine. Ultrasound meets two very specific needs in sports medicine created by the pressure in professional athletics to return the athlete to competition as quickly as possible. First, it allows immediate identification of problems, thereby avoiding many diagnostic surgical procedures. Secondly, it allows the study of problems which are only manifest during physical activity. These same attributes also enhance the study of inflammatory conditions including infections, traumatic conditions including fractures, and dislocation and neoplastic conditions.

Drs. van Holsbeeck and Introcaso, two of the premier authorities on ultrasound, have provided a text equally valuable to the clinician and to the radiologist. In a concise manner, the book describes the clinical indications for ultrasound imaging. The authors also provide information about theory and technique for the benefit of the practicing radiologist or technician. The book is a timely and valuable text in an important and expanding field. I compliment Drs. van Holsbeeck and Introcaso for an excellent job and a fine accomplishment.

David J. Collon, M.D.
Chairman, Bone and Joint Center
Henry Ford Health System
Detroit, Michigan

Foreword

The practice of medicine has always been a balance of art and science. Examination of the soft tissues of the musculoskeletal system has been the privilege of the clinician for centuries. Those clinicians gifted with exceptionally skilled hands and other senses of clinical observation are fortunate. This clinical information formed the basis for their therapeutic decisions and professional renown. However, these data are subjective and not comparable among various examiners. The development of high resolution real-time ultrasound imaging tips the balance toward more objective and quantitative measures.

Development of the sonographic evaluation of the musculoskeletal system has in large part been limited by technology. Current state-of-the-art equipment has broken down these technological barriers. This text demonstrates the broad spectrum of applications of diagnostic ultrasound to evaluate the musculoskeletal system. It will have a profound impact on the practice of medicine in rheumatology, orthopedics, sports medicine, and traumatology. I have personally had the pleasure of seeing these techniques develop and grow in our rheumatology-orthopedic unit while Dr. van Holsbeeck was with us.

Ultrasound is the ideal modality for the examination of soft tissues because of its multiplanar and real-time capabilities. Sonography yields anatomic information during active and passive mobilization that is unattainable with other modalities. In addition, synovial and cartilage thickness can be accurately quantitated, providing an objective means of following patients with inflammatory arthritides. Ultrasound examination of deep seated joints such as the hip and shoulder is especially valuable. Joint effusions, loose bodies, tendonitis, and tendon and muscle ruptures can all be demonstrated sonographically. The noninvasive nature of the examination and lack of ionizing radiation make it very well accepted by patients, especially children.

This book is a necessity for rheumatologists, orthopedists, traumatologists, and sports medicine, physical medicine, and rehabilitation physicians. These physicians will quickly learn to utilize musculoskeletal ultrasound as an extension of the clinical diagnostic skills with which they are already so familiar.

Jan Dequeker, M.D., Ph.D.
Professor Emeritus of Rheumatology
Former Head, Division of Rheumatology
Department of Internal Medicine
Arthritis and Metabolic Bone Disease Research Unit
Katholieke University Leuven
Belgium

Preface

Since the publication of the first edition of this text, significant improvements in ultrasound equipment, a better understanding of sonographic musculoskeletal soft tissue anatomy, and changes in health care reimbursement have contributed to growing interest in ultrasound of the musculoskeletal system. The time was right to publish a follow-up to our initial work.

Soft tissues such as fibroconnective tissue, fat, and muscle contribute more than 50 percent of mass of the human body. Despite the importance of the soft tissues of the musculoskeletal system, the pathology of these tissues remains poorly understood. Magnetic resonance imaging (MRI) has improved the diagnosis of musculoskeletal pathology and has resolved some of the difficulties in diagnosis of internal joint derangement. However, the diagnosis of chronic repetitive injury, work-related injury, inflammation, and infection in soft tissues has not changed significantly during the explosive growth of MRI. Ultrasound shows great promise in this realm, but its ultimate role must still be explored.

Ultrasound shows us musculoskeletal anatomy from a new and unique perspective. The backbone of fibroconnective tissue consists of a collagenous framework. This matrix can be viewed as the microskeleton of muscles, tendons, ligaments, and nerves. Reflection of the sound beam by this collagenous framework displays structure that is imperceptible with other imaging techniques. Lesions that disrupt this framework become very obvious when examined sonographically.

A better understanding of the principles of musculoskeletal ultrasound has led to anisotropic imaging (i.e., image reconstruction based on anisotropic characteristics of collagen in connective tissue). In addition to tissue anisotropy, musculoskeletal anatomy is singular in its capability to form fluid through the synovial membrane. Ultrasound shows fluid because of the uniformity of its acoustic impedance. The capability of ultrasound to demonstrate fluid with great sensitivity and specificity proves extremely useful in the diagnosis of osteoarticular diseases. Anisotropic imaging characteristics of mesoderm and unique acoustic impedance of fluid represent the physical principles on which successful musculoskeletal ultrasound is based.

With the diagnostic success of ultrasound so tightly related to the demonstration of internal tissue architecture, we have organized the text according to anatomy. As in the first edition, we divided the text into chapters on pathology according to tissue type (histology) and according to a more regional anatomy (topographic anatomy). This new edition emphasizes the use of color Doppler and power color Doppler imaging. Important new insights in the mechanisms of disease have been grouped in Chapter 7 as a new addition to this volume. Chapter 14, on interventional musculoskeletal ultrasound, covers a subject that represents the fastest growing share of our ultrasound referrals—invasive procedures under ultrasound guidance. This chapter will be useful to those who have already started musculoskeletal ultrasound but would like to expand their scope of services.

This second edition contains more information on ultrasound anatomy, indications for musculoskeletal ultrasound examinations, and information on pathology and ultrasound signs of disease. Positioning represents the most dynamic aspect of musculoskeletal ultrasound, and more advanced techniques develop continuously. Those just starting in the field should be aware that it is vital to stay in touch with the latest developments. An excellent way to stay current on the latest techniques is to participate in the activities of the Musculoskeletal Ultrasound Society (telephone and fax: 313-973-7462 or 800-221-0058). You will also find updated material on imaging protocols and technique on the society's website (www.musoc.com).

Eleven years have passed since the publication of our first edition. A number of findings in the first edition have aged, but most information contained there has survived the test of time. This new edition shows more maturity. The steady growth of this technique and evidence of an ever-increasing number of followers prove that musculoskeletal ultrasound represents an important tool in the hands of the modern musculoskeletal practitioner.

Marnix T. van Holsbeeck, M.D.
Joseph H. Introcaso, M.D., D.M.D.

Acknowledgments

We would like to thank all who have contributed to this project. Special thanks are due to our parents and families, whose patience, understanding, and countless years of tuition payments have made this work possible. Contributions of several prominent doctors in the field enrich the content of this book and are greatly appreciated. Our orthopedic surgeons, our plastic surgeons, and our sports physicians provided superb clinical and surgical correlation for many of the cases presented here. This assistance was invaluable in confirming our sonographic impressions. Dr. Christian Hessler contributed greatly in the constructive review of our work and this manuscript. Mrs. Kidney at Codonics assisted us with the printing of color images at the last minute. Lisette Bralow, our executive editor, provided an extraordinary amount of freedom to us in the preparation of the manuscript, as well as valuable guidance. Mr. Kristo van Holsbeeck performed the statistical analysis for a number of studies presented in this text. Dr. Roeland Lysens performed clinical examinations of the patients who were included in our control groups. Finally, but not least, we thank our teachers who have shaped us over the years.

We thank you for your support!

Marnix T. van Holsbeeck, M.D.
Joseph H. Introcaso, M.D., D.M.D.

NOTICE

Contents

Chapter 1
Physical Principles of Ultrasound Imaging 1

Fundamental Principles *1*
Equipment *3*
Imaging *4*
Doppler Flow Imaging *5*
Extended Field of View Imaging *6*
Tissue Harmonic Imaging *6*
Transmission Ultrasound *6*
Conclusion *7*

Chapter 2
Artifacts in Musculoskeletal Ultrasound 9

The Good . . . *9*
The Bad . . . *15*
The Ugly . . . *21*

Chapter 3
Sonography of Muscle 23

Examination Technique *23*
Normal Sonographic Anatomy *26*
Muscle Pathology *29*

Chapter 4
Sonography of Tendons 77

Examination Technique *77*
Sonographic Tendon Anatomy *79*
Sonographic Diagnosis of Tendon Pathology *82*

Chapter 5
Sonography of Bursae 131

Examination Technique *131*
Normal Sonographic Bursa Structure *131*
Pathology of Bursae *136*

Chapter 6
Sonography of Ligaments 171

Examination Technique *171*
Normal Sonographic Structure of Ligament *171*
Ligament Pathology *175*

Chapter 7
Pathophysiology and Patterns of Disease 193

Muscle Rupture *193*
Tendon Rupture *194*
Tendinosis *221*
Chronic Overuse *224*
Ligament Tears *227*

Chapter 8
Sonography of Large Synovial Joints 235

Examination Technique *235*
Normal Sonographic Anatomy *236*
Sonography of Articular Pathology *238*

Chapter 9
Pediatric Musculoskeletal and Spinal Sonography 277
Michael A. DiPietro, M.D., and Theodore Harcke, M.D.

Developmental Dysplasia of the Hip *227*
Epiphyseal Alignment *292*
Extremity Deformities *295*
Inflammation and Infection *295*
Fibromatosis Colli *299*
The Spinal Canal *299*

Chapter 10
Sonography of the Dermis, Hypodermis, Periosteum, and Bone 325

Epidermis, Dermis, and Hypodermis *325*
Periosteum *333*

Bone *337*
Measurement to Detect Abnormal Development of the Extremities *355*
Tumors *359*

Chapter 11
Sonography of Rheumatoid Disease 373
Rethy K. Chhem, M.D., Ph.D., FRCPC, and Marnix T. van Holsbeeck, M.D.

Diagnosis *373*
Follow-up of Rheumatoid Arthritis *382*
Complications of Rheumatoid Disease *382*

Chapter 12
Evaluation of Foreign Bodies 393

Examination Technique *393*
Ultrasound Versus Radiography *395*
Diagnostic Approach to Foreign Bodies *405*
Orthopedic Implants *407*
Summary *414*

Chapter 13
Sonography of Pain Syndromes Following Arthroscopy 419

Pain Syndromes Following Therapeutic Arthroscopy *419*
Pain Following Diagnostic Arthroscopy *425*

Chapter 14
Interventional Musculoskeletal Ultrasound 427

Examination Technique *427*
Applications *428*

Chapter 15
Sonography of the Shoulder 463
Ronnie Ptasznik, MBBS, FRANZCR

Introduction *463*
Clinical Aspects *463*
Instrumentation *465*
Examination Technique *465*
Joint Fluid *473*
Rotator Cuff Disease *474*
Rotator Cuff Tears *477*
Calcific Tendinitis *488*
Acromioclavicular Joint *490*
Suprascapular Nerve Compression *491*
Fractures of the Greater Tuberosity *491*
Subacromial Bursa *492*
Postoperative Assessment *495*
Long Head of Biceps Tendon (LHB) *498*
Adhesive Capsulitis *504*
Instability *505*
Arthropathy *506*
Anatomical Variations *511*
Reporting Method *512*
Conclusion *513*

Chapter 16
Sonography of the Elbow, Wrist, and Hand 517

The Elbow *517*
The Wrist and Hand *531*

Chapter 17
Sonography of the Hip 573
David P. Fessell, M.D., and Marnix T. van Holsbeeck, M.D.

Hip Pain: Imaging Options and the Role of Ultrasound *573*
Scanning Technique *573*
Hip Pain *573*
Ultrasound of the Prosthetic Hip *580*
Hip Snaps, Locks, and Clicks *581*

Chapter 18
Sonography of the Knee 587
Ruth Y. Ceulemans, M.D., and Marnix T. van Holsbeeck, M.D.

Technical Guidelines and Scanning Technique *587*
Summary of the Routine Examination *590*
Swelling *590*
Acute Knee Injury *594*
Chronic Localized Knee Pain *598*
Limited Use in Internal Derangement *599*
Postoperative Knee *601*

Chapter 19
Sonography of the Ankle and Foot 605
David P. Fessell, M.D., and Marnix T. van Holsbeeck, M.D.

Technical Guidelines and Scanning Technique *605*
Acute Injuries of the Ankle *607*
Chronic Ankle Pain *611*
Soft Tissue Masses *619*
Heel Pain *619*
Metatarsalgia *620*

Appendix: Table of Normal Values 625

Index 629

Chapter 1 Physical Principles of Ultrasound Imaging

Ultrasound is defined as sound having a frequency greater than that which is audible by humans. The human ear functions over a frequency range of 15,000 to 20,000 cycles per second (hertz). Thus, any sound having a frequency greater than 20 kilohertz (kHz) falls into the category of ultrasound. Medical imaging today most commonly uses frequencies ranging from 2 to 12 megahertz (MHz).

The practical use of ultrasound has evolved slowly, largely due to limitations imposed by equipment. In 1912 the first significant attempt at practical application of ultrasound was made in the unsuccessful search for the wreck of the *Titanic.* Technological advances made during the Second World War led to the development of SONAR (*S*ound *N*avigation *A*nd *R*anging), which played an important role in the war at sea. Following the war, Dr. Douglas Howry applied this technology to medical applications with limited success. It was not until the development of B-mode imaging that ultrasound began to have a prominent position in medical diagnosis. Another leap forward occurred with the advent of gray scale imaging in 1972. The application of digital computers to sonographic imaging in the late 1970s led to the development of real-time gray scale imaging as we know it today.

Fundamental Principles

Sound waves and x-ray photons both are forms of energy transmission. However, that is where the similarity between the two ends. Their interactions with matter are quite dissimilar. The ways in which these two forms of energy interact with matter determines how they can be used in medical imaging. Unlike radiography, ultrasound imaging most commonly utilizes energy reflected back to the source to produce an image. This is referred to as *pulse-echo imaging.*

X-rays are best transmitted through a vacuum, but sound requires matter for its transmission. The speed at which x-ray photons travel is constant. However, the speed of sound varies with the type of matter through which it passes. Table 1–1 lists the speed of sound through a variety of substances. The factors that determine the speed of sound through a substance are density and compressibility. Materials with the greatest density and least compressibility will transmit sound at the highest velocity.

Sound is reflected at interfaces between materials. Two factors influence reflectivity: the acoustic impedance of the two materials and the angle of incidence of the sound beam. Acoustic impedance is the product of a material's density and the speed of sound within that substance. Reflectivity is greatest at interfaces between materials with dissimilar acoustic impedance, as defined by the following equation:

$$R = \left(\frac{Z_2 - Z_1}{Z_2 + Z_1}\right)^2 \times 100$$

where R is the percentage of sound beam reflected and Z_1 and Z_2 are the acoustic impedances, assuming an angle of incidence of 90 degrees.

The data in Table 1–2 indicate that interfaces between soft tissue and air should be highly reflective, which is what we observe clinically. With this in mind, it is clear why a coupling gel must be used to ensure contact between the ultrasound transducer and the patient's skin. The previous equation tells us that 99.9% of a sound beam is reflected at any tissue–air interface. In areas of poor contact with the skin, where an air gap exists, essentially no energy is available for imaging.

Reflection of a sound beam varies greatly with the angle of incidence. The least reflection occurs with the sound beam perpendicular to the reflecting interface, in other words, an angle of incidence of 90 degrees. As the angle of incidence is decreased,

Table 1–1
Speed of Sound Through Various Substances

Transmitting Substance	Speed of Sound (m/sec)
Air	331
Fat	1,450
Water	1,540
Liver	1,549
Blood	1,570
Muscle	1,585
Cortical bone	4,080

Table 1–2
Acoustic Impedance of Various Materials

Material	Acoustic Impedance (gm/cm^2 sec × 10^{-5})
Air	0.0004
Fat	1.38
Water	1.54
Blood	1.61
Muscle	1.70
Cortical bone	7.8

the percentage of the sound beam reflected increases. Beyond a certain angle, the entire sound beam is reflected. In addition, the direction of the reflected beam is determined by the angle of incidence (Fig. 1–1). This is important to keep in mind when imaging an object with a curved surface, such as the femoral condyles or the diaphysis of a long bone. As the angle of incidence is decreased, the beam will be reflected away from the transducer and will not contribute to the image (Fig. 1–2). Therefore, the optimal scanning pattern for a curved surface is an arc that keeps the beam perpendicular to the surface of the object to be imaged (Fig. 1–3).

Spatial localization will also be impaired when the angle of incidence is less than 90 degrees. This phenomenon is known as *refraction.* Refraction is a change in the direction of a sound beam occurring at an interface between two dissimilar materials when the beam is not perpendicular to the interface. A change in the wavelength of the sound beam occurs in accommodation to the different speed of sound in the new material. This acts to "bend" the beam. The magnitude of the change in direction of the sound beam is proportional to the difference of the speed of sound within the two materials and inversely proportional to the angle of incidence. In most circumstances, the error introduced by refraction is not significant. However, under certain conditions, the true location of an object will differ significantly from its imaged position.

As a sound beam passes through a material, a portion of its energy is absorbed by frictional forces. The energy is converted to heat and no longer contributes to the imaging process. Viscosity, relaxation time, and temperature of the material, along with the frequency of the sound beam, all affect absorption. Of these factors, the one that can be modified in the clinical setting is the frequency of the transducer. The degree of absorption of a sound beam in soft tissue is directly proportional to its frequency. If the fre-

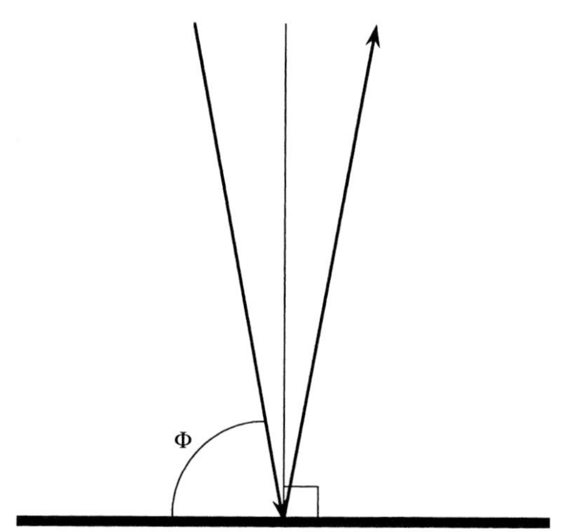

Figure 1–1 ■ Reflection of sound and angle of incidence (Φ).

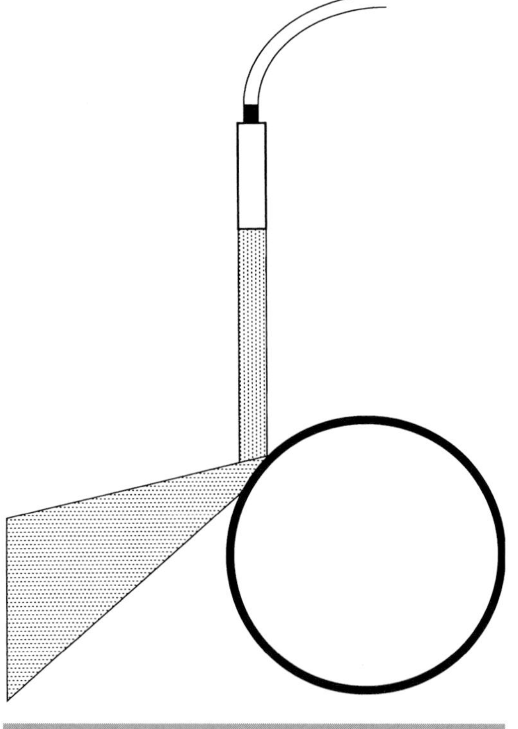

Figure 1–2 ■ Improper imaging of a curved object.

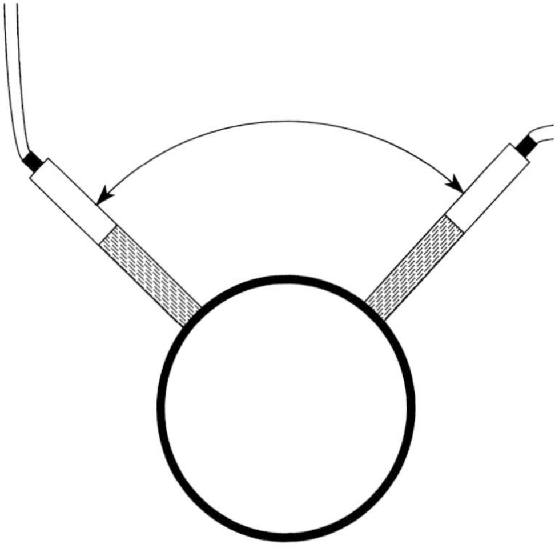

Figure 1–3 ▪ Optimal imaging of a curved object.

quency of the sound beam is doubled, absorption will double. This becomes important in selecting a transducer because spatial resolution is also proportional to frequency. The best transducer for a specific examination is one having the highest frequency that can penetrate to the desired depth within the soft tissues being examined. This will result in images with the greatest possible spatial resolution.

Equipment

Four types of ultrasound transducers are currently available: (1) sector scanners, (2) annular arrays, (3) radial arrays, and (4) linear arrays. The basic principles governing their function are identical for the four types. They differ only in how some of the components are arranged (Fig. 1–4). Annular arrays

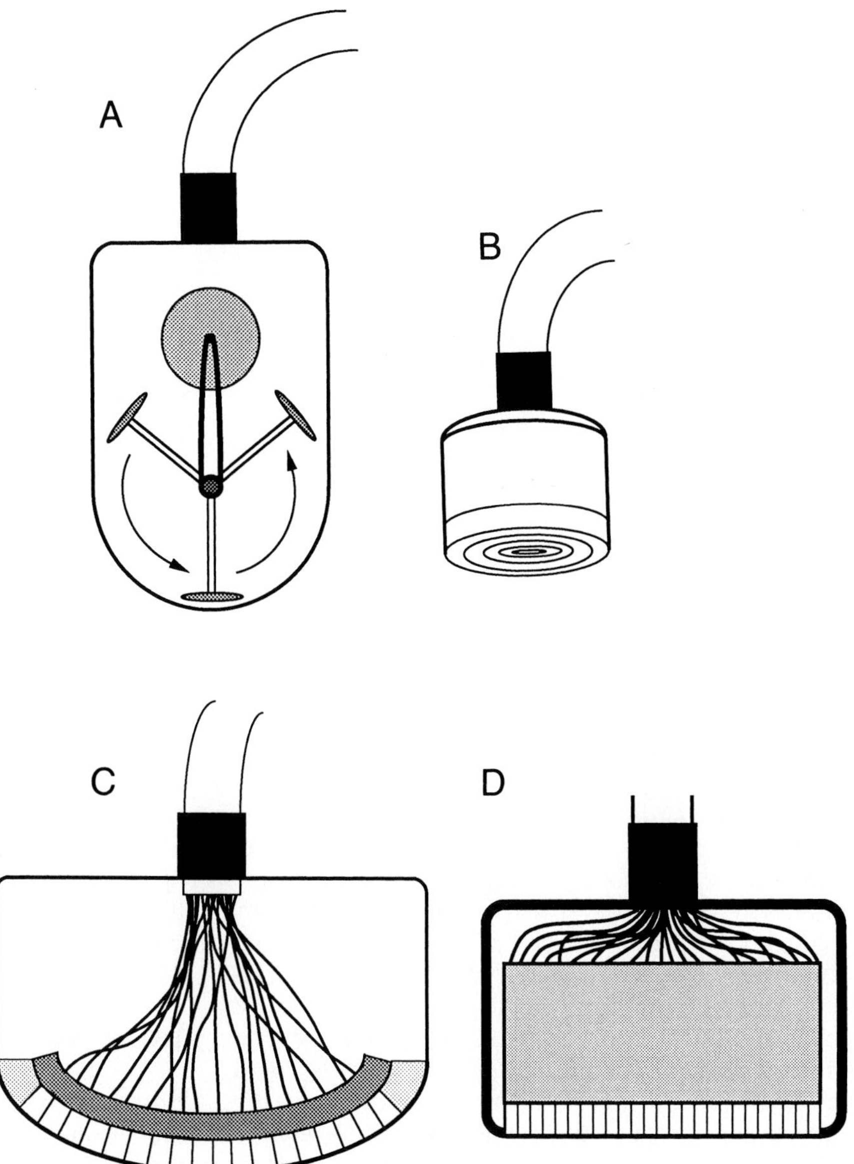

Figure 1–4 ▪ **A,** Sector scanning transducer. **B,** Annular array transducer. **C,** Radial array transducer. **D,** Linear array transducer.

are the least familiar because they are used predominantly in cardiac and ophthalmological examinations.

The heart of an ultrasound transducer is a piezoelectric crystal. These crystals, discovered by Pierre and Jacques Curie in 1880, have unique physical and electrical properties. When a voltage pulse is applied to a piezoelectric crystal, it vibrates and produces sound at a specific resonant frequency. In addition, if a mechanical force is applied to a piezoelectric crystal, an electrical potential will result. These properties make piezoelectric crystals ideal for ultrasound transducers because the same element serves as both transmitter and receiver of the ultrasound beam. The original materials described by the Curies were quartz and Rochelle salts, but these have been replaced in modern medical imaging equipment by lead zirconate titanate.

How these crystals are incorporated into an imaging transducer is demonstrated schematically in Figure 1–4A–D. Two opposing sides of the crystal are plated with a metallic conductor, usually gold, to serve as electrical contacts. Electrical leads attached to the plated surfaces deliver the electrical pulses to the crystal and conduct the potential generated by the crystal when it detects the reflected sound beam. The crystal surface facing the patient may be in contact with an acoustic lens that helps to focus the sound beam. These lenses are usually formed of polystyrene and use the principle of refraction to focus the sound beam. This unit is separated from the patient by an insulating layer that protects the patient from possible electrical shock and protects the crystal from contamination. The other side of the piezoelectric crystal is in contact with a backing block that dampens the vibration of the crystal and absorbs sound moving away from the patient. This assembly is protected from noise by a layer of acoustic insulating material and enclosed within a plastic housing.

The operating characteristics of a transducer are described by its resonant frequency and the Q factor. Two properties of a transducer are described by the Q factor: the purity of sound produced and the ring down time. *Ring down time* refers to the time required for the crystal to stop vibrating. Piezoelectric crystals with a high Q factor produce pure sound but have a long ring down time. Crystals with a low Q factor produce a sound beam containing a relatively wide variety of frequencies but have a short ring down time. Crystals with a relatively low Q factor are most desirable for use in medical imaging because they are sensitive to a wider frequency range of sound returning to the transducer, and the short ring down time reduces interference with the returning signal. Careful selection of the backing block utilized in the transducer can enhance the operating characteristics by further reducing the ring down time.

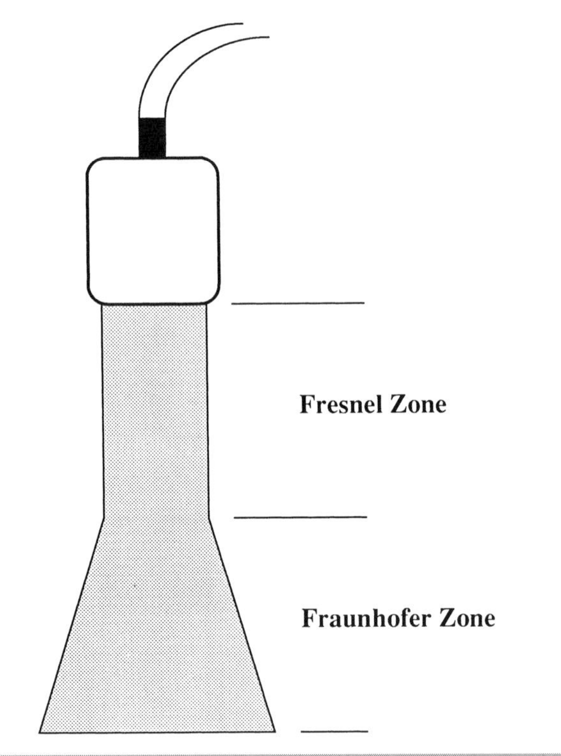

Figure 1–5 ■ Fresnel and Fraunhofer zones of a sound beam.

The sound beam emitted by the transducer has a shape that changes with its distance from the transducer (Fig. 1–5). In the near field, the borders of the sound beam are almost parallel, referred to as the *Fresnel zone.* At a certain distance from the transducer, the beam diverges, referred to as the *Fraunhofer zone.* The point of transition varies with the frequency and width of the sound beam. As the frequency and width of the beam increase, the Fresnel zone (parallel borders) becomes longer. Side lobes are also present, extending laterally from the main beam, called the *Twilight zone.* (No! Just kidding.) These side lobes are usually less than 1% of the intensity of the main beam and thus are rarely clinically significant. When they do contribute to an image, they have the same effect as beam width artifact, described in Chapter 2. Acoustic lenses and the firing sequence of an array of crystals can be used to modify the shape of the ultrasound beam.

Imaging

Ultrasound images are composed of a matrix of picture elements. Gray scale images are produced by the display of echos returning to the transducer as picture elements (pixels) varying in brightness in proportion to the intensity of the echo. The location of the echo to be displayed is determined by the location on the transducer receiving the echo and the time of flight. Time of flight is the time elapsed between initiation of the sound pulse and its return to the transducer.

In ultrasound imaging we speak of two types of resolution: axial and horizontal. *Axial resolution* is the ability to distinguish two objects as being separate when they lie directly over each other, that is, aligned sequentially along the length of the beam. The frequency of the transducer and the Q factor determine axial resolution. A higher-frequency transducer will provide greater axial resolution. Since the Q factor of the transducer is determined by the manufacturer, selection of transducer frequency is the only control the examiner has over axial resolution.

Horizontal resolution is the ability to distinguish two objects as separate when they are located side by side at the same distance from the transducer. Beam width is the determining factor in horizontal resolution. Factors determining beam width relate to focusing of the ultrasound beam, principally whether imaging is performed in the Fresnel or Fraunhofer zones. The examiner has little control over beam width, and therefore horizontal resolution, because it is largely a function of transducer design. Therefore, careful attention should be paid to transducer specifications when an ultrasound machine is purchased.

Divergence of the sound beam, absorption, and scattering all play a role in attenuation of the ultrasound beam within the body. A sound beam undergoes an exponential decrease in intensity as it passes through tissue. If uncorrected, this attenuation would result in images that are markedly decreased in diagnostic information with increasing distance from the transducer. Correction for attenuation is made by amplifying echos returning to the transducer using an exponential function based on the time of flight. This type of correction is called *time gain compensation.* The examiner may modify the correction function using controls on the ultrasound unit to optimize the information displayed.

Doppler Flow Imaging

Doppler ultrasound imaging is rapidly finding increasing application in the diagnosis of disorders of the musculoskeletal system. Local hyperemia is often associated with focal tendon lesions and a synovial reaction in inflammatory arthropathies. Granulation tissue at sites of healing is also quite vascular. These alterations in tissue vascularity can often be observed using Doppler ultrasound imaging.

The basic principle of Doppler ultrasound lies in the observation that the frequency of a sound beam reflected back to the source is altered when it encounters a moving object. The frequency increases if the object is moving toward the source and decreases if it is moving away. The change in frequency is proportional to the velocity of the object, which can be determined by the equation

$$\Delta F = (2F_T v/c) \cos\theta$$

where ΔF is the change in frequency of the sound beam, F_T is the transmitted frequency, v is the velocity of the object, c is the speed of sound within the substance, and θ is the angle of incidence of the sound beam relative to the direction of motion of the object. An important aspect of this equation to note is the effect of the angle of incidence of the sound beam on frequency shift. The greatest frequency shift occurs when the sound beam is traveling along the same trajectory as the object being evaluated. No frequency shift occurs when the angle of incidence of the ultrasound beam is 90 degrees ($\cos 90 = 0$).

In musculoskeletal imaging, the two most common ways of presenting flow-related information involve either color flow or power Doppler images. *Color flow* Doppler images present the frequency shift data by converting them into a spectrum of color, which encodes both directional and velocity information. The benefit of having both types of information is the principal advantage of color flow Doppler imaging. The disadvantages of color flow are that it is extremely sensitive to the angle of incidence of the sound beam, aliasing can occur, and noise will result in image artifacts. *Aliasing* is an artifact related to the pulsed Doppler technique when large frequency shifts occur. If the sampling frequency (pulse repetition frequency [PRF]) is too low (less than half of the frequency shift encountered), then aliasing will result. This can be dealt with by either increasing the PRF or increasing the Doppler angle, which will result in a smaller frequency shift.

Power Doppler differs from color flow in that it displays in color information on the amplitude (power) of the Doppler signal, rather than the frequency data directly. This approach has several advantages. Power Doppler is less angle dependant, no aliasing is experienced, and noise results in much less image degradation. In addition, power Doppler is much more sensitive to slow flow. The major disadvantages of this technique are that the direction and velocity information is lost. However, in musculoskeletal ultrasound, direction and velocity information is usually of little value. Therefore, power Doppler usually proves to be the more valuable technique.

Extended Field of View Imaging

One of the significant limitations of ultrasound imaging has been its limited field of view. However, recent advances in computer hardware and software have made possible extended field of view ultrasound imaging without the use of an articulated arm or special position sensors (SieScape, Siemens Medical Systems, Iselin, N.J.). High-speed video image processing hardware analyzes sequential frames acquired from a linear array transducer as it is moved slowly over the region being examined. The direction of motion is determined by dividing each image into a group of blocks of equal size and comparing sequential image frames. Each block is examined to determine a motion vector for that block, which is dependent on the degree of change occurring within that block. The individual motion vectors are then analyzed to determine the overall direction of transducer motion. If all vectors are in the same direction and have equal magnitude, then transducer motion must be linear. Transducer motion with a rotational component will yield vectors which vary in direction and magnitude. This type of imaging proves most valuable when evaluating long muscles, tendons, and vessels. Measurement across the extended field of view is accurate and proves useful in selection and preoperative assessment of soft tissue grafts.

Tissue Harmonic Imaging

Improvements in transducer technology, specifically the development of "multifrequency" transducers, have opened the door to greater tissue characterization through a technique referred to as tissue harmonics (Fig. 1–6). This technique exploits the characteristic resonant frequency of tissues, which fortunately fall in the range of diagnostic ultrasound. When a tissue is examined using ultrasound, the signal of greatest amplitude returning to the transducer is observed at the frequency of the transmitted signal. However, a second quite prominent peak is observed at a frequency approximately double that of the transmitted signal. This is called the second harmonic. Characteristics of the tissue being examined determine the exact characteristics of this second harmonic. Band-pass filtering techniques can then be employed to isolate this second harmonic, which can be used to enhance tissue contrast in diagnostic ultrasound images.

Transmission Ultrasound

Recent developments in equipment and image processing techniques have made the production of high-quality images using transmitted ultrasound possible in much the same way that computed to-

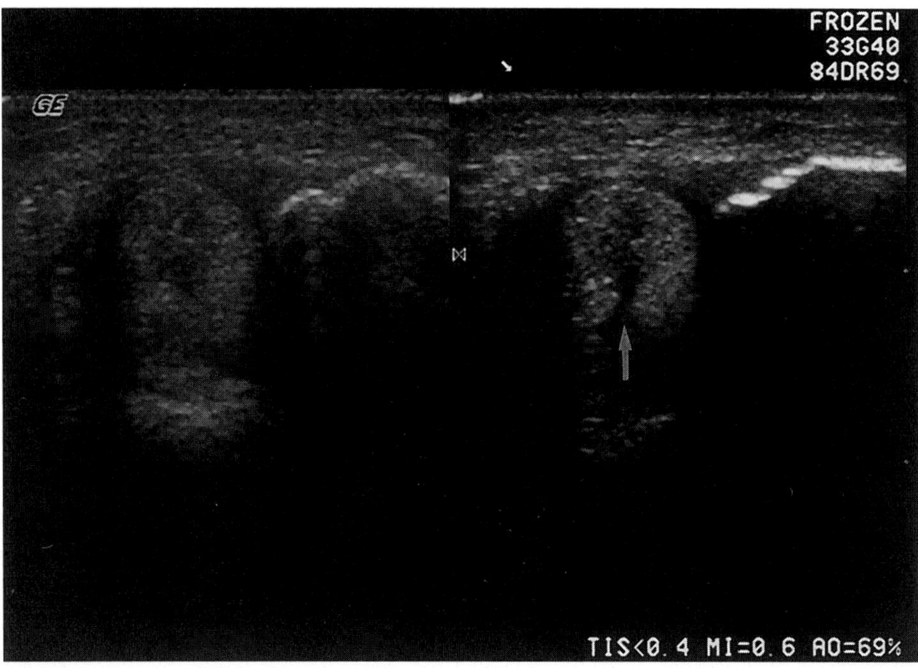

Figure 1–6 ▪ Tissue harmonic imaging. This split-screen image shows an almost identical transverse section through the same diseased posterior tibial tendon (PTT) at the level of the medial malleolus. The regular gray-scale image is displayed on the left while the image obtained with tissue harmonics shows at the right. Notice how much easier it is to visualize the partial-thickness tear (*arrow*) in the PTT with tissue harmonics. The new technique clearly shows extension of the PTT tear to the surface; this significant finding may change a conservative approach into surgical treatment. Tissue harmonics improves the visualization of the surfaces of a tear and it clears fluid from reverberation artifact—two important features in musculoskeletal ultrasound.

mography images are produced. Two transducers are utilized, positioned to face each other. One serves as the signal source, and the other is the receiver. The most recent examples have demonstrated exquisite contrast resolution and anatomical detail. Imaging is currently limited to the extremities due to the requirement of a water path. It is hoped that further development will continue, resulting in a clinical transmission ultrasound imaging system. Transmission ultrasound has proven valuable for bone densitometry. A clinical unit is now available for measurement of bone density, using the calcaneus as the standard for evaluation.

Conclusion

The purpose of this chapter is not to provide a thorough review of ultrasound physics that will enable readers to pass their specialty board examination. Its goal is to present technical information about ultrasound imaging that will allow readers to improve the diagnostic quality of images produced daily in clinical practice. Its success can be determined only by the individual reader, but if you have read it to this point, perhaps that too can be considered a success.

Bibliography

Bronzino J: *Technology for Patient Care.* St Louis, CV Mosby, 1977.

Carpenter DA: Ultrasonic transducers. *Clin Diagn Ultrasound* 5:31, 1980.

Curry TS, Dowdey JE, Murry RC: *Christensen's Introduction to the Physics of Diagnostic Radiology,* ed 3. Philadelphia, Lea & Febiger, 1984.

Goodsitt M: In Taveras J, Ferrucci JT (eds): *Radiology: Diagnosis-Imaging-Intervention,* Vol 1. Philadelphia, JB Lippincott, 1986.

Hentz VR, Green PS, Arditi M: Imaging studies of the cadaver hand using transmission ultrasound. *Skeletal Radiol* 16:474–480, 1987.

Kremkau F: *Diagnostic Ultrasound: Physical Principles and Exercises.* New York, Grune & Stratton, 1980.

Rose JL, Goldberg BB: *Basic Physics in Diagnostic Ultrasound.* New York, Wiley, 1979.

Rumack CM, Wilson SR, Charboneau JW: *Diagnostic Ultrasound,* 2nd ed. St Louis, Mosby–Year Book, 1998.

Sarti D: *Diagnostic Ultrasound,* ed 2, Chicago, Year Book Medical, 1987.

Wells PNT: *Biomedical Ultrasonics.* New York, Academic Press, 1977.

Wells PNT: Real-time scanning systems. *Clin Diagn Ultrasound* 5:69, 1980.

Chapter 2 Artifacts in Musculoskeletal Ultrasound

All imaging modalities are subject to artifacts that are unique to that system. In radiography systems, artifacts degrade images and reduce their diagnostic value. Sonographic imaging differs in that some artifacts may facilitate the ability to make the correct diagnosis. Artifacts in ultrasound can be categorized in three ways, much like an old Clint Eastwood movie: the good, the bad, and the ugly. Therefore, it is especially important to be aware of the various types of artifacts and the circumstances in which they may be encountered. We must recognize the good artifacts to optimize our diagnostic accuracy. The bad and ugly artifacts must be identified so that they may be corrected or ignored.

The Good . . .

Shadowing

At a highly reflective interface, almost all of the energy of a sound beam incident on that interface will be reflected. A minimal amount of energy will pass deep to this interface and will be available for imaging. The result is a signal void deep to the hyperreflective object. On sonographic images this signal void appears similar to the shadow cast by a building on a sunny day.

In clinical imaging, shadowing is seen at interfaces of materials that differ significantly in acoustic impedance. Classic examples of materials that produce shadowing in vivo are bone, air, calcifications, and biliary and renal calculi. *Dirty shadowing* is a characteristic exhibited by gas within the soft tissues. It is a form of reverberation artifact that produces false echos deep to the highly reflective soft tissue–gas interface. If dirty shadowing is not observed, the differential diagnosis can usually be narrowed by consideration of the region being examined. For example, shadowing from an object within muscle is usually caused by myositis ossificans, arterial calcification, or a foreign body (Figs. 2–1, 2–2). The clinical history will further narrow the list, usually allowing a definitive diagnosis to be made.

Refractile shadowing or *critical angle shadowing* is observed when objects with highly curved surfaces, such as the diaphysis of a long bone, are imaged. However, the interface need not be as highly reflective as a soft tissue–bone interface. Large arteries and the gallbladder can demonstrate refractile shadowing. The shadow is observed at the lateral margins of the object, where the sound beam contacts the interface at a very oblique angle (Figs. 2–3 through 2–5). Due to both refraction and reflection, essentially none of the incident sound beam returns to the transducer from that region. The result is an acoustic shadow. Refractile shadowing is a common finding at the ends of torn, retracted tendons. When associated with a torn tendon, refractile shadowing will almost invariably signify a full-thickness tear. The distance between the acoustic shadowing deep to the rounded edges of the proximal and distal stumps of the tendon will accurately reflect the degree of tendon retraction. In rare circumstances, one may observe this type of shadowing in partial tears when a torn flap of tendon folds back upon itself. Refractile shadowing is most obvious in musculoskeletal imaging when the surface of a tissue folds acutely along an interface with another tissue of markedly different acoustic impedance (Figs. 2–6 through 2–8).

On occasion, shadowing will not be observed deep to objects that usually shadow. This situation occurs when the object expected to shadow is small relative to the ultrasound beam width or the axial resolution of the transducer. Inappropriate positioning of the focal zone will also minimize acoustic shadows. In addition, high levels of background noise will obscure shadowing. These problems will

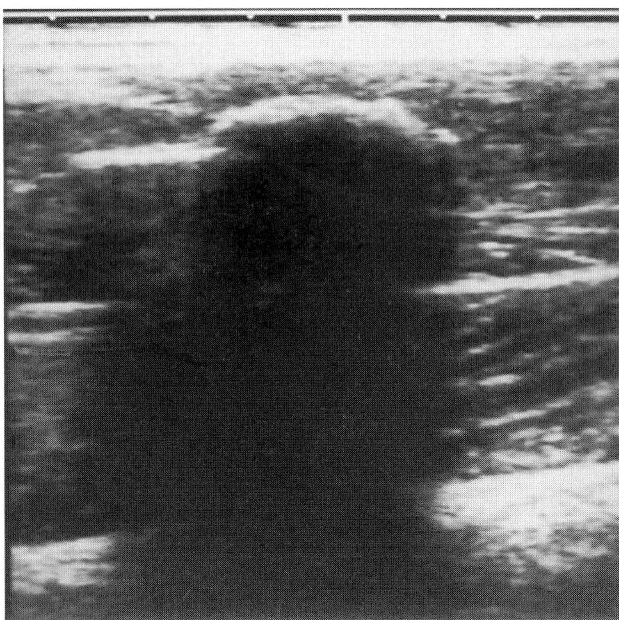

Figure 2-1 ■ Acoustic shadowing deep to myositis ossificans.

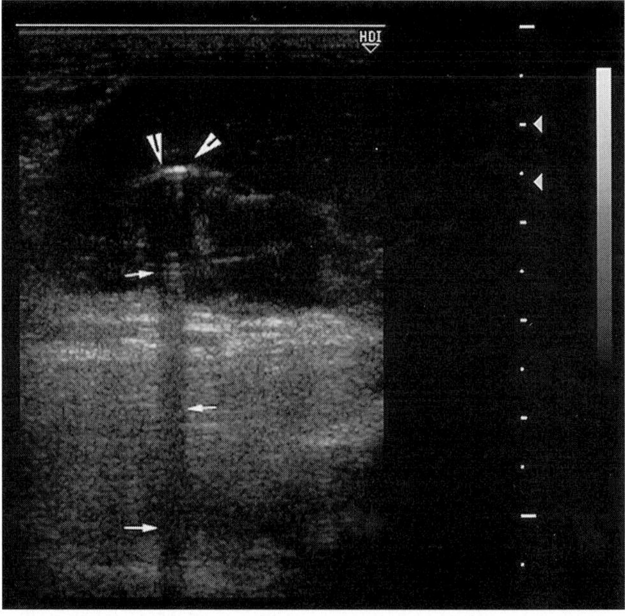

Figure 2-2 ■ Acoustic shadowing often assists us in finding foreign bodies in the soft tissues. A polyethylene drainage catheter (*arrowheads*) is demonstrated within an infected prepatellar bursa. Refraction artifact associated with curved and irregular surfaces can cast distinct acoustic shadows (*arrows*).

be discussed further in the sections on bad and ugly artifacts.

Enhanced Through-Transmission

The intensity of echos returning to the transducer decreases exponentially with increasing depth in the tissues being examined. Superficial echos may be 106 times greater in amplitude than those from the deeper tissues. If the discrepancy is uncorrected, the result will be a rapid decline in image definition with increasing depth. Time gain compensation is the primary means of correcting for this discrepancy in the image to be displayed. Echos returning to the transducer from deeper structures are amplified based on a curve that increases exponentially with time. This method of correction results in the artifact we know as *increased through-transmission.*

This method of image processing assumes that all materials attenuate sound equally—a false assumption. When a structure that does not attenuate the sound beam as much as surrounding tissues is encountered, more sound is available to image the structures at deeper levels. Therefore, echos returning to the transducer have greater amplitude. These echos are further amplified by the time gain compensation. The result is a false impression of increased echogenicity of the deeper structures. Enhanced through-transmission is most commonly seen deep to anechoic structures, usually simple fluid. A fluid-filled bursa and the urinary bladder are common examples (Figs. 2-9, 2-10). With this in mind, it is clear why enhanced through-transmission is one of the criteria used to make the diagnosis of a simple cyst.

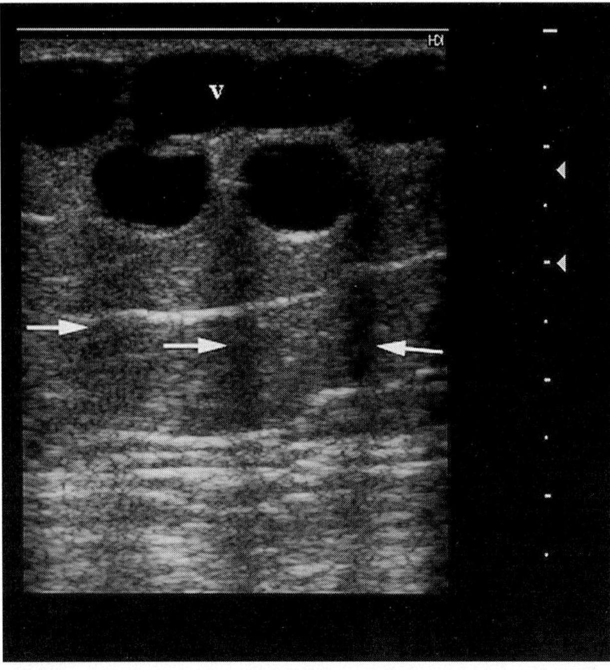

Figure 2-3 ■ Refractile shadowing (*arrows*) occurring at the edges of varices (*V*) in the subcutaneous tissues of the thigh.

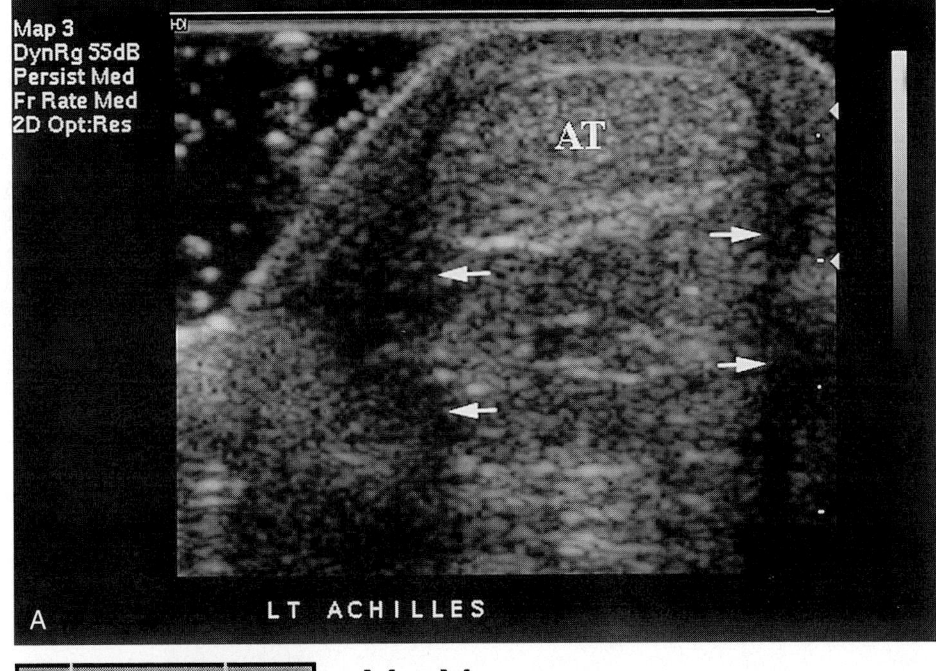

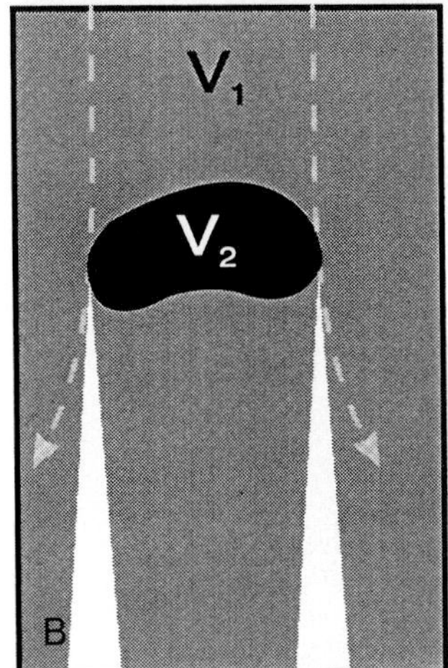

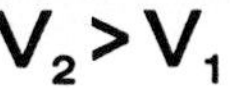

Figure 2-4 ■ **A,** Refractile shadowing (*arrows*) at the edges of the normal Achilles tendon (*AT*) on transverse imaging. **B,** Refractile shadowing is characterized by reflection of sound away from the transducer at the interface between two tissues. Refraction occurs at an interface only when there is a velocity change between two tissues and the sound beam strikes the interface at an oblique angle. V_1 = speed of sound in the fat surrounding the Achilles tendon; V_2 = speed of sound in the Achilles tendon.

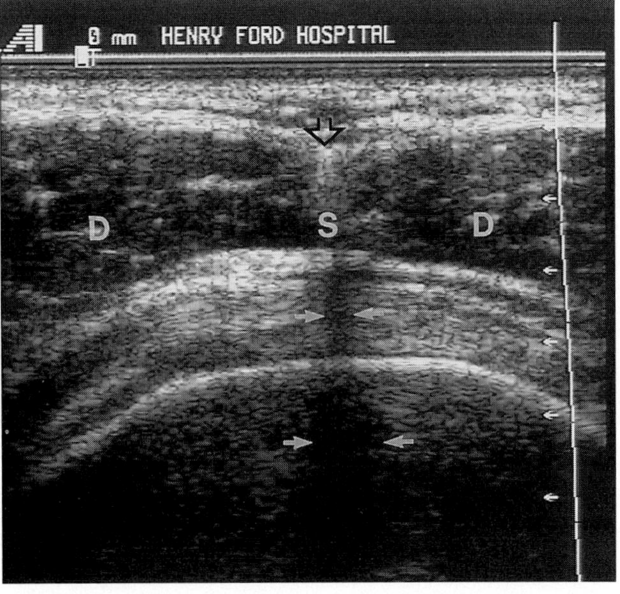

Figure 2-5 ■ Refractile shadowing (*arrows*) from a septum (*S*) within the deltoid muscle (*D*) of an athlete can mimic a rotator cuff tear. Refraction is caused at the abrupt interface between the hyperechoic septum and the hypoechoic muscle. Note the indentation (*open arrow*) of the overlying fascia.

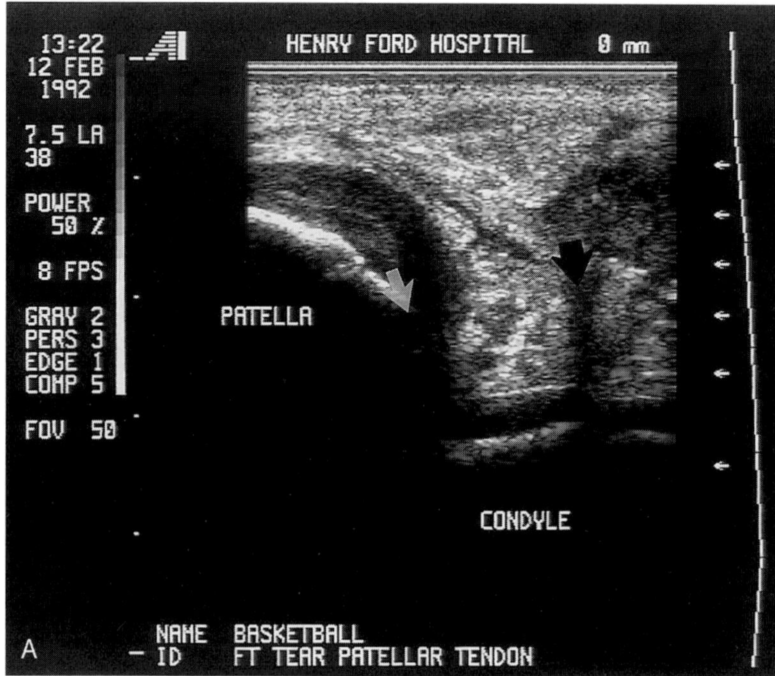

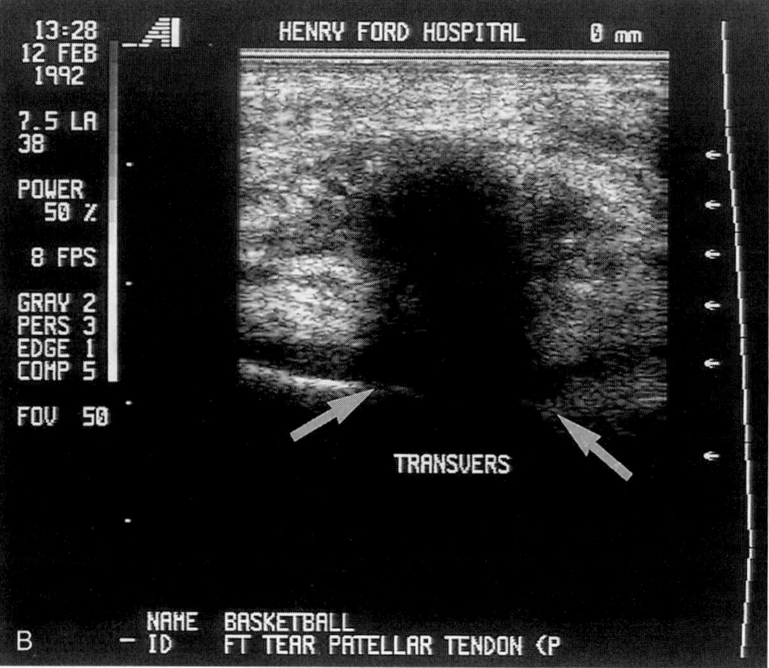

Figure 2–6 ■ **A,** Refractile shadowing is seen deep to the torn edge of the proximal (*white arrow*) and distal stumps (*black arrow*) of a full-thickness patellar tendon tear. Longitudinal image. **B,** Refractile shadowing deep to the distal end of a torn patellar tendon in transverse view. A segment (*arrows*) of the femoral condyle cannot be seen due to the broad shadow.

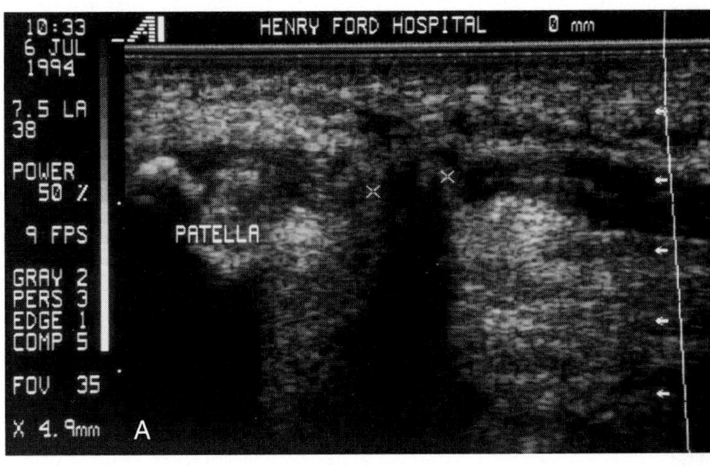

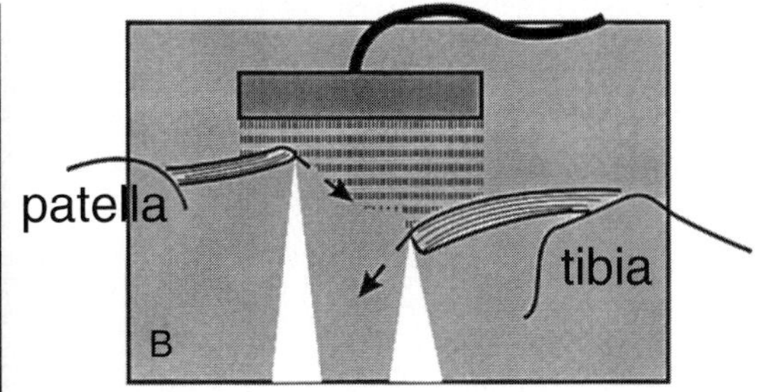

Figure 2-7 ■ **A,** Refractile shadowing seen in a full-thickness tear of the patellar tendon at its midpoint. There is little retraction of the torn tendon ends; therefore, shadowing is the only sign of rupture (*x–x*). At surgery, there was no evidence of calcification in the ends of the tendon, thus confirming refraction as the cause of acoustic shadowing. **B,** Diagram representing refractile shadowing in a full-thickness patellar tendon rupture at its midpoint. The tear disrupts the fibrillar architecture of the tendon focally. Refractile shadowing results from reflection of the sound beam in all directions by the disorganized, torn tendon fibers. Only a minimal portion of the incident sound beam is reflected back to the transducer.

Comet Tail Artifact

Metal and glass will produce characteristic bands of increased echogenicity deep to the object. These bands cross tissue boundaries, including the boundaries of tissues that produce shadowing. The intensity of these echogenic bands decreases with distance from the object, giving the appearance of the tail of a comet.

This artifact has been shown to result from reverberation occurring within the metallic or glass object. Figure 2–11 demonstrates diagrammatically how the sound beam is repeatedly reflected between the highly reflective anterior and posterior

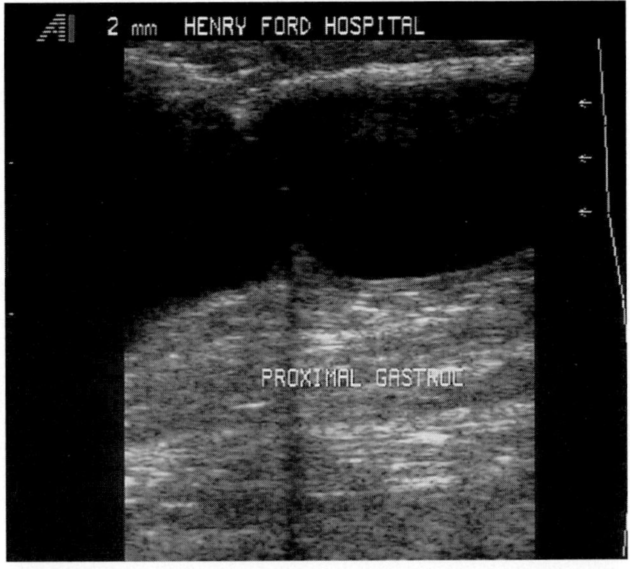

Figure 2-8 ■ Refractile shadowing due to tissue infolding. A synovial fold in the wall of a Baker cyst casts an acoustic shadow deep to the cyst. This type of shadowing frequently occurs in the musculoskeletal system. Shadowing from septae within the deltoid muscle have been observed, mimicking rotator cuff tears in very muscular athletes.

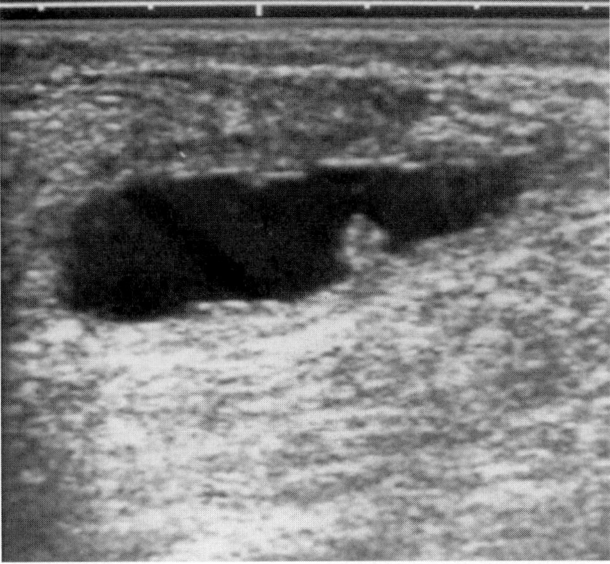

Figure 2-9 ■ Enhanced through-transmission deep to a muscle cyst.

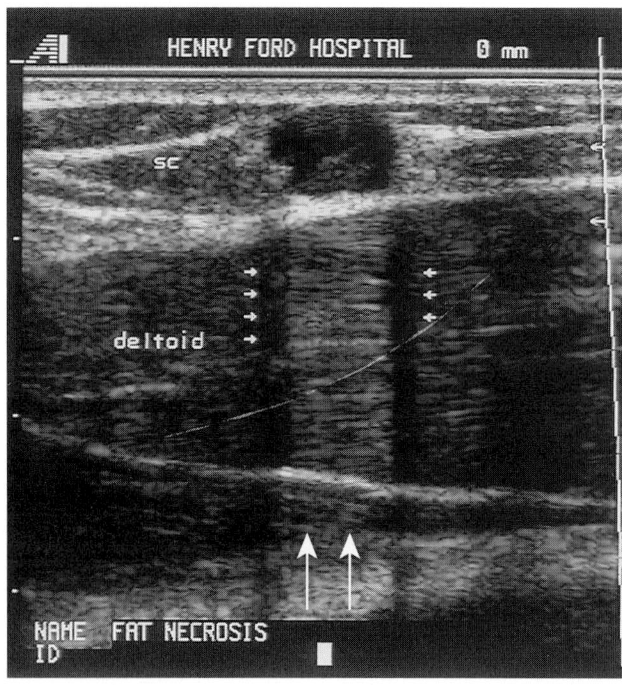

Figure 2–10 ■ Enhanced through-transmission (*large arrows*) deep to a posttraumatic seroma in the subcutaneous tissues. In addition, refractile shadowing is noted at the edges of the anechoic fluid collection (*small arrows*).

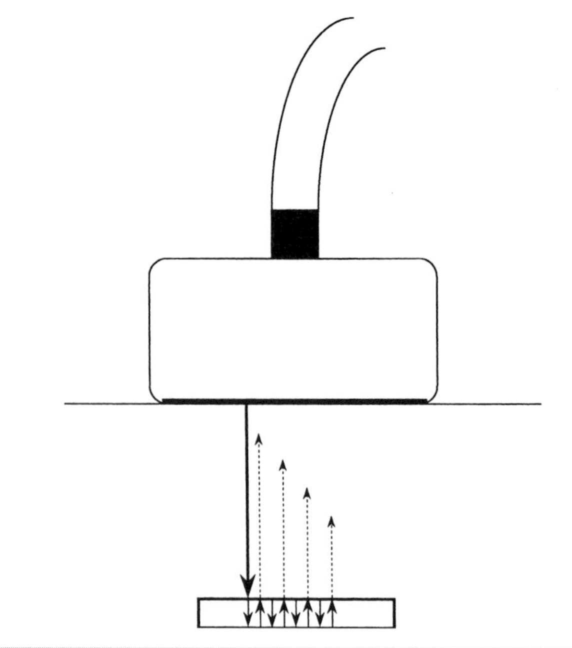

Figure 2–11 ■ Schematic representation of reverberation in a comet tail artifact.

surfaces of the object. The periodicity of the bands within the comet tail is equal to the thickness of the object (Fig. 2–12).

Recognition of this artifact allows the examiner to quickly diagnose metallic and glass foreign bodies (Fig. 2–13). The position of the object can be accurately established; however, the size of relatively small objects cannot be determined accurately. This is especially true of cylindrical metal or glass objects and is a by-product of the reverberation.

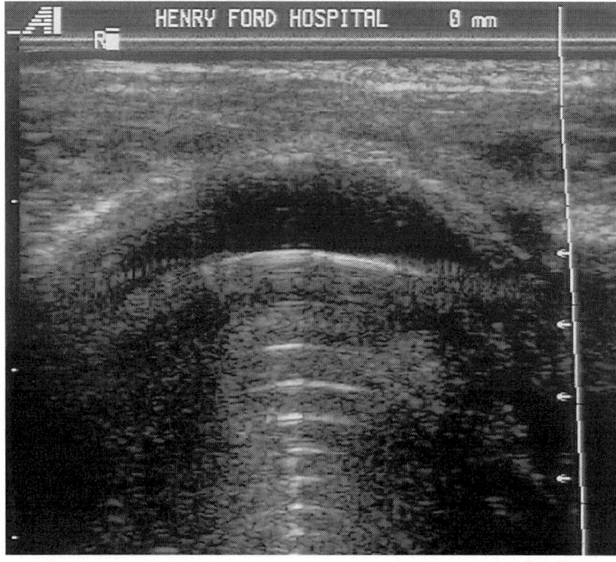

Figure 2–12 ■ Comet tail artifact deep to a femoral condyle prosthesis in a patient with a total knee arthroplasty. Note the periodicity in the artifact.

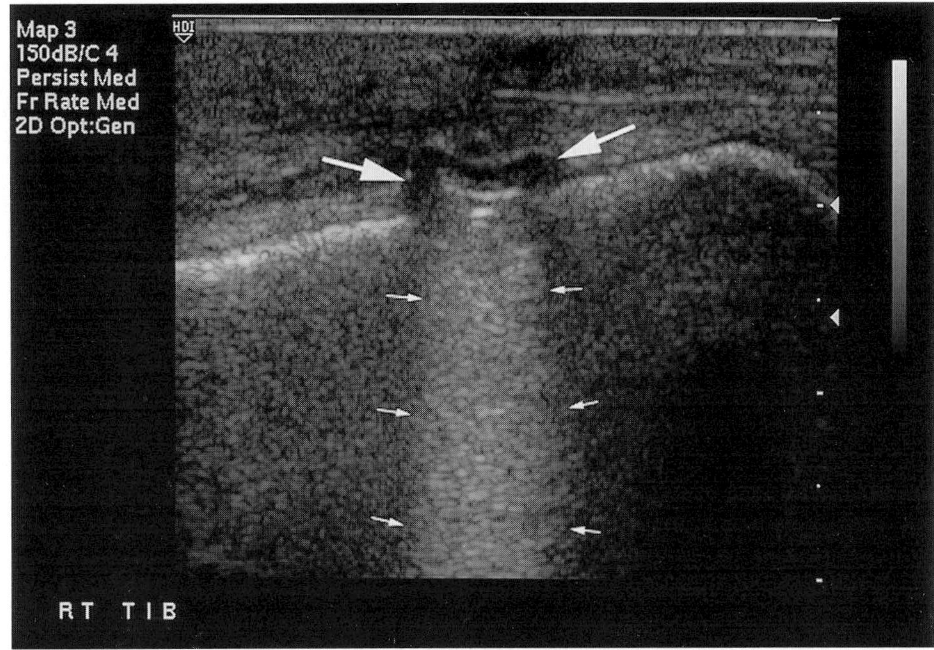

Figure 2-13 ■ Comet tail artifact associated with an interlocking screw fixation of an intramedullary rod in the tibia. The head of the screw is noted along the surface of the bone (*large arrows*). The comet tail widens distally (*small arrows*).

The Bad . . .

Refraction

An artifact resulting from refraction is the depiction of real structures in false locations. Refraction occurs at interfaces between substances that transmit sound at different velocities, such as fat (1,450 m/sec) and muscle (1,585 m/sec). The sound beam is "bent" at these interfaces in proportion to the difference in velocity of sound transmission within the two materials and the angle of incidence of the sound beam. Bending of the sound beam results in the depiction of structures deep to the interface in an incorrect location (Fig. 2-14). Since we cannot control the speed of sound in various tissues, refraction artifact must be minimized by having the angle of incidence as close to 90 degrees as possible. Figure 2-14 demonstrates schematically what can occur when one is scanning obliquely. A lesion is identified but depicted in an incorrect location. If needle aspiration were attempted using a needle guide, the lesion would be missed.

Reverberation

Earlier we discussed how a reverberation artifact, the comet tail, can be beneficial by helping to characterize foreign bodies. However, other types of reverberation artifacts can be misleading and, if unrecognized, will result in an incorrect diagnosis. Fortunately, situations in which these artifacts are encountered in musculoskeletal ultrasound are rare.

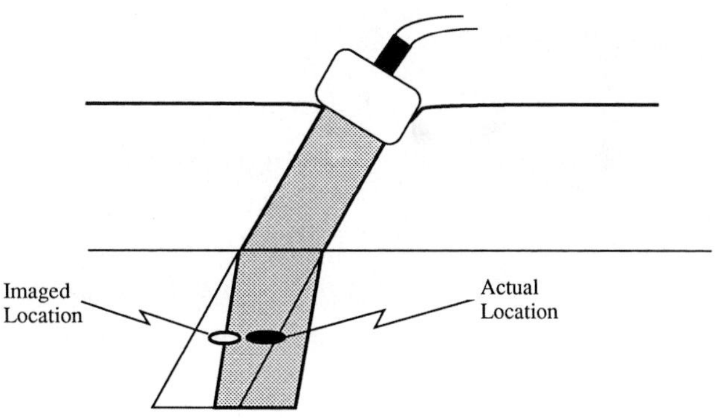

Figure 2-14 ■ Refraction artifact resulting in depiction of a real lesion in an incorrect location.

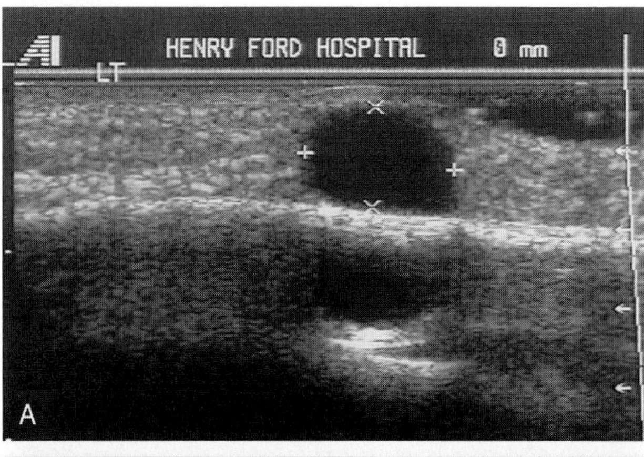

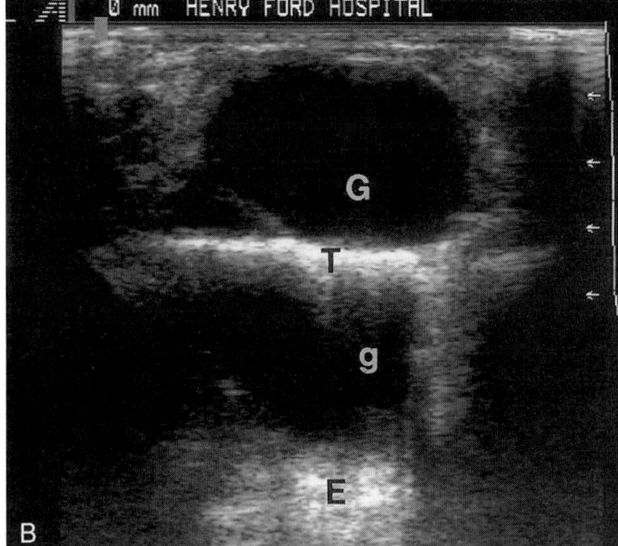

Figure 2–15 ■ **A,** Mirror image artifact of an ankle ganglion. An anechoic ganglion is noted over the cortex of the tibia (*cursors*). The mirror image is noted on the opposite side of the tibial cortex. **B,** Mirror image artifact of an ankle ganglion. The same ganglion is shown with maximum magnification. The anechoic ganglion (*G*) present over the distal tibia (*T*) is reproduced as a mirror image (*g*) behind the highly reflective surface of the bone. Acoustic enhancement (*E*) is seen deep to the phantom image.

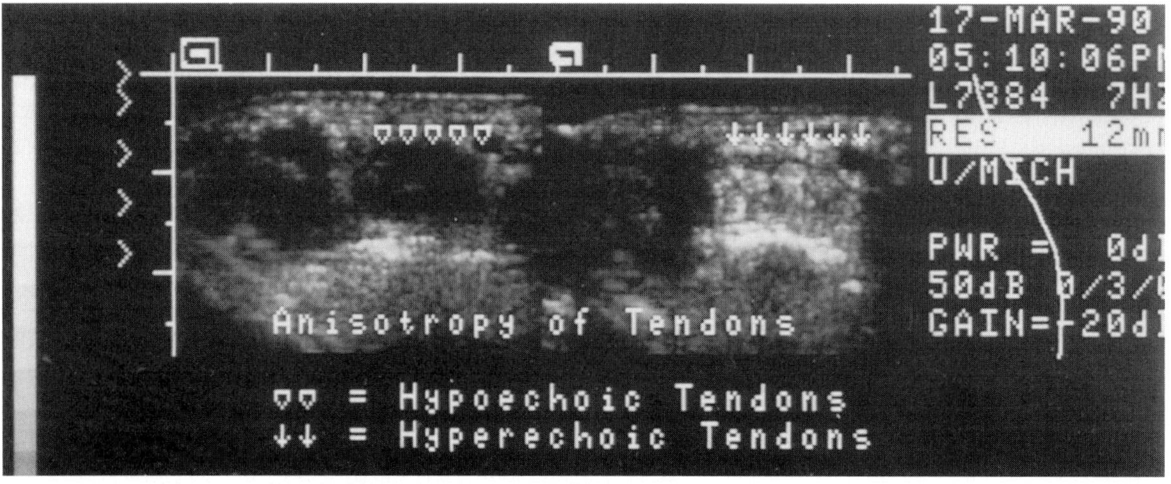

Figure 2–16 ■ Anisotropy of the flexor tendons of the wrist.

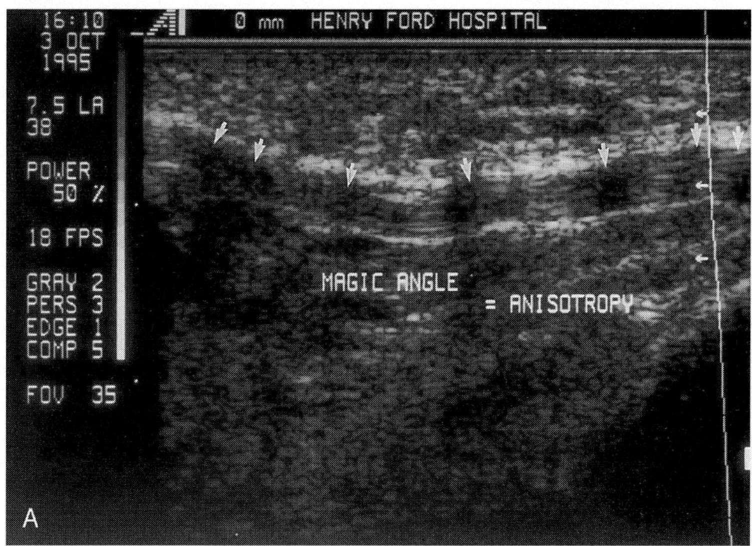

Figure 2–17 ■ **A,** Anisotropy of the patellar tendon. Each segment of the tendon imaged with an angle of incidence other than 90 degrees appears hypoechoic (*arrows*). Note that structure and outline of the tendon appear indistinct in these areas of decreased echogenicity. This decreased echogenicity is in sharp contrast to the normally hyperechoic fibrillar appearance when the tendon is imaged with the sound beam at a right angle to the long axis of the tendon. Anisotropy observed in ultrasound examination of tendons is the equivalent of the *magic angle* phenomenon in MRI, which has been observed on T_1-weighted images of tendons. **B,** This sagittal gradient echo MR image of the knee (same patient as in Figure 2–16A) demonstrates sequelae of an old quadriceps injury. Marked buckling of the patellar tendon is seen, which is the cause of anisotropy observed on the ultrasound examination (**A**). This MR image does not display the magic angle artifact.

Reverberation occurs at highly reflective interfaces, such as the diaphragm. The sound beam is reflected back and forth within the body, resulting in phantom structures, sometimes mirror images. The intensity of the echos decreases exponentially with the increasing number of iterations. The sites at which these artifacts are most frequently encountered are the pelvis, the diaphragm, and the tibia. In musculoskeletal exams, phantom echos should always be kept in mind when scanning the pelvis and calf (Fig. 2–15).

Anisotropic Reflectors

An *anisotropic* substance is one that displays different properties, depending on the direction of measurement. In abdominal imaging the kidney is the only anisotropic reflector. Its anisotropic reflectivity is often subtle in vivo and therefore is often unappreciated. Musculoskeletal ultrasound involves imaging of strongly anisotropic reflectors such as tendons (Fig. 2–16). Muscles, ligaments, and nerves demonstrate anisotropy as well, but their anisotropic features are much less pronounced than that of the tendon (Figs. 2–17 through 2–20). Figure 2–16 demonstrates the anisotropic character of the flexor tendons of the wrist. The image on the right was obtained with the sound beam perpendicular to the surface of the tendons, and they appear rather echogenic. Immediately after this image was obtained, the transducer was positioned slightly oblique without changing the position of the face of the transducer. The resulting image is displayed on the left. Now the same tendons appear markedly hypoechoic. The decrease in echogenicity is accompanied by loss of definition of the tendons' surface and lack of delineation of the fibrillar internal architecture. Obviously, this is not desirable when evaluating the integrity of tendons. Imaging tendons with an oblique transducer position will markedly increase image contrast. This technique is beneficial only to distinguish tendons from surrounding fat when the echogenicity of fat approximates that of tendon. An example is the peroneal tendons at the level of the lateral malleolus and the posterior tibial tendon below the medial malleolus. Examination of

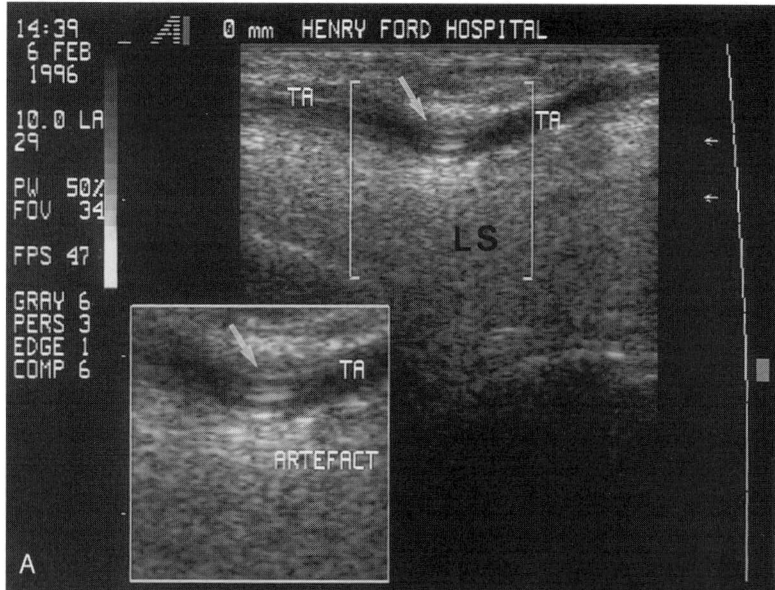

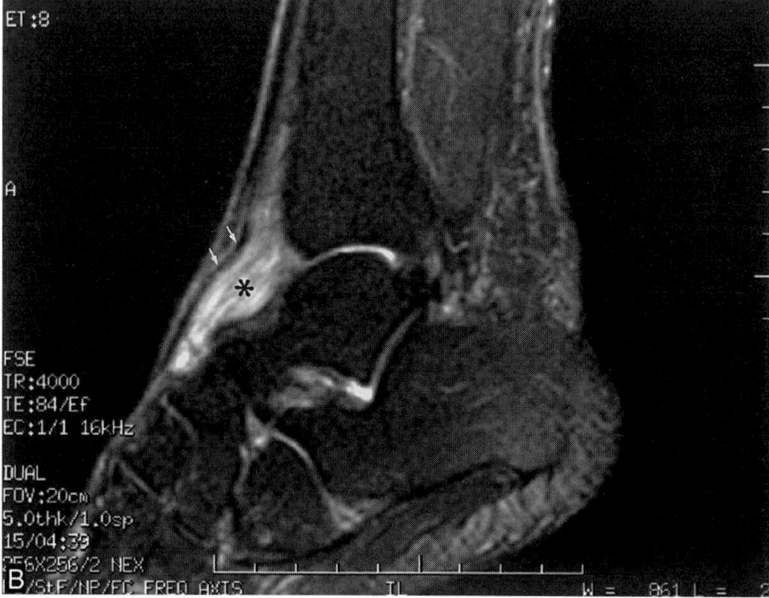

Figure 2-18 ▪ **A,** Anisotropy of the tibialis anterior tendon. A liposarcoma (LS) is present deep to the extensor tendons of the ankle. The tibialis anterior tendon (*TA*) is pushed away from the ankle by the mass. Proximal and distal ends of the tendon (*TA*) appear markedly hypoechoic due to the oblique angle of the incident sound beam. The only segment of the tendon displaying normal echogenicity is the tibialis anterior tethered to the tibia by the extensor retinaculum. **B,** Anisotropy of the tibialis anterior tendon. Same patient as in **A.** On the MRI scan, the liposarcoma (*asterisk*) causes similar signal intensity changes in the tendon (*arrows*) because of the magic angle phenomenon.

the integrity of tendons should always be performed with the sound beam perpendicular to the surface of the tendon. Images obtained with a 90 degree angle of incidence of the sound beam will optimally demonstrate the tendon surface and internal architecture, with the characteristic periodicity made up by interfaces between tendon fascicles and endotendineum. Keeping a perpendicular alignment to the long axis of the tendon during real-time examination is not as difficult as it may appear.

Speed of Sound Artifact

Ultrasound equipment determines the distance of an object from the transducer by measuring the time elapsed between the origination of the sound pulse and its return to the transducer. This is referred to as the *time of flight.* In calculating distance, the machine assumes a constant speed of sound. However, as we discussed in the previous chapter (see Table 1–1), this is a false assumption. Although the speed of sound within human tissues does not vary greatly, it may still produce a significant artifact. The image in Figure 2–21 was obtained while scanning the liver of a patient with retroperitoneal lipomatosis. The apparent rent in the diaphragm is an artifact created by the difference in the speed of sound passing through two different tissues (liver and fat). In this example, refraction also plays a role. This type of artifact may also be encountered at

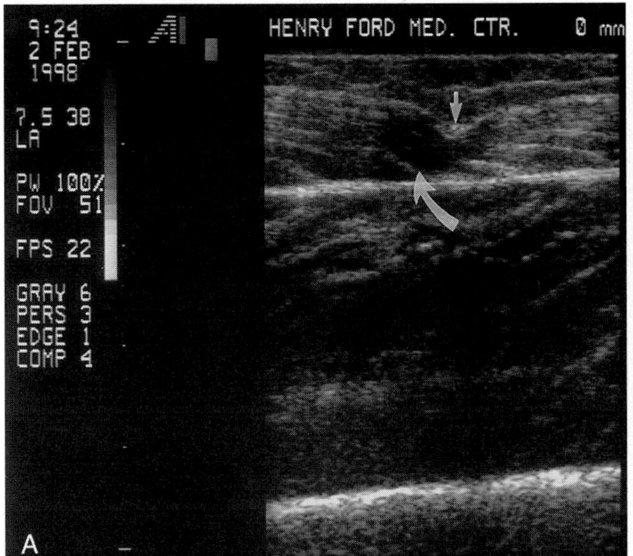

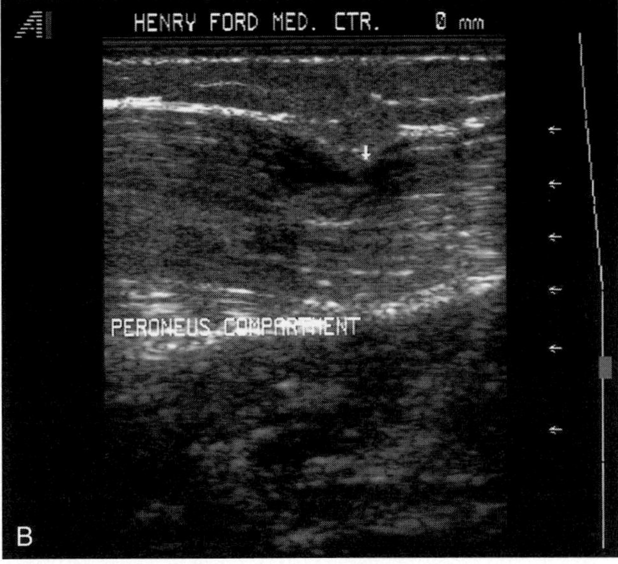

Figure 2–19 ■ **A,** Anisotropy of muscle. Scar tissue deeply indents the fascia (*arrow*) of the peroneal compartment of the lateral calf. Note that the muscle appears hypoechoic (*curved arrow*) in the region distorted by the scar. **B,** Anisotropy of muscle. This magnified view of the muscle shown in **A** was obtained with a 10-MHz transducer. The muscle architecture is preserved, and normal fibroadipose septae are present deep to the scar (*arrow*). The tissue on either side of the indentation appears hypoechoic. Normal echogenicity is observed remote from the scar where muscle fibers and fibroadipose septae resume a parallel orientation relative to the footprint of the transducer.

Figure 2–20 ■ **A,** Anisotropy of muscle. About a 40 degree difference in the inclination of the transducer causes a significant change in the echogenicity of the biceps brachii muscle. The same muscle appears hyperechoic on the left side and hypoechoic on the right side of the split screen. The transducer was not repositioned but just angled differently. **B,** Anisotropy of nerves. This image is an in vitro sonogram of an excised human sciatic nerve suspended in a saline bath. The tibial (*t*) and peroneal (*p*) nerves appear hyperechoic when imaged with the incident sound beam at a right angle to the long axis of the nerve (left side of the split screen). The same nerves appear less echogenic when imaged obliquely (right side of the split screen). Most tissues of the extremities display features of anisotropy. This artifact is observed in tendon, muscle, ligament, fibrocartilage, and nerve imaging. Tendons are the strongest anisotropic reflectors.

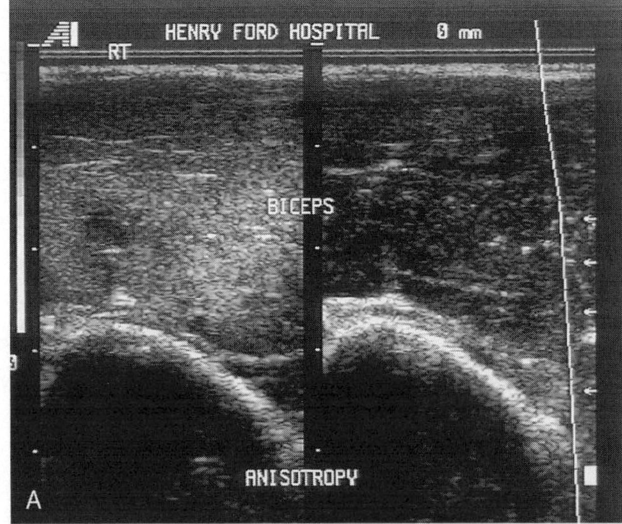

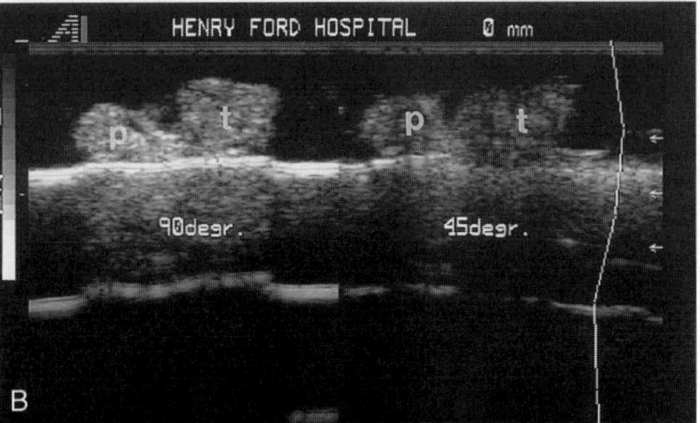

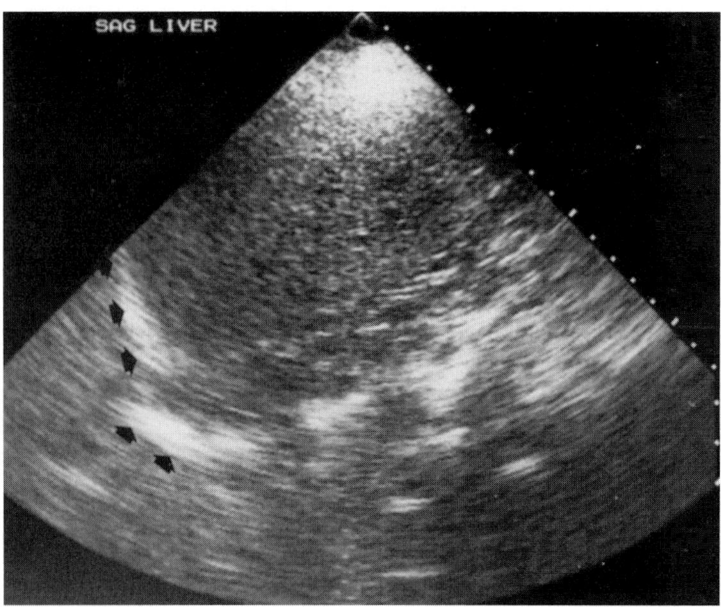

Figure 2–21 ■ Speed of sound artifact. A false discontinuity in the diaphragm (*arrows*) is imaged due to the speed of sound artifact and refraction in this patient with retroperitoneal lipomatosis. (Courtesy of Dr. Jonathan Rubin, University of Michigan Hospitals, Ann Arbor, Michigan.)

muscle–fat interfaces in the extremities of obese patients.

Beam Width Artifact

An ultrasound beam has a width that varies according to the design characteristics of the transducer. Therefore, like other cross-sectional imaging modalities, ultrasound images a volume of tissue. When an object is smaller than the width of the ultrasound beam, echos depicted at that location are a combination of the echos from the object and the surrounding tissues. This *volume averaging,* as it is called in computed tomography (CT) and magnetic resonance imaging (MRI), can give the appearance of echos within simple cysts, as well as eliminating shadowing deep to small calcifications. Normally, this does not interfere with the diagnosis. However, in musculoskeletal ultrasound, we are often dealing with very small structures, so this artifact is seen much more frequently than in abdominal imaging. The examiner must always remember that a highly echogenic focus may be a calcification despite the lack of acoustic shadowing (Fig. 2–22).

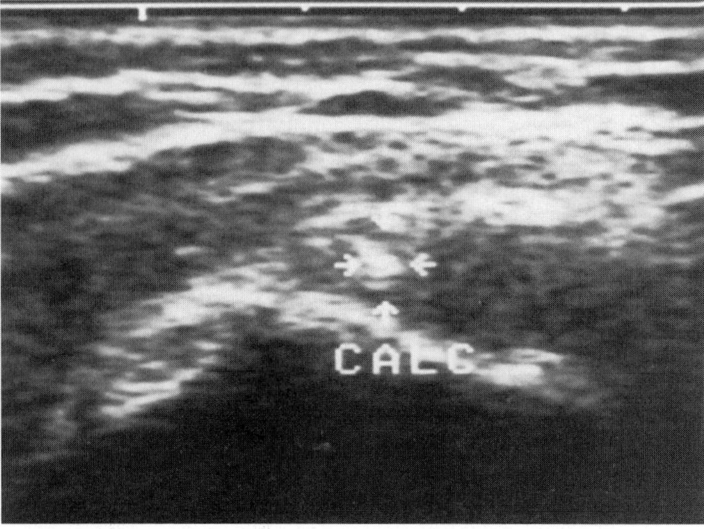

Figure 2–22 ■ Beam width artifact resulting in lack of acoustic shadowing deep to a calcification in the rotator cuff.

The Ugly . . .

Motion Artifact

Patient motion can degrade ultrasound images as well as radiographs. The displayed image on an ultrasound machine is an average of several data acquisitions. When movement occurs, the image is blurred, sometimes severely limiting its diagnostic value. State-of-the-art machines provide cine-loop functions that can help in some cases. On other machines, the degree of persistence (i.e., the number of acquisitions averaged) can be reduced.

Electrical Noise

Ultrasound machines are generally well insulated from electronic noise. However, some circumstances may arise in which electromagnetic interference from high-voltage transformers or other equipment degrades images (Fig. 2–23). If you are ever requested to perform a portable examination on a patient in the MRI holding area, you may be confronted with a bizarrely distorted image. Strong magnetic fields don't like cathode ray tubes. These types of artifacts are never diagnostic problems but rather minor annoyances.

Frame Buffer Dropout

All modern ultrasound machines use digital image processing. The displayed image is stored in a matrix of computer memory. When a memory chip fails, a number of pixels that compose the image will be missing. The pattern of loss will depend on the design of the display circuitry. Once again, this is not a difficult artifact to recognize but merely a sign that a call for maintenance is required.

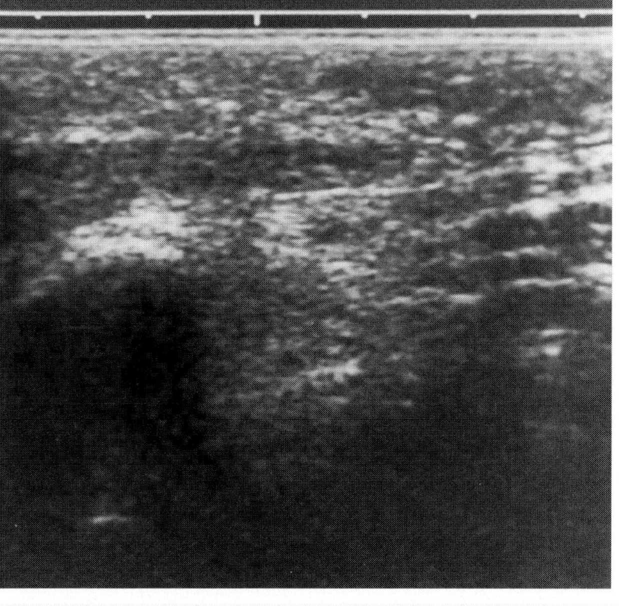

Figure 2–23 ■ Electrical noise artifact caused by electrocautery equipment. The dotted lines running obliquely downward from left to right are the result of electrocautery equipment used during this intraoperative ultrasound.

Bibliography

Fornage BD: Achilles tendon. US examination. *Radiology* 159:759–764, 1986.

Fornage BD: The hypoechoic normal tendon—a pitfall. *J Ultrasound Med* 6:19–22, 1987.

Laing FC: Commonly encountered artifacts in clinical ultrasound. *Semin Ultrasound CT MR* 4:27–43, 1983.

Metreweli C: *Practical Abdominal Ultrasound.* Chicago, Year Book Medical, 1978.

Rubin JM, Carson PL, Meyer CR: Anisotropic ultrasonic backscatter from the renal cortex. *Ultrasound Med Biol* 14:507–511, 1988.

Rumack CM, Wilson SR, Charboneau JW: *Diagnostic Ultrasound,* 2nd ed. St Louis, Mosby–Year Book, 1998.

Thickman DI, et al: Clinical manifestations of the comet-tail artifact. *J Ultrasound Med* 2:225–230, 1983.

Ziskin MC, et al: The comet-tail artifact. *J Ultrasound Med* 1:1–7, 1982.

Chapter 3
Sonography of Muscle

Ultrasound was the first imaging modality available for the evaluation of muscle pathology. Xeroradiography and low-kilovoltage radiography lack sufficient contrast resolution for the evaluation of muscle injury. Even CT cannot define muscle structure sufficiently to detect the most common types of muscle pathology. Intravenous (IV) contrast enhancement does not improve the performance of CT in this area. In addition, the transverse axial plane of section provided by CT is usually unsuitable for evaluation of muscle injury. Muscle retracts along its long axis when injured, making it difficult to visualize on transverse axial images.

The multiplanar capability and improved tissue characterization provided by MRI have made it quite suitable for the evaluation of muscle pathology. Traumatic and ischemic injury can be well demonstrated using T_1-, proton density, and T_2-weighted images. In addition, MR 31P spectroscopy allows detailed analysis of the metabolic state of muscle (Zochmodne et al., 1988; Lenkinski et al., 1988; Kuhl et al., 1994). However, MRI lacks the ability to perform a real-time dynamic examination. Cost and availability factors further limit the utility of MRI in the diagnosis of muscle pathology.

Sonography can provide all of the information available with MRI and more with regard to muscle pathology. Its spatial resolution and definition of muscle structure are usually superior to those provided by MRI. Real-time examination available only with ultrasound elucidates some types of muscle lesions that are occult on static examinations (Graf and Schuler, 1988). The degree of functional deficit resulting from fibrosis, muscular cysts, or myositis ossificans can be fully assessed using real-time sonography. This information may have a major impact on decision making in competitive athletics, disability, and medicolegal cases. Currently, the only role we see for MRI of muscle is in the diagnosis of muscular dystrophies and inflammatory lesions of muscle (Huang et al., 1994; Park et al., 1995; Schedel et al., 1995). These lesions are rare, with the exception of diabetic myonecrosis (Scully et al., 1997).

The availability, ease of examination, and low cost of sonography in contrast to MRI make follow-up of healing lesions practical. The majority of patients referred for evaluation of muscle lesions are athletes. Several studies have demonstrated that approximately 30% of all sports injuries are muscular in origin (Peterson and Renstrom, 1986). In these patients the decision on when to return to training or competition is extremely important (Box 3–1). Reinjury resulting from premature resumption of activity can be costly for both the athlete and the team. Serial sonographic examinations can accurately evaluate the rate and stage of healing, significantly decreasing the likelihood of reinjury.

Examination Technique

Muscles can be relatively large structures, some extending over two joints. The longest can measure more than 50 cm. A muscle tear tends to be a long fusiform lesion. In cases of complete rupture, the severed ends of the muscle may retract more than 10 cm. With these factors in mind, it is clear that we must have the ability to examine a long anatomical segment. Therefore, long linear array transducers are

Box 3–1
Ultrasound of Muscle Injury

- Approximately 30% of sports injuries affect muscles
- Ultrasound useful in staging—determines date of return to competition

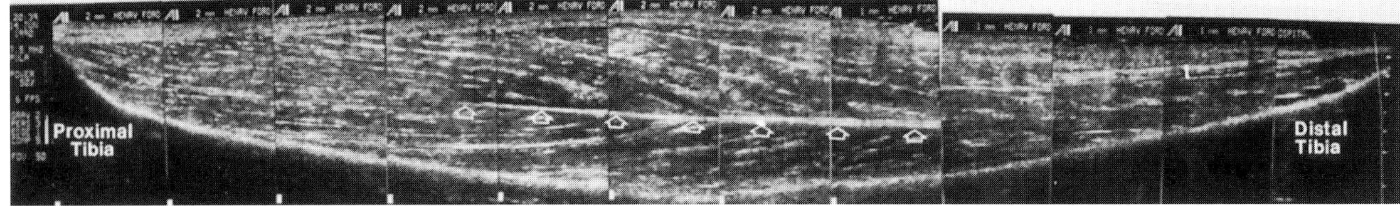

Figure 3–1 ■ Normal muscular anatomy of the anterior tibial compartment: composite longitudinal image. This image demonstrates the normal muscular anatomy of the anterior tibial compartment in a young athlete. Serial longitudinal images were obtained and then juxtaposed to produce a composite image demonstrating the entire length of the tibialis anterior muscle. This is a circumpennate muscle that functions in dorsiflexion of the foot. Note the feather-like appearance of the muscle created by the convergence of the fibroadipose septa upon the aponeurosis (*open arrows*). Abbreviation: tibialis anterior tendon (*t*).

the most desirable for the examination of muscles. The majority of exams can be performed using a long 7.5-MHz linear array. This will provide excellent resolution. Obese patients may require a 5-MHz transducer for better penetration. In addition to a long linear transducer, a machine that has the ability to display two images side by side is essential. This ability allows the examiner to provide a composite image demonstrating a longer segment of muscle (Fig. 3–1). However, conventional ultrasound techniques are suboptimal because of their limited field of view (FOV). The image FOV is determined by the probe width, even with the use of a side-by-side dual-image mode. Linear-array transducers, which are the most useful for examination of muscle, have a width of 2 to 4 cm. Fortunately, research has provided several possible solutions for overcoming the problem of limited FOV (Detmer et al., 1994; Kossoff et al., 1994; Wong et al., 1996; Weng et al., 1997). Transmission ultrasound is one solution, but this technique is in the very early stages of development and therefore will not be discussed further. Two other technical developments have emerged recently; three-dimensional (3-D) sonography and extended FOV imaging. Three-dimensional sonography is not very different from 3-D MRI or 3-D CT data acquisition. A series of images are stacked in memory and reconstructed as a volume. One method uses images from a single sweep with the transducer. Another method uses a bulky transducer which contains a curved array of piezoelectric crystals. The array of crystals can make a scanning sweep within the large container holding the elements. This transducer is held over the area of interest and cannot be moved until the translation movement of the array is complete. The enhanced computing power of newer digital ultrasound equipment provides fast 3-D volumetric reconstruction almost in real time. A recent technical advance is ultrasonic volume imaging. This technique allows real-time 3-D imaging with conventional B-mode equipment. A cylindrical silicone rubber lens is applied to a conventional linear or curved-array transducer. The lens defocuses the beam and insonates a volume of tissue. Three-dimensional imaging is attained when a structure reflects all of the incident energy. The necessity for total reflection is a major limitation of this technique. Total reflection has been attained by examining structures at highly inclined angles, such as a baby's face in utero. All current 3-D methods still have a fairly limited FOV. In addition, real-time ultrasound is a freehand technique, and the 3-D images are often fraught with error because of motion- and position-related artifacts. Extended-FOV imaging (Siescape, Issaquah, WA) is

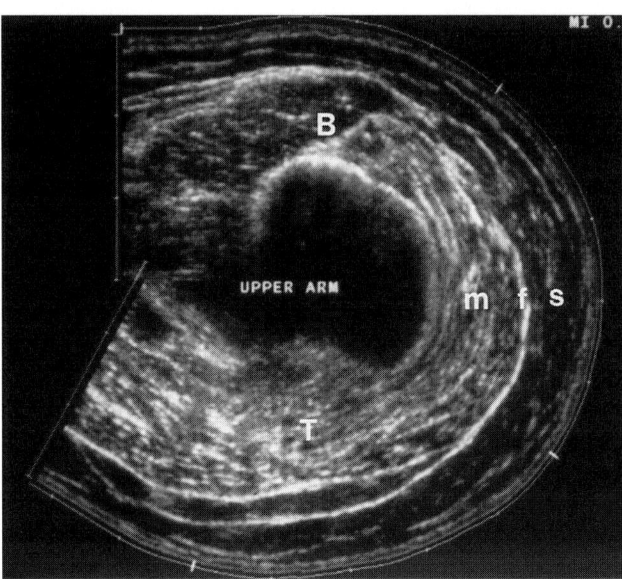

Figure 3–2 ■ Extended FOV image of the normal anatomy of the upper arm: transverse ultrasound. This Siescape image of a normal upper arm shows the biceps muscle (*B*) covering the anterior humerus and the triceps (*T*) over the posterior surface. Ultrasound shows a clear distinction between the subcutaneous tissues (*s*), fascia (*f*), and muscle (*m*) of the upper arm. Siescape imaging facilitates the teaching of ultrasound anatomy.

currently the best method of displaying musculotendinous anatomy using ultrasound (Weng et al., 1997). This technique is now rapidly gaining popularity. Images are more easily interpretable by the novice. It is a valuable teaching tool which will also improve cross-specialty communication. Extended-FOV imaging uses image registration between sequentially acquired image frames for motion estimation (Weng et al., 1997). A large panoramic view is constructed in real time (Fig. 3–2). The image looks somewhat like the image provided by static B-mode ultrasound scanning. Large high-resolution images up to 60 cm long can be obtained (Weng et al., 1997). This technique allows sonographic demonstration of lower-extremity muscles extending across joints. The Siescape technology can be applied to any transducer or image format. It requires a fast parallel processor computer because of its high computational demands. Current equipment which allows Siescape imaging is capable of executing 4 billion operations per second (Weng et al., 1997). The new technology incorporates the advantages and eliminates the disadvantages of both real-time and static B-mode scanners. Fuzzy-logic technique is applied in extended-FOV imaging, allowing detection of and correction for small-scale tissue motion, such as arterial pulsation, muscle contraction, heartbeat, and respiration. Probe off-plane motion, a significant problem in conventional 3-D imaging, is less of an issue with this technique. Extended-FOV imaging allows the operator to track along the length of a structure without being confined to a single plane (Weng et al., 1997). This technique is applicable to many structures in the extremities (Fig. 3–3). A large number of musculotendinous structures and neurovascular bundles cross conventional anatomic planes. The oblique course of the sartorius muscle is a good example. An additional benefit of this technique is accuracy of measurement over long distances. The majority of measurement errors are less than 2% of the measured distance (Weng et al., 1997).

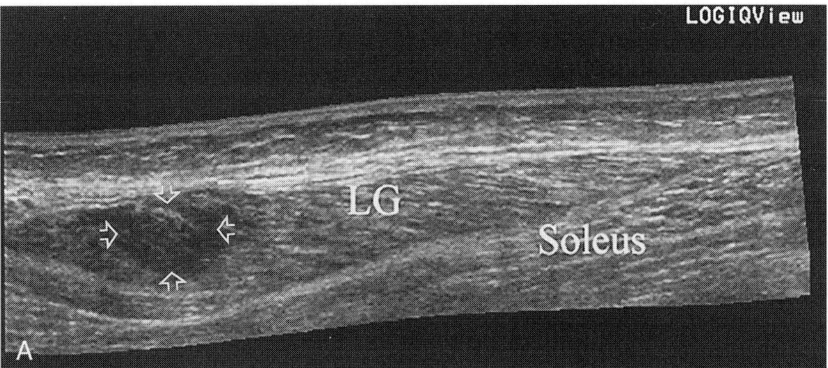

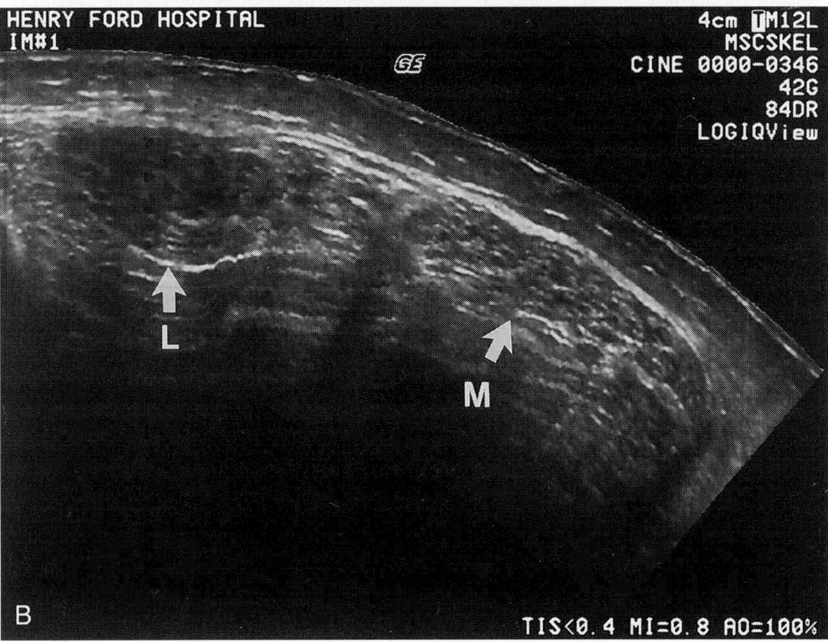

Figure 3–3 ▪ Focal muscle mass. **A,** Longitudinal sonogram with extended-FOV technique. Over a three-week period, pain and swelling developed in the calf of this 50-year-old woman. This longitudinal image of the calf demonstrates a focal hypoechoic area (*open arrows*) within the lateral gastrocnemius (*LG*). Extended-FOV imaging allows the examiner to track the anatomy along the length of a structure. In this case, ultrasound shows the anatomy along the oblique course of the gastrocnemius muscle belly. With this picture in hand, it was easy to explain to the clinician how this lesion affects the proximal lateral gastrocnemius only. The lesion respects fascial boundaries, as clearly demonstrated on the image. Extended-FOV imaging improves the ability to interpret static images by providing greater perspective. However, the technique does not significantly improve diagnostic accuracy for the examiner who scans in real time. The type of information that the extended imaging adds is that which the examiner has in mind during the real-time examination. Therefore, the principal benefit of the technique is to improve communication with referring physicians. **B,** Transverse sonogram with extended-FOV technique. Same patient as in **A.** By sliding the transducer over the calf, making a sweep from side to side, one notices the significant swelling and edema of the lateral gastrocnemius (*L*) when compared with the medial gastrocnemius (*M*). Two weeks later, biopsy of the muscle shows bone formation compatible with myositis ossificans.

A standoff cushion may be required for the examinations of muscles. This allows optimal visualization of the superficial fascia and the musculotendinous junction. Fascial defects, muscle hernias, and superficial muscle tears will be missed if a standoff cushion is not utilized. Standoff cushions will also facilitate the production of composite images by conforming to the irregular contours of the skin surface. If a radial array or sector scanner must be used because a high-frequency linear array is not available, a standoff cushion will help by reducing the obliquity of the beam in the region of interest. Regardless of the transducer utilized, a standoff cushion will help to place the region of interest within the optimal focal zone of the transducer. Companies have made great efforts to improve the near-field resolution of most transducers. Those adjustments have been implemented for small parts and breast ultrasound. Abdominal sonography has benefited indirectly from this change, and the muscular abdominal wall can now be studied routinely in great detail. The benefits of musculoskeletal sonography have been many. Superficial tendons, ligaments, bursae, and cartilage are now visible with resolution unmatched by that of any other noninvasive imaging method (Erickson, 1997). Higher and higher frequencies are now utilized in clinical applications. Most companies have multifrequency transducers with center frequencies above 10 MHz. Modern linear array and curved array transducers can now move the depth of focus electronically to the skin level. Popular for musculoskeletal use are transducers that have frequency ranges from 10 or 12 to 5 MHz.

Pain resulting from muscle injury is generally well localized, unlike chest or abdominal pain. Therefore, the examination is designed to find the point of maximal tenderness. This technique is called *sonographic palpation.* The patient is directed to point to the symptomatic region or the referring physician may mark a specific region of interest on the skin. Systematic examination of the indicated area is then performed by gentle compression with the ultrasound transducer. During the examination, the degree of compression should be as consistent as possible. Fascia and fibroadipose septa are the most echogenic elements of muscle structure. When these elements are approximated more closely by increased compression, the overall echogenicity of the muscle appears to be increased. If no abnormality is clearly evident at the point of maximal tenderness, comparison with the corresponding area on the asymptomatic side is mandatory.

Muscles are dynamic structures; therefore, they cannot be properly evaluated with static images alone. Real-time sonography allows examination of muscle structure under dynamic conditions. Ultrasound machines with cine-loop capability are very helpful during dynamic examinations. A videocassette recorder may also be valuable during this portion of the examination. Identification of muscles is made by location, origin, insertion, and function. This can easily be established under sonographic observation. Initial observation is performed without stress, followed by increasing graded isometric contraction. Small muscle tears may be occult on images obtained during relaxation but clearly visible during isometric contraction.

The examination is started with the transducer oriented in the long axis of the muscle using sonographic palpation. After the area of abnormality is established, images are obtained during relaxation and isometric contraction. Then the transducer is rotated 90 degrees, and the process is repeated for transverse imaging. Comparable images of the asymptomatic side are obtained to facilitate detection of subtle abnormalities.

Normal Sonographic Anatomy

Individual skeletal muscle fibers are enveloped by the *endomysium,* which consists of an extensive network of capillaries and nerves (Moore, 1980). These muscle fibers are grouped into bundles surrounded by the *perimysium,* which is composed of connective tissue, blood vessels, nerves, and adipose tissue (Clemente, 1985). Some authors refer to the perimysium as *fibroadipose septa* (Graf and Schuler, 1988; Fornage, 1989). A sheath of dense connective tissue called the

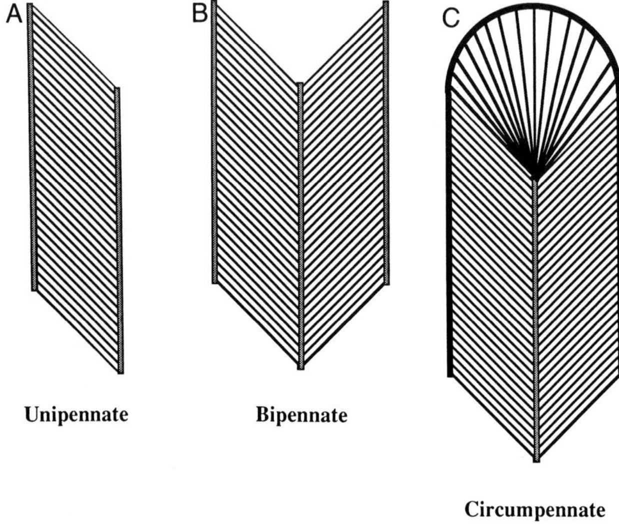

Figure 3-4 ■ Pennate structure of muscles. The diagrams depict the most common arrangements of muscle fibers in the extremities. These arrangements allow greater weight to be lifted over a shorter distance. Parallel arrangements of muscle fibers, seen more commonly in the abdomen, head, and neck, are more suitable for lifting less weight over long distances.

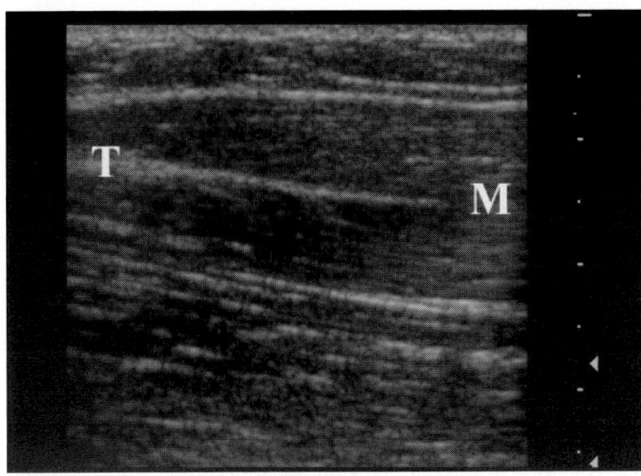

Figure 3-5 ▪ Circumpennate muscle arrangement: longitudinal ultrasound. This image along the longitudinal axis of the distal biceps brachii muscle demonstrates the circumpennate arrangement of muscle fibers (*M*) relative to the distal biceps tendon (*T*) and its central aponeurosis. The proximal muscle is displayed at the right side of the image, and the distal muscle is displayed at the observer's left.

epimysium surrounds the entire muscle. A fascial layer may separate single muscles or groups of muscles.

The internal architecture of skeletal muscle varies, depending on its designated function. Muscles with fibers arranged parallel to the long axis of the muscle are best suited for movement over a long distance. Unipennate, bipennate, and circumpennate configurations are better suited for lifting greater weight over shorter distances (Fig. 3-4). Attachment of muscles to the bones is accomplished by tendons and the fibro-osseous junction (Sharpey's fibers). Each muscle has at least one belly, or venter, and two tendons. However, a muscle may have more than one belly with fibrous intersections separating them, such as the rectus abdominus. Multiple origins of a muscle with a single belly, another possible configuration, is seen in the biceps, triceps, and quadriceps muscles.

These different arrangements can easily be observed sonographically (Fig. 3-5). Variations from these systematic arrangements are easily detected with a thorough ultrasound examination. Muscle bundles have a hypoechoic appearance. The fibroadipose septa of the perimysium are seen as hyperechoic lines separating the muscle bundles (Figs. 3-6 through 3-9). Epimysium, nerves, investing fascia, tendons, and fat also appear hyperechoic relative to the muscle bundles. These features allow easy recognition of the pennate structure of muscle. Fat planes between muscles will aid in differentiation of separate muscles. The pennate structure is most easily identified in longitudinal images. In transverse images, muscle will have a speckled appearance. Muscle tissue is occasionally mistaken for a disease process. Accessory muscle tissue in the wrist or ankle can appear mass-like or may mimic tenosynovitis. We have observed such pseudo-

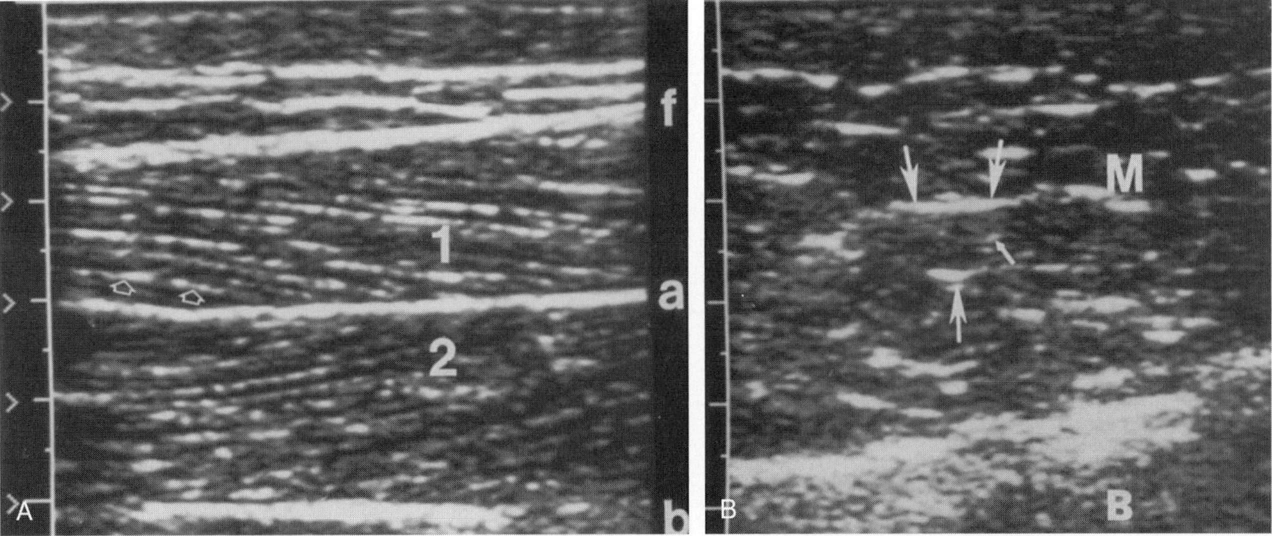

Figure 3-6 ▪ **A,** Normal anterior thigh muscles: longitudinal sonogram. This image was obtained in a normal 27-year-old man. The fibroadipose septa (*open arrows*) are seen as hyperechoic lines separating the hypoechoic muscle bundles. These septa converge on the highly reflective aponeurosis (*a*), giving the appearance of a feather. The aponeurosis divides the rectus femoris (*1*) and vastus intermedius (*2*) muscles. Two highly reflective lines bound the muscles: the fascia (*f*) superficially and the bone (*b*) deep to the muscles. Subcutaneous fat lies superficial to the fascia. **B,** Normal anterior thigh muscles: transverse sonogram. Same patient as in A. In transverse images the fibroadipose septa (*arrows*) appear as hyperechoic lines of varying lengths. The pennate arrangement seen in longitudinal images is not evident on oblique or transverse images. Abbreviations: muscle (*M*), femur (*B*).

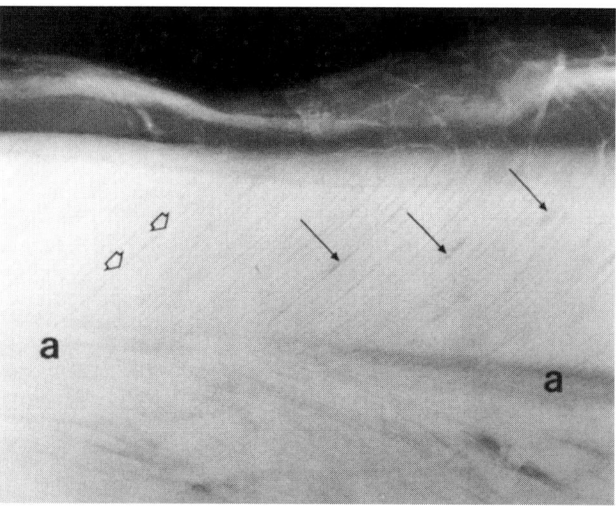

Figure 3-7 ■ Specimen radiograph of the rectus femoris muscle: longitudinal anatomical section. This radiograph was obtained using mammographic technique on a specimen 1 cm thick. Note the pennate structure of the muscle defined by the radiolucent fibroadipose septa (*open arrows*) converging on the thick fibrous aponeurosis (*a*) or intermuscular septum. These septa contain collagen, nerves, and blood vessels in addition to fat. A periodicity can be seen in the presence of thicker septa (*long arrows*).

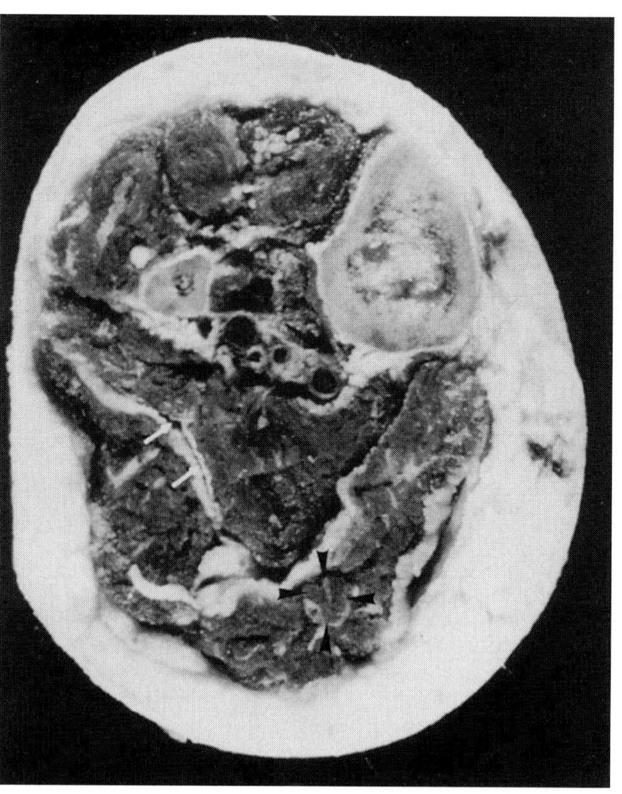

Figure 3-8 ■ Cross-sectional anatomical specimen of the lower leg: photograph. Muscles are divided into compartments by fibrous septa, which contain vessels (*white arrows*). Compare the appearance of the fibroadipose septa cut transversely with the sonographic image in Figure 3-6B. The *arrowheads* indicate a muscle bundle surrounded by septa.

masses in the hand with accessory extensor musculature over the knuckles and an accessory soleus appearing as a mass above the heel. Palmaris longus muscle tissue in the wrist and aberrant peroneus brevis and peroneus quartus muscles in the ankle are among the common normal pseudomasses encountered. In the adolescent rotator cuff, muscle of the supraspinatus is longer than its counterpart in the adult shoulder (Petersson, 1984). This may result in hypoechoic areas within the cuff. Knowledge

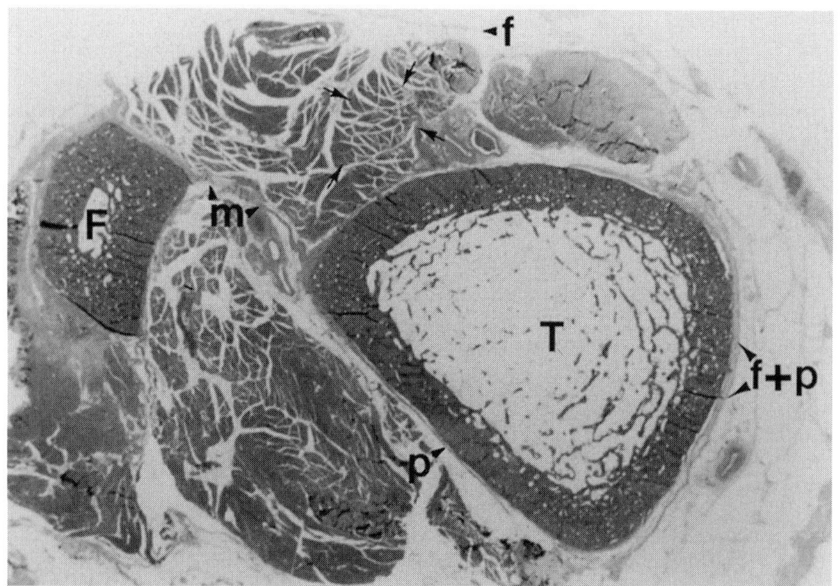

Figure 3-9 ■ Normal muscle architecture: transverse histological section (10 mm thick). This hematoxylin and eosin preparation was made from a specimen proximal to the one depicted in Figure 3-8. The fibroadipose septa are seen as clefts due to the histological preparation. *Arrows* indicate a muscle bundle similar to the one seen in Figure 3-8. Note the further division within the bundle by finer septa. The interosseous membrane (*m*), fascia (*f*), and periosteum (*p*) are composed of dense fibrous tissue, seen as hyperechoic lines sonographically. Fascia of the lower leg is intimately related to the periosteum covering the anterior medial surface of the tibia (*f* + *p*). Abbreviations: tibia (*T*), fibula (*F*).

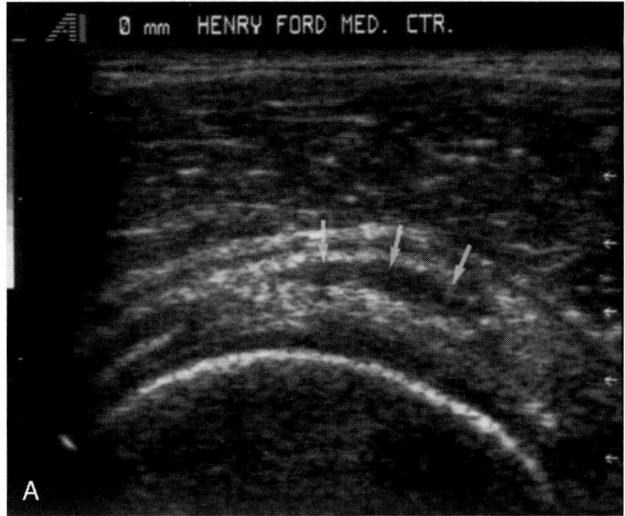

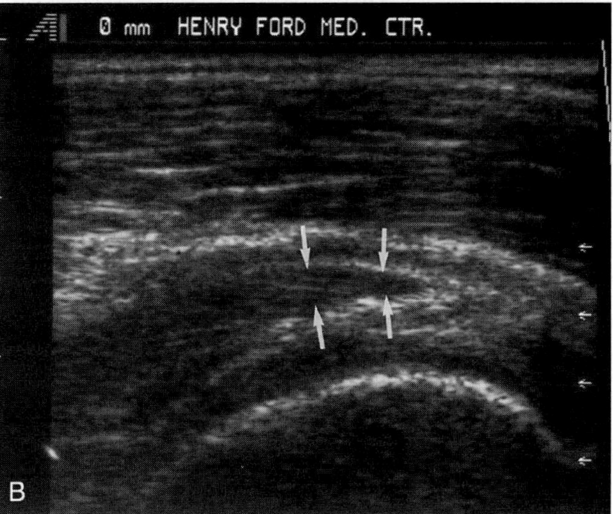

Figure 3-10 ■ A, Normal rotator cuff of the adolescent: transverse sonogram. This transverse image of the rotator cuff of a young athlete demonstrates a hypoechoic area (*arrows*) within the supraspinatus tendon. Normal hyperechoic tendon surrounds this unusual area within the cuff. **B,** Normal rotator cuff of the adolescent: longitudinal sonogram. Examining the supraspinatus tendon longitudinally, one notes that the hypoechoic area seen on transverse images is triangular in shape, with well-defined margins (*arrows*). The internal structure demonstrates the pennate architecture of muscle. Muscle tissue appearing lateral to the acromion has been observed only in patients under the age of 20 years.

of this phenomenon will avoid the mistake of identifying muscle as a rotator cuff tear. Identification of the pennate structure of the muscle will help avoid an erroneous diagnosis and will allow the operator to distinguish reliably between muscle tissue and pathology (Fig. 3-10).

Images obtained during isometric contraction will demonstrate an apparent increase in muscle mass. This is due to the thickening of muscle bundles during contraction. Since these muscle bundles appear hypoechoic, the overall echogenicity of the muscle decreases during isometric contraction. Hypertrophy of muscle bundles in a well-conditioned athlete will also result in decreased echogenicity. This may prove to be a valuable tool in evaluating the level of conditioning in athletes. Conversely, during relaxation, firm compression with the transducer will result in a more echogenic appearance of the muscle.

Another aspect of muscle physiology that must be kept in mind is blood flow. Although muscle comprised approximately 40% of body mass, it receives only 15% of total body blood flow at rest (Guyton, 1982). However, exercise can increase blood flow by 20-fold, resulting in a volumetric increase in muscle size by 10% to 15% (see Fig. 3-52). For example, tiptoe exercise performed over several minutes will increase the volume of the posterior compartment of the calf sufficiently to cause anterior and lateral bowing of the interosseous membrane. The volume of the compartment will return to normal within approximately 10 to 15 minutes following exercise.

Muscle Pathology

The overwhelming majority of muscle pathology is traumatic in origin, either occupational or sports related. Lesions can be further categorized as intramuscular or muscle boundary lesions. We consider the intramuscular lesions to involve the muscle belly or venter. Muscle boundary lesions are those involving the muscle–fascia/tendon interface.

Intramuscular Pathology

There are many etiologies of muscle pain, and not all of them are associated with an identifiable lesion. Delayed muscle soreness and muscle cramps are two well-recognized entities that are frequently encountered clinically. In exceptional cases, it may be difficult to distinguish these causes of muscle pain from the sequelae of muscle rupture. Sonography is extremely valuable in these cases to exclude anatomic lesions (Takebayashi, 1995).

Delayed muscle soreness is typically characterized by pain, by tenderness, and frequently by swelling of the involved muscle groups. Onset of symptoms is usually observed approximately 12 to 24 hours following strenuous exercise. The symptoms slowly resolve over several days. Everyone has experienced delayed muscle soreness at some time. Usually this occurs after playing three sets of tennis on the first day of a vacation. The remainder of the vacation is spent in a sedentary manner recuperating from the injury. Studies conducted with athletes and military recruits have demonstrated acute elevation of muscle enzyme levels measured in serum (Nicholas and Hershman, 1986; Peterson and Renstrom, 1986). These changes are highly suggestive of microruptures and myofibrillar lysis. Histologic evidence of this injury has been observed. However, MRI and sonography have failed to demonstrate the microscopic lesions in these cases.

Muscle cramps affect a broad spectrum of people, ranging from well-conditioned athletes to the elderly. They are caused by a focus of spontaneous muscle activity that results in muscle spasm and pain (Nicholas and Hershman, 1986). The pathogenesis of muscle cramps remains unknown, but multiple predisposing factors have been identified. Prolonged exercise, dehydration, extremes of tempera-ture, lactic acidosis, chronic hemodialysis, atherosclerotic disease, and varicose veins are among the factors cited as predisposing to muscle cramps. Muscle rupture may also result in muscle cramps, often leading the clinician away from the correct diagnosis. In the past, the correct diagnosis came to light only when the symptoms did not resolve after 3 to 4 days. The role of ultrasound in the evaluation of prolonged muscle cramp is to diagnose the underlying muscle rupture so that appropriate therapy may be instituted. Therapy for muscle cramps often includes passive stretching of the muscle. In simple cases, this maneuver will result in alleviation of pain and resolution of the cramp. However, this diagnostic/therapeutic maneuver will result in increased pain and progression of the lesion in cases where there is underlying muscle or tendon injury.

Muscle Rupture

A muscle rupture may be caused by either compression (direct trauma) or distraction (indirect trauma). In compression injuries, the muscle is crushed against the underlying bone by an external force. This type of injury is frequent in contact sports and motor vehicle accidents. The collision of two football players, with the impact of one player's helmet on the quadriceps muscle of the other, is an example of how this injury may result. The involved muscle fibers are macerated along with the associated vessels, usually resulting in hematoma formation. The investing fascia may also be torn, with extension of the hematoma beyond the muscle belly, possibly involving multiple compartments. Healing of these lesions takes place slowly with considerable reparative tissue, which evolves into extensive scar tissue. This invariably results in a considerable long-term functional deficit.

Sonography is well suited for the evaluation of compressive muscle ruptures (Lehto and Alanen, 1987). These lesions are characterized by an irregular cavity with shaggy borders (Fig. 3–11). When imaged acutely, the echogenicity of the hematoma may limit evaluation of the extent of the lesion, resulting in an underestimation of its size. Approximately 48 to 72 hours following injury the collection becomes essentially anechoic, allowing measurement of the true extent of the injury. Follow-up examinations to evaluate healing will demonstrate progressive filling in of the lesion from the periphery with echogenic tissue. Scar tissue will appear hyperechoic, and acoustic shadowing will be seen deep to regions of myositis ossificans. Areas of myositis ossificans will have a pseudotumor appearance, which is detected significantly earlier with sonography than with conventional radiographs.

Distraction muscle ruptures differ from compression ruptures in both their pathogenesis and their morphology. They are the result of the intrinsic force generated by sudden forceful contraction of a muscle (Peterson and Renstrom, 1986). Sports that have a high incidence of distraction muscle ruptures are track and field, weight lifting, football, and gymnastics. Muscles of the lower extremity are most frequently affected, particularly those muscles that span two joints (Genety et al., 1980; Bouvier et al., 1982; Nicholas and Hershman, 1986). The most susceptible are the hamstrings, rectus femoris, and triceps surae muscles. Distraction injury in the upper extremities and trunk is seen far less frequently (see Fig. 3–19).

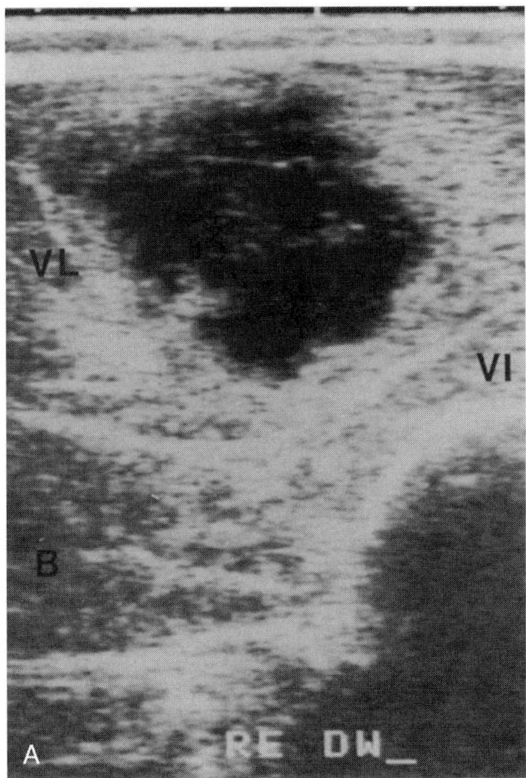

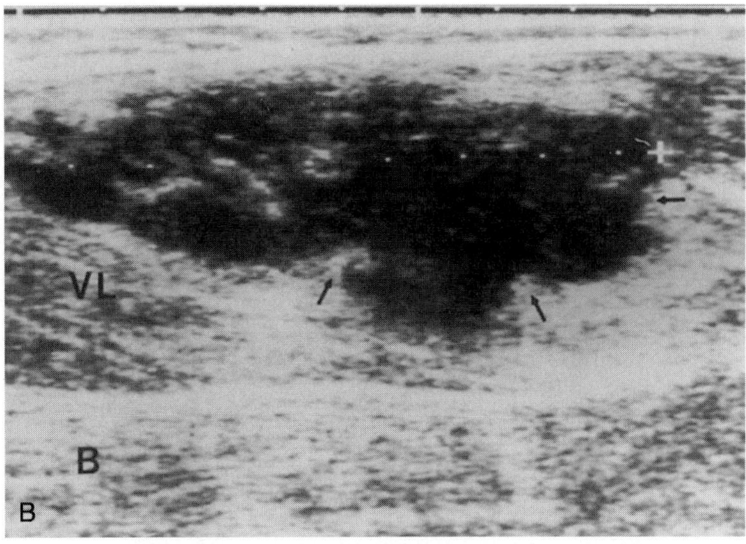

Figure 3-11 ■ **A,** Compression rupture of the vastus lateralis: transverse sonogram. The patient is a 23-year-old football player who was kicked in the lateral thigh 6 days earlier. This transverse image was obtained over the lateral aspect of the midthigh. A large, hypoechoic fluid collection with very irregular borders is identified within the substance of the vastus lateralis muscle (*VL*). The irregular border of the lesion is characteristic of compressive muscle rupture. Approximately 20% of significant compression ruptures progress to myositis ossificans. Abbreviations: biceps muscle (*B*), vastus intermedius muscle (*VI*). **B,** Compression rupture of the vastus lateralis: longitudinal sonogram. Same patient as in **A**. The compressive injury is again identified within the substance of the vastus lateralis muscle (*VL*). Compressive force applied to the muscle results in diffuse injury with irregular borders in the region of rupture (*arrows*). Measurement of the rupture site is important for comparison with follow-up examinations. Abbreviation: biceps muscle (*B*).

At the time of injury, the patient experiences a sharp stabbing pain in the region of the injured muscle. Pain dissipates slightly with the involved muscle at rest but can be reproduced by contraction of the muscle. Loss of function is proportional to the extent of injury. A complete rupture results in total loss of function in the region served by that muscle. The extremity is swollen secondary to both the inflammatory reaction and hemorrhage. In cases of superficial muscle rupture, skin discoloration may be observed approximately 24 hours following injury (Peterson and Renstrom, 1986). The area of skin discoloration should not be mistaken for the site of injury because blood will track inferiorly as it makes its way toward the subcutaneous tissues. Therefore, the site of rupture invariably lies superior to the region of skin discoloration. In contrast to compressive injury, distraction ruptures are subdivided into three groups based on sonographic findings: elongation injury (grade I), partial rupture (grade II), and complete rupture (grade III) (Peetrons and Sintzoff, 1987) (Fig. 3-12). Elongation injury occurs when a muscle is stretched to its elastic limit. Patients report severe pain throughout the muscle,

MUSCLE DISTRACTION

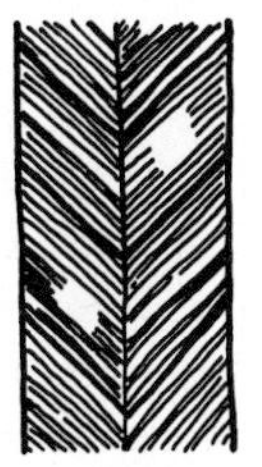
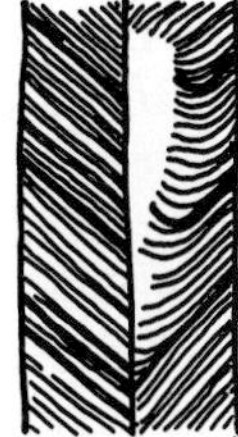
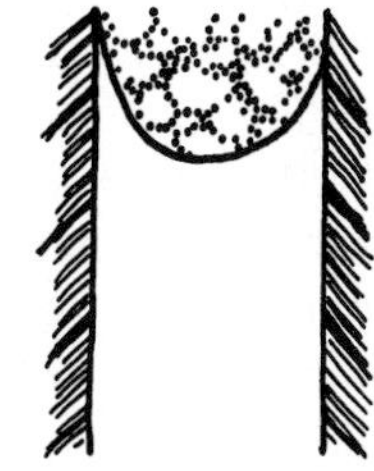

ELONGATION **PARTIAL TEAR** **COMPLETE TEAR**

Figure 3-12 ■ Diagram of muscle distraction. Three major categories of distraction injury can be identified sonographically. Elongation injuries have the best prognosis. Partial tears of muscle are associated with longer recovery times. Full-thickness tears carry the worst prognosis because scar tissue replaces muscle mass during the healing process. The white areas in this diagram represent muscle tears. Torn muscle fills with hemorrhage in the acute phase. At the time of the first ultrasound examination, most tears will appear as hypoechoic or anechoic spaces within the muscle.

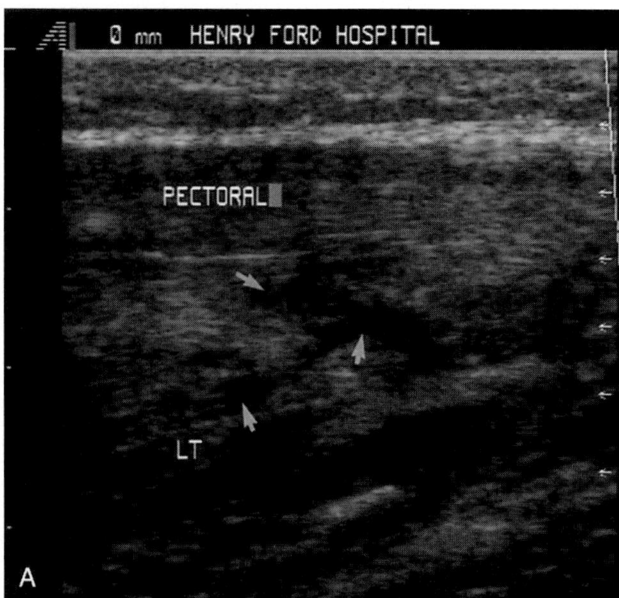

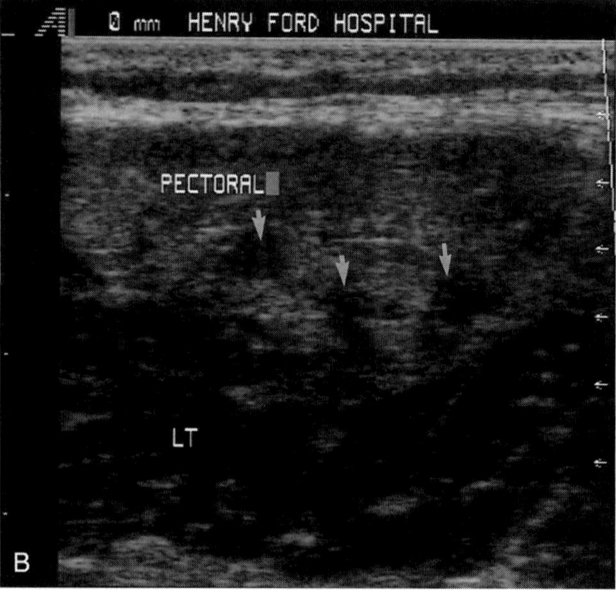

Figure 3–13 ▪ **A,** Elongation injury of the pectoralis major: longitudinal ultrasound. A 28-year-old policeman felt a pop when he was bench pressing 405 pounds. The orthopedic surgeon evaluating him referred him for ultrasound examination because he was concerned that the pectoralis tendon may have been avulsed. The tendon appears intact, but the superficial pectoralis muscle contains hypoechoic patches (*arrows*), which are changes compatible with elongation injury. A torn tendon would have required immediate surgery, while an elongation injury of muscle is treated conservatively. Abbreviation: left arm (*LT*). **B,** Elongation injury of the pectoralis major: transverse ultrasound. Same patient as in **A.** The hypoechoic regions (*arrows*) are also seen in the superficial pectoral muscle when the muscle is examined with the transducer oriented transversely over the belly of the pectoralis major. After 3 weeks of rest, the policeman returned to his routine weight-lifting activity.

without point tenderness. This entity is clinically indistinguishable from muscle cramp. Anatomically, the lesions are predominantly microscopic, with injury involving less than 5% of muscle substance. On gross pathologic examination, small cavities containing serosanguinous fluid are identified (Fig. 3–13). The cavities range from 3 to 7 cm and have a cross-sectional diameter ranging from 2 mm to 1 cm. These areas are believed to represent small fluid collections that fill voids created by myofibrillar retraction following rupture (Zuinen et al., 1982; Peterson and Renstrom, 1986). Ultrasound demonstrates these cavities as flame-shaped, hypoechoic areas in the muscle belly. Examination in multiple planes is necessary in some cases to differentiate subtle lesions from artifact. Follow-up examination performed 2 weeks following injury will demonstrate restoration of normal muscle architecture. Therapy for elongation injury consists of rest of the involved muscle and palliation of pain.

Partial muscle rupture (grade II) is a more extensive injury, with the muscle stretched well beyond the limit of its elasticity. It involves more than 5% of muscle substance but less than the entire muscle cross section (Fig. 3–14). At the time of injury, the patient often experiences a "snap" accompanied by the sudden onset of sharp focal pain (Fig. 3–15). Acutely, muscle function is completely absent. Partial function returns slowly over several days. Unlike elongation injury, point tenderness and focal swelling are present. Ecchymosis may develop if the muscle is located superficially. This usually develops

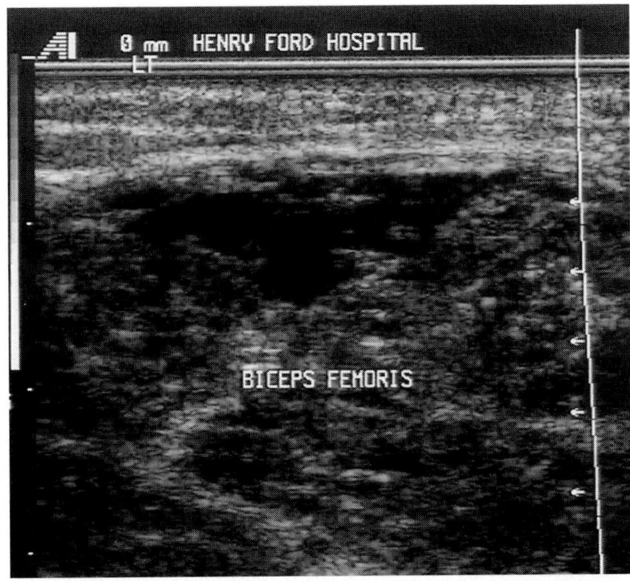

Figure 3-14 ■ Partial rupture of the superficial biceps femoris tendon: transverse sonogram. Three weeks ago, this 27-year-old soccer player sustained an injury to his left leg. A triangular hypoechoic defect is seen in the superficial layer of the biceps femoris muscle. It took several months before this athlete could perform at full strength again. Hamstring injuries are often very resistant to treatment.

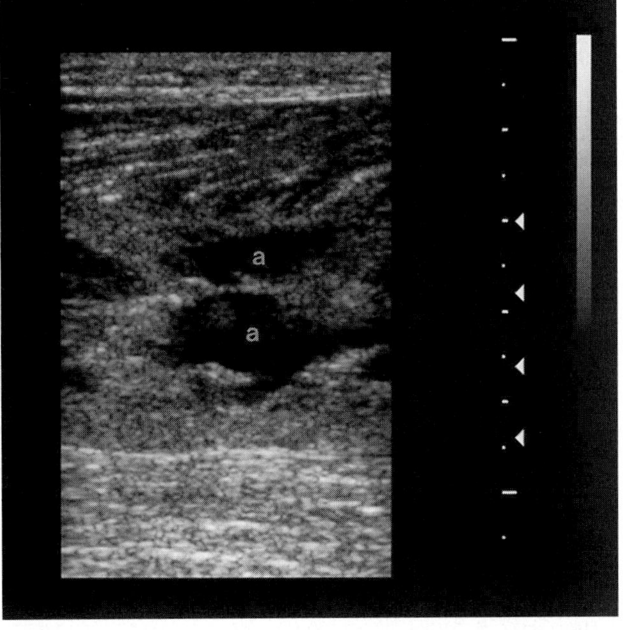

Figure 3-15 ■ Partial-thickness tear of the hamstring: longitudinal ultrasound. This professional football wide receiver felt a sudden stabbing pain in his posterior thigh while sprinting. He was unable to finish the game. Fifty percent of the biceps femoris muscle is replaced by hematoma. Anechoic spaces (*a*) surround irregular, torn muscle tissue.

2 to 24 hours following injury and is found distal to the site of rupture. Rarely, the rupture is detected clinically as a palpable defect.

Sonography clearly demonstrates the discontinuity in the muscle, with disruption of the fibroadipose septa (Fig. 3-16). A hypoechoic gap is identified within the muscle substance. Fragments of torn muscle originating from the walls of the cavity can be identified within the hematoma, which fills the gap. Gentle pressure applied with the transducer will demonstrate these torn muscle fragments to be free floating, referred to as the *bell clapper sign* (Fig. 3-17) (Wagner et al., 1980; Fornage et al., 1983; Harcke et al., 1988). The proportion of intact muscle can be evaluated accurately by imaging in multiple planes. A mass effect displacing adjacent perimysium, fascia, and tendons may also be observed. Follow-up examinations will show a hyperechoic wall (Fig. 3-18) that corresponds to granulation tissue and regenerating muscle fibers. This wall thickens progressively and fills in the cavity. The

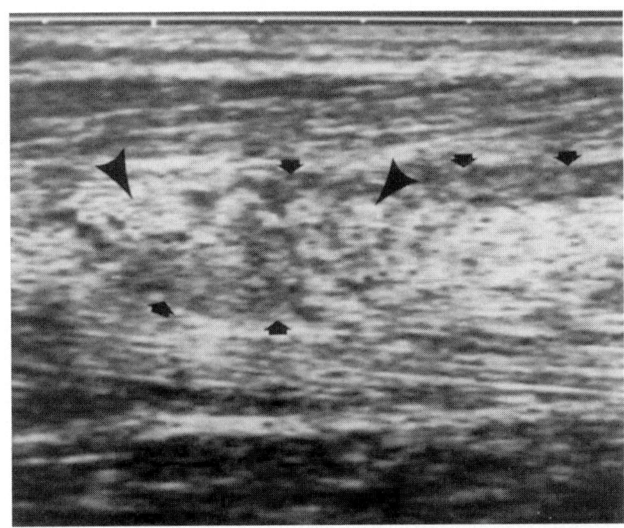

Figure 3-16 ■ Fresh partial hamstrings rupture: longitudinal sonogram. This 24-year-old sprinter had acute onset of sharp pain in the posterior right leg during a 100-m race. Pain increased progressively throughout the day. This examination was performed the same day, with the transducer aligned along the length of the biceps. The normal pennate structure of the muscle is disrupted, with slightly rounded ends of the ruptured muscle bundles (*large arrowheads*) separated by slightly hypoechoic hemorrhage (*small arrows*).

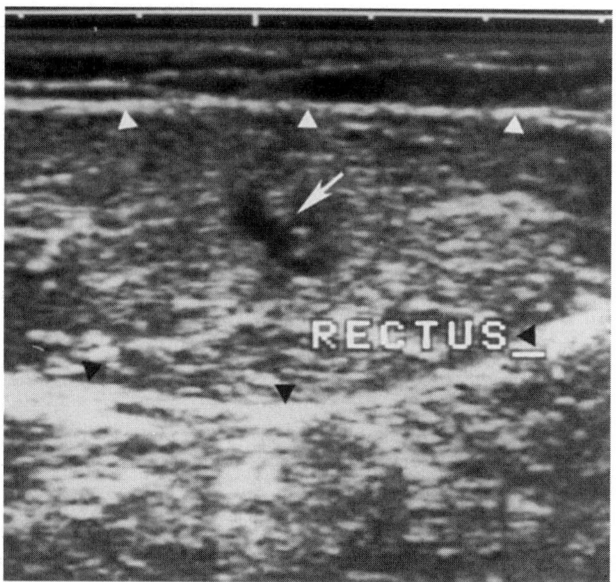

Figure 3-17 ▪ Partial rectus muscle tear: transverse sonogram. This 20-year-old football player presented 2 days after experiencing sharp pain in the anterior right thigh. A flap of torn muscle tissue (*white arrow*) with one end freely floating is seen in the rupture defect (a bell clapper sign). The torn end of the muscle flap is clearly identified as moving freely within the hematoma on real-time imaging. Fascia (*white arrowheads*), aponeurosis (*black arrowheads*).

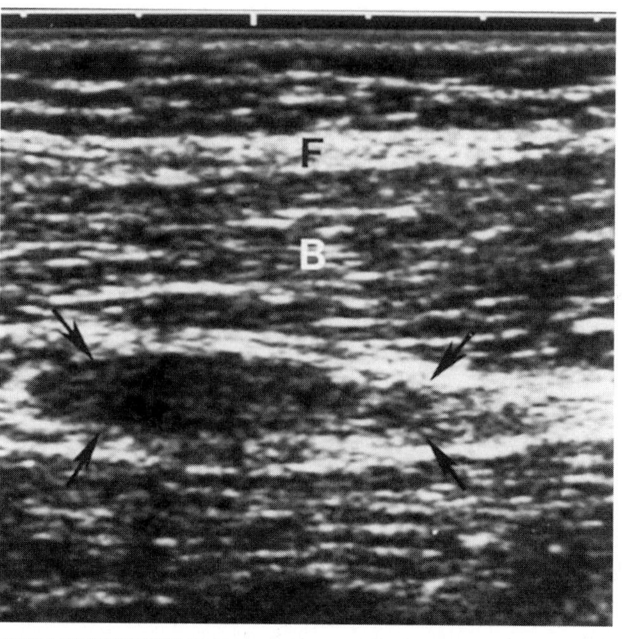

Figure 3-18 ▪ Healing partial hamstrings tear: longitudinal sonogram. Three weeks ago, this 25-year-old professional soccer player experienced sharp pain in the posterior right thigh during a game. He has experienced persistent pain and has been unable to exercise since the injury. The transducer is positioned over the mid-posterior thigh along the length of the biceps (*B*). An ovoid, hypoechoic lesion with thick, echogenic borders (*arrows*) is identified within the substance of the hamstrings, consistent with a healing partial muscle rupture. Abbreviation: fascia (*F*).

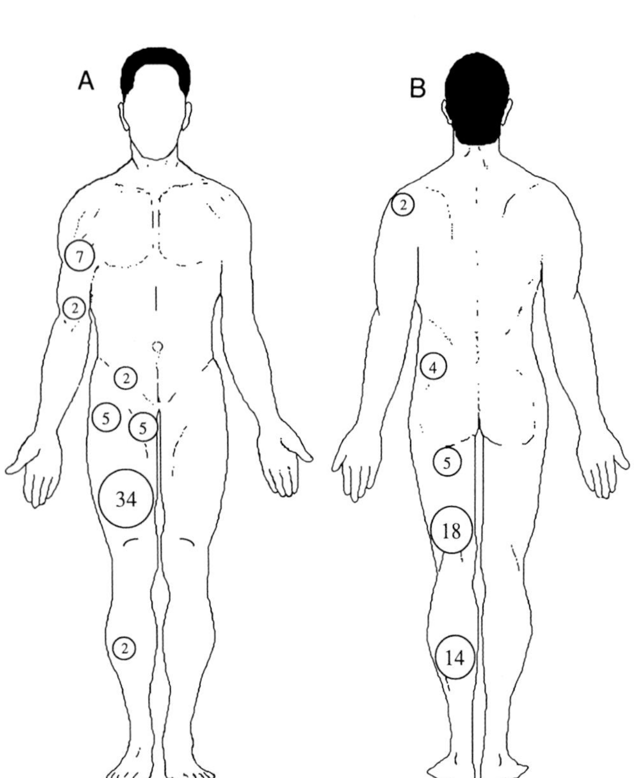

Figure 3-19 ▪ Frequency of muscle ruptures by site.

sonographic triad of a hypoechoic cavity within the muscle substance, a thick hyperechoic wall of the cavity, and the bell clapper sign are pathognomonic for muscle rupture. In extensive injury, therapy may include surgical repair of the ruptured segment. Management of the accompanying hematoma will be discussed later.

Complete muscle rupture (grade III) is seen less frequently than either elongation injury or partial rupture. The initial clinical presentation is quite similar to that of partial rupture, although associated syncope has also been reported (Peetrons and Sintzoff, 1987). In complete rupture, total functional impairment persists. When the muscle is superficially located, the gap between the retracted ends of the ruptured muscle can usually be palpated. Ecchymosis is also more common in cases of complete rupture. Figure 3-19 shows the frequency of muscle ruptures by site as observed in our practice.

Complete separation and retraction of the severed muscle are apparent on sonographic examination (Figs. 3-20 through 3-22). The distal portion of the retracted muscle may "bunch up," resembling a soft tissue mass (Peterson and Renstrom, 1986)

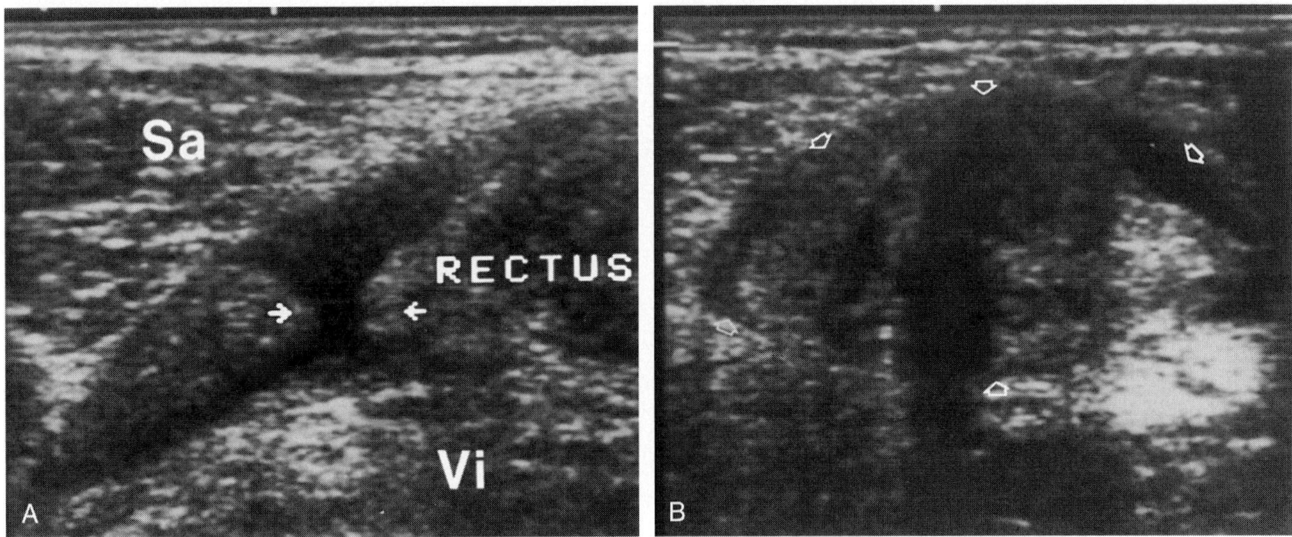

Figure 3-20 ▪ **A,** Complete rectus muscle rupture by distraction: longitudinal sonogram. The patient is a 21-year-old soccer player who felt a pop and a sharp, stabbing pain while running. This longitudinal image of the proximal anterior thigh was obtained 5 days after injury. The rounded proximal and distal ends of the ruptured muscle (*arrows*) are separated by hematoma throughout the cross section of the muscle. Distraction injury of the rectus femoris is the most commonly observed muscle rupture. Abbreviations: sartorius muscle (*Sa*), vastus intermedius muscle (*Vi*). **B,** Complete rectus muscle rupture by distraction: transverse sonogram. Same patient as in A. The transducer is positioned transversely over the point of maximal tenderness, just proximal to the site of rupture. A finding characteristic of complete rupture is fluid within the epimysium (*open arrows*) surrounding the entire circumference of the muscle.

(Figs. 3-23 and 3-24). Hematoma fills the void created by the retracted muscle ends. The investing fascia may be intact. However, extension of hematoma through a rent in the investing fascia is observed in the majority of cases. Several days following injury, enhanced through-transmission will be noted deep to the hematoma. Nerve involvement may also be noted sonographically. However, electromyographic evaluation is indicated when a neurological deficit is evident clinically, despite identification of an intact nerve on sonographic images.

Hematoma

Hematoma formation is a hallmark of muscle rupture. The magnitude of the hematoma generally indicates the extent of the underlying injury. However, muscle hematoma may be out of propor-

Figure 3-21 ▪ Complete vastus intermedius rupture by distraction: longitudinal sonogram. A 27-year-old male soccer player presented with a complaint of stabbing pain in the anterior right thigh, which developed suddenly while playing. This image was obtained with the transducer placed along the length of the rectus (*R*) at the point of maximal tenderness. A 2-cm gap (*open arrows*) is present in the vastus intermedius (*VI*) throughout its cross section. Compare the smooth, distinct margins of this distraction injury with the rough margins of the compression injury seen in Figure 3-11.

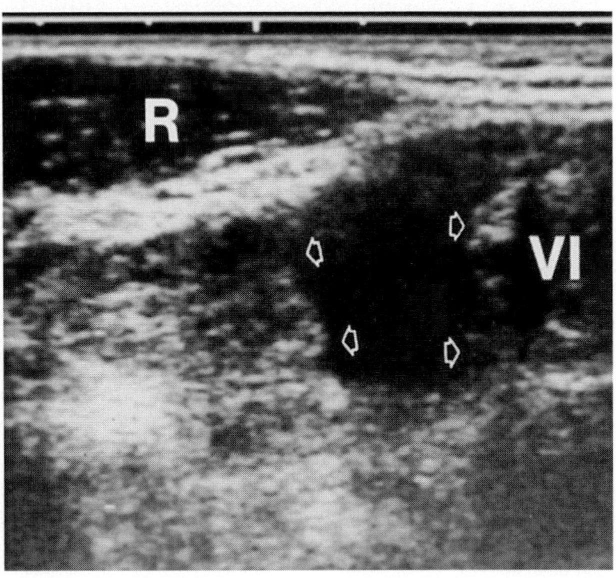

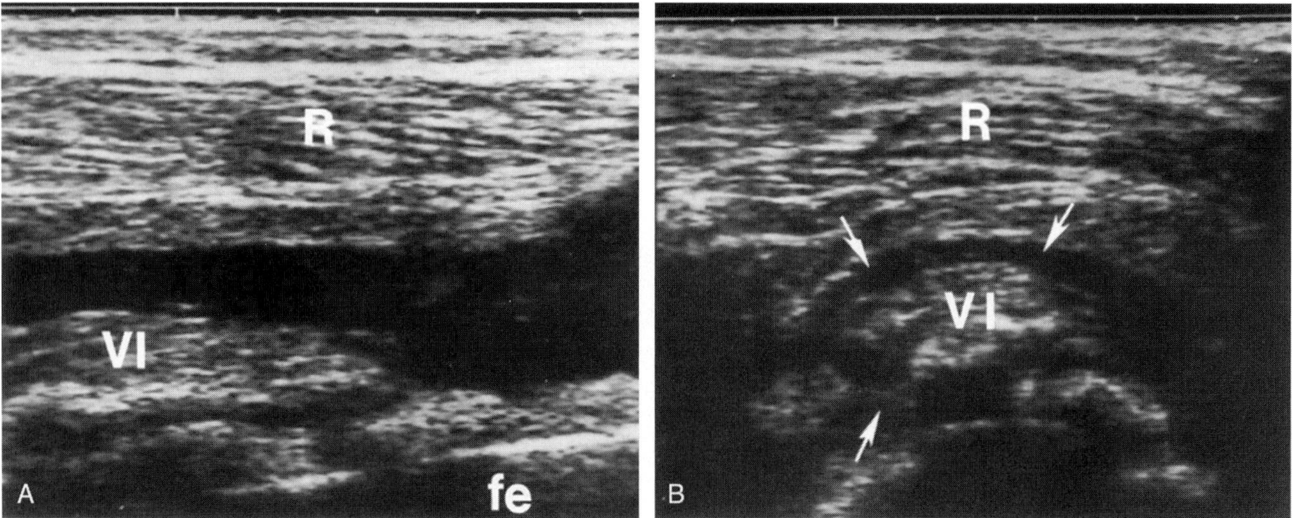

Figure 3-22 ■ A, Bell clapper sign: longitudinal sonogram. The patient is a 20-year-old football player who experienced a sudden onset of sharp pain in the anterior right midthigh. No definite clinical signs of complete rupture were present. The transducer position is just superior to that in Figure 3-20. A complete tear of the vastus intermedius (*VI*) is present. Pressure applied with the transducer demonstrated free movement of the torn muscle ends. The bell clapper sign is present in both partial and complete ruptures. Abbreviations: rectus muscle (*R*), femur (*fe*). B, Bell clapper sign: transverse sonogram. Same patient as in A. The transducer is positioned transversely just proximal to the site of rupture. Hemorrhage (*arrows*) completely surrounds the vastus intermedius (*VI*) immediately beneath the rectus (*R*).

tion to the associated injury in patients with hemophilia or on anticoagulant therapy. Direct trauma will result in contusion of the highly vascular fibroadipose septa. These septa are markedly thickened on sonographic images (Fig. 3-25), and diffuse hemorrhage leads to increased echogenicity (Figs. 3-26 through 3-28). Elongation injury may also cause contusion of the fibroadipose septa. In these cases, disruption of vessels in the epimysium may also occur, producing intermuscular hematoma. Intermuscular hematoma is characterized by blood dissecting within the fascial planes between muscles (see Fig. 3-25). More extensive injury will result in formation of intramuscular fluid collections that are

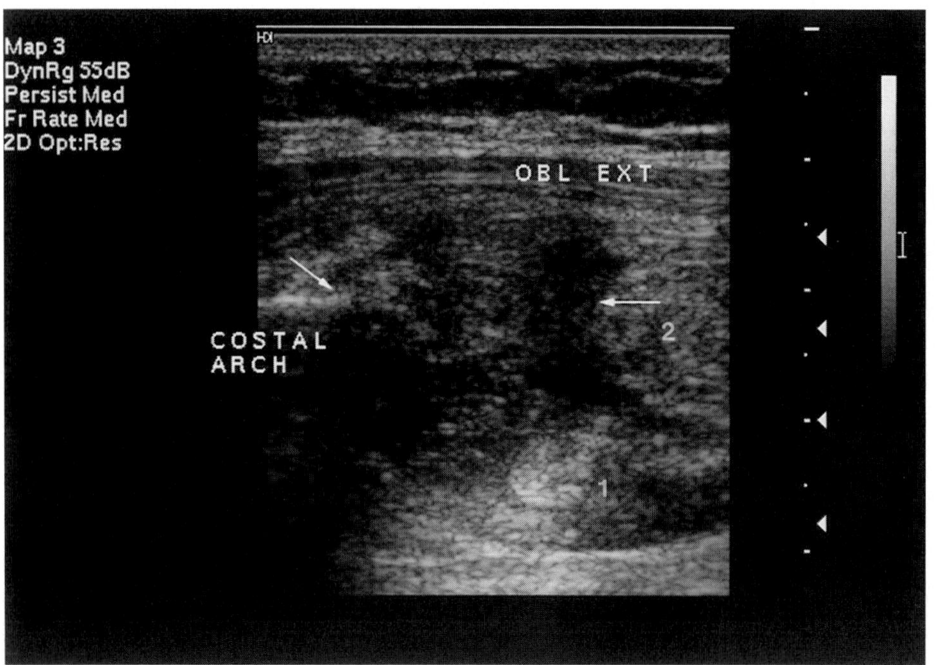

Figure 3-23 ■ Rupture of the internal oblique and transverse abdominis musculature: obliquely oriented image along the fibers of the external oblique muscle. This professional football quarterback had upper abdominal pain and was unable to throw the ball after an injury in the prior game. The external oblique muscle fibers of the anterior abdominal wall are intact. Both the transverse (*1*) and internal oblique (*2*) muscles have been avulsed from the lower rib cage (*COSTAL ARCH*). Hypoechoic hematoma separates (*arrows*) the muscles from the tenth rib. Note the rounded edge of the two torn muscles.

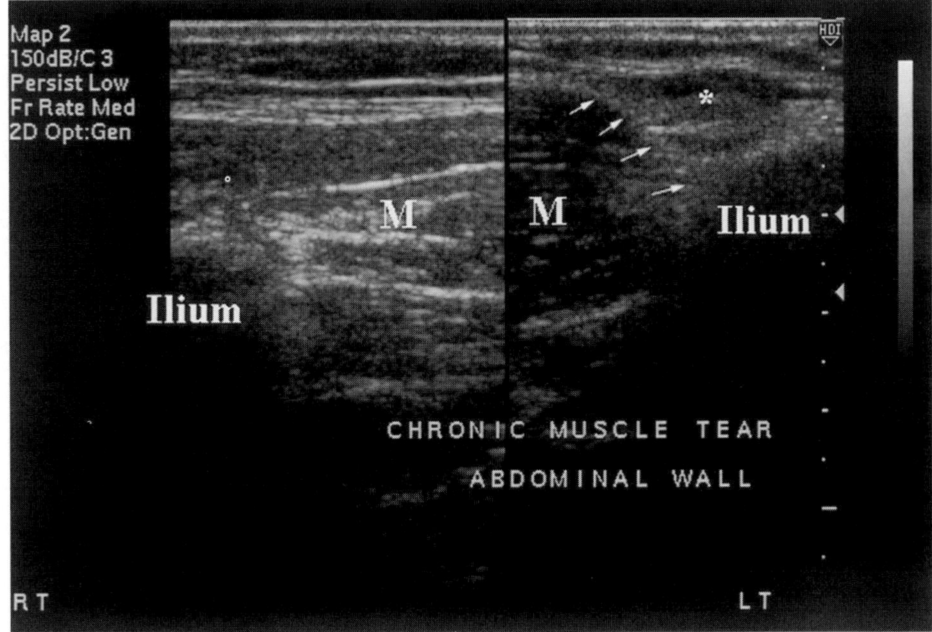

Figure 3-24 ■ Avulsion of abdominal musculature: transverse ultrasound scan with split-screen technique. A young athlete presents with a left iliac fossa mass 6 months after an abdominal wall injury. The three layers of the normal abdominal wall (*M*) are noted on the left side of the split screen and the avulsed abdominal muscles (*M*) on the right. Scar or granulation tissue (*) separates the retracted abdominal muscles from the iliac wing. The avulsed muscles have a rounded, retracted lateral border (*arrows*).

easily identified on ultrasound images. In cases of complete rupture, these collections may exceed 100 mL and extend beyond the investing fascia. Large hematomas may exhibit considerable mass effect (Fig. 3–29). The resulting compartment syndrome will further compromise the condition of surrounding muscles and nerves. Prompt evacuation of large hematomas is recommended in patients with increased compartment pressure.

The evolution and resolution of intramuscular hematoma do not differ from those of hematomas elsewhere in the body. Active hemorrhage may be hyperechoic; within a few hours, the bleeding will appear homogeneously hypoechoic. Several hours later, serum, cellular elements, and fibrin elements will separate out (see Fig. 3–29), resulting in an identifiable fluid-fluid level. As a result of further changes occurring over several days, the collection

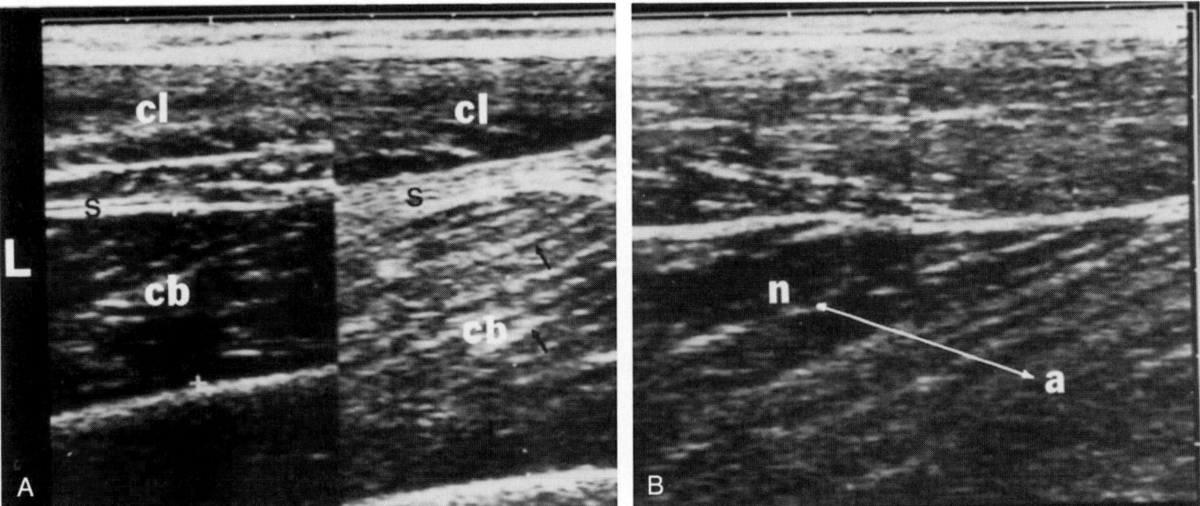

Figure 3-25 ■ **A,** Muscular contusion: longitudinal sonogram. Two hours after being hit in the right posterior thigh with the helmet of another player, this 20-year-old football player presented for sonographic examination. The transducer is positioned over the midportion of the hamstrings, along its length. In the image on the right, the short head of the biceps muscle (caput breve, *cb*) on the symptomatic leg is markedly swollen. Thickening and increased echogenicity are noted in the fibroadipose septa (*arrows*) and intermuscular septum (*s*). Compare this with the appearance of the asymptomatic side, shown on the left. Long head of the biceps muscle (caput longum, *cl*). **B,** The transducer is moved slightly superiorly to demonstrate the transition point from normal to contused muscle. Abbreviations: normal (*n*), abnormal (*a*).

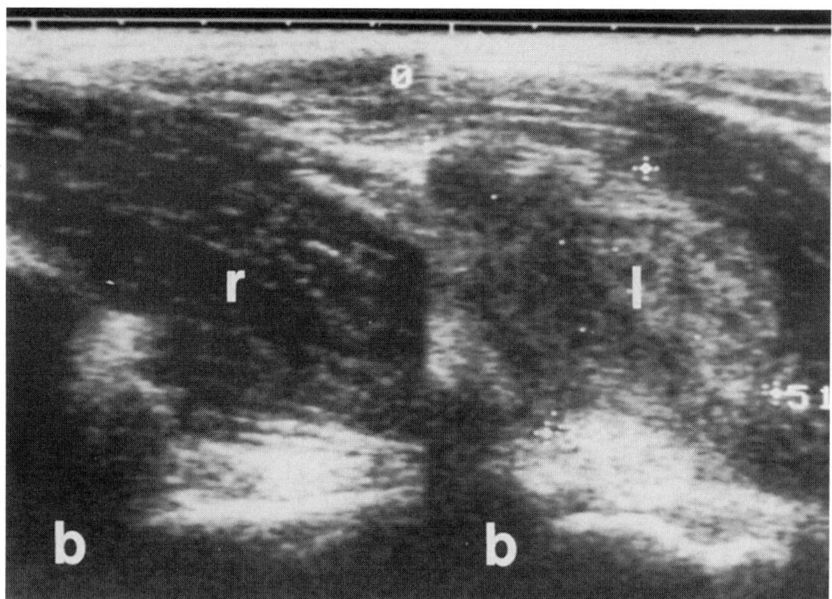

Figure 3-26 ▪ Recent iliopsoas contusion: longitudinal sonogram. At a local carnival, this 20-year-old man was injured by the steering wheel while driving one of the "bump cars." He complained of pain just medial to the left anterior-superior iliac spine and walked with a limp. The transducer is positioned along the length of the iliacus muscle, with the proximal side of the transducer at the anterior superior iliac spine. Comparison with the asymptomatic right side (*r*) is provided. The left (*l*) iliacus is markedly swollen and diffusely increased in echogenicity. Normal fibroadipose septa can no longer be identified at the site of injury, but no gap in the muscle substance is identified. Aspiration yielded approximately 20 ml of blood. Abbreviation: iliac bone (*b*).

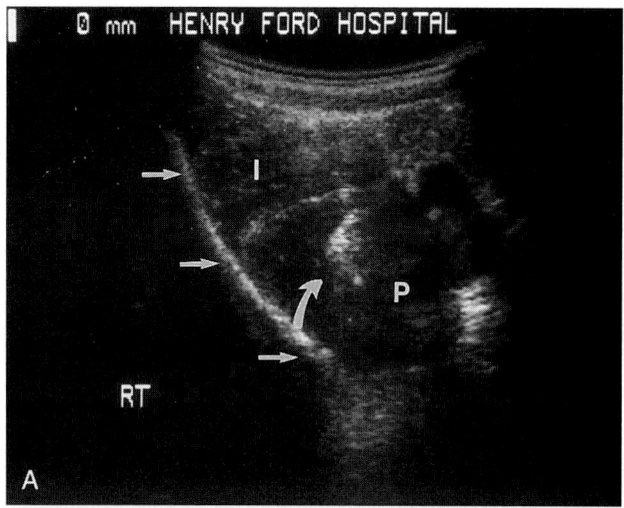

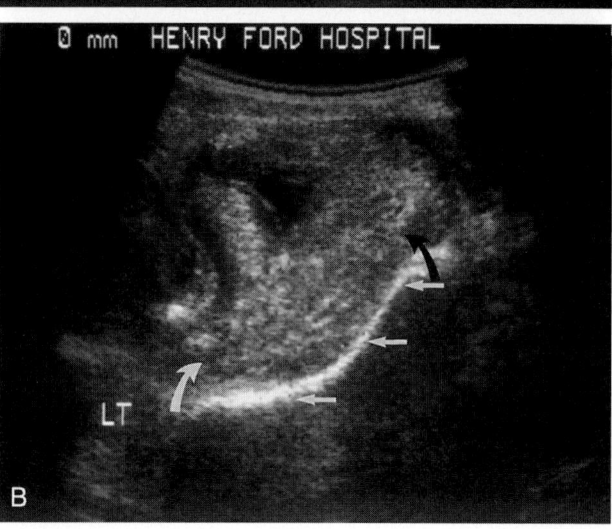

Figure 3-27 ▪ **A,** Recent iliopsoas contusion: transverse sonogram. This 20-year-old soccer player took a hard hit on his left hip. His left leg felt paralyzed for the rest of the game. A joint aspiration was performed because of a positive leg roll test, but the aspirate had been negative. The aspiration procedure was very painful. This transverse image of the asymptomatic right (*RT*) side of the pelvis shows normal psoas (*P*) and iliacus (*I*) muscles located along the curved surface of the ilium (*arrows*). The more echogenic tendon (*curved arrow*) is noted deep to the musculature. **B,** Recent iliopsoas contusion: transverse sonogram. Same patient as in **A.** The symptomatic left (*LT*) hip had no joint effusion on ultrasound examination. The painful aspiration could have been avoided had sonography been performed first. A simple explanation was found for the positive leg roll test by observing the pelvic musculature. Comparison of the abnormal left side with the normal right side (A) reveals swelling of the left pelvic musculature and abnormally increased echogenicity of the psoas (*curved white arrow*) and iliacus (*curved black arrow*) muscles. Note the sloped surface of the iliac wing which forms the lateral border of the pelvis (*arrows*).

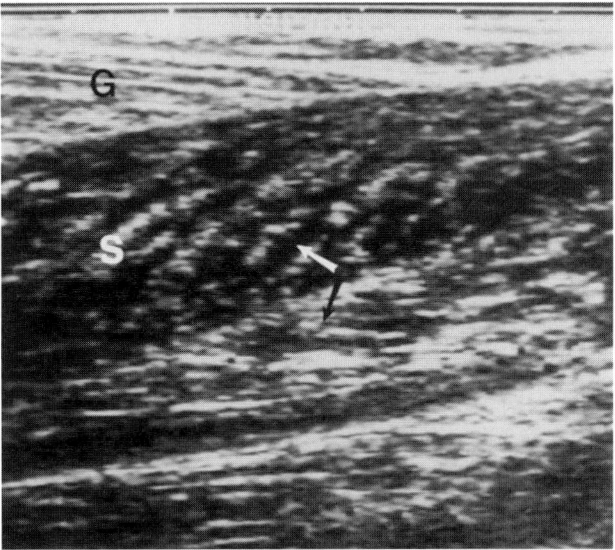

Figure 3-28 ■ Resolving muscular contusion of the calf muscles: longitudinal sonogram. Two weeks ago, this patient sustained a blow to the posterior calf. Muscle bundles (*white arrow*) and fibroadipose septa of the soleus (*s*) are markedly thickened and decreased in echogenicity. Compare this appearance with that of the flexor hallucis longus (*black arrow*) deep to the soleus. Abbreviation: normal gastrocnemius (*G*).

will become uniformly anechoic (Fig. 3-30). Fluid aspirated from the collection at this stage of evolution will have the characteristic "crank case oil" appearance. These collections will be resorbed slowly, over a period of weeks, without intervention. Spontaneous hematomas can occur in patients who receive anticoagulants. However, one should be aware of the fact that soft tissue sarcoma, particularly malignant fibrous histiocytoma, can present with acute bleeding of the tumor. A hemorrhage in the thigh of an older individual which does not resorb within the normal time period should be considered with suspicion. Biopsy of the lesion will then be necessary for diagnosis.

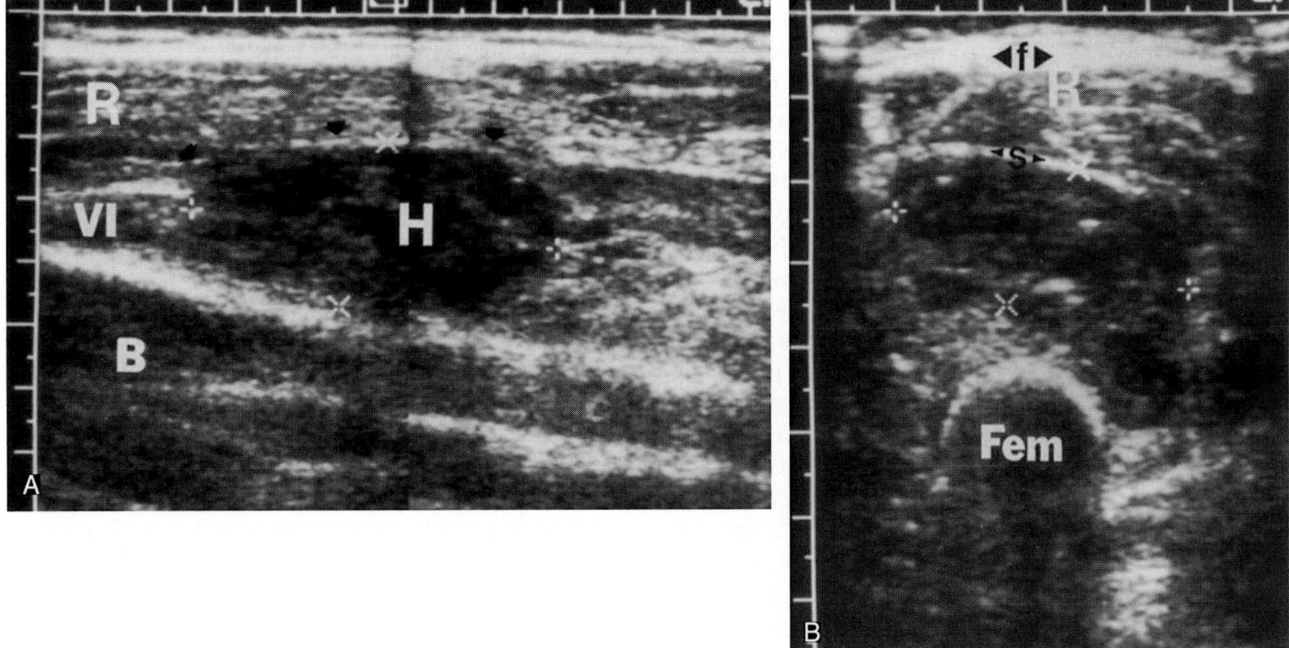

Figure 3-29 ■ **A,** Quadriceps hematoma: longitudinal sonogram. This 30-year-old man developed a distraction rupture of the quadriceps during a soccer game 3 days ago. A hypoechoic fluid collection (*H*) is identified within the vastus intermedius (*VI*) dorsal to the rectus (*R*). The intramuscular hematoma elevates the intermuscular septum (*small arrows*). Fibrin clots are seen floating within the hematoma. Abbreviation: femur (*B*). **B,** Quadriceps hematoma: transverse sonogram. Same patient as in A. Anterior bowing of the intermuscular septum (*s*) is better appreciated on this transverse image through the hematoma (×). Note the three hyperechoic arcs identified in this image: the fascia cruris (*f*), intermuscular septum (*s*), and femoral cortex (*Fem*).

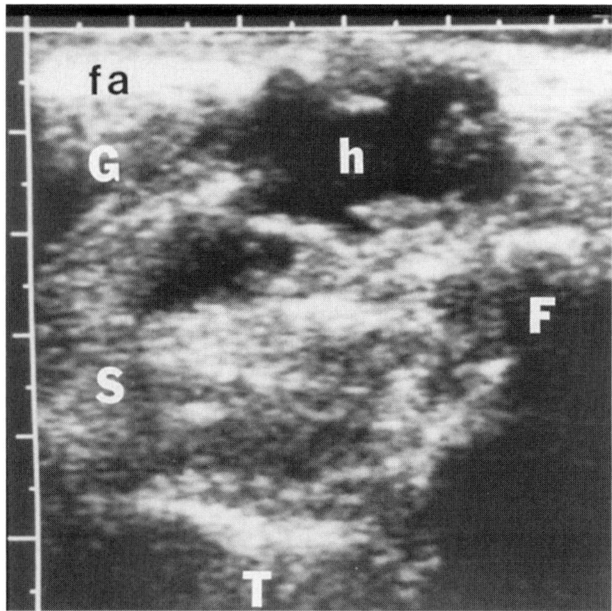

Figure 3-30 ■ Intramuscular hematoma after compression injury: transverse sonogram. An ecchymosis developed at the posterior-superior aspect of the left calf of this 40-year-old man after a horse kicked him. At the time of presentation 12 days following injury, he was unable to walk on his left leg. The transducer is positioned transversely over the calf muscles just below the knee. A characteristic compression rupture is identified. An anechoic hematoma (*h*) with markedly irregular borders is present, involving both the gastrocnemius (*G*) and the soleus (*S*). Note that the superficial fascia (*fa*) and the intermuscular septum are ruptured. This type of multiple compartment involvement is frequently associated with compression injury but is unheard of in distraction injury. Abbreviations: fibula (*F*), tibia (*T*).

Healing of Muscle Rupture

Healing of muscle rupture occurs slowly, taking 3 to 16 weeks to complete. The time required for healing is proportional to the extent of injury and is related to the location of the lesion. Lesions in the calf tend to heal more slowly than others. Surprisingly, muscle has a very strong capacity for regeneration. If the sarcolemmal sheaths are intact, complete regeneration of normal muscle architecture will occur by regeneration of myocytes (Bullough and Vigorita, 1984). This is typically seen in elongation injury and following infection. More extensive injury requires two different types of repair: regeneration and scar formation. These processes compete with each other. The objective of therapy is to ensure that regeneration predominates. In gross muscle rupture, regeneration occurs by growth of undamaged muscle fibers at the wound margin and formation of new fibers. These new fibers are formed by recruiting reserve cells found in the endomysium (Bullough and Vigorita, 1984). Formation of scar tissue will inhibit the process of regeneration.

The role of sonography in the evaluation of healing muscle rupture lies in three areas. First is the assessment of the extent of injury and measurement of the separation of wound margins. These two factors are the best predictors of the proportion of scar formation that can be measure sonographically. The greater the percentage of muscle substance involved and the larger the distraction gap, the highed the proportion of scar tissue. This information will guide the clinician in determining what intervention, if any, is indicated.

After initial evaluation, the role of sonography is to determine the stage of healing. The earliest detectable change toward healing is increased echogenicity of the margins of the wound (Figs. 3-31 through 3-33). This hyperechoic band will increase progressively in thickness as healing proceeds. Echogenicity of the inner aspect of this band will be slightly less than at the periphery. Eventually, the entire cavity will be filled in. Over a period of weeks this region will demonstrate further organization, and more normal muscle architecture with fibroadipose septa can be identified (Fig. 3-34). These serial follow-up examinations are extremely valuable in determining when it is safe for the patient to resume limited athletic activity. In our experience, resumption of training at the time when the lesion has filled in but further organization is not evident will lead to a high incidence of recurrent injury. Premature resumption of athletic activity will therefore prolong the recovery period and increase scar formation, to the detriment of both the individual athlete and his or her team.

The final role of ultrasound in the evaluation of healing muscle rupture is assessment of the magnitude of scar formation (Fig. 3-35). Fibrosis is evident sonographically as hyperechoic tissue (Figs. 3-36 and 3-37). Following distraction rupture, the fibrous scar is usually linear in contrast to compressive ruptures, in which the scar is usually nodular or triangular. Fibrous scar from superficial tears will result in focal retraction of the fascia or intermuscular septum (Fig. 3-38) toward the center of the lesion (see Fig. 3-37). Evaluation of the extent of

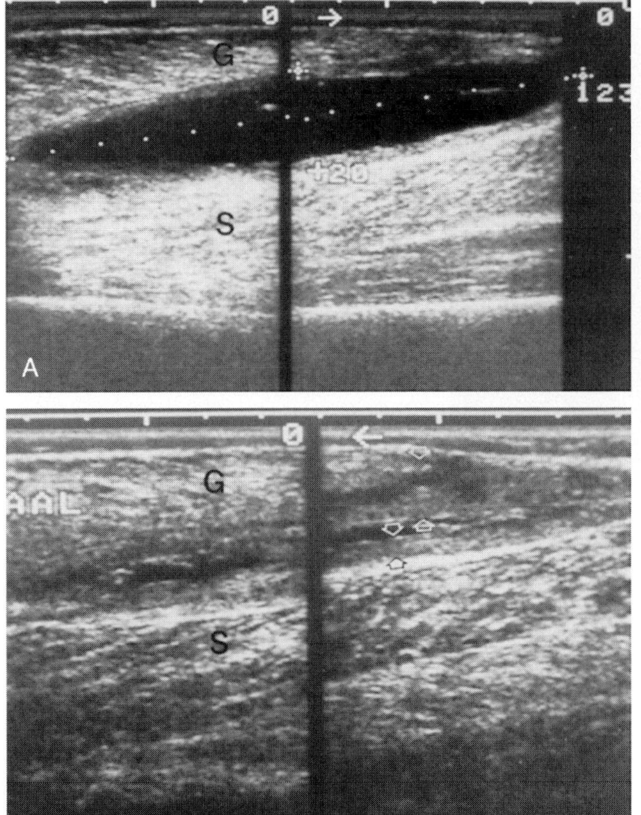

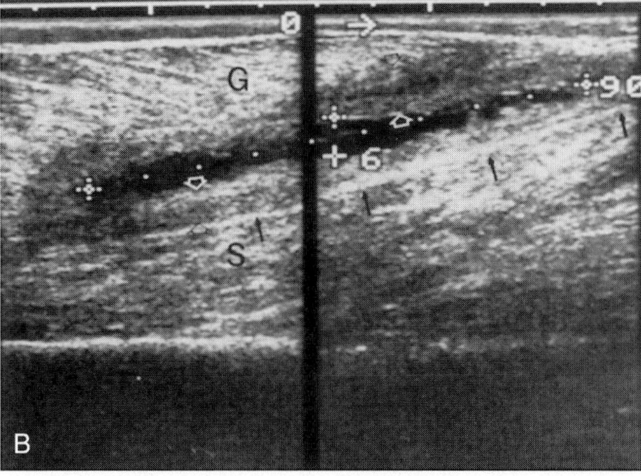

Figure 3-31 ■ **A,** Healing muscle rupture in the calf: longitudinal sonogram. A long jumper felt a sudden snap in the left calf during a jump. He experienced increased pain and swelling over the next 10 days and then finally presented for treatment. This longitudinal image demonstrates the long axis of the gastrocnemius (*G*) and soleus (*S*). A 12.5-cm fusiform hematoma separates the gastrocnemius and soleus along the intermuscular septum. This is the typical site of distraction injury in the lower leg. A thin rim of tissue lines the cavity, consistent with an early reparative response. The soleus appears hyperechoic relative to the gastrocnemius due to increased through-transmission. **B,** This image was obtained 7 weeks after injury. Note the marked interval decrease in the size of the hematoma. The reparative reaction (*open arrows*) is markedly increased, and the intermuscular septum (*black arrows*) is better visualized. Abbreviations: medial gastrocnemius (*G*), soleus (*S*). **C,** Twelve weeks after the injury healing continues normally, as demonstrated by further filling in of the lesion by reparative tissue (*open arrows*). Normal muscle architecture begins to be seen at the periphery of the lesion.

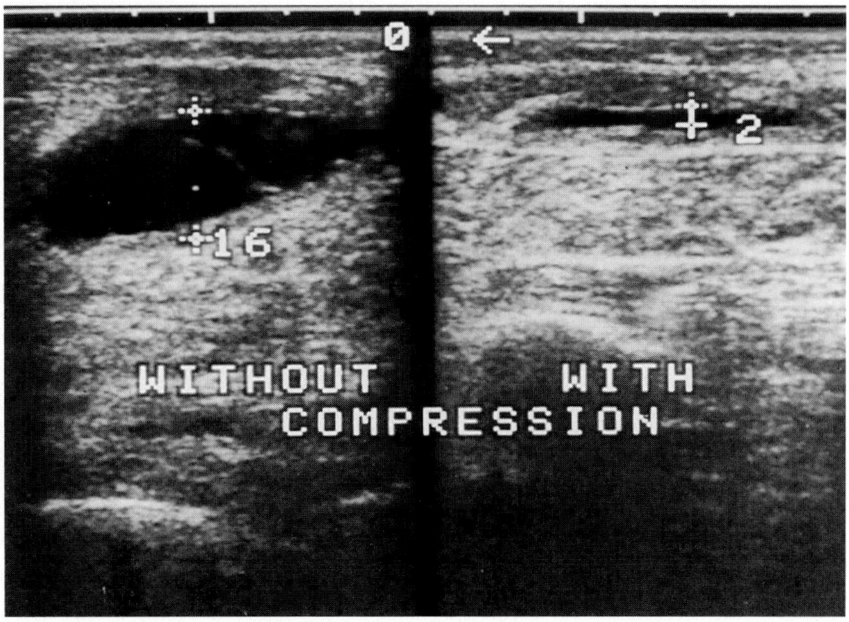

Figure 3-32 ■ Healing muscle rupture: transverse sonogram. This sonogram of the proximal left calf was obtained during the first examination of the patient in Figure 3-31. The compression image demonstrates without question that this is a fluid collection. Reparative tissue along the walls of the cavity does not change in dimension.

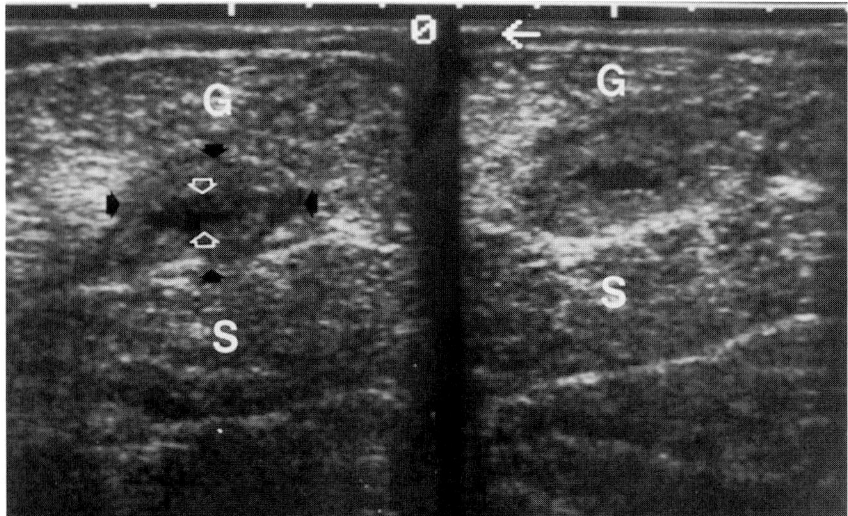

Figure 3-33 ■ Healing muscle rupture in the calf: transverse sonograms. Same patient as in Figures 3-31 and 3-32 12 weeks after trauma. Note the concentric appearance of the reparative tissue that fills in the lesion (*black arrows*). Residual hematoma (*white arrows*) is seen centrally within the lesion. The compression image on the right demonstrates that soft tissue of the reparative reaction is not compressible, unlike fluid (see Fig. 3-32). Abbreviations: medial gastrocnemius (*G*), soleus (*S*).

fibrosis is a direct indicator of the loss of a muscle's ability to produce tension. In addition, the risk of recurrent injury is proportional to the amount of residual fibrous scar (Nicholas and Hershman, 1986; Peterson and Renstrom, 1986) (Fig. 3-39).

An infrequent complication seen in cases of healing muscle rupture is the formation of a muscle cyst (Fig. 3-40). In our experience, the calf is the most common location of these cysts. The appearance of these cysts may vary slightly from the classic sonographic characteristics of a simple cyst. A perceptible thin wall may be identified, with focal areas of nodular thickening (Fig. 3-41). Septations may also be present (Zuinen et al., 1980, 1982). Little, if any, change occurs in the size of these lesions over observation periods as long as 3 years. Muscle cysts may cause chronic muscle pain, and surgical excision is indicated in such cases. At surgery these lesions are demonstrated to be cysts with a synovial lining filled with synovial fluid. They probably arise from pluripotential reserve cells found in the epimysium.

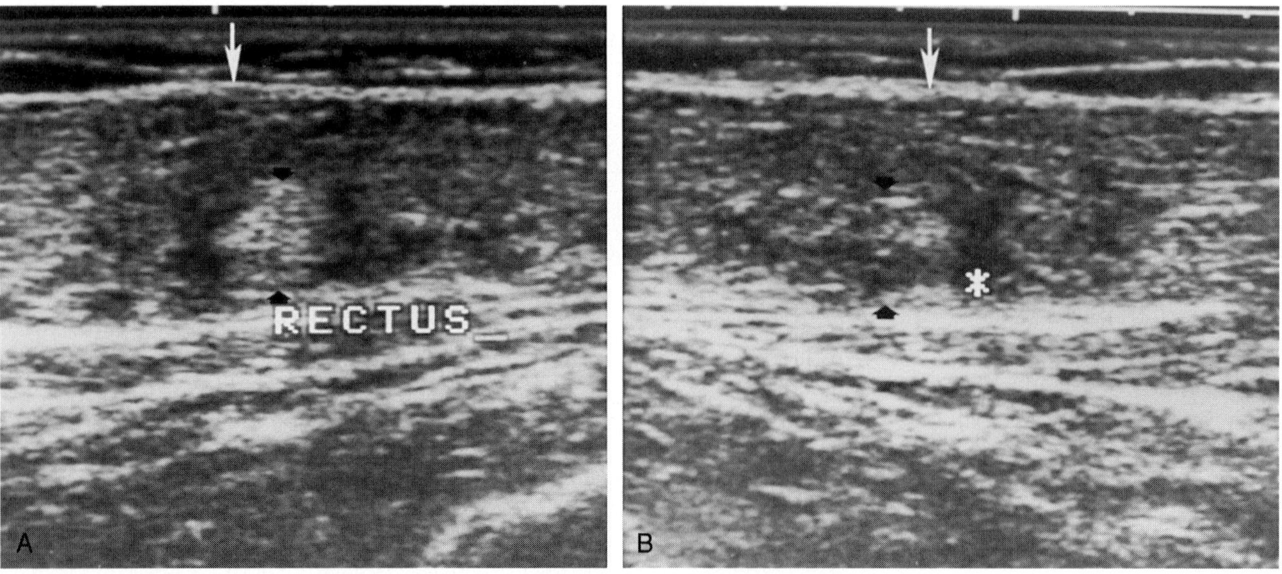

Figure 3-34 ■ **A,** Healing rectus muscle tear: longitudinal sonogram. Two gaps with an intervening segment of retracted muscle (*black arrows*) are identified within the rectus femoris of this 25-year-old basketball player 4 weeks after injury. The overlying fascia is slightly elevated (*white arrow*). **B,** Six weeks after injury, regeneration of muscle bundles is observed in the proximal gap, restoring continuity with the middle segment (*black arrows*). The distal gap (*asterisk*) remains visible. Elevation of the fascia (*white arrow*) is less prominent.

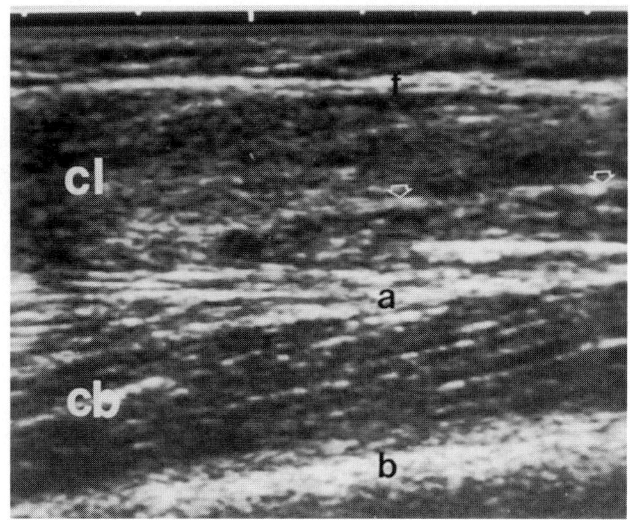

Figure 3-35 ■ Reparative tissue in the hamstrings: longitudinal sonogram. Seven weeks after a complete hamstrings rupture, the gap is filled in with homogeneous, hypoechoic tissue. A long hyperechoic line (*open arrows*) is identified running almost perpendicular to the axis of normal fibroadipose septa of the long head of the biceps (caput longum, *cl*). This is consistent with a fibrous scar. Note the normal pennate structure of the short head of the biceps (caput breve, *cb*). Abbreviations: aponeurosis (*a*), fascia (*f*), femur (*b*).

Myositis Ossificans

Muscular contusion with intramuscular hematoma may calcify and then ossify (Fig. 3-42). This lesion, called *myositis ossificans*, is a frequent finding in athletes involved in contact sports (Box 3-2). Often the inciting trauma is not extensive. In 40% of the cases, the lesion cannot be linked to a specific traumatic event. These lesions are most common in the thigh and pelvis. Identification of myositis ossificans is important because these lesions can cause chronic pain as they enlarge. Surgical removal may be required for palliative reasons. In addition, documentation of these lesions may prevent misdiagnosis at a later date. A young person may present with a painful extremity, and radiographs demonstrate an ossified mass in the diaphyseal region adjacent to the cortex. If the lesion is misinterpreted as a tumor, the pathologist will probably interpret the histologic specimen as a low-grade periosteal or parosteal sarcoma. Previous sonographic documentation of the size and location of myositis ossificans will prevent this unfortunate occurrence.

The evolution of myositis ossificans is easily followed with sonography. Maturation of these lesions takes approximately 5 to 6 months. Initially, within 3 weeks of injury, the lesion is identified as a soft tissue mass with disorganized, inhomogeneous internal architecture. At this stage, the lesion is indistinguishable sonographically from a soft tissue neoplasm. Clinicians may refer to this lesion as *gelosis*, a palpable, firm mass within muscle. This term comes from the Latin *gelare*, meaning "to freeze" (Figs. 3-43 and 3-44).

Three to 4 weeks following injury, the first calcifications appear. Early calcification may follow the

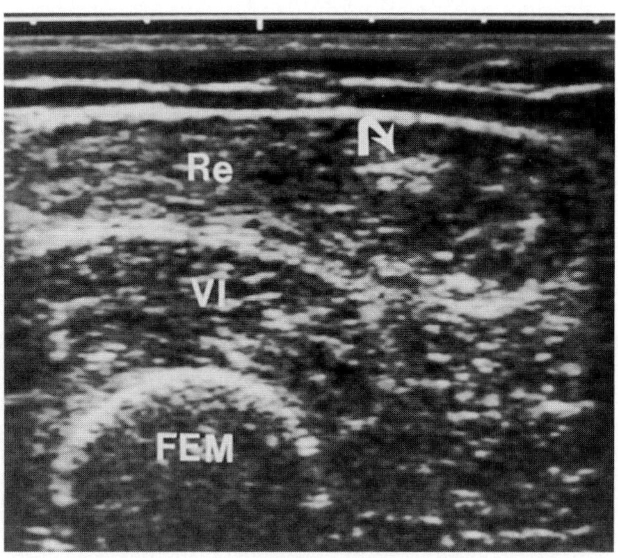

Figure 3-36 ■ Rectus scar after distraction injury: transverse sonogram. The patient experienced continued weakness of the right leg after distraction injury 3 months earlier. The transducer is positioned transversely over the anterior midthigh, demonstrating two divisions of the quadriceps: the rectus femoris (*Re*) and the vastus intermedius (*VI*). An echogenic ovoid area (*curved arrow*) within the substance of the rectus represents residual scar from prior rupture. Abbreviation: femur (*FEM*).

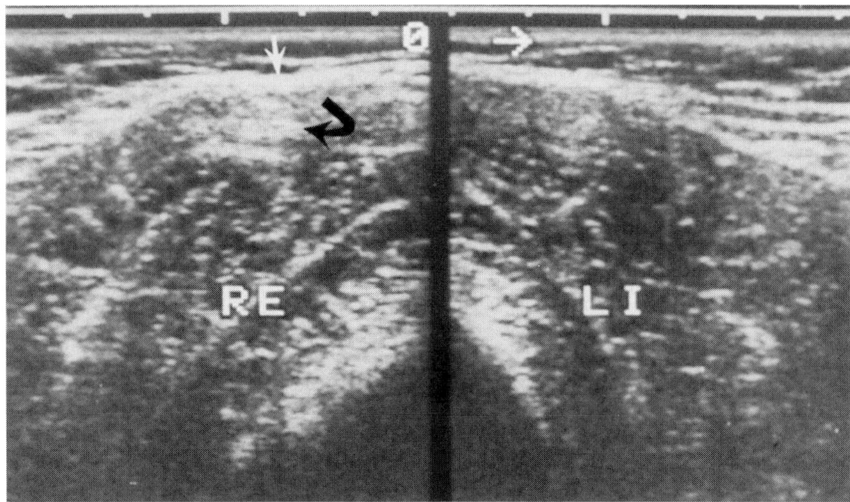

Figure 3–37 ■ Scar in the gluteus muscle: transverse sonogram. This 16-year-old female victim of a motor vehicle accident was struck on the right gluteal region 3 months ago. She complained of continued pain in the right gluteal region (*RE*) during normal activity. Side-by-side comparison demonstrates a region of increased echogenicity (*curved arrow*) in the right gluteus maximus deep to the fascia (*white arrow*), which appears retracted. Increased echogenicity and focal retraction are hallmarks of scar formation. Abbreviation: left gluteus maximus (*LI*).

feather-like structure of the muscle (Fig. 3–45). These calcifications are identifiable sonographically well before they are evident on conventional radiographs. The predominantly peripheral distribution of these calcifications is characteristic of myositis ossificans (see Figs. 3–42 and 3–45). This is soon followed by ossification (Kramer et al., 1979). During this process of maturation, acoustic shadowing will become evident. At this stage, it is important to note that no abnormal soft tissue extends beyond the borders defined by the shadowing calcifications. This helps to differentiate myositis ossificans from parosteal sarcoma. Further evidence to exclude parosteal sarcoma can be obtained by examination of the tissues deep to the calcifications. This requires careful angling of the transducer to direct the sound beam between shadowing calcifications. If normal periosteum adjacent to the cortex can be demonstrated, parosteal sarcoma has been excluded.

Heterotopic bone formation following total joint replacement, burns, or neurologic injury will demonstrate sonographic features similar to those of myositis ossificans. In these disorders, the distribution of ossification is predominantly periarticular, and the clinical history will clinch the diagnosis. Sonographic follow-up of these patients can be quite valuable, especially in patients with ankylosing spondylitis or Forestier's disease undergoing total hip arthroplasty, due to their predilection for heterotopic bone formation. Although satisfactory therapy is not yet available, clinical trials with diphosphonates have shown promise in reducing the formation of heterotopic bone.

Congenital myositis ossificans is an extremely rare disorder also referred to as *myositis ossificans progressiva*. In this idiopathic disorder, muscle ossification is symmetrical and bilateral. Systemic diseases such as dermatomyositis and scleroderma are also characterized by muscle calcifications. However,

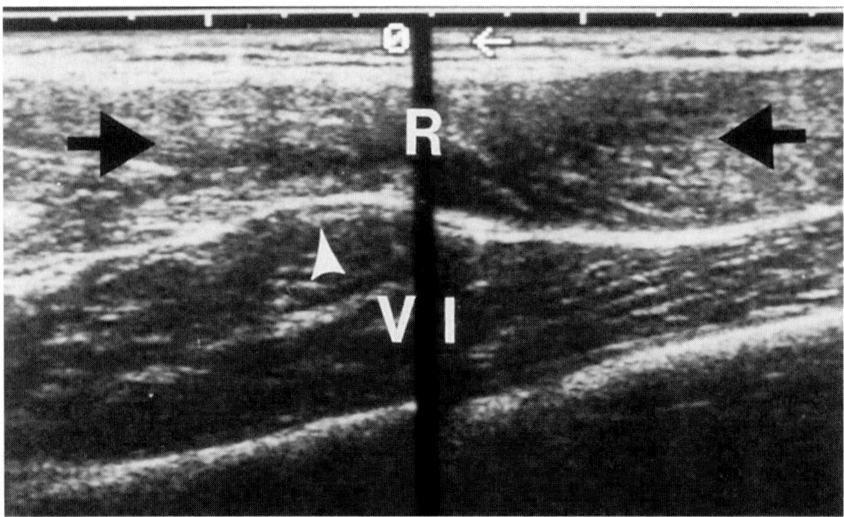

Figure 3–38 ■ Volume loss after rectus tear: longitudinal sonogram. One and one-half years ago, this 24-year-old football player suffered a complete rectus tear. He presented for sonographic evaluation after being unable to attain his previous level of performance. The normal pennate structure of the rectus (*R*) is replaced with inhomogeneous tissue (*large black arrows*). Marked retraction due to scarring of the healing rectus results in anterior bowing of the aponeurosis (*arrowhead*) and bulging of the vastus intermedius (*VI*).

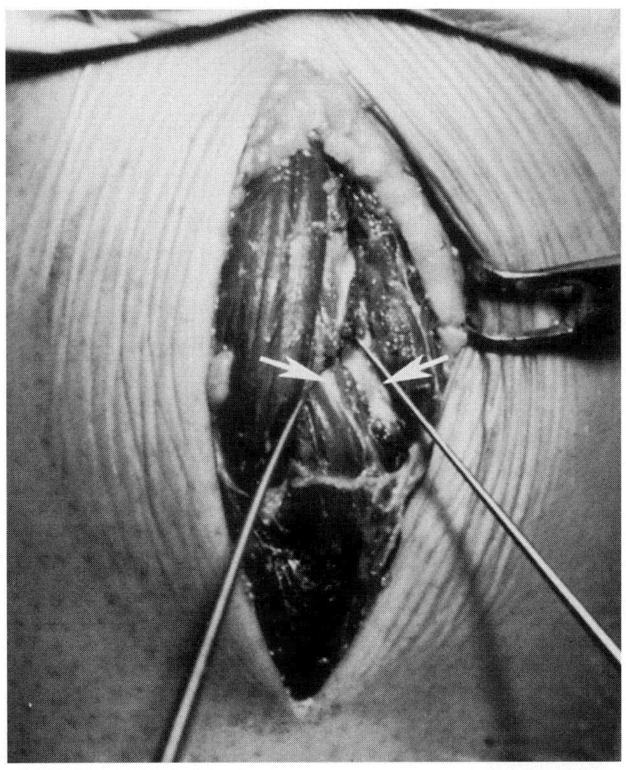

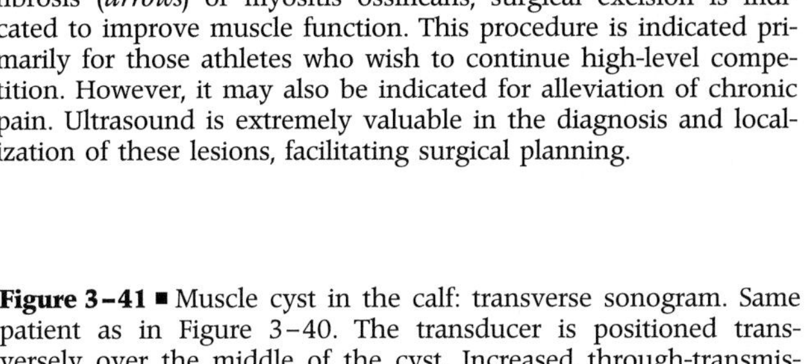

Figure 3–39 ■ Rectus fibrosis: surgical findings. In severe cases of fibrosis (*arrows*) or myositis ossificans, surgical excision is indicated to improve muscle function. This procedure is indicated primarily for those athletes who wish to continue high-level competition. However, it may also be indicated for alleviation of chronic pain. Ultrasound is extremely valuable in the diagnosis and localization of these lesions, facilitating surgical planning.

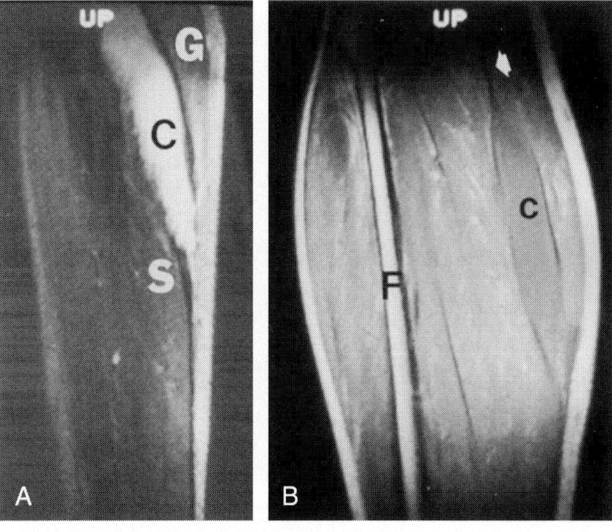

Figure 3–40 ■ A, Muscle cyst in the calf: sagittal MR image. This middle-aged man experienced blunt trauma to the right calf 4 months earlier. In this sagittal T_2-weighted spin-echo image, a large fluid collection of high-signal intensity (*C*) is identified between the gastrocnemius (*G*) and the soleus (*S*). The margin of the cyst adjacent to the soleus appears frayed. The location suggests a muscle-aponeurosis lesion. The duration of the lesion indicates markedly delayed healing, often seen in calf muscle rupture. B, Muscle cyst in the calf: coronal MR image. Same patient as in A. The cyst is identified as a fusiform collection of slightly decreased signal intensity on this coronal T_1-weighted spin-echo image. The location of the lesion (*c*) between the gastrocnemius and the soleus along the aponeurosis (*arrow*) is confirmed. Abbreviation: fibula (*F*).

Figure 3–41 ■ Muscle cyst in the calf: transverse sonogram. Same patient as in Figure 3–40. The transducer is positioned transversely over the middle of the cyst. Increased through-transmission deep to the cyst (*Cy*) is noted. This image demonstrates a torn muscle bundle (*arrow*) along the deep margin of the lesion, accounting for the frayed appearance of this border on the MRI examination. Abbreviations: gastrocnemius (*G*), soleus (*S*).

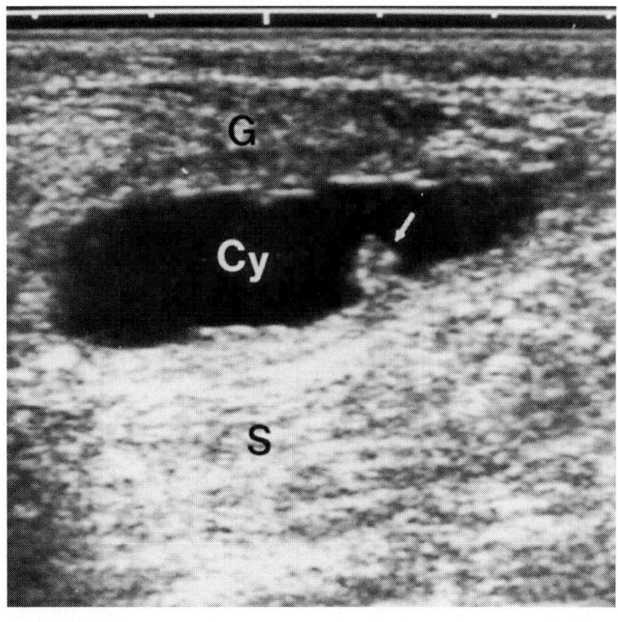

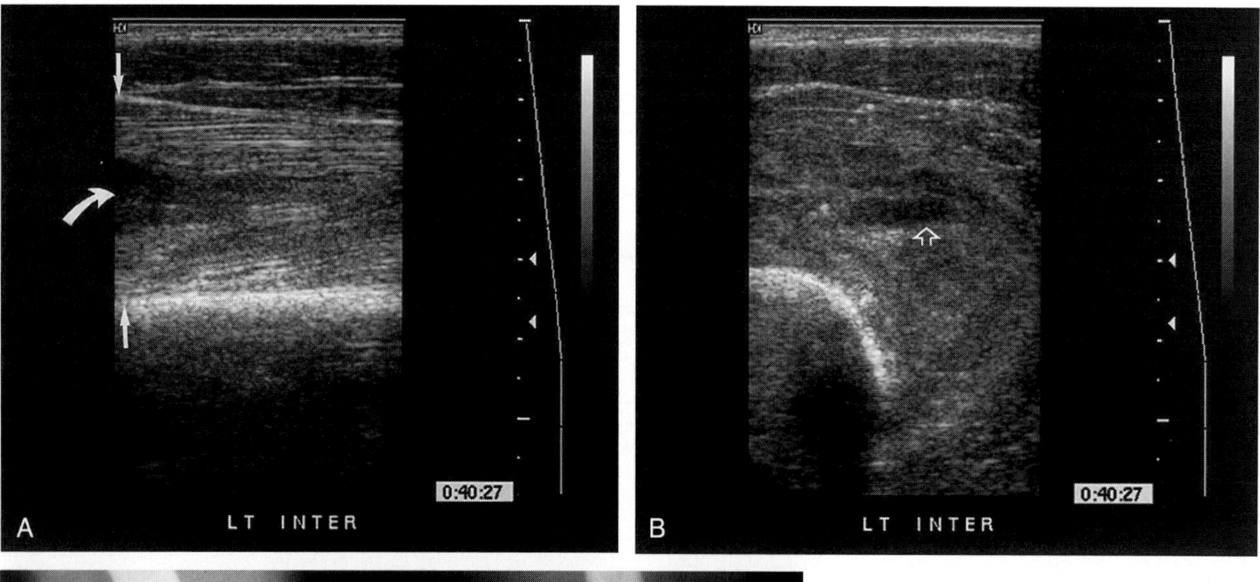

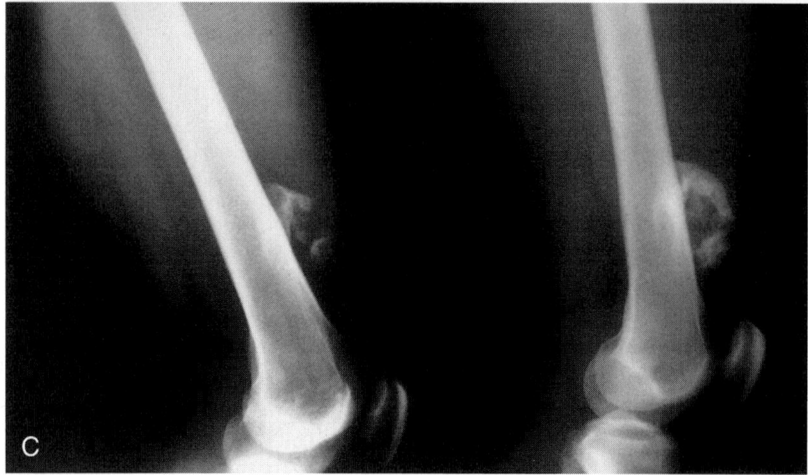

Figure 3–42 ■ **A,** Stages of myositis ossificans: longitudinal ultrasound. After a direct hit on the thigh, this 23-year-old soccer player had little strength in his left leg. The clinician palpated a firm mass and was concerned that a sarcoma might be growing in the thigh. An ultrasound exam was done 1 week after the injury. With the transducer over the distal thigh and aligned along the quadriceps, swelling (*between the arrows*) of the extensor musculature was noted. There was focal disruption (*curved arrow*) of the normal muscle architecture. **B,** Stages of myositis ossificans: transverse ultrasound. Same patient as in A. The examination demonstrated that the injury affected vastus intermedius tissue predominantly. The change in echogenicity suggested a fluid-fluid level (*open arrow*) compatible with hemorrhage. Conventional radiographs were negative at this time. Myositis ossificans frequently affects the vastus intermedius, and hemorrhage is often observed in the early stages of disease. **C,** Stages of myositis ossificans: lateral radiographs of the thigh. Same patient as in **A.** Conventional radiographs at 3 (at left side of picture) and 9 months (at right side of picture) at follow-up show maturing myositis ossificans. The zonal phenomenon with central lucency surrounded by peripheral ossification is supposed to be a specific sign of myositis ossificans.

calcifications will also be identified in the subcutaneous tissues of patients with these diseases.

Myositis

Myositis is a general term used to denote inflammation of muscle. It can occur as a result of trauma, infection, or systemic disease. Viral infection is frequently accompanied by muscle involvement characterized by myalgia. A classic example of this type of muscle pain is epidemic pleurodynia, or

Box 3–2
Myositis Ossificans

- No distinct trauma in 40% of cases
- Common in the vastus intermedius
- Appears as a mass initially
- Takes 3–4 weeks for calcification to appear

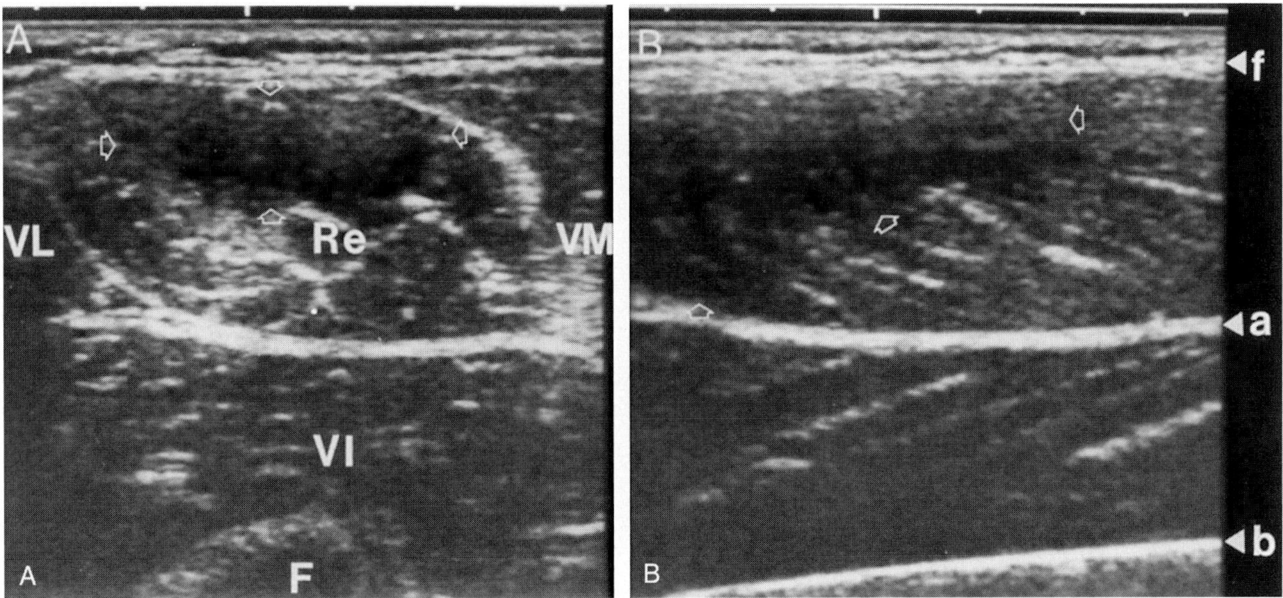

Figure 3-43 ■ **A,** Gelosis of the rectus muscle: longitudinal sonogram. A basketball player presented for sonographic examination 3 weeks after being hit in the anterior thigh by another player. The clinician palpated a firm mass in the rectus muscle. This transverse image was obtained over the rectus approximately 20 cm superior to the patella. A hypoechoic area (*open arrows*) composed of soft tissue is identified within the rectus (*Re*) corresponding to the clinically palpable abnormality. No fibroadipose septa are seen in this region. Abbreviations: vastus lateralis (*VL*), vastus medialis (*VM*), vastus intermedius (*VI*), femur (*F*). **B,** Gelosis of the rectus muscle: transverse sonogram. Same patient as in A. The transducer has been rotated to lie along the length of the quadriceps. A region of hypoechoic soft tissue replaces the normal muscle architecture. Note that this appearance differs from that of a healing muscle rupture. Abbreviations: aponeurosis (*a*), bone (*b*), fascia (*f*).

Bornholm disease. This is associated with coxsackie virus infection. Viral inclusions in muscle have been demonstrated by electron microscopy in association with viral infection (Resnick and Niwayama, 1988), but we have been unable to identify any sonographic changes.

Bacterial infection involving muscle is a serious condition that is most common in children and young adults. Although rare in temperate climates, pyogenic myositis is quite common in tropical regions (Resnick and Niwayama, 1988). It accounts for 4% of all surgical admissions in East Africa. Muscles of the lower extremities are most commonly involved; however, any muscle may become infected. In the majority of cases, the infection remains contained within a single fascial compartment. The involved muscle initially feels hard to palpation, and induration of the skin makes it resemble the texture of wood (Resnick and Niwayama, 1988). Subsequently, the mass becomes fluctuant, and regional adenopathy is palpable.

Ultrasound is particularly valuable in the early diagnosis of bacterial myositis, when the clinical picture is still nonspecific. The sonographic appearance of the involved muscle is the opposite of that of normal muscle. Muscle fibers become relatively hyperechoic. The fibroadipose septa are distended with inflammatory exudate and appear relatively hypoechoic (Figs. 3-46 and 3-47). Comparison with the asymptomatic side will demonstrate an increase in the diameter of the involved muscle. Given time, this lesion will evolve into a frank abscess with central necrosis and formation of a collection of purulent material (Fig. 3-48). Once the infection has reached this point, its appearance may be quite similar to that of an organizing hematoma. A hypoechoic fluid collection containing echogenic debris is identified. In some cases, a fluid-fluid level may be observed (Harcke et al., 1988). The clinical picture of high fever, chills, leukocytosis, and an elevated erythrocyte sedimentation rate will ensure the diagnosis. Echogenic foci with characteristic dirty shadowing can be seen if gas-forming organisms are present.

An abscess resulting from pyogenic myositis can usually be distinguished from one secondary to osteomyelitis. In cases of pyogenic myositis, the abscess is clearly centered in muscle. However, in muscle abscess resulting from osteomyelitis, purulent material will be seen tracking along the bony

Text continued on page 52

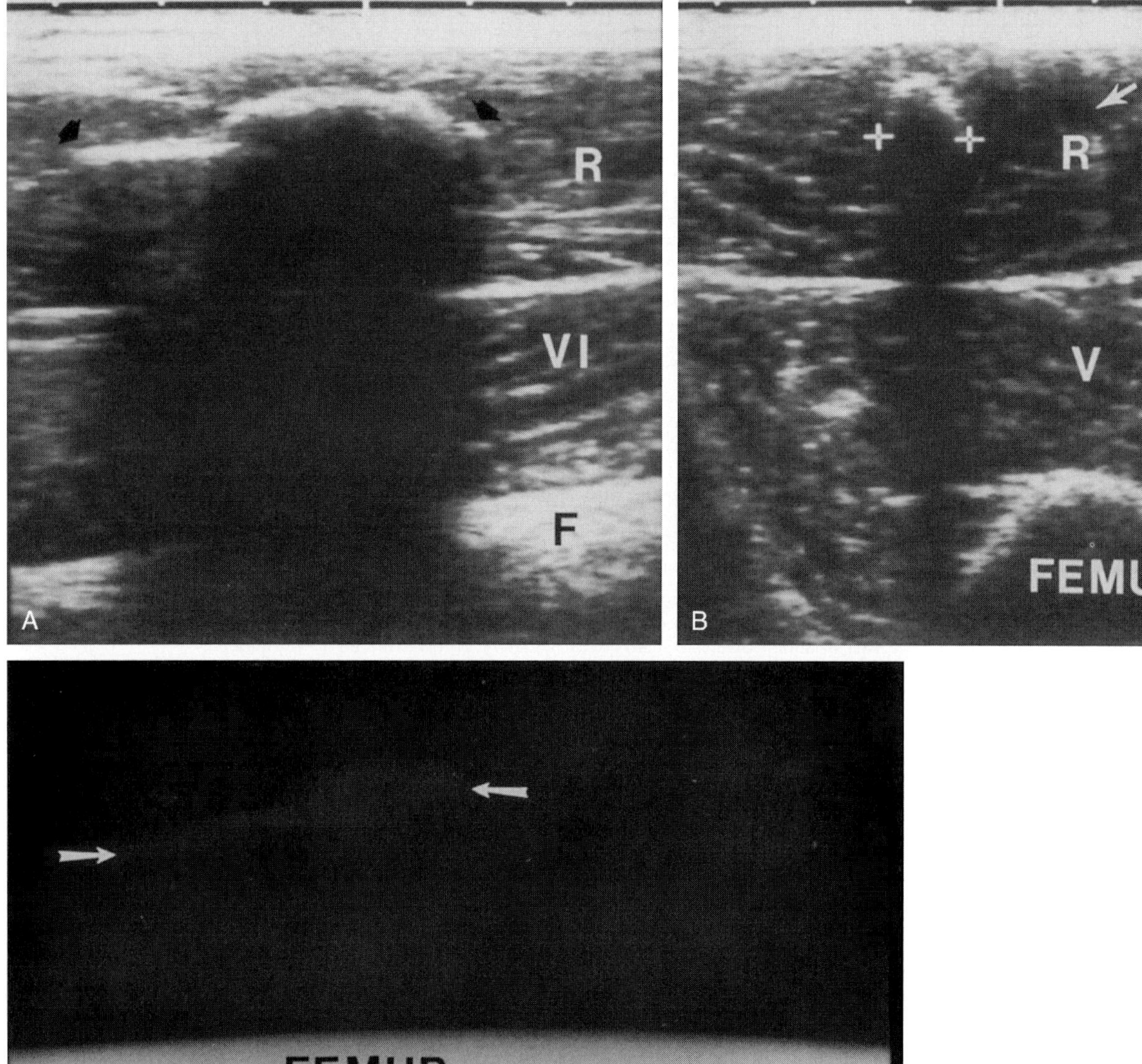

Figure 3-44 ■ A, Gelosis progressing to myositis ossificans in the rectus muscle: longitudinal sonogram. Same patient and transducer position as in Figure 3-43B 3 months following injury. A linear-curvilinear hyperechoic line (*arrows*) with acoustic shadowing is identified within the rectus in the same location as the previously noted abnormality. Incomplete shadowing is noted deep to the linear segment due to volume averaging. Shadowing makes evaluation of the depth of the lesion difficult. Scanning obliquely will help to demonstrate the deep extent of myositis ossificans. Abbreviations: femur (*F*), rectus (*R*), vastus intermedius (*VI*). **B,** Myositis ossificans in the rectus muscle: transverse sonogram. Same patient as in Figures 3-43 and 3-44A. The region of ossification is shown to be much narrower than it is long. A hypoechoic region (*arrow*) adjacent to the ossification represents reparative tissue. Abbreviations: rectus (*R*), vastus intermedius (*V*). **C,** Myositis ossificans in the rectus muscle: conventional radiograph. Same patient as in Figures 3-43, 3-44A, and 3-44B. This low-kilovoltage radiograph demonstrates a subtle area of myositis ossificans (*arrows*). Two small, round areas of ossification that were outside the sonographic FOV are also noted. Ultrasound more clearly demonstrates lesions of myositis ossificans. Sonographic identification of ossification is much less dependent on technique, than radiographic identification, since radiographs may be overpenetrated. Localization of the ossification to a specific muscle is also far more precise with ultrasound than with conventional radiography. As shown in this case, ultrasound demonstrates the soft tissue abnormality that will lead to myositis ossificans.

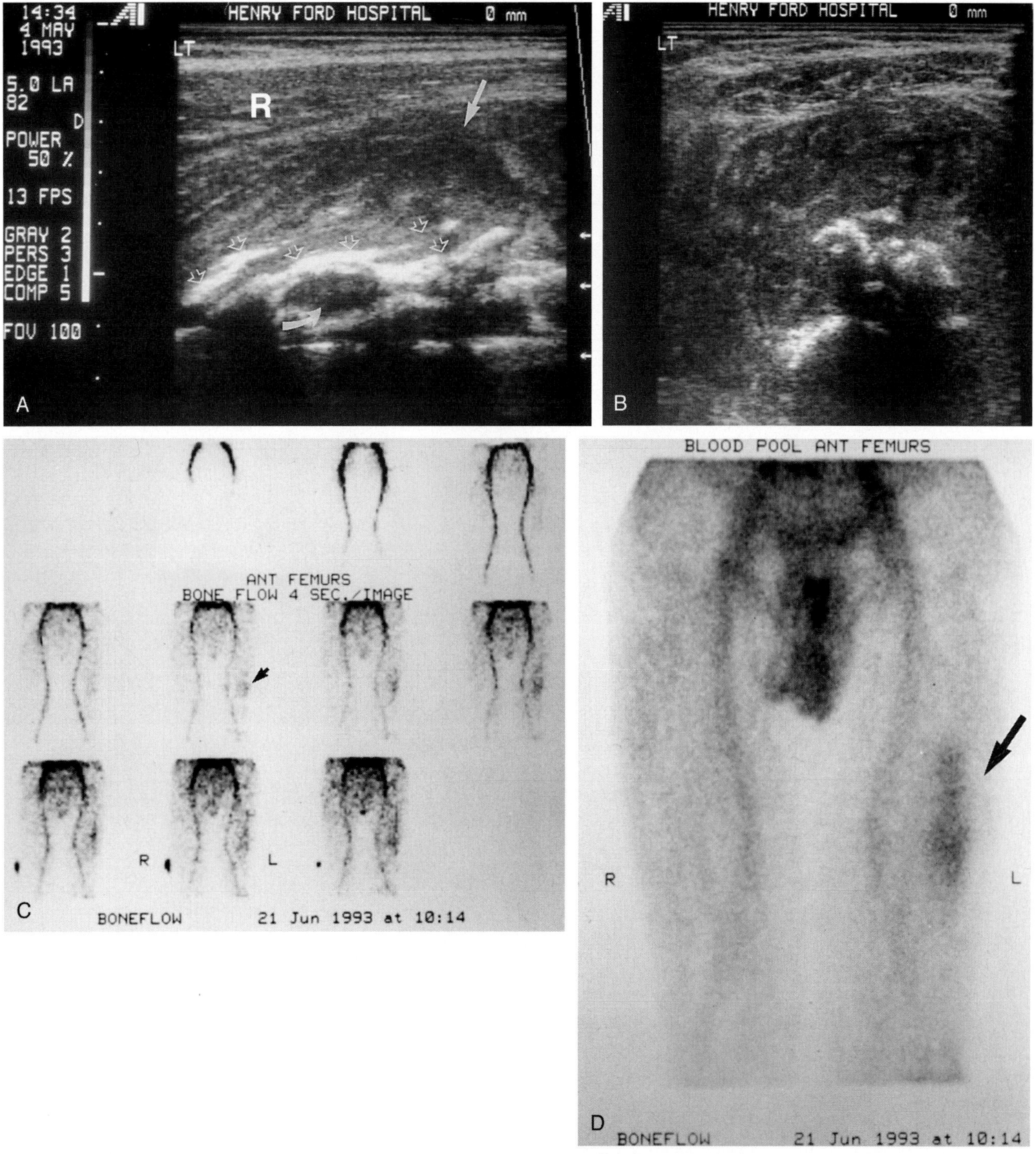

Figure 3–45 ■ **A,** Ultrasound detection of myositis ossificans: longitudinal ultrasound. Because of a solid mass in the thigh, this 38-year-old man consulted his primary care physician. The patient was an alcoholic. He did not recall injuring that leg, and he reported that the mass first presented about $1\frac{1}{2}$ weeks earlier. Radiographs taken at the time of the visit are negative. The ultrasound shows a normal rectus muscle (*R*) but gross change throughout the vastus intermedius muscle (*arrow*). Linear hyperechoic strands (*open arrows*) deep in the vastus intermedius may represent ossification along the fibrofatty septa. It is interesting how the ossification casts only a partial shadow, which does not impair visualization of the lesion. The zonal phenomenon (*curved arrow*) in the center of the lesion suggests myositis ossificans. **B,** Ultrasound detection of myositis ossificans: transverse ultrasound. Same patient as in **A.** The transverse ultrasound scan over the midthigh shows nodular, hyperechoic masses in the deep layers of the vastus intermedius. **C–E,** Ultrasound detection of myositis ossificans: bone scan findings. Same patient as in Figure **A.** Three-phase bone scan performed on the same day as the ultrasound scan shows abnormal uptake (*arrows*) in the left thigh on all three phases of the scan.

Figure continued on following page

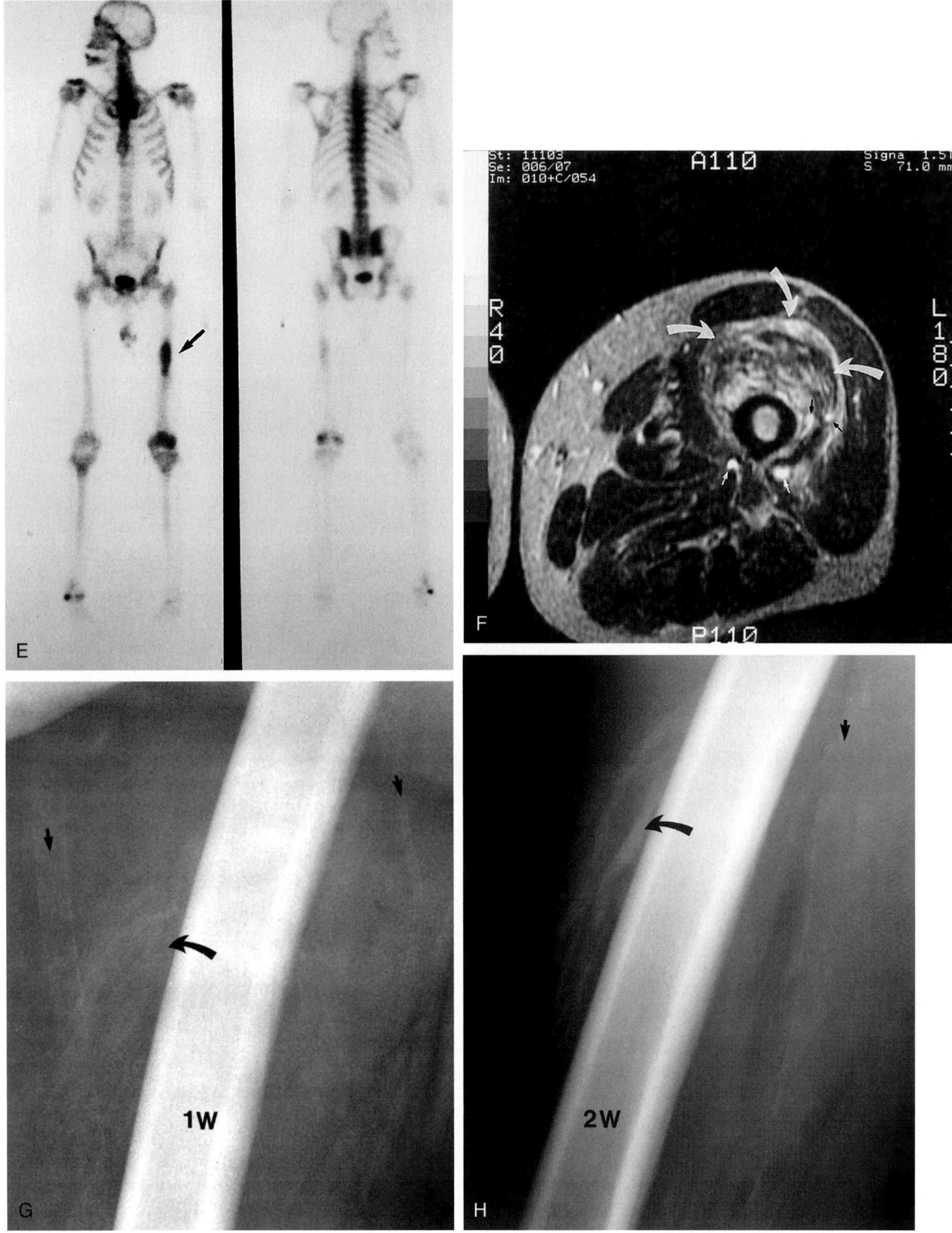

Figure 3–45 *Continued* ■ *See legend on opposite page*

Figure 3-45 *Continued* ▪ **F,** Ultrasound detection of myositis ossificans: MRI study. Same patient as in **A.** With the bone scan findings read as being positive for tumor or infection, a MRI study was performed. The multiple sequences showed a very large mass (*curved arrows*) in the quadriceps. The T_1-weighted sequence showed blood within the vastus intermedius; the postgadolinium images demonstrated diffuse enhancement of the mass. The T_2-weighted showed diffuse high signal throughout the vastus intermedius. Several dilated veins that had been seen on a vascular sequence appeared in the capsule or pseudocapsule of the lesion (*small arrows*). There was increased marrow signal. The most likely diagnosis on MRI, similar to the bone scan findings, was tumor. **G,H,** Ultrasound detection of myositis ossificans: radiographic follow-up. Same patient as in **A.** Soft tissue radiographs at 1 week (*1W*) and at 2 weeks (*2W*) after the initial workup. Calcifications first appear as woven bone 1 week after ultrasound depicted them. More mature bone is seen on the second follow-up (*2W*). The patient felt perfectly well after this follow-up, and he refused to come in for further study. The initial ultrasound diagnosis of myositis ossificans was confirmed by radiographic and clinical follow-up. Characteristic findings in this case include the history of alcoholism, the rapid-onset swelling, the location in the vastus intermedius, the hemorrhage on MRI, the speed of maturation of the bone, and the favorable clinical outcome.

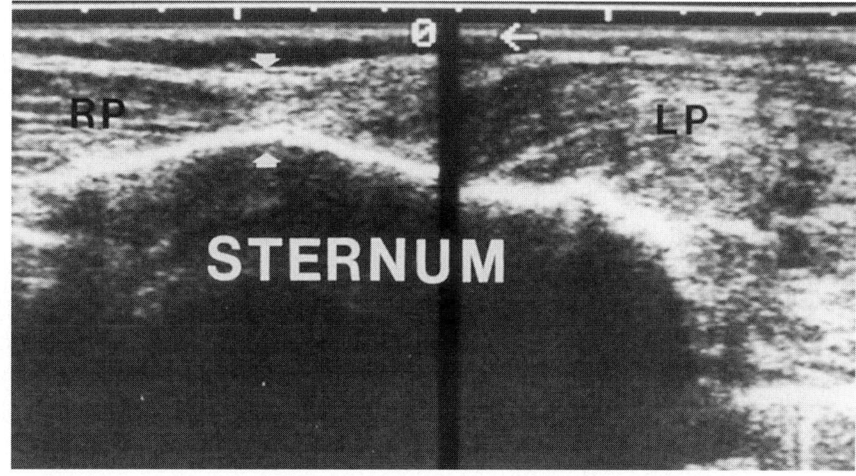

Figure 3-46 ▪ Pyogenic myositis of the pectoral muscle: longitudinal sonogram. A 50-year-old man was admitted with fever and pain in the left upper thorax. A posteroanterior chest x-ray film demonstrated a marked ill-defined opacity in the left suprahilar region. This opacity could not be localized on the lateral projection. Ultrasonography was performed to exclude chest wall pathology. The transducer was positioned along the length of the pectoralis muscles in the midline of the chest. The orientation is similar to that of a CT section, with the patient's left at the observer's right. The *small white arrows* indicate the origin of the pectoralis muscles at the midline of the sternum. Note the marked anterior bulge of the left pectoralis muscle (*LP*) compared with the right (*RP*). Fibroadipose septa are less well defined in the left pectoralis muscle.

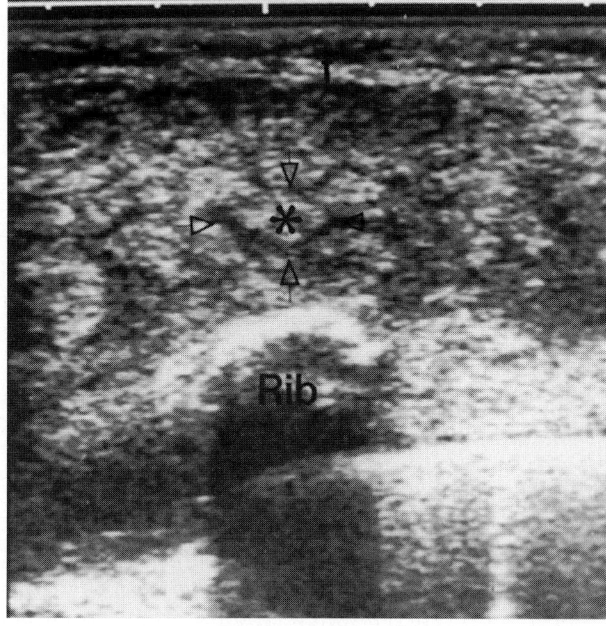

Figure 3-47 ▪ Pyogenic myositis: transverse sonogram. Same patient as in Figure 3-46. The transducer has been rotated 90 degrees, parallel to the sternum, and moved laterally to yield a cross-sectional image of the pectoralis muscle. The pectoralis muscle is inhomogeneous, and a reversal in the echo texture of the muscle is seen. Fibroadipose septa (*arrows*) appear hypoechoic relative to the involved muscle bundles (*asterisk*). Edema fluid is noted beneath the fascia (*f*). Aspiration and culture revealed *S. aureus* to be the causative organism.

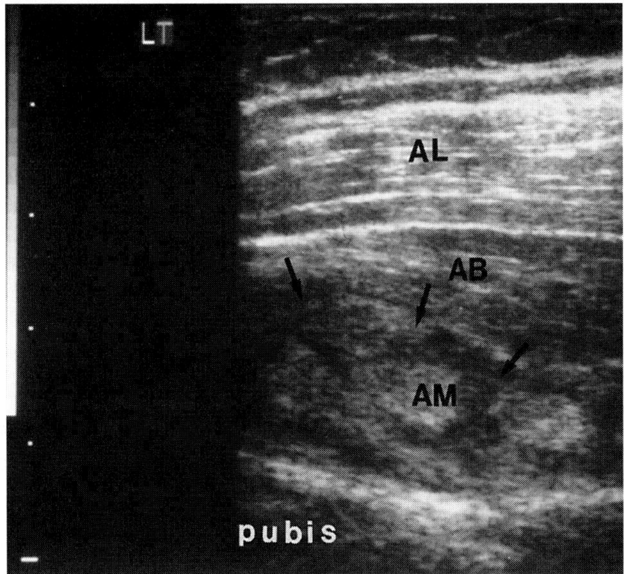

Figure 3-48 ▪ Pyomyositis of the adductor magnus: transverse image of the left groin. Acute onset of left groin pain prompted this 39-year-old retired professional football player to seek treatment. A necrotic (*arrows*) adductor magnus (*AM*) is present deep to the adductor longus (*AL*) and adductor brevis (*AB*). Aspiration of the muscle yielded pus. The fluid cultured positive for *S. aureus*. This pyomyositis was the first clinical sign of acquired immunodeficiency syndrome (AIDS) in this human immunodeficiency virus (HIV) positive individual.

contours, and a cloaca may be identified. Elevation of the periosteum, with fluid separating the periosteum from the cortex, will also be noted (van Sonnenberg et al., 1987; Abiri et al., 1988).

Compartment Syndrome

Muscle ischemia and ischemic necrosis are often difficult to diagnose clinically when they are not the result of atherosclerotic disease. A compartment syndrome is the most frequent cause of muscle ischemia in patients less than 50 years old. Compartment syndromes are characterized by elevated pressure within a muscle group surrounded by investing fascia (Anderson, 1983). Elevated interstitial pressure in an anatomically confined compartment results in impaired capillary perfusion. Although blood flow at the capillary level is severely compromised, major arteries remain patent. Therefore, normal pulses are observed distal to the involved compartment in the vast majority of cases. This frequently misleads the clinician.

Muscle edema is a frequent cause of increased pressure within a compartment. Due to the limited elasticity of the investing fascia, intracompartmental pressure may be significantly increased, with slight edema. This edema often results from strenuous exercise or blunt trauma. A tightly fitting plaster cast can have the same effect.

Acute Compartment Syndrome

Compartment syndromes are divided into two categories: acute and chronic. Acute compartment syndrome is the result of a single insult, either exercise-induced muscular overload or trauma. It is characterized clinically by increasing pain associated with movement, particularly passive stretching. If it is exercise induced, the pain usually starts during exercise, but its onset may be delayed as much as 12 hours following exercise. Swelling of the involved compartment may be clinically detectable. Paresthesia in the sensory distribution of nerves running through the compartment will also be observed (Nicholas and Hershman, 1986). Most frequently affected are the anterior, posterior, and lateral compartments of the lower leg. A high priority must be placed on confirming the diagnosis of compartment syndrome because delay in treatment will result in a permanent neurological and functional deficit. Surgical fasciotomy is the only treatment available. Fascial release adversely affects the strength of a muscle group, making it more than a benign procedure. This further increases the importance of accurate diagnosis (Garfin et al., 1981).

Until now, the only way to confirm the diagnosis of a compartment syndrome was direct pressure measurement. A catheter was inserted into the suspect compartment using sterile technique and local anesthesia, and pressure measurements were obtained. Evaluation of chronic compartment syndrome required pressure measurement at rest, during exercise, and following recovery (Mubarak, 1981). A pressure difference of 30–40 mm Hg between the compartment and the subcutaneous tissues will result in significant tissue damage. Noise introduced by muscle contraction and limb motion significantly reduces the accuracy of this test. In addition, the invasive nature of the test makes it less desirable.

CT provides little assistance in making the diagnosis of compartment syndrome. Edema attributable to compartment syndrome may appear slightly lower in attenuation (20–30 Hounsfield units) following bolus contrast administration (Weissman and Sledge, 1986). However, this is subject to all of the variables inherent in IV contrast administration. This technique has not demonstrated a high degree of sensitivity or specificity.

The noninvasive nature of ultrasound makes it an attractive alternative to direct pressure measurement. Sonography also has the ability to exclude other entities that must be considered in the differential diagnosis of compartment syndrome. Posttraumatic hematoma, abscess, deep venous thrombo-

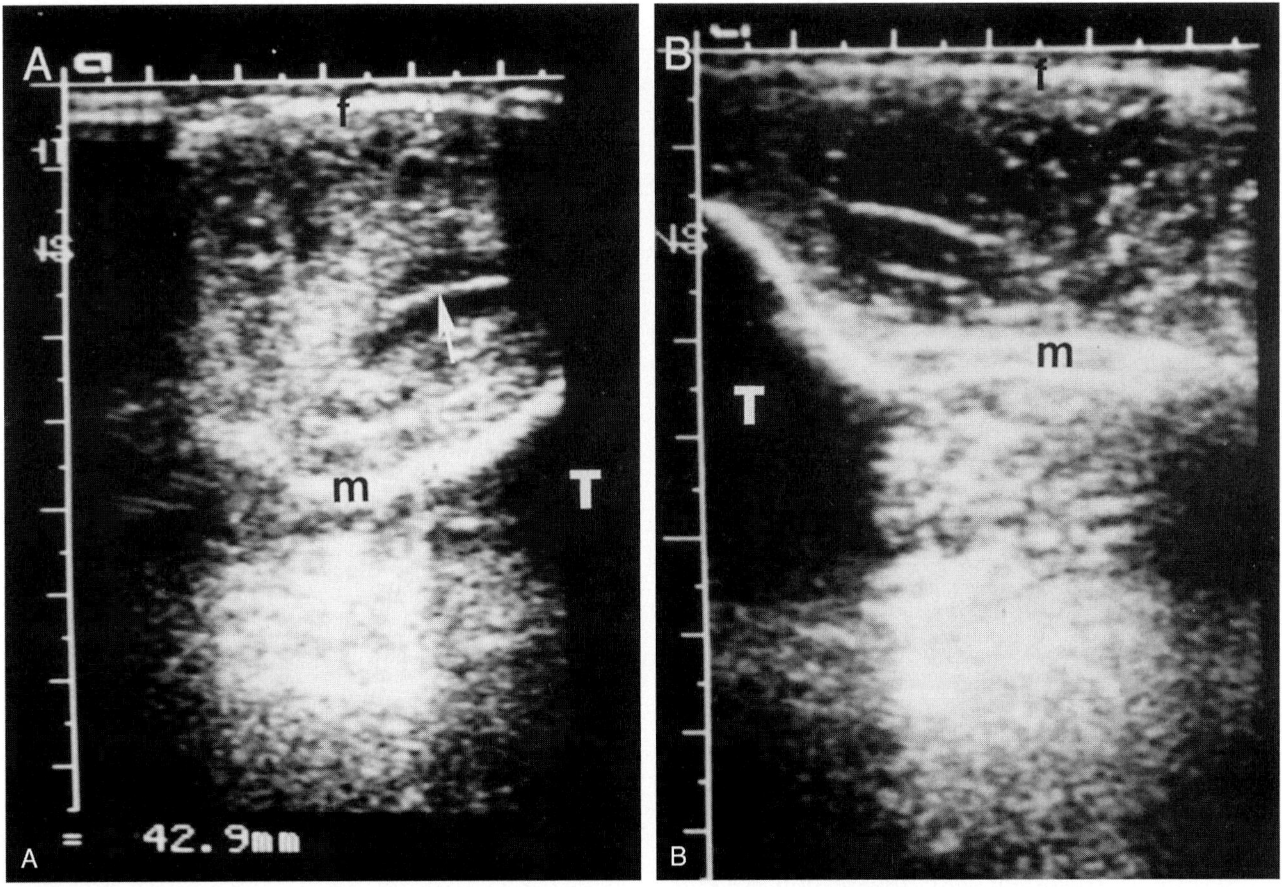

Figure 3–49 ■ **A,** Acute anterior compartment syndrome of the lower leg: transverse sonogram. The patient was a 55-year-old male tennis player who usually played one set each week. This past weekend he played in a tournament. One match lasted for 4 hours. Several hours after the match, he experienced a gradual onset of pain in the anterior lateral aspect of the right lower leg, which reached a peak 2 days later. After 7, days he could no longer tolerate the pain and presented to the hospital's emergency room. He was admitted with a clinical diagnosis of deep venous thrombosis. The right lower leg was edematous, erythematous, and warm. Distal pulses were intact. Contrast venography was normal. Ultrasound examination confirmed the presence of normal veins and excluded a ruptured Baker cyst. This image was obtained at the level of the midtibia (*T*). The anterior tibial compartment of the right leg was markedly distended and increased in echogenicity. Superficial fascia (*f*) and the interosseous membrane (*m*) were bulging due to a mass effect. Note the relative sparing of muscle architecture immediately adjacent to the larger fibroadipose septa (*arrow*). The anterior tibial compartment on the right measures 42.9 mm, 30% greater than the asymptomatic side. CT confirmed the presence of edema in the anterior compartment by demonstrating decreased attenuation within the compartment and absence of enhancement with bolus contrast administration. **B,** Acute anterior compartment syndrome of the lower leg: transverse sonogram. Same patient as in **A.** This image depicts the anterior tibial compartment of the asymptomatic left leg at the same level. Compare the normal appearance of this compartment with that seen in **A.** Note the straight appearance of the superficial fascia (*f*) and interosseous membrane (*m*).

sis, and ruptured Baker's cyst are all well evaluated with ultrasound (Lawson and Mittler, 1978; Gompels and Darlington, 1979; Magnussen et al., 1988).

Acute compartment syndrome is characterized sonographically by diffusely increased echogenicity of the muscles within the compartment (Figs. 3–49 through 3–51). Unlike pyogenic myositis, the fibroadipose septa remain hyperechoic. In some cases, sparing of the periseptal muscle bundles may be observed. These spared muscle bundles will maintain their normal hypoechoic appearance, accentuating the feather-like structure of the muscles (Graf and Schuler, 1988). The explanation for this pattern of injury is the distribution of the vascular supply, which enters along the fibroadipose septa. Another sign of compartment syndrome is the increased dimension of the compartment compared with the asymptomatic side. Bowing and displacement of the investing fascia will be evident.

Some investigators have observed an irregular sonographic pattern in compartment syndrome, with both solid and cystic components (Auerbach and Bowen, 1981; Peterson and Renstrom, 1986). This represents a later stage in the evolution of compart-

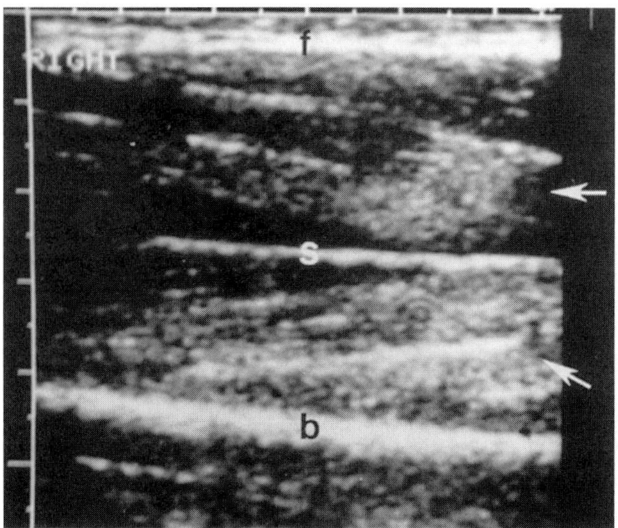

Figure 3-50 ▪ Acute anterior compartment syndrome of the lower leg: longitudinal sonogram. Same patient as in Figure 3-49. This image is a longitudinal section obtained over the symptomatic anterior compartment. The muscles of the anterior compartment are markedly increased in echogenicity (*arrows*). Note that the region adjacent to the intermuscular septum (*s*) is relatively spared, probably due to the proximity to larger vessels in the septum. Abbreviations: fascia (*f*), tibia (*b*).

ment syndrome. The loss of recognizable muscle architecture is consistent with progression beyond ischemia to frank infarction. Hypoechoic cystic areas will progress and may contain some material of higher echogenicity. Their sonographic appearance may resemble that of extensive rhabdomyolysis. At this stage, the diagnosis comes too late. Extensive tissue damage has already occurred. Foot drop, nerve palsy, and Volkmann's contracture are common sequelae of compartment syndrome when it is not treated promptly. Muscle necrosis will heal with extensive fibrosis and ossification, which will also involve the surrounding fascia (Resnick and Niwayama, 1988). Aggressive treatment with fasciotomy early in the development of compartment syndrome is still the best treatment available. A recent study has shown that patients who are treated surgically immediately after the onset of symptoms show virtually no change in muscle architecture when examined with sonography (Kullmer et al., 1997). The degree of muscle disorganization increases with the interval between the onset of symptoms and the time of fascial release.

Chronic Compartment Syndrome

Chronic compartment syndrome is associated with recurrent pain during exercise. It usually results from a rapidly increased muscle mass following rigorous athletic conditioning. Muscle mass is increased significantly in a short period of time, too rapidly for the nonelastic fascia to adapt. The result is a pathological increase in intracompartmental pressure during exercise because the compartment cannot expand to accommodate the transient increase in volume required secondary to increased blood flow (Nicholas and Hershman, 1986). The diagnosis of chronic compartment syndrome is more difficult than that of acute compartment syndrome. The pain is intermittent, occurring predominantly during exercise. It may be characterized as sharp, cramp-like, or burning. The level of exercise that brings on symptoms may vary considerably, from running a 4-minute mile to walking several blocks. Often the patient can continue to exercise but at a reduced level due to the discomfort. At the end of exercise the pain usually resolves quickly, but it may persist for hours or even days. Symptoms are bilateral in 70% of patients (Mubarak, 1981; Martens et al., 1984).

Clinical examination during an active episode of chronic compartment syndrome reveals pain on movement of the extremity. Pain is most commonly associated with plantar flexion and dorsiflexion of the foot, as the anterior and posterior compartments of the lower leg are most often involved. Sensation in the distal portion of the extremity may be al-

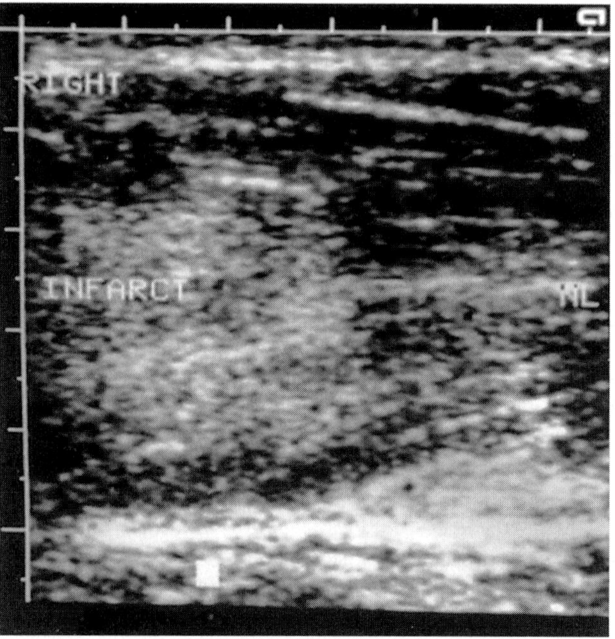

Figure 3-51 ▪ Infarcted muscle: longitudinal sonogram. Same patient as in Figures 3-49 and 3-50. A gradual transition is seen from the abnormal infarcted muscle at the left and the viable muscle (*NL*) on the right. Unfortunately, the patient refused surgery for 7 days. When he finally consented to fasciotomy, irreversible damage to the deep peroneal nerve had already occurred. Considerable muscle necrosis was also present. As a result of the delay in treatment, this patient had a significant permanent motor and neurologic deficit.

tered, but this is not a constant finding. Distal arterial pulses are always normal (Brahim and Zaccardelli, 1986). The differential diagnosis includes shin splints, stress fractures, periostitis, popliteal entrapment, and true claudication. It is easy to see why the diagnosis of chronic compartment syndrome is so difficult.

Pathological examination has demonstrated increased water content within the involved compartment. This would explain the increased intracompartmental pressure that results in decreased perfusion. Decreased xenon-133 clearance and increased accumulation of lactate (Nicholas and Hershman, 1986) have demonstrated the decrease in perfusion. Phosphorus MR spectroscopy has also been used to demonstrate a decrease in muscle adenosine triphosphate.

An increase in dimension of approximately 10% has been demonstrated by sonographic measurement of the anterior tibial compartment following dorsiflexion exercise of the foot (Gershuni et al., 1982; Brahim and Zaccardelli, 1986). These investigators postulated that the limitation of further expansion by inelastic fascia results in ischemia and chronic compartment syndrome.

We examined the compartments of the lower leg in a large group of patients including normal young people, normal athletes, and athletes with the clinical diagnosis of chronic compartment syndrome. The greatest dimension of the compartment was measured using a standardized technique. The transducer was positioned transversely at a point equidistant from the tibiofemoral joint space and the medial or lateral maleolus, depending on the compartment to be measured. A line perpendicular to the interosseous membrane was established to measure the distance from the membrane to the compartmental fascia. The position utilized for measurement was marked on the skin along with an identical position on the other leg. Measurements of the anterior compartment are most important in patients who present with pain lateral to the anterior border of the tibia. In patients with pain posterior to the tibia and fibula, both the superficial and deep posterior compartments must be examined. Peroneal compartment syndrome is rare. We did not encounter a patient with peroneal compartment syndrome in this series. Dimensions of the compartments were obtained at rest, immediately following exercise, and after a 10-minute recovery period.

In our patients, exercise consisted of plantar flexion and dorsiflexion of the foot with a 4-kg load at a rate of 60 cycles/minute. This was performed for 15 minutes or until symptoms forced the patient to stop. In all of these patients, direct pressure measurements were obtained at the same time that sonographic measurements were taken.

Normal nonathletes and athletes demonstrated normal compartmental pressures. In these patients, an increase in the dimension of the compartments immediately following exercise ranging between 10% and 15% was observed. The appearance of the compartments was slightly less echogenic immediately following exercise compared with the sonograms taken at rest (Fig. 3–52). These changes can be attributed to increased blood flow during exercise. Sonographic measurement following the 10-minute recovery period demonstrated a return to normal dimension and echogenicity. These findings

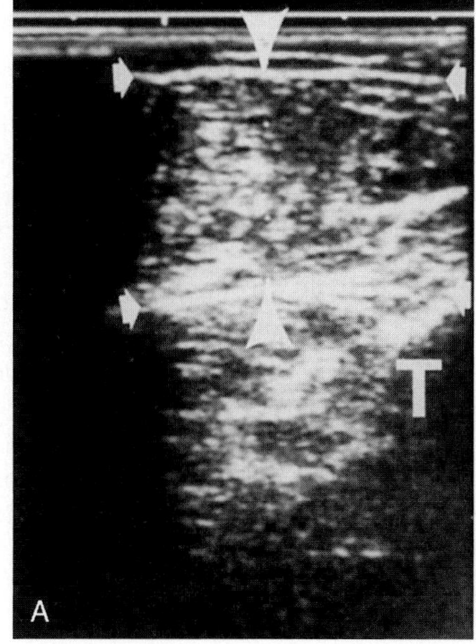

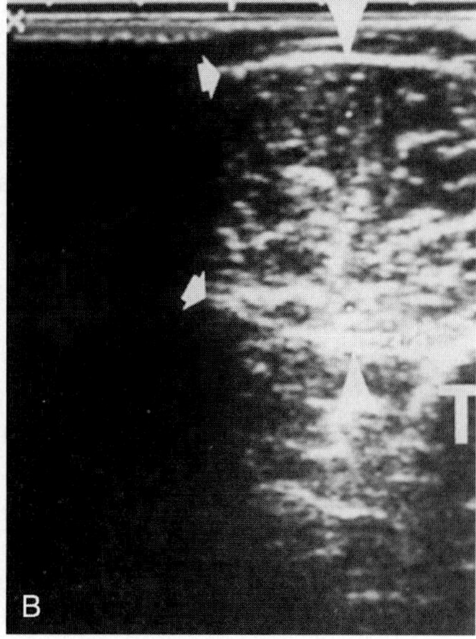

Figure 3–52 ■ Compartment measurement: transverse sonogram of the anterior tibial compartment. A normal 26-year-old male athlete. The image on the left of the anterior tibial compartment was obtained at rest, and the image on the right was obtained after 15 minutes of strenuous dorsiflexion of the foot. Note the increased dimension (*arrowheads*) of the compartment, as demonstrated by displacement of the fascia and the interosseous membrane (*arrows*). In a normal exercise test, the compartment volume should increase 10% to 15%. The muscles of the compartment are decreased in echogenicity following exercise. This is normal, probably the result of increased blood flow to the muscle. Abbreviation: tibia (*T*).

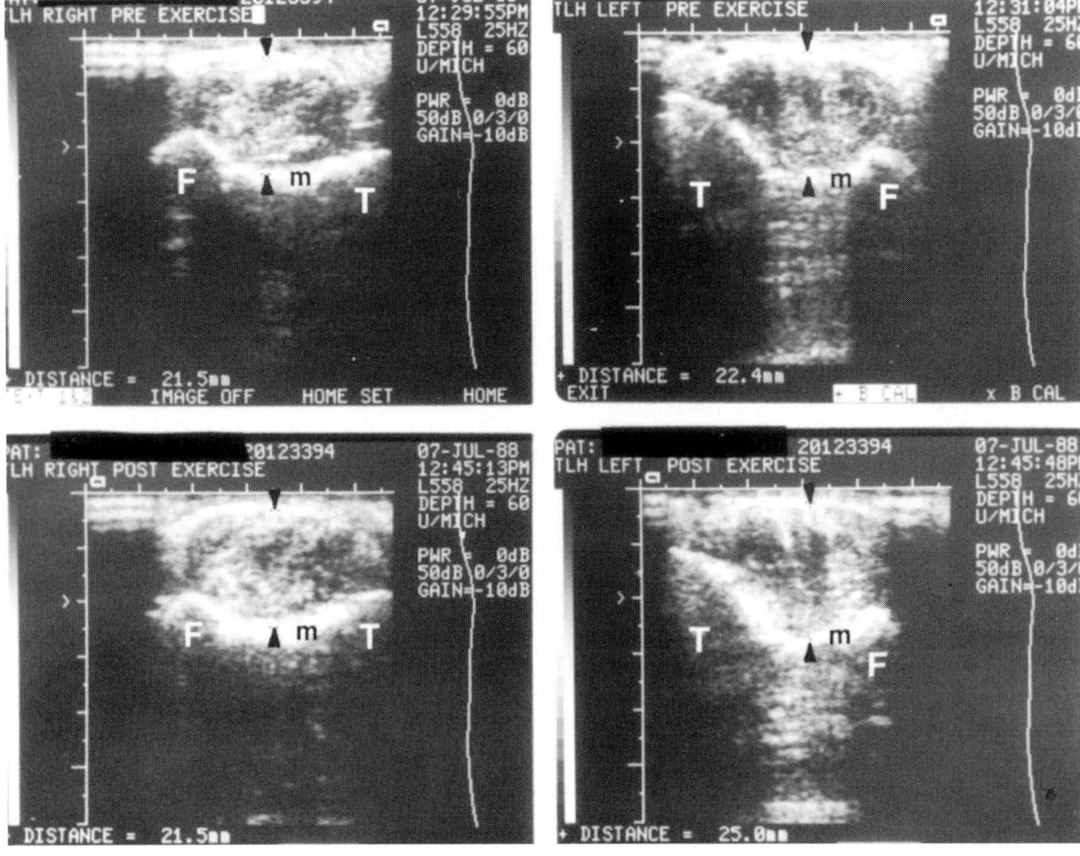

Figure 3–53 ■ Compartment measurement: transverse sonogram of the anterior tibial compartment. Each time after sprinting 50 yards, this football player experienced shooting pain in the anterior tibia. At the observer's left are images of the anterior tibial compartment of the patient's right leg. The left leg is at the observer's right; note the preexercise and postexercise labels. The interosseous membrane (*m*) in the right leg is thickened. Dimensions of this compartment do not change with exercise, consistent with chronic compartment syndrome. A normal increase of slightly more than 10% is noted in the left leg. Abbreviations: fibula (*F*), tibia (*T*).

were observed bilaterally in normal individuals. Patients with the clinical diagnosis of chronic compartment syndrome were divided into two groups based on the sonographic findings. All of these patients demonstrated elevated compartment pressures: peak pressure with exercise was elevated more than 30 mm Hg over extracompartmental pressure. The first group, which constituted approximately one-third of the symptomatic patients, did not demonstrate any detectable increase in compartmental volume. Thickening and rigidity of the interosseous membrane were evident (Fig. 3–53). In 5% of these patients, herniation of muscle through the fascia cruris was observed.

The second group, comprising two-thirds of the symptomatic patients, demonstrated normal expansion of the compartment, a 10% to 15% increase in volume. This finding was quite unexpected in light of the clearly abnormal intracompartmental pressure. However, return to the normal compartmental dimension was markedly delayed. In some patients, the recovery period was as long as 1 hour, six times the upper limit of normal. One percent of patients demonstrated increased echogenicity of the muscle, similar to that seen in acute compartment syndrome (Fig. 3–54).

Although unexpected, the discovery of two different sonographic patterns of presentation in chronic compartment syndrome is not inconsistent with the presumed etiology. Clearly, in the first group, fascial rigidity is responsible for increased intracompartmental pressure during exercise. However, the second group demonstrated a normal degree of compartmental expansion with exercise. It is possible that although the amount of expansion observed was within the normal range, it was insufficient for these athletes undertaking a rigorous training regimen. This would explain increased intracompartmental pressures at high levels of exercise and increased recovery times. More detailed data are needed to confirm this hypothesis.

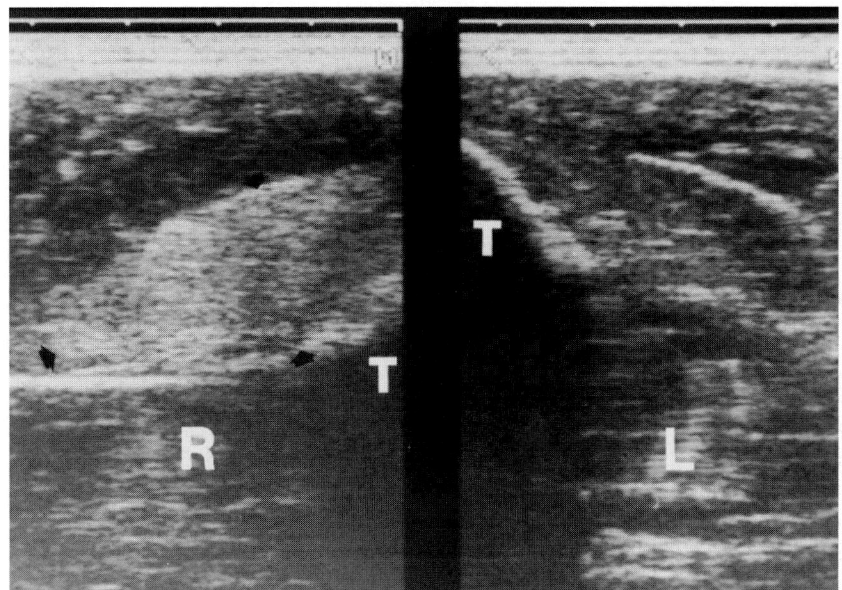

Figure 3–54 ■ Subacute anterior tibial compartment syndrome: transverse sonogram. One day following a tough soccer match, this 30-year-old man presented with intense pain in the right lower leg. He also experienced limitation of dorsiflexion of the foot and paresthesia. Anterior tibial compartment measurements were increased on the right side compared with the asymptomatic left side. The right flexor hallucis muscle (*black arrows*) is increased in both dimension and echogenicity. This patient was followed sonographically. Over the course of 2 days, he improved both clinically and sonographically. An exercise stress test of the leg performed 2 weeks later demonstrated increased echogenicity of the flexor hallucis longus rather than the normal decrease in echogenicity. Abbreviations: left (*L*), right (*R*), tibia (*T*).

Rhabdomyolysis

Rhabdomyolysis is a general term denoting skeletal muscle necrosis. It is considered an entity separate from compartment syndromes (Box 3–3). Many etiologies of rhabdomyolysis have been documented. These have been divided into five groups: (1) primary muscle injury, (2) abnormalities of energy production (McArdle's disease, carnitine palmityl transferase deficiency), (3) infection, (4) hypoxia, and (5) miscellaneous causes (drugs and toxins) (Knochel, 1981). The most common causes seen today are primary muscle injury and hypoxia. Primary muscle injury consists largely of exertional rhabdomyolysis (see Fig. 3–54) seen in athletes and military recruits, as well as crush injury secondary to trauma (Kaplan, 1980). Hypoxic injury frequently results from peripheral vascular disease (Fig. 3–55). Unfortunately, an alarming increase in severe rhabdomyolysis has been observed in drug addicts, particularly those who abuse cocaine and heroin (Kaplan, 1980; Roth et al., 1988). Clinical signs indicative of rhabdomyolysis are myoglobinuria, hyperuricemia, hyperuricosuria, and elevated serum levels of muscle enzymes.

Box 3–3
Etiology of Rhabdomyolysis

- Injury
- Errors in metabolism
- Infection/inflammation
- Hypoxia/infarct
- Drugs/toxins

Prompt diagnosis is extremely important because significant rhabdomyolysis will result in acute renal failure, secondary hyperkalemia, and disseminated intravascular coagulation (Kaplan, 1980; Nicholas and Hershman, 1986).

A region of rhabdomyolysis will appear as a hypo- or hyperechoic area deep within the muscle (Kaplan, 1980; Vukanovic et al., 1983). Multiple lesions may be observed, and the muscle may be diffusely enlarged. The gluteal muscles are most involved in drug addicts and patients with epilepsy. A multiplicity of lesions and their deep location are characteristic of rhabdomyolysis (Kaplan, 1980). Sonographic features will differentiate rhabdomyolysis from distraction injury, but these lesions may strongly resemble abscesses. A clinical history of fever and leukocytosis will help make the diagnosis. However, noninfected regions of rhabdomyolysis can produce fever. Aspiration of the lesion is indicated when the diagnosis is not clear. Uncomplicated areas of rhabdomyolysis will yield clear serous fluid on aspiration. Hematomas may also appear similar to rhabdomyolysis immediately following injury. However, hematomas are not usually associated with myoglobinuria and elevated serum levels of muscle enzymes. Several hours following injury, the diagnosis of hematoma will be clear sonographically.

Contrast-enhanced CT shows nonspecific findings of circumscribed regions of decreased attenuation within the muscle (Kaplan, 1980; Vukanovic et al., 1983). Gross examination of the pathological

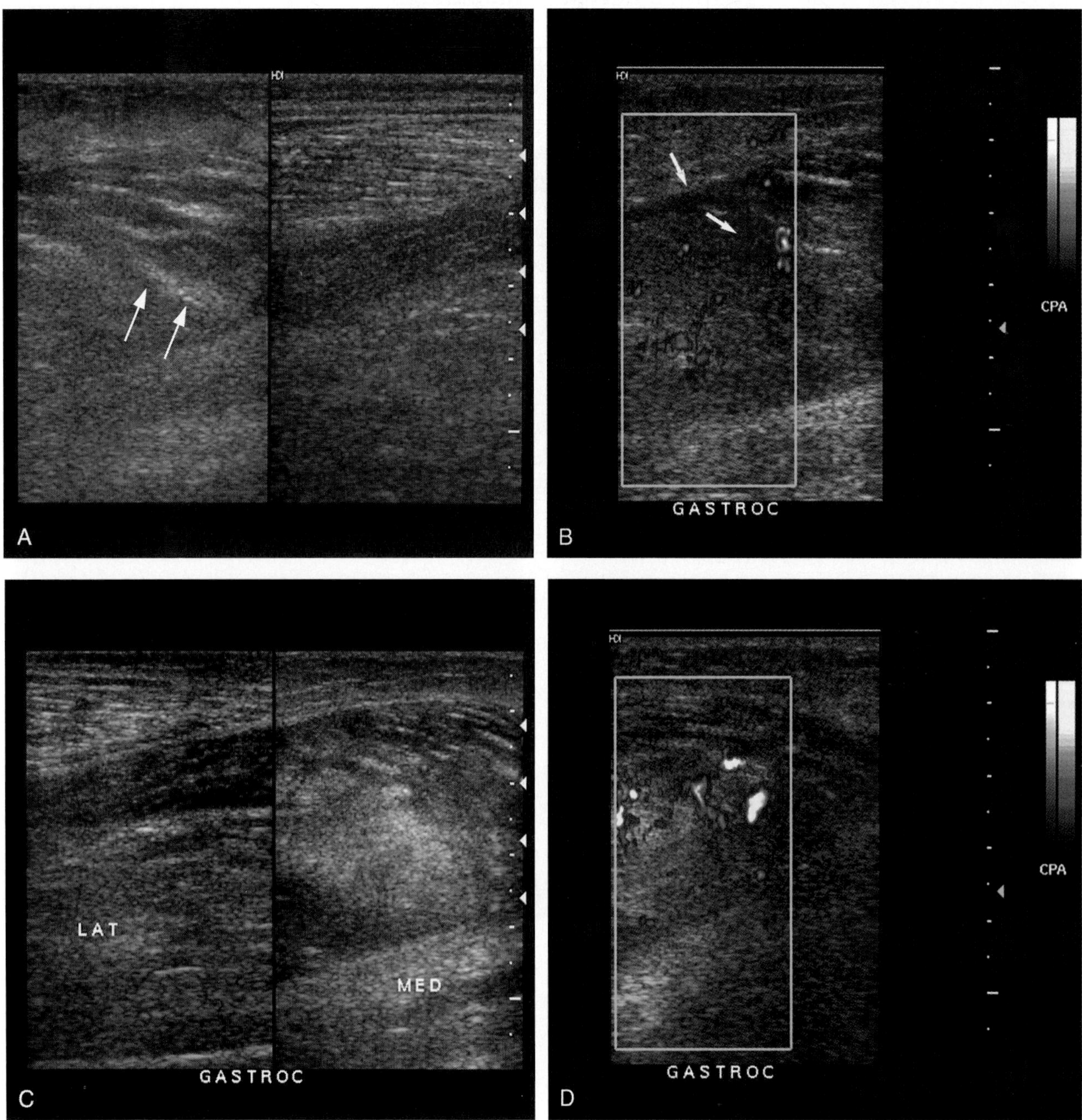

Figure 3–55 ■ **A,** Combined diabetic muscle infarct and diabetic pyomyositis: longitudinal sonogram with split-screen technique. A 62-year-old diabetic woman experienced swelling and pain in her calf for 3 weeks. There is a 6-cm discrepancy in the circumference of the calves, with the tender right calf being larger. The abnormal medial gastrocnemius is on the left side of the split screen; the muscle has a diffuse abnormal echo texture, with alternating hypo- and hyperechoic segments of muscle. The fibroadipose septa (*arrows*) seem thickened and hyperechoic. Compare the texture of the abnormal muscle to that of the normal left medial gastrocnemius shown on the right. **B,** Combined diabetic muscle infarct and diabetic pyomyositis: longitudinal sonogram with power Doppler sonography. Same patient as in **A.** The inhomogeneous muscle tissue demonstrates areas of hyperemia mixed with areas of decreased flow (*arrows*). The examination was interpreted as muscle infarction. **C,** Combined diabetic muscle infarct and diabetic pyomyositis: longitudinal sonogram with split-screen technique through the margin of the lesion. Same patient as in **A.** A section through a more peripheral part of the lesion is presented on the right side of this split-screen image. A markedly swollen, hyperechoic medial gastrocnemius (*MED*) is very different from the normal-appearing adjacent lateral gastrocnemius (*LAT*). **D,** Combined diabetic muscle infarct and diabetic pyomyositis: longitudinal sonogram with power Doppler through the margin of the lesion. Same patient as in **A.** The periphery of the muscle mass is markedly hyperemic.

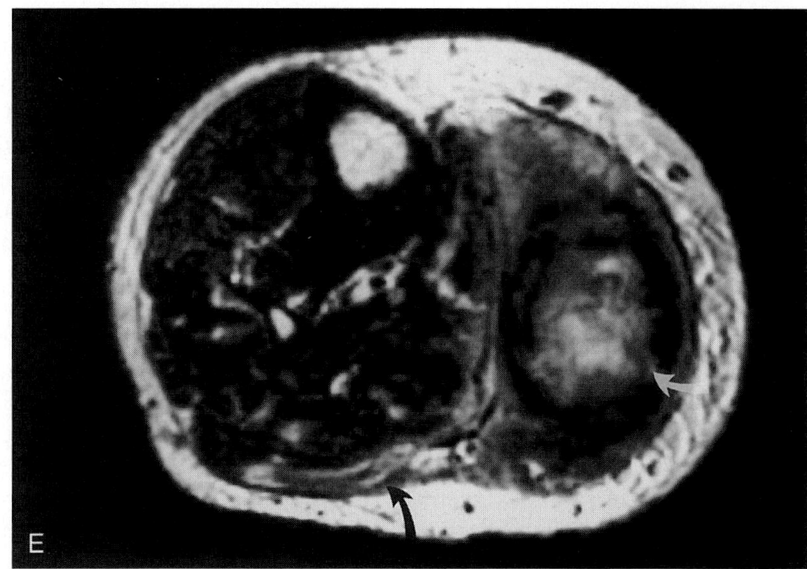

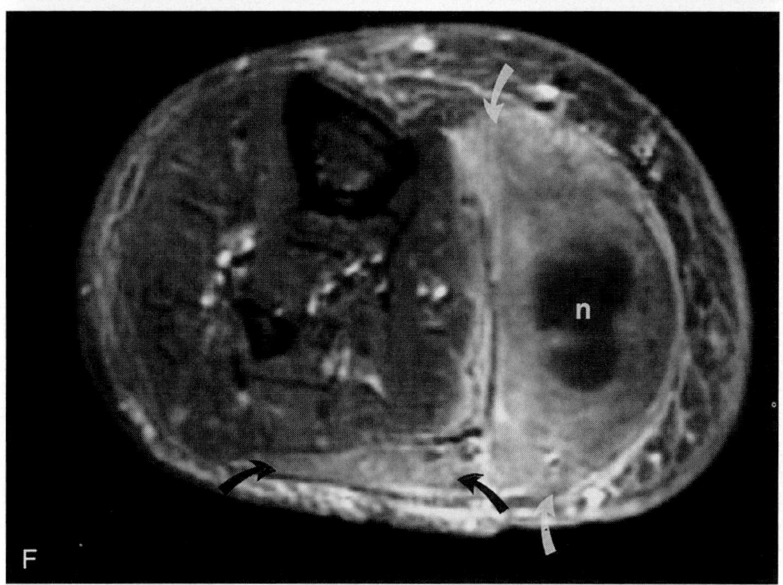

Figure 3-55 *Continued* ■ **E,** Combined diabetic muscle infarct and diabetic pyomyositis: axial T_1-weighted spin-echo MRI. Same patient as in **A.** The patient's condition then deteriorated. She developed sepsis a few days after the ultrasound examination, and an MRI scan was performed 1 week later. The transverse MRI images with T_1 weighting show increased signal intensity in the center of the medial gastrocnemius. The lesion has a bulls-eye appearance. This appearance and the high signal intensity on the T_1-weighted sequence have been observed in myositis ossificans and in diabetic myonecrosis. Compare the size of the abnormal medial gastrocnemius (*curved white arrow*) with that of the normal lateral gastrocnemius (*curved black arrow*). **F,** Combined diabetic muscle infarct and diabetic pyomyositis: axial T_1-weighted spin-echo technique with fat suppression after intravenous gadolinium administration. Same patient as in **A.** The dark ring noted in E enhances after contrast injection. A central necrotic component within the medial gastrocnemius does not enhance. Muscle biopsy revealed necrosis of muscle (*n*); cultures after evacuation of a central fluid pocket were positive for *S. aureus.* The infected medial gastrocnemius (*curved white arrows*) is over five times the size of the normal lateral gastrocnemius (*curved black arrows*).

specimen reveals a swollen, firm, pale muscle. Histopathological findings include muscle cell swelling, hyaline degeneration with loss of characteristic striation, and areas of interstitial inflammation (Geller, 1973; Kaplan, 1980). The inflammatory exudate surrounding necrotic muscle cells explains the hypoechoic appearance seen on sonographic images.

Diabetic myonecrosis (Box 3-4) is a relatively common cause of leg swelling in diabetics. In published case reports, the age of the patients has ranged from 19 to 64 years (mean, 36.7 years). Women are affected 1.3 times more often than men. The infarction is usually preceded by severe pain that develops over a period of several days to weeks. Over time, the swelling diminishes and a well-defined mass-like lesion becomes apparent (Barohn and Kissel, 1992; Rocca et al., 1993; Chason et al., 1996). The patient typically presents with an exquisitely tender muscle in the absence of trauma or fever. The patient's range of motion is limited, but muscle strength is normal. Pain is present at rest and is exacerbated with muscle contraction. In our experience, these lesions occur most

Box 3-4
Most Common Causes of Rhabdomyolysis

- Exertional rhabdomyolysis
- Diabetic myonecrosis
- Pyomyositis (tropical disease)

commonly in muscles of the pelvis and lower extremities. The exact cause of this condition is unclear (Banker and Chester, 1973; Chester and Banker, 1986). Poorly controlled diabetes mellitus is the major predisposing factor, typically in patients with nephropathy, neuropathy, and hypertension. Occlusive atherosclerosis has been postulated to have a major role in diabetic muscle infarction (Banker, 1973). A number of investigators believe that these patients have a hypercoagulable state and that their fibrinolytic pathway is impaired. As in other cases of rhabdomyolysis, the muscle appears to be hypoechoic. The echo pattern is often very inhomogeneous. We have observed hyperechoic speckles centrally in the hypoechoic mass in a number of cases. The hyperechogenicity may be related to gas bubbles within regions of necrosis. Muscle biopsy under ultrasound guidance typically reveals regions of hemorrhage and necrosis, with evidence of myocytic infiltration. MRI demonstrates the edema of muscle on T_2-weighted images with great sensitivity. Large, bright areas are noted on fat-suppressed T_2-weighted sequences. In some infarcts, the lesion has a bull's-eye appearance on both T_1- and T_2-weighted sequences. This appearance may mimic the early stage of myositis ossificans. The findings lack specificity. Traumatic muscle lesions, myositis, infection, and tumor in muscle have a similar appearance on MRI scans. In a few cases, postgadolinium images show an enhancing rim around a dark central area (Vande Berg et al., 1996). The combination of ultrasound and MRI is often needed to reach a definitive diagnosis. The ultrasound images may be degraded because of the subcutaneous changes, that accompany these lesions (Fig. 3–56). However, ultrasound shows that the central dark, nonenhancing region does not represent fluid or pus, but rather necrotic muscle (see Fig. 3–55). The myonecrotic area loses its normal fibrillar architecture (Fig. 3–57), but it is not fluctuant upon palpation. We have observed a muscle diameter increase of up to five times its normal dimension.

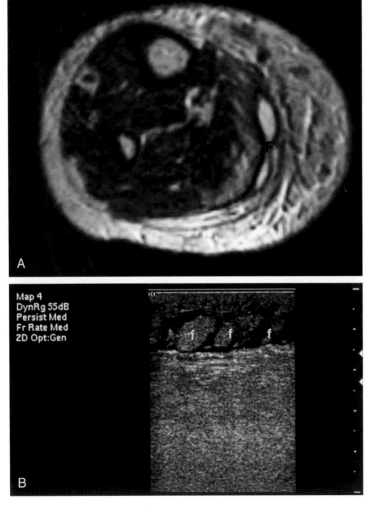

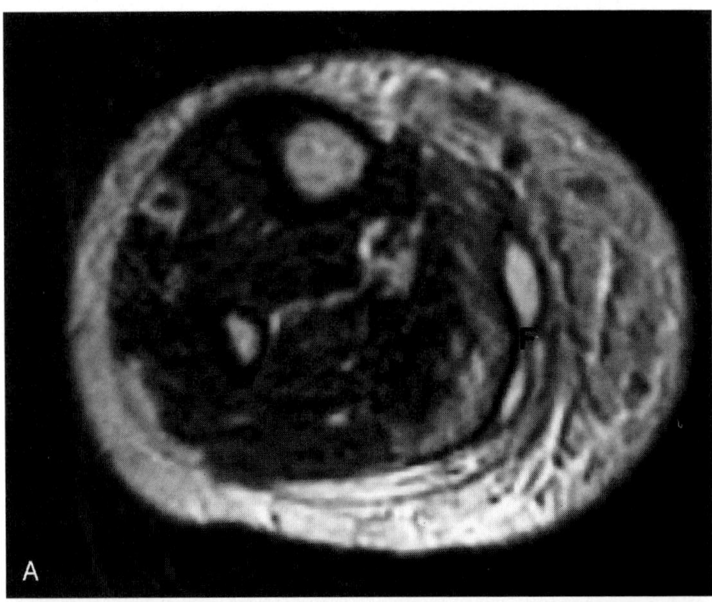

Figure 3–56 ■ **A,** Subcutaneous and fascial changes in myositis: axial proton-density MRI. Inflammatory changes are obvious in the subcutaneous tissues, around the fascia, and in the muscle of this diabetic patient who had *S. aureus* cultured from the interfascial fluid (*F*). **B,** Subcutaneous changes in myositis: transverse ultrasound of the calf. Same patient as in **A.** Fat lobules (*f*) are surrounded by edema. The structural changes in the subcutaneous tissues obscure the underlying tissues, and it is difficult to observe changes in the muscle. We have observed this in muscle infarcts, pyomyositis, and AIDS-related myositis. In cases with extensive subcutaneous edema, it is often better to use MRI rather than ultrasound to evaluate the muscles.

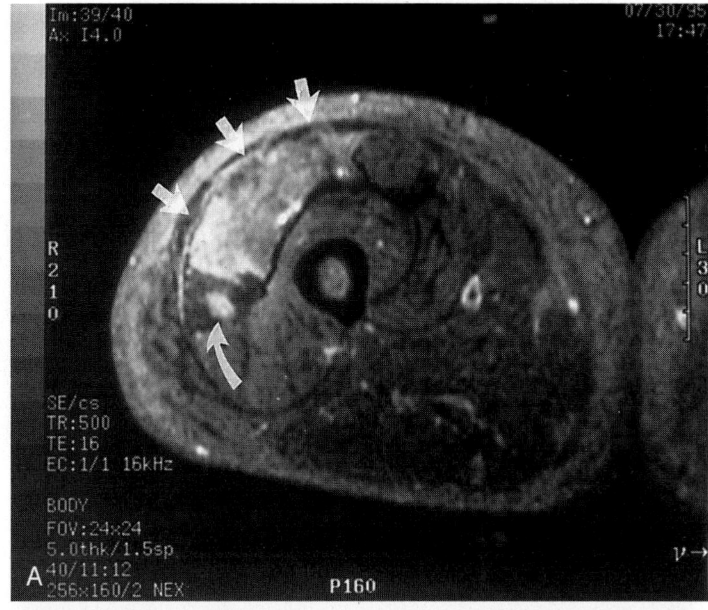

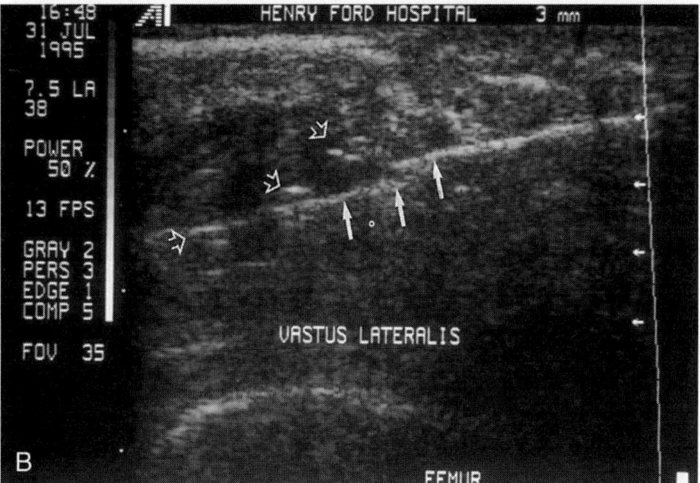

Figure 3–57 ▪ **A,** Muscle infarct: axial MRI sequence. Swelling and pain in the thigh of this 49-year-old diabetic man developed over a 1-week period. Axial images of a fat-suppressed T_1-weighted sequence were obtained after gadolinium administration. The vastus lateralis muscle enhances diffusely (*arrows*). The posterior segment of the muscle, which was exquisitely tender, enhances and has a bull's-eye appearance (*curved arrow*). **B,** Muscle infarct: transverse ultrasound. Same patient as in **A.** The patient is lying on his side. A biopsy needle is guided into the tender zone of the muscle. The needle is visualized in the open position; note the step-off at the indented part of the needle (*arrows*). The muscle architecture is diffusely abnormal, with small flecks (*open arrows*) of hyperechogenicity throughout the abnormal muscle. The hyperechogenicities might represent gas bubbles; however, we have never been able to show this on radiographs.

The differential diagnosis with pyomyositis is most challenging. This disease can occur in diabetics as well (Scully et al., 1997). In a review of 84 cases of pyomyositis in the United States, 15% of the patients had diabetes mellitus. Patients with diabetes have an increased frequency of colonization with *Staphylococcus aureus*, local defects in muscle tissue, and impaired host defenses, which may predispose them to the development of pyomyositis (Scully et al., 1997). Pyomyositis is similar in appearance to a diabetic muscle infarct, with a painful swollen muscle group, often in the groin (see Fig. 3–48) or thigh. Interestingly, serum levels of muscle enzymes are usually normal or only slightly elevated (Scully et al., 1997). Fever may or may not be present. *S. aureus* is the causative organism in about 90% of cases (Chiedozi, 1979). As in myonecrosis, the erythrocyte sedimentation rate will be elevated, and systemic leukocytosis will be observed. The MRI image of end-stage pyomyositis will resemble that of myonecrosis, but ultrasound shows fluid centrally within the mass, while solid necrotic muscle is present in myonecrosis. Ultrasound-guided biopsy is often necessary to make the diagnosis in the early stages of the disease (see Fig. 3–57).

Muscle Boundary Lesions

Muscle-Aponeurosis Avulsion

We consider muscle boundary lesions to be pathology involving investing fascia, an aponeurosis, or the myotendinous junction. Muscle tears of the calf frequently fall into this category. Distraction lesions involving the gastrocnemius and soleus muscles typically occur along their attachment to the aponeurosis (Fig. 3–58). Similar ruptures are seen along the soleus and flexor hallucis longus muscles (Fig. 3–59). These muscle-aponeurosis avulsions are

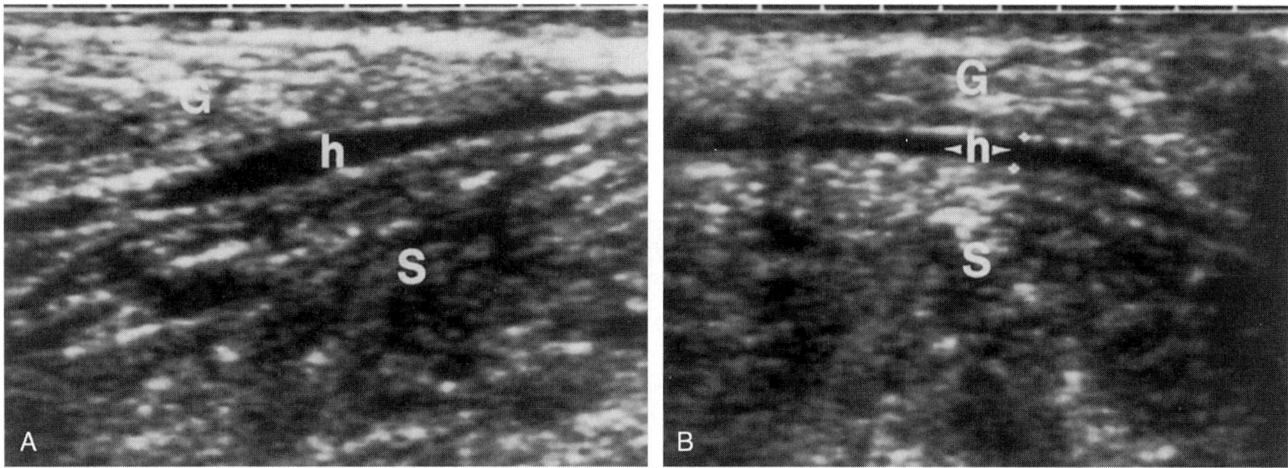

Figure 3–58 ■ Muscle-aponeurosis avulsion: longitudinal (**A**) and transverse (**B**) sonograms of the calf. An anechoic cleft (*h*) along the aponeurosis between the gastrocnemius (*G*) and soleus (*S*) represents a resolving hematoma. This is the classic location and appearance of a muscle-aponeurosis avulsion in the calf.

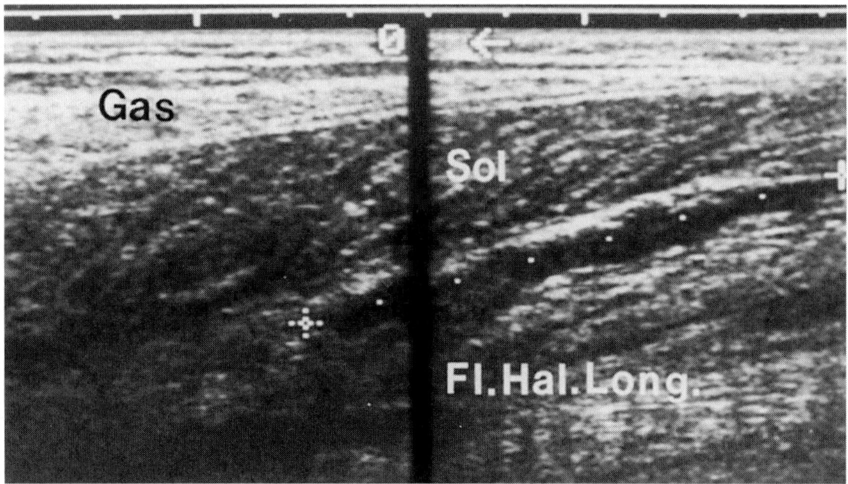

Figure 3–59 ■ Muscle-aponeurosis avulsion: longitudinal sonogram of the calf. After 1 week of pain and swelling of the right calf, this 38-year-old man presented for sonographic evaluation. The transducer is aligned along the proximal portion of the flexor hallucis longus muscle. An avulsion of the flexor hallucis longus from the aponeurosis is present (+). The aponeurosis is seen as a hyperechoic line superficial to the hematoma. Abbreviations: gastrocnemius (*Gas*), soleus (*Sol*).

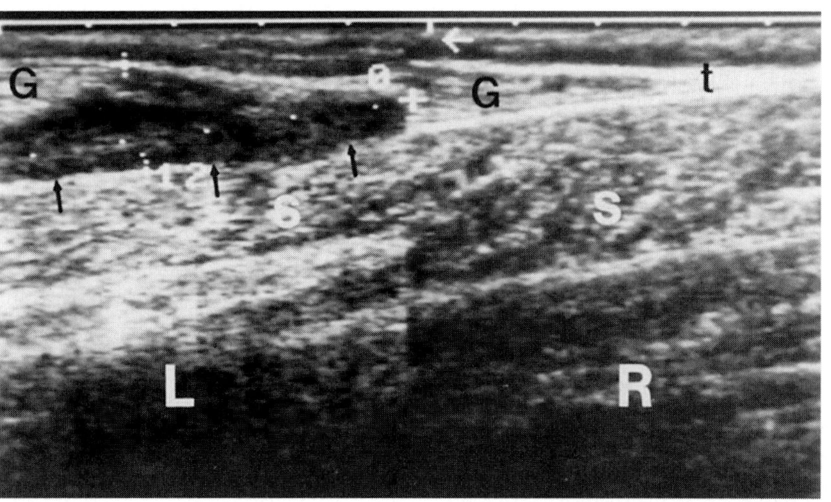

Figure 3–60 ■ Rupture of the gastrocnemius musculotendinous junction: longitudinal sonogram. A 25-year-old sprinter experienced sudden sharp pain in the distal left calf at the start of a race. He has limited plantar flexion of the foot associated with severe pain. The transducer is positioned over the musculotendinous junction of the medial head of the gastrocnemius. Side-to-side comparison is provided in this split-screen image. On the left, the tendon is retracted out of the FOV. A hematoma (*arrows*) is seen in the usual location of the musculotendinous junction. The retracted gastrocnemius is noted at the left corner of the image. A normal gastrocnemius musculotendinous junction is shown on the right. Abbreviations: gastrocnemius (*G*), proximal Achilles tendon (*t*), soleus (*S*), left (*L*), right (*R*).

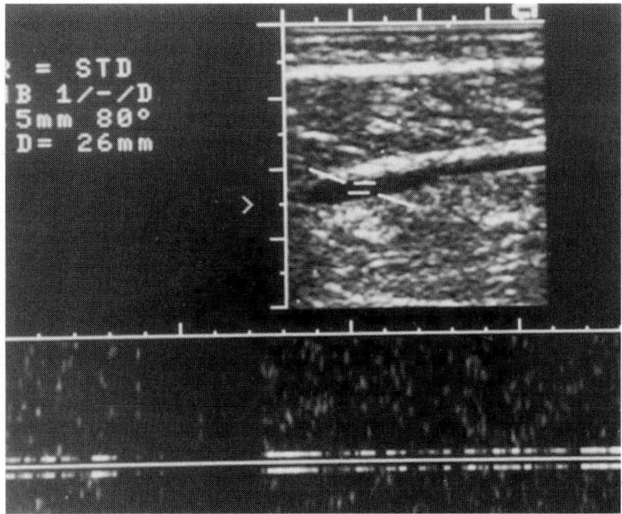

Figure 3–61 ■ Muscle-aponeurosis avulsion in the calf: Doppler study. Occasionally, a muscle-aponeurosis avulsion in the calf will have an appearance similar to that of ectatic veins. In these cases, the diagnostic problem is easily solved with Doppler flow analysis. The avulsion of the soleus from the aponeurosis shown here demonstrates this problem. No Doppler signal is observed from the lesion.

commonly seen in athletes whose sports require speed: sprinting, soccer, football, baseball, and hockey (Fig. 3–60). Sonography demonstrates a linear (Figs. 3–59 and 3–61) rupture filled with blood that extends along the aponeurosis. A characteristic feature of muscle-aponeurosis avulsion is a change in the orientation of the fibroadipose septa on either side of the aponeurosis in longitudinal images (Fig. 3–62). The most common traumatic tear in the calf is the distal medial gastrocnemius tear, known as *tennis leg* (see Fig. 3–53). These tears may be difficult to distinguish from plantaris tendon tears. Some medial gastrocnemius tears may be associated with tears of the plantaris; muscle tears can be com-

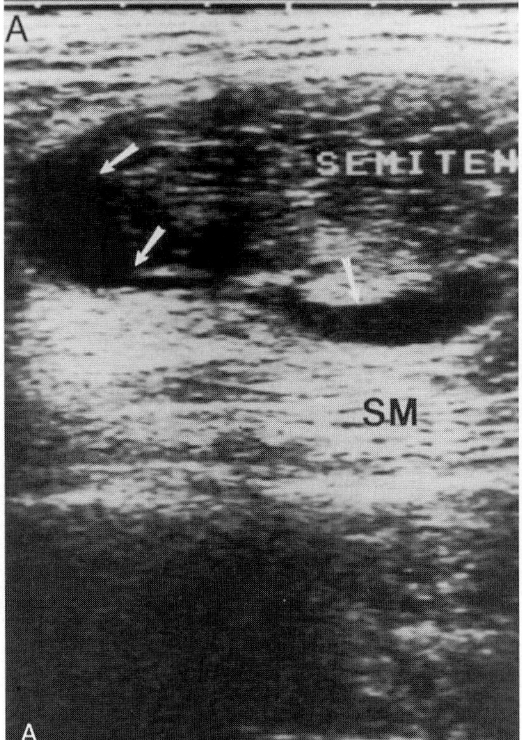

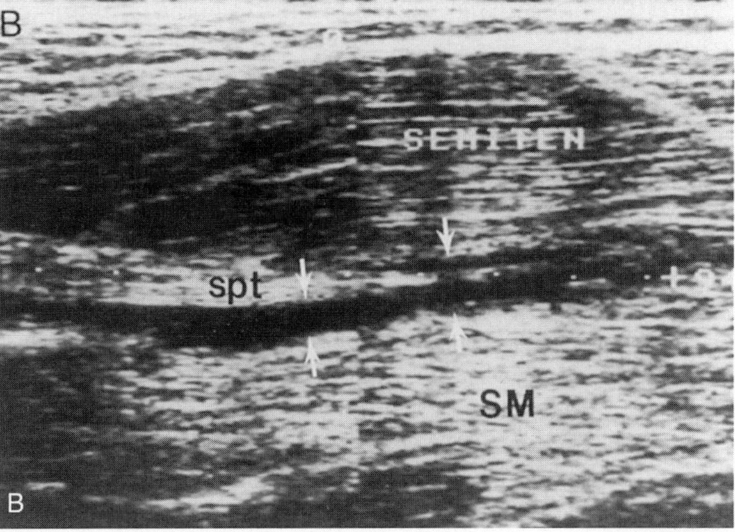

Figure 3–62 ■ **A,** Semitendinosus muscle-aponeurosis avulsion: transverse sonogram. This 20-year-old soccer player was kicked in the back of the calf while flexing his knee to attempt a kick. He felt a snap in the posterior right thigh accompanied by immediate function loss. At presentation 2 days later, the posterior thigh was markedly swollen. The transducer is positioned transversely over the posterior medial aspect of the upper thigh. Hematoma (*arrows*) surrounds the deep portion of the semitendinosus muscle. The avulsion has occurred between the semimembranosus (*SM*) and semitendinosus muscles. **B,** Semitendinosus muscle-aponeurosis avulsion: longitudinal sonogram. Same patient as in **A.** A plate-like hematoma (*arrows*) is seen on both sides of the fibrous septum (*spt*), which separates the two muscles; the orientation of the fibroadipose septa changes on either side of the hematoma. No intramuscular rupture is noted.

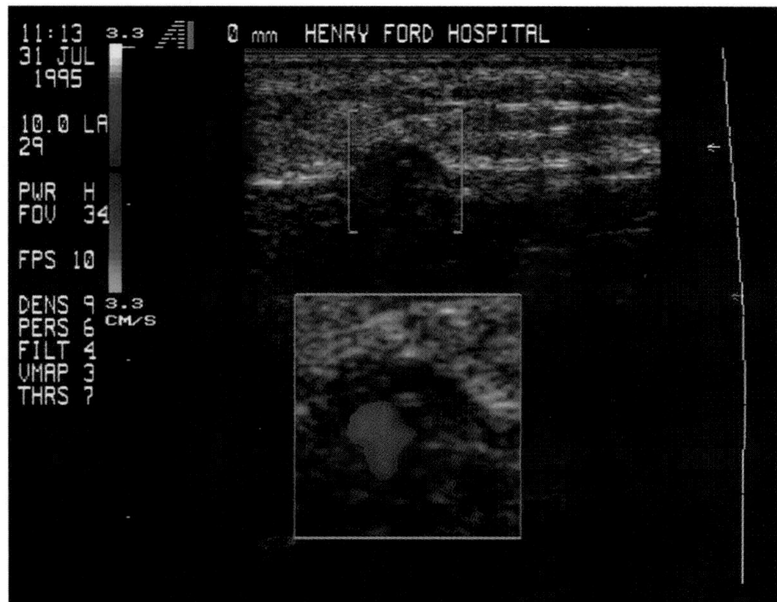

Figure 3–63 ■ Small muscle hernia with color Doppler signal: longitudinal ultrasound. A painful mass was present over the tibialis anterior muscle. The image on top shows bulging of the muscle into the subcutaneous tissues. The insert demonstrates vascularity within the mass. The muscle often protrudes through the fascia along neurovascular pedicles. This anatomic relationship explains why hernias can be painful.

plicated with venous thrombosis as well. Different combinations of soft tissue injuries can be very confusing clinically.

Muscle Hernia

Fascial defects with associated herniation of muscle are uncommon lesions. Chronic compartment syndrome is the most frequent cause of muscle hernias, but they may also be found following trauma or surgery. In chronic compartment syndrome, herniation occurs through weak areas in the fascia as a result of increased intracompartmental pressure. Often herniation occurs only during strenuous exercise and is reduced with rest. Therefore, examination should be performed immediately following strenuous exercise that reproduces the pain. Muscle her-

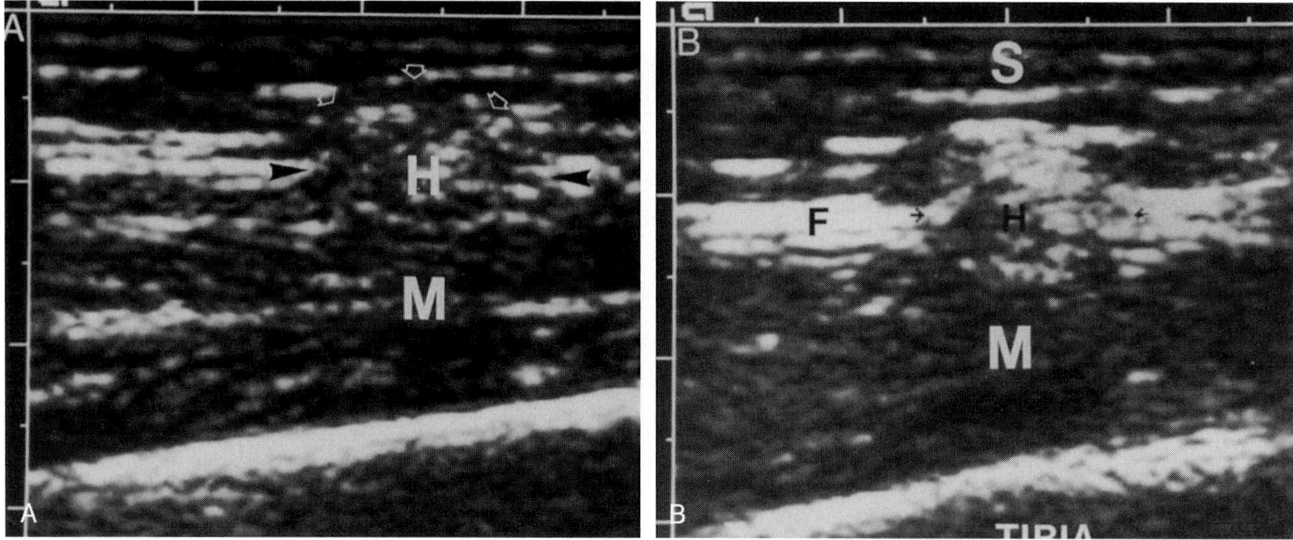

Figure 3–64 ■ **A,** Small muscle hernia of the anterior tibial muscle: longitudinal sonogram. A 19-year-old soccer player experienced pain in both calves during play. He reported being able to palpate painful nodules lateral to the tibia at the end of exercise. Sonographic examination was performed immediately after the patient had run several miles. The transducer is positioned over the midportion of the anterior compartment along its length. A portion of the anterior tibial muscle (*M*) herniates through a rent in the fascia (*arrowheads*) of the anterior compartment, bulging into the subcutaneous tissues (*open arrows*). **B,** Slight angling of the transducer provided better visualization of the fascial defect (*arrows*). The fascia (*F*) is seen as a hyperechoic layer 3 to 4 mm thick separating the muscle compartment (*M*) from the subcutaneous tissues (*S*). Small hernias (*H*) tend to have a hyperechoic appearance compared with that of normal muscle.

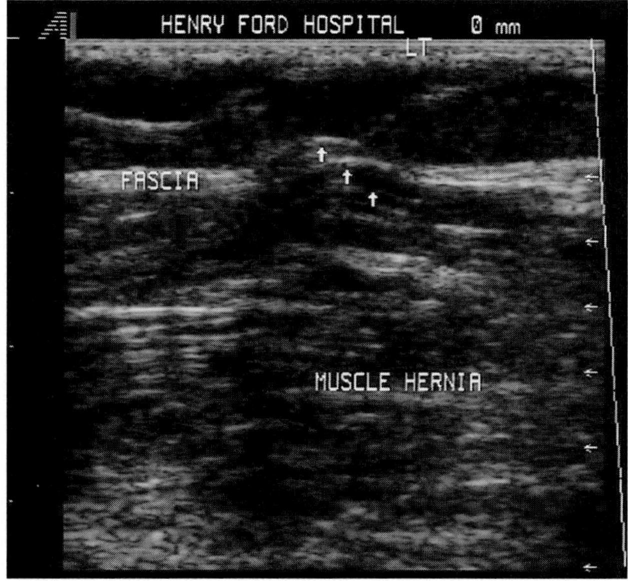

Figure 3-65 ■ Small muscle hernia in the popliteal fossa: longitudinal sonogram. A small mass is noted in the popliteal fossa of this 42-year-old woman who was exercising vigorously in a rehabilitation program. Pain occurred when pressure was applied on the mass with the transducer. The image was obtained with minimal pressure. The transducer is aligned along the fibroadipose septa. Septa (*small arrows*) protrude through the defect. Muscle hernias are usually very small lesions. They are rarely seen with imaging modalities other than ultrasound.

nias may be unilateral, bilateral, single, or multiple. They are frequently palpable clinically. Pain may be due to ischemia of the herniated muscle or irritation of an adjacent nerve. Neuroma formation is a rare complication.

Sonography will demonstrate the fascial defect, as well as the extent of muscle herniation. The most common site of muscle hernia is the lower third of the calf overlying the anterior intermuscular septum between the anterior and lateral compartments. At this site, a branch of the superficial peroneal nerve exits through the fascia cruris (Nicholas and Hershman, 1986). Herniation along small neurovascular pedicles is quite common in muscle hernias (Fig. 3-63). Acutely, the herniated muscle will have a hyperechoic appearance due to crowding of the fibroadipose septa (Figs. 3-64 and 3-65). However, if the hernia is not intermittent, it will become hypoechoic as the involved muscle becomes edematous and eventually necrotic. The lesion will remain hypoechoic as the muscle is replaced by reparative tissue (Figs. 3-66 and 3-67). Do not apply much pressure with the transducer if you suspect a muscle hernia. Pressure may reduce the hernia, making it invisible during the sonographic examination. Optimal scanning conditions include a thick layer of gel, almost no transducer pressure, the highest-frequency transducer available, and the focal zone directed as superficially as possible. The small mass may not demonstrate much contrast with the surrounding hypoechoic fat. The diagnosis can be made easily if the fascial defect is identified. This

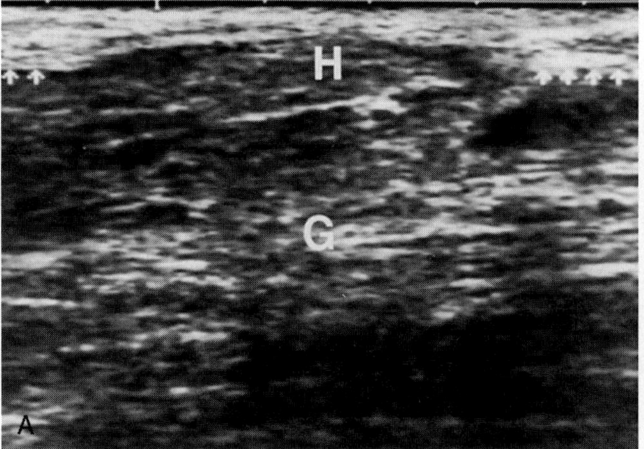

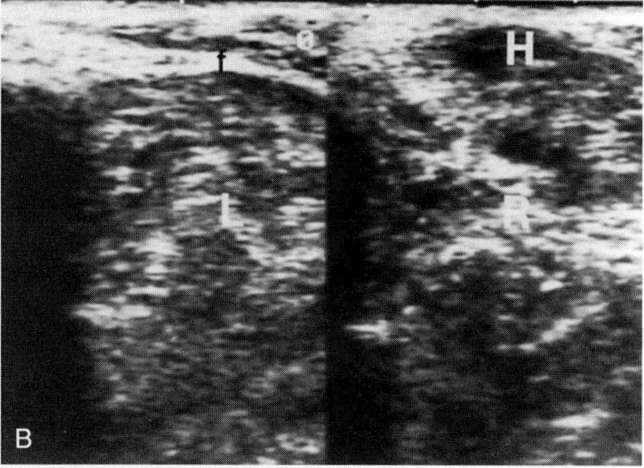

Figure 3-66 ■ **A,** Large muscle hernia of the proximal gastrocnemius: longitudinal sonogram. The patient is a 25-year-old football player with chronic posterior compartment syndrome of the right leg. He experienced pain and swelling over the medial aspect of the proximal gastrocnemius, which was most severe following exercise. A 4.5-cm defect is noted in the fascia cruris, with the gastrocnemius (*G*) herniating through the gap (*H*). Normal hyperechoic fascia (*arrows*) is seen defining the extent of the lesion. **B,** Large muscle hernia of the proximal gastrocnemius: transverse sonogram. Same patient as in **A.** In this split-screen display, the image on the left demonstrates the normal left calf. Fascia (*f*) completely covers the gastrocnemius. On the right, the gastrocnemius protrudes through the large fascial defect. Abbreviations: left (*L*), right (*R*), hernia (*H*).

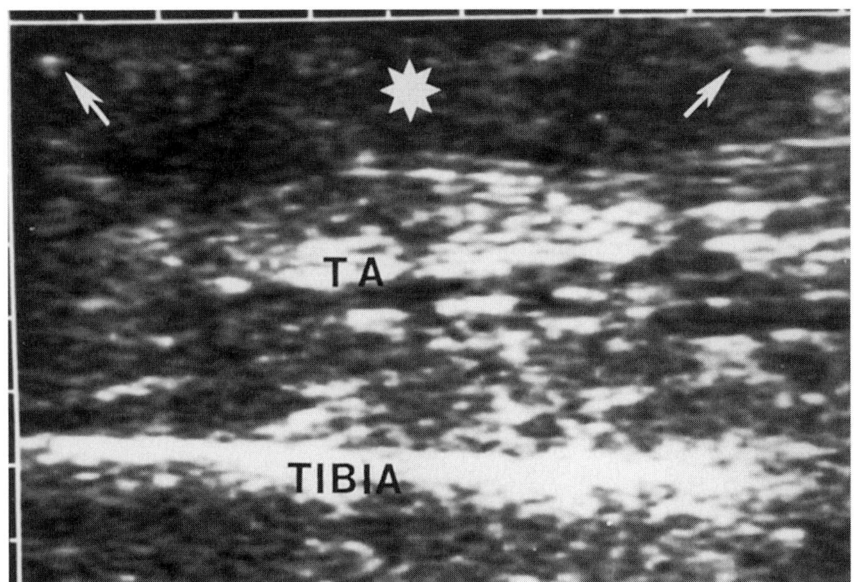

Figure 3-67 ■ Traumatic muscle hernia: longitudinal sonogram. A large fragment of glass ruptured the anterior tibial muscle after this 35-year-old woman dropped a vase. The fragment was surgically removed, and the ruptured muscle was repaired. Edema of the muscle prevented closure of the fascial defect. Two months following this injury, the patient presented with limited dorsiflexion of the foot. The transducer is positioned over the middle segment of the anterior tibial muscle. A large, hypoechoic segment of the muscle (*asterisk*) herniates through the remaining fascia (*arrows*). Normal fibroadipose septa are not present in this region. During dorsiflexion of the foot, this segment was akinetic. A hypoechoic appearance of herniated muscle is rare. It can be seen in cases of muscle necrosis or, as in this case, may represent muscle undergoing regeneration following rupture. Abbreviation: anterior tibial muscle (*TA*).

defect appears as a hypoechoic gap in the highly reflective fascial sheath (Bianchi et al., 1995). Patients are often quite alarmed when they find these small, tumor-like swellings, which characterize a muscle hernia. CT and MRI are not well suited for detection of these lesions and these examinations are reported as negative, adding to the patient's anxiety. The small size of the lesion and the intermittent character of the swelling are challenges best met by ultrasound examination.

A weak fascia can also allow fat or bowel to protrude between muscle layers. Direct and indirect inguinal and femoral hernias, which can be congenital or acquired, are typical examples. Hernias can cause hip or groin pain, and the lesions may develop in athletes because of increased abdominal pressure during sports activity (Fig. 3-68). Ultrasound can assist in the diagnosis of hernias which cause equivocal clinical findings. Spigelian hernias form in athletes as well. One must have a good

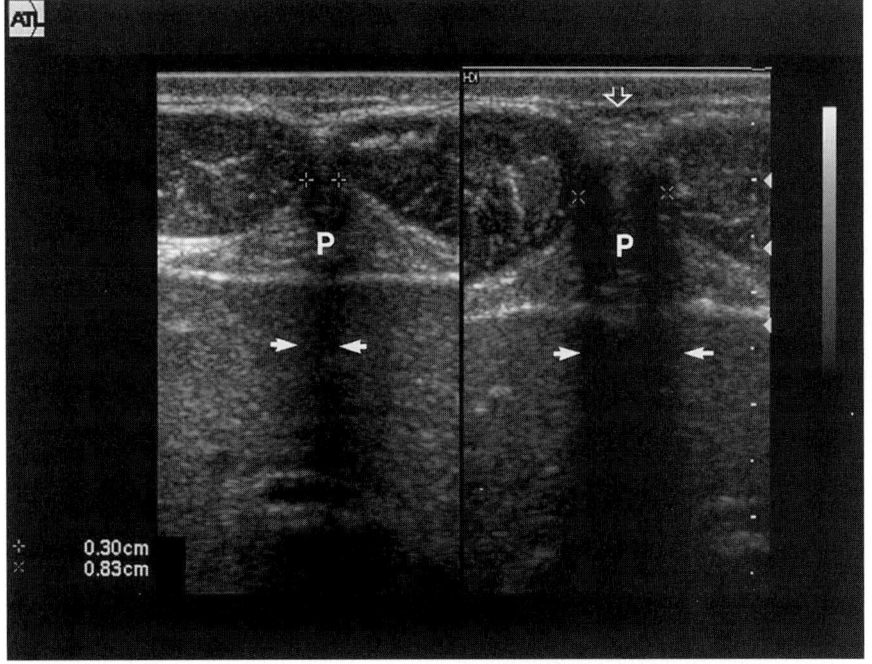

Figure 3-68 ■ Epigastric hernia: transverse ultrasound with split-screen technique. This high school athlete feels a painful swelling in the epigastrium when he practices sit-ups. The transverse ultrasound scan taken in the supine position is displayed on the left side of the split screen. The ultrasound scan on the right side of the split screen shows the diastasis of the linea alba during a sit-up exercise. The calipers measure the distance between the rectus muscles. Refraction artifact off the medial aspect of the rectus muscles casts a shadow (*between the arrows*) over the abdomen. Properitoneal fat (*P*) extends through the linea alba defect and protrudes subcutaneously (*open arrow*).

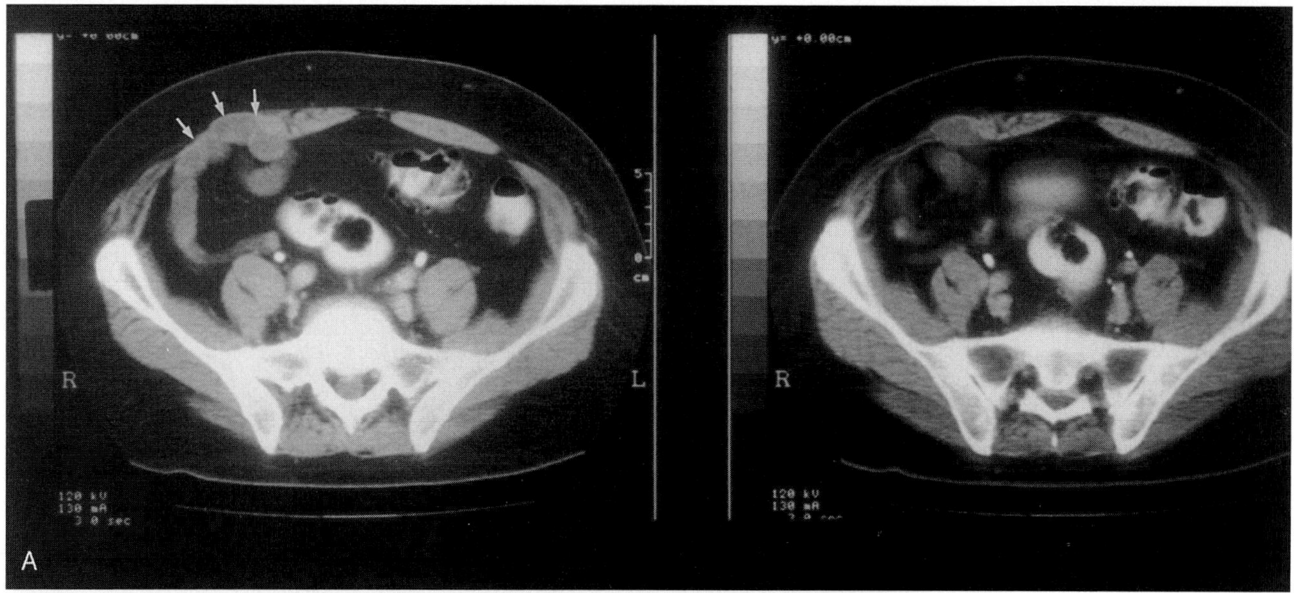

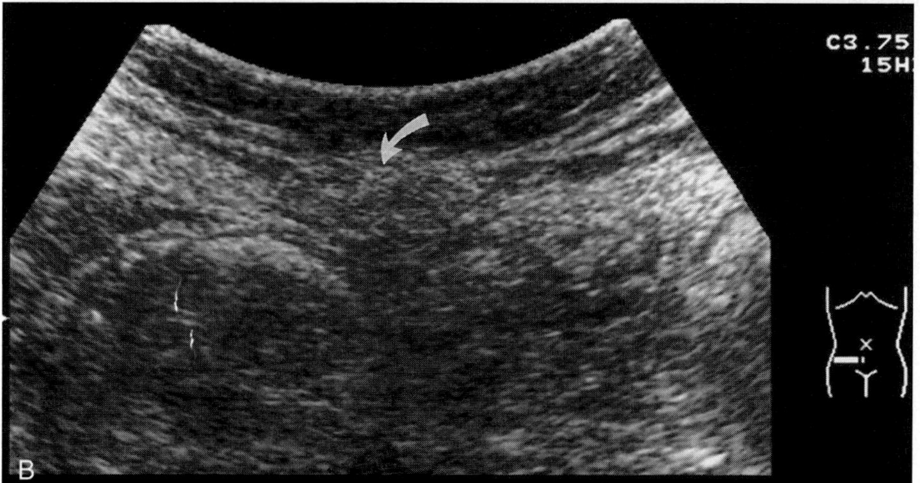

Figure 3-69 ■ **A,** Spigelian hernia containing small bowel: CT exam of the lower abdomen. This patient complains of pain in the right iliac fossa. A loop of small bowel (*arrows*) extends into the subcutaneous fat. (Courtesy of Dr. Christian Hessler, CHUV, Switzerland) **B,** Spigelian hernia containing small bowel: transverse ultrasound of the lower abdomen. Same patient as in **A.** Transverse ultrasound imaging reveals displacement of small bowel (*curved arrow*) subcutaneously, without the interposition of abdominal wall musculature. (Courtesy of Dr. Christian Hessler, CHUV, Switzerland)

understanding of the local anatomy in order to find small lesions (Figs. 3-69 and 3-70).

Shin Splints

Chronic changes in the fascia may also affect muscle function. Fascial thickening may result from infection of muscles, joints, or osteomyelitis. It may also be caused by trauma or exercise-induced overload. The American Medical Association's (AMA) standard nomenclature defines *shin splints* as "pain and discomfort in the legs from repetitive running on hard surfaces or forceful excessive use of the foot flexors." The AMA suggests that the diagnosis be limited to musculotendinous inflammation, excluding fatigue fractures and ischemic disorders such as compartment syndrome. The patient typically presents with pain and tenderness lateral to the tibia and along the posteromedial border of the middle to lower tibia. The pain is characterized as a dull ache that varies in intensity. Onset of symptoms occurs after rhythmic, repetitive exercise. Physical examination reveals pain on active movement of the ankle.

Fascial thickening over the facies medialis of the tibia (Figs. 3-71 through 3-75) is observed on ultrasound examination. Thickening is also noted at the anchor points of the muscle compartment to the periosteum along the posteromedial and lateral borders of the tibia. Minimal focal thickening of the periosteum may be observed at these attachment sites. Although the etiology of pain in shin splints is not known, these findings suggest that the cause may be traumatic inflammation of the fascia and adjacent periosteum (Fig. 3-76).

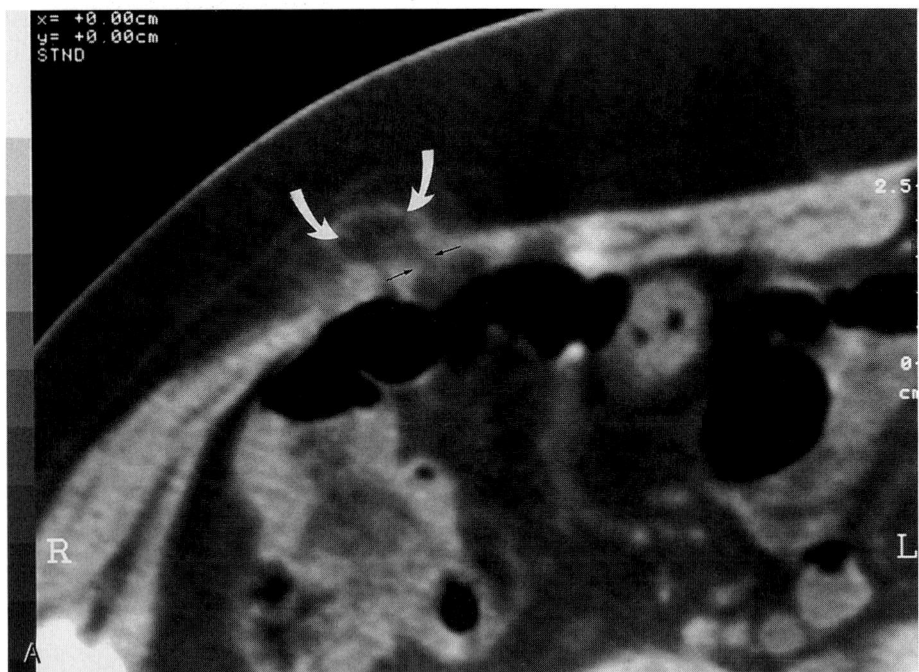

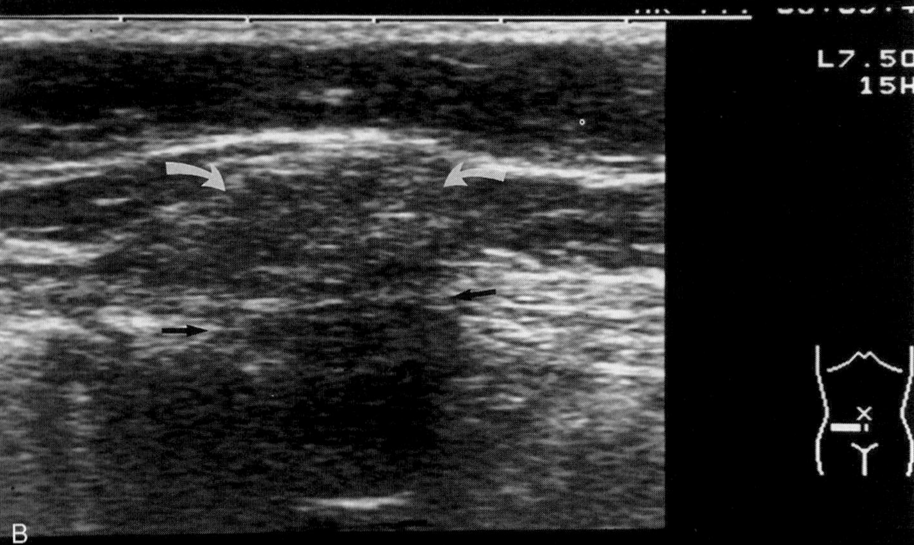

Figure 3–70 ▪ **A,** Spigelian hernia containing fat: CT of the abdominal wall. Localized pain over the abdominal wall was present. Properitoneal fat (*curved arrows*) herniates into the subcutaneous tissues through a small area of fascial weakness (*arrows*) between the rectus and the lateral abdominal wall musculature. The fat has an hourglass appearance across the abdominal wall. (Courtesy of Dr. Christian Hessler, CHUV, Switzerland) **B,** Spigelian hernia containing fat: ultrasound of the abdominal wall. Same patient as in **A.** The fat-filled, hernia sac (*curved arrows*) is seen in the subcutaneous tissues. Widening in between abdominal musculature (*between the arrows*) is demonstrated as an area of relative hypoechogenicity. (Courtesy of Dr. Christian Hessler, CHUV, Switzerland)

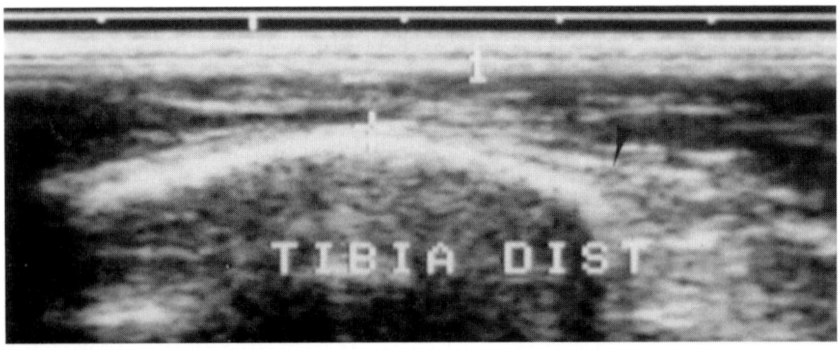

Figure 3–71 ▪ Periosteum and fascia: transverse ultrasound image of a specimen. This transverse image of the distal third of the tibia was obtained on an autopsy specimen. The fascia (*arrowhead*) joins the periosteum of the anterior tibia to form a hyperechoic layer (+) 1 mm thick overlying the anterior medial tibial cortex.

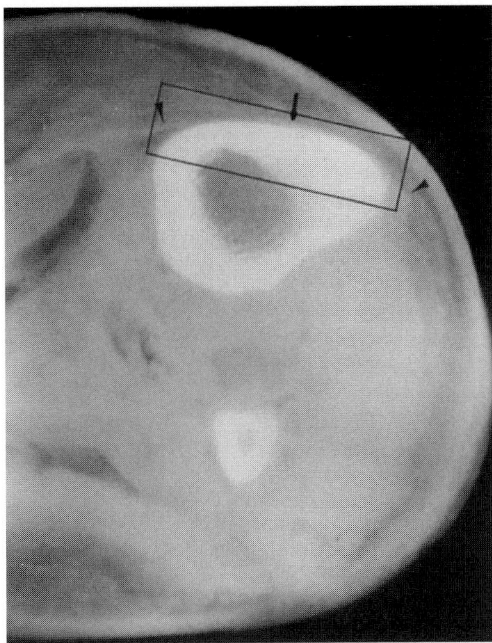

Figure 3-72 ▪ Radiography of a specimen of the distal tibia: transverse section. A specimen radiograph was obtained through the same region shown in Figure 3-71. The specimen was 6 mm thick. Within the rectangular area is the region depicted in Figure 3-71. Fascia (*arrowheads*) is again seen fusing with the periosteum (*arrow*) of the anteromedial tibia, providing a firm point of anchorage.

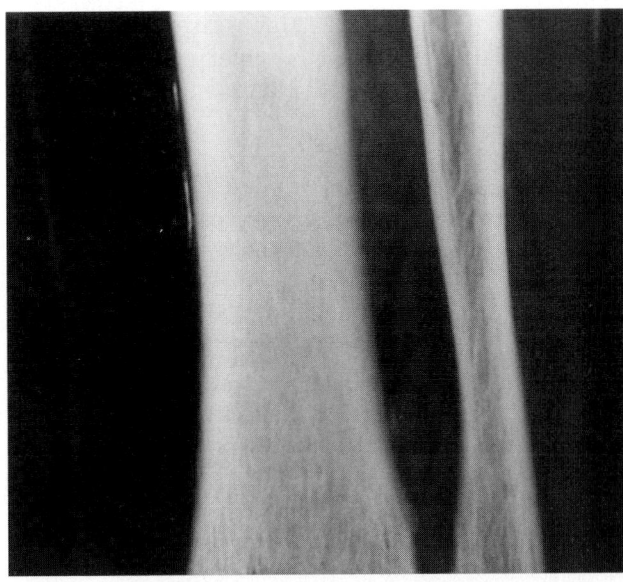

Figure 3-73 ▪ Anteroposterior radiograph of a distal leg specimen. Under sonographic guidance, a needle was placed under the hyperechoic fascial and periosteal layer covering the anterior medial tibia in Figure 3-71. Barium sulfate was then injected, and this radiograph was obtained. The barium sulfate is seen layering adjacent to the tibial cortex. Histological sections were then obtained.

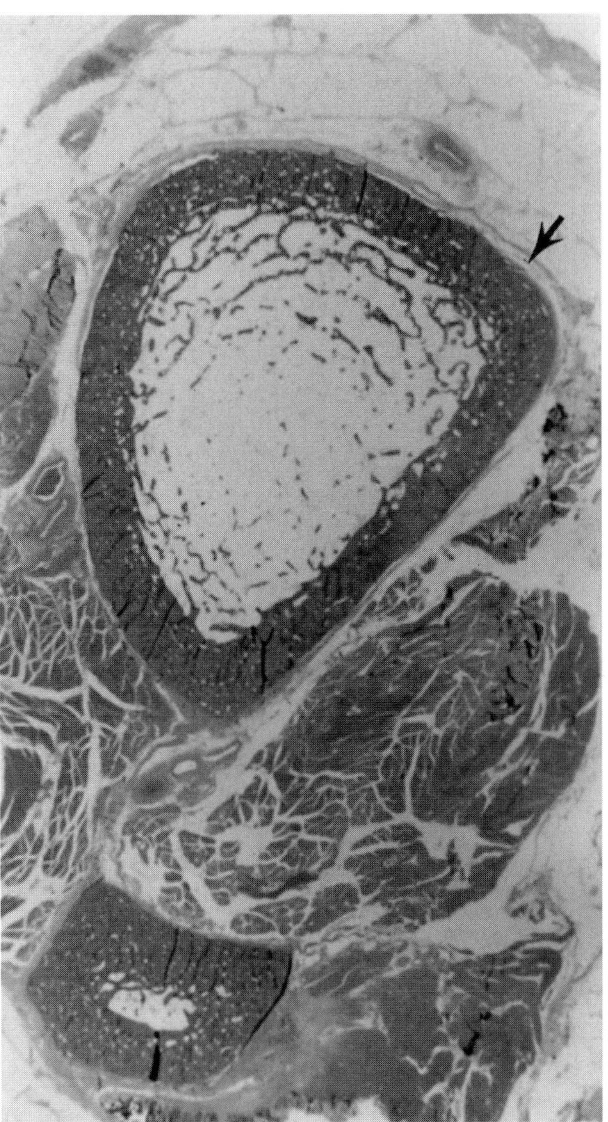

Figure 3-74 ▪ Histological section through the distal tibia: hematoxylin and eosin stain. A section 6 mm thick was obtained through the tibia in the region of barium injection. Barium sulfate particles (*arrow*) are identified beneath the fascial periosteal layer, which was dissected off of the cortex by the barium injection. This confirms the anatomical relationship demonstrated on the sonographic images.

Runner's Knee

Iliotibial band friction syndrome is another traumatic fascial lesion, also referred to as *runner's knee.* The syndrome is characterized by pain over the lateral aspect of the knee, particularly in the region of the lateral femoral condyle anterior to the origin of the lateral collateral ligament (Nicholas and Hershman, 1986). Runners with excessive pronation of the feet and those who run on cambered roads are at increased risk. Patients with hip abduction contracture, genu varum, tight heel cords, and inter-

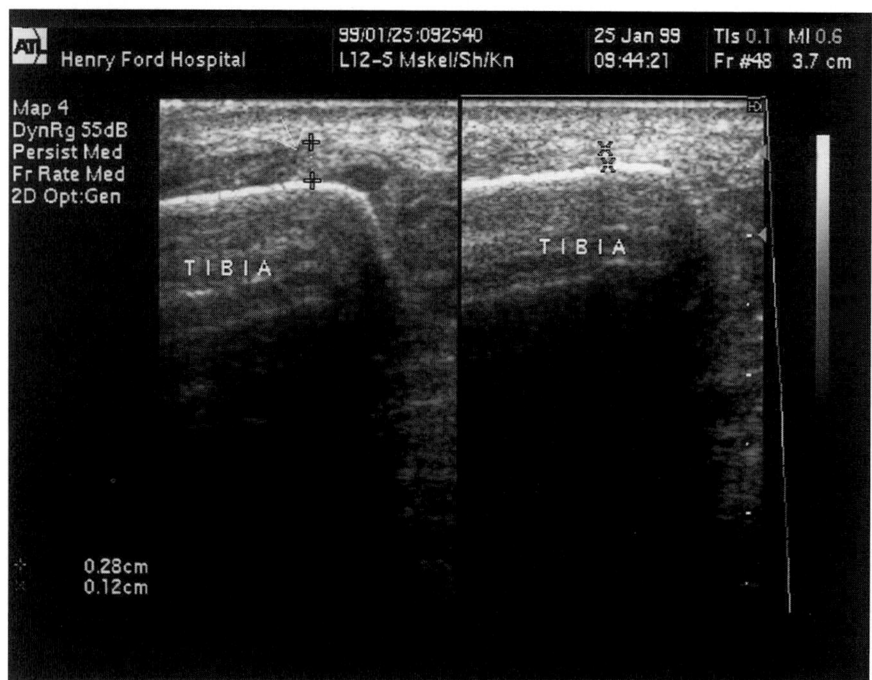

Figure 3–75 ■ Periostitis of the tibia: transverse ultrasound. After a long period of inactivity, this 42-year-old individual starts playing competitive soccer again. Pain develops over the anterior tibia, and the patient notices swelling over the shin. The conventional radiographs are negative; an ultrasound study is ordered to evaluate the mass. The transverse ultrasound scan over the anterior tibia compares the abnormal right tibia on the left side of the split screen with the normal left tibia on the right side. The periosteal envelope (*between the calipers*) is twice as thick as that on the symptomatic side. This layer appears more hypoechoic as well.

nal tibial torsion are also predisposed to develop runner's knee. No clinical signs of internal derangement of the knee are present. Renne was first to recognize that this form of lateral knee pain was a distinct syndrome (Renne, 1975). He attributed it to inflammation of the synovium due to movement of the iliotibial tract over a prominent lateral femoral condyle (Cravers, 1978; James et al., 1978; Noble, 1980; Sutker et al., 1981).

Fascia forming the iliotibial tract is seen as a hyperechoic lamellar structure adjacent to the lateral femoral condyle. Ultrasound examination is usually normal unless performed immediately following exercise that reproduces the pain. Following exercise, the fascia is swollen and decreased in echogenicity (Figs. 3–77 and 3–78). In some cases, edema is so prominent that it gives the appearance of a fluid-filled bursa. No synovial thickening is observed.

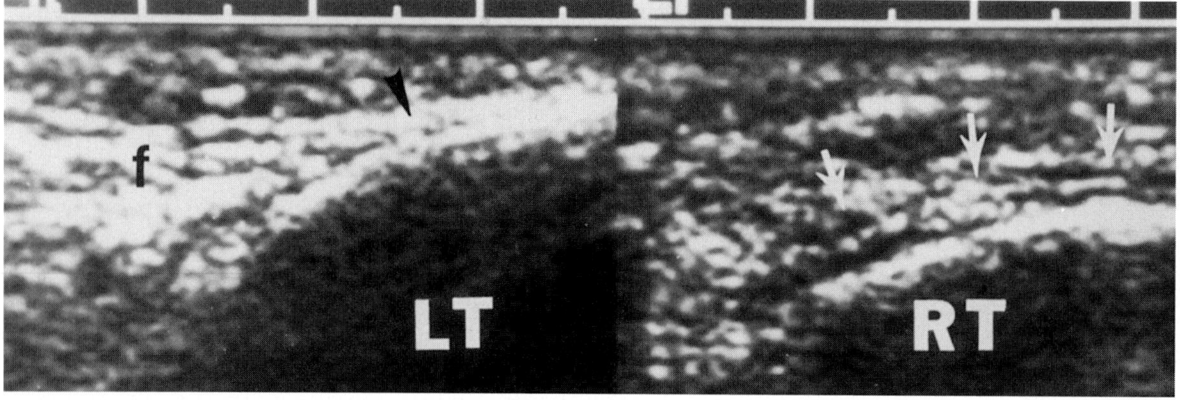

Figure 3–76 ■ Shin splint: transverse sonogram. This 20-year-old female volleyball player complained of pain over the lateral margin of the middle third of the right tibia during play. The point of maximal tenderness is established at the junction of the fascia cruris with the tibia. A transverse image over the point of maximal tenderness is shown side by side with a comparable image of the asymptomatic left leg. The image of the left side has been reversed to make the two images superimposable. On the right, the fascia–tibia junction (*white arrows*) is thickened and hypoechoic relative to the normal left side (*arrowhead*). The subcutaneous tissues overlying the abnormal fascia–tibia junction are thickened as well. Abbreviation: normal fascia (*f*).

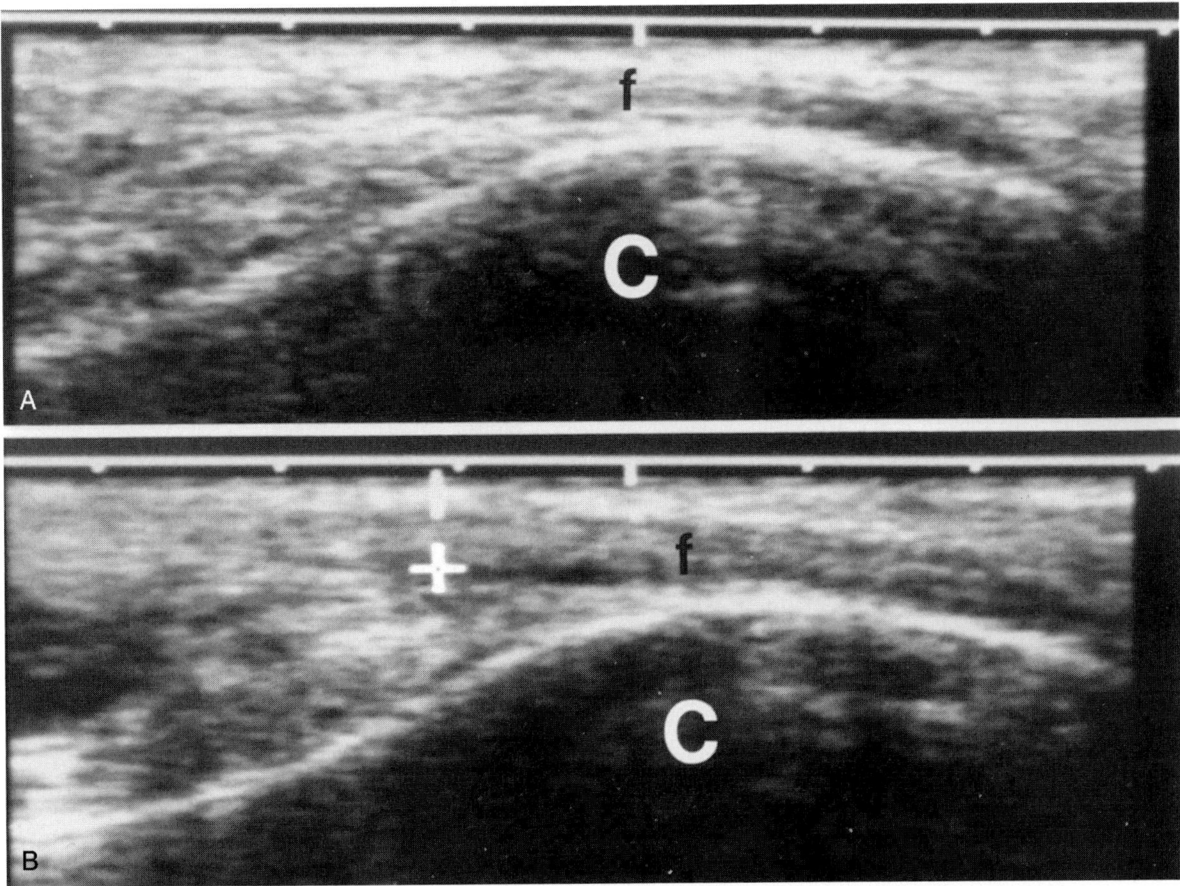

Figure 3-77 ■ A: Runner's knee: coronal sonogram. This 28-year-old jogger increased his exercise routine from 5 miles to 10 miles daily. After several weeks, he developed pain over the lateral aspect of the knee, which forced him to stop after 9 miles. Pain recurred after 1 week of rest. This coronal image was obtained over the lateral femoral condyle anterior to the lateral collateral ligament prior to exercise. Fascia (*f*) overlying the lateral femoral condyle (*C*) appears hyperechoic, particularly the peripheral margins. **B,** Runner's knee: coronal sonogram after exercise. Same patient and transducer position as in **A**. Immediately after running to his limit, the fascia (*f*) is thickened and hypoechoic.

Therapy for iliotibial tract syndrome is conservative. Rest, cold compresses, and anti-inflammatory medication are the mainstays of treatment. These may be combined with therapeutic ultrasound. Local steroid injection may be of value in advanced cases. Stretching of the iliotibial tract and orthotics may be useful in preventing recurrence. A change in running habits is also beneficial. Patients should be advised to shorten their stride and alternate sides of the road while running. If these conservative measures fail, an effective release operation is available. This involves horizontal incision of the iliotibial band.

Plantar Fascia Rupture

Long-distance runners often suffer from chronic foot pain. Heel pain is frequently due to plantar fasciitis (see Fig. 19-23), which may be accompanied by a plantar spur (Resnick and Niwayama, 1988). Obesity is a predisposing factor as well. The swelling in this disease typically occurs at the origin of the plantar fascia. Maximal swelling is noted over the calcaneal tuberosity. Right-left comparisons are not very useful because the disease is often bilateral and symmetric. However, the fascia demonstrates decreased echogenicity and markedly increased thickness at its origin compared with the middle and distal thirds (Gibbon, 1992; Cardinal et al., 1996). Normal plantar fascia does not thicken at its origin, remaining even in thickness throughout the foot. Generalized and more severe pain may result from rupture of the plantar fascia (Nicholas and Hershman, 1986; Peterson and Renstrom, 1986). These lesions tend to heal poorly, with abundant granulation tissue. Casts and special taping are usually not helpful. Surgical repair is often required; therefore, the diagnosis must be certain.

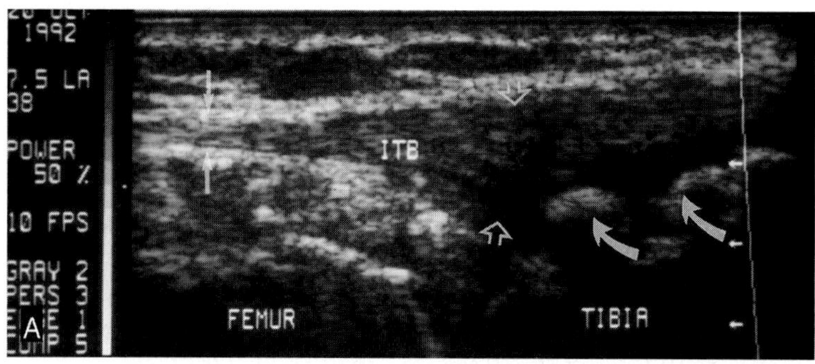

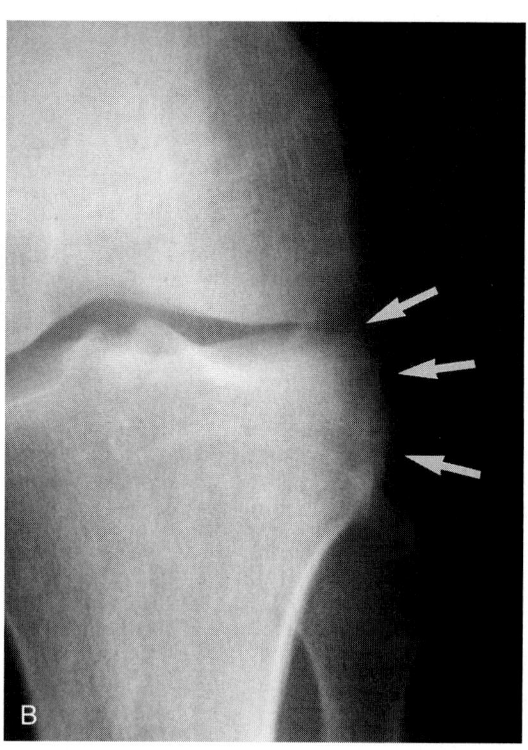

Figure 3-78 ■ **A,** Distal iliotibial tract syndrome: coronal sonogram. Prior trauma had injured the patellar tendon in this middle-aged man. The injury had not been recognized, and a defect in the extensor mechanism persisted. The patient now experiences lateral knee pain. Chronic overload of the iliotibial band resulted in edema of the distal iliotibial band (*ITB*). The proximal band has a normal thickness (*arrows*), but the distal band is hypoechoic and widened (*open arrows*). Gerdy's tubercle at the distal insertion of the iliotibial tract shows bone proliferation (*curved arrows*). **B,** Distal iliotibial tract syndrome: anteroposterior radiograph of the knee. Same patient as in **A.** Bone proliferation is noted at the lateral tibial condyle (*arrows*).

The majority of ruptures are found at the middle to posterior third of the fascia. Ultrasound usually demonstrates a hypoechoic, thick, fusiform lesion between the parallel fascicles of the plantar fascia or aponeurosis (Fig. 3-79). Rarely, discontinuity of the fascia will be observed because the patient usually presents well after rupture occurs. Sonography is essential to exclude bursitis of the bursa subcutanea calcanea. Painful nodular masses develop in the medial plantar fascia in patients with plantar fibromatosis. These lesions may be difficult to distinguish from chronic rupture sonographically. However, the clinical presentation and the pathology are quite different. The lesions often occur in patients with a family history of palmar and/or plantar fibromatosis or in patients who have other superficial fibromatoses, including Dupuytren's disease, Peyronie's disease, or knuckle pads. The lesions are located more distal than the traumatic fascial rupture. The masses are typically hypoechoic, and in contrast with tears, fibromas will infiltrate the fascia; ultrasound may be able to demonstrate fascial fibers through the lesion (Fig. 3-80). The swelling is fusiform and has its longest dimension

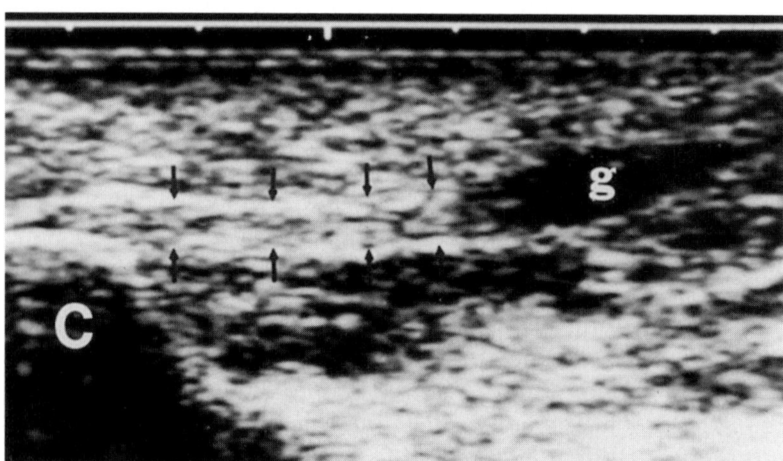

Figure 3-79 ■ Plantar fascia rupture: longitudinal sonogram. A marathon runner with intractable pain in the sole of the right foot presents for sonographic examination. The transducer is aligned along the length of the foot, touching the lateral tuberosity of the calcaneus (*C*) at the observer's left. The plantar fascia (*arrows*) is seen as a hyperechoic band attached to the lateral tuberosity. A gap (*g*) in the fascia is noted in its midportion. At surgery 3 weeks later, a discontinuity filled with granulation tissue was found.

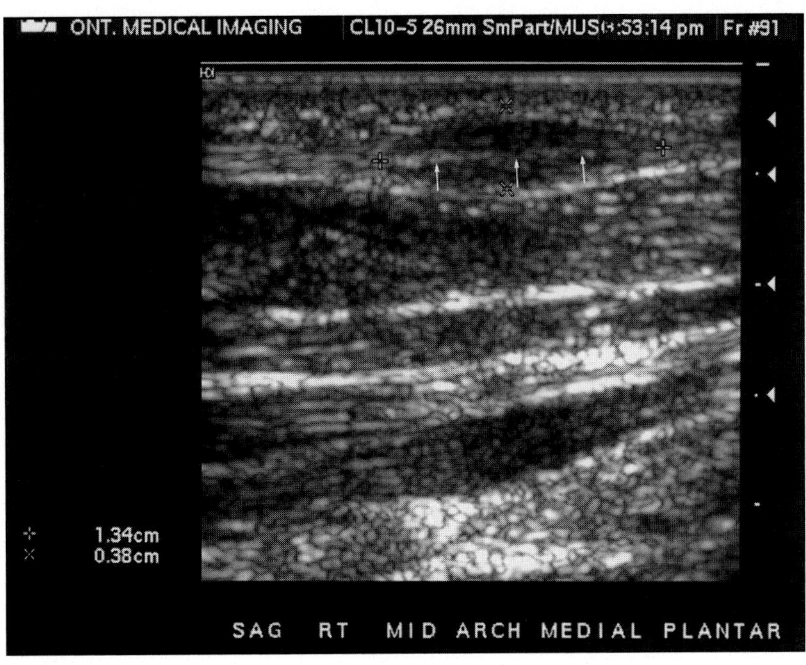

Figure 3-80 ■ Plantar fibromatosis: longitudinal sonogram. Hard nodules can be found in the midfoot and within the medial rim of the plantar aponeurosis in patients with plantar fibromatosis. Most patients have a family history of superficial fibromatosis; some have diabetes or may be taking anticonvulsant medication. Trauma and excessive use of alcohol sometimes play a role in the development of this disease. This longitudinal sonogram through the plantar aponeurosis is aligned with the orientation of the medial plantar fascia. The 1-cm-long lesion (*between the calipers*) is hypoechoic, fusiform, and blends with the fascia both proximally and distally. Continuity of fascial fibers within the lesion suggests a cellular fibroma lesion rather than a chronic fascial tear, as seen in Figure 3-79. (Courtesy of Jag Dhanju, RDMS, Ontario Medical Imaging, Canada)

in the length of the fascia plantaris (plantar aponeurosis). Several nodules can develop, and the lesions are bilateral in up to 25% of cases (Enzinger and Weiss, 1995). Repetitive trauma can be a factor contributing to the development of this condition; however, genetic predisposition, and hormonal and drug-related etiologies, seem far more important. Plantar fibromatosis, also called *Ledderhose's disease*, consists pathologically of fibroblasts, glycosaminoglycans, and collagen. The cellularity of the lesions and the number of mitotic figures depend on the stage development of the lesion at the time of biopsy. Benign plantar fibromas have sometimes been mistaken for fibrosarcoma pathologically, and amputations have been performed based on this incorrect diagnosis. As is so often the case, it is important to recognize Ledderhose disease as an entity and to remember: "first, do no harm" (Enzinger and Weiss, 1995).

Summary

Ultrasound is a reliable means of diagnosing intramuscular and muscle boundary lesions. Its real-time capability is unique in providing a means to evaluate structures under dynamic conditions. This allows diagnosis of lesions that would otherwise remain occult. Serial follow-up examinations provide valuable information about healing and about the prognosis for recurrent injury. These factors, as well as reasonable cost, make ultrasound the examination of choice for the evaluation of muscle pathology.

References

Abiri MM, Kirpekar M, Ablow RC: Osteomyelitis: Detection with ultrasound. *Radiology* 169:795–797, 1988.

Anderson JE: *Grant's Atlas of Anatomy*. Baltimore, Williams & Wilkins Co, 1983.

Auerbach DN, Bowen A III: Sonography of the leg in posterior compartment syndrome. *AJR* 136:407–408, 1981.

Banker BQ, Chester CS: Infarction of thigh muscle in the diabetic patient. *Neurology* 23:667–677, 1973.

Barohn RJ, Kissel JT: Painful thigh mass in a young woman: Diabetic muscle infarction. *Muscle Nerve* 15:850–855, 1992.

Bianchi S, et al: Sonographic examination of muscle herniation. *J Ultrasound Med* 14:357–360, 1995.

Bouvier JF, Chassain AP, Veyriras E: Place de l'echotomographie dans les accident musculaires des membres inferieurs du footballeur. *Cinesiologie* 21:274–278, 1982.

Brahim F, Zaccardelli W: Ultrasound measurement of the anterior leg compartment. *Am J Sports Med* 14:300–302, 1986.

Bullough PG, Vigorita VJ: *Atlas of Orthopedic Pathology*. New York, Gower Medical, 1984.

Cardinal E, et al: Plantar fasciitis: Sonographic evaluation. *Radiology* 201:257–259, 1996.

Chason DP, et al: Diabetic muscle infarction: Radiologic evaluation. *Skeletal Radiol* 25:127–132, 1996.

Chester CS, Banker BQ: Focal infarction of muscle in diabetics. *Diabetes Care* 9:623–630, 1986.

Chiedozi LC: Pyomyositis: Review of 205 cases in 112 patients. *Am J Surg* 137:255–259, 1979.

Clemente CD: *Gray's Anatomy*. Philadelphia, Lea & Febiger, 1985.

Cravers S: Iliotibial tract friction syndrome in athletes. *Br J Sports Med* 12:69, 1978.

Detmer PR, et al: 3D ultrasonic image feature localization based on magnetic scanhead tracking: In vitro calibration and validation. *Ultrasound Med Biol* 20(9): 923–936, 1994.

Enzinger FM, Weiss SW: *Soft Tissue Tumors*, ed 3. St. Louis, Mosby-Yearbook, 1995.

Erickson SJ: High-resolution imaging of the musculoskeletal system. *Radiology* 205:593–616, 1997.

Fornage BD, et al: Ultrasonography in the evaluation of muscular trauma. *J Ultrasound Med* 2:549–554, 1983.

Fornage BD: Ultrasonography of muscles and tendons, in *Examination Technique and Atlas of Normal Anatomy of the Extremities*. New York, Springer-Verlag, 1989.

Garfin SR, et al: Role of fascia in maintenance of muscle tension and pressure. *J Appl Physiol* 51:317, 1981.

Geller SA: Extreme exertion rhabdomyolysis. *Hum Pathol* 4:241–245, 1973.

Genety J, et al: Pathologie musculaire du sportif. *La Vie Medicale* 1:1607–1612, 1980.

Gershuni DH, et al: Ultrasound evaluation of the anterior musculo-fascial compartment of the leg following exercise. *Clin Orthop* 167:185–190, 1982.

Gibbon WW: Plantar fasciitis: Ultrasound imaging. *Radiology* 182:285, 1992.

Gompels BM, Darlington LG: Gray scale ultrasonography and arthrography in the evaluation of popliteal cysts. *Clin Radiol* 30:539–545, 1979.

Graf R, Schuler P: *Sonographie am Stutz und Bewegungsapparat bei Erwachsenen undKindern*. Weinheim, Edition Medizin VCH, 1988.

Guyton AC: *Textbook of Medical Physiology*, ed 6. Philadelphia, WB Saunders Co, 1982.

Harcke HT, Grissom LE, Finkelstein MS: Evaluation of the musculoskeletal system with sonography. *AJR* 150: 1253–1261, 1988.

Huang Y, et al: Quantitative MR relaxometry study of muscle composition and function in Duchenne muscular dystrophy. *J Magn Reson Imaging* 4:59–64, 1994.

James SL, et al: Injuries to runners. *Am J Sports Med* 6:40, 1978.

Kaplan GN: Ultrasonic appearance of rhabdomyolysis. *AJR* 134:375–377, 1980.

Knochel JP: Rhabdomyolysis and myoglobinuria. *Semin Nephrol* 1:75, 1981.

Kossoff G, Griffiths KA, Warren PS: Real time quasi three-dimensional viewing in sonography with conventional, gray-scale volume imaging. *Ultrasound Obstet Gynecol* 4:211–216, 1994.

Kramer FL, et al: Ultrasound appearance of myositis ossificans. *Skeletal Radiol* 4:19–20, 1979.

Kuhl GK, et al: Mitochondrial encephfalomyopathy: Correlation of P-31 exercise MR spectroscopy with clinical findings. *Radiology* 192:223–230, 1994.

Kullmer K, et al: Das traumatisch bedingte kompartmentsyndrom des unterschenkels. Ultraschalldiagnostik zur qualitativen beurteilung von spatfolgen der muskulatur nach dermatofasziotomie. *Unfallchirurgie* 23: 87–91, 1997.

Lawson TL, Mittler S: Ultrasonic evaluation of extremity soft tissue lesions with arthrographic correlation. *J Assoc Can Radiol* 29:58–61, 1978.

Lehto M, Alanen A: Healing of muscle trauma. Correlation of sonographical and histologic findings in an experimental study in rats. *J Ultrasound Med* 6:425–429, 1987.

Lenkinski RE, et al: Integrated MR imaging and spectroscopy with chemical shift imaging of P-31 at 1.5T. *Radiology* 169:201–206, 1988.

Magnussen PA, Crozier AE, Gregg PJ: Detecting hematomas by ultrasound. *J Bone Joint Surg* 70(B): 150, 1988.

Martens MA, et al: Chronic leg pain in athletes due to recurrent compartment syndrome. *Am J Sports Med* 12(2):148–151, 1984.

Moore K: *Clinically Oriented Anatomy*. Baltimore, Williams & Wilkins Co, 1980.

Mubarak SJ: *Compartment Syndromes and Volkmann's Contracture*. Philadelphia, WB Saunders Co, 1981.

Nicholas JA, Hershman EB: *The Lower Extremity and Spine in Sports Medicine*. St Louis, CV Mosby Co, 1986.

Noble CA: Iliotibial band friction syndrome in runners. *Am J Sports Med* 8:232, 1980.

Park JH, et al: Use of magnetic resonance imaging and P-31 magnetic resonance spectroscopy to detect and quantify muscle dysfunction in the amyopathic and myopathic variants of dermatomyositis. *Arthritis Rheum* 38(1):68–77, 1995.

Peetrons P, Sintzoff S: Les accidents du membre inferieur chez les sportifs: Integration des differents modes d'imagerie (abstract). *J Francophone Radiol* 1987.

Peterson L, Renstrom P: *Sports Injuries*. Chicago, Year Book Medical, 1986.

Petersson CJ: Ruptures of the supraspinatus tendon. Cadaver dissection. *Orthop Scand* 55:52–56, 1984.

Petersson CJ, Gentz CF: Ruptures of the supraspinatus tendon. The significance of distally pointing acromioclavicular osteophytes. *Clin Orthop* 174:143–148, 1983.

Renne JW: The iliotibial band friction syndrome. *J Bone Joint Surg* 57(A):1110, 1975.

Resnick D, Niwayama G: *Diagnosis of Bone and Joint Disorders*. Philadelphia, WB Saunders Co, 1988.

Rocca PV, Alloway JA, Nashel DJ: Diabetic muscle infarction. *Semin Arthritis Rheum* 22:280–287, 1993.

Roth D, et al: Acute rhabdomyolysis associated with cocaine intoxication. *N Engl J Med* 319:673–677, 1988.

Schedel H, et al: Muscle edema in MR imaging of neuromuscular diseases. *Acta Radiol* 36:228–232, 1995.

Scully RE, et al: Weekly clinicopathological exercises—Case 29. *N Engl J Med* 337(12):839–845, 1997.

Sutker AN, et al: Iliotibial band friction syndrome in distance runners. *Physiol Sports Med* 9:69–73, 1981.

Takebayashi S, et al: Sonographic findings in muscle strain

injury: Clinical and MR imaging correlation. *J Ultrasound Med* 14:899–905, 1995.

Vande Berg B, et al: Idiopathic muscular infarction in a diabetic patient. *Skeletal Radiol* 25:183–185, 1996.

Van Sonnenberg E, et al: Sonography of thigh abscess: Detection, diagnosis and drainage. *AJR* 149:769, 1987.

Vukanovic S, Hauser H, Curati WL: Myonecrosis induced by drug overdose: Pathogenesis, clinical aspects and radiological manifestations. *Eur J Radiol* 3:314–318, 1983.

Wagner P, et al: L'Echotomographie dans les accidents musculaires du sportif. *Ultrasons* 1:277–287, 1980.

Weissmann BN, Sledge CB: *Orthopedic Radiology.* Philadelphia, WB Saunders Co, 1986.

Weng L, et al: US extended-field-of-view imaging technology. *Radiology* 203:877–880, 1997.

Wong J, et al: Accuracy and precision of in vitro volumetric measurements by three-dimensional sonography. *Invest Radiol* 31(1):26–29, 1996.

Zochmodne DW, et al: Metabolic changes in human muscle denervation: Topical 31P NMR spectroscopy studies. *Magn Reson Med* 7:373–383, 1988.

Zuinen C, Carlier L, Gaudissart JL: L'echotomographie en traumatologie musculaire. *Med Sport* 54:379–382, 1980.

Zuinen C, et al: Echotomographie du muscle. *Med Sport* 56:396–404, 1982.

Chapter 4
Sonography of Tendons

In this chapter, we will discuss the examination of tendons, with and without synovial sheaths, using ultrasound. Prior to the application of ultrasound to the evaluation of the musculoskeletal system, clinicians relied on low-kilovoltage radiography and xeroradiography to aid in the diagnosis of tenomuscular injury (Bock et al., 1981). These techniques provided little information beyond indicating the site of soft tissue swelling. Ultrasound now provides detailed information about the involved anatomy and the nature of the pathology.

MRI and ultrasound are competing modalities in the diagnosis of tendon pathology. Ultrasound has a significant advantage over MRI. Tissues with few mobile protons emit little or no signal and, therefore, the internal architecture of the tendon is not well demonstrated. In contrast, ultrasound shows the fine internal structure of tendons (Fig. 4–1). The ultrasonographer can make use of the dynamic real-time character of sonography, so that tendons will be studied throughout their range of motion. Side-to-side comparison is always available during the ultrasound study. MRI requires complex surface coils to attain maximal spatial resolution. It is much easier to change to a higher-frequency ultrasound transducer to obtain greater spatial resolution. In fact, the spatial resolution of ultrasound is much better than that of MRI if both studies are performed with the most modern equipment (Erikson, 1997).

A synovial sheath is a tubular sac wrapped around the tendon (Warwick and Williams, 1980). The inner layer is tightly applied to the tendon and has a smooth inner surface juxtaposed with the outer layer. A minute amount of viscous mucoid fluid separates the two layers. Synovial sheaths are found in areas of stress in the hand, wrist, and ankle. These sheaths facilitate the examination of individual tendons sonographically. In the shoulder, the long biceps tendon is an example of a tendon with a synovial sheath that plays an important role in shoulder disease. Tendons without a synovial sheath are slightly more difficult to examine using ultrasound. They are enveloped by loose areolar connective tissue called the *paratenon* (Fornage et al., 1984; Fornage, 1986). It is possible to examine long tendons, especially if they are surrounded by fat. The Achilles, patellar, proximal gastrocnemius, and semimembranosus tendons are a few examples. All tendinous insertions, including those hidden by bony structures and short tendons, may be examined by the experienced musculoskeletal ultrasonographer. In these cases, side-to-side comparison is essential.

Examination Technique

Equipment

The evolution of musculoskeletal ultrasound was delayed, in part, by limitations imposed by equipment. Examination of tendons requires relatively high spatial and contrast resolution. This is achieved through the use of high-frequency transducers (7.5–20 MHz). Axial resolution increases with transducer frequency. However, a trade-off between resolution and depth of field exists (Box 4–1). Penetration of sound through soft tissues decreases as frequency increases. The depth of field may be limited to only 3 to 4 cm using a 12-MHz transducer. Selection of an appropriate frequency transducer is dependent on the region to be examined and the body habitus of the patient. When superficial tendons are examined, a standoff pad or a bag of IV fluid can be used to position the tendon of in-

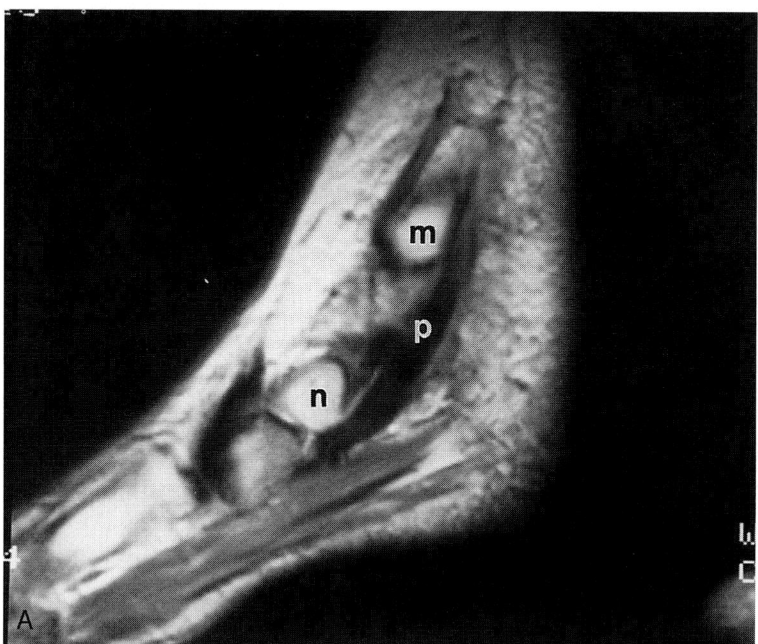

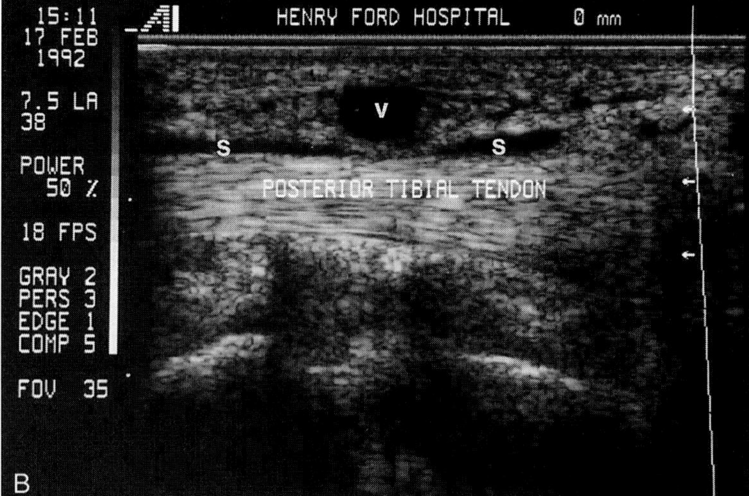

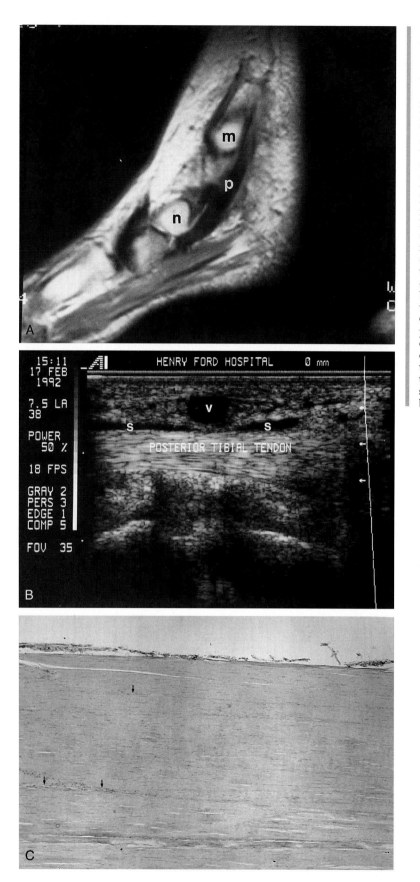

Figure 4–1 ■ **A,** Posterior tibial tendon tenosynovitis: sagittal proton density MRI. MRI fails to demonstrate the internal architecture of tendons. On this proton density image, the posterior tibial tendon (*p*) appears as a homogeneous low-signal structure. Abbreviations: medial malleolus (*m*), navicular (*n*). **B,** Posterior tibial tendon tenosynovitis: longitudinal sonogram. Ultrasound demonstrates the exquisite detail of anatomical structures within an FOV, which is usually limited by the width of the linear array transducer. Extended FOV ultrasound imaging allows a broader overview of musculoskeletal anatomy. The internal architecture of tendons is clearly depicted, revealing echogenic linear striations. The fluid-filled synovial sheath (*s*) is identified over the entire length of the tendon. In this case, minimally increased fluid within the sheath is consistent with tenosynovitis, which correlated with the patient's posterior tibial tendon dysfunction. When the volume of fluid within the tendon sheath is sufficient to be seen as an anechoic collection, the diagnosis of tenosynovitis can be made. An internal control within this image is the anechoic blood within the adjacent vein (*v*). **C,** Normal tendon histology: longitudinal low-power view. The collagen within most tendons is oriented along the long axis of the tendon. Vascular spaces (*arrows*) within these tendons parallel the tendon fibers. The monotonous repetition of the tendon architecture contributes to its fibrillar sonographic image and its anisotropic behavior in both MRI and sonographic imaging.

Box 4–1
Tendon Ultrasound System Requirements

- Transducer frequency >7 MHz
- Linear array transducer
- Split-screen or extended FOV

terest in an optimal position within the transducer's field of view (Fornage et al., 1984).

Dynamic real-time imaging is needed to examine tendons throughout their physiological range of motion. Sector scanners have the disadvantages of a narrow near FOV, near-field unsharpness, and obliquity of the sound beam when tendons are examined in their longitudinal axis. Linear array transducers provide optimal images, having their sound beam perpendicular to the tendon throughout the imaging field. In our experience, state-of-the-art ultrasound machines with high-frequency linear array transducers (7.5, 10, and 12 MHz) provide the best combination of FOV, resolution, and depth of field with electronic focusing of the sound beam. Using the transducer with the highest frequency that will penetrate to the desired depth eliminates the need to change to a higher-frequency transducer in the middle of an examination, thus reducing the examination time.

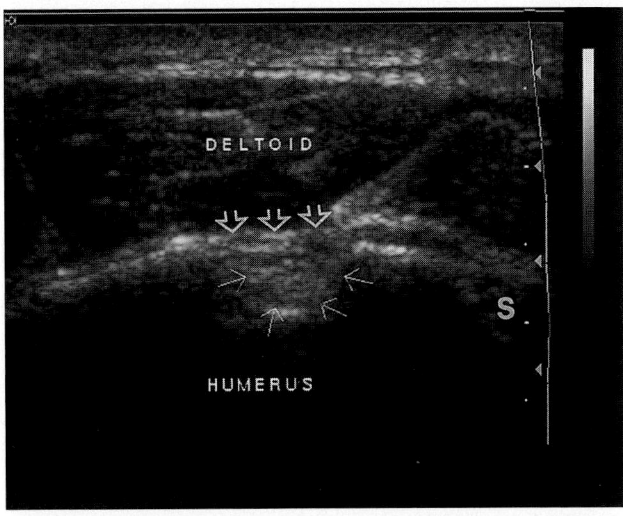

Figure 4–2 ▪ Normal biceps tendon: transverse sonogram. Examination of an asymptomatic young man. This image was obtained with the right shoulder in the neutral position. The medial aspect is at the observer's right. The bicipital groove (*arrows*) is identified at the anterior aspect of the humeral head. The transducer is positioned perpendicular to the long axis of the humerus over the proximal metaphysis. The long biceps tendon is located in the middle of the bicipital sulcus and has a hyperechoic appearance. A small sonolucent area separates the tendon from the transverse ligament (*open arrows*). This represents a normal amount of fluid in the synovial sheath. Abbreviation: subscapularis muscle (*S*).

Scanning Technique

The location of the tendon is established relative to easily recognized bony landmarks (Fig. 4–2). In the majority of cases, scanning is started in the longitudinal axis of the tendon. Longitudinal images allow the examiner to distinguish separate tendons more clearly. Exceptions to this procedure concern the proximal insertion of the long biceps tendon in (Fig. 4–2) both the upper and lower extremities and the proximal posterior tibial tendon. These tendons are difficult to detect when scanning in the longitudinal axis. In these cases, transverse imaging is primarily used and careful side-to-side comparison is made throughout the study. Simple tricks like imaging the bone surface deep to the long biceps and posterior tibial tendons, parallel to the face of the transducer, will provide optimal visualization of these tendons. Applying pressure to the distal end of the transducer for better visualization of the long biceps tendon in the shoulder will significantly improve visualization of pathology during longitudinal scanning due to reduced anisotropic artifact.

Sonographic Tendon Anatomy

Tendons are composed largely of parallel running fascicles of collagen fibers that interweave and interconnect (Warwick and Williams, 1980; Dillehay et al., 1984). These fascicles are large enough to be visible to the naked eye as well as sonographically (Fornage et al., 1984; Fornage, 1986; Martinoli et al., 1993). It is still not clear whether the ultrasound reflection occurs at interfaces between fascicles of collagen, between subfascicles, or at interconnections of interfascicular ground substance (Martinoli et al., 1993; Miles et al., 1996). The number of linear reflecting lines within tendons, such as the Achilles tendon, increase with the frequency of the transducer. This fibrillar pattern, which is not visible on MRI, is distorted in torn tendons examined by ultrasound. Very subtle changes in the architecture can be seen in intrasubstance tendon degeneration and partial-thickness tears. Reflectivity, attenuation, and backscatter of the ultrasound signal are highly anisotropic characteristics in tendons. These parameters depend on the orientation of the ultrasound beam relative to the tendon structure (Miles et al., 1996). The chemical composition of tendons, i.e.,

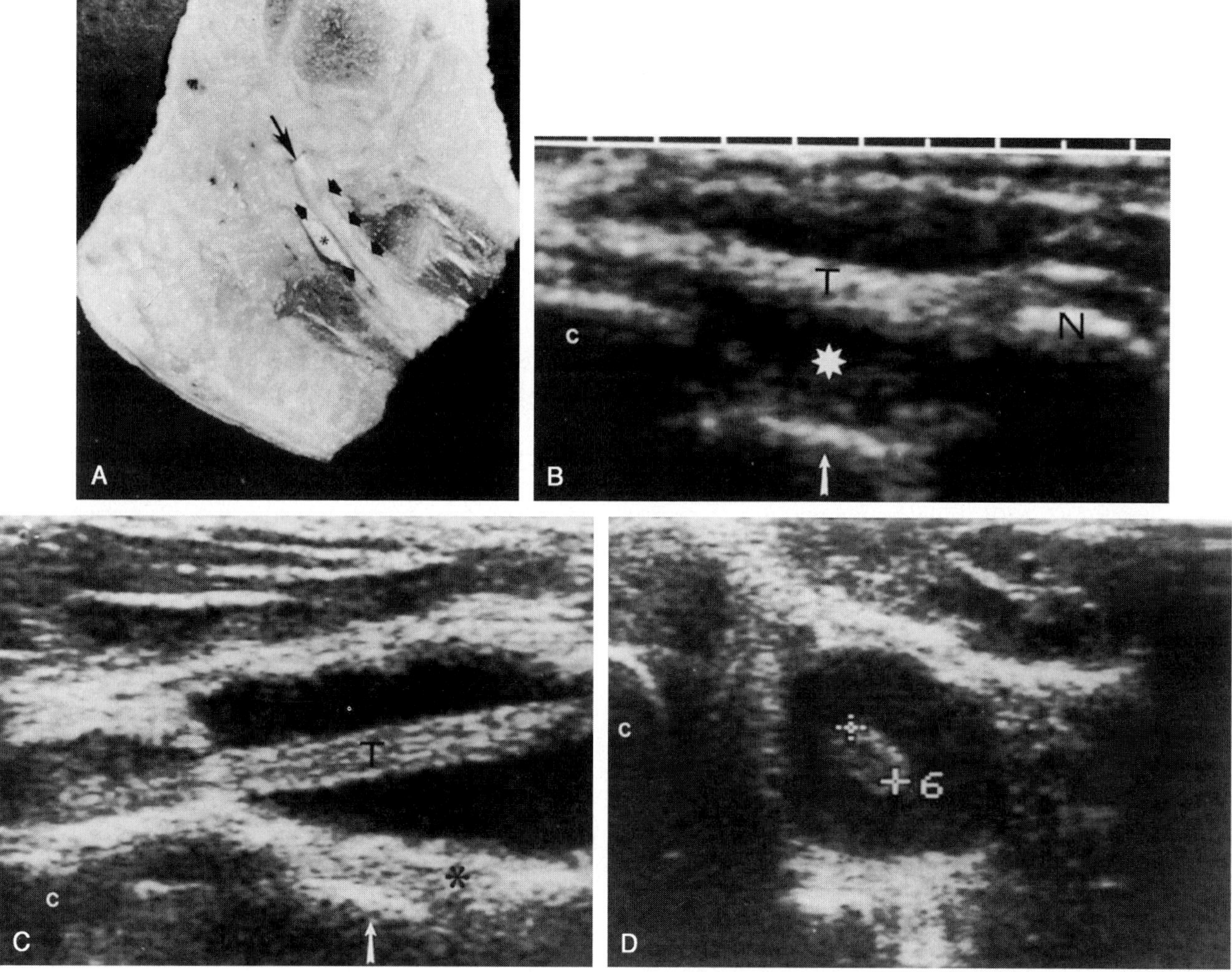

Figure 4–3 ■ **A**, Anatomical section through the medial aspect of the ankle that bisects the tibialis posterior tendon sagittally. The tibialis posterior tendon (*arrow*) has a separate tendon sheath. A normal tendon sheath has a very small quantity of synovial fluid. This is seen as a membrane wrapped around the tendon (*small arrows*). A small part of the flexor digitorum longus tendon is seen posterior to the tibialis posterior tendon (*asterisk*). **B**, Normal tibialis posterior tendon: longitudinal sonogram. The position of the transducer is at the medial plantar surface of the foot, overlying the talonavicular region. It is oriented along the long axis of the foot, with the distal portion of the foot at the observer's right. The tibialis posterior tendon (*T*) is adjacent to the sustentaculum tali (*white arrow*) and inserts on the navicular bone (*N*). Normal fat surrounding the tendon appears hypoechoic (*asterisk*). Abbreviation: calcaneus (*c*). **C**, Longitudinal sonogram through an inflamed tendon sheath of the tibialis posterior tendon. The patient is a soccer player with pain and swelling over the medial aspect of the foot. Pain was localized to the region overlying the tibialis posterior tendon, with maximal tenderness on palpation focused over the sustentaculum tali (*white arrow*). The transducer position and orientation are identical to those in **B**. The tibialis posterior tendon is surrounded by a large amount of fluid in the tendon sheath. Individual fibers are visualized more clearly due to this pathological fluid collection. The surrounding fat is now hyperreflective (*asterisk*). Abbreviation: calcaneus (*c*). **D**, Transverse image through the inflamed tibialis posterior tendon. Same patient as in **C**. The transducer is rotated 90 degrees and is now perpendicular to the long axis of the foot. The thickness of the tendon sheath exceeds the diameter of the tendon itself (greater than 6 mm). Abbreviation: calcaneus (*c*).

the proportion of water, collagen, glycosaminoglycans, and DNA does not influence tendon echogenicity to any significant degree. This was shown in an in vitro study of normal animal tendons (Miles et al., 1996). This may explain why ultrasound is more sensitive in detecting structural changes than chemical changes in tendons. It may also explain why ultrasound has fewer problems than MRI in differentiating tendinosis from partial-thickness tears.

During postnatal growth, tendons increase in length interstitially (Warwick and Williams, 1980). At the musculotendinous junction, growth is especially rapid due to the increased cellularity in this region, which allows for rapid elaboration and maturation of collagen. Tendon growth is slowest at the attachment of the tendon to bone. Vascular networks within the tendon are sparse. Therefore, minimal bleeding is seen sonographically after tendon rupture (Zuinen et al., 1983).

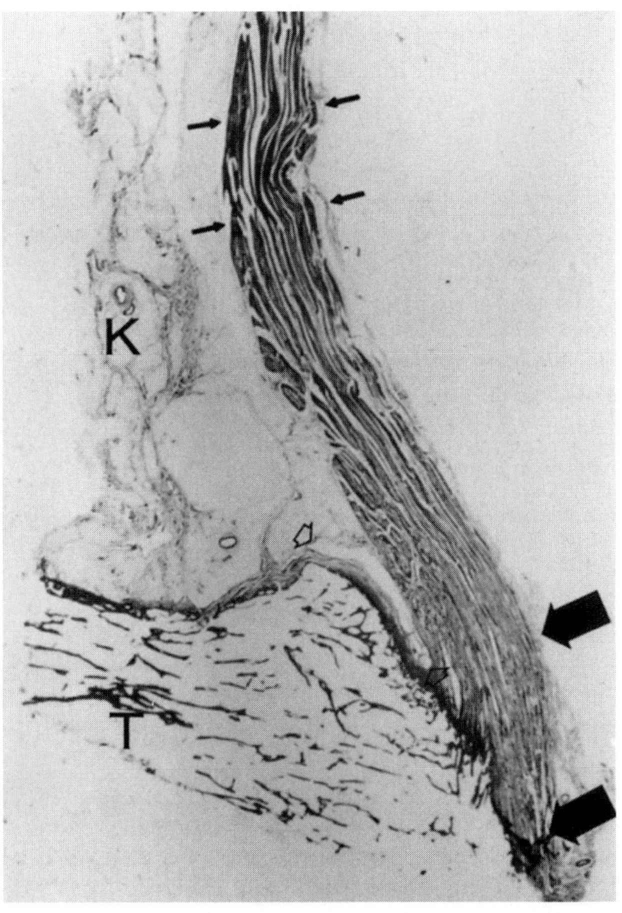

Figure 4–4 ■ Photomicrograph of an anatomical specimen of the Achilles tendon insertion: sagittal section. In the distal 1 cm of the tendon (*area between the black arrows*) the fibers are more densely arranged, and cartilage cells are found at higher magnification. Between the tendon and the superoposterior angle of the calcaneus, a small boomerang-shaped bursa is present (*open arrows*). The wall of the bursa is microscopically thin, but the lumen is relatively large. In vivo the bursa is filled with a small amount of serous fluid. Around the tendon there is a paper-thin rim of connective tissue known as the *peritenon* (*small arrows*). The dorsal aspect of the peritenon is thicker than the ventral aspect. Achilles tendon fat pad, Kager's fat pad (*K*), trabecular bone of the calcaneus (*T*). (Courtesy of Dr. E. Verbeken, K.U. Leuven, Belgium)

Surrounding the tendon is either a synovial sheath or a dense connective tissue layer called the *epitendineum.* The synovial sheath, as previously described, contains a capillary film of fluid that serves as a lubricant. This fluid is seen as a dark halo surrounding the tendon on ultrasound images (Fig. 4–3). The thickness of the sheath usually does not exceed a couple of millimeters. However, in acute tendon disease it may exceed the thickness of the tendon that it surrounds (see Fig. 4–3D).

In tendons without a synovial sheath (Fig. 4–4), the epitendineum, a dense connective tissue layer, is tightly bound to the tendon. Connective tissue fibers permeate the fascicles, making the epitendineum adherent to the tendon. Blood vessels and nerves enter the tendon along these fibers. Loose areolar connective tissue, the paratenon, envelops the epitendineum. Sonographically, the epitendineum is seen as a reflective line surrounding the tendon (Fornage, 1986).

The cross-sectional profile of a tendon is round (long biceps tendon; see Fig. 4–2), oval (Achilles tendon), or rectangular (patellar tendon). This cross-sectional profile can change after athletic conditioning. A round Achilles tendon is found in nonconditioned subjects, and a more ovoid Achilles tendon is found in athletes.

A narrow band of fibrocartilage joins the tendon to bone (Cooper and Misol, 1970; Niepel and Sit, 1979). This is referred to as the *tendon insertion.* The tendon insertion is an avascular structure. For example, the insertion of the Achilles tendon is approximately 1 cm long. The sonographic appearance is a relatively well-defined hypoechoic zone in the distal portion of the tendon (Fig. 4–5). It has a triangular shape when scanned longitudinally. The hypoechoic character of this fibrocartilaginous insertion is similar to the sonographic appearance of cartilage elsewhere in the body (Aisen et al., 1984). It is uncertain whether the hypoechogenicity of the tendon enthesis is related to the cartilage in its substance or to the anisotropic characteristics of the curved fibers of the tendinous attachment. Thickening of the tendon insertion is seen in traumatic disease (Merkel et al., 1982).

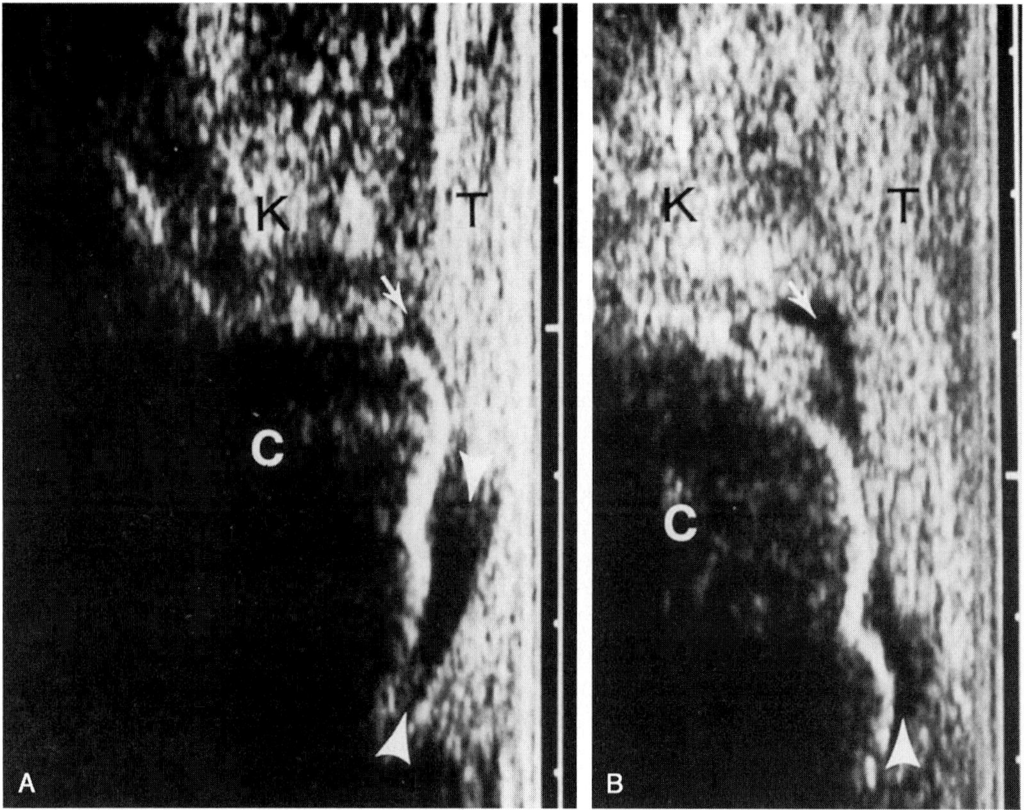

Figure 4–5 ■ **A**, Achilles tendon insertion. Longitudinal sonogram of the specimen in Figure 4–4 prior to sectioning with an identical orientation. The sonographic architecture of the Achilles tendon (*T*) changes in the distal portion at its insertion (*white arrow*). The insertion (*arrowheads*) is markedly hypoechoic, nearly anechoic. This region is approximately 1 cm long and consists of densely packed connective tissue with a structure similar to that of fibrocartilage (see Fig. 4–4). This hypoechoic appearance is similar to that seen in cartilage elsewhere in the body. A normal retrocalcaneal bursa is seen as a hypoechoic, boomerang-shaped cleft approximately 5 mm in the craniocaudal dimension (*small white arrow*). Abbreviations: Kager's fat pad (*K*), calcaneus (*C*). **B,** Retrocalcaneal bursitis: longitudinal sonogram. The orientation is identical to that in **A**. This is a patient with pain in the heel after a direct blow to the posterior surface of the Achilles tendon. There is tenderness localized over the area immediately proximal to the tendon insertion. The retrocalcaneal bursa (*arrow*) is enlarged. Bursitis, with production of nonviscous fluid, in an athlete is called *frictional bursitis*. The tendon insertion (*arrowhead*) is considerably shorter than the insertion seen in **A**. Variability in the length of the tendon insertion is great, but there is a strong correlation with the patient's height. Abbreviations: Kager's fat pad (*K*), Achilles tendon (T), calcaneus (C).

Sonographic Diagnosis of Tendon Pathology

Tendons with a Synovial Sheath

Tendinitis

Acute tendinitis or tenosynovitis is detected by increased fluid within the synovial sheath. The increased fluid within the sheath is seen as an anechoic halo around the tendon on transverse images (Figs. 4–3D, 4–6, and 4–7). This differs from the normal synovial sheath, in which the capillary fluid film appears as a hypoechoic halo (Fig. 4–8). On longitudinal views, the tendon is bounded on both sides by anechoic lines. Often the width of this fluid collection exceeds the diameter of the tendon that it surrounds. Fluid within a tendon sheath is not always anechoic. Debris may be present within the fluid. This debris may be composed of cellular elements or metabolic by-products. Substances causing increased echogenicity of synovial fluid include aggregates of white cells, fibrin (Fig. 4–9), cholesterol, clusters of uric acid, and calcium pyrophosphate or hydroxyapathite crystals. Differentiation between fluid, which can be aspirated, and inflamed synovium may not always be straightforward (see Fig. 4–8). When in doubt, one should use percussion of the tendon sheath under ultrasound observation. Fluid containing debris will exhibit swirling movement of debris within the liquid. Clearly, fluctuation and swirling are not observed in cases of synovial edema or chronic inflammation.

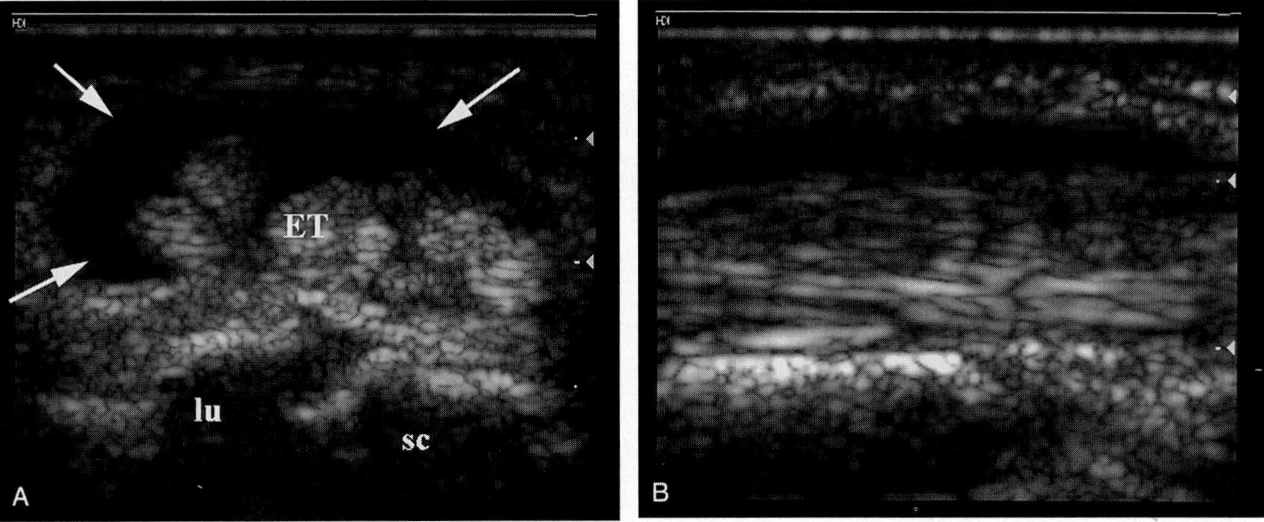

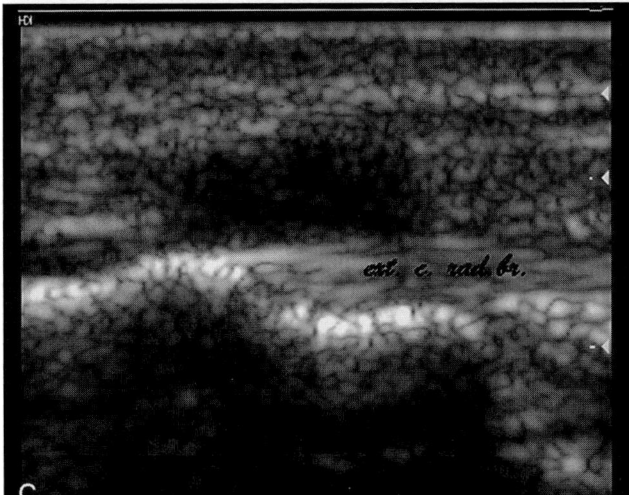

Figure 4–6 ■ **A**, Extensor tendons of the wrist: transverse sonogram. A 46-year-old male auto assembly line worker presented with repetitive stress syndrome involving the left wrist. The common extensor tendon sheath is markedly distended with anechoic fluid (*arrows*), consistent with tenosynovitis. Normally, the fluid film within the tendon sheath is 1–2 mm thick. Abbreviations: extensor tendons (*ET*), dorsal aspect of the lunate (*lu*), dorsal aspect of the scaphoid (*sc*). **B**, Extensor tendons of the wrist: longitudinal sonogram. Same patient as in **A**. With the 12-MHz transducer along the long axis of the tendon, the fibrillar pattern shows clearly. Fluid layers out as a hypoechoic sheet over the dorsal aspect of the tendon. This layer of fluid is characteristic of tenosynovitis. **C**, Ganglion over finger extensor: longitudinal sonogram. Different patient from the one in **A** and **B**. An oval-shaped ganglion is noted over the extensor carpi radialis brevis insertion. A ganglion is more focal than that seen in tenosynovitis; the fluid accumulates in the shape of a mass. The communication with the synovium is typically narrow. Characteristically, the radiologist drew thick, gelatinous fluid from this mass.

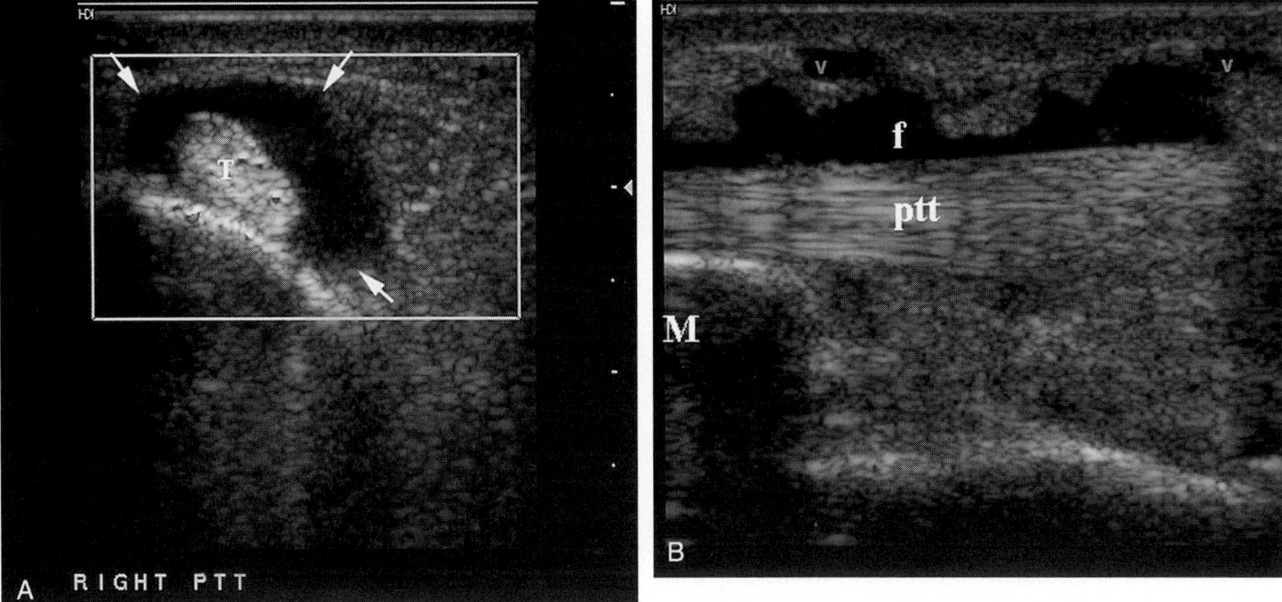

Figure 4–7 ■ **A**, Posterior tibial tendon tenosynovitis: transverse sonogram. This image of the posterior tibial tendon (*T*) at the level of the medial malleolus shows increased fluid within the tendon sheath (*arrows*), approximately four times normal. The box surrounding the tendon indicates that the region was examined using power Doppler. In acute tenosynovitis there is no hypervascularity of the synovium, as seen here. This is in contrast to chronic tenosynovitis, which may demonstrate marked hypervascularity of the synovium. **B,** Posterior tibial tendon tenosynovitis: longitudinal sonogram. Same patient as in **A**. Often, a tendon sheath distended with fluid (*f*) will have an undulating outer contour, as seen here. Abbreviations: medial malleolus (*M*), posterior tibial tendon (*ptt*), veins (*v*).

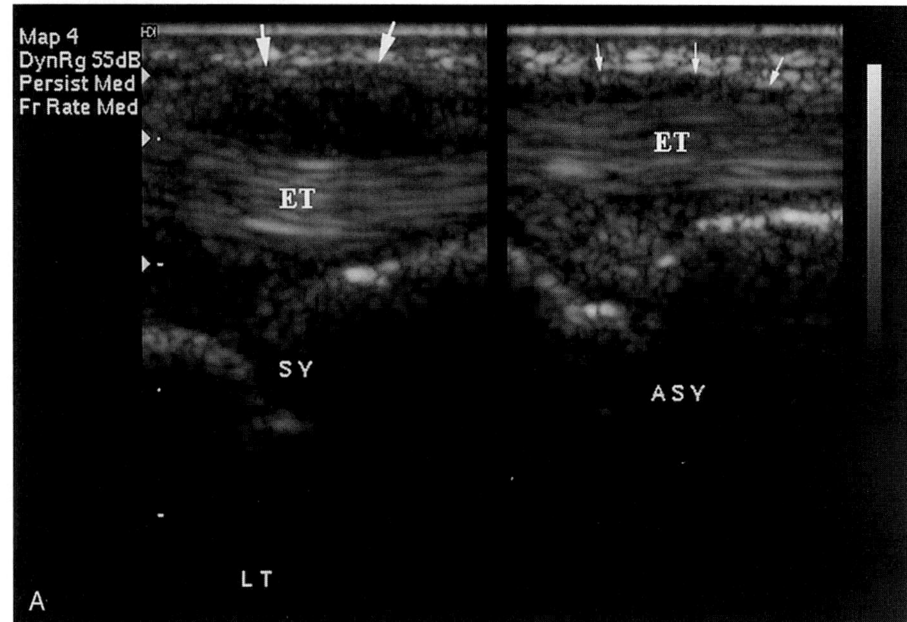

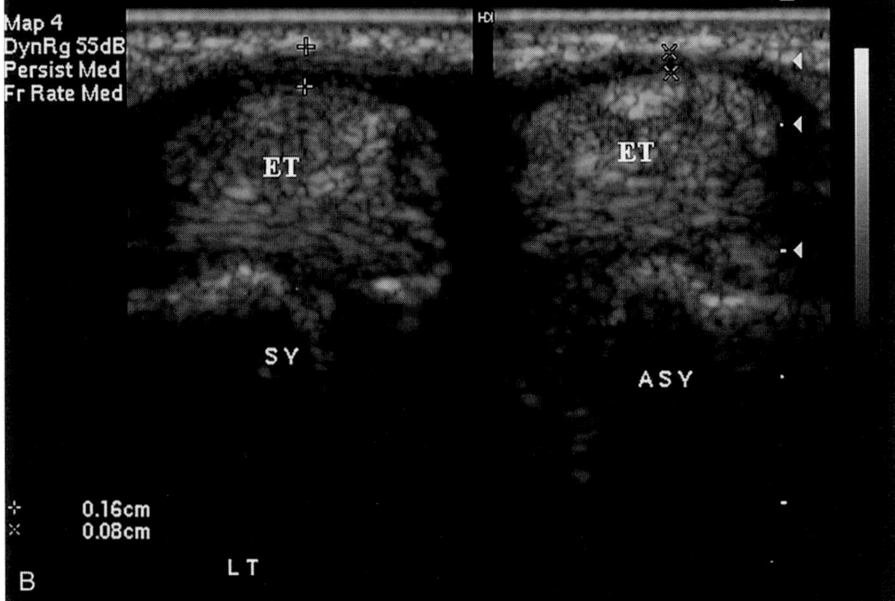

Figure 4-8 ■ **A,** Chronic tenosynovitis: longitudinal sonogram. In this split-screen comparison image, a normal extensor tendon (*ET*) of the wrist is seen on the right. Note the appearance of the normal tendon sheath (*small arrows*). On the left (*LT*), the tendon sheath is markedly distended by hypoechoic material with definite internal echoes (*large arrows*). This appearance is characteristic of chronic tenosynovitis. **B,** Chronic tenosynovitis: transverse sonogram. Same patient as in **A**. Side-by-side comparison of the extensor tendons in this split-screen transverse image confirms thickening of the synovial sheath on the left. It is twice the normal thickness observed on the right. Abbreviations: symptomatic wrist (*SY*); asymptomatic wrist (*ASY*).

Synovium is often thick and hypoechoic but not hyperemic, as in pannus. Increased cellularity within the synovium and fibrosis in the subsynovium might be the cause of this type of chronic hypoechoic swelling.

In subacute cases of tendinitis, tendon thickening can be observed. We have seen this most commonly in the long biceps tendon of swimmers with a shallow bicipital groove (Fig. 4-10). In these patients, tendon dislocation may be seen (see Fig. 4-10C). De Quervain's tendinitis is a common form of subacute tendinitis and synovitis in the wrist (Fig. 4-11). Passive stretching of the involved tendons with the wrist in maximal ulnar deviation (Finkelstein test) will result in intense pain over the radial styloid. This test is sensitive but not specific for tendinitis. Ultrasound confirms swelling of the abductor pollicis longus and extensor pollicis brevis tendons. Intrasubstance changes and synovitis will be striking when the affected side is compared with the asymptomatic side. Ultrasound can aid in the intrasynovial injection of steroids, which is the initial treatment of this disease. It has been shown that treatment fails if the extensor pollicis brevis is located in a separate anatomical compartment and injection fails to distend that compartment (Zingas et al., 1998). Therefore, ultrasound can increase the success of treatment by appropriately targeting the therapeutic injection.

Chronic tendinitis is often difficult to diagnose sonographically. Frequently there is no increase in synovial fluid. The most common finding is thickening of the tendon itself (Middleton et al., 1985b, 1986a). Comparison with the asymptomatic side is essential to make the diagnosis of chronic tendinitis (Bruce et al., 1982; Crass et al., 1984, 1986; Demarais et al., 1984; Dillehay et al., 1984; Blei et al., 1986; Fornage, 1986).

The differential diagnosis in cases with these findings includes rheumatoid disease. However, this can usually be distinguished from other disease processes by irregular thickening of the synovial lining (Fig. 4–12). This will result in echos within the abnormally increased synovial fluid collection (see Fig. 11–20). Inflammatory synovium is very rich in lymphatic vessels and capillaries. Power Doppler sonography shows hyperemia more accurately than does color Doppler ultrasound (Fig. 4–12). The color blush in conventional color Doppler overestimates the flow in the synovium. Power Doppler depicts vessels with a closer approximation of their actual size.

Tendon Rupture

The biceps tendon is a common site in which tendon rupture can be observed. Predisposing lesions are rotator cuff tendinitis and inflammation of the long biceps tendon (Middleton et al., 1986b). These

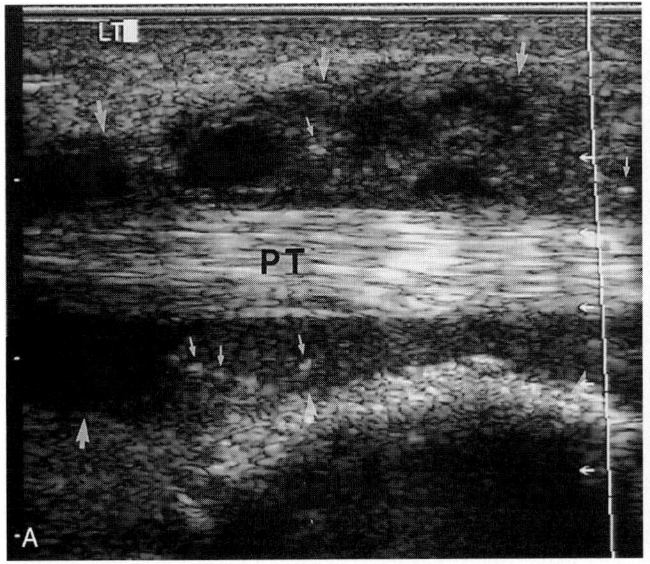

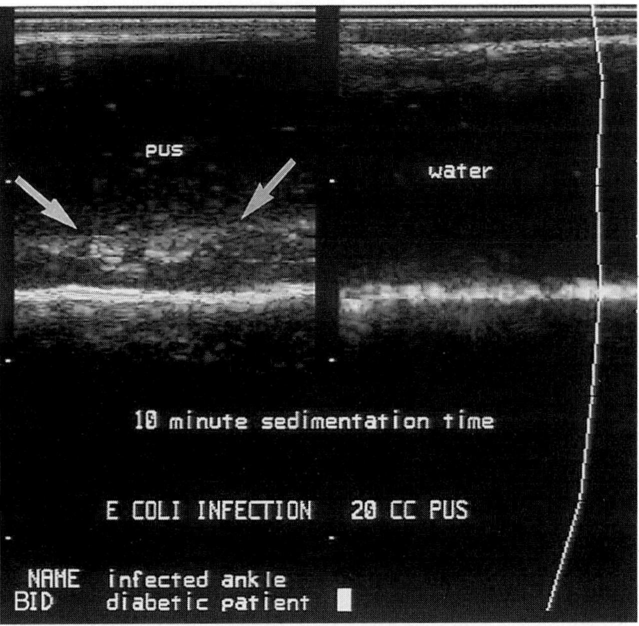

Figure 4–9 ■ **A,** Septic posterior tibial tendon tenosynovitis: longitudinal sonogram. Sudden swelling of the ankle in a 55-year-old diabetic patient prompts an ankle ultrasound study. Fluid is shown in the ankle joint and around the PTT (*PT*). The distention (*arrows*) of the PTT sheath appears inhomogeneous and compartmentalized. The tendon sheath's content presents as a mixture of anechoic, hypoechoic, and hyperechoic material. The hyperechogenicity shows as small dots (*small arrows*) in the fluid; this appearance has been found to be quite characteristic of sepsis. The dotted appearance of synovial fluid is a fairly specific but not especially sensitive feature of infection. **B,** Septic posterior tibial tendon tenosynovitis: split-screen comparison of aspirated fluid. The syringe with aspirated fluid from the tendon sheath illustrated in **A** was examined 10 minutes after aspiration. The fluid in the syringe was left in the horizontal position to allow sedimentation. A 7.5-MHz transducer was placed over the plastic syringe, and the picture on the left side of the split screen shows the content of the tendon sheath aspirate. The fluid on the right side of the split screen represents tap water in a comparison syringe, which had been resting in an identical position and for the same length of time. Hyperechoic material shows as sediment (*arrows*) in the syringe with pus. Microscopically, it consists of cellular debris and fibrinous elements. The control tube shows no sedimentation. This patient proved to have an *Escherichia coli* septic tenosynovitis. Surgery was necessary to debride the tendon sheath and the adjacent tibiotalar and subtalar joints. The patient did well until he needed a below-knee amputation for osteomyelitis caused by a subsequent staphylococcus-induced infection of the foot.

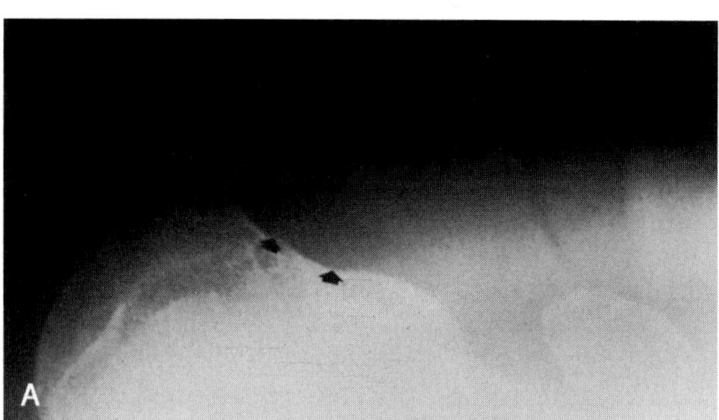

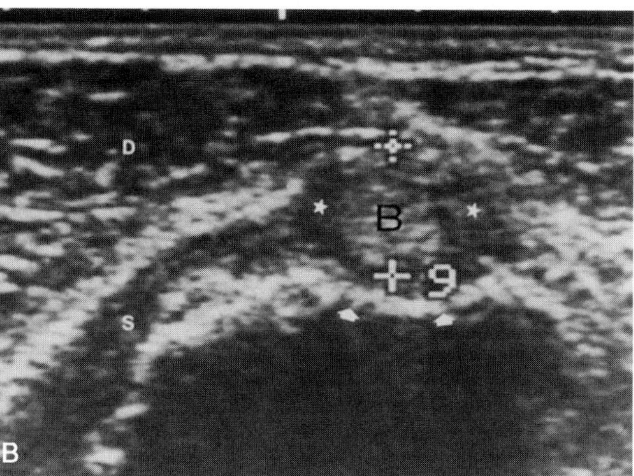

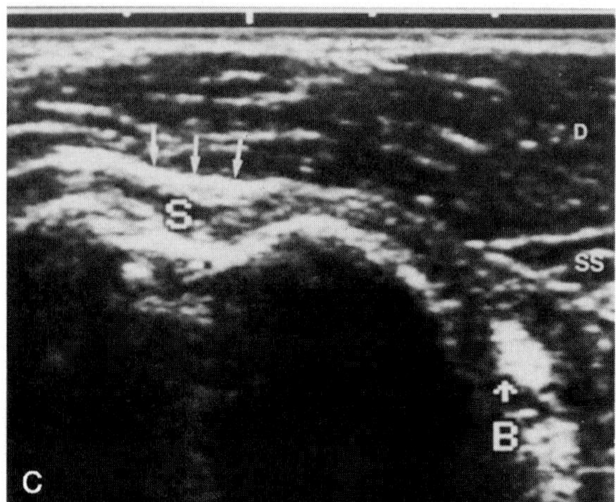

Figure 4-10 ■ **A**, Investigation of a shallow bicipital groove. Conventional radiograph of the bicipital groove. A shallow bicipital groove (*arrows*) is a normal variant seen in about 8% of the population. The most frequent sequela is tendinosis involving the long biceps tendon. **B**, Ultrasound scan of the bicipital groove. The transducer is positioned perpendicular to the long axis of the humerus over the anterior aspect of the humeral epiphysis. The arm is in neutral position. The diameter of the tendon is significantly increased, measuring 9 mm instead of the normal 2 to 4 mm. Fluid within the synovial sheath is also increased (*asterisk*). Compare this image with Figure 4-2. Abbreviations: deltoid muscle (*D*), subscapularis muscle (*S*), long biceps tendon (*B*). Bicipital groove (*small white arrows*). **C**, Ultrasound/scan of the bicipital groove: biceps tendon dislocation. The patient is a swimmer with right anterior shoulder pain. An infrequent finding in athletes with a shallow bicipital groove is dislocation of the long biceps tendon. The transducer's position is identical to that in **B**, the bicipital groove or sulcus (*S*) is empty. The transverse ligament settles within the groove (*arrows*), and the long biceps tendon is seen medially beneath the subscapularis muscle (*ss*). Abbreviation: deltoid muscle (*D*).

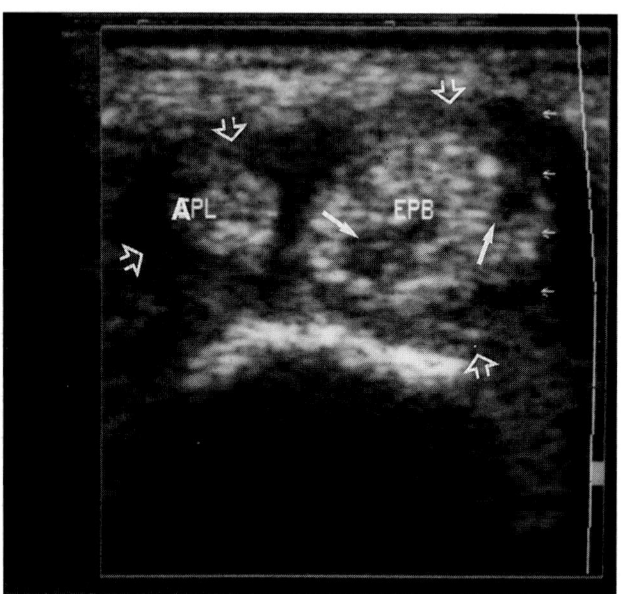

Figure 4-11 ■ De Quervain's tendinitis: transverse sonogram over the first extensor compartment. This wheelchair-bound patient with a history of poliomyelitis develops weakness and swelling in his right wrist. The abductor pollicis longus (*APL*), the extensor pollicis brevis (*EPB*), and their tendon sheath (*open arrows*) appear swollen. The extensor pollicis brevis shows evidence of more advanced disease; the tendon is almost three times the size of the abductor pollicis longus, and distinct areas of hypoechoic tendon degeneration (*arrows*) are seen within its substance.

lesions are frequently found in athletes involved in baseball, tennis, squash, and field events (javelin throwing, discus, etc.). Clinicians usually refer to lesions involving tendons of the shoulder with edema as *shoulder impingement* (Jobe and Jobe, 1983). Patients who suffer from shoulder impingement usually develop tears of the long biceps tendon and rotator cuff many years later (Neer, 1983).

Sonographic findings in rupture of the biceps tendon are an empty bicipital groove and a fusiform muscle mass located distally (Fig. 4–13). It is important to recognize this pair of findings to avoid misinterpretation of the muscle mass as a soft tissue neoplasm (Chui, 1988). Loss of the fibrillar pattern (Fig. 4–13) of the biceps tendon in the bicipital groove is always a sign of tear. The actual tear may be difficult to see for a number of reasons. In some cases, torn long biceps tendons will reattach within the bicipital groove, and fibrous scar will replace the torn and retracted tendon. Scar tissue is similar to the mesenchymal tissue of tendons, and the two tissues may look alike sonographically. Often, a difference between scar and tendon can be detected. The lack of an organized fibrillar architecture and the

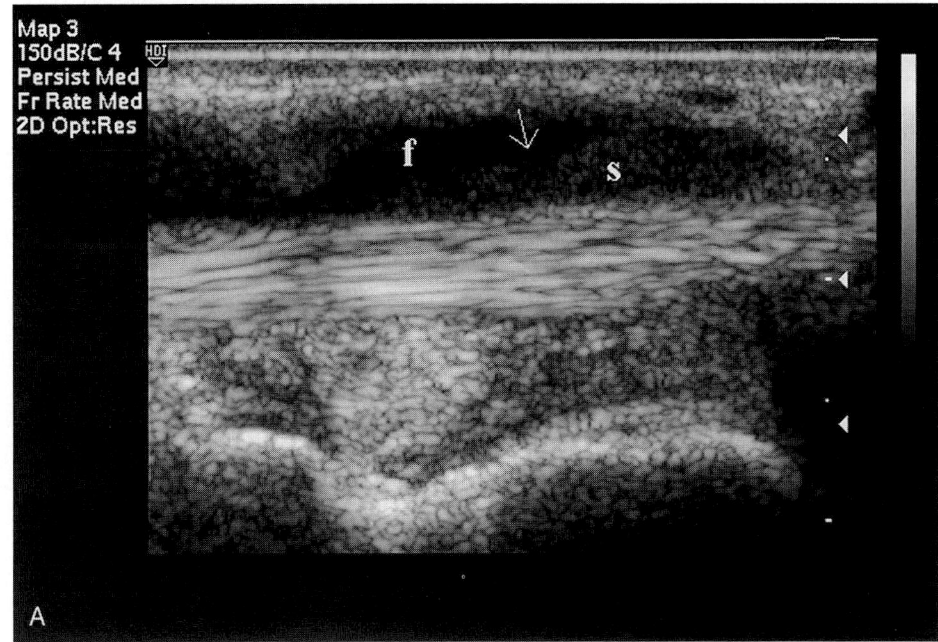

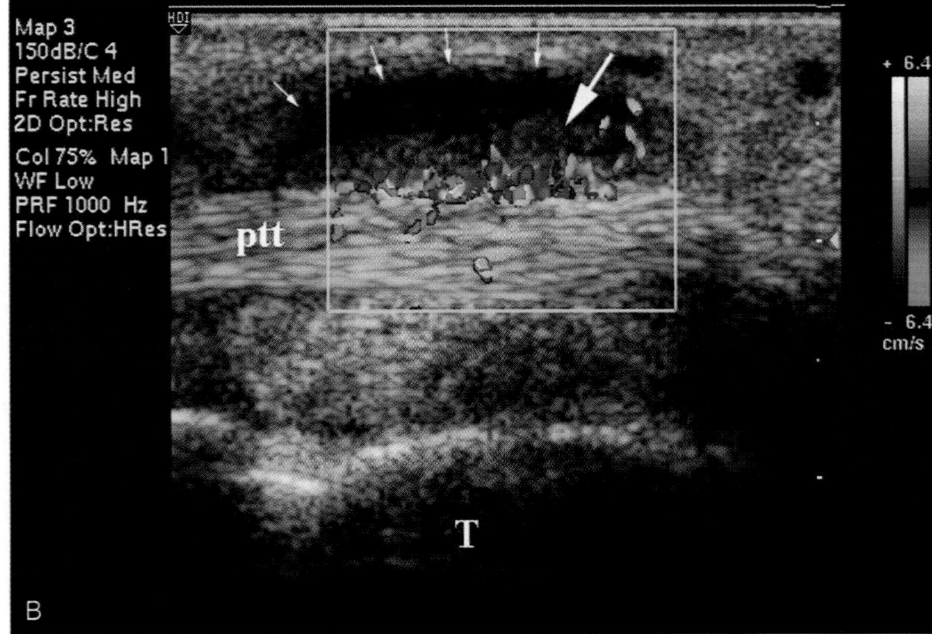

Figure 4–12 ■ **A,** Rheumatoid synovitis: longitudinal sonogram. This 50-year-old woman presented with acute flat foot deformity. Irregular synovial thickening (*s*) and increased fluid (*f*) are present within the sheath of the posterior tibial tendon. There is a clear demarcation (*arrow*) between the hypoechoic synovial thickening and the anechoic fluid. **B,** Rheumatoid synovitis: longitudinal sonogram with color Doppler. Same patient as in **A**. Note the marked hypervascularity of the synovial component (*arrow*). Synovial sheath distended with fluid (*small arrows*). Abbreviations: posterior tibial tendon (*ptt*), talus (*T*).

Figure continued on following page

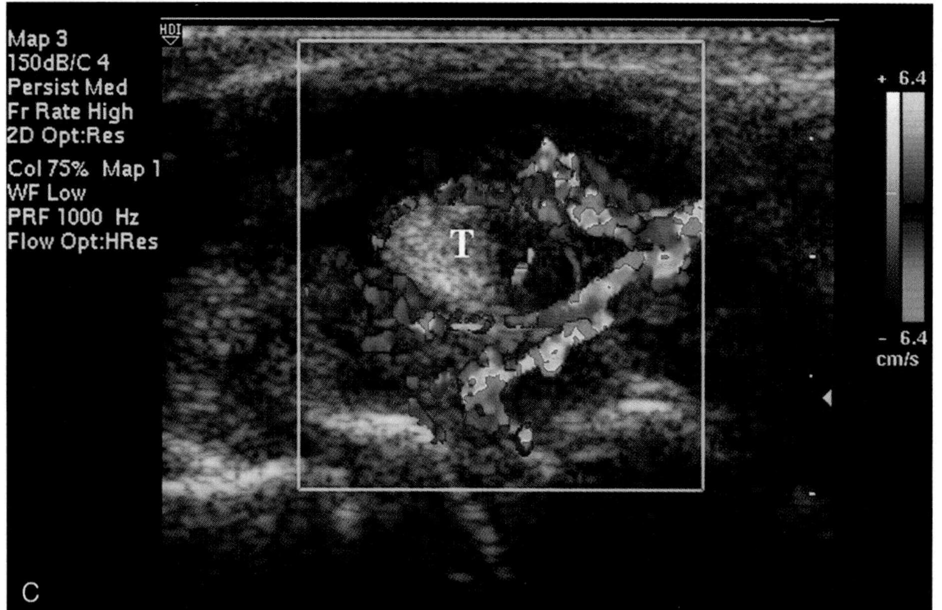

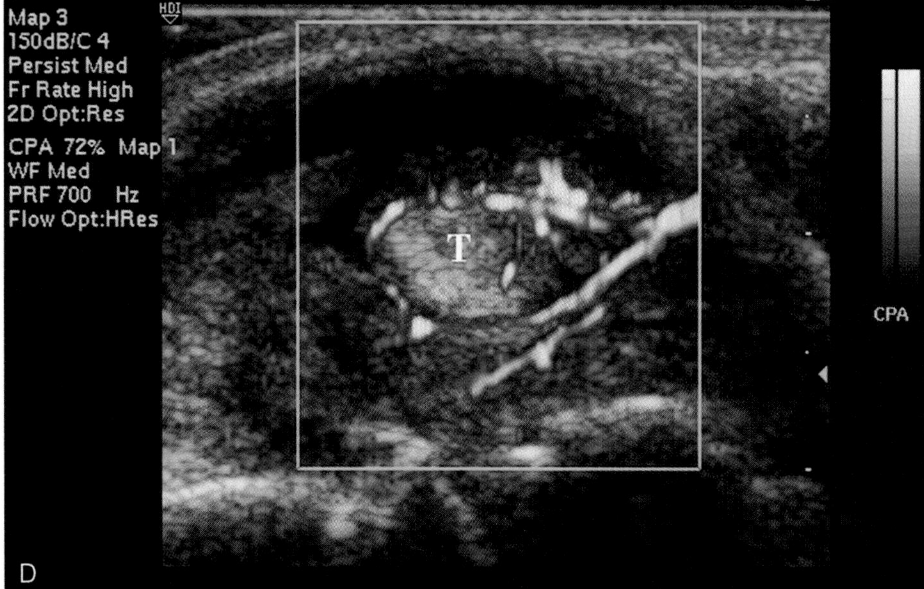

Figure 4-12 *Continued* ■ **C,** Rheumatoid synovitis: transverse sonogram with color Doppler. Same patient as in **A**. Hypervascularity is seen within the synovial component of the distended tendon sheath and along the surface of the tendon (*T*). **D,** Rheumatoid synovitis: longitudinal sonogram with power Doppler. Same patient as in **A**. A vascular pattern identical to that seen with color Doppler is observed with power Doppler. However, power Doppler more accurately represents the size of vessels. Abbreviation: posterior tibial tendon (*T*).

lack of anisotropic characteristics of scar will aid in differentiation. Scar does not have collagenous layers oriented in parallel bundles, as tendons do (Ptasznik and Hennessy, 1995). Proximal biceps tendon reattachment may not be associated with the typical clinical "Popeye" sign. In those cases, discontinuity in the fibrillar pattern will be diagnostic of a bicipital tear even in the absence of typical clinical signs of tear.

The posterior tibial tendon (PTT) in the ankle is also prone to injury and rupture (Fig. 4-14). Patients with this injury develop a painful flat foot, often a unilateral finding (Box 4-2). The foot will further deform with hindfoot valgus, midfoot abduction at the midtarsal joints, and forefoot pronation. However, this foot deformity is not pathognomonic, and degenerative arthritis, neuropathic arthropathy, traumatic collapse, and unilateral tarsal coalition can all mimic a torn PTT (Crenshaw, 1996). The definitive diagnosis of PTT rupture as the cause of the foot deformity must be established before treatment is initiated. An expensive diagnostic workup has

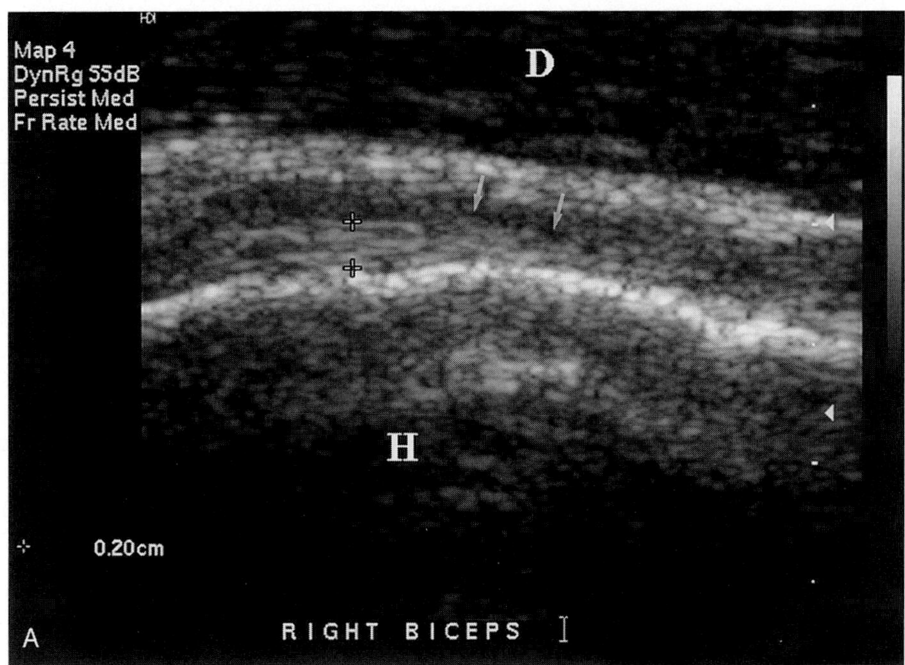

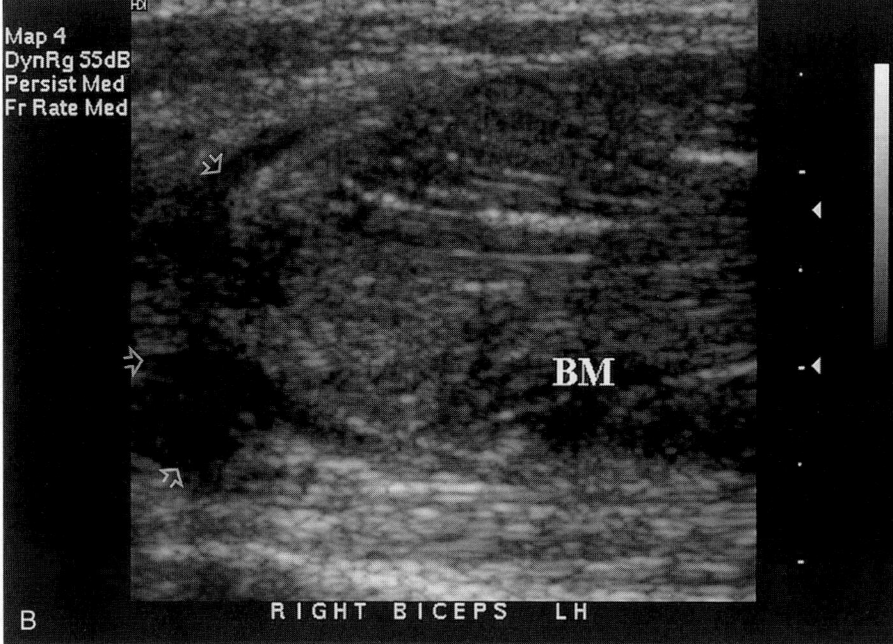

Figure 4–13 ■ **A**, Rupture of the long biceps tendon: longitudinal sonogram through the biceps tendon groove. While docking his boat, this 59-year-old man felt a sudden sharp pain in his right upper arm. A longitudinal sonogram of the biceps tendon groove demonstrates a linear cleft (*arrows*) in the hyperechoic structure of the long biceps tendon. The normal fibrillar pattern of the tendon is seen just proximal to the tear in the tendon portion marked with the calipers. Abbreviations: proximal humerus (*H*), deltoid muscle (*D*). **B**, Rupture of the long biceps tendon: longitudinal sonogram through the myotendinous junction. Same patient as in **A**. Tendon tears of the biceps humeri have a tendency to retract significantly. It is not always clear whether the proximal or distal tendon has torn. With the 12-MHz transducer aligned with the long axis of the biceps muscle (*BM*), one notices the proximal rounded end (*open arrows*) of the retracted muscle.

Box 4–2
Presentation of PTT Tear

- *Predisposition*: woman over 40, obese persons and those with rheumatoid arthritis
- *Symptoms*: painful flat foot, often a unilateral finding
- *Results in*: hindfoot valgus, midfoot abduction at midtarsal joints, forefoot pronation

been proposed (Crenshaw, 1996). A number of institutions use MRI for the diagnosis. Ultrasound has gained wide acceptance for the diagnosis of PTT pathology, however, due to both its cost effectiveness and its diagnostic accuracy (van Holsbeeck and Powell, 1995; Miller et al., 1996; Hsu et al., 1997). PTT rupture can occur in athletes, but this type of tendon rupture is seen predominantly in females over the age of 40 with a predisposition for rupture, i.e., obese individuals or patients with rheumatoid arthritis. Posttraumatic PTT rupture can occur and should be suspected if medial ankle pain persists after a pronation injury, in particular after medial malleolar fracture.

Ultrasound is a valuable asset in the differential diagnosis of PTT dysfunction. This functional deficit is characterized by limited plantar flexion and ankle inversion. Ultrasound can differentiate surgically correctable dysfunction due to tendon rupture from dysfunction that requires conservative treatment. Mechanical blockage of the tendon in its pulley system, attributable to tendon subluxation, intrasubstance tear, and tenosynovitis, is the etiology of dysfunction in the group often requiring conservative treatment (see Fig. 4–14B). The purpose of the treatment is to reduce swelling. The treatment consists of rest, nonsteroidal anti-inflammatory agents, and a short leg walking cast (Crenshaw, 1996). Occasionally, a steroid is injected into the tendon sheath proximal to the medial malleolus. Ultrasound can be used to select the proper patients for this therapy. The injection can be done under ultrasound guidance, which will avoid injecting a diseased tendon.

The sonographic diagnosis of acute rupture is simple. A gap is identified within the tendon in the early stages of rupture. A small fluid collection within the tendon sheath separates the retracted ends of the tendon (see Fig. 4–14A). The continuity of the synovial sheath of the PTT can be followed despite the full-thickness tendon tear. The sheath will often collapse when the tendon retracts. Longitudinal views show discontinuity of the fibrillar

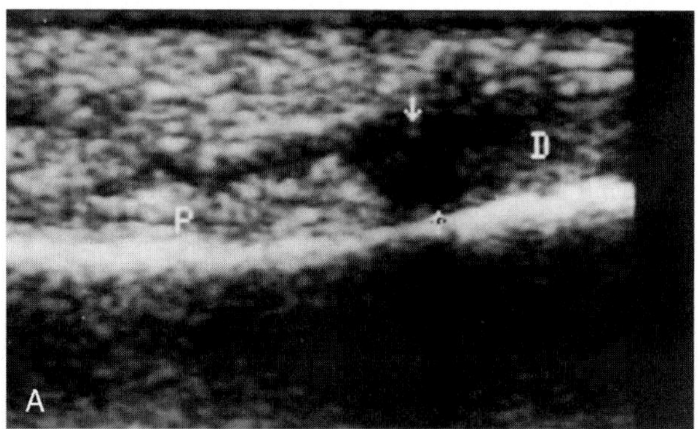

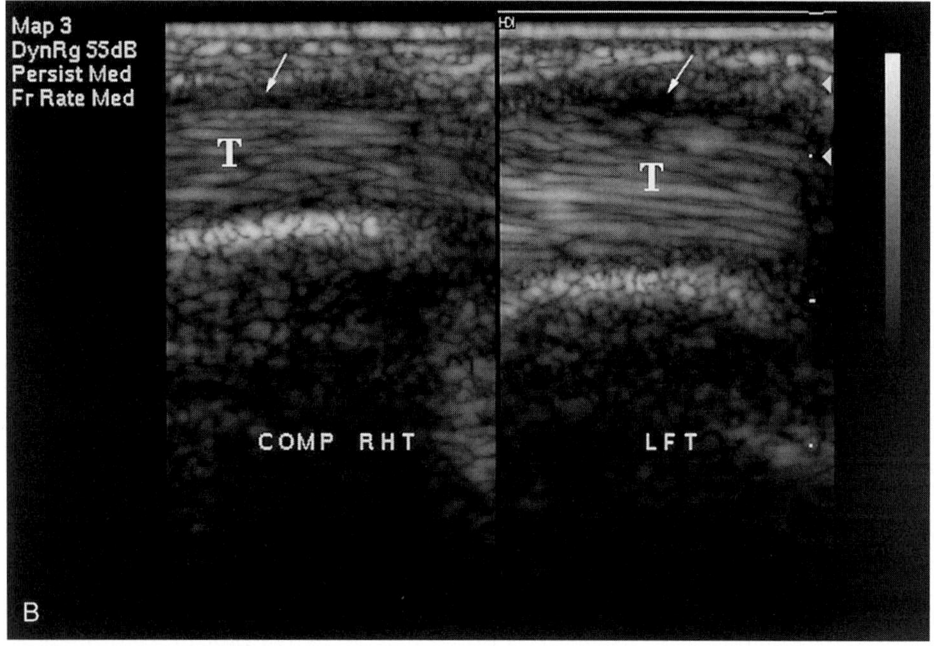

Figure 4–14 ■ **A**, Complete rupture of the PTT: longitudinal sonogram. The patient is a 75-year-old man who plays tennis once a week. Five months ago, he felt a snap pain in a lateral aspect of his foot during accidental ankle eversion. He presents today after having sought treatment from many clinicians for painful swelling of the ankle without relief. The patient is found to have significant weakness when inverting his ankle. This image was obtained along the length of the PTT immediately posterior and superior to the medial malleolus. A discontinuity (*arrows*) is noted in the tendon. Fluid fills the gap created by the retracted ends of the tendon and tracks along the synovial sheath. Abbreviations: proximal PTT (*P*), distal PTT (*D*). **B**, Tenosynovitis of the PTT: split-screen longitudinal sonograms. A story of trauma and weak ankle inversion similar to that in **A**. The clinical diagnosis in this 62-year-old woman was PTT tear as well. The longitudinal images show a normal right PTT (*COMP RHT*) just above the tip of the medial maleolus and a thickened left PTT (*LFT*). The thickening involves tendon tissue and surrounding synovium. The clinical test that measures ankle inversion cannot distinguish between the weakness caused by a torn tendon and the weakness caused by tendon swelling, which causes impaired gliding in the tarsal tunnel. Abbreviation: tendon (*T*). Synovium (*arrow*).

pattern, and the gap between the torn ends can be measured (see Fig. 4–14A). A tear with only a few centimeters of retraction will be reparable by end-to-end suturing of the tendon. In some cases, the proximal and distal ends of the tendon may recoil and overlap. The segment of overlap will be observed sonographically as a bulbous end of the tendon with deformed or absent fibrillar architecture. Acoustic shadowing may be seen deep to the overlapping segment.

Late-stage ruptures present particular diagnostic and therapeutic challenges. The proximal end of the tendon can retract into the calf and may not be discernible (Fig. 4–15) (van Holsbeeck and Powell, 1995). Simple suturing cannot repair these tendons, and tendon grafting is often required. The flexor digitorum, which is often used as a graft, can be mistaken for the PTT during the diagnostic workup (van Holsbeeck and Powell, 1995). It is important that the sonographer understand the regional anatomy. Demonstration of the posterior tibial and flexor digitorum tendons should be part of a complete diagnostic workup. The diameter of the flexor digitorum tendon is less than half the diameter of the PTT; therefore, the experienced sonographer has no difficulty distinguishing these two structures. Left–right comparison can be helpful if there is any doubt (van Holsbeeck and Powell, 1995). Complete rupture at this stage is revealed by an empty tibial groove at the level of the medial malleolus. The distal end of the torn PTT typically demonstrates a wavy fibrillar pattern on the longitudinal views (Fig. 4–15) (van Holsbeeck and Powell, 1995; Miller et al., 1996; Hsu et al., 1997). Long-standing pronation can result in impingement of the anterior surface of the lateral process of the talus upon the floor of the sinus tarsi. Soft tissue swelling can be seen sonographically in some patients. The symptoms may be difficult to interpret for the clinician, as these patients will have lateral pain away from the area of rupture. Patients in this stage of the disease benefit from subtalar arthrodesis (Crenshaw, 1996).

Partial tears of the PTT may also be observed. These injuries will be recognized as clefts that extend into the synovial surface of the tendon (Fig. 4–16). Longitudinal clefts occur quite often around the medial malleolus. Ultrasound's ability to show small partial-thickness tears is currently unequaled (Fig. 4–17) (Erickson, 1997). The sonographer can pinpoint the site of tear. Chronic PTT tears often show signs of hyperemia, and they are relatively easy to find with ultrasound (Figs. 4–16 and 4–18). When conservative treatment fails, ultrasound will facilitate surgery, allowing more closely targeted surgical access and smaller scars. Partial-thickness tears are treated by surgical imbrication of the tendon overlying the diseased segment (Fig. 4–19).

Incomplete tears of the peroneal tendons are common. An example of incomplete tendon rupture is seen in Figures 4–20A and 4–20B. These images demonstrate a partial tear of the peroneus tendon (Hardaker et al., 1985). They are typically oriented along the longitudinal axis of the peroneus brevis and longus. The brevis is affected far more often than the longus (Figs. 4–20 and 4–21). Proximity to the bone surface and rupture mechanism (see Chapter 7) have been blamed for the peroneus brevis's predisposition to tear (Sobel et al., 1991; Geppert et al., 1993). Anechoic clefts are seen within the tendon, and fluid is also present within the tendon sheath. Both findings are probably secondary to functional overload. It is unusual to see a large amount of hemorrhage within the sheath following tendon rupture due to the hypovascularity of tendons. Occasionally, the peroneus longus can tear completely and transversely relative to its long axis. Ankle inversion may cause a tear and a fracture through the os peroneale, the sesamoid which is often observed lateral to the cuboid on radiographs (Fig. 4–22).

Tendon Luxation

Luxation of the long biceps tendon is a rare finding but is easily diagnosed sonographically (O'Donoghue, 1982). Scanning is initiated in the transverse plane with the arm in neutral position. The bicipital groove is identified on the anterior aspect of the humeral head. This serves as a landmark that helps to distinguish the subscapularis muscle from the supraspinatus. The diagnosis of luxation of the long biceps tendon can be made when the bicipital groove is empty and there is concavity of the transverse ligament. The long biceps brachii tendon can dislocate if the attachment of the transverse ligament is torn (Petersson, 1986). Identifi-cation of the medially displaced long biceps tendon confirms the diagnosis. It is most frequently seen under the subscapularis tendon (see Fig. 4–9C) (Petersson, 1986). Primary stabilization of the biceps tendon is provided by the coracohumeral ligament (Clark and Harryman, 1992). Dislocation may be initiated by rupture of this important ligament. Dislocation of the biceps is rarely observed as an isolated finding. Most commonly, luxation is seen in combination with rotator cuff tear. Those tears are typically large or massive and involve the subscapularis in the majority of patients. Dislocation of the long biceps tendon can occur intermittently. Subluxable tendons are de-

Text continued on page 95

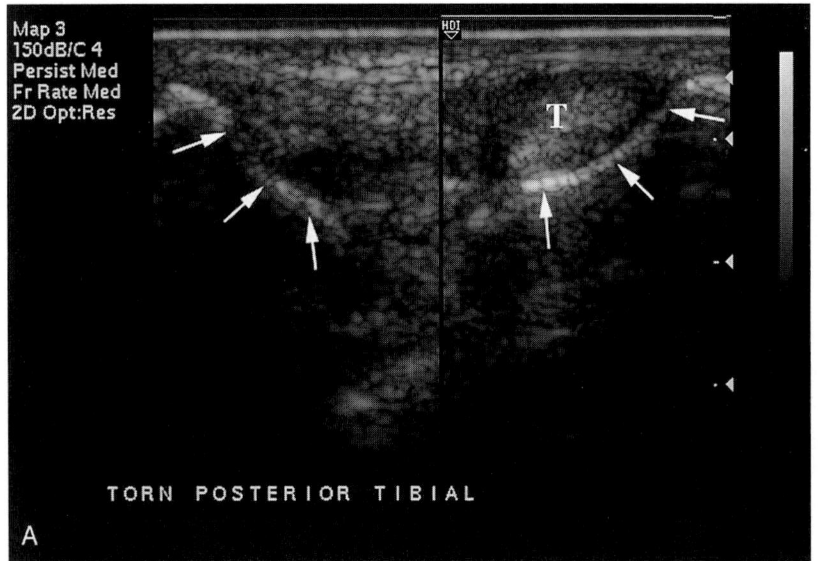

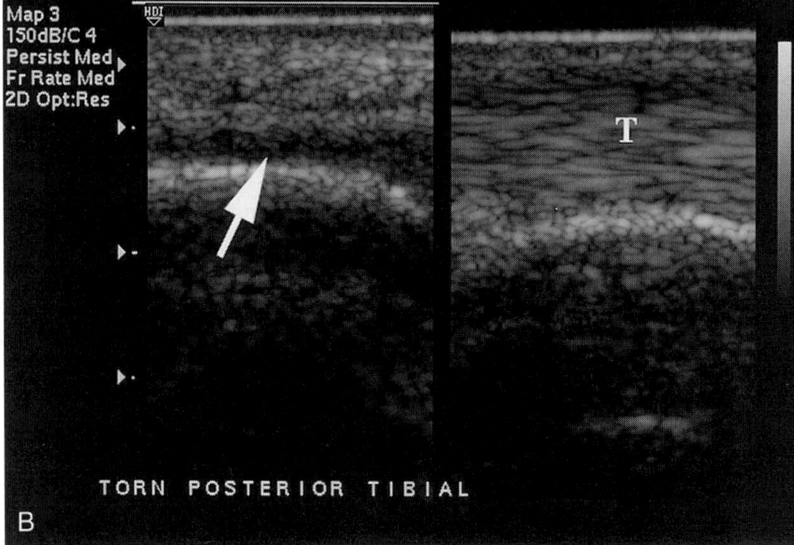

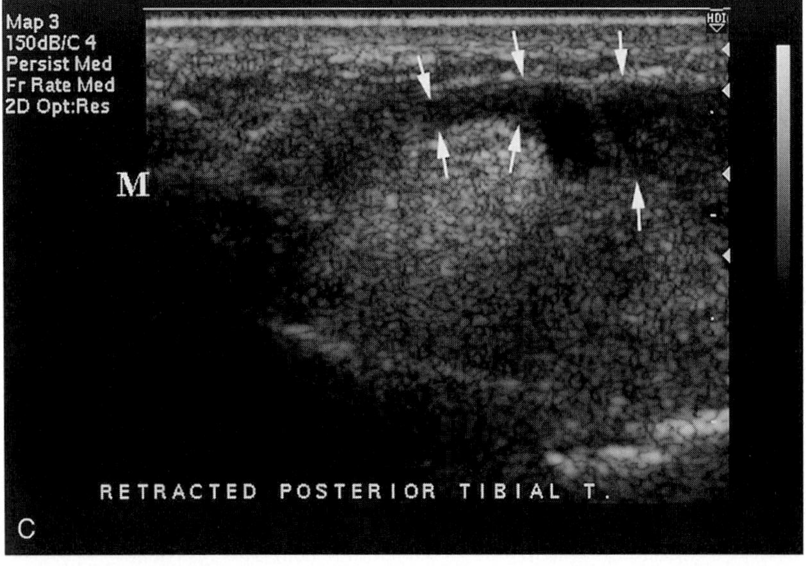

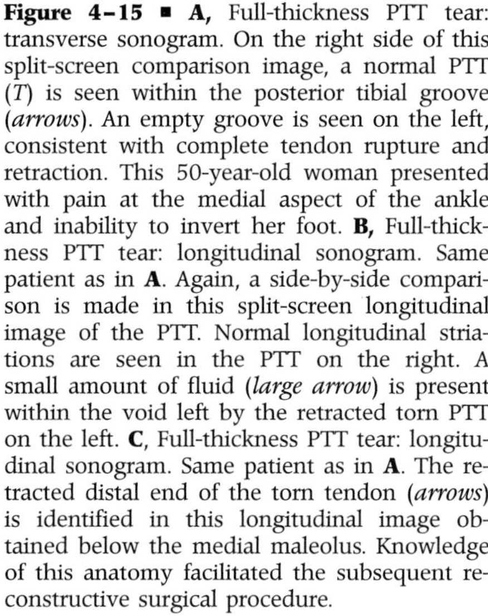

Figure 4-15 ■ **A,** Full-thickness PTT tear: transverse sonogram. On the right side of this split-screen comparison image, a normal PTT (*T*) is seen within the posterior tibial groove (*arrows*). An empty groove is seen on the left, consistent with complete tendon rupture and retraction. This 50-year-old woman presented with pain at the medial aspect of the ankle and inability to invert her foot. **B,** Full-thickness PTT tear: longitudinal sonogram. Same patient as in **A**. Again, a side-by-side comparison is made in this split-screen longitudinal image of the PTT. Normal longitudinal striations are seen in the PTT on the right. A small amount of fluid (*large arrow*) is present within the void left by the retracted torn PTT on the left. **C,** Full-thickness PTT tear: longitudinal sonogram. Same patient as in **A**. The retracted distal end of the torn tendon (*arrows*) is identified in this longitudinal image obtained below the medial maleolus. Knowledge of this anatomy facilitated the subsequent reconstructive surgical procedure.

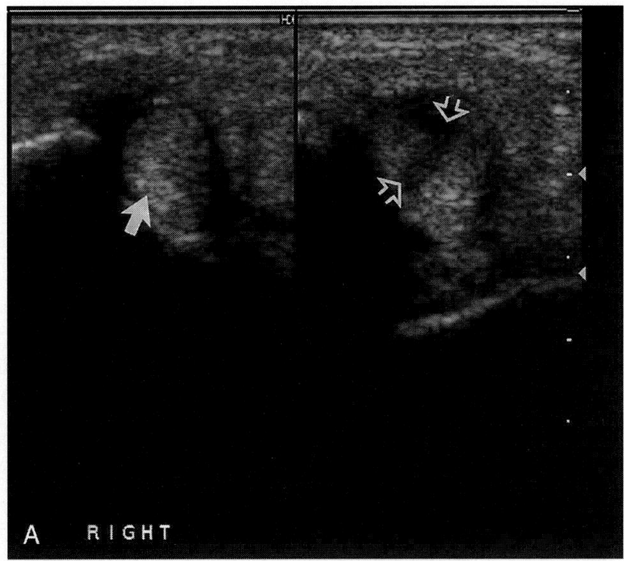

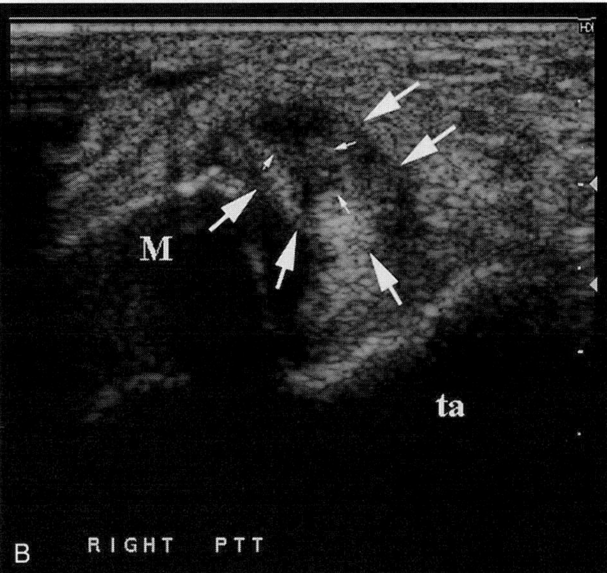

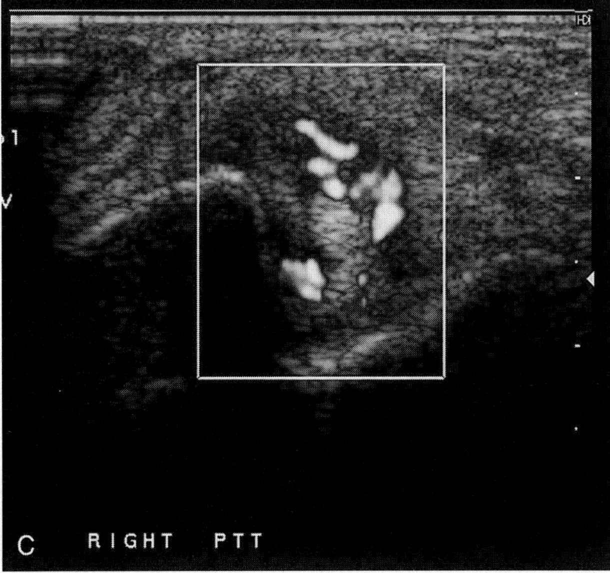

Figure 4–16 ■ **A,** Partial longitudinal split of the PTT: transverse sonograms. An ankle injury that occurred 5 months earlier never really healed, and this 51-year-old woman has been having right medial malleolar pain with ankle swelling ever since. She also noticed flattening of the arch of the injured right foot. The split screen shows a normal right PTT (*arrow*) at and proximal to the medial malleolus, demonstrated on the left side of the split screen. A sudden change in the tendon structure is noted around the medial malleolus and in the tendon distal to the malleolus, demonstrated on the right side of the split screen. The distal tendon shows a central split (*open arrows*) consistent with a partial-thickness tear. **B,** Partial longitudinal split of the PTT: transverse sonogram. Same patient as in **A**. This image was obtained at the tip of the medial malleolus (*M*). An irregular tendon surface (*large arrows*) is noted. A laceration (*small arrows*) extends from the medial side of the tendon into the tendon substance. The tear extends about halfway through the tendon. Abbreviation: talus (*ta*). **C,** Partial longitudinal split of the PTT: transverse power Doppler sonogram. Same patient as in **A**. The transducer position is unchanged from that in **B**. Hyperemia is noted within the tendon defect. The vessels seem to be continuous with the synovium.

Figure continued on following page

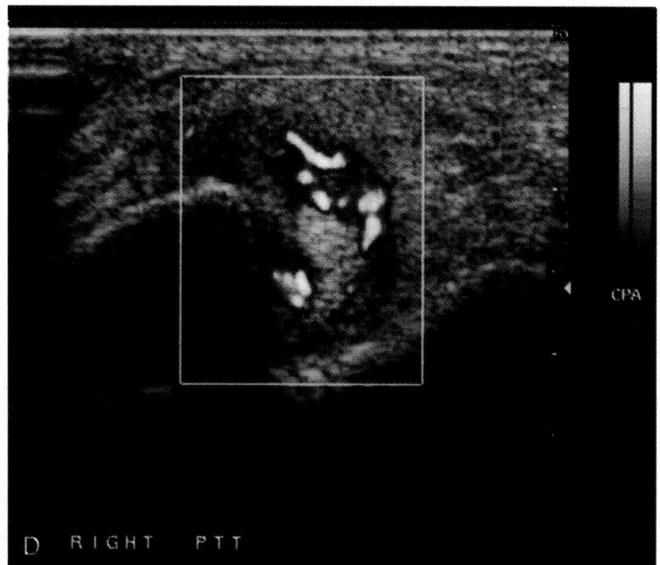

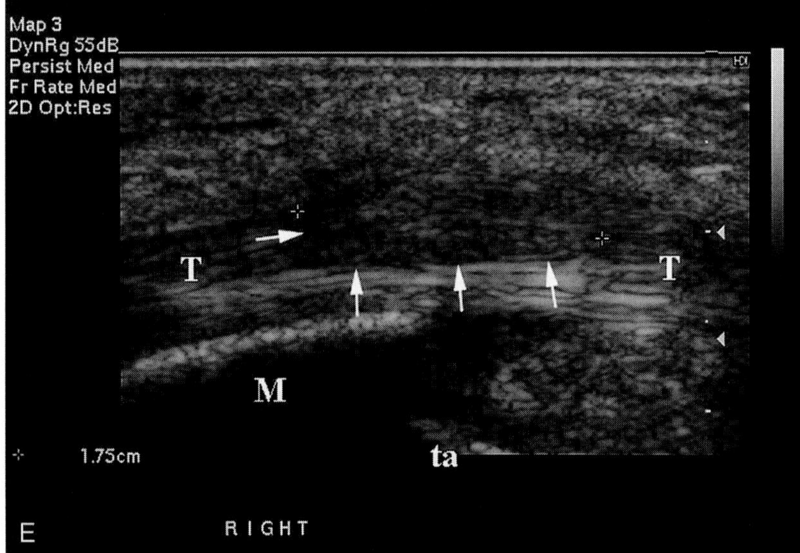

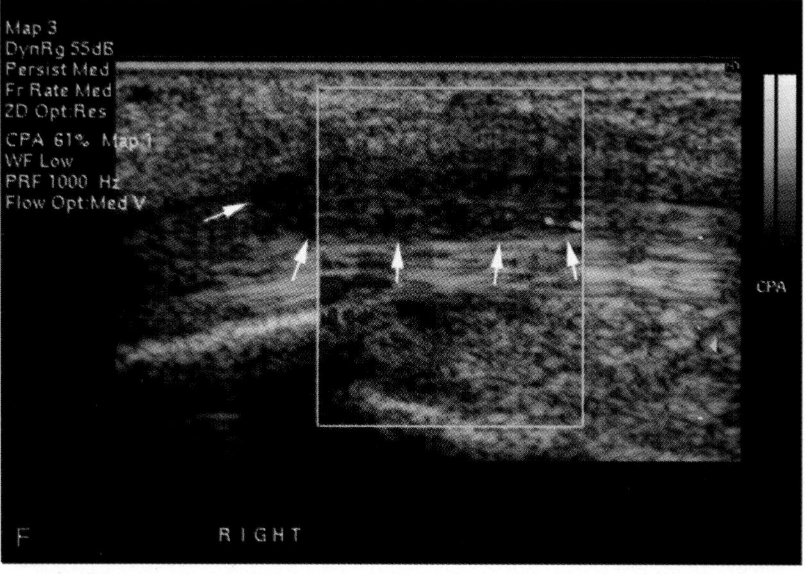

Figure 4-16 *Continued* ■ **D**, Partial longitudinal split of the PTT: transverse power Doppler sonogram. Same figure as in **C** but with the actual color. **E**, Partial longitudinal split of the PTT: longitudinal sonogram. Same patient as in **A**. The transducer is aligned with the long axis of the PTT (*T*). The proximal aspect of the tear starts at the level of the medial malleolus (*M*), and the tear extends along the tendon over a distance of 1.75 cm (*between the calipers*). This tear is called *longitudinal* because of its prolongation in the length (*arrows*) of the tendon, and it is called *partial* because it does not transect the tendon. Abbreviation: talus (*ta*). **F**, Partial longitudinal split of the PTT: longitudinal power Doppler sonogram. Same patient as in **A**. A vessel penetrates in the tendon through the tendon defect. Normal tendons do not have vascular flow that is discernible with power Doppler sonography. The longitudinal tear is marked with arrows.

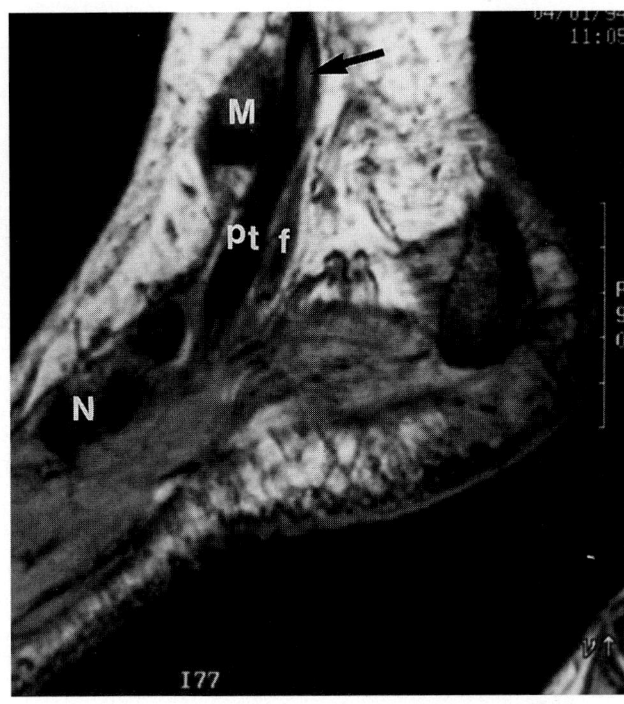

Figure 4–17 ■ Partial longitudinal split of the PTT: sagittal MRI scan. Different patient but with the same type of pathology as in Figure 4–16. The sagittal gradient MRI sequence shows the PTT (*pt*) in close proximity to the medial malleolus (*M*) and the navicular (*N*). Abnormally increased signal intensity (*arrow*) corresponded with a longitudinal tear in the tendon found at surgery. This tear is located more proximally in the tendon than the tear in Figure 4–16. The signal changes were mistakenly attributed to the magic angle phenomenon at first. Notice the close proximity of the flexor digitorum tendon (*f*), which is also a potential pitfall in this type of tear. Ultrasound of the PTT is easier than MRI. Power Doppler sonography assists in demonstrating symptomatic tears. The hyperemia shown in symptomatic lesions distinguishes them from artifacts and asymptomatic variants.

tected by adding routine dynamic maneuvers to the standard shoulder examination. Active external rotation of the arm with the elbow flexed 90 degrees and adducted will accentuate subluxation or cause dislocation in patients with intermittent abnormalities (Farin et al., 1995).

Luxation of the peroneus tendons (Church, 1977; McConkey and Favero, 1987; Oden, 1987) is often attributable to the chronic trauma (Eichelberger et al., 1982) seen in athletes involved in football, soccer, gymnastics, and dancing (Fig. 4–23). A standoff or water bath may be necessary for sonographic examination of the lateral malleolar region (Box 4–3). The examination is conducted with the foot everted against resistance to accentuate the dislocation. The transducer is placed just inferior to the lateral malleolus, scanning in the transverse plane. Passive dorsiflexion and eversion of the foot is often necessary to evoke subluxation (Fig. 4–23). If luxation is present, the tendon will be seen overlying the lateral malleolus. Excess fluid surrounding the tendon may also be noted. Patients with this condition are treated surgically, and a torn superior peroneal retinaculum has been found in all cases (Das and Balasubramaniam, 1985). The instability of tendons caused by trauma to the superior peroneal retinaculum may result in peroneal tendon damage and partial-thickness tears (Fig. 4–24) (Geppert et al., 1993; Davis et al., 1994).

Tendons without a Synovial Sheath

Tendinitis

Tendinitis (syn.: tendinosis, tendinopathy) is almost always attributable to chronic trauma and a high level of athletic activity (Roels and Martens, 1978; Feretti et al., 1985). Plain film findings can be detected only in advanced cases and only if the examiner uses low-kilovoltage technique (Fig. 4–25). The sonographic findings are identical in all locations. Focal thickening of the tendon (van Holsbeeck, 1987) and widening of the distance between the longitudinal fascicles are invariably present (Fig. 4–26). Focal hypoechoic areas within the tendon are also present (Fig. 4–27). Most tendons show uniform thickness and echogenicity over their course from origin to insertion (Fig. 4–28). It is therefore not difficult to detect an abnormality, especially if the examiner uses systematic left–right comparison during routine screening (Fig. 4–29). Edema, myxoid degeneration, and vascular proliferation may all contribute to tendon hypoechogenicity (Fig. 4–30). Fat surrounding the tendon has increased echogenicity, as seen in Figure 4–30 (Hoffa's fat pad, Kager's triangle). A number of longitudinal tendon fibers are seen to be intact (Fig. 4–30). In some cases, hypoechoic foci are seen around the tendon (Figs. 4–30 through 4–33). These were shown to be fibromyxoid tissue on his-

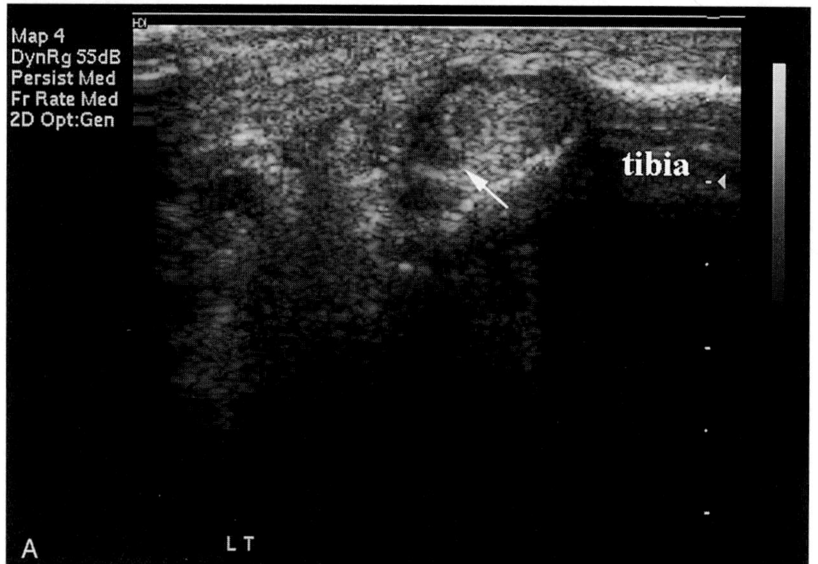

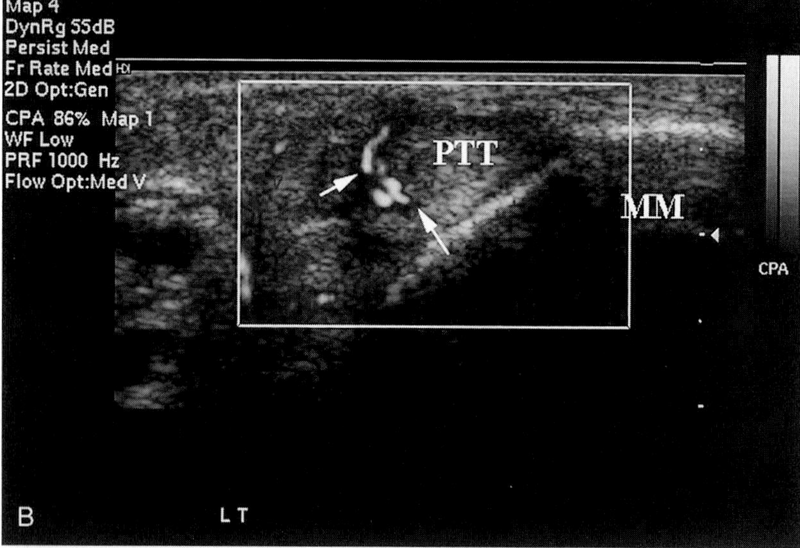

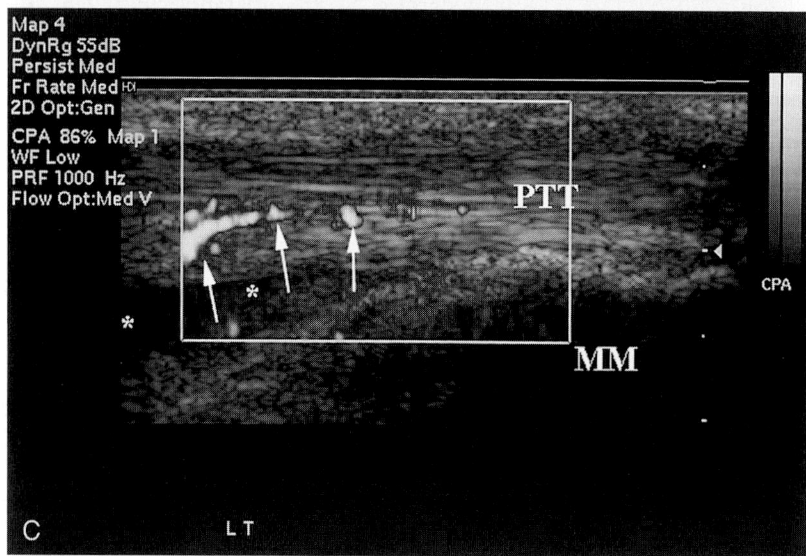

Figure 4-18 ■ **A,** Surface erosion of the PTT: transverse sonogram. An ankle injury that occurred during jogging causes persistent pain in this 38-year-old woman. With the transducer above the medial maleolus and transversely oriented over the long axis of the tibia, one can distinguish a cleft (*arrow*) in the surface of the tendon. The tear is no larger than 3 mm. **B,** Surface erosion of the PTT: transverse sonogram with power Doppler sonography. Same patient as in **A**. The transducer position is unchanged, but the power Doppler system has been activated. A synovial vessel penetrates the tendon defect (*arrows*). The patient experiences maximal tenderness at this site. Abbreviations: posterior tibial tendon (*PTT*), medial maleolus (*MM*). **C,** Surface erosion of the PTT: longitudinal sonogram with power Doppler sonography. Same patient as in **A**. Abnormal color flow enters (*arrows*) the tendon above the medial malleolus (*MM*). The tendon sheath appears distended with fluid (*asterisks*). Abbreviation: posterior tibial tendon (*PTT*).

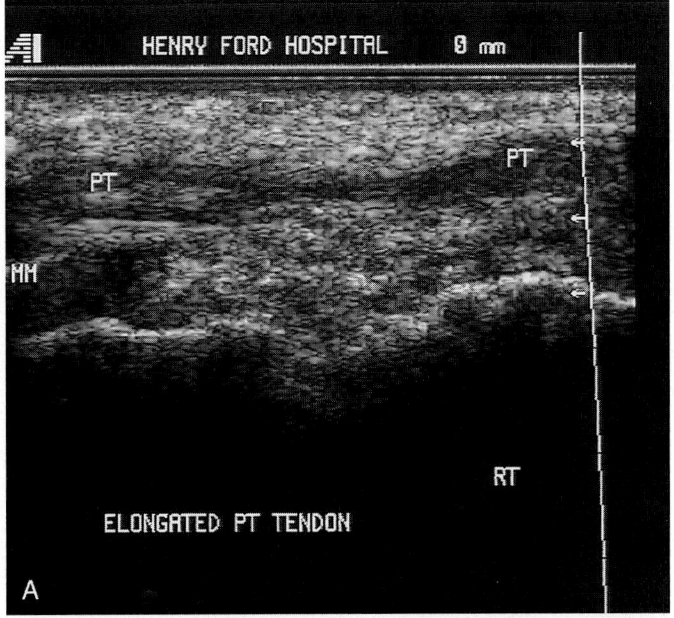

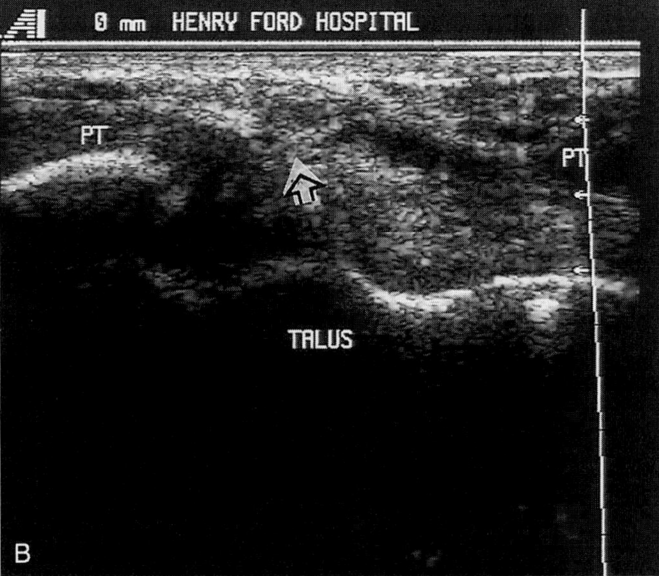

Figure 4–19 ▪ **A**, Partial- versus full-thickness tear: longitudinal sonogram. A painful collapse of the foot arch prompts this patient's visit to the foot clinic. The patient, who is 70 years old, has rheumatoid arthritis. Ankle valgus and foot pronation are noted by the clinician. With the 7.5-MHz transducer aligned along the PTT below the medial maleolus (*MM*), one can discern thinning of the PTT (*PT*); however, note the continuity of the tendon despite the thinning. Surgical treatment requires imbrication of the tendon. **B**, Partial- versus full-thickness tear: longitudinal sonogram. This 71-year-old woman presents 2 years after injury. The transducer is in a similar position below the medial maleolus and adjacent to the talus. Complete interruption (*arrow*) of the PTT (*PT*) is seen 0.5 cm distal to the maleolus. Surgical treatment requires a flexor digitorum graft to restore the anatomy.

tological analysis of 53 cases. The tendon itself may have a nodular appearance (Fig. 4–31). Bony enthesophytes (Figs. 4–32 and 4–33) may be seen at the tendon insertion in cases of prolonged tendinitis. In some patients, tendinitis persists for years, with episodic flare-ups during the sports season. Rarely, calcium deposits may be detected within the tendon. Calcium is deposited preferentially in the cartilaginous tendon insertion (Fig. 4–34).

In patients with the sonographic diagnosis of patellar tendinitis who underwent surgery, all were found to have an intact epitendineum. On longitudinal sectioning of the tendon, degenerating or

Box 4–3
Swollen Lateral Ankle with Painful "Clicking"

- Assess peroneal tendons for flattening and splitting
- Assess superior retinaculum for rupture (hypoechogenicity) or avulsion (bone fragment)
- Assess for tendon instability

Text continued on page 103

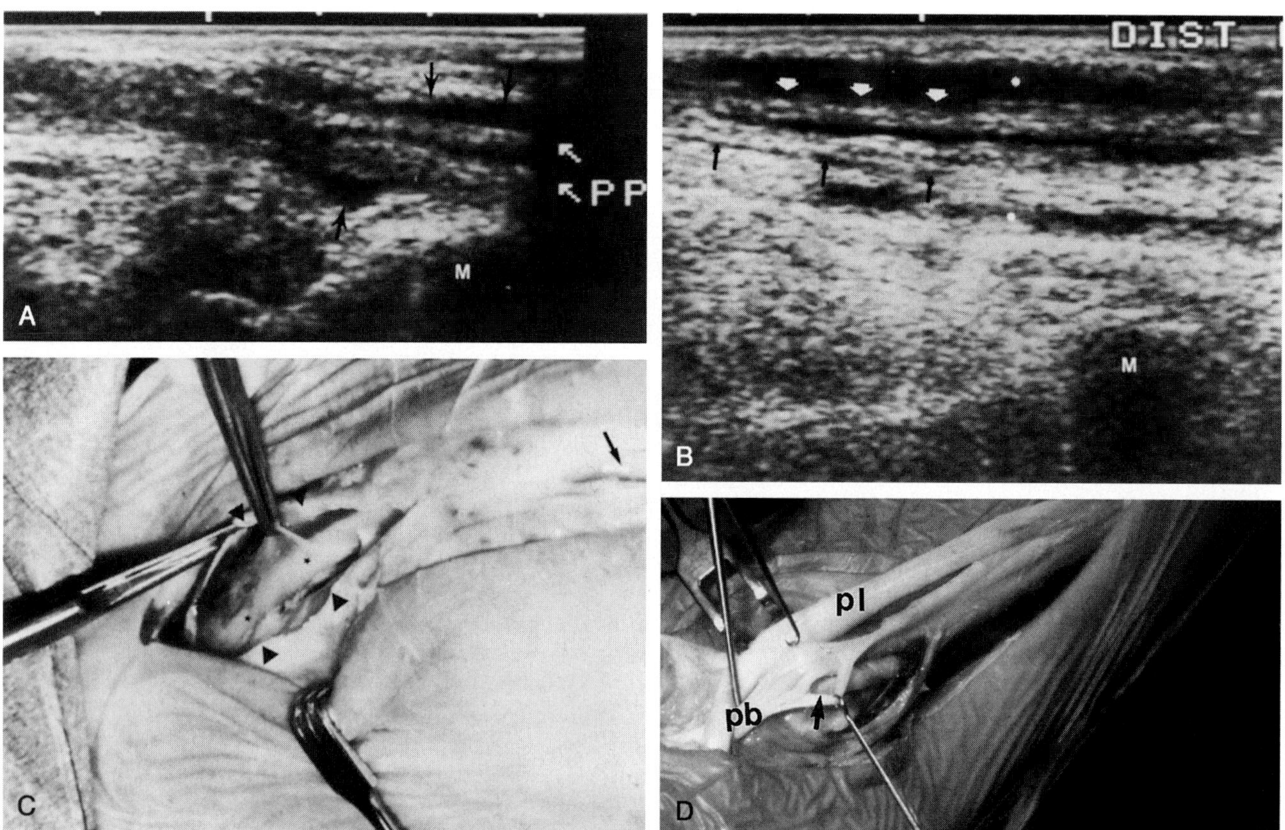

Figure 4–20 ▪ **A**, Tendinosis of the peroneus tendons progressing to incomplete rupture: sonogram. This ballet dancer has persistent ankle pain. The pain is localized to the lateral aspect of the ankle and is worsened by eversion of the foot. The transducer is positioned posterior to the lateral malleolus, parallel to the tibia. An increased amount of fluid (*black arrows*) is found in the sheath of the peroneus tendons (*PP*). Abbreviation: lateral malleolus (*M*). **B**, Incomplete rupture of the peroneus tendons: longitudinal sonogram taken 5 months later. The position of the transducer is identical to that in **A**. Fluid within the tendon sheath has increased (*white asterisk*). A hypoechoic gap seen centrally within the peroneus brevis tendon represents a fluid collection within the tendon (*black arrows*). Individual tendon fibers are visualized more clearly due to this pathological fluid collection. The peroneus longus tendon is frayed, and a large defect is seen in the posterior aspect (*white arrows*). **C** and **D**, Intraoperative photographs: peroneus tendinosis. Same patient as in **A** and **B**. The skin incision is made longitudinally, posterior to the lateral malleolus. The skin is retracted anteriorly, revealing the opened tendon sheath (*black arrowheads*) and the peroneus tendon (*stars*). When the tendon sheath was incised, a pathological collection of synovial fluid was found, as seen sonographically. Its reflection is indicated by the *black arrow* at the right. **D**, The surgeon moves the peroneus longus tendon anteriorly (*pl*), and the peroneus brevis (*pb*) is exposed. Fine hook retractors reveal the defect in the tendon (*arrow*).

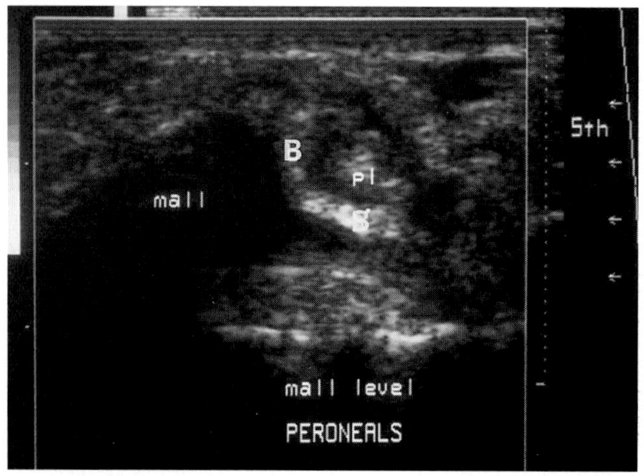

Figure 4–21 ▪ Longitudinal split of the peroneus brevis: transverse sonogram. A 42-year-old woman presents with a similar case history and with the same operative findings as the patient in Figure 4–20. More characteristic findings are typically observed on the transverse images of patients with peroneus brevis tears. The 10-MHz transducer is placed behind the lateral maleolus (*mall*), oriented transversely over the long axis of the fibula. Instability of the peroneal tendons leads to flattening of the peroneus brevis (*B*) as it rolls over the fibula. The peroneus longus (*pl*) retains its shape early on (as illustrated here), but the tendon will eventually deform if the process is not corrected by surgery. This patient underwent an elective repair of the peroneus brevis and was back at her job as a truck unloader 3 months after surgery.

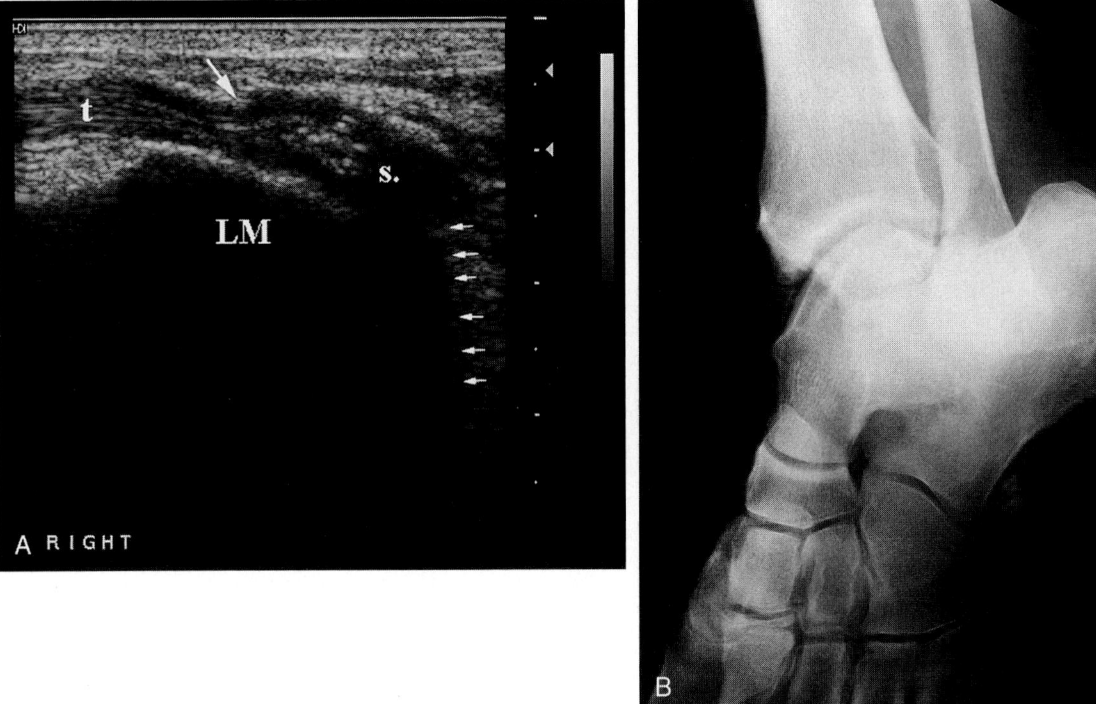

Figure 4–22 ■ **A**, Transverse full-thickness tear of the peroneus longus: longitudinal sonogram. Four months after injury, this 53-year-old woman keeps complaining of lateral ankle pain and tenderness over the lateral Achilles tendon. The ultrasound exam was requested to exclude a partial tear of the Achilles tendon and to evaluate the lateral collateral ligaments of the ankle. The longitudinal scan over the peroneal tendons indicated complete disruption of the peroneus longus tendon (*t*). The retracted tendon undulates (*arrow*), and an abrupt stop of its fibrillar pattern is noted distal to the os peroneale (*s*). An acoustic shadow (*arrows*) is noted deep to the sesamoid. **B**, Transverse full-thickness tear of the peroneus longus: oblique ankle radiograph. Same patient as in **A**. The displaced sesamoid bone is noted at the lateral aspect of the foot.

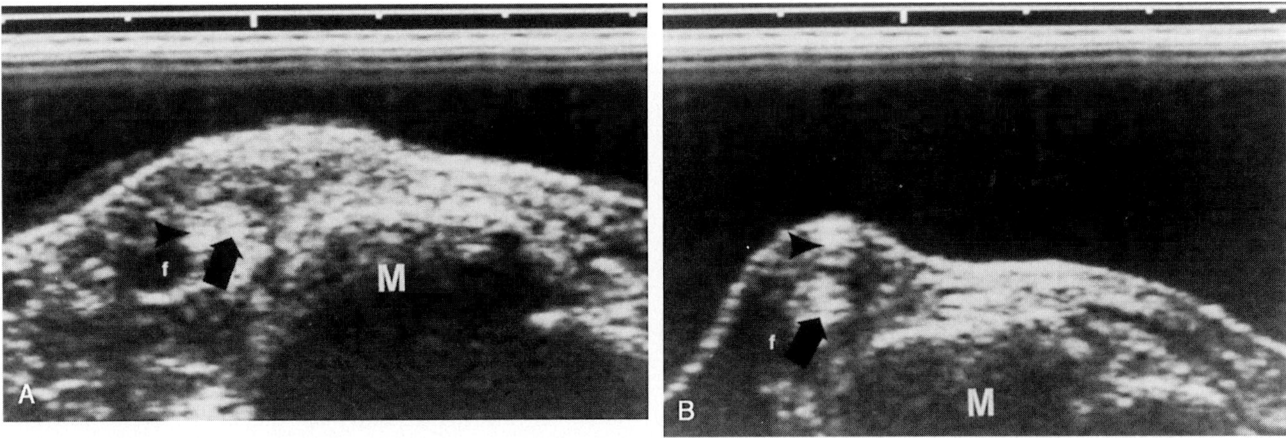

Figure 4–23 ■ **A**, Peroneus tendon luxation: transverse sonogram through the common peroneus tendon sheath. A ballet dancer presented with pain and swelling over the distal fibula. She could reproduce the pain by dorsiflexion and eversion of the foot. Examination of the lateral malleolus required a standoff. The position of the transducer is perpendicular to the long axis of the tibia, posterior to the lateral malleolus. There is a slightly increased amount of fluid (*f*) in the peroneus tendon sheath. The peroneus brevis tendon (*black arrow*) is located anteriorly near the lateral malleolus (*M*). The peroneus longus tendon (*arrowhead*) is located more posteriorly. **B**, Peroneus tendon luxation: transverse sonogram with the foot in dorsiflexion and eversion. Same patient as in **A**, with identical positioning of the transducer. With the patient's foot in dorsiflexion and everted, the peroneus longus tendon dislocates laterally and anteriorly, overriding the peroneus brevis tendon (*black arrow*). This type of instability is considered the cause of the abnormalities shown in Figures 4–20 and 4–21.

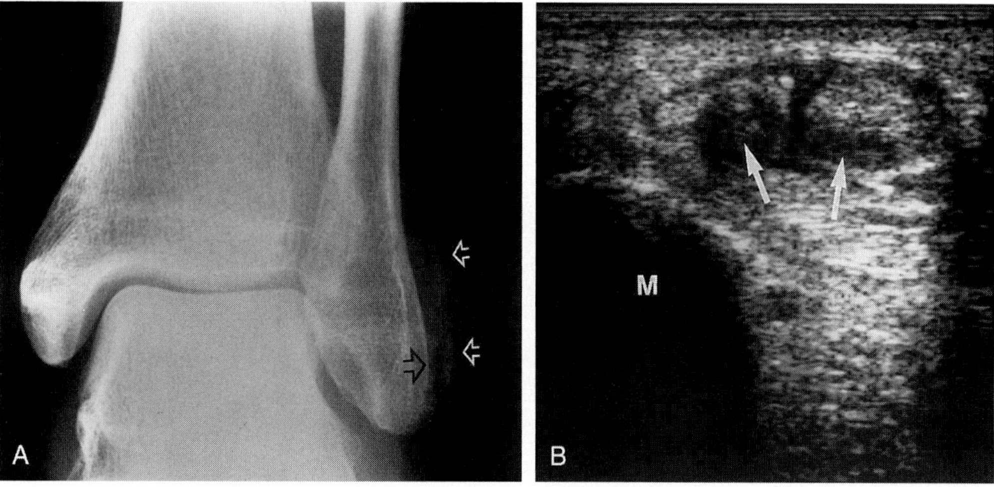

Figure 4–24 ■ **A**, Disruption of the superior peroneal retinaculum: anteroposterior radiograph of the ankle. Ultrasound-diagnosed chronic instability and longitudinal tears of both peroneal tendons in this 56-year-old man. The radiograph shows avulsion and heterotopic bone formation (*open arrows*) in the region of the superior peroneal retinaculum. Injury to this ligament causes tendon instability, as depicted in Figure 4–23, and peroneal tears, as illustrated in Figures 4–20 and 4–21. (Reproduced with permission from Diaz GC, van Holsbeeck M, et al: Longitudinal split of the peroneus longus and peroneus brevis tendons with disruption of the superior peroneal retinaculum. *J Ultrasound Med* 17:525–529, 1998.) **B**, Disruption of the superior peroneal retinaculum: transverse ultrasound. Same patient as in **A**. With the transducer placed transversely over the lateral maleolus, erosions (*arrows*) are detected at the surface of both peroneal tendons. Note the unusual lateral position of the tendons relative to the lateral maleolus (*M*). The subluxation would not be possible without a tear of the superior peroneal retinaculum.

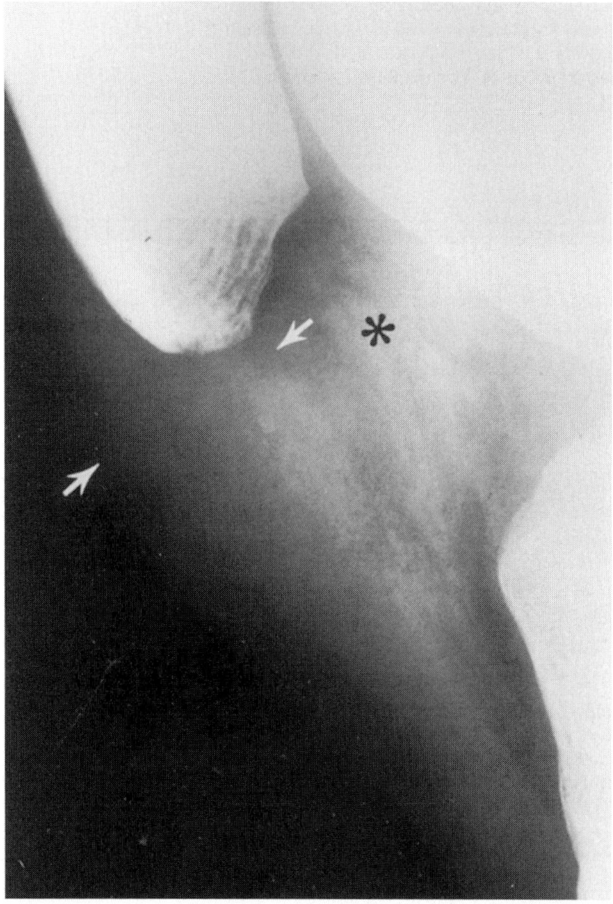

Figure 4–25 ■ Jumper's knee: conventional radiograph with soft tissue contrast. A soccer player presented with knee pain at the beginning and end of exercise. Pain and tenderness were localized under the apex of the patella. The top image is a lateral view of the knee produced using a Gevaert MRL cassette and mammography film. Thickening of the patellar tendon is seen in the infrapatellar region (*white arrows*). The adjacent infrapatellar fat pad (Hoffa's fat pad) is infiltrated and is less radiolucent (*black asterisk*) than the rest of the infrapatellar fat. A small calcification is seen within the posterior third of the patellar tendon at its point of maximal thickening.

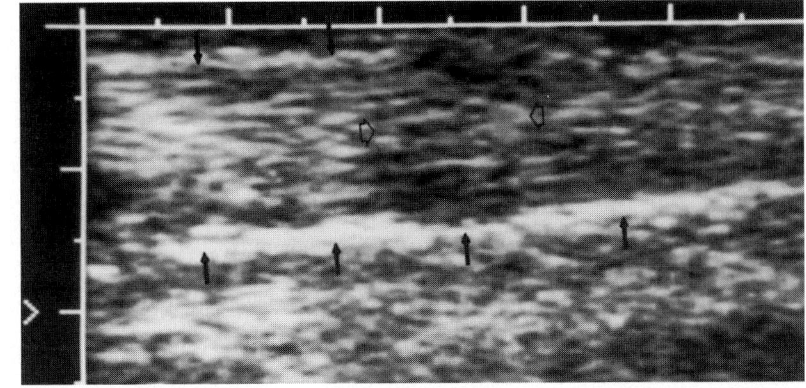

Figure 4–26 ■ Achilles tendinosis: longitudinal sonogram. A long-distance runner with a 3-month history of pain in the Achilles tendon. The pain is located 5 cm above the tendon insertion. The transducer is positioned over the heel, dorsal to the Achilles tendon, oriented along the long axis of the tendon. The lesion (*open arrows*) is identified sonographically as a hypoechoic focal swelling of the tendon, with increased distance between the individual longitudinal fibers. The longitudinally oriented fibers of the Achilles tendon can easily be identified. There is no synovial sheath and no fluid surrounding the tendon. The hyperreflective area (*black arrows*) surrounding the tendon corresponds to the epitendineum.

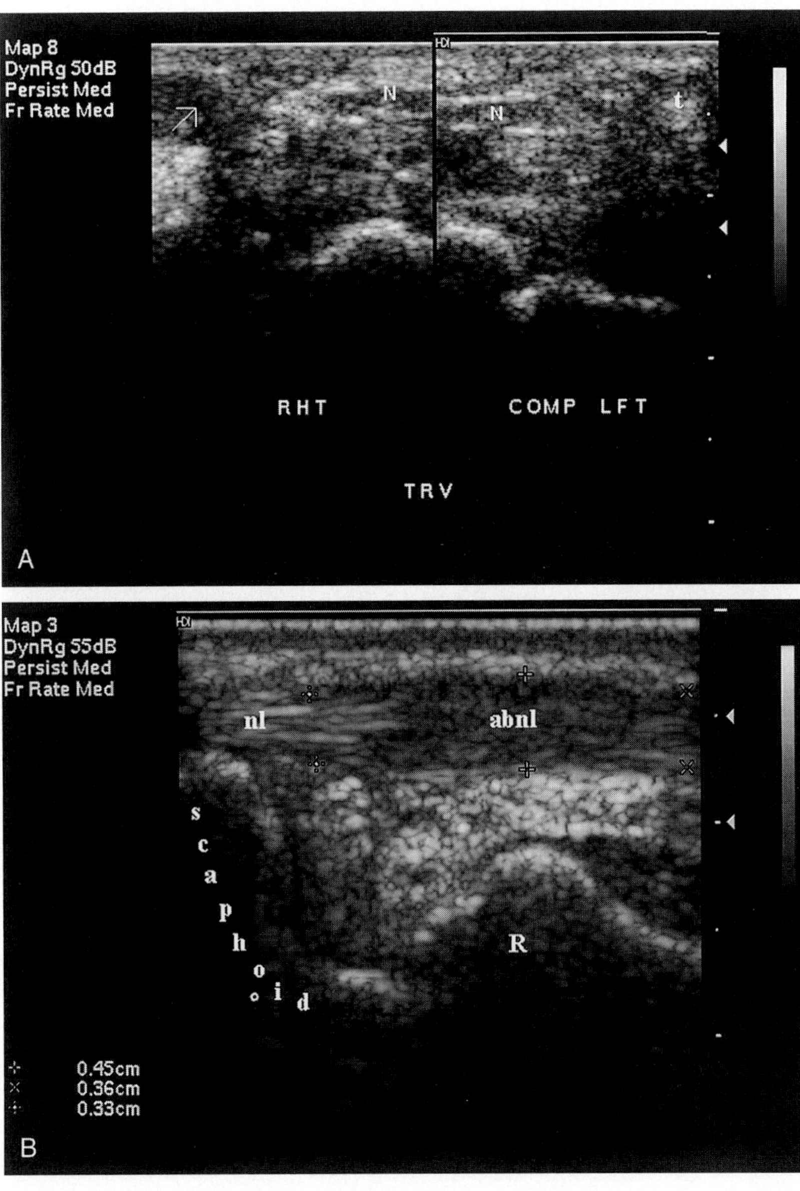

Figure 4–27 ■ **A,** Flexor carpi radialis tendinosis: transverse sonogram. During a rehabilitation program after myocardial infarction, this 62-year-old Korean notices a mass developing in his right wrist (*RHT*). The wrist pain that accompanies the mass was interpreted as carpal tunnel disease by the referring physician. The ultrasound study was requested to rule out a ganglion as the cause of the condition. Split-screen transverse sonograms of both carpal tunnels show that the mass (*arrow*) in the right wrist is located outside the carpal tunnel boundaries. The median nerves (*N*) appear symmetric and unaffected. The palpable soft tissue mass appears hypoechoic and solid. The location corresponds to that of the flexor carpi radialis over the proximal scaphoid. The contralateral normal tendon (*t*) is noted in the left wrist (*LFT*). Abbreviation: transverse (*TRV*). **B,** Flexor carpi radialis tendinosis: longitudinal sonogram. Same patient as in **A**. With the transducer aligned along the flexor carpi radialis tendon, one notices the focal thickening of the tendon. Compare the distance between the middle calipers with the distances between the proximal and distal calipers. The fibrillar pattern (*abnl*) appears more disorganized in the swollen segment of the tendon. The normal distal tendon shows the typical linear interfaces (*nl*). The proximal wrist is displayed on the right side of the image. Abbreviation: radius, (*R*).

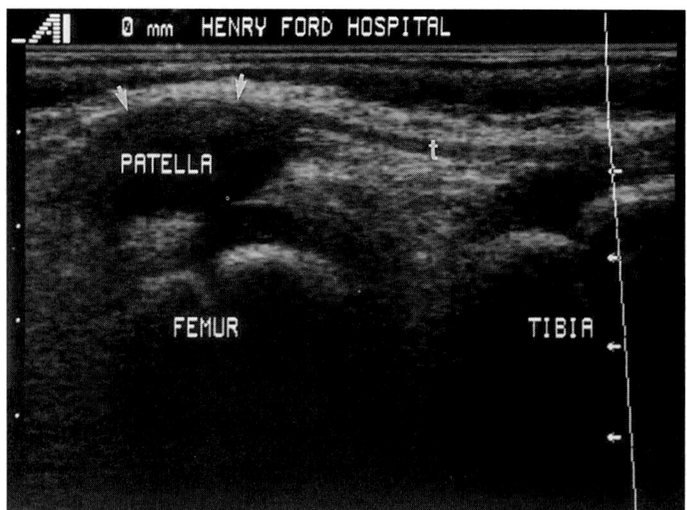

Figure 4-28 ▪ Normal patellar tendon in a child: longitudinal ultrasound. The extensor mechanism of the knee in this 3-year-old child blends imperceptibly with the cartilages of the patella and tibial tuberosity. Thin prepatellar fibers (*arrows*) may be responsible for the increased echogenicity of the anterior surface of the patella. The physes and the epiphyseal cartilages of the proximal tibia and distal femur are clearly discernible. Note the equal thickness of the proximal and distal patellar tendons (*t*) in the normal knee.

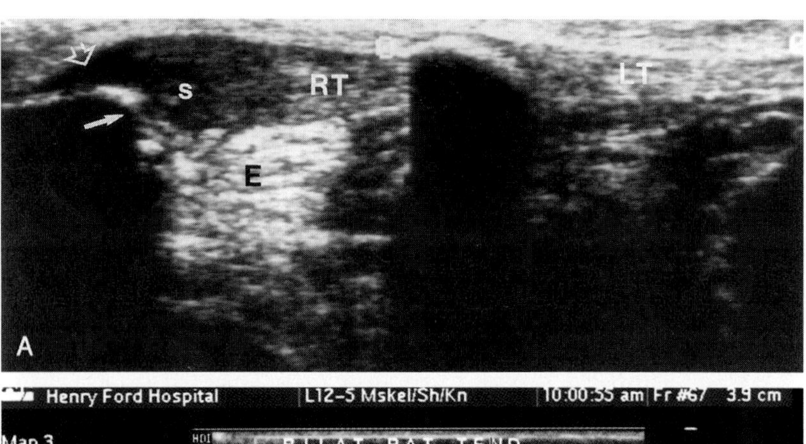

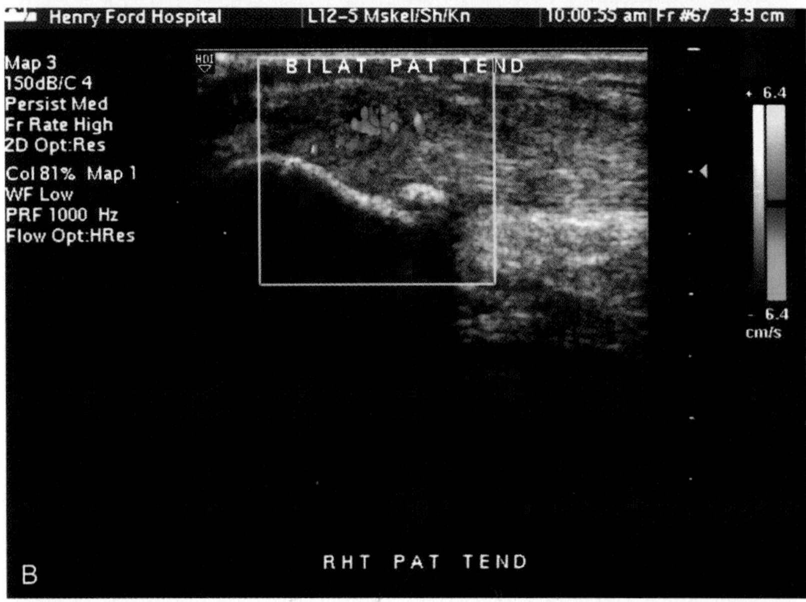

Figure 4-29 ▪ **A**, Unilateral proximal patellar tendinitis: longitudinal sonograms with split-screen comparison technique. Intense anterior knee pain plagues this 31-year-old long-distance runner. A bone scan shows intense uptake at the apex of the patella. With the ultrasound transducer aligned along the patellar tendons, one notices significant hypoechoic swelling (*S*) of the right patellar tendon (*RT*) when compared with the normal left patellar tendon (*LT*). The bone surface of the patellar apex shows irregularity (*arrow*). Acoustic enhancement (*E*) appears deep to the tendinitis. Characteristic swelling of the prepatellar fibers (*open arrow*) of the extensor mechanism is noted as well. Compare this finding with the normal left patellar tendon. **B**, Unilateral proximal patellar tendinosis: color Doppler sonography. Same patient as in **A**. Small vessels are seen in the affected tendon distal to the patellar apex. Hyperemia is quite common in segments of tendon affected by tendinosis.

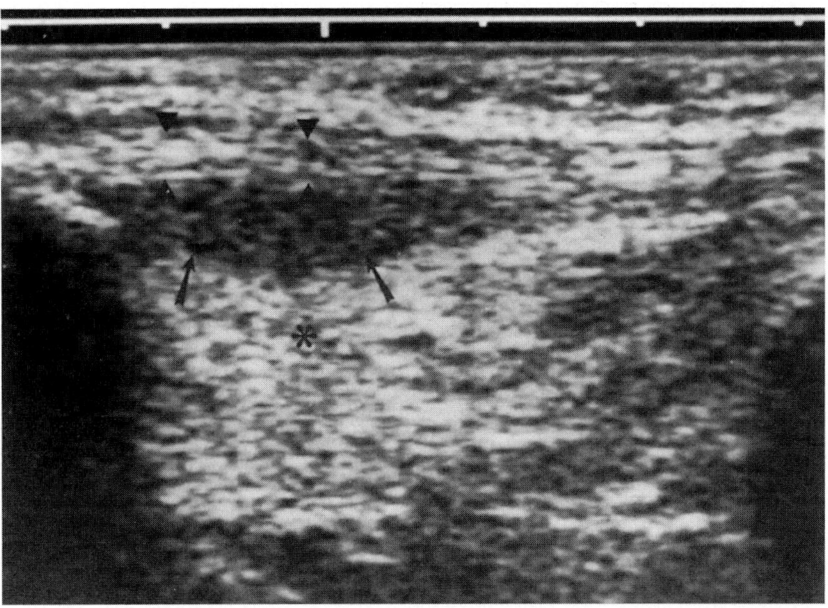

Figure 4–30 ■ Jumper's knee: longitudinal sonogram. A volleyball player experienced anterior knee pain at the end of the season. The pain was worse during practice, especially on flexion, and disappeared after warmup. The transducer is positioned in the long axis of the right patellar tendon. The fibers of the tendon (*arrowheads*) are continuous and have a normal appearance throughout their length. Hypoechoic fibromyxoid tissue (*black arrows*) surrounds the proximal portion of the tendon. Hoffa's fat pad, deep to this hypoechoic fibromyxoid tissue, is hyperechoic (*black asterisk*).

necrotic tissue was identified just below the patellar apex. The superficial tendon fibers in this region were grossly normal. Histological examination revealed mucoid degeneration, fibrinous necrosis, clefts, and microtears. Areas of regeneration with reparative and granulation tissue were also seen (Roels and Martens, 1978). The widened distance between longitudinal fascicles seen sonographically proved to be ruptured collagen fibers under light microscopy, especially those cross-linking the fascicles. Focal thickening of the tendon was the result of tiny pockets of necrotic debris. Hypoechoic foci were attributable to edema and mucoid degeneration. The nodular appearance of tendons was due to collections of granulation and scar tissue.

Merkel et al. (1982) described the pathological findings in traumatic tendinitis using electron microscopy. They reported rupture of collagen bundles as well as a decrease in the mean diameter of collagen fibrils (from 450 Å to 345 Å). The fibrils also displayed a disordered arrangement. Merkel et al. (1982) also noted an increase in the quantity of acid mucopolysaccharide ground substance. They

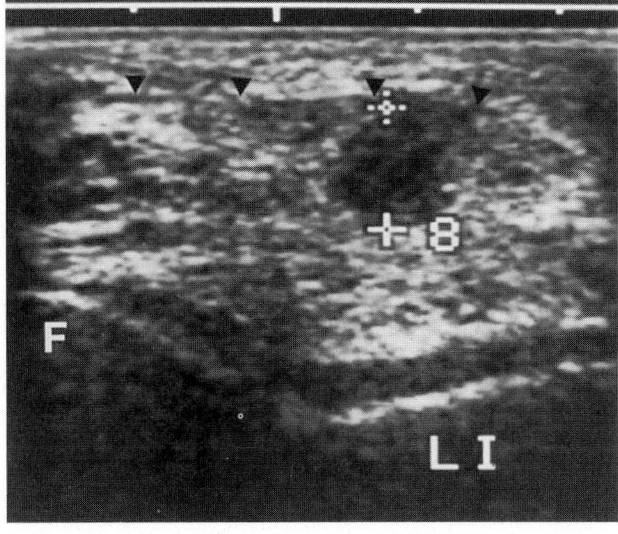

Figure 4–31 ■ Jumper's knee: transverse sonogram. A soccer player had chronic knee pain for almost 1 year. The exercise-induced pain prevented him from participating in professional sports. The left patellar tendon is scanned transversely, with the transducer positioned perpendicular to its longitudinal axis. The patellar tendon is convex anteriorly (*black arrowheads*). A nodule (*crosses*) is seen within the deep aspect of the tendon. The articular cartilage of the femoral condyles is seen deep to the tendon. Abbreviation: lateral femoral condyle (*F*).

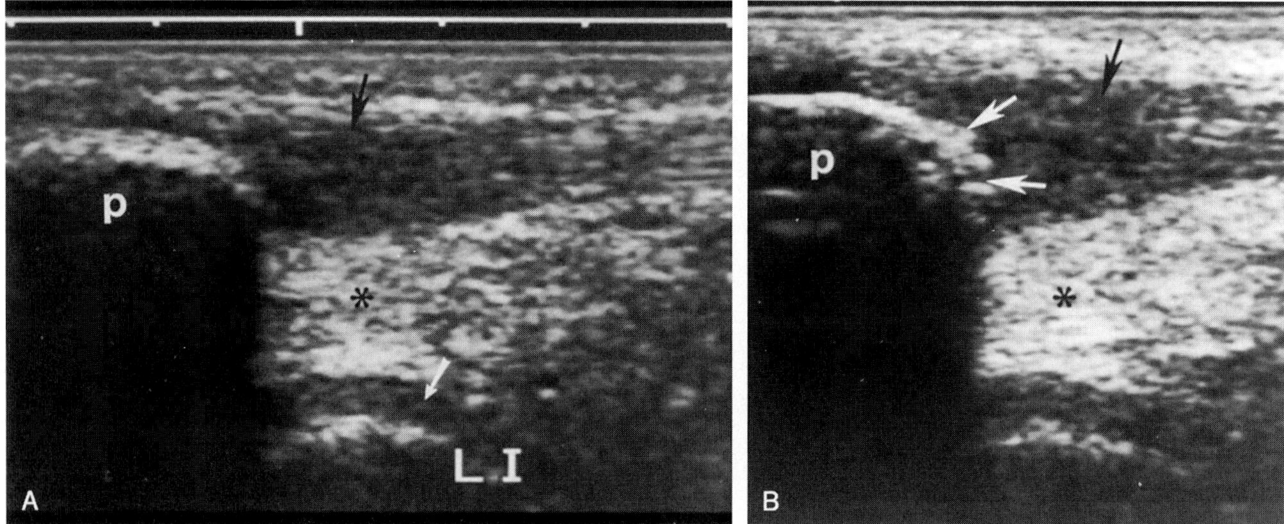

Figure 4-32 ■ **A,** Progression of subacute patellar tendinosis to chronic tendinosis. The sonogram was taken 7 months after the onset of symptoms, including infrapatellar pain during training. The transducer is positioned in the long axis of the tendon over the patellar apex. The hypoechoic lesion is located inferior to the patellar apex (*p*). Only a few tendon fibers remain intact in this hypoechoic region (*black arrow*). The portion of Hoffa's fat pad deep to the area of tendinosis is hyperechoic (*black asterisk*). Cartilage of the femoral condyle (*white arrow*) is seen. **B,** Two years after the onset of symptoms. The position of the transducer is identical to that in **A**. There is increased infrapatellar swelling (*black arrow*). A sign of the chronicity of patellar tendinosis is the irregular new bone formation (*white arrows*) identified as inhomogeneous hyperreflectivity. Symbol: hyperechoic fat (*asterisk*).

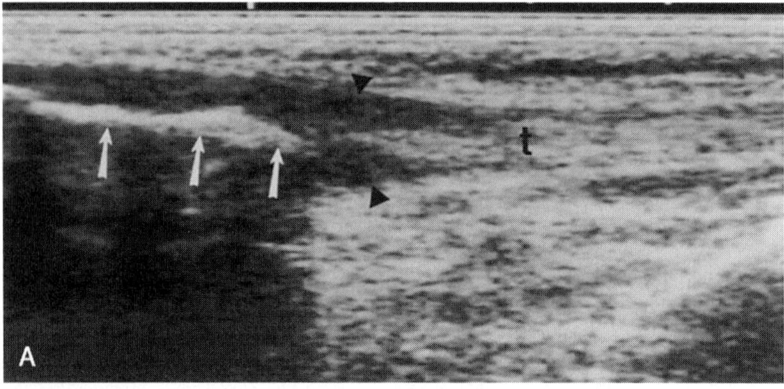

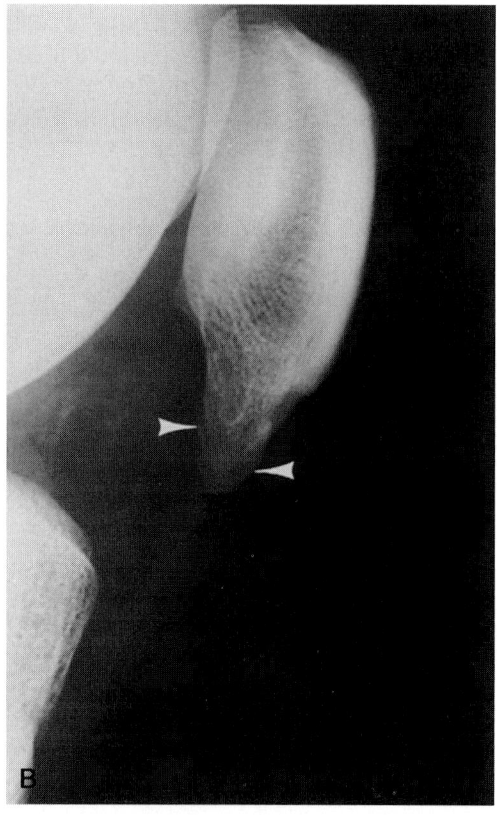

Figure 4-33 ■ **A,** Chronic recurrent patellar tendinosis: longitudinal sonogram. In each of the past 4 years, this patient experienced symptoms of patellar tendinosis at the end of the sporting season. The transducer is positioned along the length of the patellar tendon over the patellar apex. Lengthening of the patellar apex (*white arrows*) is seen. The patellar tendon (*t*) shows the characteristic lesion of patellar tendinosis (*black arrowheads*). **B,** Chronic recurrent patellar tendinosis: conventional radiograph. Same patient as in **A**. Patellar lengthening with well-organized new bone formation (*white arrowheads*) is a characteristic feature of chronic recurrent patellar tendinosis.

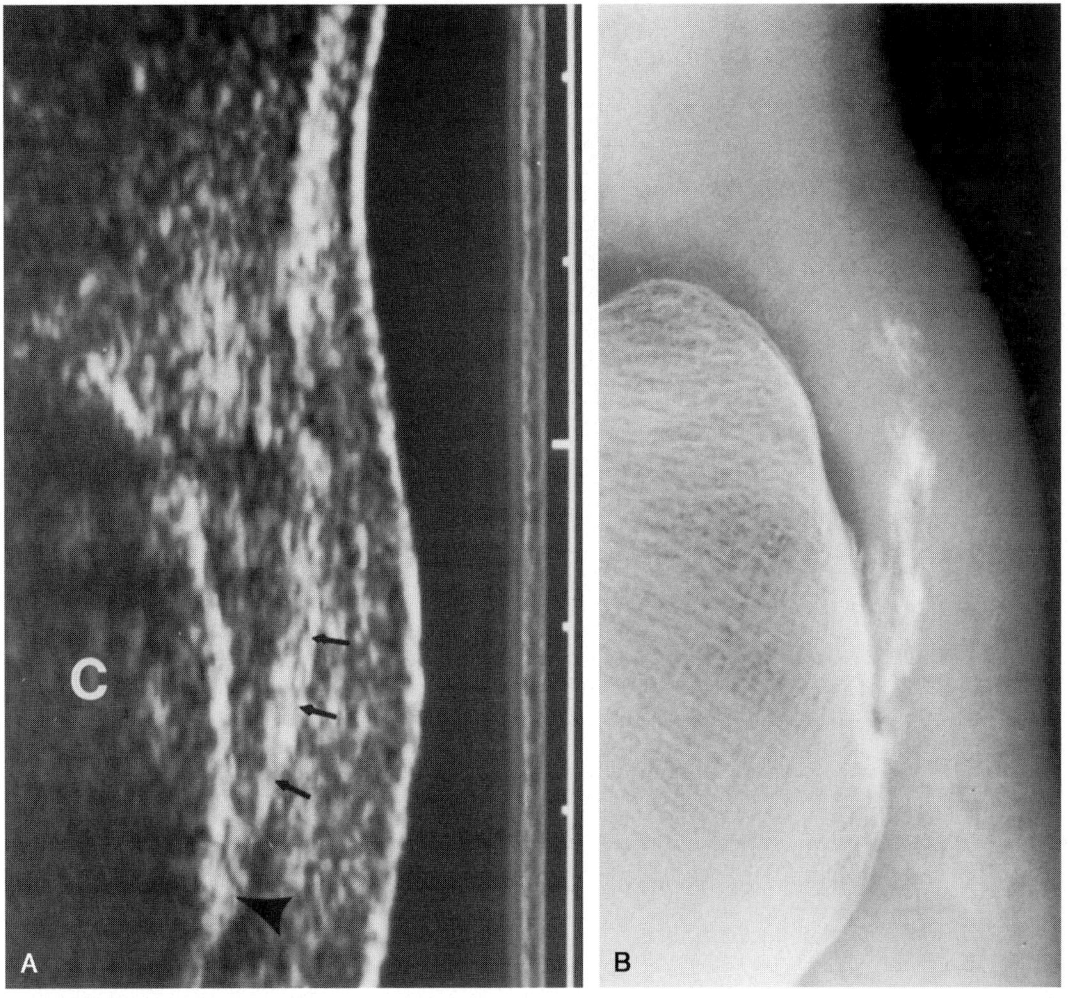

Figure 4-34 ■ **A,** Calcifying tendinitis: sagittal sonogram. A long-distance runner with pain and swelling over the Achilles tendon insertion. A few days prior to the examination, he experienced an acute exacerbation of symptoms. The area of tenderness is now markedly swollen and erythematous. The transducer is oriented in the long axis of the Achilles tendon, overlying its insertion. The triangular fibrocartilaginous insertion demonstrates increased reflectivity. The most hyperechoic areas are the distal part of the insertion (*black arrowhead*) and the marginal areas of the insertion (*black arrows*). Small areas of acoustic shadowing correspond to calcifications within the tendon. Abbreviation: calcaneus (*C*). **B**, Calcifying tendinitis: Gevaert MRL radiograph. Same patient as in **A**. Conventional radiograph of the heel (*lateral view*) demonstrates calcifications within the triangular tendon insertion surrounded by soft tissue swelling.

concluded that the increased ground substance and edema interfered with nutrient transport, compounding the metabolic disturbance caused by trauma.

Patellar tendinitis (jumper's knee) is frequently found in people who participate in sports that require repetitive activity of the extensor mechanism of the knee. Examples include football, soccer, basketball, and track and field (Roels and Martens, 1978; Martens et al., 1982). However, focal patellar tendinitis can also be seen in patients who do not participate in athletics. These patients usually have a history of blunt trauma to the patellar tendon. In rare cases, the cause may be iatrogenic. Lesions identical to those found in blunt trauma can be seen following arthroscopy. When a transtendinous approach is chosen, granulation tissue and tendinitis can be observed at the puncture site (Chapter 13).

Presenting symptoms include pain on climbing stairs, pain on long walks, and pain when sitting with the knees bent. Patellar hypermobility, quadriceps wasting, and local tenderness are frequent findings on physical examination. Localized swelling over the apex of the patella was noted clinically in approximately 5% of our patients. The mean age of our patients with patellar tendonitis is 20 years of age.

Unfortunately, many cases of patellar tendinitis are completely overlooked or misdiagnosed as bursitis or chondromalacia. Correct diagnosis is impera-

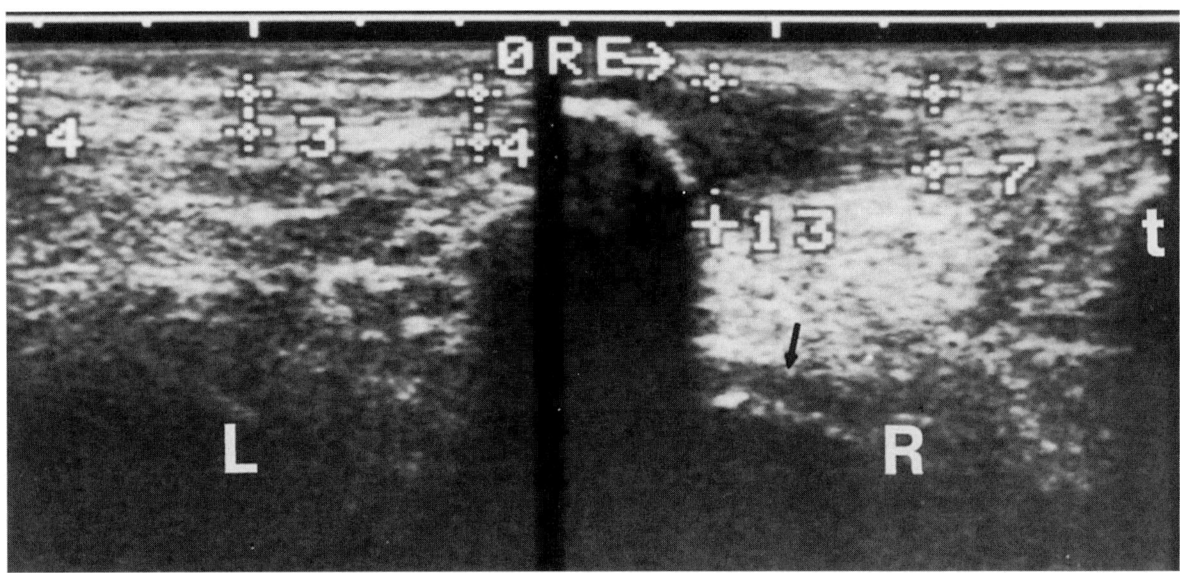

Figure 4–35 ■ Measurement in patellar tendinosis: sagittal sonograms. The patient's normal left knee is seen to the left (*L*). The infrapatellar portion of the patellar tendon is on the left side of the image, and the tibial insertion is on the right. The sagittal diameters are expressed in millimeters. Normal tendons have a sagittal diameter between 3 and 5 mm. Comparison with the asymptomatic side is very helpful. The patient's symptomatic right knee is seen on the right (*R*). Traumatic lesions in the patellar tendon are located under the patellar apex in more than 90% of cases. The infrapatellar portion of the tendon is hypoechoic and enlarged. The sagittal diameter is more than three times the normal diameter. Hoffa's fat pad is increased in echogenicity, which allows better visualization of the condylar cartilage (*black arrow*). Abbreviation: tibia (*t*).

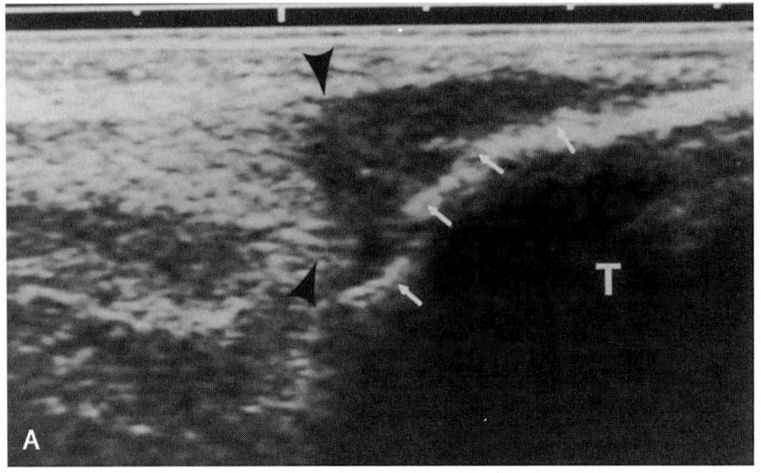

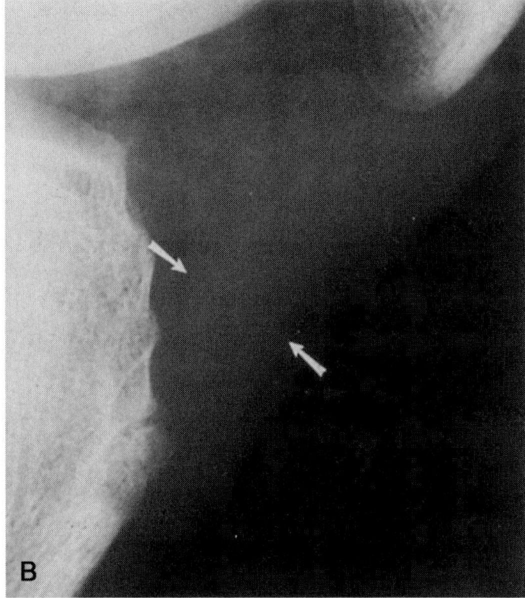

Figure 4–36 ■ **A**, Atypical patellar tendinosis: longitudinal sonogram. This 27-year-old basketball player presented with chronic pain in his knee. As a child, he was treated for Osgood-Schlatter disease. The image is a longitudinal sonogram through the patellar tendon. The distal end of the patellar tendon and the insertion on the tibia have a hypoechoic appearance. The diameter of the tendon is markedly increased (*black arrowheads*). The insertion on the tibia (*T*) has a highly irregular surface (*white arrows*). **B**, Atypical patellar tendinosis: conventional radiograph depicting a lateral view of the knee. Swelling (*white arrows*) of the distal end of the patellar tendon and irregularity of the patellar tendon insertion are present.

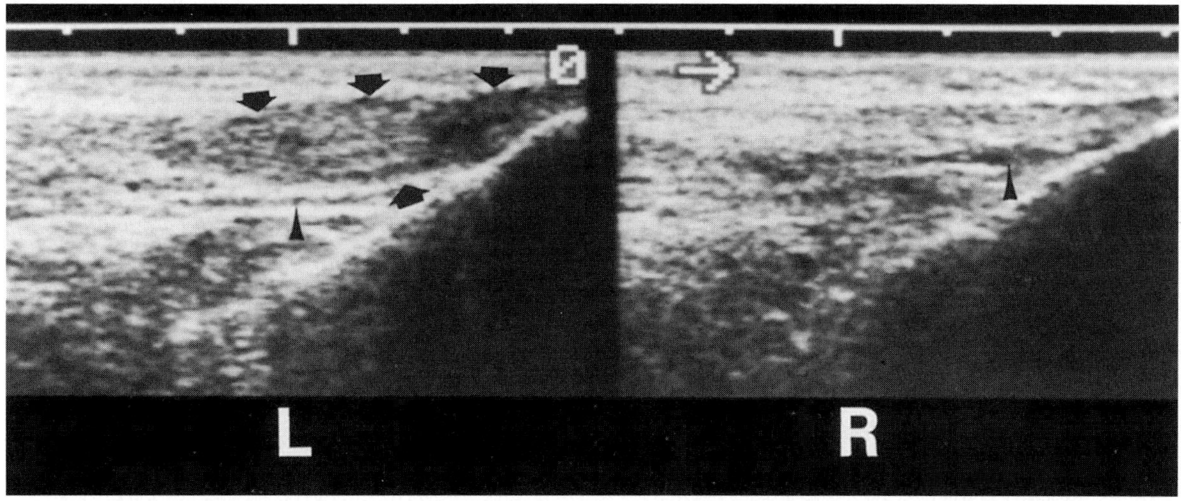

Figure 4–37 ■ Distal patellar tendinosis with incomplete rupture: longitudinal sonograms. A 40-year-old man with chronic pain in the left knee after blunt trauma to the anterior aspect of the knee. Longitudinal sonograms through the patellar tendons. The entire distal half of the left patellar tendon is swollen and hypoechoic (*arrows*). Some of the fibers are interrupted in the most distal 2 cm of the tendon. The right patellar tendon is normal. Normal deep infrapatellar bursa (*arrowheads*) are seen.

tive for institution of adequate therapy. Sonography can be especially important in selecting those cases that are best suited for surgical treatment.

In patellar tendinitis, two patterns may be seen sonographically: focal or global tendon thickening. Focal tendon thickening was observed in 91.5% of our cases. In the majority of these cases (97%), the site of thickening was proximal (Martens et al., 1982) near the apex of the patella (Fig. 4–35). The remaining 3% of cases of focal thickening demonstrated the lesion near the tibial tuberosity (Figs. 4–36 and 4–37).

Global tendon thickening comprised 8.5% of our cases. This was the result of very long-standing disease and is frequently a precursor to tendon rupture. Figure 4–38 demonstrates the

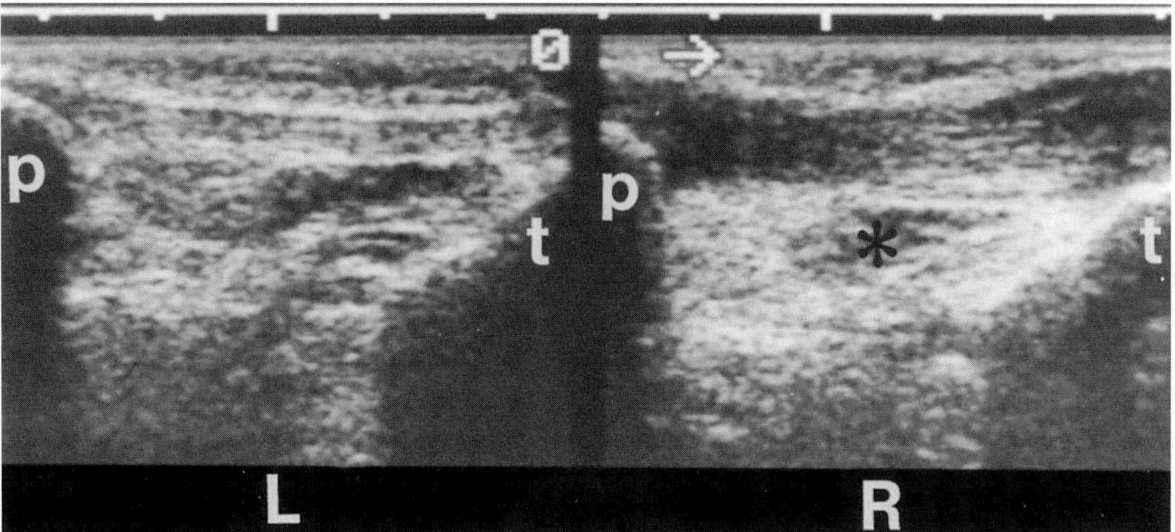

Figure 4–38 ■ Global patellar tendinosis: longitudinal sonograms. A patient with right patellar tendinosis for more than 4 years. He played volleyball, but due to constant pain, he stopped all sports activity. The transducer is positioned along the length of the patellar tendon between the apex of the patella (*p*) at the left and the insertion on the tibia (*t*). The entire tendon is thickened and hypoechoic in appearance. Hoffa's fat pad is markedly hyperreflective throughout (*black asterisk*).

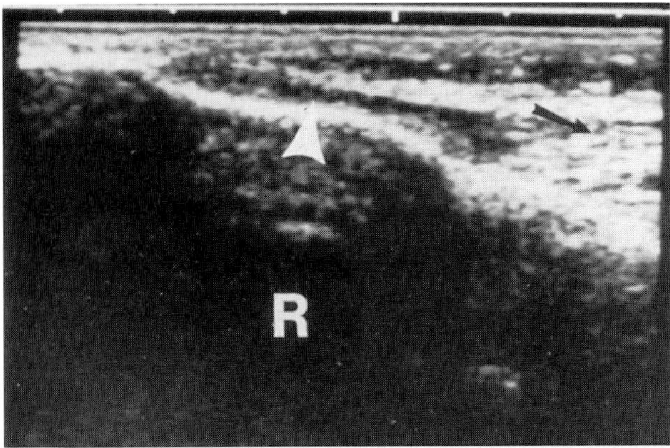

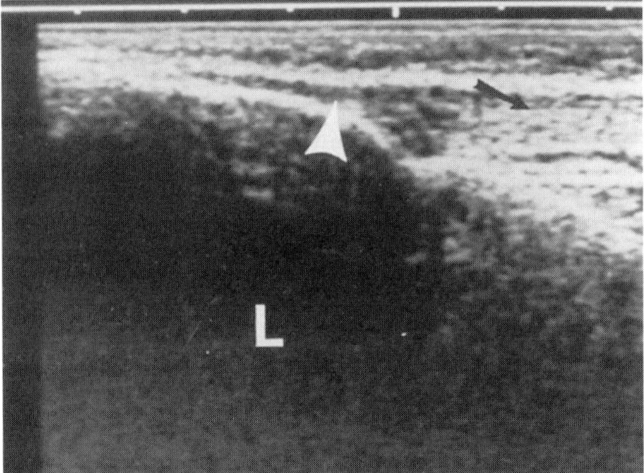

Figure 4–39 ▪ Insertion tendinopathy of the distal patellar tendon: longitudinal sonograms. A 23-year-old soccer player with pain over the tibial tuberosity. The transducer is positioned in the longitudinal axis of the patellar tendon. The distal patellar tendon lies on the observer's left. Thickening and decreased echogenicity are seen in the tendon insertion of the right knee (*R*). The tendon insertion on the left is normal. At surgery, the condition was found to be edema of cartilage and inflammation of the perichondrium. No necrosis was present. It did not require surgical treatment. Tendon insertion (*arrowhead*) and tendon fibers (*arrow*).

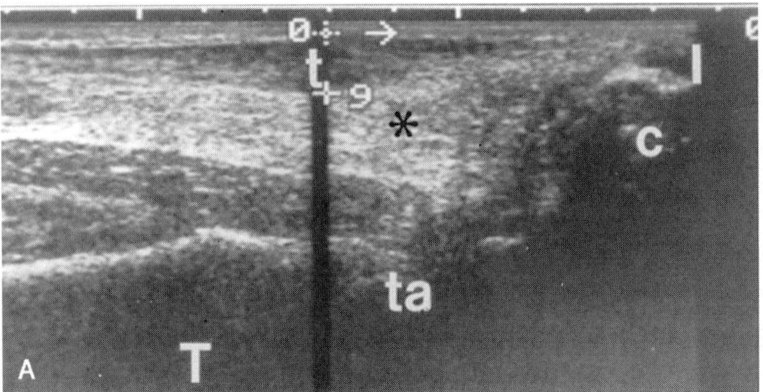

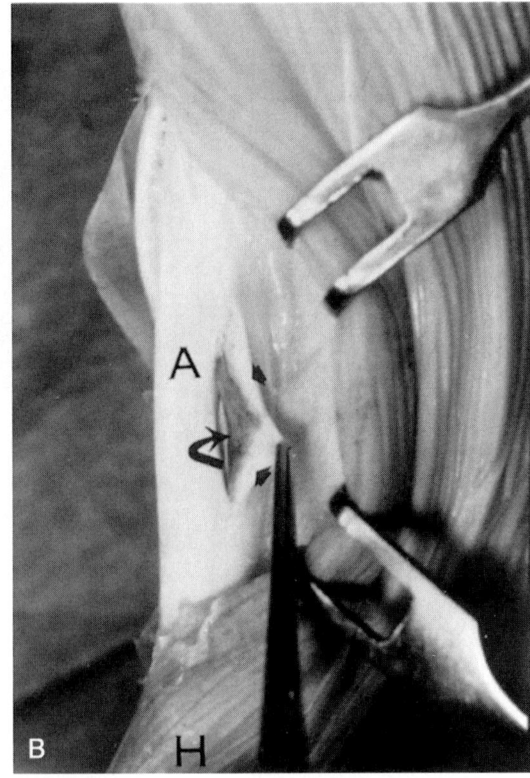

Figure 4–40 ▪ **A**, Achilles tendinosis, proximal type: longitudinal sonogram. A 24-year-old long-distance runner with pain in the Achilles tendon at the beginning of exercise, which persisted. Swelling of the tendon after exercise was evident. The transducer is positioned posteriorly over the Achilles tendon. An image is constructed of the entire Achilles tendon using image memory to juxtapose two images. Maximal thickening of the tendon (*t*) is seen 6 cm above the tendon insertion (*I*). The tendon has a hypoechoic appearance with a maximal thickness of 9 mm. Kager's fat pad appears hyperechoic (*black asterisk*). Abbreviations: tibia (*T*), talus (*ta*), calcaneus (*c*). **B**, Intraoperative photograph of Achilles tendinosis. Same patient as in **A**. The peritenon has been incised (*short arrows*) and is being retracted with a pair of toothed forceps. Within the tendon, fibromyxoid and necrotic tissue is seen (*curved arrow*). Abbreviations: heel (*H*), Achilles tendon (*A*).

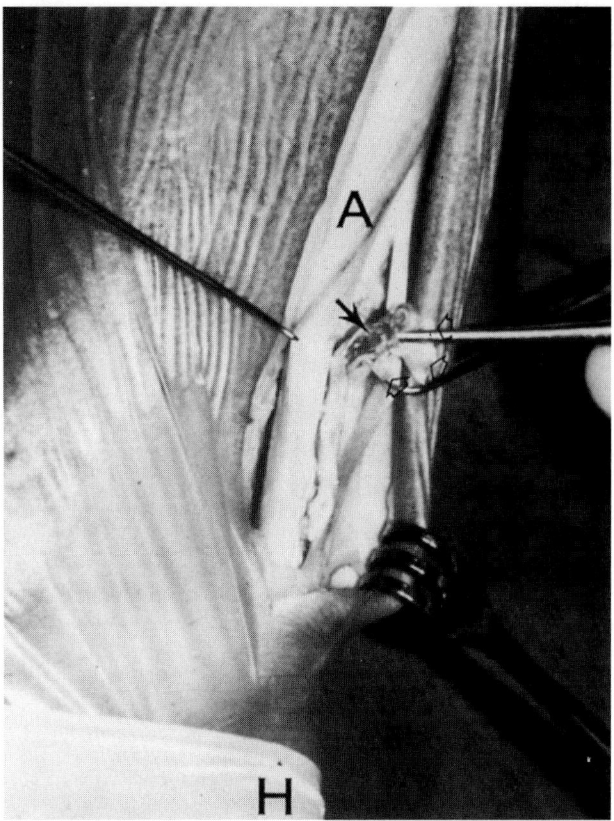

Figure 4–41 ■ Intraoperative photograph of another patient with Achilles tendinosis. Again, the peritenon has been incised and retracted. Granulation tissue is seen within the tendon (*black arrow*). Several ruptured fiber bundles are reflected posteriorly (*open arrows*). Abbreviations: heel (*H*), Achilles tendon (*A*).

sonographic appearance of global tendon thickening. Patients with global tendon thickening or foci of amorphous material within the tendon are candidates for surgical treatment. However, it should be noted that symptoms are not related directly to sonographic tendon morphology. A recent study of female athletes showed that a hypoechoic tendon abnormality can predate the development of symptoms or persist for some time after the symptoms of jumper's knee resolve. The investigators in

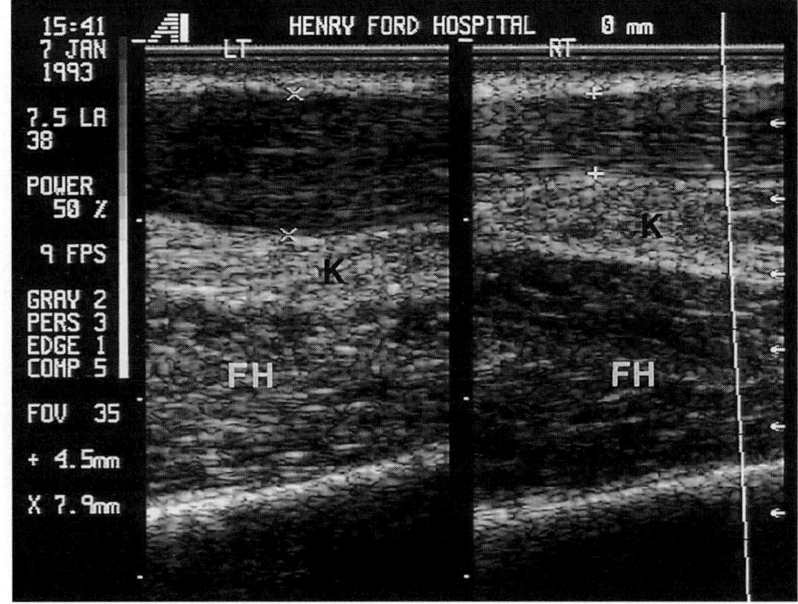

Figure 4–42 ■ Achilles tendinosis, proximal type: split-screen comparison. A jogger with continuous pain in the Achilles tendon. The image on the left of the split screen is a detail of a longitudinal sonogram through the symptomatic left Achilles tendon (*LT*) at the level of the distal tibia and approximately 6 cm above the insertion. There is fusiform swelling of the tendon (*between the cursors*). The tendon has a hypoechoic appearance, and the distance between the longitudinal tendon fascicles is widened. The surrounding fat of Kager's fat pad (*K*) is hyperechoic and compressed between the tendon and the flexor hallucis longus muscle (*FH*). The flexor hallucis on the symptomatic side appears more echogenic because of increased through-transmission. Compare the abnormal left (*LT*) with the normal right (*RT*) Achilles tendon. The cursors measure the anteroposterior diameter of both Achilles tendons.

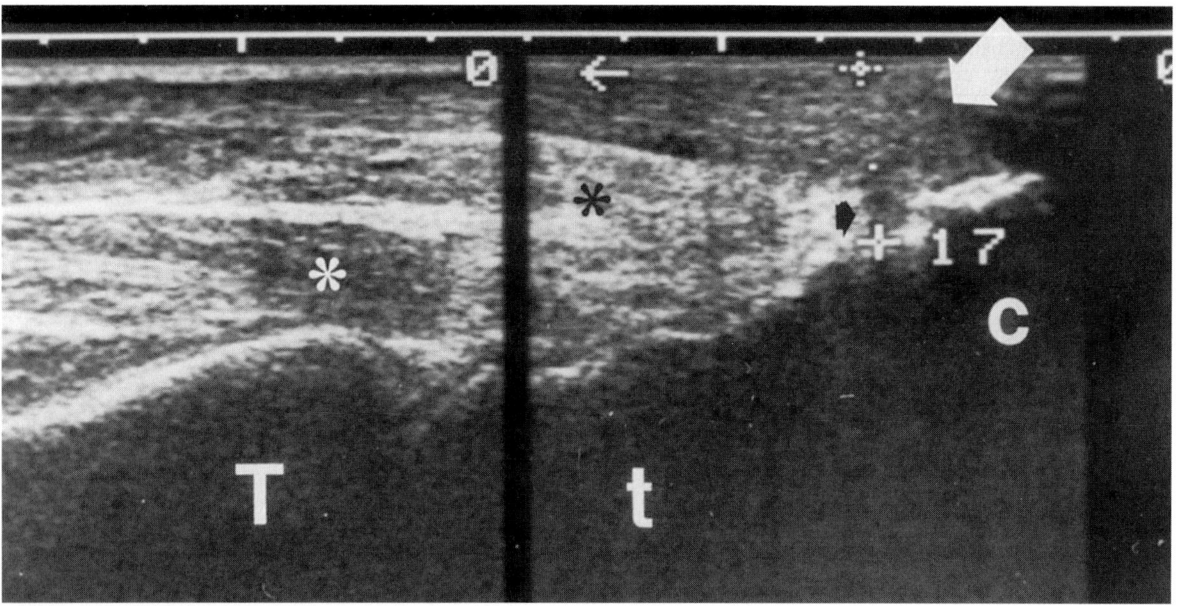

Figure 4–43 ■ Achilles tendinosis, distal type: longitudinal sonogram. After minor injury to the posterior aspect of the heel, this 20-year-old long-distance runner developed pain located at the distal insertion of the Achilles tendon. The pain was worse at the beginning and end of exercise. The transducer is positioned dorsally over the Achilles tendon. An image of the entire tendon is produced using image memory to juxtapose two images. Maximal thickening of the Achilles tendon is seen just superior to the calcaneus (*white arrow*). In addition, there is inflammation of the retrocalcaneal bursa (*black arrow*). The normal retrocalcaneal bursa is flat. Here it has an ovoid appearance. Abbreviations and symbols: pretendinous fat pad (*black asterisk*), tibia (*T*), talus (*t*), calcaneus (*c*), flexor hallucis longus muscle (*white asterisk*).

this study stress that conservative treatment is the first-line therapy for patellar tendinitis and that surgery should be contemplated only when appropriate conservative treatment fails (Khan et al., 1997).

The differential diagnosis of patellar tendinitis includes two other disease processes that can elicit identical clinical symptoms. Bursitis involving one of the peritendinous bursae is a frequent cause of localized tenderness over the patella or tibial tuberosity (Bywaters, 1979). This is easily differentiated from patellar tendinitis sonographically. An oval, anechoic, fluid-filled structure is identified adjacent to the patellar tendon. These lesions dif-

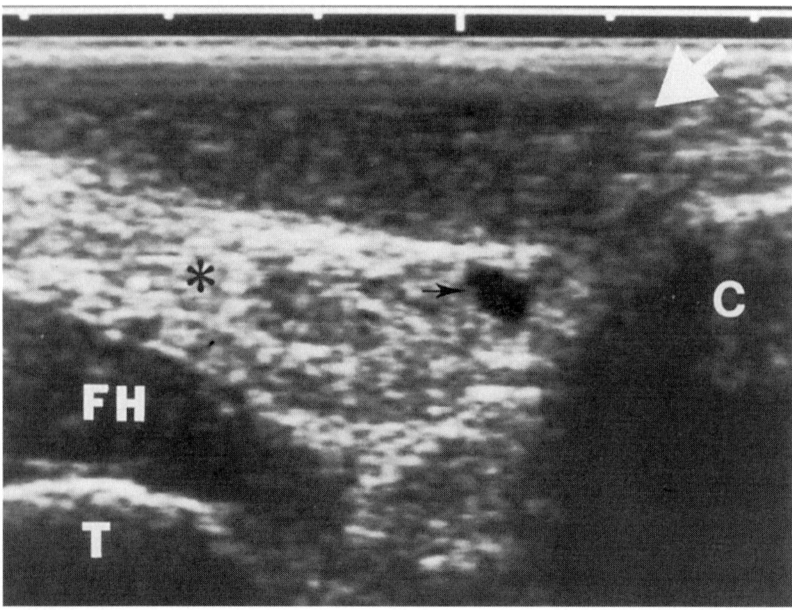

Figure 4–44 ■ Achilles tendinosis, distal type: longitudinal sonogram. Pain, erythema, and swelling were present over the Achilles tendon insertion in this 20-year-old basketball player. The image is a detail of a longitudinal sonogram through the Achilles tendon (*white arrow*) at the level of the calcaneus (*C*). Fusiform swelling of the distal 5 cm of the tendon is present. The retrocalcaneal bursa is enlarged (*black arrow*). Note the increased echogenicity of Kager's fat pad (*black asterisk*). Abbreviations: tibia (*T*), flexor hallucis longus muscle (*FH*).

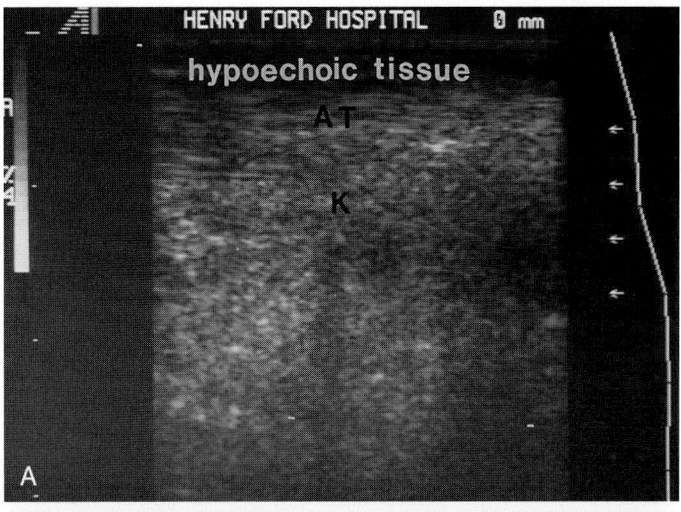

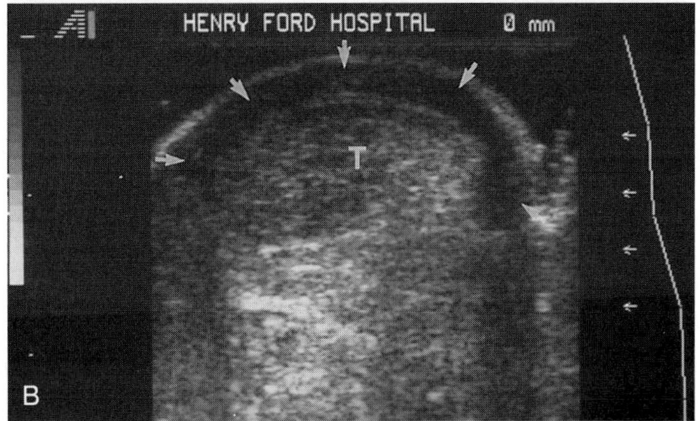

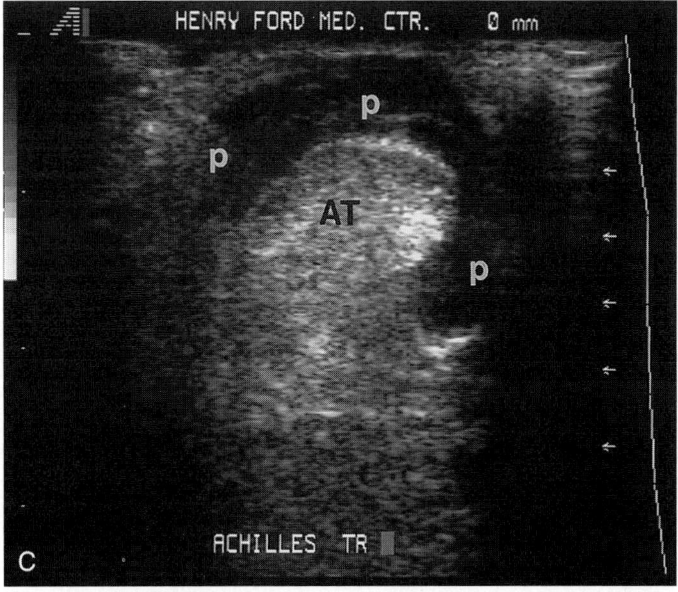

Figure 4–45 ■ **A**, Peritendinitis of the Achilles tendon: longitudinal sonogram. This 58-year-old woman has had rheumatoid arthritis for 2 years. Heel pain developed recently. The pain intensifies toward the end of the day, especially when she is on her feet for a long time. The transducer is positioned in the long axis of the Achilles tendon over the dorsal aspect of the heel. Posterior to the tendon, an abnormal hypoechoic tissue layer is seen; this tissue causes increased through-transmission. Abbreviations: Achilles tendon (*AT*), Kager's fat pad (*K*). **B**, Peritendinitis of the Achilles tendon: transverse sonogram. Same patient as in **A**. The transverse image of the tendon (*T*) demonstrates posterior, medial, and lateral thickening of the peritenon (*arrows*). **C**, Peritendinitis of the Achilles tendon: transverse sonogram. Another middle-aged woman with rheumatoid arthritis and ankle pain. The transverse ultrasound scan, which was performed with a 7.5-MHz linear array transducer, shows the hoof-shaped, hypoechoic swelling of the peritenon (*p*) around the Achilles tendon (*AT*); the finding is characteristic of peritendinitis. Peritendinitis occurs in rheumatoid arthritis, but the changes can occur in tendon disease induced by overuse as well.

fer in both prognosis and therapeutic management. Therefore, a definitive diagnosis is mandatory. Bursitis will be discussed in more detail in Chapter 5.

Insertion tendonopathy (Merkel et al., 1982) is another entity included in the differential diagnosis of patellar tendinitis. This disease occurs almost exclusively in athletes. It is limited to the fibrocartilaginous insertion of the tendon. The diagnosis of insertion tendonopathy is made if enlargement of the cartilaginous insertion is identified (Fig. 4–39). Differentiation of this disease process from tendinitis is very important because there is no indication for surgery in insertion tendonopathy.

Achilles tendinitis is found somewhat less frequently than patellar tendonitis. The population at greatest risk is once again athletes (Palvalgyi and Balint, 1981; Clement et al., 1984). In our institution, the mean age of those afflicted with Achilles tendinitis is 33.5 years, 13.5 years older than the population with patellar tendinitis. However, closer examination of the data reveals a bimodal age distribution of individuals with Achilles tendinitis.

The older group, with a mean age of 35 years, demonstrates tendon thickening in the proximal portion of the tendon. This comprises 85% of all cases of Achilles tendinitis (Figs. 4–40 through 4–42). Individuals with lesions in the distal 5 cm of the tendon fall into the second age peak, which has a mean age of 25 years. These patients represent 14.8% of all cases. An associated retrocalcaneal bursitis (Canoso, 1984) is almost always present in these cases (Figs. 4–43 and 4–44). The prognosis for patients with distal lesions is significantly worse than that for patients with proximal lesions. Proximal lesions in Achilles tendinitis are amenable to treatment by surgical release. In our experience, surgical therapy has not been successful in treating distal lesions.

The remaining 0.2% of cases of Achilles tendinitis affect only the epitendineum and surrounding loose areolar tissues (Clement et al., 1984). This diagnosis is made when edema is seen surrounding the tendon. The tendon itself appears normal (Fig. 4–45). Surgical pathology demonstrates edema and inflammation affecting the epitendineum and adjacent mesenchymal tissues (Fig. 4–46).

The differential diagnosis of Achilles tendinitis includes metabolic causes of tendinosis, Haglund's disease, retrocalcaneal bursitis, and insertion tendonopathy. Gout and hypercholesterolemia (Fig. 4–47) can cause swelling of the Achilles tendon through deposition of uric acid and cholesterol deposition, respectively. This deposition is often symmetric in both Achilles tendons, and calcifications can occur in the deposits. The pump-bump of Haglund's disease is due to thickening of the dermis and hypoderm (Fig. 4–48). This is often accompanied by a bony excrescence on the posterosuperior aspect of the calcaneus. During exacerbations, a retrocalcaneal or subcutaneous bursitis develops. This is easily differentiated sonographically and is discussed further in Chapter 5 (see Figs. 5–12 and 5–13).

Isolated disease of the retrocalcaneal bursa will emulate Achilles tendinitis clinically. This condition can result from trauma, psoriasis, Reiter's disease, or rheumatoid arthritis (see Fig. 5–32). In cases of in-

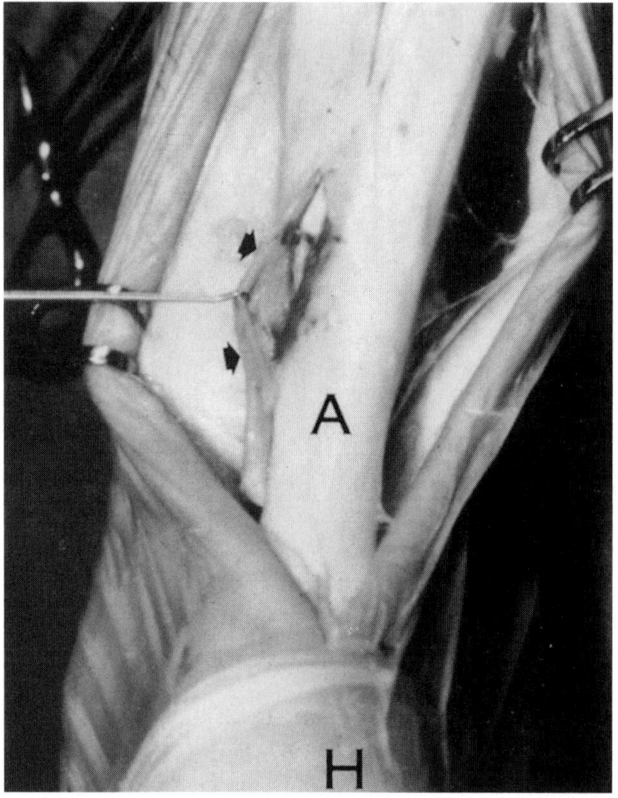

Figure 4–46 ▪ Intraoperative photograph of peritendinitis of the Achilles tendon. The hypoechoic layer surrounding the posterior portion of the Achilles tendon (*A*) represents the incised band of fibrous tissue being retracted laterally (*short arrows*). This is secondary to a chronic inflammatory reaction in the peritenon. Abbreviation: heel (*H*).

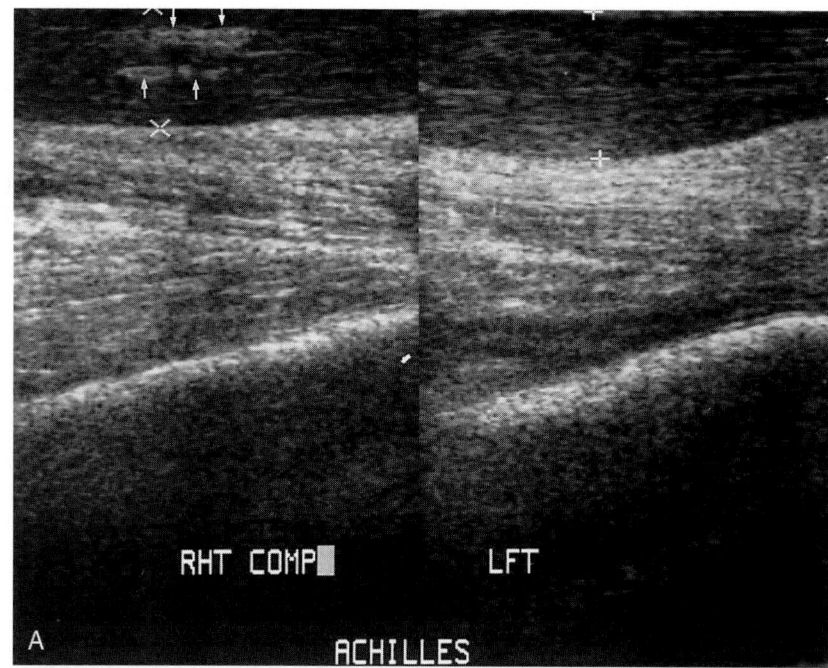

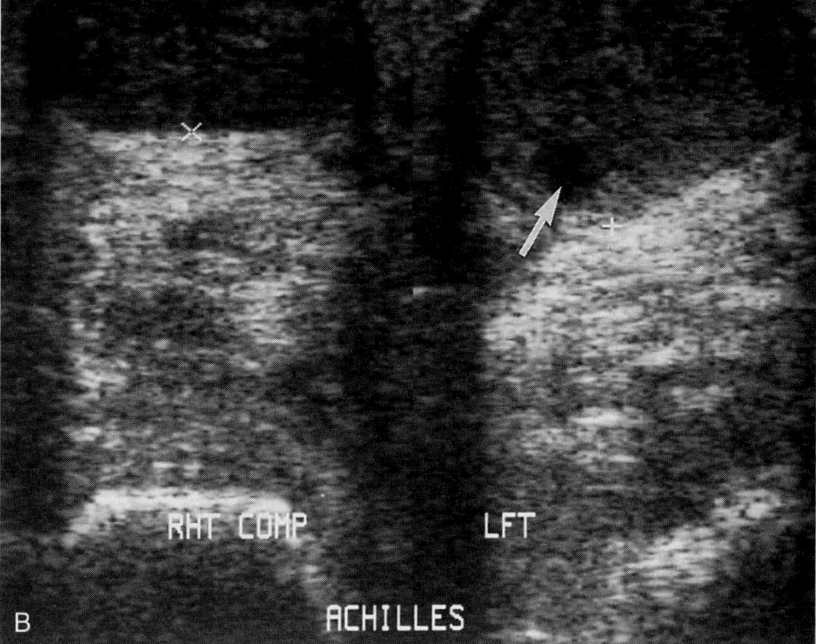

Figure 4-47 ■ **A**, Tendinosis in a patient with hypercholesterolemia: split screen with comparison of longitudinal sonograms. A 78-year-old woman with hypothyroidism presents with bilateral posterior ankle pain and swelling. Both Achilles tendons (*between the calipers*) are fusiformly swollen, inhomogeneous, and predominantly hypoechoic. Linear streaks (*arrows*) of hyperechogenicity are noted in the central aspect of the right Achilles tendon. The sonographer suggests the diagnosis of hypercholesterolemia because of the bilateral Achilles swelling despite the patient's lack of physical activity. **B**, Tendinosis in a patient with hypercholesterolemia: split screen with comparison of transverse sonograms. Same patient as in **A**. The transverse images show that both Achilles tendons have lost their normal kidney shape. The left tendon (*LFT*) is more affected, and the shape of its cross section is almost round. Both tendons are hypoechoic. A patch (*arrow*) in the left tendon appears nearly anechoic. Focal anechoic and hypoechoic lesions have been reported frequently in hypercholesterolemia.

Figure continued on following page

flammatory bursitis, irregular thickening of the wall of the bursa can often be detected sonographically. Traumatic bursitis carries a better prognosis than tendinitis or inflammatory bursitis.

An insertion tendonopathy is another possibility in the differential diagnosis of Achilles tendinitis. It usually results from traumatic overload of the tendon. The lesion is restricted to the fibrocartilage at the insertion of the Achilles tendon on the calcaneus. This region appears as a hypoechoic triangle at the junction of the tendon with the calcaneus. In cases of insertion tendinopathy, sonography shows thickening of the cartilaginous insertion of the Achilles tendon; in some cases, calcific deposits are detected in an inflamed cartilaginous insertion (see Fig. 4-34). Therefore, we believe that the insertion tendinopathy of the Achilles tendon is closely related to calcific tendinitis. This type of lesion is not an indication for surgery (Fiamengo et al., 1982).

Tendinitis in other locations can be demonstrated sonographically. In the upper extremity, the

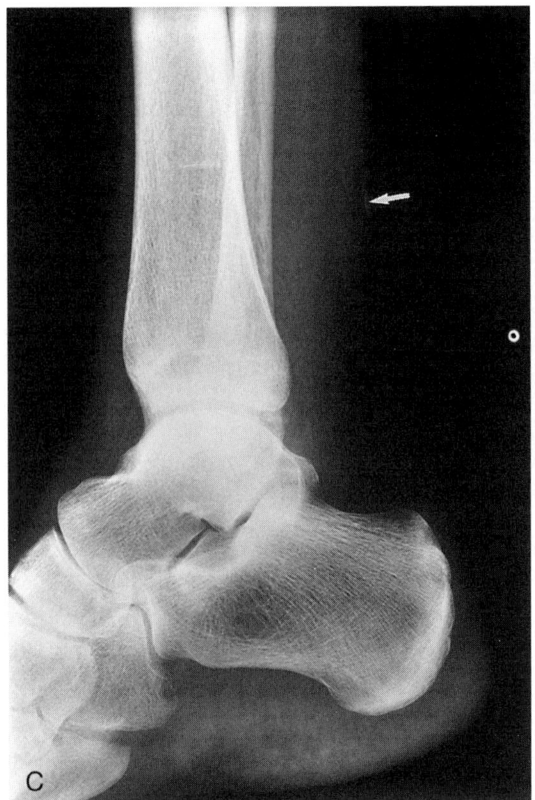

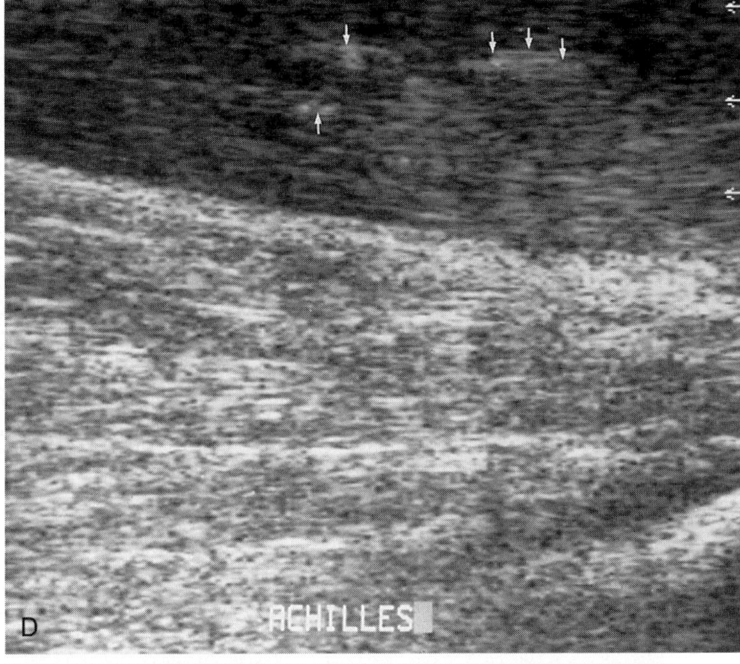

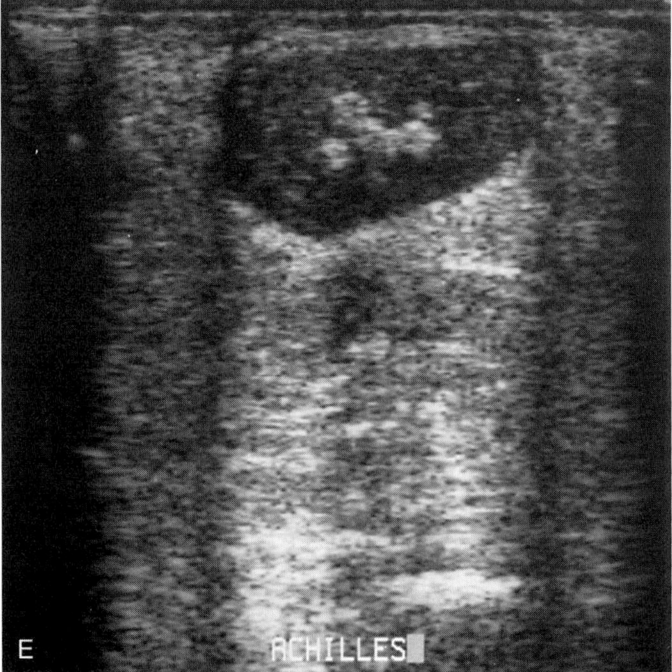

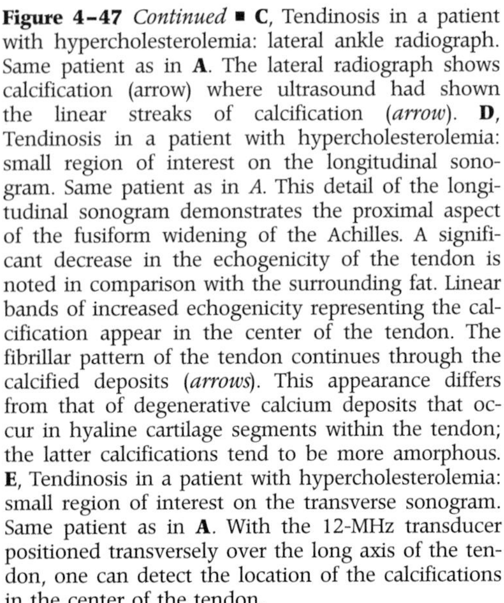

Figure 4–47 *Continued* ■ **C**, Tendinosis in a patient with hypercholesterolemia: lateral ankle radiograph. Same patient as in **A**. The lateral radiograph shows calcification (arrow) where ultrasound had shown the linear streaks of calcification (*arrow*). **D**, Tendinosis in a patient with hypercholesterolemia: small region of interest on the longitudinal sonogram. Same patient as in *A*. This detail of the longitudinal sonogram demonstrates the proximal aspect of the fusiform widening of the Achilles. A significant decrease in the echogenicity of the tendon is noted in comparison with the surrounding fat. Linear bands of increased echogenicity representing the calcification appear in the center of the tendon. The fibrillar pattern of the tendon continues through the calcified deposits (*arrows*). This appearance differs from that of degenerative calcium deposits that occur in hyaline cartilage segments within the tendon; the latter calcifications tend to be more amorphous. **E**, Tendinosis in a patient with hypercholesterolemia: small region of interest on the transverse sonogram. Same patient as in **A**. With the 12-MHz transducer positioned transversely over the long axis of the tendon, one can detect the location of the calcifications in the center of the tendon.

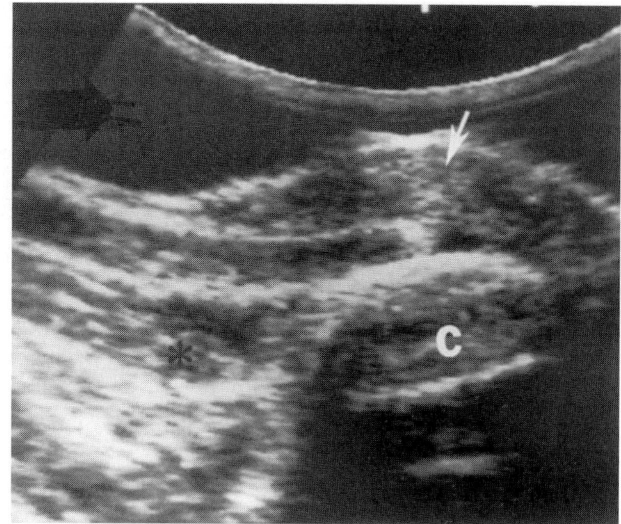

Figure 4–48 ▪ Haglund's disease: longitudinal sonogram. An 18-year-old girl with pain and chronic swelling over the distal Achilles tendon. For this examination, a 5-MHz radial array transducer with a standoff pad was utilized (*black arrow*). The FOV is larger than that of a 5-MHz linear array transducer, but the images of the Achilles tendon and the tendon insertion suffer from decreased spatial resolution and anisotropy. The characteristic pump-bump of Haglund's disease is seen as thickening of the skin and subcutaneous tissues (*white arrow*). Abbreviation and symbol: prominent calcaneus (*C*), fat pad (*black asterisk*).

tendons of the brachial flexors and extensors may be examined. Tendinitis is common at the tendon origins over the medial and lateral epicondyles of the elbow. The best-known example of tendinitis in the arm is edema and swelling of the proximal extensor carpi radialis, known as *tennis elbow*. The quadriceps (suprapatellar) tendon, tendon of the hamstrings, adductor tendons, and pes anserinus can be examined in the lower extremity. Careful side-to-side comparison of identical segments is essential in these cases. In our experience, the sensitivity of the sonographic examination in these regions is less than that in other, more accessible areas. Hypoechoic swelling is seen in the majority of the cases. Echogenic foci with or without acoustic shadowing are present in cases of calcific tendinitis.

Tendon Rupture

Rotator cuff tears are a frequent finding in the elderly and may be entirely asymptomatic. Autopsy studies of individuals more than 55 years old have discovered rotator cuff tears in 32% (Petersson and Gentz, 1983). However, a true traumatic tear is a rare finding. These lesions are found in athletes

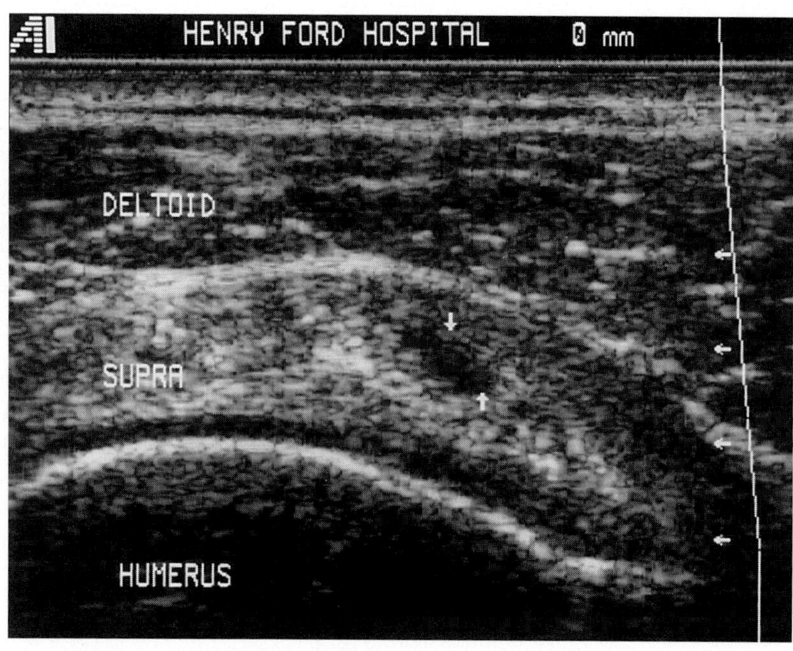

Figure 4–49 ▪ Intratendinous tear: transverse ultrasound. A 52-year-old tennis player with pain in the right shoulder worsened by elevation. Clinical examination demonstrated a painful arc. The transducer is positioned horizontally lateral to the acromion. The shoulder anatomy in this area is seen as a bilayered structure. The most superficial part is the deltoid muscle (*DELTOID*). Directly overlying the hyperechoic bone and the hypoechoic cartilage is the supraspinatus tendon (*SUPRA*), which is slightly more reflective than the deltoid. In the anterior portion of the tendon is a hypoechoic region representing a partial tear (*arrows*) in the substance of the tendon.

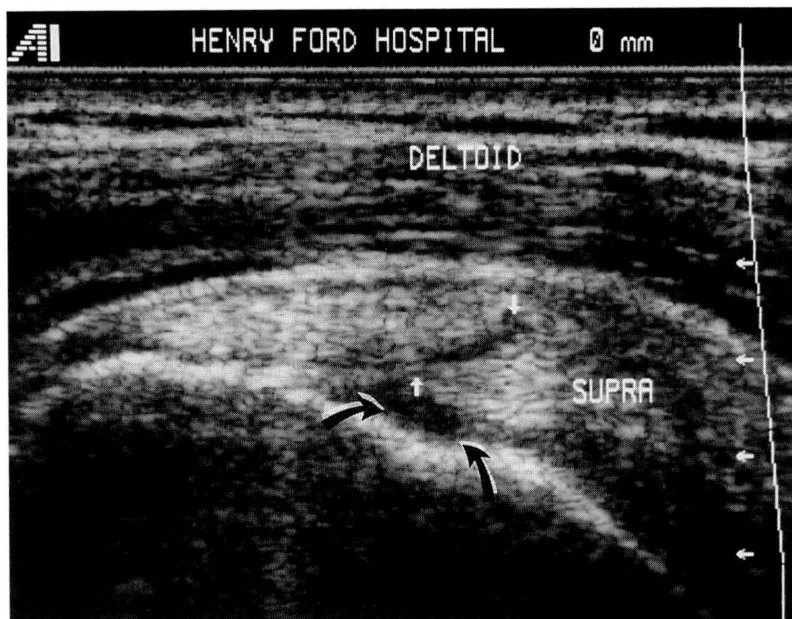

Figure 4–50 ▪ Partial tear: longitudinal ultrasound. Pain in the shoulder of this 47-year-old man started after an episode of intense weight-lifting activity. A linear lesion appeared in this patient's supraspinatus tendon 8 months before the current ultrasound examination. The longitudinal ultrasound scan demonstrates a linear hypoechoic cleft (*arrows*) which was unchanged from the prior study. The lesion was considered an articular side partial-thickness tear of the tendon because of its broad extension (*curved arrows*) over the anatomical neck of the humerus.

who repeatedly perform a throwing motion (e.g., baseball pitchers, javelin throwers, and football quarterbacks) and in contact sports after shoulder dislocation.

The principal sonographic findings of full-thickness tears (Bretzke et al., 1985; Mack et al., 1985) are fluid-filled clefts in the supraspinatus in axial images (Middleton et al., 1985a) with increased fluid in the subdeltoid bursa or retraction of the supraspinatus from the very lateral edge of the lateral tuberosity, with associated pitting of the cortical surface (Wohlwend et al., 1998). In some chronic cases of rotator cuff tear, the supraspinatus muscle layer may be completely absent (Mack et al., 1985). The diameter of the tear measured sonographically is always smaller than that observed with arthroscopy, plain film arthrography, or CT/MRI arthrography (Beltran et al., 1986). In all of these invasive diagnostic modalities, the joint is distended with fluid, air, or both. This leads to an exaggeration of the dimensions of the tear and the degree of muscle retraction (Ahovuo et al., 1984). Tendon tears can be very small. In some cases, they do not extend through the joint capsule or into the subacromial-subdeltoid bursa. These intrasubstance tears are interesting for diagnostic purposes. They can be debrided, but they cannot be repaired surgically. In the early phase of tear by rotator cuff fiber failure, changes appear in the substance of the tendon. Intrasubstance degeneration appears as a hypoechoic focus (Figs. 4–49 and 4–50) within the rotator cuff, and some lesions are characterized by vascular ingrowth and hyperemia (Fig. 4–51). In all likelihood, these partial-thickness changes represent the precursors of full-thickness tears. Sonography, being entirely noninvasive, demonstrates the true extent of the lesion in vivo (Fig. 4–52). This allows the surgeon to plan the procedure preoperatively more accurately.

In cases of small tendon tears, the repair is often made by simple approximation of the two ends with sutures. The prognosis in these lesions is quite good. Large tears, greater than 5 cm, require more extensive procedures. Certain situations may require graft material. In these cases, the prognosis is poor.

Other disease processes are included in the differential diagnosis of painful soft tissue lesions of the shoulder. These include biceps tenosynovitis, biceps tendinosis (Fig. 4–53), biceps tendon dislocation (see Fig. 4–9C), and edema of the rotator cuff (Jobe and Jobe, 1983). Biceps tendon lesions have already been discussed in detail. The diagnosis of rotator cuff edema (Fig. 4–54) can be made sonographically when there is swelling of the rotator cuff, sometimes in association with distention of the subacromial-subdeltoid bursa. Edema of the supraspinatus tendon is seen as enlargement of the affected tendon, with a decrease in its echogenicity. This phenomenon has been described as the initial phase of the impingement syndrome (see Chapter 15). Patients with chronic impingement may eventually develop rotator cuff tears, some

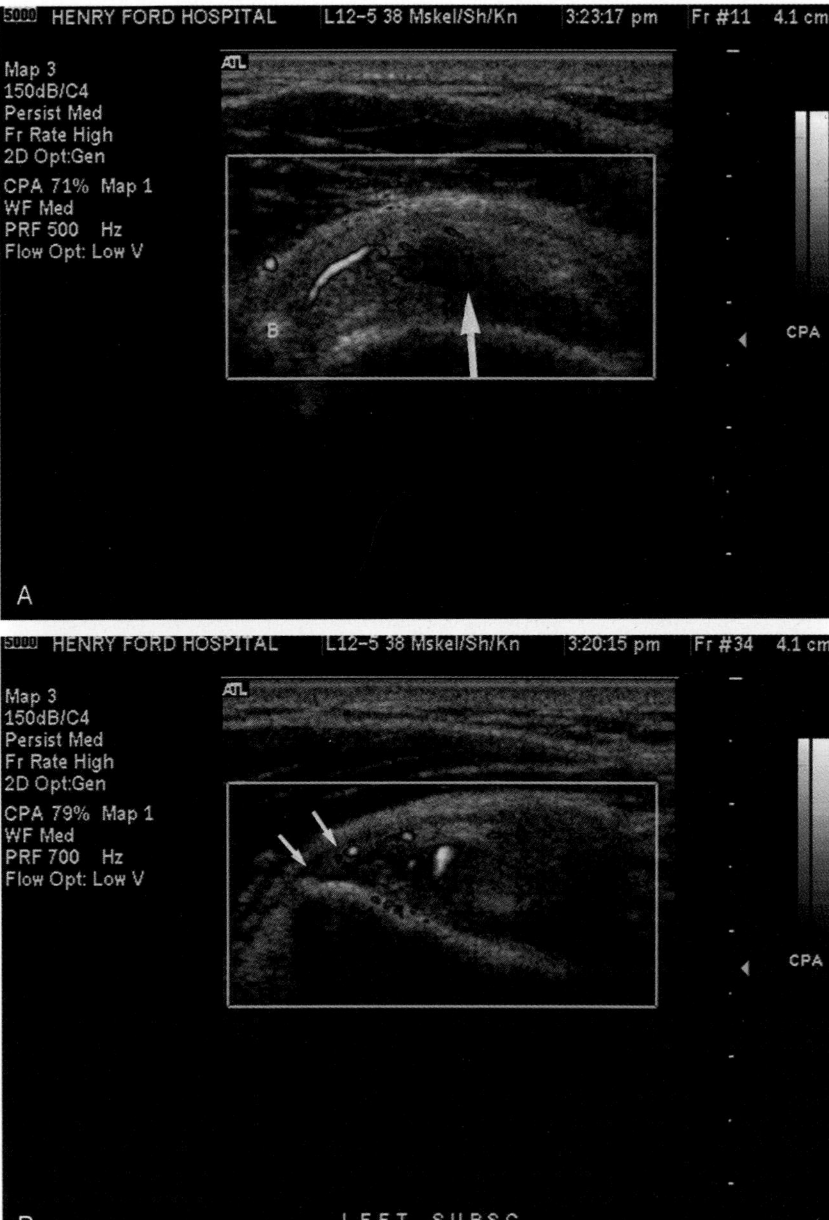

Figure 4–51 ■ **A,** Intratendinous tear: power Doppler sonography in the long axis of the supraspinatus. This 36-year-old man complains of shoulder pain, which started 3 months ago. A vessel penetrates the supraspinatus tendon from the rotator cuff interval, the space surrounding the long biceps tendon (*B*), and is directed toward a hypoechoic focus (*arrow*) within the tendon. **B,** Intratendinous tear: power Doppler sonography in the long axis of the supraspinatus. Same patient as in **A**. The longitudinal tomogram through the hypoechoic tear in the supraspinatus insertion demonstrates several vessels in cross section. Observe that in this partial-thickness tear, the bursal interface (*between the arrows*) can be followed without interruption as far as the lateral edge of the greater tuberosity.

times after 10 to 15 years of shoulder pain (Jobe and Jobe, 1983; Neer, 1983).

Acute shoulder pain and swelling in weight lifters may relate to tears of the rotator cuff and biceps tendon or traumatic lesions of the lateral clavicle and acromioclavicular joint. However, lesions of the pectoralis muscle and tendon should be considered as well. Tears of the myotendinous junction of the pectoralis, lesions that are treated conservatively, must be distinguished from lesions of the pectoralis tendon proper. The true tendon tear is an indication for surgery (Fig. 4–55).

In contrast to rotator cuff tears, rupture of the Achilles tendon is almost always traumatic in origin. These lesions may be found in athletes engaged in high-level competition. The diagnosis is usually made clinically, but it may be overlooked if the rupture is incomplete. Radiographic findings are nonspecific (Fig. 4–56). In a series of 14 cases of Achilles tendon ruptures, 3 were referred to us with the clinical diagnosis of tendinitis. Early diagnosis is imperative, as delay can lead to permanent functional impairment.

Sonographic findings in acute cases of Achilles

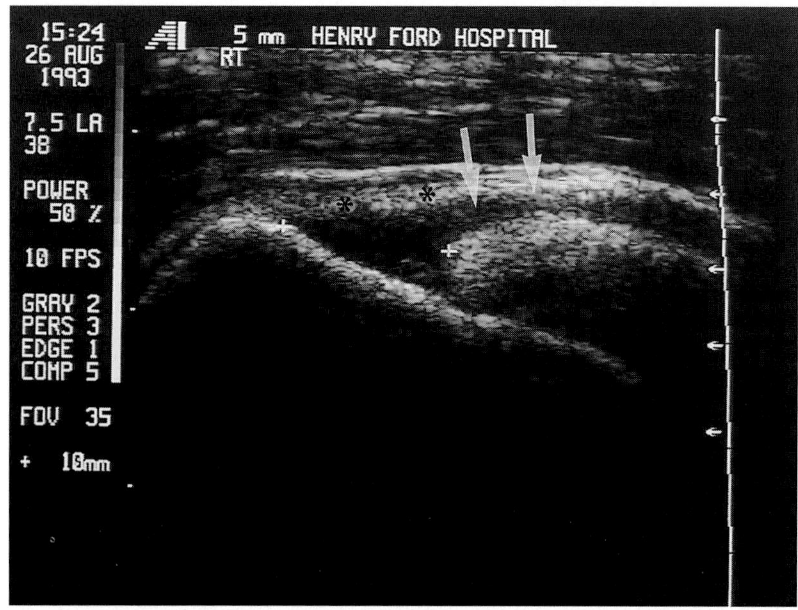

Figure 4–52 ■ Full-thickness tear retracted over the greater tuberosity: longitudinal sonogram. Shoulder pain started 20 years ago when the patient was a 17-year-old baseball pitcher. Now, at age 37, the patient notices pain with throwing, lifting, and overhand activity. Night pain in his shoulder wakes him occasionally. A 7.5-MHz transducer placed over the longitudinal axis of the supraspinatus tendon images the tendon insertion. The bursal interface with the tendon (*between the arrows*) ends over the greater tuberosity and does not extend to the lateral edge, as seen in Figure 4–51B. These findings are consistent with a full-thickness tear. The torn tendon is retracted 1 cm, equal to the distance between the calipers. A full-thickness tear appeared at surgery. Unexperienced examiners mistake the peribursal fat (*asterisks*) for normal tendon all too often.

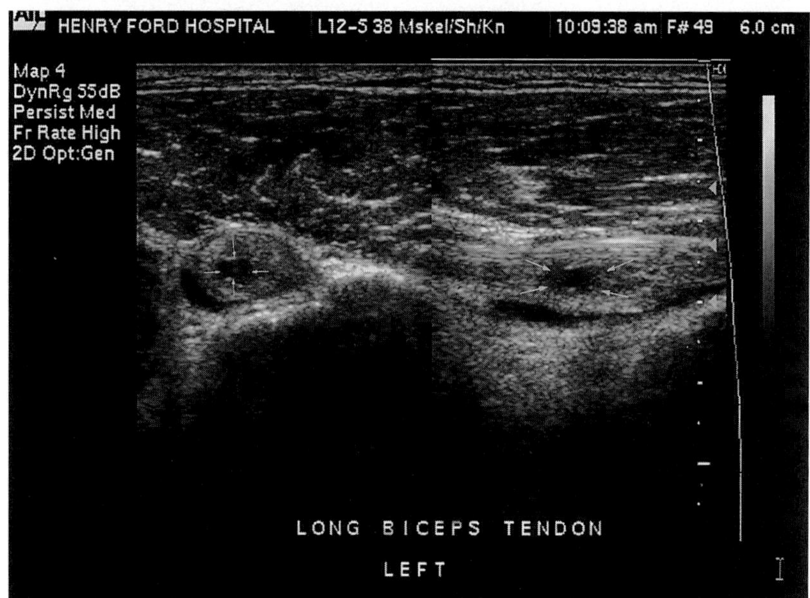

Figure 4–53 ■ Intrasubstance tear of long biceps tendon: split-screen transverse and longitudinal images. In this 38-year-old man, localized pain over the anterior shoulder is aggravated when he lifts heavy objects from a shelf. The patient is unemployed and receives workman's compensation for a back injury. He claims to have no injury. The rotator cuff exam shows no abnormality. The transverse image (left side of the split screen) and the longitudinal image (right side of the split screen) demonstrate a hypoechoic defect (*small arrows*) in the center of the tendon. The tenderness experienced by the patient was elicited by putting transducer pressure on the lesion. It is important to realize that intratendinous tears in the rotator cuff and long biceps tendon are common and are not visible by direct inspection of the surface of the tendon during arthroscopy or open surgery.

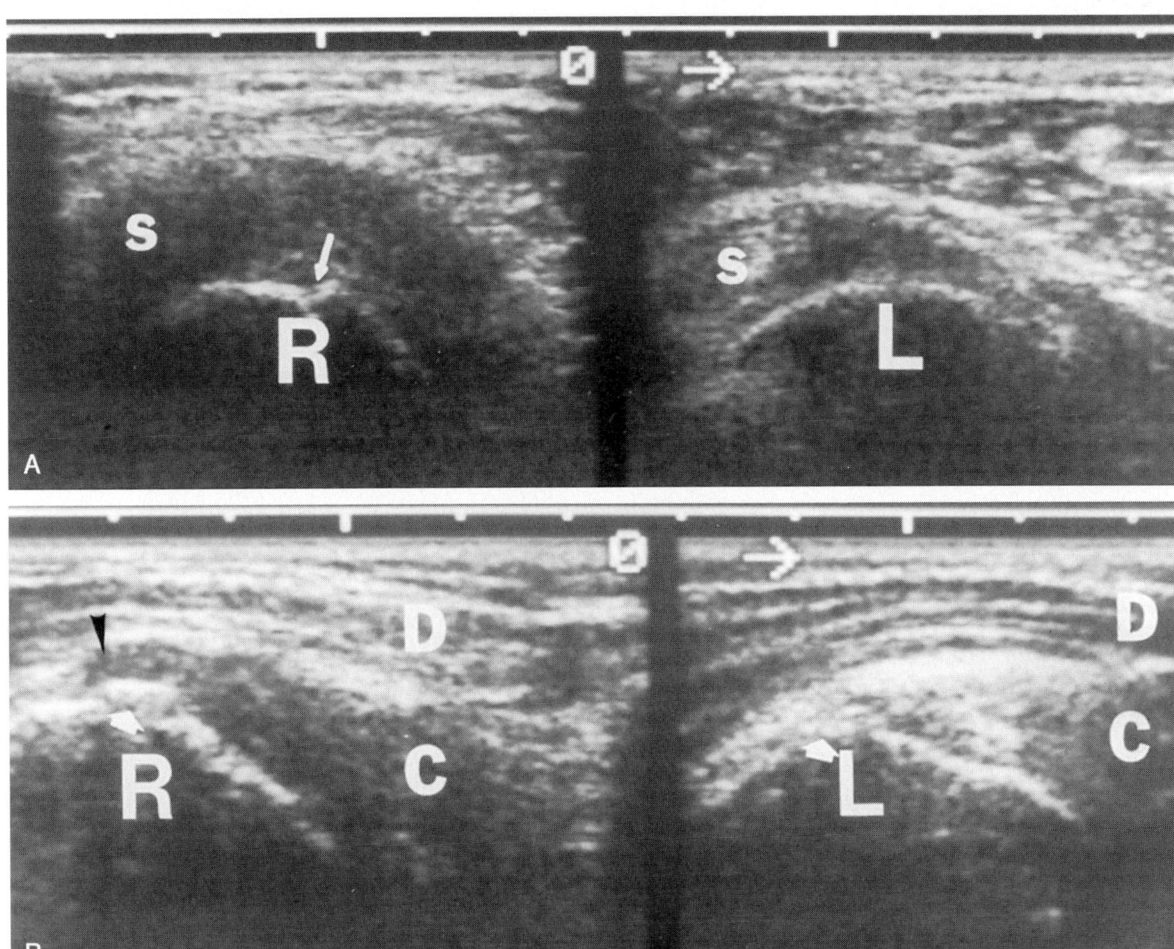

Figure 4–54 ■ **A**, Impingement syndrome with edema of the rotator cuff: transverse sonograms. An axial sonogram of the right (*R*) and left (*L*) shoulders. The patient is a house painter with pain in his right shoulder. Clinically, he has a painful arc and is tender over the rotator cuff. The transducer is positioned lateral to the acromion. The supraspinatus tendon (*s*) of the symptomatic right shoulder is swollen and is more than 1 cm in diameter. The edematous supraspinatus tendon has a hypoechoic appearance relative to the deltoid and the contralateral supraspinatus tendon. The right humeral head has an irregular outline (*arrow*). **B**, Impingement syndrome with edema of the rotator cuff: coronal sonogram. Same patient as in **A**. The transducer is positioned perpendicular to the one used in **A** to obtain coronal images of the shoulder. The normal left rotator cuff has a triangular shape. It is slightly more reflective than the overlying deltoid muscle (*D*), and the cuff inserts on the greater tuberosity (*arrow*). The edematous right rotator cuff (*C*) is hypoechoic and swollen. The insertion bulges over the insertion area on the greater tuberosity (*black arrowhead*) and has a more irregular appearance. The insertion is more rounded, losing its triangular shape. The greater tuberosity (*arrow*) on the right is more irregular in shape. Abbreviations: right (*R*), left (*L*).

tendon rupture are interruption of tendon fibers and fluid-filled clefts within the tendon (Fig. 4–57). In most cases, the cleft is located approximately 6 to 10 cm proximal to the tendon insertion (Figs. 4–58 and 4–59). Surrounding hematoma is minimal due to the poor vascularity of the tendon. The plantaris tendon is often intact, even in cases of complete Achilles tendon rupture. This tendon is identified as a small strand at the medial aspect of the Achilles tendon (Fig. 4–60). Occasionally, fusiform contracture of the distal portion of the tendon can be seen (Fig. 4–61). This is often misinterpreted as tendinitis. On making this finding, the examiner should always check for a more proximal interruption in the tendon. Acoustic shadows are often noted at the edges of the rupture. Previously, we felt that this represented injury to the surrounding fat occurring at the time of tendon rupture. However, recent cases of partial tear without fat injury suggest that this artifact is probably related to refraction or critical angle shadowing of the edges of the torn tendon. This artifact is a pathognomic finding of tear, and it

Text continued on page 122

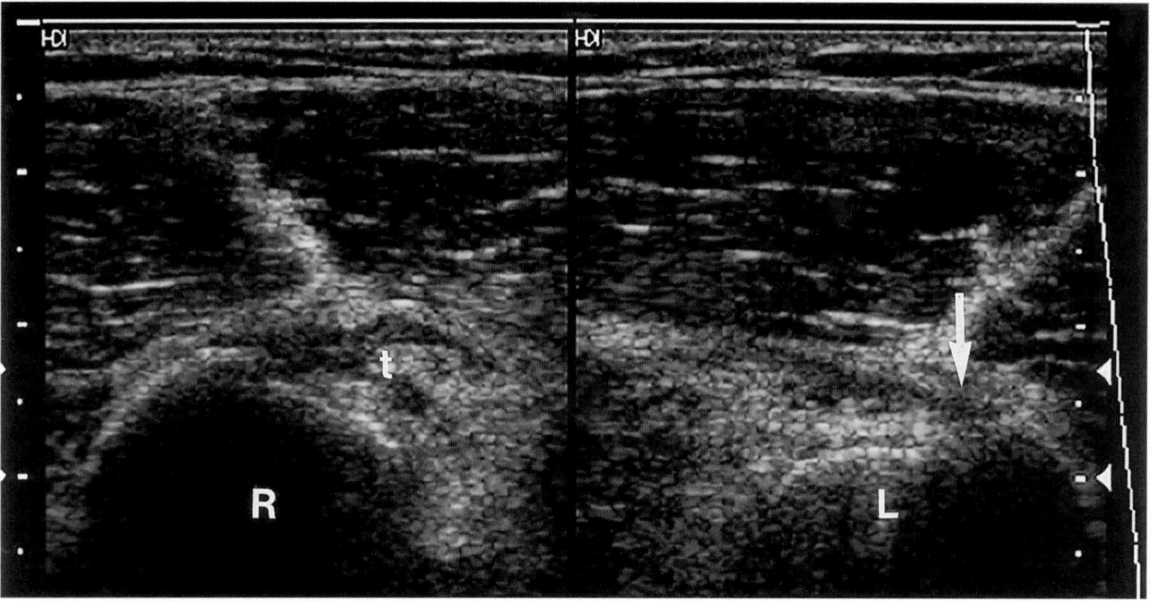

Figure 4–55 ▪ Pectoralis tendon tear: transverse ultrasound with split-screen comparison. A sudden sharp pain in the shoulder of this 24-year-old man occured during weight lifting. The examination was performed with a 12-MHz linear array transducer. Comparison of the normal left (*L*) with the abnormal right (*R*) pectoralis insertion shows the curled end of the torn pectoralis tendon (*t*) surrounded by a small hematoma on the symptomatic side. The normal left tendon–bone junction (*arrow*) with the lateral lip of the intertubercular groove is noted on the observer's right. Surgical repair of the torn pectoralis tendon was necessary to restore normal function.

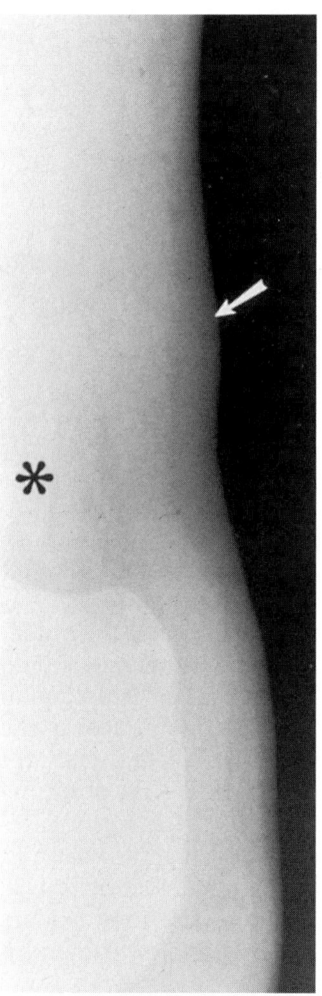

Figure 4–56 ▪ Tendon rupture: Gevaert MRL radiograph. A patient with known tendinosis has increasing pain in his right Achilles tendon. He cannot stand on the tips of his toes. The Thompson sign was inconclusive, and a gap could not be palpated in the tendon. A lateral radiograph demonstrates thickening of the Achilles tendon (*arrow*), and Kager's fat pad (*black asterisk*) appears fuzzy. With radiography, it is not possible to differentiate between tendinosis and tendon rupture.

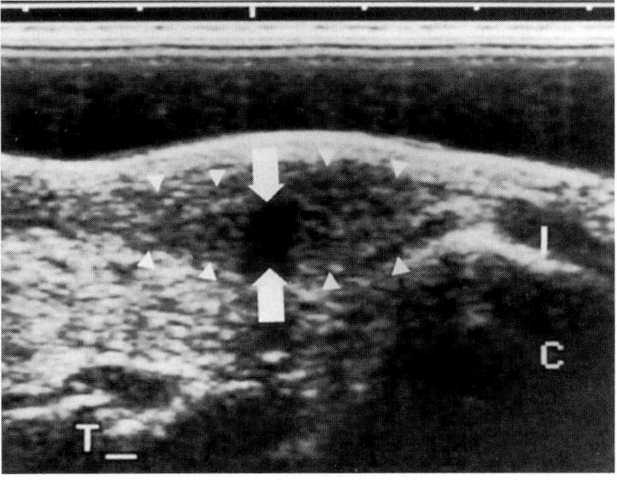

Figure 4–57 ■ Complete Achilles tendon rupture: longitudinal sonogram. Same patient as in Figure 4–56. The 7.5-MHz linear array transducer is positioned dorsally over the Achilles tendon. The distal portion of the tendon, the insertion (*I*), is at the observer's right. Tendon rupture is seen as a hypoechoic gap in the tendon (*white arrows*). There is fusiform contraction of the tendon segments, which is greater in the distal portion (*white arrowheads*). Abbreviations: tibia (*T*), calcaneus (*c*).

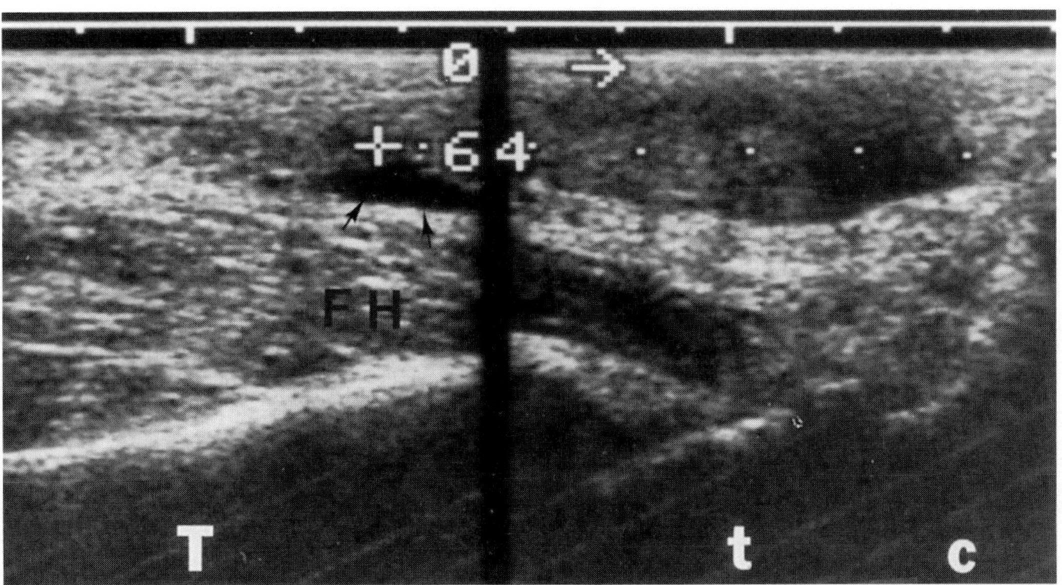

Figure 4–58 ■ Complete Achilles tendon rupture: longitudinal sonogram. A 50-year-old woman with asthma taking corticosteroids for chronic therapy felt a sudden sharp pain in the Achilles tendon while walking upstairs. Physical examination revealed absence of plantar flexion and a positive Thompson sign. The clinician palpated a gap in the Achilles tendon. The transducer is positioned dorsally over the Achilles tendon. Using the image memory, an image was constructed of the entire Achilles tendon. Ultrasound determines the exact location of the tendon rupture (*white cross*), and the distance from the rupture to the tendon insertion can be accurately measured. The distance is 64 mm in this case. Fusiform contraction of the distal tendon fragment is also seen. A small amount of blood surrounds the area of rupture (*small arrows*). Oblique white lines in the lower portion of the figure are artifacts due to electrical interference. Abbreviations: tibia (*T*), talus (*t*), calcaneus (*c*), flexor hallucis longus muscle (*FH*).

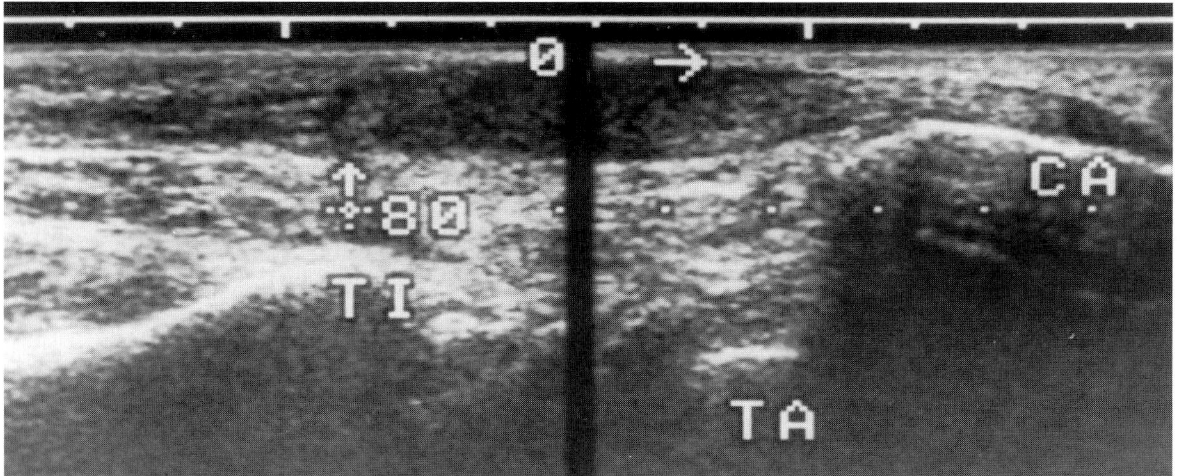

Figure 4–59 ▪ Complete Achilles tendon rupture: longitudinal sonogram. This 40-year-old tennis player felt a crack in his heel during a vigorous vertical jump. Clinical examination revealed some swelling of the Achilles tendon, but the clinician could not palpate a gap in the tendon. The Thompson sign was positive. The examination technique was identical to that used in Figure 4–58. An interruption in the tendon fibers is seen 80 mm proximal to the tendon insertion. There was minimal bleeding, and therefore the tendon rupture is seen as a small, hypoechoic band (*white arrow*). Most of the tendon ruptures occur at the level of the tibial epiphysis (*TI*). Abbreviations: talus (*TA*), calcaneus (*CA*).

allows us to measure the degree of retraction with great accuracy (Fig. 4–62). Changes in the echotexture of the fat can be seen during and after healing of the tendon, sometimes months following trauma (Figs. 4–63 and 4–64).

Herniation of fat through the site of the rupture may occur in chronic cases. This is seen as a small, hyperechoic nodule protruding through the cleft in the tendon (Figs. 4–65 through 4–69). A high-quality conventional radiograph of the soft tissues

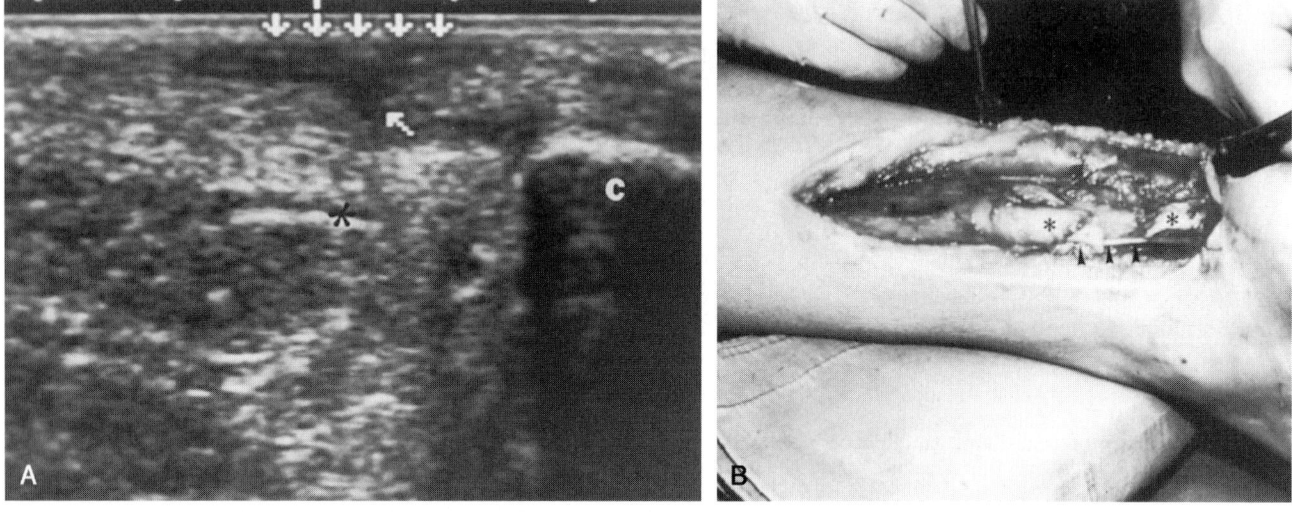

Figure 4–60 ▪ **A**, Complete Achilles tendon rupture: longitudinal sonogram. This figure is a magnification sonogram of the site of a complete tendon rupture. The rupture of the tendon (*oblique arrow*) was considered complete by the surgeon, although the plantaris tendon was intact (*small arrows*). Symbols and abbreviations: fat pad (*asterisk*), calcaneus (*c*). **B**, Complete Achilles tendon rupture: intraoperative photograph. Same patient as in **A**. The operative site is viewed from the medial aspect, with the skin retracted laterally. Contracted proximal and distal segments of the ruptured Achilles tendon are seen centrally in the surgical field (*asterisk*). The intact plantaris tendon just medial and deep to the ruptured Achilles tendon is seen (*arrowheads*).

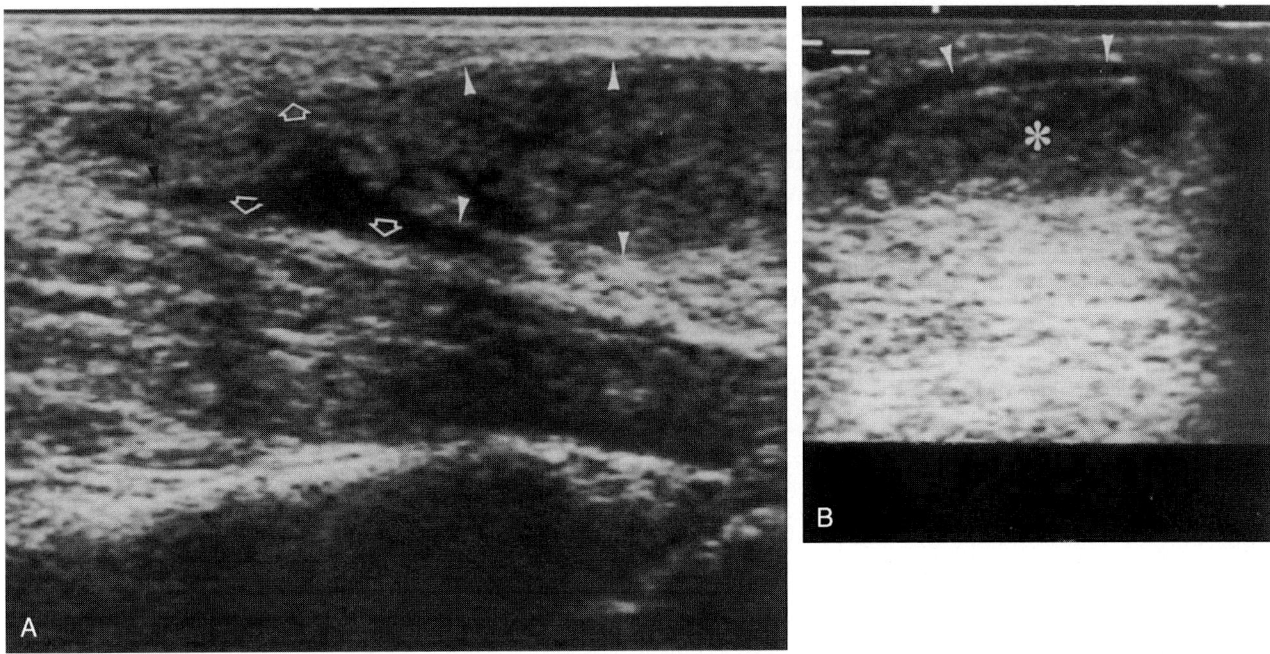

Figure 4–61 ■ **A,** Complete rupture of the Achilles tendon: longitudinal sonogram. This is a detailed sonogram of the site of the rupture. The retracted distal portion (*solid white arrowheads*) is generally thicker than the retracted proximal portion (*black arrowheads*). Hematoma surrounds the two ends of the ruptured tendon. In this case, the hematoma is confined within the peritenon (*open white arrows*). **B,** Complete rupture of the Achilles tendon: transverse sonogram. Same patient as in **A**. The transducer is oriented perpendicular to the long axis of the tendon. This is a detailed view of the proximal portion of the tendon above the site of rupture. The retracted, thickened proximal tendon (*white asterisk*) is seen surrounded by hematoma within the peritenon (*arrowheads*).

Figure 4–62 ■ Complete Achilles tendon rupture: longitudinal sonogram. A detail of the rupture site demonstrates the hypoechoic gap in the tendon (*white arrowheads*), which seems to continue in the peritendinous fat as a hypoechoic band (*black arrowheads*). This is a frequent finding in complete tendon rupture. It seems to represent a sonographic artifact rather than a true gap in the fat pad. Abbreviation and symbol: tibia (*T*), contracted distal portion of the tendon (*white asterisk*).

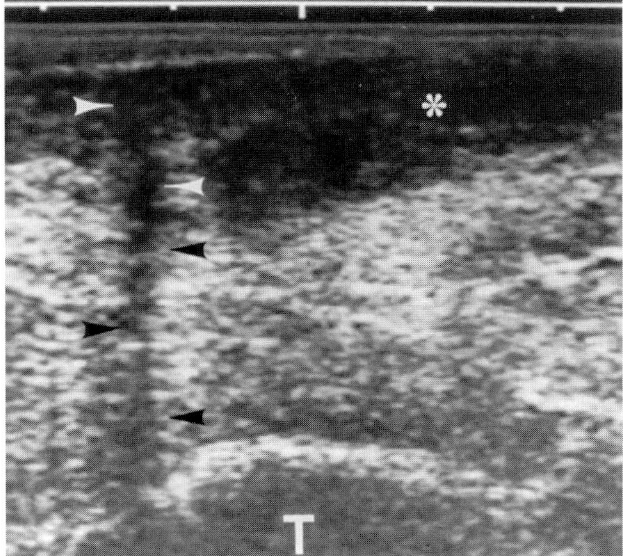

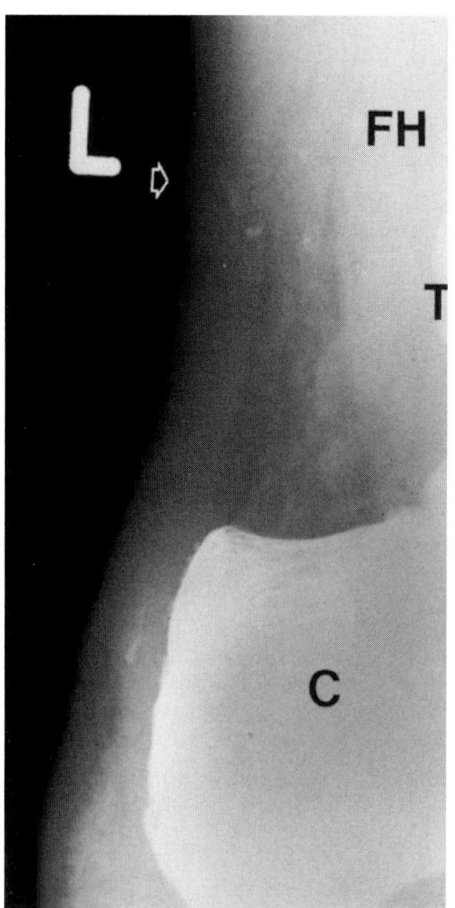

Figure 4-63 ■ Healing Achilles tendon: Gevaert MRL radiograph (lateral view). The patient sustained a tendon rupture 6 months earlier. He was treated conservatively with cast immobilization. The area of tendon rupture is still swollen (*open arrow*). Calcifications are present at the site of the rupture and also at the tendon insertion. Abbreviations: flexor hallucis longus (*FH*), tibia (*T*), calcaneus (*c*).

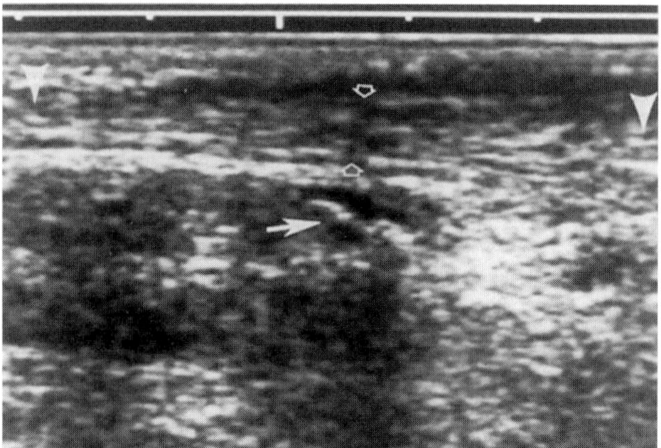

Figure 4-64 ■ Achilles tendon healing: longitudinal sonogram. Same patient as in Figure 4-63. The image is a detail of a longitudinal sonogram of the Achilles tendon 6 months following injury. The hypoechoic cleft (*open arrows*) is still seen, but now some tendon fibers cross the cleft. The structure of the tendon in this area is hypoechoic compared with the more normal proximal and distal tendon segments (*white arrowheads*). In this image, the calcifications (*white arrow*) appearing in Figure 4-63 lie within the fat pad. Tendon rupture appears to result in damage to the fat pad as well.

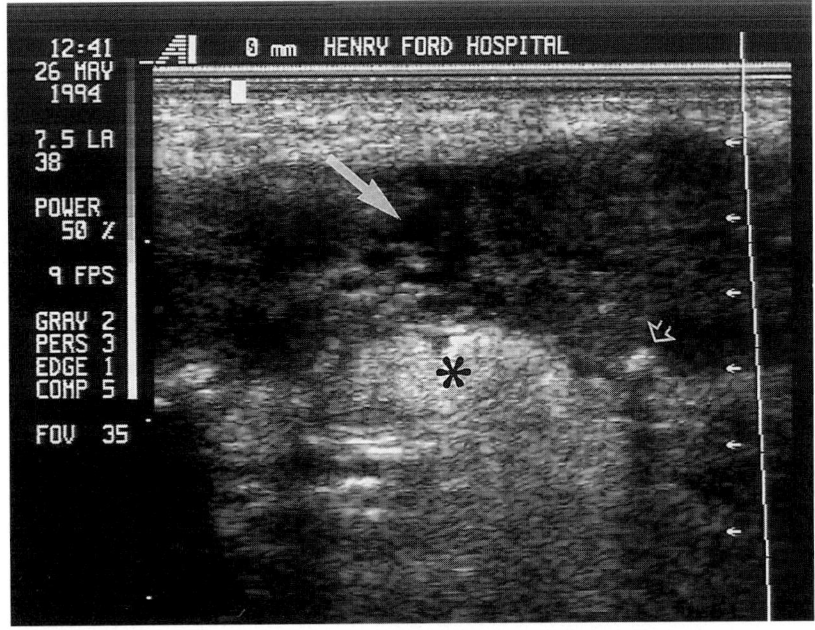

Figure 4-65 ▪ Achilles tendon rerupture: longitudinal sonogram. Sudden weakness and ankle swelling developed in this 43-year-old renal transplant patient who had torn his Achilles tendon years ago. This detail of a longitudinal ultrasound scan which was performed with a 7.5-MHz transducer shows the complete disruption of tendon continuity (*arrow*). Several calcifications (*open arrow*) were noted in and around the tendon during real-time scanning. The fat of Hoffa's fat pad protrudes (*asterisk*) into the anterior aspect of the gap.

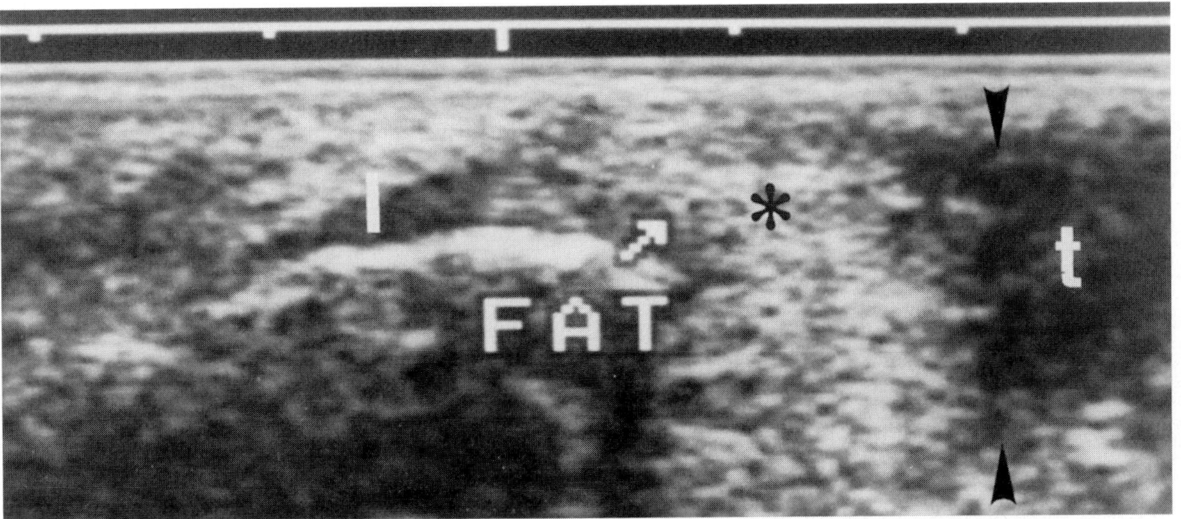

Figure 4-66 ▪ Chronic Achilles tendon rupture: longitudinal sonogram. This patient ruptured his left Achilles tendon 1 year ago. The rupture was not recognized immediately, and treatment was started 1 month after the accident. Now, 1 year later, the patient is unable to plantarflex his foot. A longitudinal sonogram was obtained by positioning the transducer over the dorsal aspect of the tendon. The insertion (*I*) is seen on the left, and the proximal part of the tendon is at the right. The ruptured tendon is widened and appears hypoechoic (*black arrowheads*). Compared to the ruptured tendon, the surrounding fat is hyperechoic (*black asterisk*). This fat has herniated through the gap in the tendon at the site of rupture (*arrow*), impairing healing. A retracted proximal portion of the tendon (*t*) is also seen.

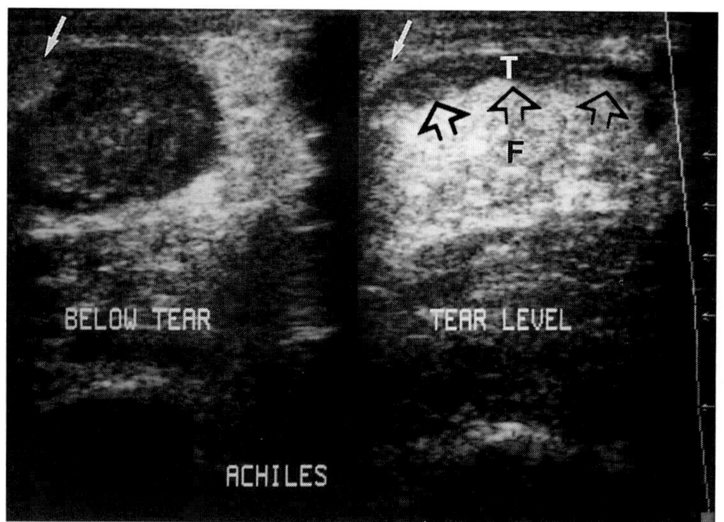

Figure 4-67 ■ Chronic Achilles tendon rupture: transverse sonogram. Same patient as in Figure 4-66. The transducer is now positioned perpendicular to the long axis of the tendon. The image on the left depicts the site of tendon retraction in cross section at the level below the tear. The plantaris tendon appears unaffected (*arrow*). The image on the right was obtained at the level of the tear. Centrally, in the proximal portion of the ruptured tendon (*open arrows*), hyperechoic fat is found (*F*). A small rim of torn tendon tissue (*T*) is left at the posterior aspect of the heel.

will demonstrate this as radiolucent deposits within the Achilles tendon. These lesions heal only after removal of the interposed fat.

Quadriceps tendon rupture (Figs. 4-70 and 4-71) is a rare finding even in athletes (Roels and Martens, 1978). Tendon rupture after trauma is more common in Afro-Americans. A fall on ice is a classic mechanism of injury. The quadriceps tendon can rupture spontaneously in patients with knee arthroplasty. Degeneration of the tendon substance

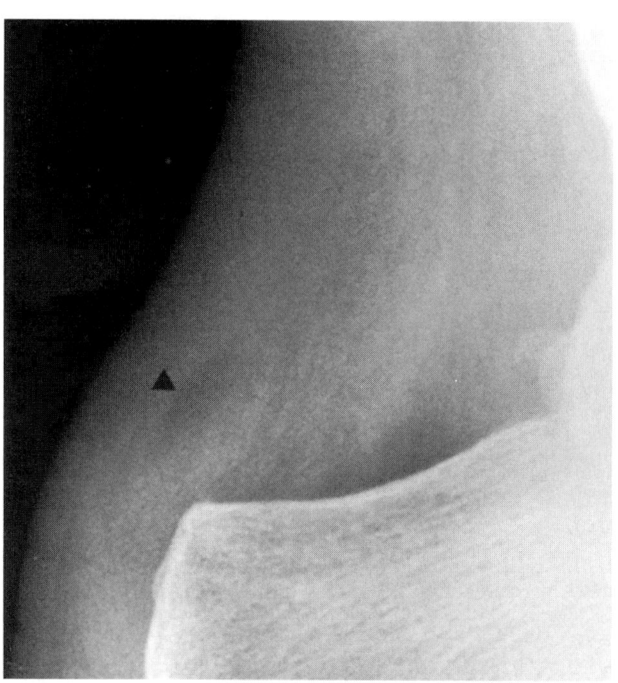

Figure 4-68 ■ Chronic Achilles tendon rupture: Gevaert MRL radiograph (*lateral view*). Same patient as in Figures 4-66 and 4-67. Fat is seen as a radiolucent area (*arrowhead*) in the substance of the distal tendon.

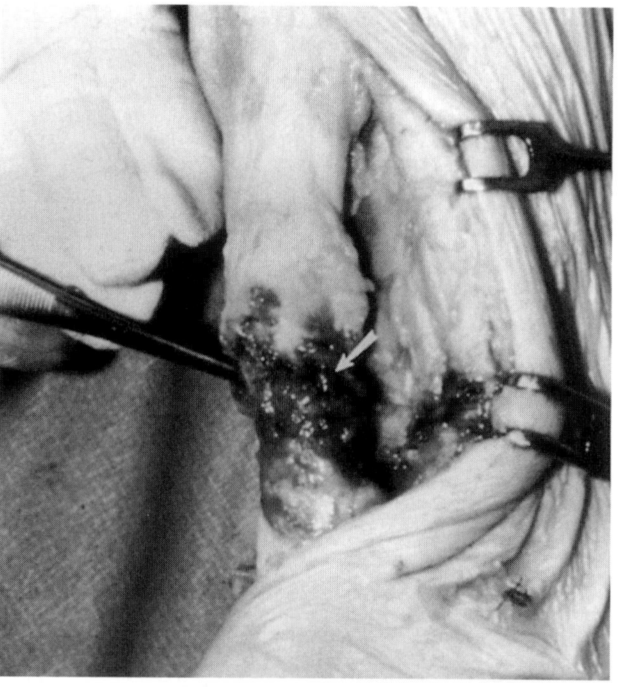

Figure 4-69 ■ Chronic Achilles tendon rupture: intraoperative photograph. Same patient as in Figures 4-66, 4-67, and 4-68. Fat was found separating the ends of the ruptured tendon at the time of surgery (*arrow*). Necrotic debris was also present at the rupture site.

has been cited as the etiology for these spontaneous ruptures (Kannus and Jozsa, 1991). We have observed areas of myxoid degeneration and calcification sonographically in a significant percentage of spontaneous ruptures of lower extremity tendons. Systemic disease may result in bilateral tendon rupture, systemic lupus erythematosus weakens tendons considerably, and bilateral ruptures are relatively common.

A complete rupture of the tendon is often the end stage of patellar tendinitis, especially if further overload and weakening of the tendon are caused by corticosteroid injections. Prior to the use of ultrasound in the evaluation of musculoskeletal pathology, only arthrography (Aprin and Broukhim, 1985) or even more invasive exploratory surgery were able to prove this diagnosis. Now sonography can demonstrate the discontinuity with an exami-

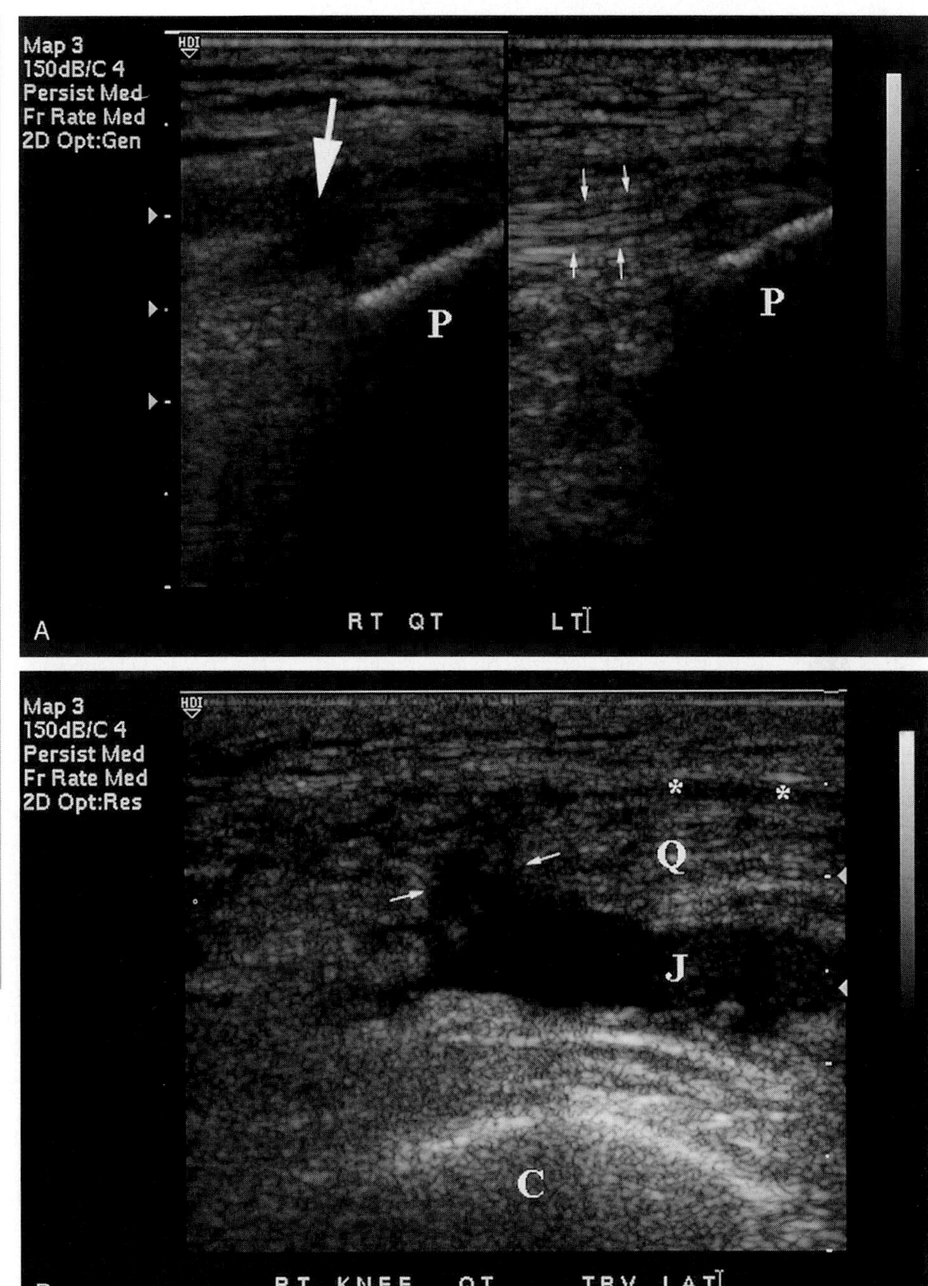

Figure 4–70 ▪ **A**, Full-thickness quadriceps tendon tear: split-screen longitudinal sonogram. A fall on the ice injured this 46-year-old police officer, who was unable to extend his knee. He kept limping for a week before seeking medical attention. The split-screen images were obtained with the transducer aligned along the fibers of the quadriceps tendon. The normal tendon attachment (*between the small arrows*) on the base of the patella is noted in the left knee (*LT*). Loss of the fibrillar pattern is noted in the right knee (*RT*) at the site of the tear (*big arrow*). Abbreviation: patella (*P*). **B**, Full-thickness quadriceps tendon tear: transverse sonogram. Same patient as in **A**. The transverse image of the distal quadriceps demonstrates a full-thickness (*arrows*) defect in the lateral aspect of the tendon. The tendon tear forms a communication between the joint (*J*) and the synovial space of the prepatellar bursa (*asterisks*). Transverse images are crucial in the workup of quadriceps tears. This tear was staged as a full-thickness tear but was incomplete, as it was only 1 cm in cross-sectional diameter. The treatment therefore was conservative. Complete tears that extend from the medial to the lateral expansion of the tendon, in contrast, must be treated surgically. Abbreviations: quadriceps (*Q*), lateral femoral condyle (*C*).

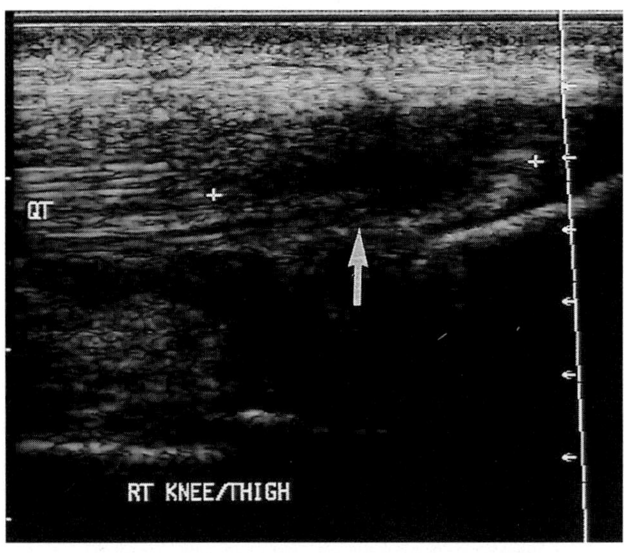

Figure 4–71 ■ Partial-thickness quadriceps tendon tear: longitudinal sonogram. After a fall from the roof of a three-floor building, this 39-year-old man is unable to perform a straight-leg raise with his right lower leg. However, the clinical exam proceeds with great difficulty because of a paresis associated with a lumbar burst fracture. The longitudinal scan through the distal quadriceps tendon shows a 2-cm-long tear (*calipers*). The tear is superficial, and normal fibers (*arrow*) are still visible deep to the lesion. With the ultrasound results indicating a partial rather than a full-thickness tear, the patient was treated conservatively.

nation that is fast, noninvasive, cost effective, and reliable.

References

Ahovuo J, Paavolainen P, Slatis P: The diagnostic value of arthrography in rotator cuff tears. *Acta Orthop Scand* 55:220–223, 1984.

Aisen AM, et al: Sonographic evaluation of the cartilage of the knee. *Radiology* 153:781, 1984.

Aprin H, Broukhim N: Early diagnosis of acute rupture of the quadriceps tendon by arthrography. *Clin Orthop* 195:185–190, 1985.

Beltran J, et al: Rotator cuff lesions of the shoulder: Evaluation by direct sagittal CT arthrography. *Radiology* 160:161–165, 1986.

Blei CL, Nirschl RP, Grant EG: Achilles tendon: Ultrasound diagnosis of pathologic conditions. *Radiology* 159: 765–767, 1986.

Bock E, et al: Xeroradiography of tenomuscular traumatic pathologic conditions of the limbs. *Diagn Imag Clin Med* 50:235–248, 1981.

Bretzke LA, et al: Ultrasonography of the rotator cuff: Normal and pathologic anatomy. *Invest Radiol* 20: 311–315, 1985.

Bruce RK, Hale TL, Gilbert SK: Ultrasonographic evaluation for ruptured Achilles tendon. *J Am Pediatr Med Assoc* 72:15–17, 1982.

Bywaters EGL: Lesions of the bursae, tendons and tendon sheaths. *Clin Rheum Dis* 5:885, 1979.

Canoso JJ: Aspiration of the retrocalcaneal bursa. *Ann Rheum Dis* 43:308–312, 1984.

Chui MT: Shoulder ultrasound finds more than just cuff tears. *Radiol Today* 5:20, 1988.

Church CC: Radiographic diagnosis of acute peroneal tendon dislocation. *AJR* 129:1065–1068, 1977.

Clark JM, Harryman DT: Tendons, ligaments and capsule of the rotator cuff. *J Bone Joint Surg Am* 74: 713–725, 1992.

Clement DB, Taunton JE, Smart GW: Achilles tendonitis and peritendonitis: Etiology and treatment. *Am J Sports Med* 12:179–187, 1984.

Cooper RR, Misol S: Tendon and ligament insertion. A light and electron microscopic study. *J Bone Joint Surg Am* 52:1–20, 1970.

Crass JR, Craig EV, Feinberg SB: Sonography of the postoperative rotator cuff. *AJR* 146:561–564, 1986.

Crass JR, et al: Ultrasonography of the rotator cuff: Surgical correlation. *J Clin Ultrasound* 12:487–491, 1984.

Crenshaw AH: *Campbell's Operative Orthopaedics*, CD-ROM ed. Philadelphia, Mosby–Year book, 1996.

Das De S, Balasubramaniam P: A repair operation for recurrent dislocation of peroneal tendons. *J Bone Joint Surg Br* 67:585–587, 1985.

Davis WH, et al: The superior peroneal retinaculum: An anatomic study. *Foot Ankle Int* 15(5):271–275, 1994.

Demarais Y, et al: Echoscannographie dans les tendinites achilleennes et rotuliennes specialement chez le sportif. *Cinesiologie* 23:249–256, 1984.

Dillehay GL, et al: The ultrasonographic characterization of tendons. *Invest Radiol* 19:338–341, 1984.

Eichelberger RP, Lichtenstein P, Brogdon BG: Peroneal tenography. *JAMA* 247:2587–2591, 1982.

Erickson S: High-resolution imaging of the musculoskeletal system. *Radiology* 205:593–618, 1997.

Farin PU, et al: Medial displacement of the biceps brachii tendon: Evaluation with dynamic sonography during maximal external shoulder rotation. *Radiology* 195: 845, 1995.

Feretti A, et al: The natural history of jumper's knee. Patellar or quadriceps tendonitis. *Int Orthop* 8:239–242, 1985.

Fiamengo SA, et al: Posterior heel pain associated with a calcaneal step and Achilles tendon calcification. *Clin Orthop* 167:203–211, 1982.

Fornage B: Achilles tendon: US examination. *Radiology* 159:759–764, 1986.

Fornage B, et al: Sonography of the patellar tendon: Preliminary observations. *AJR* 143:179–182, 1984.

Geppert MJ, Sobel M, Bohne WHO: Lateral ankle instability as a cause of superior peroneal retinacular laxity: An anatomic and biochemical study of cadaveric feet. *Foot Ankle Int* 14(6):330–334, 1993.

Hardaker WT Jr, et al: Foot and ankle injuries in theatrical dancers. *Foot Ankle Int* 6(2):59–69, 1985.

Hsu T, et al: Ultrasonographic examination of the posterior tibial tendon. *Foot Ankle Int* 18(1):34–38, 1997.

Jobe FW, Jobe CM: Painful athletic injuries of the shoulder. *Clin Orthop* 173:117–124, 1983.

Kannus P, Jozsa L: Histopathological changes preceding spontaneous rupture of a tendon. *J Bone Joint Surg Am* 73(10):1507, 1991.

Khan KM, et al: Patellar tendon sonography and jumper's knee in female basketball players: A longitudinal study. *Clin J Sport Med* 7(3):200–205, 1997.

Mack LA, et al: US evaluation of the rotator cuff. *Radiology* 157(1):205–209, 1985.

Martens M, et al: Patellar tendinitis: Pathology and results of treatment. *Acta Orthop Scand* 53:445–450, 1982.

Martinoli C, et al: Analysis of echotexture of tendons with ultrasound. *Radiology*, 186:839–843, 1993.

McConkey JP, Favero KJ: Subluxation of the peroneal tendons within the peroneal tendon sheath. *Am J Sports Med* 15:511–513, 1987.

Merkel KHH, Hess H, Kunz M: Insertion tendonopathy in athletes. *Pathol Res Pract* 173:303–309, 1982.

Middleton WD, et al: Pitfalls of rotator cuff sonography. *AJR* 146:555–560, 1986a.

Middleton WD, et al: Sonographic detection of rotator cuff tears. *AJR* 144:349–353, 1985a.

Middleton WD, et al: Ultrasonic evaluation of the rotator cuff and biceps tendon. *J Bone Joint Surg Am* 68:440–450, 1986b.

Middleton WD, et al: US of the biceps tendon apparatus. *Radiology* 157(1):211–215, 1985b.

Miles CA, et al: Factors affecting the ultrasonic properties of equine digital flexor tendons. *Ultrasound Med Biol* 22(7):907–915, 1996.

Miller SD, et al: Ultrasound in the diagnosis of posterior tibial tendon pathology. *Foot Ankle Int* 17(9):555–558, 1996.

Neer CS: Impingement lesions. *Clin Orthop* 173:70–77, 1983.

Niepel GA, Sit AJ: Enthesopathy. *Clin Rheum Dis* 5:857–872, 1979.

Oden RR: Tendon injuries about the ankle resulting from skiing. *Clin Orthop* 216:63–69, 1987.

O'Donoghue DH: Subluxing biceps tendon in the athlete. *Clin Orthop* 164:26–29, 1982.

Palvalgyi R, Balint BJ: Radiographic examination of the large tendons of the knee and ankle joints. *Arch Orthop Trauma Surg* 98:19–24, 1981.

Petersson CJ: Spontaneous medial dislocation of the tendon of the long biceps brachii. *Clin Orthop* 211: 224–227, 1986.

Petersson CJ, Gentz CF: Ruptures of the supraspinatus tendon. The significance of distally pointing acromioclavicular osteophytes. *Clin Orthop* 174:143–148, 1983.

Ptasznik R, Hennessy OF: Abnormalities of the biceps tendon of the shoulder: Sonographic findings. *AJR* 164:409, 1995.

Roels J, Martens M: Patellar tendonitis (jumper's knee). *Am J Sports Med* 6:362–368, 1978.

Sobel M, et al: Longitudinal splitting of the peroneus brevis tendon: An anatomic and histologic study of cadaveric material. *Foot Ankle Int.* 12(3):165–170, 1991.

van Holsbeeck M: Medische beeldvorming en diagnose van sportletsels, in *Praktische Behandeling van Sportletsels,* chapter 3. Leuven, Samson, 1987.

van Holsbeeck M, Powell A: Ankle and foot, in Musculoskeletal ultrasound, Clin Diagn Ultrasound 30: 221–237, Naperville, IL, Churchill-Livingstone, 1995.

Warwick R, Williams PL: *Gray's Anatomy,* ed 36. Philadelphia, WB Saunders Co, 1980.

Wohlwend J, et al: Simultaneous changes in tendon and bone: A sonographic study of alteration of the greater tuberosity associated with rotator cuff tear. A study of the normal population. *AJR* 171:229–233, 1998.

Zingas C, Failla JM, van Holsbeeck M: Injection accuracy and clinical relief of de Quervain's tendinitis. *J Hand Surg [Am]* 23(1):89–96, 1998.

Zuinen C, et al: Les lesion chirurgicales du tendon d'Achille. *Sports Med* 25:7–11, 1983.

Chapter 5
Sonography of Bursae

The word *bursa* is derived from the Greek, meaning "wine skin." In modern usage, *bursa* refers to a variety of structures that have several features in common. They are all sac-like structures with a lining similar to that found in diarthrodial joints. In addition, they are situated to facilitate movement of musculoskeletal structures (Canoso, 1981). Bursae are found in areas where a considerable degree of motion is required, yet a cartilaginous joint is not necessary.

The analogy of a wine skin is quite appropriate; both bursae and wine skins have their greatest dimensions in length and width. This provides a large surface area occupying little volume under normal circumstances (Codman, 1931). When positioned between two structures, this configuration allows mobility and gliding of one structure on the other. Bursae can develop de novo in response to friction and pressure. Examples are the bursae that occur over the bony prominence of a hallux valgus, exostosis, or an irregular spinous process (Baastrup's and Pott's diseases).

Some anatomists (Gray, Piersol) believe that bursae are sacs filled with fluid. This is a misconception resulting from studies performed by injecting bursae with various materials (Figs. 5–1 and 5–2). Physicians who perform bursography and bursoscopy often share this misconception because they distend the bursae with contrast material or irrigation fluid. In reality, bursae contain only a thin film of viscous fluid, which serves as a lubricant. The walls are separated by a fluid film approximately 1 mm thick. Therefore, bursae are really potential spaces (see Fig. 5–2), becoming fluid-filled sacs only under pathological conditions (van Holsbeeck and Introcaso, 1989).

Bursae are divided into two groups, communicating and noncommunicating, depending on their relationship to a joint space. Noncommunicating bursae are more common in humans. Bursae may be categorized further on the basis of their location: subcutaneous or deep (Table 5–1) (Canoso, 1981). Subcutaneous bursae are located between a bone and the overlying skin, such as the prepatellar and olecranon bursae. Deep bursae are located in various places deep to the investing fascia. They separate the joint capsule, tendons, ligaments, and fascial planes (iliotibial tract).

Examination Technique

Selection of a transducer is based on the location of the bursa being examined. Subcutaneous bursae are best examined using 10-, 12-, 15-, or 20-MHz transducers. In addition, these superficial bursae may require a standoff for optimal evaluation. In obese patients, a 5-MHz transducer may be required. Deep bursae usually require a 5-MHz transducer. On rare occasions, a 3-MHz transducer is required due to the patient's body habitus, limiting the examination. In all cases, a linear array transducer is utilized. Peritendinous bursae are most easily examined by scanning in the long axis of the tendon, an example being the retrocalcaneal bursa (Fig. 5–3). The quantity of fluid within the bursa is best assessed relative to the asymptomatic side.

Normal Sonographic Bursa Structure

All bursae share the fundamental attributes described earlier. A thorough knowledge of the anatomical location of the major bursae is essential. Otherwise, when pathologically enlarged, they may be mistaken for soft tissue tumors (Baudrillard et al., 1986). In our discussion of normal bursa structure, we will use the prepatellar bursa as a prototype. This is a superficial noncommunicating bursa. Figure 5–4 is a sagittal section through an anatomical

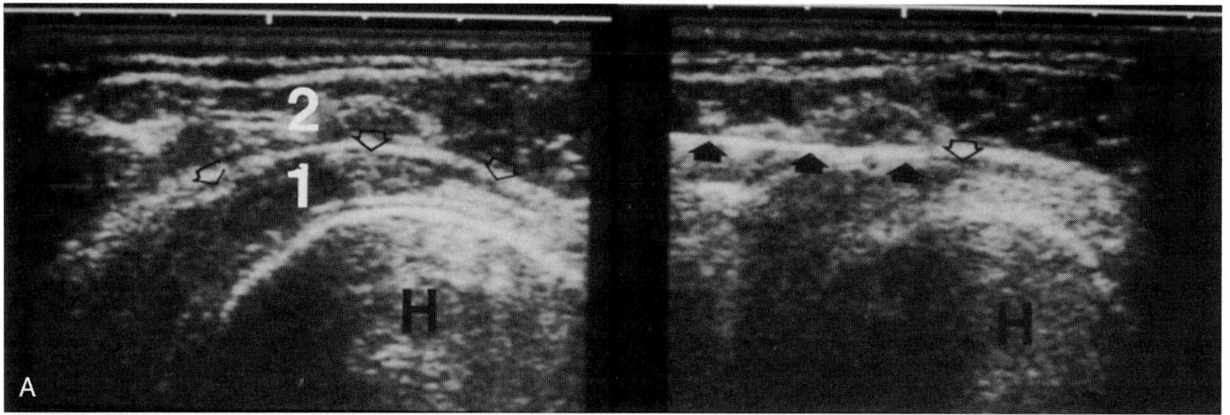

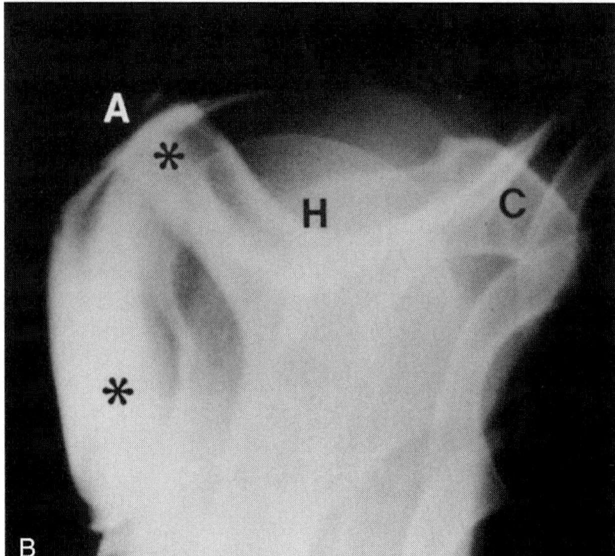

Figure 5-1 ■ **A,** Normal bursa: transverse sonogram. One of the largest bursae in humans is the subacromial-subdeltoid bursa. The surfaces of this bursa separate a large area between the rotator cuff, the acromion, and the deltoid muscle. The cross-sectional diameter of the bursa is only 1 to 2 mm and is seen as a hypoechoic line (*open arrows*) between the supraspinatus tendon (*1*) and the deltoid muscle (*2*). The cross-sectional image at the right shows a spinal needle (*solid arrows*) advanced with its tip in the bursa (*open arrow*). **B,** Normal bursa: bursogram. A bursogram was obtained in the same patient as in **A** after injection of 10 mL of water-soluble iodinated contrast medium. The bursa (*asterisks*) appears as a sac due to its distention with contrast medium. Sonography demonstrates the bursa in its natural state, a potential space (*A*). Abbreviations: humerus (*H*), coracoid (*C*), acromion (*A*). (From van Holsbeeck M, Introcaso J: Sonography of the postoperative shoulder. *AJR* 152:202, 1988. Used by permission)

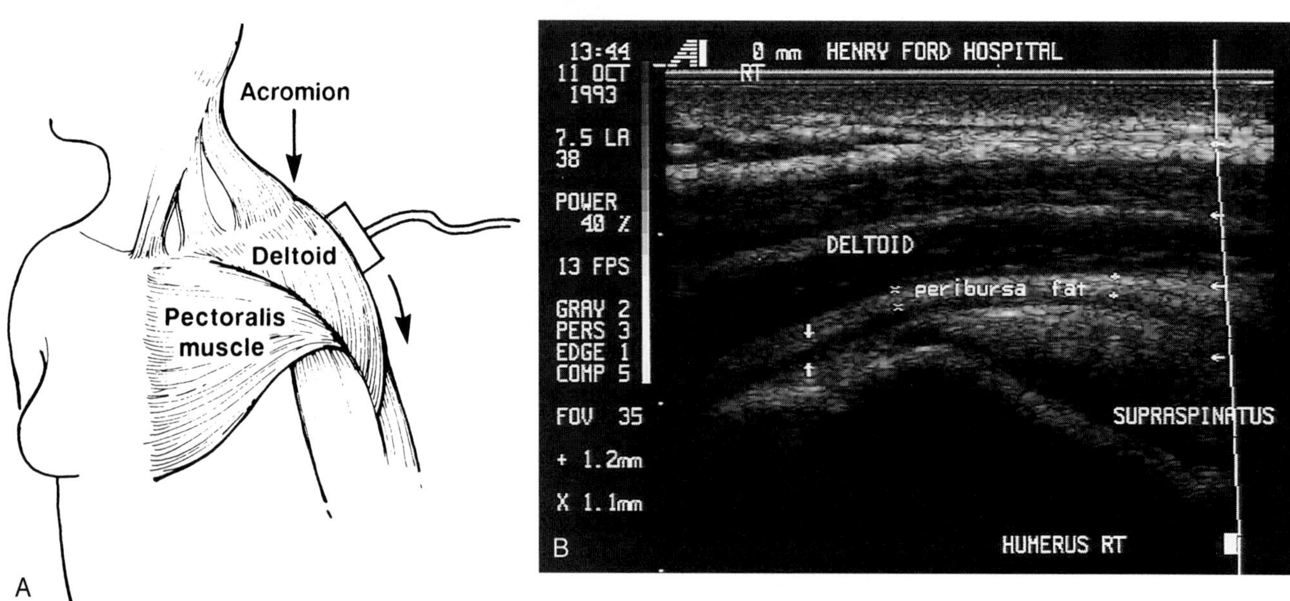

Figure 5-2 ■ **A,** Diagram of the longitudinal examination of the subacromial-subdeltoid bursa. A careful exam of the bursa must include the most dependent part, which is located deep to the deltoid muscle and extends over the proximal humerus beyond the tuberosity. **B,** Normal subdeltoid segment of the bursa: longitudinal sonogram. The normal subdeltoid bursa is a virtual space located deep to the deltoid muscle. The proximal part covers the rotator cuff, and the distal part adheres to the bone of the proximal humeral diaphysis, just distal to the greater tuberosity (*between small arrows*). Hyperechoic fat is located superficial and deep to the bursa. The fat, which is located around the bursa, appears more distinctly (*between calipers*).

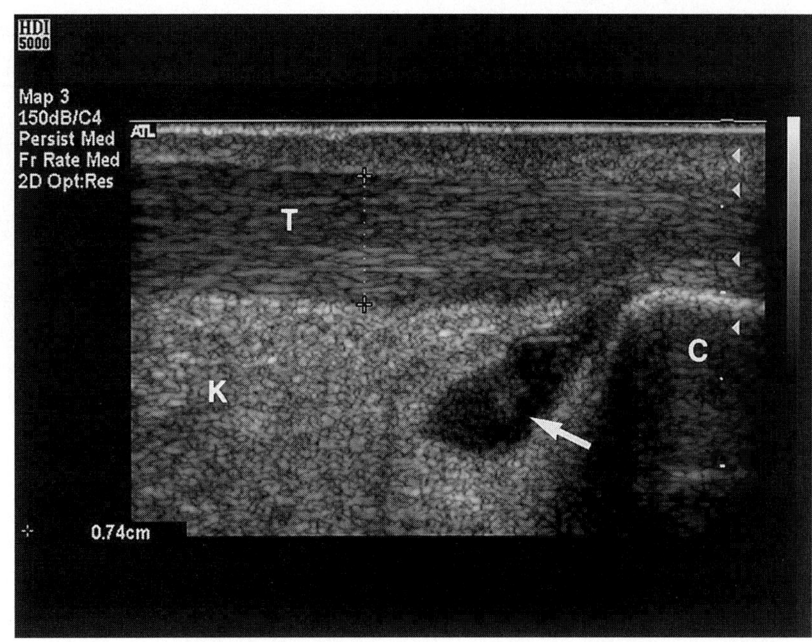

Figure 5-3 ■ Retrocalcaneal tendinobursitis: longitudinal sonogram. The patient is a 58-year-old female tennis player who suffered 6 months of continuous ankle pain, which caused her to stop all athletic activity. The transducer is oriented along the length of the Achilles tendon, with the caudal extent touching the bursal projection of the calcaneus. Swelling and decreased echogenicity are noted in the distal 4 cm of the tendon. The maximal anteroposterior dimension of the tendon is 7.4 mm. The retrocalcaneal bursa (*arrow*) is seen as a hypoechoic, fluid-filled sac between the Achilles tendon (*T*) and the calcaneus (*C*). Abbreviation: Kager's fat pad (*K*).

Table 5-1
Sites of Bursitis Detected with Sonography

Subcutaneous bursae	
Elbow:	Olecranon bursa
Spine:	Baastrup's bursa
Hip:	Subcutaneous trochanteric bursa
Knee:	Prepatellar bursa, subcutaneous infrapatellar bursa, subcutaneous tibial tuberosity bursa
Ankle:	Subcutaneous Achilles tendon bursa
Foot:	First metatarsal bursa
Deep bursae	
Shoulder:	Subacromial bursa,* subdeltoid bursa,* subscapular bursa†
Hip:	Obturator internus bursa, iliopsoas bursa,* deep trochanteric bursa
Knee:	Iliotibial tract bursa, fibular collateral ligament bursa, tibial collateral ligament bursa, subfascial prepatellar bursa, anserine bursa, popliteus bursa,* deep infrapatellar bursa, gastrocnemius-semimembranosus bursa,† suprapatellar bursa†
Ankle:	Retrocalcaneal bursa

*Communication with the joint found in less than 50% of autopsies.
†Communication with the joint found in greater than 50% of autopsies.

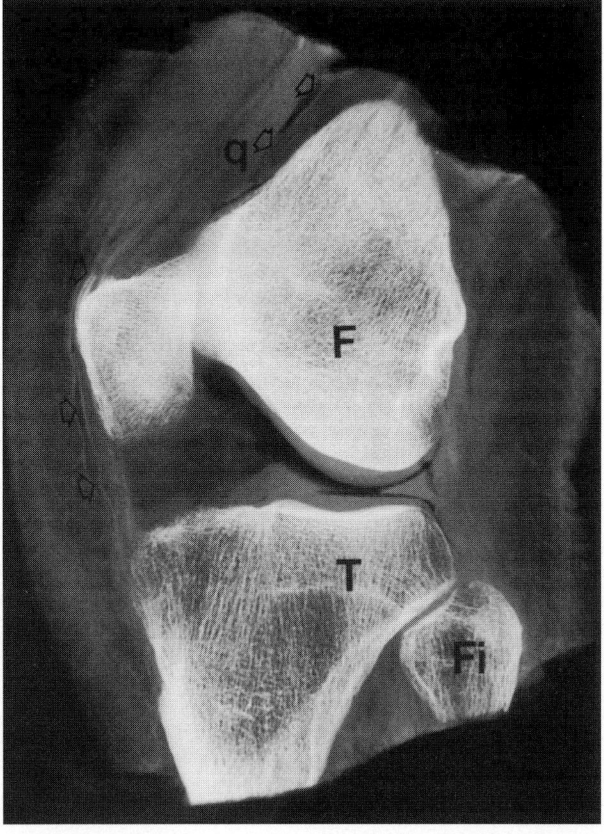

Figure 5-4 ■ Anatomical section through the lateral third of the knee: sagittal section. Two bursae are visualized on this section (*open arrows*): the suprapatellar and prepatellar bursae. The suprapatellar bursa is located deep to the quadriceps tendon (*q*). This is a communicating bursa that is continuous with the knee joint. The prepatellar bursa is a noncommunicating bursa separating the skin from the patella and the patellar tendon. Abbreviations: femur (*F*), tibia (*T*), fibula (*Fi*).

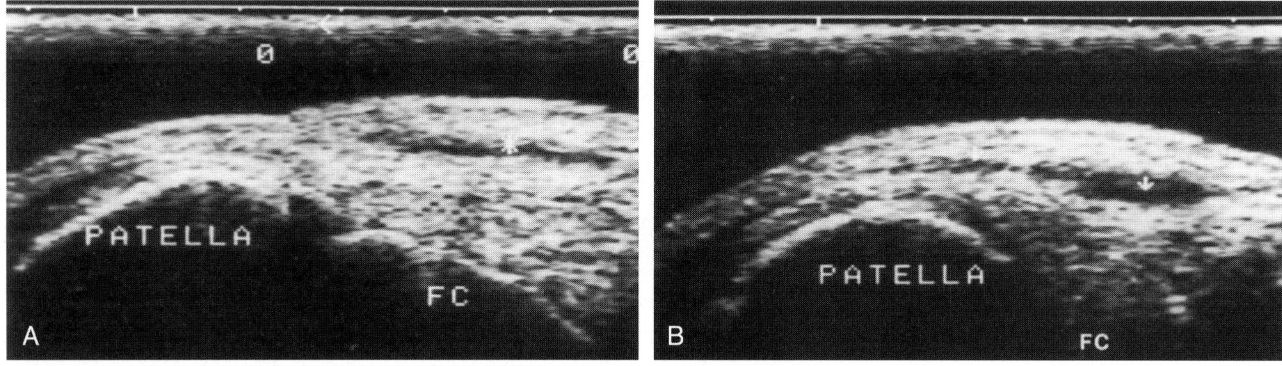

Figure 5–5 ■ **A,** Normal prepatellar bursa: longitudinal sonogram. It is not always possible to image the normal prepatellar bursa using ultrasound. In this longitudinal image, the transducer is positioned over the patella 5 mm lateral to the patellar tendon. The fluid film within the bursa (*asterisk*) measured 1.5 mm in thickness. Abbreviation: lateral femoral condyle (*FC*). **B,** Inflamed prepatellar bursa: longitudinal sonogram. The patient is a 19-year-old long jumper with pain in the right knee and point tenderness over the patellar tendon. He was given the clinical diagnosis of patellar tendonitis. The position of the tranducer is identical to that in **A.** The amount of fluid within the bursa is abnormally increased consistent with frictional bursitis (*arrow*). The patellar tendon is normal.

specimen of the knee. The prepatellar bursa lies anterior to the patella, with its base firmly fixed to the cortex of the base of the patella. The opposing wall is tightly bound to the deep surface of the skin. These thin walls of synovial tissue separated by a minute amount of viscous fluid allow the skin to glide smoothly over the bony prominence of the patella.

Sonographic images depict a bursa as a hypoechoic cleft in the soft tissues, often bounded by a hyperechoic line. This is demonstrated in Figure 5–5A, which is a sonogram of the specimen in Figure 5–4. The hyperechoic boundaries of the bursa do not correspond directly to the synovial lining (Figs. 5–5 through 5–7). Synovial tissue forming

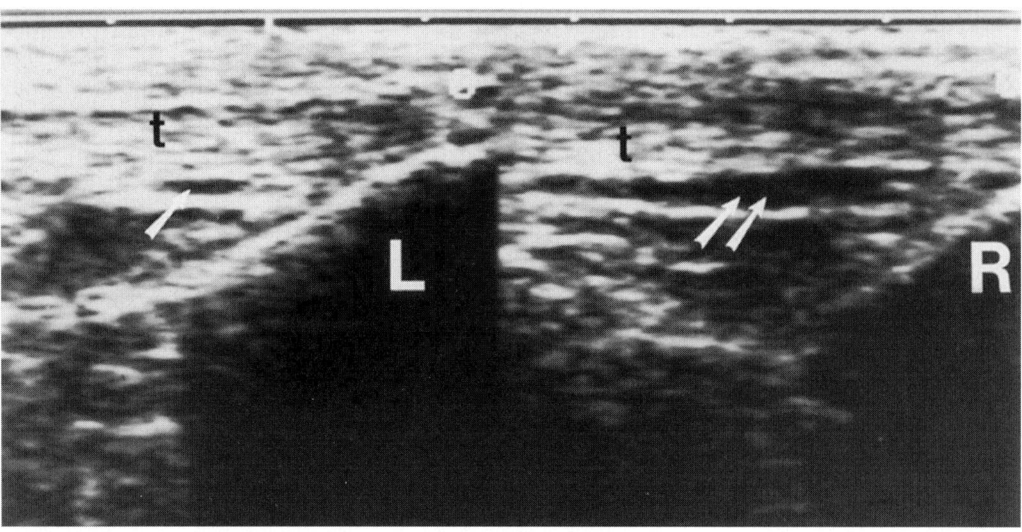

Figure 5–6 ■ Bursitis of the deep infrapatellar bursa: longitudinal sonogram. A 23-year-old soldier had right knee pain following a long march. The transducer is positioned in the long axis of the patellar tendon, with the caudal aspect touching the tibial tuberosity at the observer's right. The normal deep infrapatellar bursa (*single white arrow*) is on the left, located dorsal to the patellar tendon (*t*). It demonstrates the normal fluid film within the bursa, which is 1 to 2 mm thick. On the right, an inflamed bursa (*two white arrows*) appears larger, containing an abnormally increased amount of fluid. Note that the fluid is anechoic, and the bursal walls are not thickened in this case of frictional bursitis. The borders of the bursa are well defined by a hyperechoic line. Abbreviations: left tibial tuberosity (*L*), right tibial tuberosity (*R*).

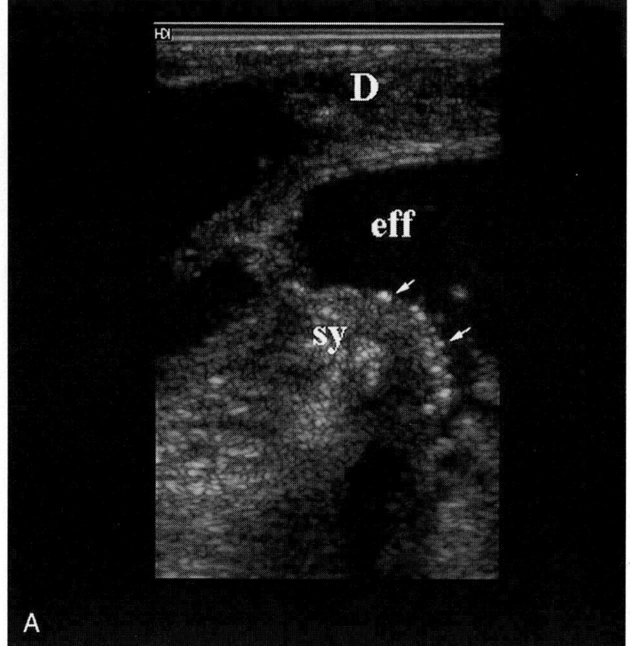

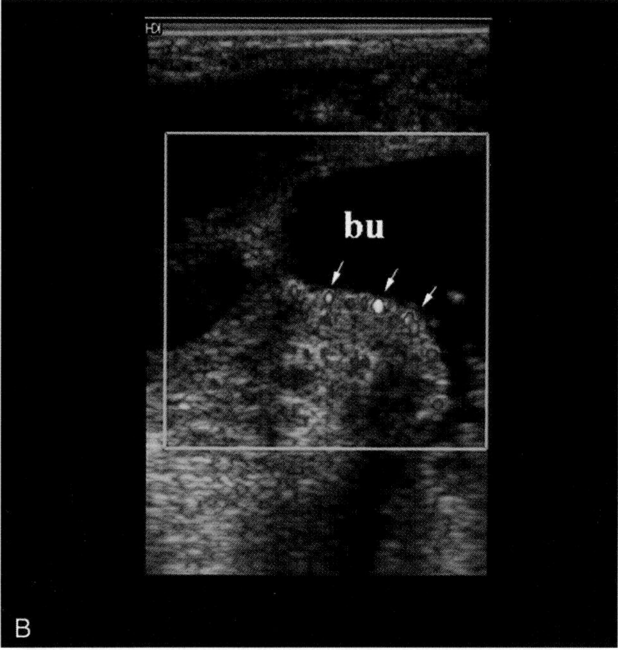

Figure 5–7 ■ **A,** Synovial hyperemia: transverse sonogram. Painful shoulder swelling in a 58-year-old hemodialysis patient. The man's joint complaints were suspected to indicate osteoarticular amyloidosis. The transverse image shows a multiloculated bursal effusion (*eff*) deep to the deltoid muscle (*D*). The inner lining of the bursa has a nodular, hyperechoic pattern (*arrows*). Subsynovial mesenchyma (*sy*). **B,** Synovial hyperemia: transverse power Doppler sonogram. Same patient as in **A.** Power Doppler demonstrates hypervascularity (*arrows*) within the subsynovium. This case illustrates that it is impossible to see the normal synovial membrane. Normal synovium is only a few cell layers thick. The synovial membrane, if visible, would be seen between the vessels and the fluid. Abbreviation: subdeltoid bursa (*bu*).

Figure continued on following page

the walls of a bursa is microscopically thin, beyond the resolution of clinical ultrasound units. Therefore, these hyperechoic lines represent the tissue–fluid interfaces of the bursa (van Holsbeeck and Introcaso, 1989). The viscous fluid that separates the walls of the bursa forms a lubricating film approximately 1 mm thick and is seen as a hypoechoic line. Side-to-side comparison (Fig. 5–6) is the best way to evaluate subtle variations in the quantity of bursal fluid. However, in rare cases, the examiner may be misled by bilateral disease. The hypoechoic fluid film within a normal bursa should not exceed 2 mm. Current technology allows visualization of hyperemia within the synovial membrane. Inflammatory lesions of the synovium demonstrate prominent feeding vessels and dilated veins in the

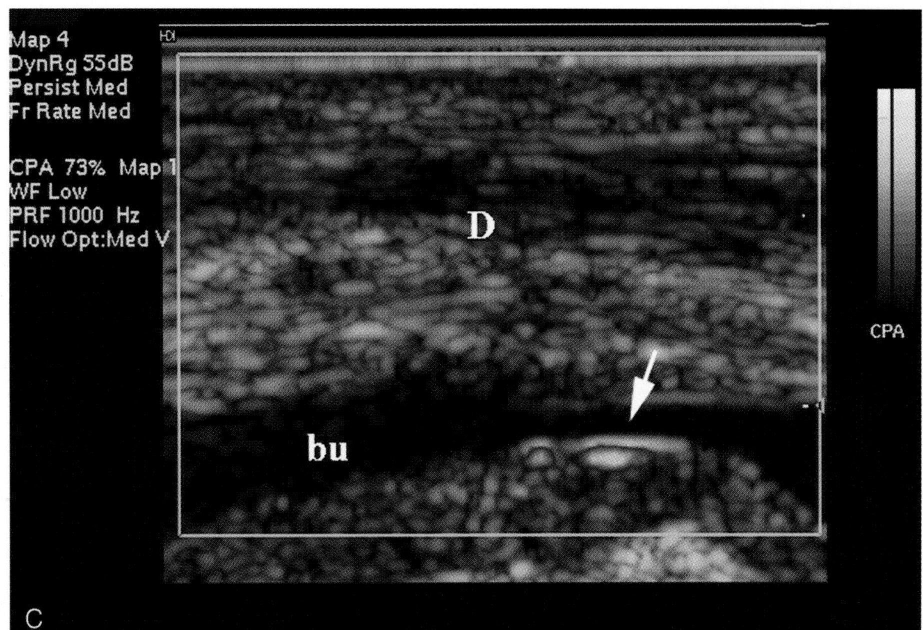

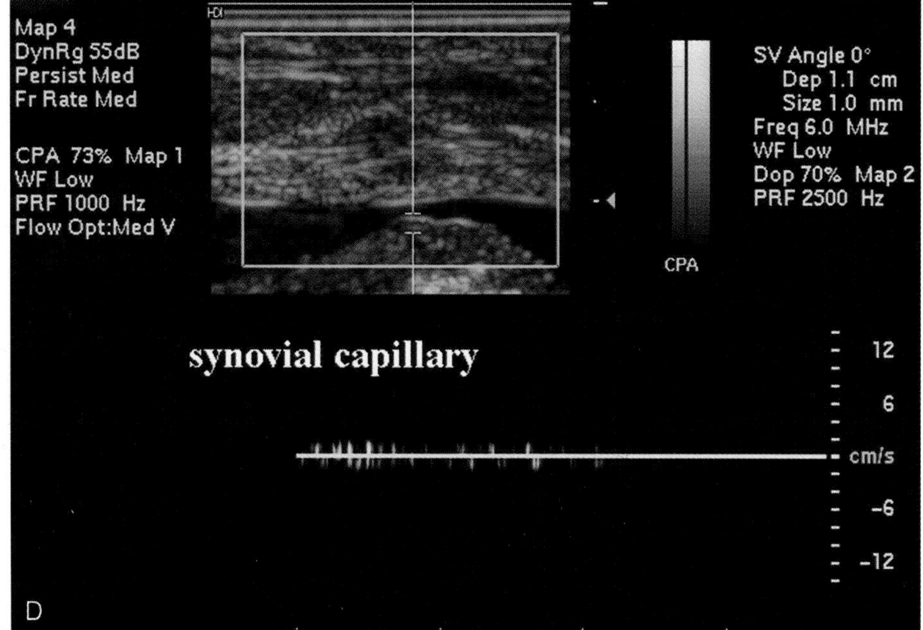

Figure 5-7 *Continued.* ■ **C,** Synovial hyperemia: longitudinal power Doppler sonogram. Same patient as in **A.** This scan along one of the larger vessels shown on cross section in **B** demonstrates flow in a synovial venule 1 mm in diameter. The bright linear interface does not correspond to the thickness of the synovium. Abbreviations: subdeltoid bursa (*bu*), deltoid muscle (*D*). **D,** Synovial hyperemia: duplex Doppler sonogram. Same patient as in **A.** Venous flow within the very small vessel is noted.

synovial wall (Newman el al., 1994). Power Doppler sonography can show vessels within normal synovium on occasion (Fig. 5-7).

Pathology of Bursae

Noncommunicating Bursae

Acute Traumatic Bursitis

A bursa may become acutely inflamed and symptomatic from either direct pressure or excessive repetitive activity of adjacent structures (Fig. 5-8). This condition is called *acute traumatic bursitis* or *frictional bursitis.* It is frequently found in athletes whose sports require repetitive motion, such as runners, tennis players, and oarsmen. Bursae adjacent to joints with irregular bony contours and hypertrophic tendon insertions are predisposed to the development of frictional bursitis. In the upper extremity, the subacromial-subdeltoid and olecranon bursae (Fig. 5-9) are most frequently involved. The trochanteric bursa (Figs. 5-10 and 5-11) is the most common site of frictional bursitis of the hip.

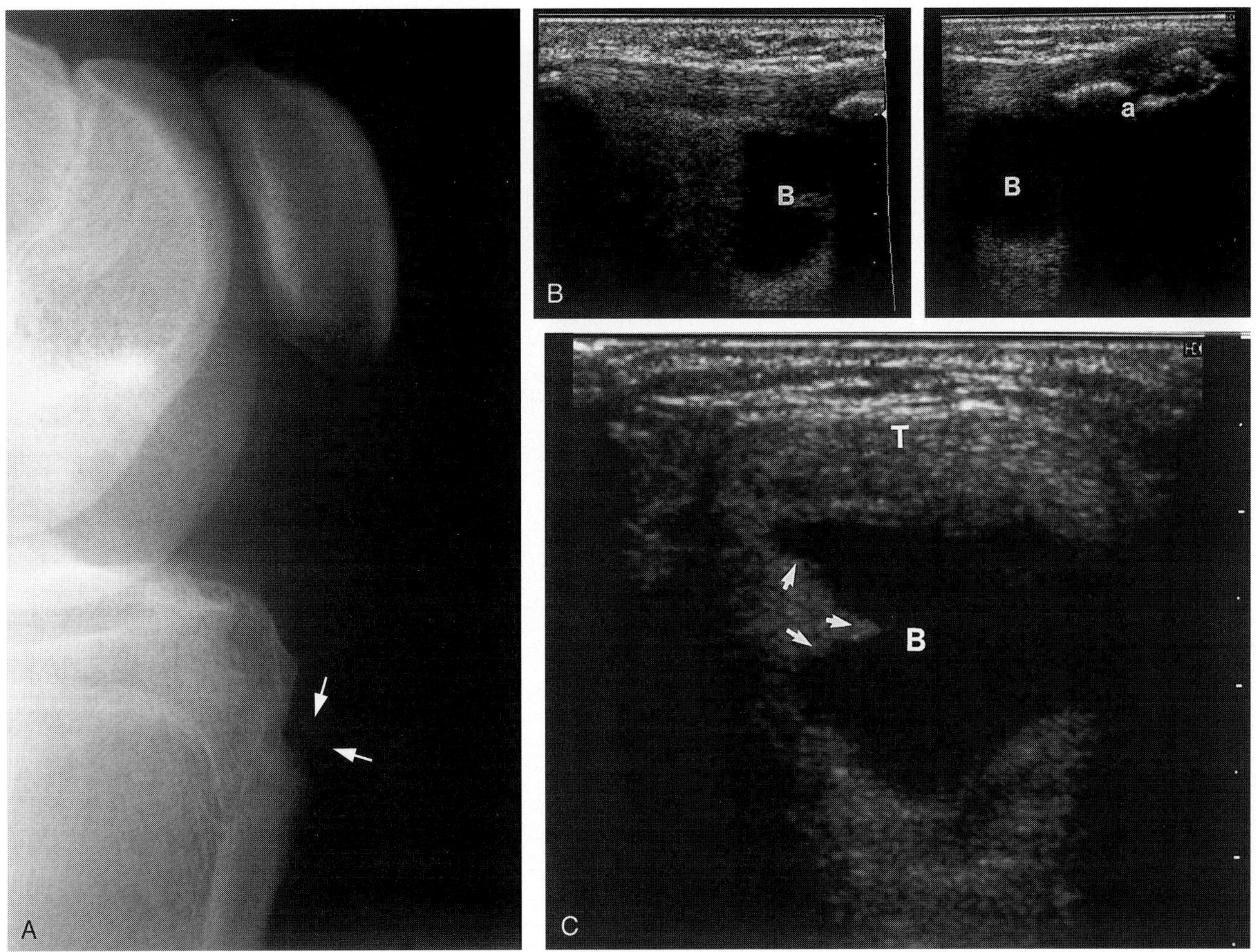

Figure 5–8 ■ **A,** Frictional bursitis of the deep infrapatellar bursa: conventional lateral knee radiograph. This 15-year-old girl, who wants to become a dancer, practiced relentlessly. Recently, she developed pain in her knee. She complains of stiffness in the knee and difficulty climbing stairs. An irregular apophysis (*A*) with a separate ossification center is noted at the distal patellar tendon insertion (*arrows*). **B,** Frictional bursitis of the deep infrapatellar bursa: longitudinal sonograms, split-screen display. Same patient as in **A.** The left side of the split screen displays the patellar tendon stretched between the apex of the patella and the tibial tuberosity. A large, distended bursa (*B*) extends adjacent to the tuberosity and the tendon. The image on the right side of the split screen is a detail of the tibial tuberosity and the large bursa, which covers the bone just proximal to the fragmented apophysis (*a*). Fluid in frictional bursitis often appears anechoic. **C,** Frictional bursitis of the deep infrapatellar bursa: transverse sonogram. Same patient as in **A.** Located deep to the patellar tendon (*T*), the anechoic fluid collection in the deep infrapatellar bursa (*B*) is indented by Hoffa's fat pad (*arrows*).

The bursae of the knee most commonly involved are the prepatellar and deep infrapatellar bursae (see Fig. 5–8). In the foot, the superficial Achilles tendon bursa, retrocalcaneal bursa, and calcaneal bursa are the most frequent sites of frictional bursitis (Figs. 5–12 and 5–13).

The pathophysiology is that of a typical acute inflammatory reaction. Initially there is a brief period of vasoconstriction followed by hyperemia. The hyperemia results from dilatation of arterioles, capillaries, and postcapillary venules. This hyperemic state leads to transudation and exudation. The bursa becomes painful and distended with a watery or mucoid fluid unlike the viscous fluid normally found within the bursa (Nicholas and Hershman, 1986) and very different from the thick gelatinous mucoid substance found in ganglia.

Ultrasound provides the clinician with a noninvasive means of examining the bursae. In acute traumatic bursitis, the primary purpose of sonography is to confirm that disease is limited to the bursa. Associated tendons, ligaments, and joint space are easily examined to exclude bursitis secondary to pathology originating in these structures (Fig. 5–14).

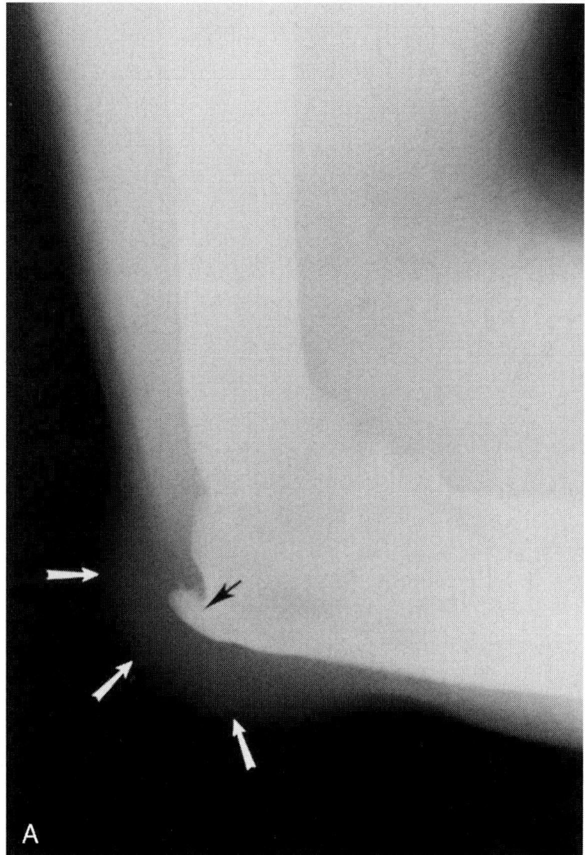

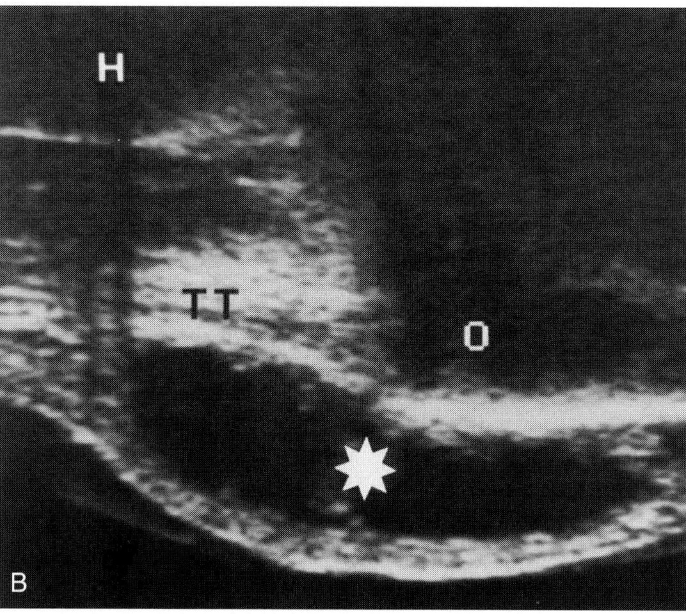

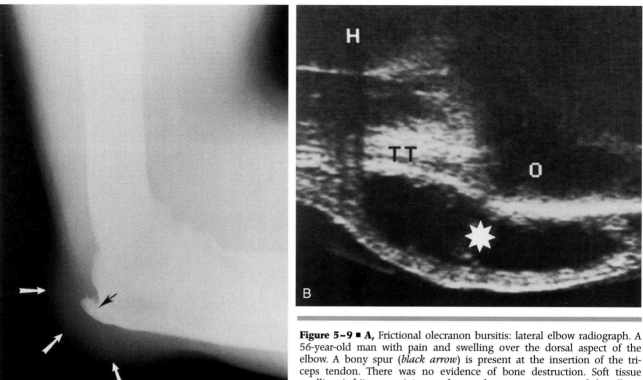

Figure 5-9 ■ **A,** Frictional olecranon bursitis: lateral elbow radiograph. A 56-year-old man with pain and swelling over the dorsal aspect of the elbow. A bony spur (*black arrow*) is present at the insertion of the triceps tendon. There was no evidence of bone destruction. Soft tissue swelling (*white arrows*) is noted over the posterior aspect of the elbow. **B,** Frictional olecranon bursitis: longitudinal sonogram. Same patient as in **A.** The forearm is extended, straightening the elbow. A standoff pad was employed, with the transducer oriented along the triceps tendon. Proximal lies to the observer's left, and the dorsal aspect of the elbow is at the bottom of the image. The triceps tendon (*TT*) inserts on the olecranon at the center of the image. A concave, spheroidal olecranon bursa (*asterisk*) overlies the olecranon and the distal triceps tendon. The fluid is essentially anechoic. Abbreviations: humerus (*H*), olecranon (*O*).

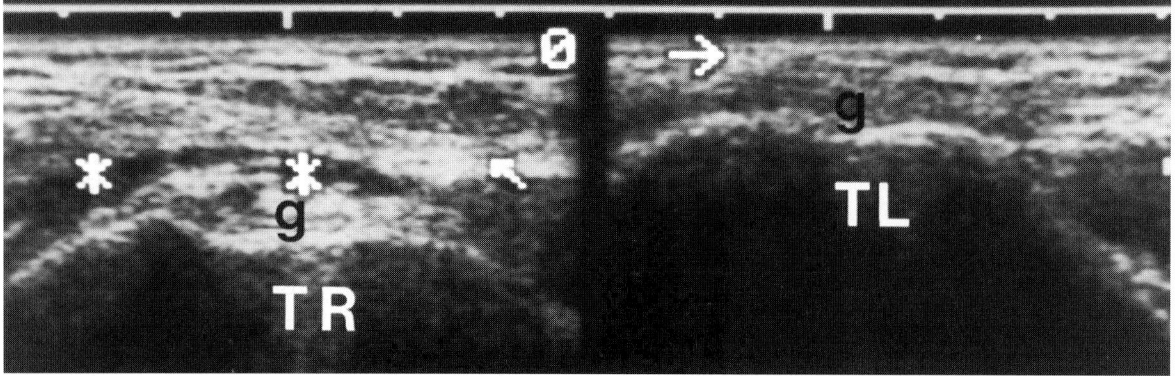

Figure 5-10 ■ Frictional bursitis of the trochanteric bursa: coronal sonogram. A 22-year-old medical student training for a marathon experienced persistent right hip pain and was instructed to discontinue training. The exam was performed with the patient in the lateral decubitus position. Scanning was performed in the coronal plane over the greater trochanter. The symptomatic right side is displayed on the left half of the image; the asymptomatic left side is to the right. An abnormal fluid-filled superficial trochanteric bursa (*asterisk*) is noted on the patient's right. This bursa is located between the tendon of the gluteus muscles (*g*) and the fascia (*arrow*). Abbreviations: right greater trochanter (*TR*), left greater trochanter (*TL*).

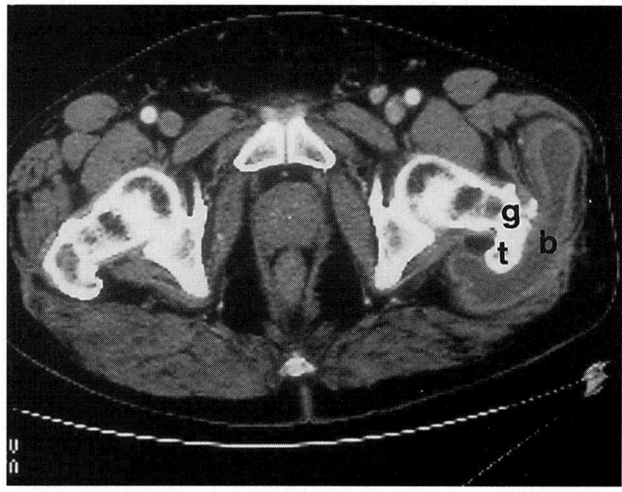

Figure 5-11 ■ Frictional bursitis of the trochanteric bursa: CT scan through the hips. Unilateral trochanteric bursitis similar to the bursitis illustrated in Figure 5-10. The surface of the greater trochanter (*gt*) is the perfect landmark to find the bursa. However, the bursa must be scanned with very light pressure, as fluid will move away from the transducer if too much pressure is applied. Superficial bursae are typically located over bony prominences. A thin film of fluid covers a large area of irregular bone. As a rule, fluid in these bursae will be shown only when the focal zones are moved to the level of the subcutis and when they are scanned with copious gel and light transducer pressure. Note that the contralateral normal bursa is perceptible only with distention. Abbreviation: trochanteric bursa (*b*).

Acute traumatic bursitis is easily recognized by an increase in the volume of the bursa, with no other changes in bursa structure. As stated previously, comparison with the asymptomatic side is extremely valuable. The character of the fluid within the bursa differs markedly from that found in a normal bursa. In acute traumatic bursitis, the fluid is most often anechoic or markedly hypoechoic compared with normal bursal fluid. Fluctuation is noted when pressure is applied on the fluid collection (Fig. 5-15). Acoustic enhancement deep to the inflamed bursa is commonly seen. The appearance of the walls of the bursa is unchanged. This is an important factor in differentiating acute traumatic bursitis from the chronic form.

Chronic Traumatic Bursitis

If the inciting factor persists, acute traumatic bursitis may become chronic. In the process of evolution, the synovial walls of the bursa become thick-

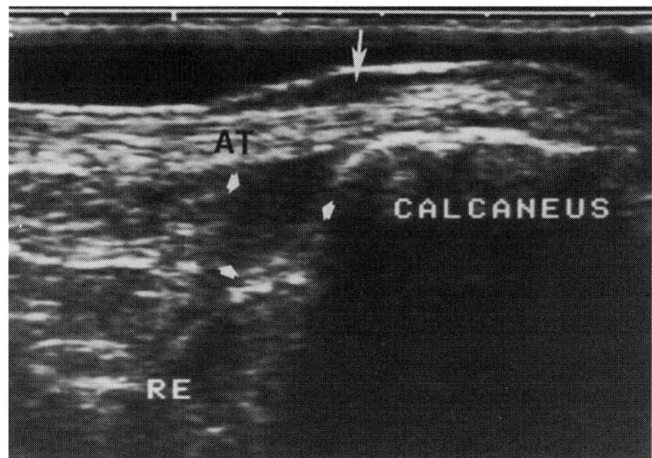

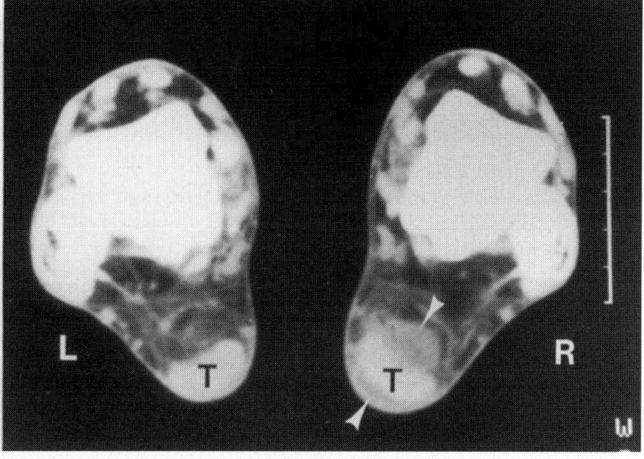

Figure 5-12 ■ **A**, Chronic ankle bursitis: longitudinal sonogram. A 30-year-old woman who frequently wore tight-fitting high heel shoes. She presented with chronic right ankle pain and a pump-bump deformity. The position of the transducer is identical to that in Figure 5-3. Two inflamed bursae surround the Achilles tendon (*AT*). The retrocalcaneal bursa (*short arrows*) lies deep to the Achilles tendon, and the superficial Achilles tendon bursa (*large arrow)* lies superficially. Multiple inflamed bursae at the same site are findings characteristic of chronic bursitis. We cite this example at this point because it nicely demonstrates the bursae of the ankle most frequently involved in traumatic bursitis. Abbreviation: Right *(RE*). **B**, Chronic ankle bursitis: CT findings. Same patient as in **A**. This is a transverse axial image of the ankles at the level of the distal Achilles tendon. The Achilles tendon (*T*) is identified between the distended, fluid-filled retrocalcaneal and superficial Achilles tendon bursae (*arrowheads*). Although smaller than the retrocalcaneal bursa, the superficial Achilles tendon bursa can cause significant ankle swelling. Abbreviations: patient's left (*L*), right (*R*).

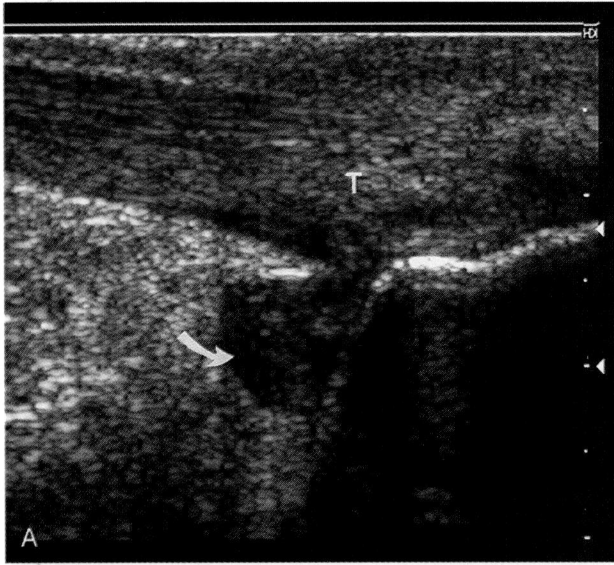

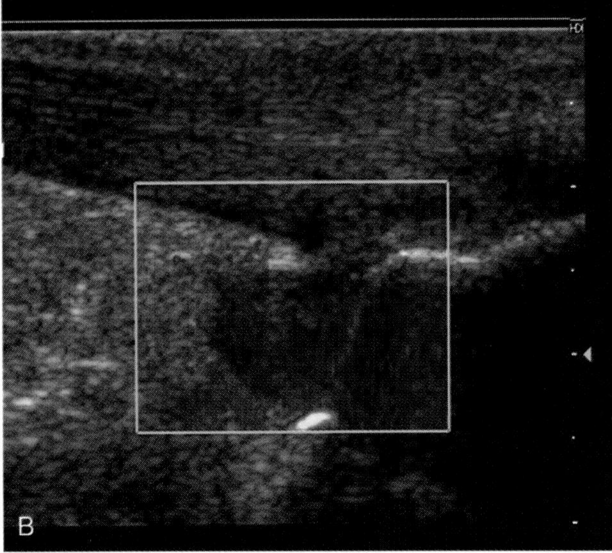

Figure 5–13 ■ **A**, Frictional bursitis: longitudinal sonogram. An athletic 33-year-old woman experienced episodes of heel pain. She noticed that it occurred every time she exchanged her sneakers for high-heeled shoes. Hypoechoic swelling of the retrocalcaneal bursa (*curved arrow*) is noted deep to a thickened distal Achilles tendon (*T*). **B**, Frictional bursitis: power Doppler sonography. Same patient as in **A**. In frictional bursitis, there is no significant hyperemia of the synovium. This finding is in sharp contrast with the increased vascularity of the synovium observed in inflammatory arthritides.

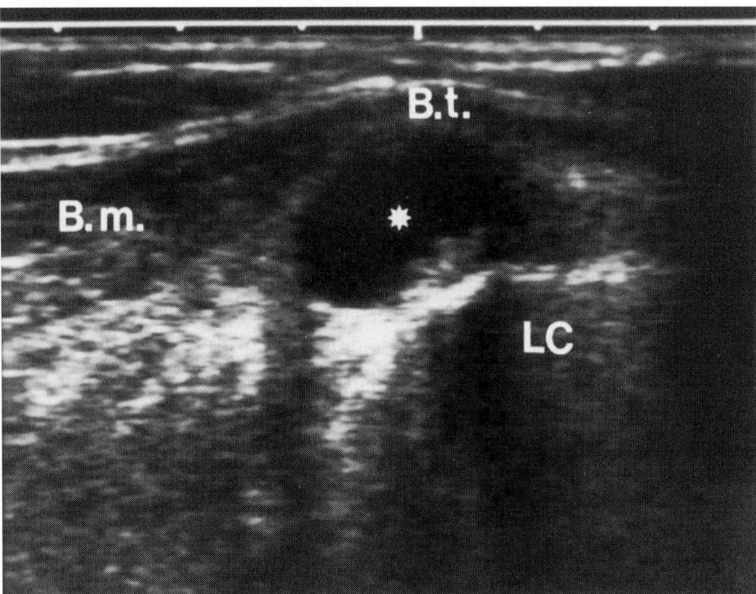

Figure 5–14 ■ Bursitis at the lateral aspect of the knee: coronal sonogram. An 18-year-old soccer player with tenderness over the lateral femoral condyle following a game. The clinical differential diagnosis was biceps femoris tendinitis and tensor fascia lata syndrome. A coronal image was obtained with the transducer over the posterior medial aspect of the knee. An oval, anechoic mass elevates the biceps tendon (*B.t.*), consistent with frictional bursitis of the bursa (*asterisk*) separating the fibular collateral ligament and the biceps tendon. Abbreviations: biceps femoris muscle (*B.m.*), lateral femoral condyle (*LC*).

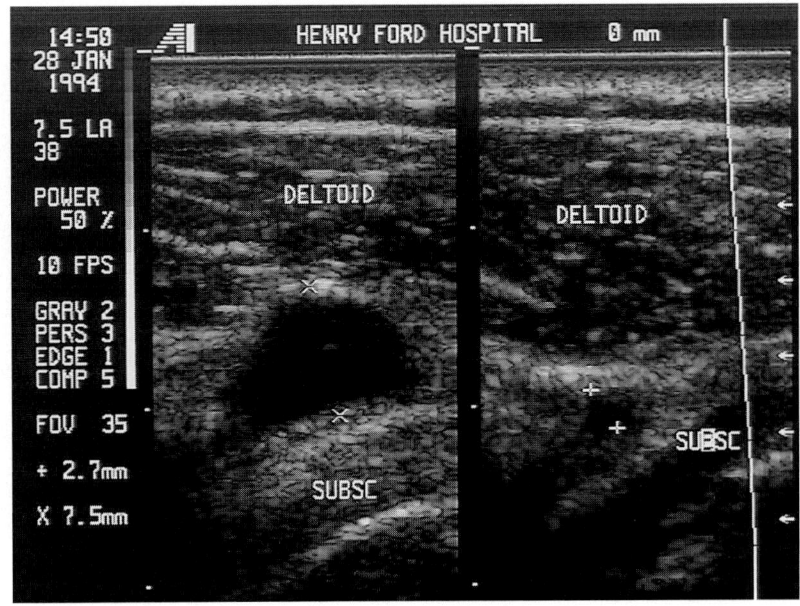

Figure 5-15 ■ Bursal effusion in subacromial-subdeltoid bursa: split-screen dynamic examination. A 74-year-old carpenter presents with pain in the shoulder and with a rotator cuff tear documented by ultrasound. Shoulder motion brings the arm from internal to external rotation. This maneuver shows expansion of the bursal lumen during external rotation (left image) and flattening (right image) of the bursa during internal rotation. This phenomenon is equivalent to fluctuation observed clinically.

ened, and it becomes filled with a fibrinous exudate. Calcifications are sometimes seen within or surrounding the chronically inflamed bursa. A subtype of chronic traumatic bursitis is the formation of an adventitious bursa in an area subjected to chronic frictional irritation. In this condition, inflammation of the adjacent areolar connective tissue forms a focus of fibrinoid necrosis (Gardner, 1965). A cystic structure filled with cellular debris, extracellular fluid, altered ground substance, and inflammatory exudate results (Nicholas and Hershman, 1986). This process is the formation of a bursa de novo (Figs. 5-16 and 5-17). In women, a common adventitious bursa is found over the first metatarsal head. It is a frequent complication of wearing narrow, pointed shoes (Fig. 5-18) (Canoso, 1981).

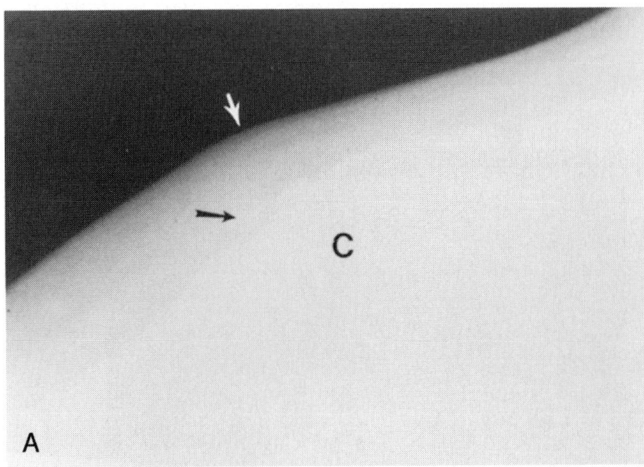

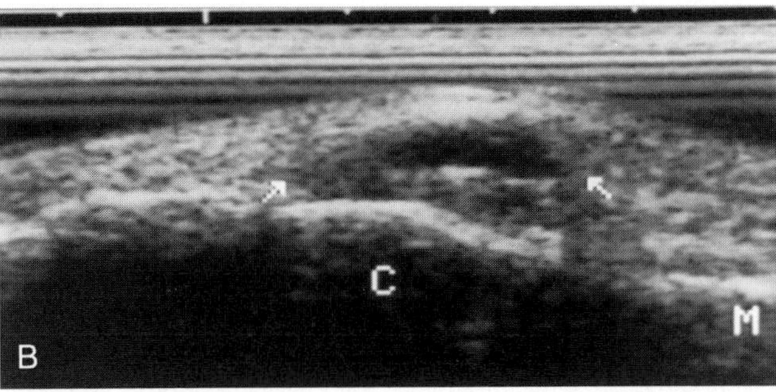

Figure 5-16 ■ **A**, Adventitious bursa on the dorsum of the foot: lateral radiograph of the left foot. A 17-year-old girl who twisted her foot 5 months ago. Initial radiographs were interpreted as normal. Pain and swelling over the dorsum of the foot persisted. This radiograph, obtained using soft tissue technique, demonstrates soft tissue swelling (*white arrow*) and an avulsed fragment (*black arrow*) over the anterior medial aspect of the medial cuneiform bone (*C*). **B**, Adventitious bursa: longitudinal sonogram. Same patient as in **A.** The transducer is positioned over the base of the first metatarsal oriented along its length. The linear, hyperechoic structure superficial to the medial cuneiform is the avulsed fragment demonstrated in **A.** Note that only faint acoustic shadowing is present due to volume averaging artifact. An ovoid bursa (*arrow*) separates the skin and the bony fragment. Surgery demonstrated a small, avulsed bone fragment with an adjacent adventitious bursa. Abbreviations: medial cuneiform (*C*), first metatarsal (*M*).

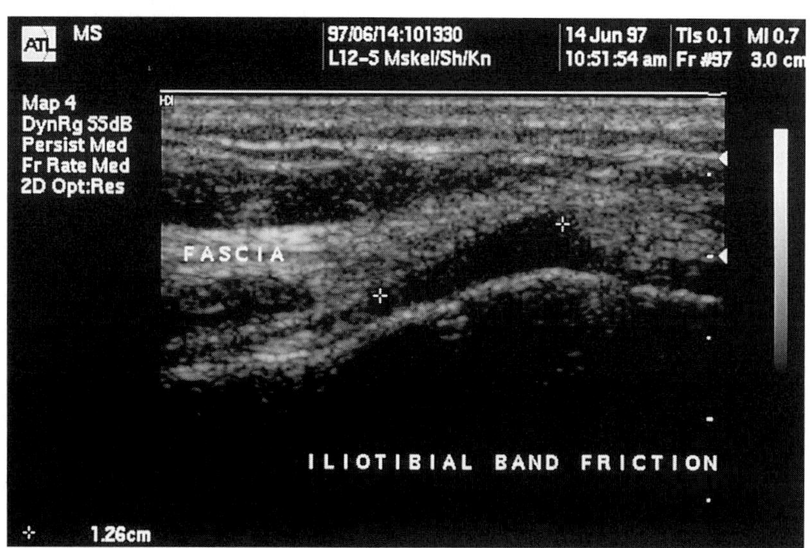

Figure 5-17 ■ Frictional bursitis in iliotibial band friction syndrome: coronal sonogram. This young woman runs half marathons. She has been following an intensive training program and was running on hard surfaces such as sidewalks. The iliotibial band is separated from the lateral femoral condyle by a distended, hypoechoic bursa (*between the calipers*).

The sonographic features of chronic traumatic bursitis are demonstrated in Figures 5-19 through 5-24. As in acute traumatic bursitis, the bursa is distended with fluid. However, the fibrinous exudate found in chronic traumatic bursitis produces definite echos within the bursa (Figs. 5-19 through 5-21). In addition, the synovial walls of the bursa are markedly thickened and easily visible as a millimeter-thick layer. The outline of the bursa is often very irregular (see Figs. 5-22 and 5-23). If present, calcifications are seen as hyperechoic foci, with or without shadowing. The presence of shadowing is dependent on the size of the calcifications and the frequency of transducer use. Adjacent bursae are often involved in chronic bursitis, as are the adjacent tendons (Fig. 5-24). Bursae having their synovium adjacent to adipose tissue may develop fatty hypertrophy of the synovium when chronically irritated. A typical example is the lipoma arborescens found in the suprapatellar bursa of the knee with chronic synovitis. This swelling may be mistaken clinically for a synovial tumor (Resnick and Niwayama, 1988).

Hemorrhagic Bursitis

A powerful blow to a bursa, fracture of an adjacent bone, or rupture of a tendon can cause hemorrhage into the bursa. If a significant amount of blood fills

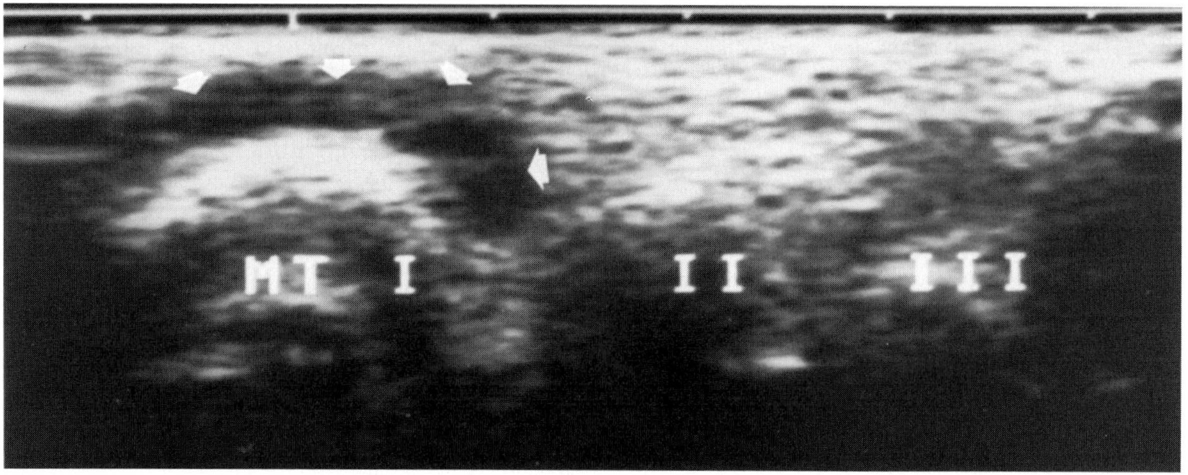

Figure 5-18 ■ Adventitious bursa over the first metatarsal head: transverse sonogram. The patient is a 35-year-old woman with a hallux valgus deformity and recurrent swelling over the head of the first metatarsal. The transducer is positioned transversely over the heads of the first through third metatarsals (*MTI–III*). An adventitious bursa (*white arrows*) is identified as a hypoechoic, curvilinear band over the first metatarsal head.

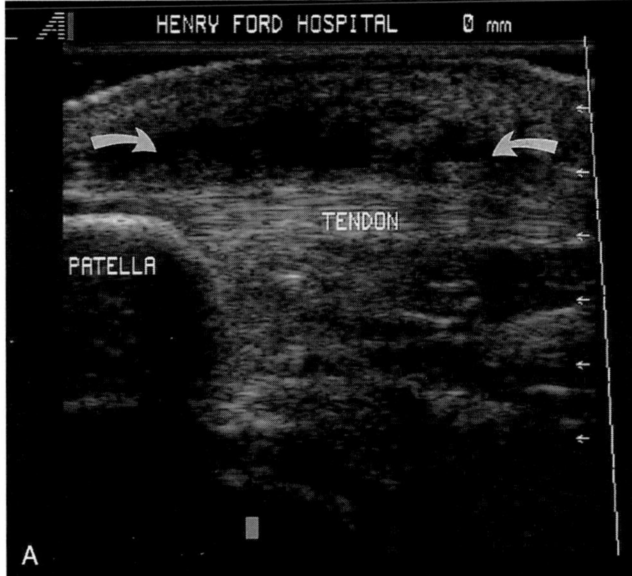

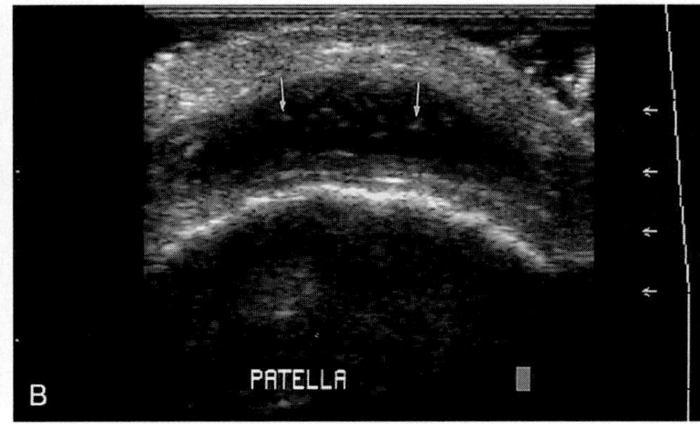

Figure 5-19 ■ **A,** Chronic prepatellar bursitis: longitudinal sonogram. This 62-year-old cleaning lady notices recurrent swelling and pain over her anterior knee. Sonography demonstrates a normal patellar tendon but swelling of the prepatellar bursa. The bursa (*curved arrows*) appears hypoechoic, with distinct echos in its lumen. The synovial lining of the bursa is irregular. **B,** Chronic prepatellar bursitis: transverse sonogram. Pathology similar to that in **A.** With the transducer gently placed over the patella, one notices the flat, sac-like structure filled with fluid and debris. The distinct internal echos (*arrows*) are often seen in chronic bursitis.

the bursa, it may form a clot (Peterson and Renstrom, 1986). Chemical irritation of the bursa during resolution of the hemorrhage will result in the formation of adhesions. Later, loose bodies and calcifications may be found within the bursa (Peterson and Renstrom, 1986).

Hemorrhagic bursitis affects bursae of the hands, knees, hips, and shoulders. This condition is frequently found in athletes who participate in sports that involve repeated contact with a hard surface, such as handball, volleyball, and football. In football players, the incidence of hemorrhagic bursitis has increased with the use of artificial surfaces. Automutilation should be suspected when hemorrhagic bursitis is diagnosed several times within a period of weeks or months. If other signs of acute

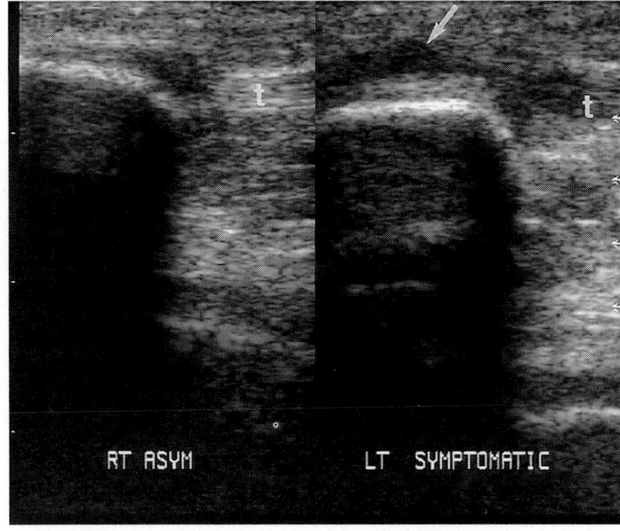

Figure 5-20 ■ Chronic prepatellar bursitis: longitudinal sonogram with split-screen technique. Pain and swelling of the left knee disabled this 46-year-old nurse. The knee swelling manifested as a hard knot overlying the apex of the patella. Therefore, she was unable to do any work that required kneeling. These longitudinal images through the proximal patellar tendon show a normal tendon and bursa of the right knee (left image). Nodular swelling (*arrow*) of the prepatellar bursa in the left knee is consistent with chronic bursitis (right image). Thickened synovium is typically hypoechoic compared to the adjacent fat and tendon. Synovial thickening can be distinguished from fluid by identification of specular echos. In addition, the synovial mass cannot be deformed by pressure, and fluid may be displaced.

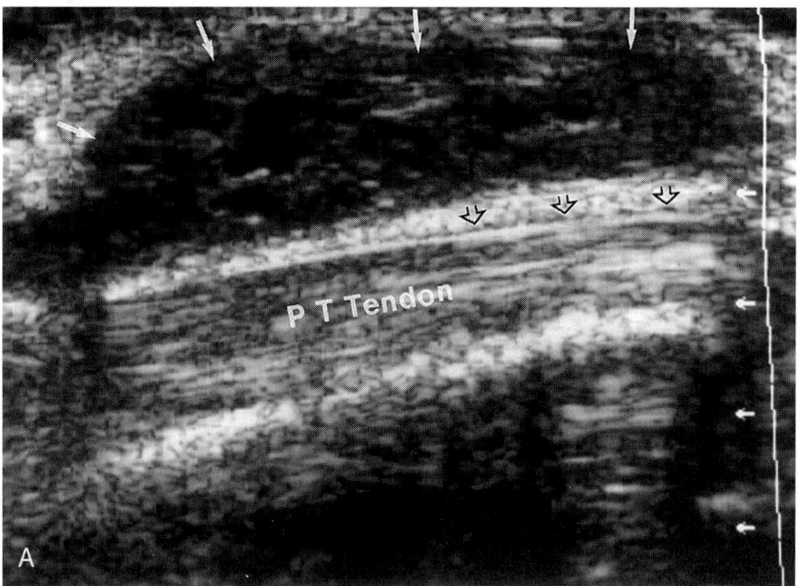

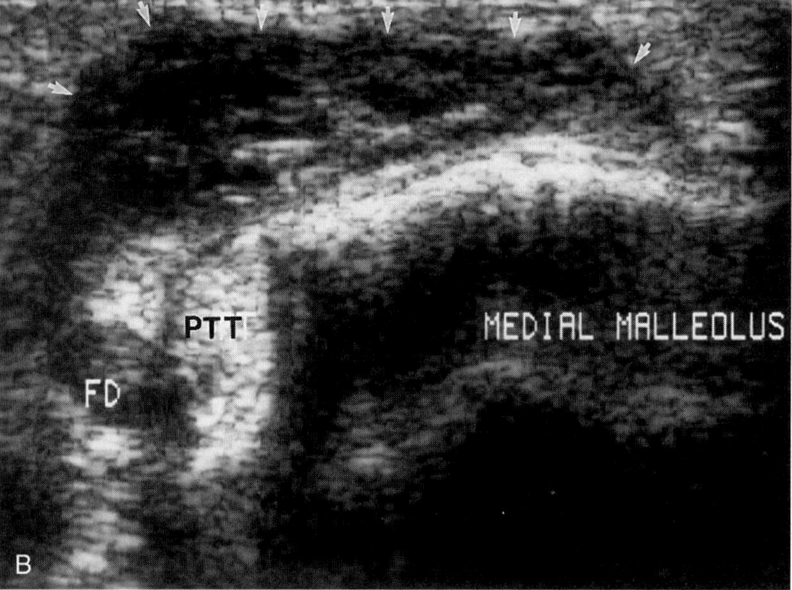

Figure 5–21 ■ **A,** Chronic bursitis over the medial malleolus: longitudinal sonogram. A middle-aged man complains of pain over the medial ankle. The clinician palpates a mass (*arrows*) and interprets the finding as an abnormal posterior tibial tendon with a swollen tendon sheath. The longitudinal image along the posterior tibial (*PT*) tendon demonstrates a normal tendon with a thin and intact tendon sheath (*open arrows*). A medial malleolar bursa (*arrows*) appears filled with tissue of mixed echogenicity. Only a small amount of fluid is present within the lumen of the bursa. Multiple interfaces within this bursa appear hyperechoic. **B,** Chronic bursitis over the medial malleolus: transverse sonogram. Same patient as in **A.** The bursa covers the medial malleolus. Posterior extension over the posterior tibial tendon (*PTT*) and over the flexor digitorum (*FD*) explains the difficulties of clinical diagnosis. Palpation of bursae is often easier over soft tissue than over bone.

or chronic trauma are found on further examination, suspicion should be increased (Fig. 5–25). Before one labels the patient a psychiatric patient, one should investigate the patient's athletic endeavors. The patient may be a rugby player. Sonography demonstrates a distended bursa forming a spheroid (prepatellar bursa), concave spheroid (olecranon bursa), bean-like (retrocalcaneal bursa), or bilobed (deep infrapatellar bursa) structure. The bursa is usually more distended than that seen in frictional bursitis. Fluid within the bursa has definite internal echos corresponding to the cellular components of blood. Immediately following injury, the bursa is filled with diffusely echogenic blood (Fig. 5–26). Blood within synovial spaces does not always clot due to the presence of enzymes within the cavity that inhibit thrombosis. However, if thrombosis occurs, clot retraction follows. Then blood and fibrin clots can be seen within the bursa as irregularly shaped, hyperechoic masses floating within the anechoic serum (Fig. 5–27). It is important to note that these masses are mobile and are not attached to the synovial walls (Fig. 5–28). No thickening of the synovial wall is present. In later stages of resolution, adhesions to the synovial walls can develop. This usually occurs several months after the initial injury.

Chemical Bursitis

Chemical bursitis results from the accumulation within the bursa of substances from metabolic dis-

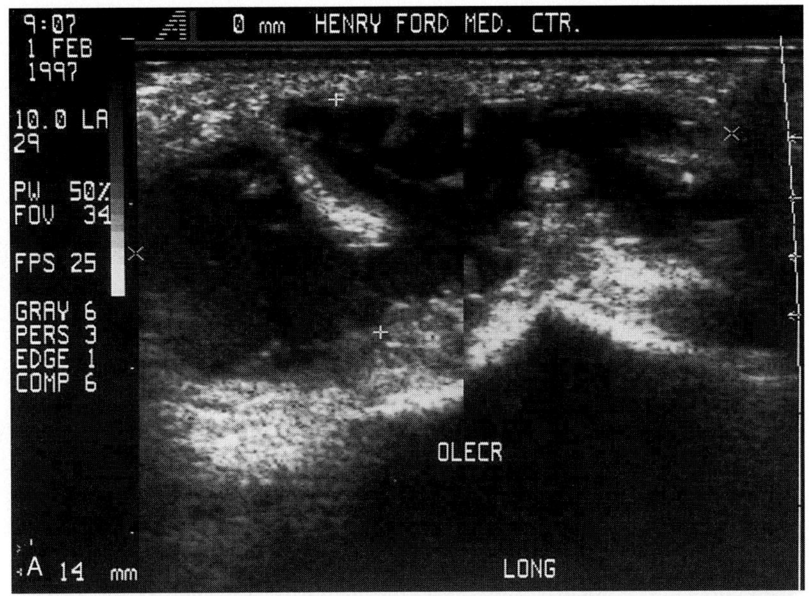

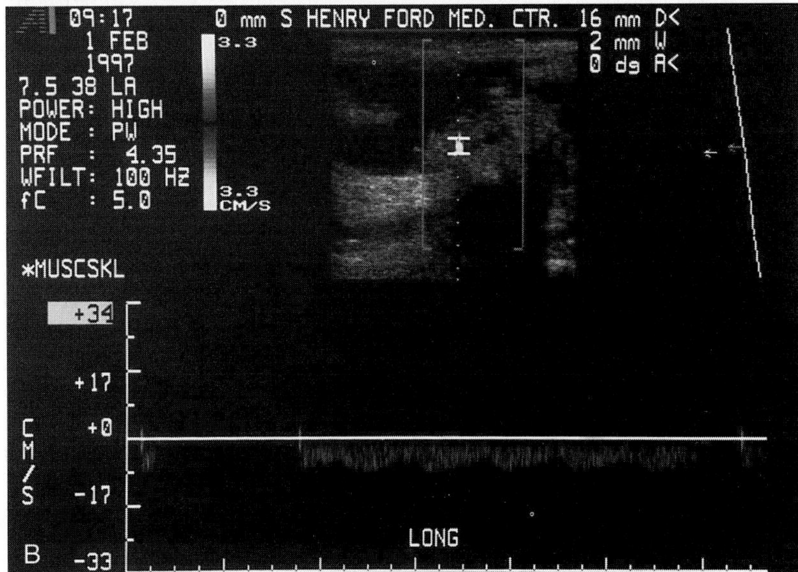

Figure 5–22 ■ **A,** Chronic traumatic olecranon bursitis: sagittal sonogram. The elbow of this 62-year-old bus driver has been traumatized several times over the course of a few months. Serosanguineous fluid has been aspirated from the elbow twice. Cultures were negative, and the fluid did not contain crystals. This split-screen image shows a distended olecranon bursa (*between the calipers*), which is over 4 cm in length. Unusual for a traumatic bursitis is the number of septations within the bursal lumen. Abbreviation: olecranon (*OLECR*). **B,** Chronic traumatic olecranon bursitis: Doppler sonography. Same patient as in **A.** Synovial septations in the bursa demonstrate arterial and venous signals. A sample of the venous signal recorded in the septal wall is illustrated here. In most cases, trauma to bursae does not cause hyperemia or result in the development of septations. This case illustrates that inflammatory changes can develop with any type of chronic bursitis.

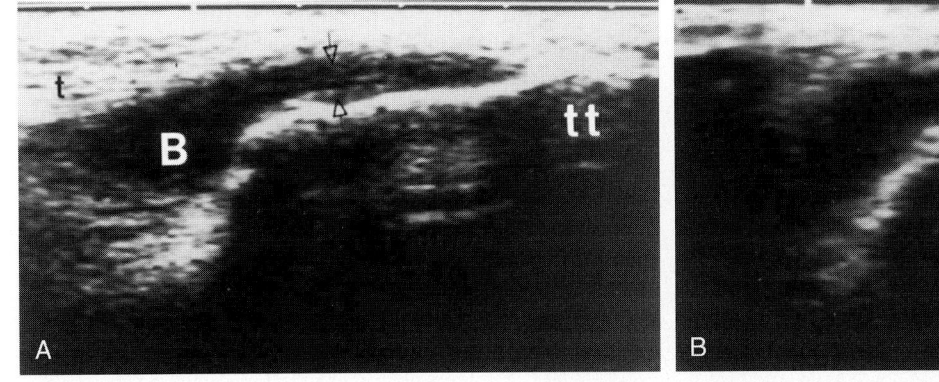

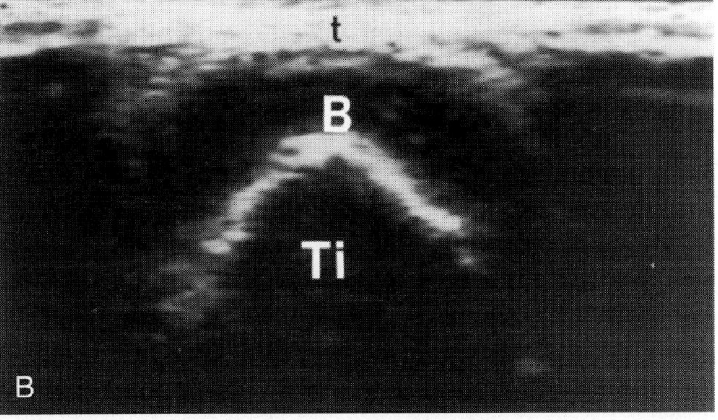

Figure 5–23 ■ **A,** Chronic bursitis of the deep infrapatellar bursa: longitudinal sonogram. A 17-year-old soccer player with pain, tenderness, and swelling over the tibial tuberosity. He was previously diagnosed as having Osgood-Schlatter disease. The transducer is oriented in the longitudinal axis of the patellar tendon (*t*). Distal structures are at the observer's right. The inflamed bursa (*B*) has a bilobed appearance, measuring approximately 5 cm long. Relative to the surrounding fat and tendon, the bursa appears essentially anechoic. Synovial wall thickening is also observed (*arrows*). Abbreviation: tibial tuberosity (*tt*). **B,** Chronic bursitis of the deep infrapatellar bursa: transverse sonogram. Same patient as in **A.** The transducer is rotated 90 degrees to give a transverse image. In this image, the bursa has a hypoechoic, bean-shaped configuration positioned between the tibia (*Ti*) and the patellar tendon (*t*). A rim of synovial thickening is again seen around the bursa.

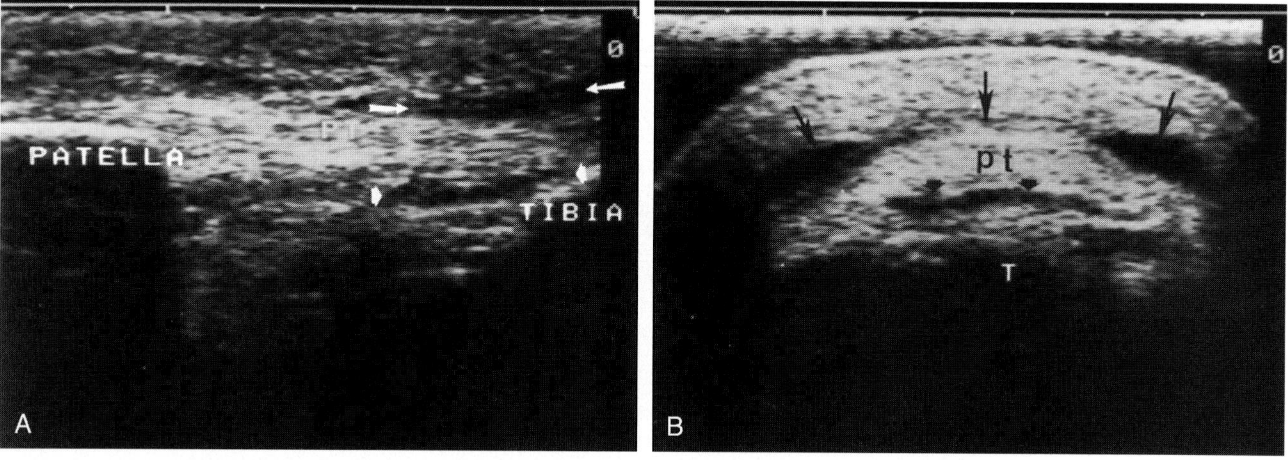

Figure 5-24 ■ **A,** Chronic bursitis around the distal patellar tendon: longitudinal sonogram. A 62-year-old man had chronic knee pain following a below-knee amputation. The transducer is positioned over the patellar tendon in the longitudinal axis of the knee. A normal patellar tendon (*PT*) is seen. Two distended, fluid-filled bursae are noted around the distal patellar tendon. These are the deep infrapatellar bursa (*short arrows*) and the subcutaneous tibial tuberosity bursa (*long arrows*). **B,** Chronic bursitis around the distal patellar tendon: transverse sonogram. Same patient as in **A.** The transducer is now positioned transversely over the distal patellar tendon (*pt*). The inflamed subcutaneous tibial tuberosity (*long arrows*) and deep infrapatellar bursae (*short arrows*) surround the patellar tendon. Essentially all of the fluid in the subcutaneous tibial tuberosity bursa is seen in the lateral recesses of the bursa. Abbreviation: proximal tibia (*T*).

orders, inflammatory processes, or degenerative processes of the surrounding tendons (Peterson and Renstrom, 1986). A resolving hemorrhagic bursitis may also be categorized as a chemical bursitis. The deposition of urate crystals within bursae, seen in gout, is the most common metabolic disorder causing chemical bursitis. Gout most frequently involves the subcutaneous bursae of the dorsal aspect of the elbows and the ventral aspect of the knees.

Inflammatory and degenerative causes of chemical bursitis occur most often in the fifth and sixth decades of life. The subdeltoid bursa is most commonly involved. Crystals found most frequently are composed of calcium hydroxyapatite (Fig. 5-29).

On ultrasound images, the bursa is distended with fluid that appears markedly hypoechoic or anechoic. Hyperechoic foci may be seen within the bursa or in the surrounding tendons corresponding

Text continued on page 151

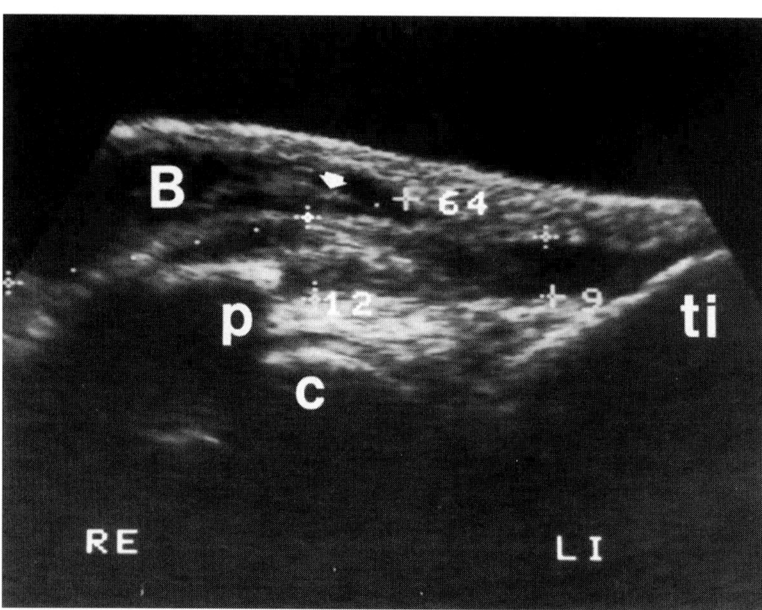

Figure 5-25 ■ Chronic hemorrhagic bursitis of the prepatellar bursa: longitudinal sonogram. This patient is a 16-year-old girl with chronic psychosis. She was admitted with a red, swollen knee, and the clinical concern was infection. The transducer is positioned in the longitudinal axis of the knee, with proximal at the observer's left. A standoff pad was utilized for optimal visualization of this superficial bursa. The swollen prepatellar bursa (*B*) is seen as an oval-shaped, hypoechoic mass overlying the patella. Free-floating, hyperechoic debris (*small arrow*) was identified within the bursa during real-time imaging. Aspiration of the bursa yielded blood, and observation of the patient confirmed the diagnosis of automutilation. Thickening of the patellar tendon was also noted, with the tendon measuring 12 mm at its thickest point, twice the normal thickness. The tendon was hypoechoic relative to the surrounding fat pad, consistent with the diagnosis of tendonitis. Abbreviations: femoral condyle (*c*), patella (*p*), tibia (*ti*), right (*RE*), left (*LI*).

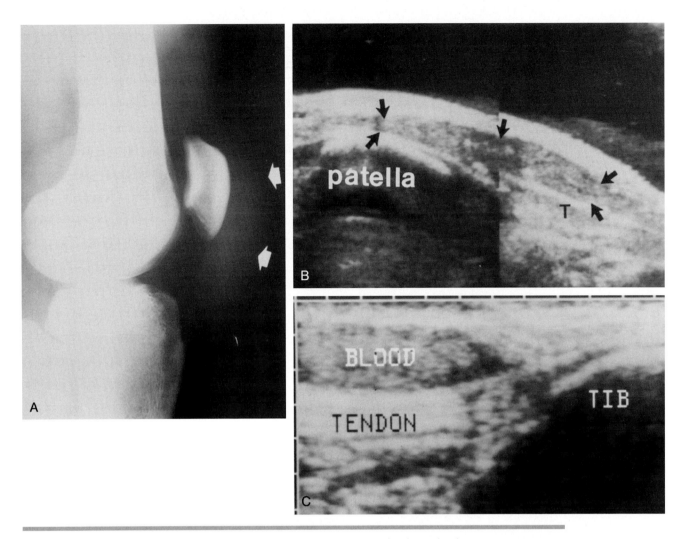

Figure 5–26 ▪ **A,** Hemorrhagic bursitis of the prepatellar bursa: conventional radiograph. The patient is a 21-year-old football player who was hit on the knee by a helmet and presented with pain and swelling over the patella. No fractures are present, but marked soft tissue swelling is noted over the patella (*white arrows*). **B,** Hemorrhagic bursitis of the prepatellar bursa: longitudinal sonogram. Same patient as in **A.** Ultrasound examination performed 3 hours following injury revealed swelling of the prepatellar bursa (*arrows*), which is filled with homogeneous hypoechoic material. Surrounding subcutaneous tissue is diffusely decreased in echogenicity compared with the normal subcutaneous tissues. Abbreviation: patellar tendon (*T*). **C,** This image of the same patient is a detail demonstrating a normal patellar tendon inserting on the tibial tuberosity (*TIB*), with the inferior aspect of the prepatellar bursa filled with blood.

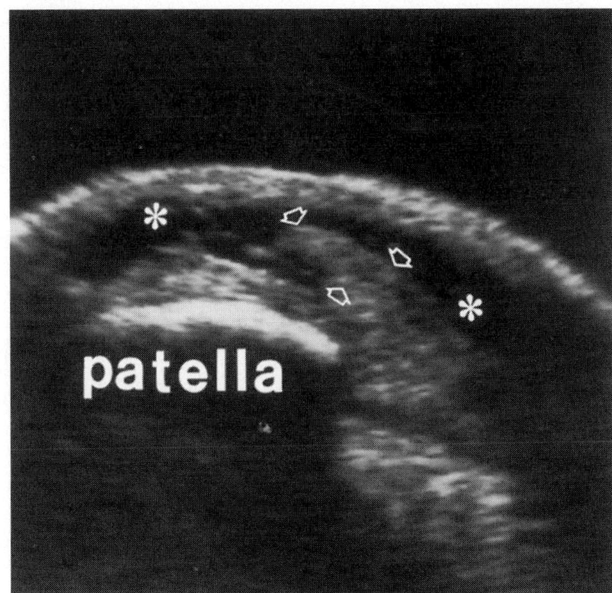

Figure 5–27 ▪ Hemorrhagic bursitis of the prepatellar bursa: longitudinal sonogram. Same patient as in Figure 5–25. After blood clot retraction, the lumen is filled with anechoic fluid (*asterisks*) and fibrin clots (*open arrows*).

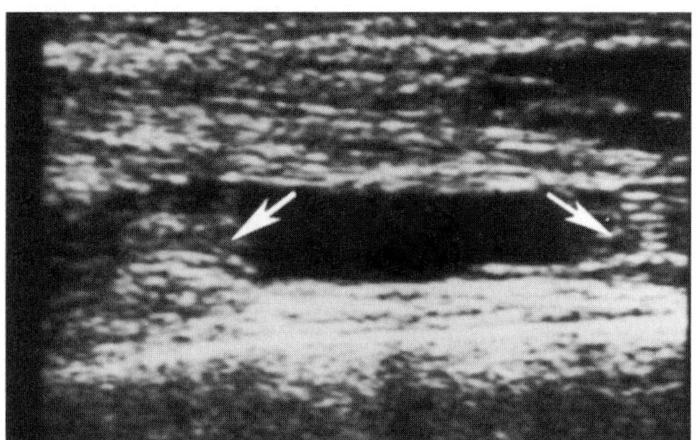

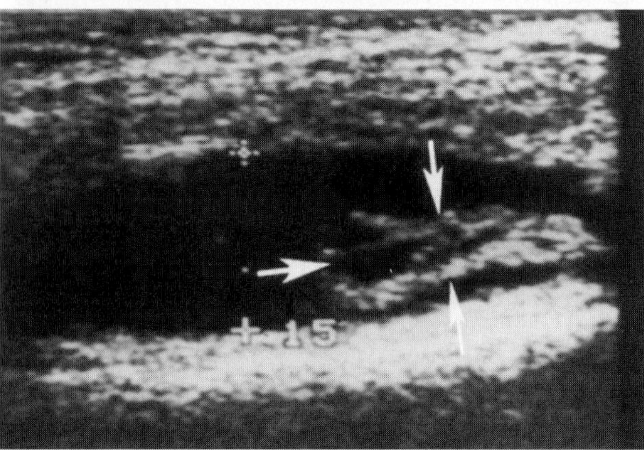

Figure 5-28 ■ Hemorrhagic bursitis of the deep trochanteric bursa: coronal sonogram. A 23-year-old man with pain and swelling over the right greater trochanter following direct trauma to this region. The patient was examined in the left lateral decubitus position, with the transducer placed over the right greater trochanter in the coronal plane. Anechoic fluid is seen within the bursa in the top image. Clumps of debris are noted within the bursa (*arrows*). Reduced pressure applied with the transducer and compression of the lateral recesses of the bursa by the examiners freehand demonstrated free-floating clots within the bursa (bottom image). The diameter of the bursa is increased to 15 mm.

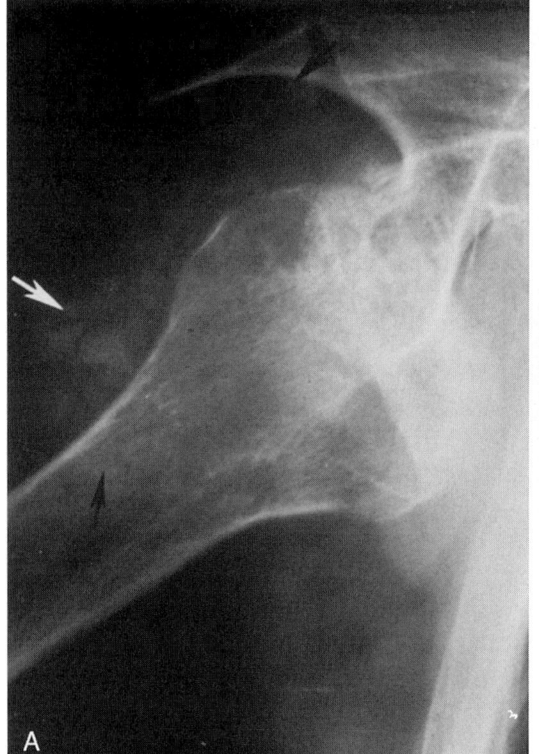

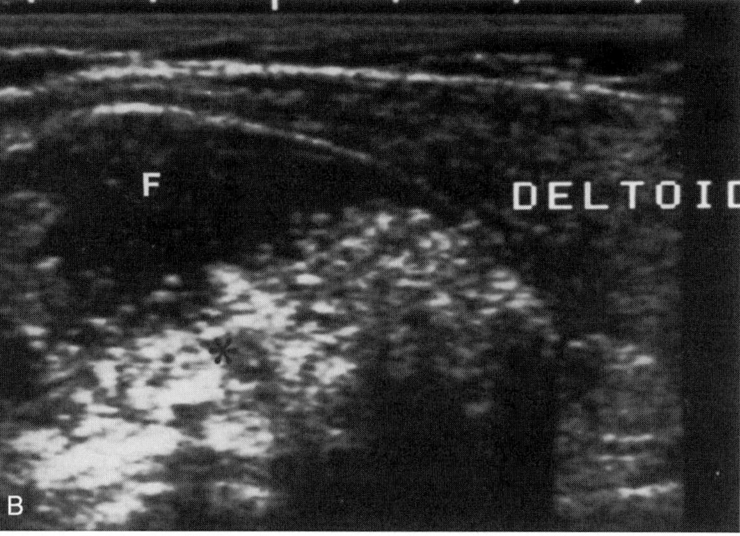

Figure 5-29 ■ **A,** Calcific bursitis of the subdeltoid bursa: conventional anteroposterior radiograph of the right shoulder. The patient is a 61-year-old man with a 20-year history of rheumatoid arthritis treated with steroids. He has known osteonecrosis of the right shoulder and both hips. Flattening of the right humeral head is noted, consistent with osteonecrosis. An oval region of calcification is seen overlaying the humerus, extending lateral and superior to the humeral head (*arrows*). **B,** Calcific bursitis of the subdeltoid bursa: coronal sonogram. Same patient as in **A.** The transducer is positioned along the length of the humerus, with the acromion just out of the field to the left. An anechoic fluid collection (*F*) is present in the subdeltoid bursa. Numerous calcifications (*asterisk*) are noted dependently in the bursa, some demonstrating acoustic shadowing.

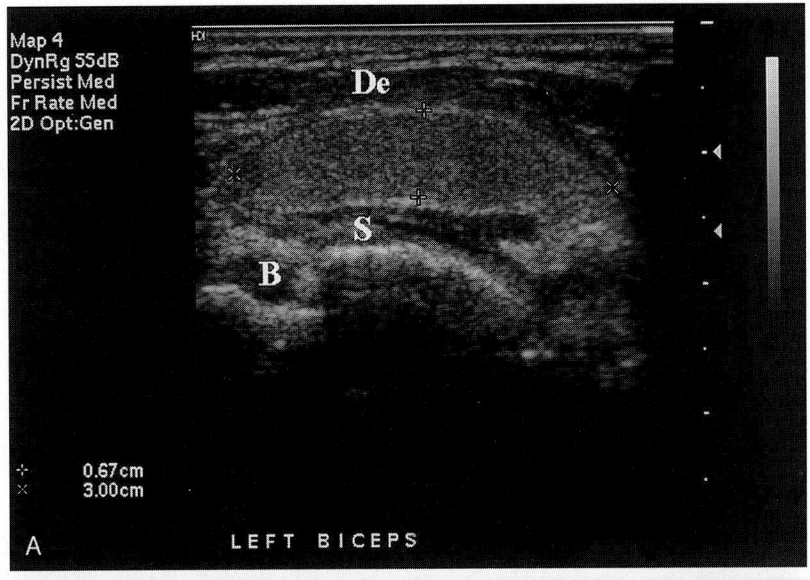

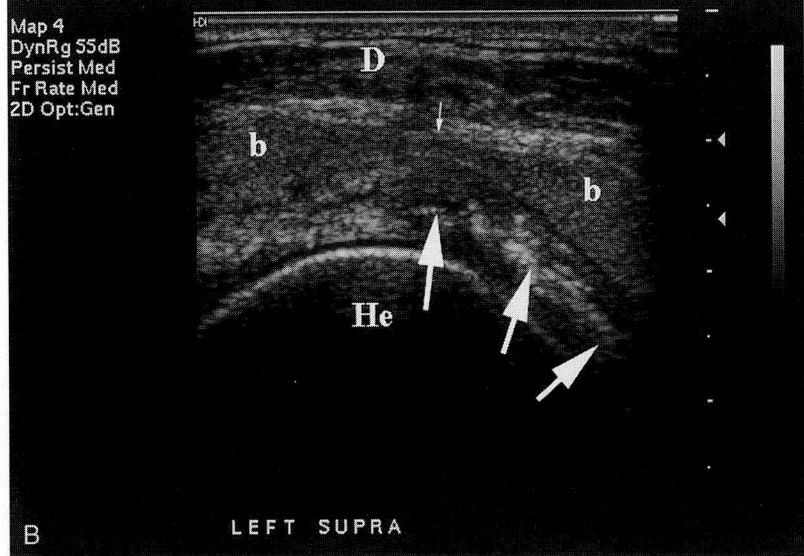

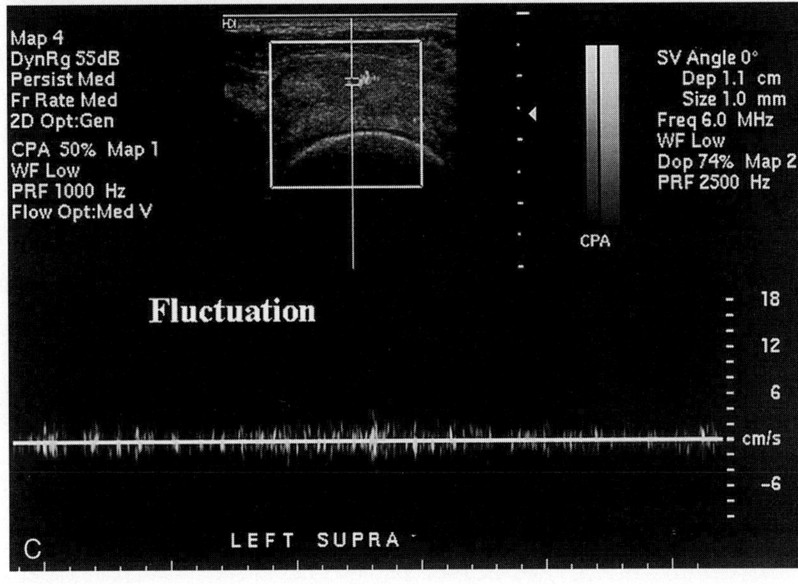

Figure 5-30 ■ **A,** Hydroxyapatite synovitis: transverse sonogram through the anterior shoulder. Acute-onset pain in the left shoulder brings this 46-year-old nurse to the orthopedic clinic with her arm in a sling. The subacromial-subdeltoid bursa is filled with hyperechoic material, which appears very homogeneous and does not demonstrate acoustic shadowing. The bursa appears as a mass sandwiched between the deltoid muscle (*De*) and the subscapularis tendon (*S*). Abbreviation: long biceps tendon (*B*). **B,** Hydroxyapatite synovitis: transverse sonogram through the supraspinatus tendon. Same patient as in **A.** When hydroxyapatite deposition causes shoulder pain, one will often find calcification within the tendon (*large arrows*) and bursa (*b*). The calcific material within the bursa is suspended in a calcium milk solution. Compression of the bursa results in displacement of the fluid (*small arrow*). Abbreviations: deltoid (*D*), humeral epiphysis (*He*). **C,** Hydroxyapatite synovitis: duplex Doppler scan through the bursa and rotator cuff in the transverse plane. Same patient as in **A.** Fluctuation can be demonstrated in the hyperechoic fluid of the subdeltoid bursa. This fluctuation is visible by movement on the Doppler scale and a color flow pattern within the bursa.

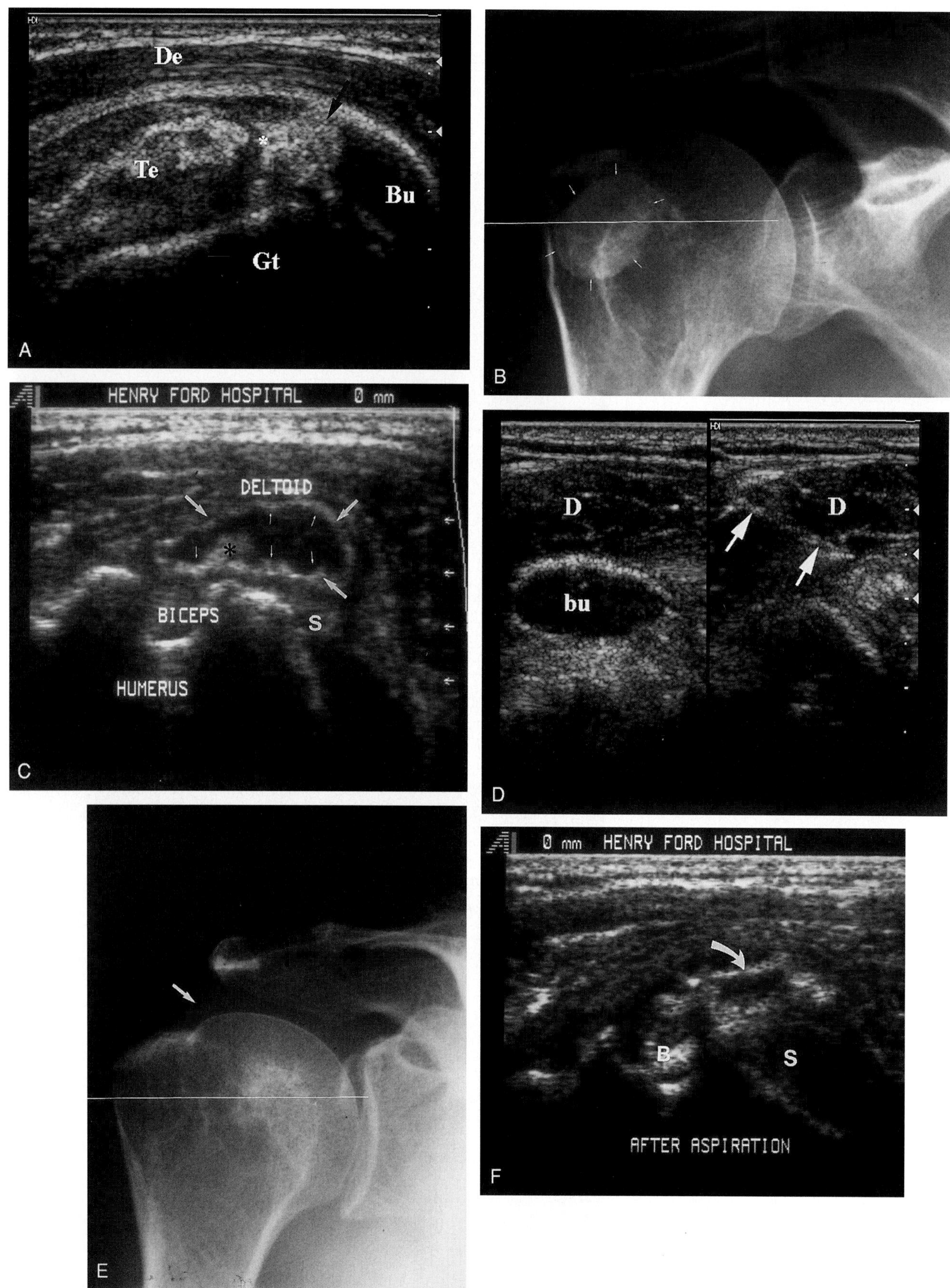

Figure 5–31 ■ *See legend on opposite page*

Figure 5-31 ■ **A,** Hydroxyapatite synovitis: longitudinal sonogram through the supraspinatus tendon. This middle-aged woman presented with acute shoulder pain. The longitudinal view shows how tendon (*Te*) calcifications can erode into the subdeltoid bursa. A large calcific mass (*black arrow*) has broken away from the tendon (*asterisk*) and protrudes into the bursa (*Bu*). Abbreviations: greater tuberosity (*Gt*), deltoid muscle (*De*). **B,** Hydroxyapatite synovitis: initial shoulder radiograph. Same patient as in **A.** A large ovoid mass (*arrows*) with calcification projects over the proximal humerus. **C,** Hydroxyapatite synovitis: transverse shoulder sonography. Same patient as in **A.** The examiner positions the transducer over the anterior shoulder along the plane indicated by the thin white line on **B.** The ovoid mass (*arrows*), which represents a distended anterior component of the subdeltoid bursa, appears over the subscapularis (*S*) and the biceps tendon and deep to the deltoid muscle. Note the anechoic fluid mixed with more echogenic material (*asterisk*) in the bursal lumen. The bursa has a distinct hyperechoic wall (*small arrows*). **D,** Hydroxyapatite synovitis: transverse sonogram with split-screen technique during bursal aspiration. Same patient as in **A.** The left side of this split-screen image demonstrates increased fluid within the distal part of the bursa. Note the hyperechoic wall which surrounds the anechoic bursal fluid (*bu*). The right side of the split screen shows the bursa during aspiration. An 18-gauge spinal needle (*arrows*) is used to aspirate the bursal fluid. Five cubic centimeters of thick white fluid which contained calcium hydroxyapatite was easily aspirated from the bursal lumen. Pain relief was instantaneous, suggesting increased pressure in the subacromial space as the cause of pain in this patient. Abbreviation: deltoid muscle (*D*). **E,** Hydroxyapatite synovitis: radiograph after aspiration. Same patient as in **A.** The large opacity is almost entirely gone after bursal aspiration. Calcifications (*arrow*) are still visible in the supraspinatus tendon. **F,** Hydroxyapatite synovitis: transverse sonogram after aspiration. Same patient as in **A.** The position of the transducer follows the thin white line drawn on the radiograph of **E.** The bursal lumen has collapsed. A hyperechoic line (*curved arrow*) may represent the residual content of the bursa or perhaps the opposed hyperechoic surfaces of synovium impregnated with calcium. Compare this image with **C.** Abbreviations: long biceps tendon (*B*), subscapularis tendon (*S*).

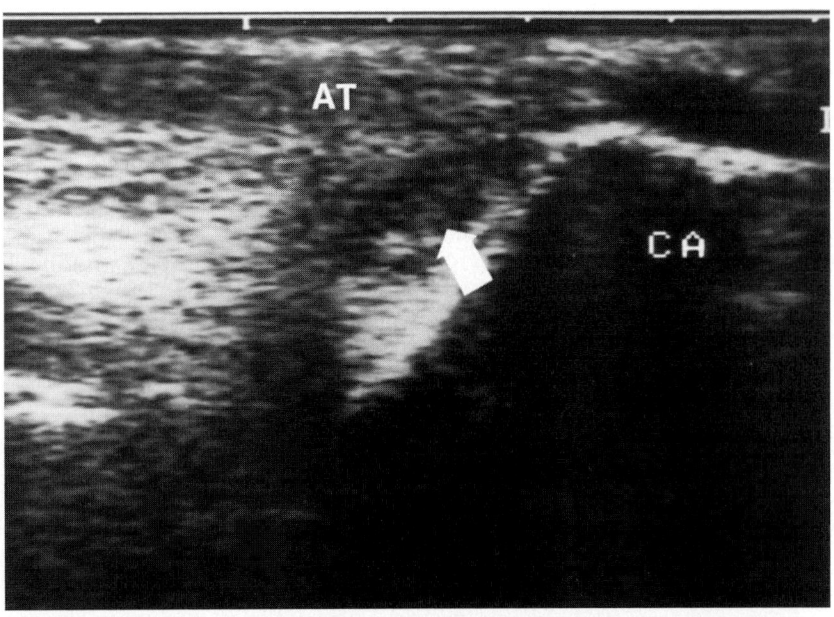

Figure 5-32 ■ Rheumatoid bursitis of the retrocalcaneal bursa: longitudinal sonogram. This 53-year-old woman presented with a 12-year history of symmetrical polyarthritis, and she is rheumatoid factor positive. Her current complaint is bilateral pain in the heels of 2 months' duration. The transducer is oriented along the Achilles tendon (*AT*). The distal Achilles tendon and its insertion (*I*) on the calcaneus (*CA*) are normal. The retrocalcaneal bursa (*arrow*) is enlarged and contains definite internal echos. The anterior synovial wall is thickened.

Box 5-1
Hyperechoic Foci within Synovium

- Crystals (uric acid—calcium precipitates)
- Infection (cellular elements and fibrin)
- Corticosteroids (recent injection)
- Bone fragments (neuropathic joint)
- Rarely in normal joints—probably related to nitrogen ("vacuum")

to calcifications (Box 5-1). Once again, shadowing may or may not be observed, depending on the size of the calcifications and the frequency of transducer use. Calcium hydroxyapatite in the shoulder sometimes homogenizes with synovial fluid in cases of painful inflammatory synovitis (Fig. 5-30). The bursal calcium may originate from deposits in surrounding tendons. The erosion of calcium hydroxyapatite into the bursal lumen is often accompanied by an excruciating pain of acute onset (Fig. 5-31). The bursal walls appear hyperechoic in the cases

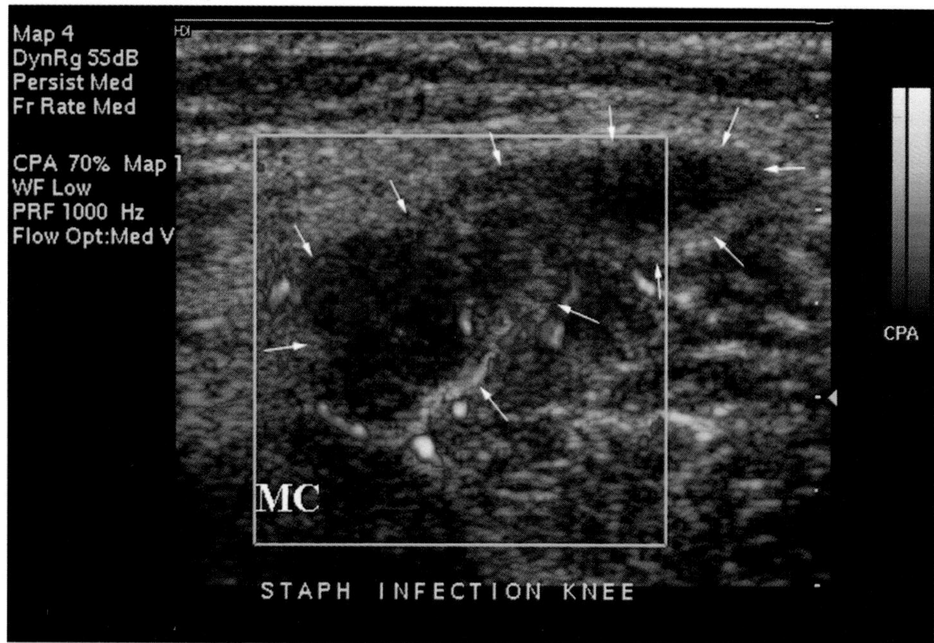

Figure 5–33 ■ Infected Baker's cyst: transverse sonogram through the medial popliteal space. The knee of this 52-year-old diabetic had been swollen for 2 weeks prior to presentation. Septic arthritis induced by *Staphylococcus aureus* infection had been confirmed by aspiration 1 week earlier. Surgical debridement and antibiotic therapy were performed for treatment of the infection. This ultrasound follow-up demonstrated residual inflammatory change within a Baker's cyst. Aspiration revealed persistence of infection in this pocket of fluid. Abbreviation: medial condyle (*MC*).

we've observed. Aspiration of the bursa results in instantaneous pain relief (see Fig. 5–31). Corticosteroids injected in small quantities may provide prolonged relief of joint pain. Small, hyperechoic foci of variable size have been identified within the bursa in some cases of chemical bursitis. These bursal effusions were positive for uric acid crystals on aspiration. We speculate that larger uric acid crystals may be visible sonographically. Another finding in gout is the remarkable peribursal inflammation and striking hyperemia within the surrounding tissues. The subcutaneous changes are similar to those of cellulitis. Definitive diagnosis requires ultrasound-guided aspiration and crystal analysis.

Rheumatoid and Septic Bursitis

The sonographic findings in rheumatoid bursitis (Fig. 5–32) and septic bursitis (Fig. 5–33) may be

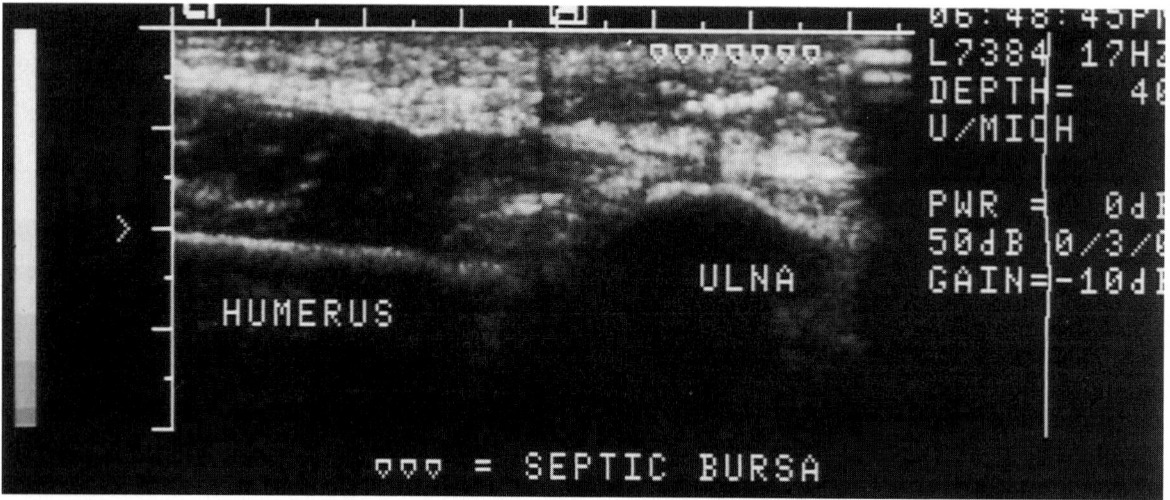

Figure 5–34 ■ Septic bursitis of the olecranon bursa: longitudinal sonogram. The patient is a 38-year-old construction worker who presented with pain and swelling of the right elbow. The transducer is positioned in the long axis of the arm over the olecranon process. A distended olecranon bursa (*arrowheads*) containing hypoechoic fluid is noted. Numerous hyperechoic foci with dirty shadowing are seen within the bursa, giving the definitive diagnosis of septic bursitis. The bursa was aspirated, and *Staphylococcus epidermidis* was cultured.

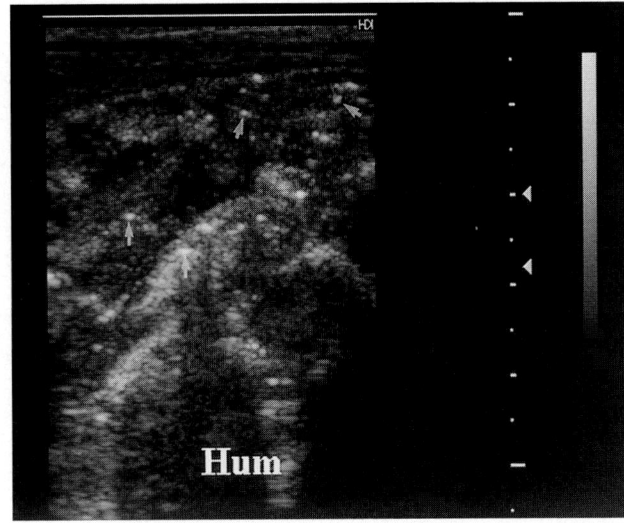

Figure 5-35 ■ Septic subacromial-subdeltoid bursa: transverse sonogram. Shoulder swelling occurred suddenly in this 50-year-old diabetic patient. Ultrasound examination of the shoulder was performed because the patient was febrile. A bursal effusion is present containing material of mixed echogenicity. Small, hyperechoic foci (*arrows*) within the synovial cavity suggest purulent material. Aspiration revealed *Staphylococcus aureus* infection of the subdeltoid bursa. Abbreviation: humerus (*Hum*).

identical to those seen in chronic traumatic bursitis. The contents of the bursa are turbid, definite internal echos are observed, and the synovial walls are often thickened and hyperemic (see Fig. 5-33). Therefore, the differential diagnosis of these three entities cannot always be narrowed using sonographic criteria alone. Sometimes multiple punctate, hyperechoic foci within the lumen of the bursa suggest infection (Figs. 5-34 and 5-35). Cases of septic bursitis with gas-producing organisms demonstrate the characteristic gas bubbles with dirty shadowing. Otherwise, clinical criteria and diagnostic aspiration of the bursal fluid must be utilized to establish a definitive diagnosis. Septic bursitis involving the subdeltoid bursa is common in patients who are intravenous drug abusers using "skin popping" as their method of injection. In chronically ill patients, such as those with rheumatoid arthritis or chronic renal failure, septic bursitis can rapidly lead to systemic sepsis and death. Early diagnosis of septic bursitis in individuals with compromised immune function is essential.

Communicating Bursae

Bursal Fluid and Intra-articular Disease

Communicating bursae are not present at birth but are acquired during growth and develop from noncommunicating bursae (Box 5-2). The passage between the gastrocnemius-semimembranosus bursa and the knee joint is never found in children less than 10 years of age but is found in 50% of knees by the fifth decade of life (Lindgren and Willen, 1977). The accumulation of fluid in the gastrocnemius-semimembranosus bursa results in the formation of Baker cysts. The hip joint communicates with the iliopsoas bursa (unilaterally or bilaterally) in approximately 20% of adults (Chandler, 1934) (Figs. 5-36 through 5-39); however, such communication occurs in less than 2% of children under the age of 10. Communication of the subacromial bursa with the glenohumeral joint is possible only in the presence of a rotator cuff tear. Bursal fluid in shoulders with rotator cuff tear accumulates in the distal aspect of the bursa when scanning is done with the patient sitting (Fig. 5-40). The bursa distends with a teardrop shape along the long axis of the proximal humeral diaphysis. Small effusions appear first over the anterior shoulder. The fluid covers the biceps tendon sheath (Figs. 5-40 and 5-41) van Holsbeeck and Strouse, 1993). This sign is fairly characteristic of a shoulder with a torn rotator cuff. Fluid that fills two different synovial compartments suggests communication between the joint and the bursa. The incidence of rotator cuff tears in adults

Box 5-2
Occurrence of Joint Communication Over Age 50

- Gastrocnemius-semimembranosus bursa—50% with posterior and medial femorotibial joints
- Iliopsoas bursa—20% with the anterior coxofemoral joint
- Subacromial-subdeltoid bursa—13% with the glenohumeral joint

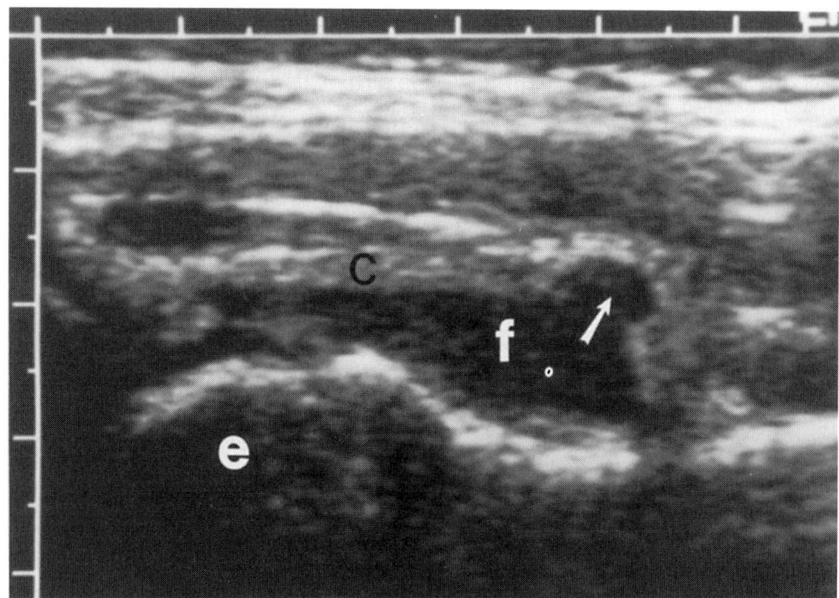

Figure 5-36 ■ Filling of the iliopsoas bursa in transient synovitis: longitudinal sonogram. A 7-year-old boy with hip pain. The transducer is positioned along the femoral neck. Fluid in the hip joint (*f*) communicates with the iliopsoas bursa (*arrow*) through an opening in the joint capsule (*C*). Communicating iliopsoas bursae are present in about 2% of joints in children less than 10 years of age. The incidence of communication increases with age, reaching 20% to 30% in patients more than 50 years old. Abbreviation: femoral epiphysis (*e*).

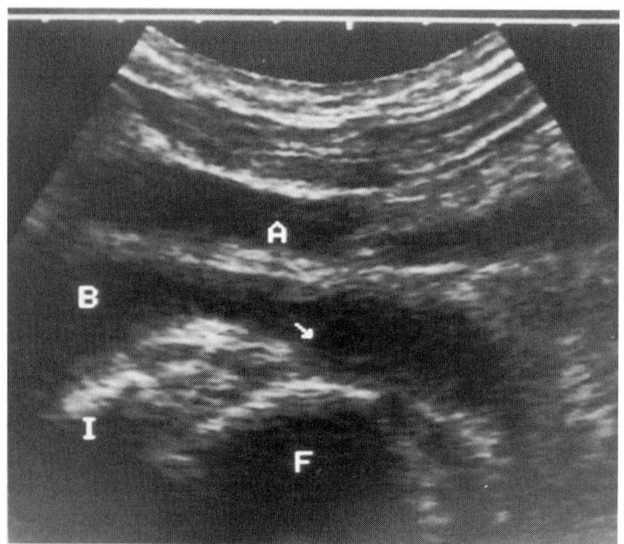

Figure 5-37 ■ Large iliopsoas bursa in an adult: longitudinal sonogram. A pulsatile mass was palpated in the left groin of this 60-year-old woman. The clinical diagnosis was femoral pseudoaneurysm. The transducer is positioned in the parasagittal plane just medial to the femoral neck. A large fluid-filled bursa (*B*) extends deep to the femoral artery (*A*) and communicates with the hip joint (*arrow*). The femoral artery is clearly normal. Abbreviations: femur (*F*), ilium (*I*).

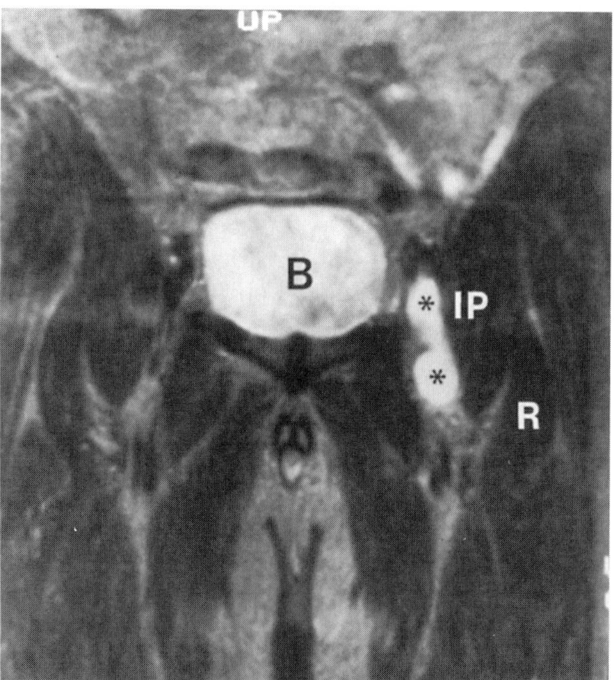

Figure 5-38 ■ Large iliopsoas bursa: MRI scan of the pelvis (coronal plane). Same patient as in Figure 5-37. The image shown is a T_2-weighted sequence in the coronal plane through the iliopsoas and the proximal rectus anterior to the hips. A bilobed iliopsoas bursa (*asterisks*) is indented by the ilioinguinal ligament. Fluid within the bursa demonstrates a very high signal, more intense than that of the urinary bladder (*B*). Abbreviations: iliopsoas (*IP*), rectus (*R*).

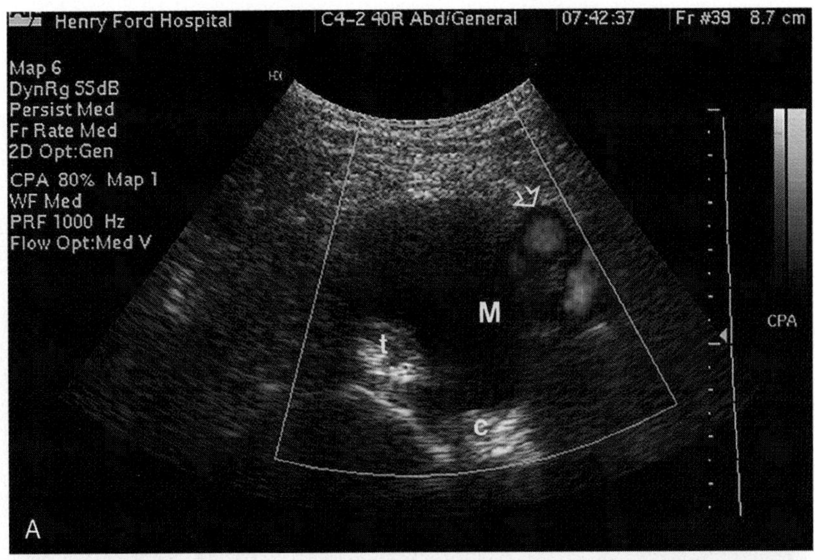

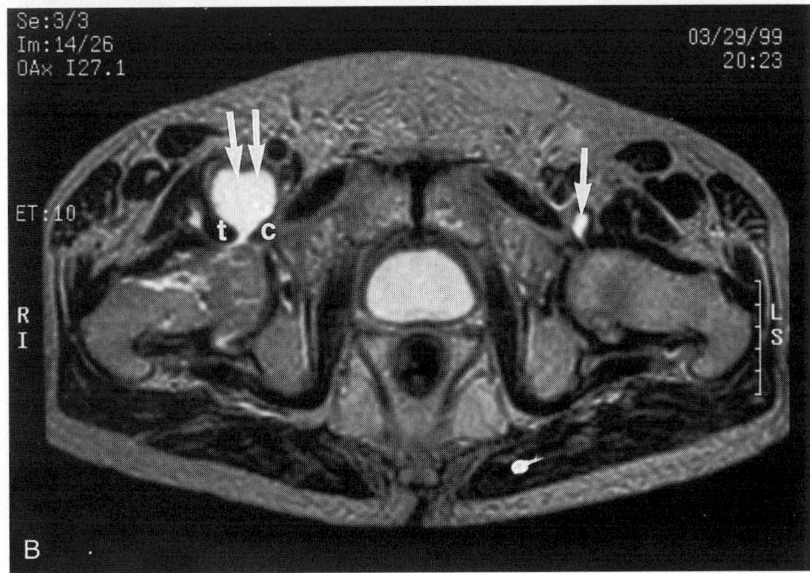

Figure 5–39 ▪ **A,** Distention of the iliopsoas bursa in crystal-related synovitis: transverse sonogram through the right groin. A large groin mass developed quickly in this 54-year-old patient who has been treated for prostate carcinoma. The patient is worried that a neoplasm is growing in his groin. The clinical diagnosis suggested an inguinal hernia, however. Transverse ultrasound with the probe over the groin shows an anechoic mass (*M*) with joint communication through a rent in the capsule between the iliopsoas tendon (*t*) and the cartilage of the anterior hip labrum (*c*). The mass extends between the capsular structures and the vessels (*open arrow*). **B,** Distention of the iliopsoas bursa in crystal-related synovitis: axial fast spin-echo T_2-weighted sequence using fat suppression. Same patient as in **A.** Right–left comparison demonstrates a distended iliopsoas bursa (*double arrows*) in the right hip and a normal iliopsoas bursa (*single arrow*) in the left hip. The defect in the anterior joint capsule, which allows communication with the bursa, is clearly visible between the iliopsoas tendon (*t*) and the cartilage (*c*) of the anterior labrum. Inflammatory changes are also noted in the joint and in the marrow of the proximal femur of the affected hip. Aspiration of the bursa with ultrasound guidance yielded 70 cc of synovial fluid. Cultures and Gram stain were negative, but the microscopic examination demonstrated calcium pyrophosphate crystals in the fluid.

more than 50 years of age is approximately 13% (De Palma, 1950) (Fig. 5–42). The communication between the joint and the bursa created by rotator cuff tears occurs significantly more often in patients with rheumatoid arthritis (Fig. 5–43). Approximately 30% of patients with long-standing rheumatoid arthritis have complete rotator cuff tears. Pannus (Fig. 5–44) due to inflammation of the glenohumeral joint erodes the undersurface of the rotator cuff. This process progresses rapidly if there is inflammation of the subacromial-subdeltoid bursa or if the patient is being treated with steroids (Resnick and Niwayama, 1988). Rarely, inflammatory processes can affect the bursa without affecting the joint. Subtle thickening of the bursa can be an early sign of subacromial impingement (Figs. 5–45 and 5–46). Isolated changes in the bursa seem to be more common in women. Adhesive capsulitis affects the tissues of the rotator cuff interval. This shoulder disease, which often affects diabetics or patients with a positive glucose tolerance test, leads to fibrosis in and around the bursa (see Fig. 5–47). In addition, synovial inflammation or a small effusion may fill the medial recess of the biceps tendon sheath (see Fig. 5–47). The normal communication between the glenohumeral joint and the long biceps tendon sheath is lost by scar tissue in the rotator cuff interval (Rakofsky, 1987).

Large bursal effusions found in communicating bursae are usually the result of synovial fluid being

Text continued on page 159

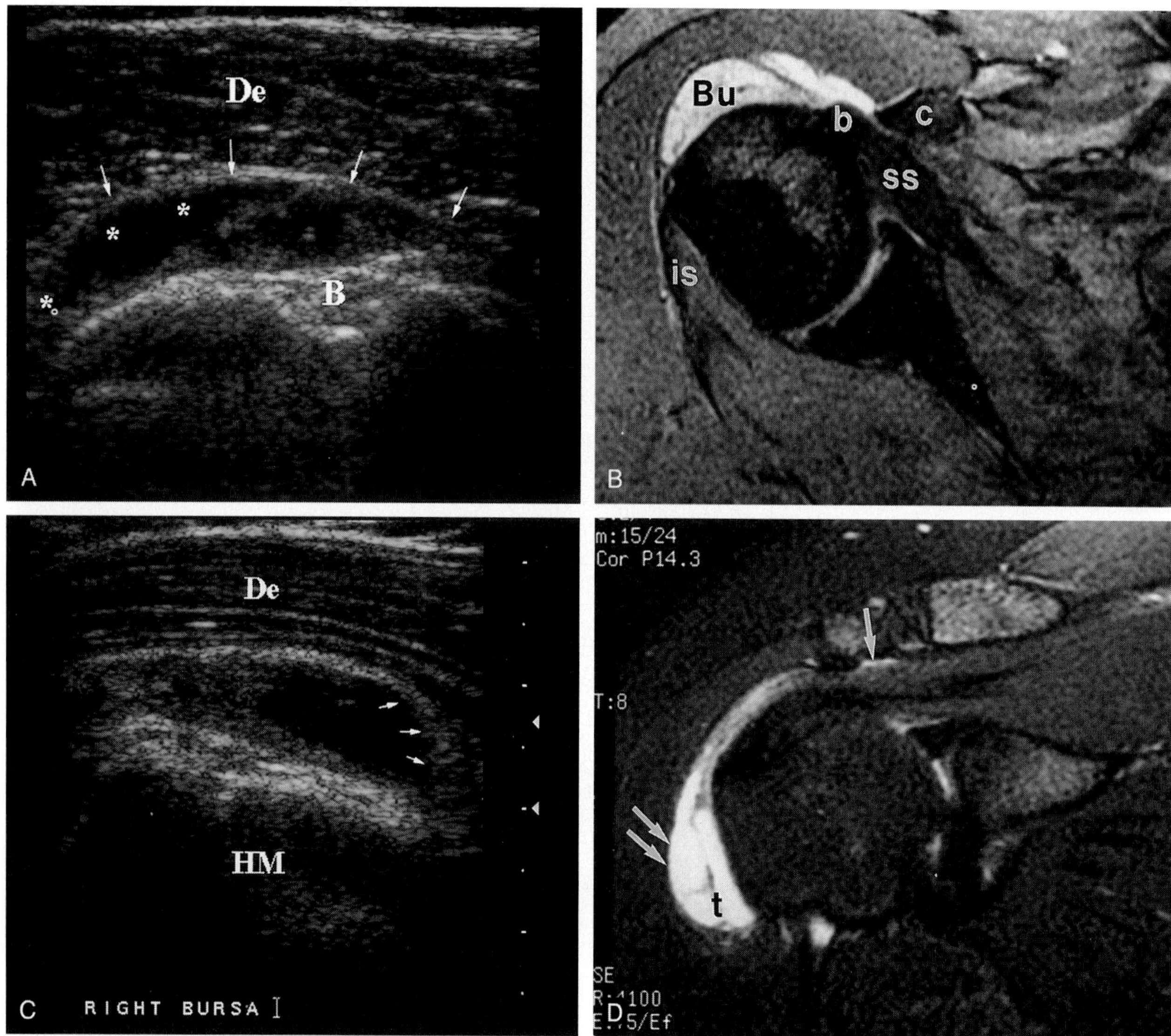

Figure 5-40 ▪ **A,** Fluid in the subacromial-subdeltoid bursa: transverse sonogram. This 67-year-old woman is unable to raise her arm. When the transducer is positioned over the anterior shoulder and the biceps tendon groove, distention of the subacromial-subdeltoid bursa by fluid of mixed echogenicity is observed (*arrows*). The bursa covers the long biceps tendon (*B*). Fluid extends far lateral (*asterisks*) to the biceps tendon groove in a soft tissue plane deep to the deltoid (*De*) muscle. **B,** Fluid in the subacromial-subdeltoid bursa: transverse gradient echo MRI. Same patient as in **A.** The fluid in the subacromial-subdeltoid bursa (*Bu*) extends as far medial as the coracoid (*c*) and covers the extracapsular long biceps tendon (*b*) and the lateral subscapularis tendon (*ss*). The bursa can be very large when distended. In this patient, the fluid reaches far lateral and posteriorly, covering the infraspinatus (*is*) tendon insertion. **C,** Fluid in the subacromial-subdeltoid bursa: coronal shoulder sonogram. Same patient as in **A.** The transducer is aligned along the fibers of the deltoid (*De*), and imaging extends beyond the distal supraspinatus. This demonstrates the typical teardrop-shaped distal end of the bursa (*arrows*). It is important to avoid application of too much pressure on the transducer. Excessive pressure may displace fluid away from the transducer, making it impossible to see the bursa. Abbreviation: humerus (*HM*). **D,** Fluid in the subacromial-subdeltoid bursa: coronal T_2 fast spin-echo MRI image. Same patient as in **A.** The bursa is divided into different components based on anatomical criteria: the subacromial portion (*arrow*) and the subdeltoid portion (*double arrows*). The distal extent of the subdeltoid portion of the bursa ends in a teardrop (*t*). This patient has a rotator cuff tear in a segment of the cuff which is not visualized in this picture, resulting in increased fluid within the bursa.

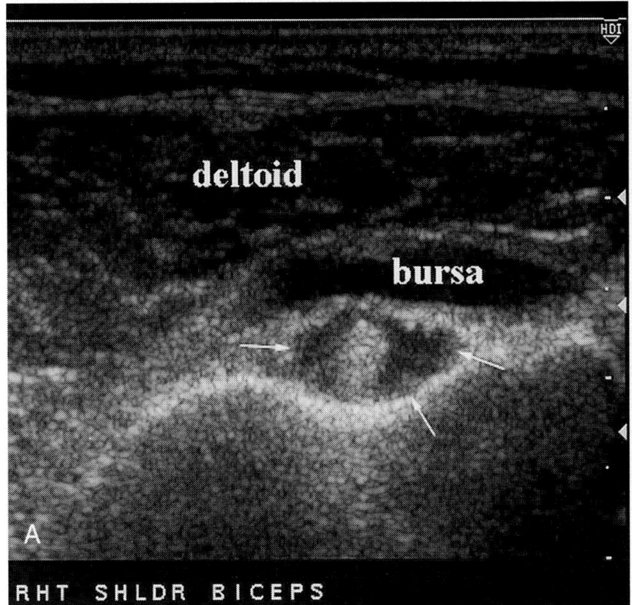

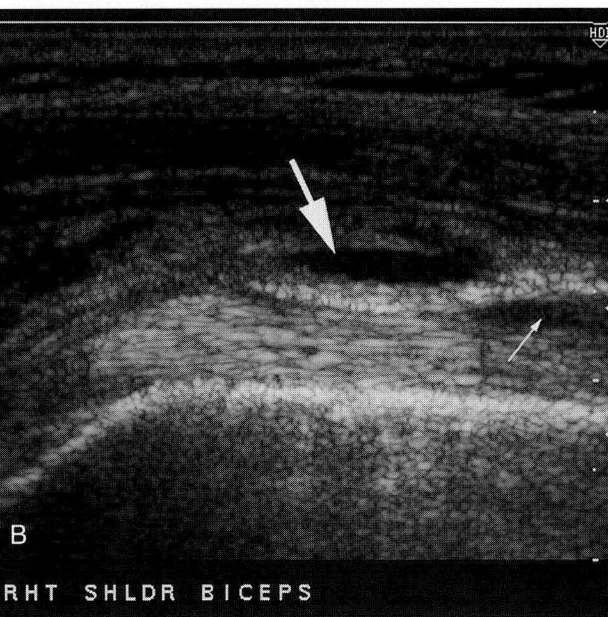

Figure 5-41 ■ A, Anatomy of the subacromial-subdeltoid bursa: transverse rotator cuff sonography. Fluid in the subacromial-subdeltoid bursa is most commonly associated with rotator cuff tear. It is therefore important to recognize increased fluid in this anatomical space. Light pressure should be applied with the transducer. Small amounts of fluid typically appear over the long biceps tendon. It may be difficult to distinguish fluid around the biceps from bursal fluid. Fluid in the biceps sheath (*arrows*) is contained within the bone of the biceps tendon groove, while fluid in the bursa extends beyond the groove both laterally and medially. The fluid in the joint and bursa of this patient is of different echogenicity. **B,** Anatomy of the subacromial-subdeltoid bursa: longitudinal view through the long biceps tendon. A thin membrane separates the synovial sheath of the biceps (*small arrow*) and that of the subacromial-subdeltoid bursa (*large arrow*). In this region of the shoulder, the joint synovium and bursal synovium are more closely approximated than in any other anatomical region of the shoulder. Again, note the difference in echogenicity in the lumen of the bursa and the tendon sheath.

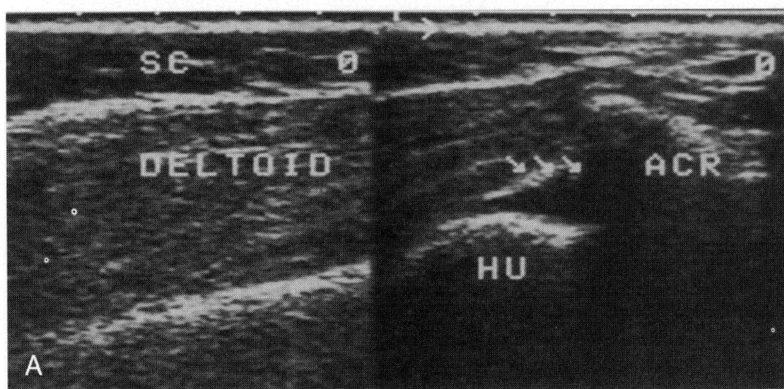

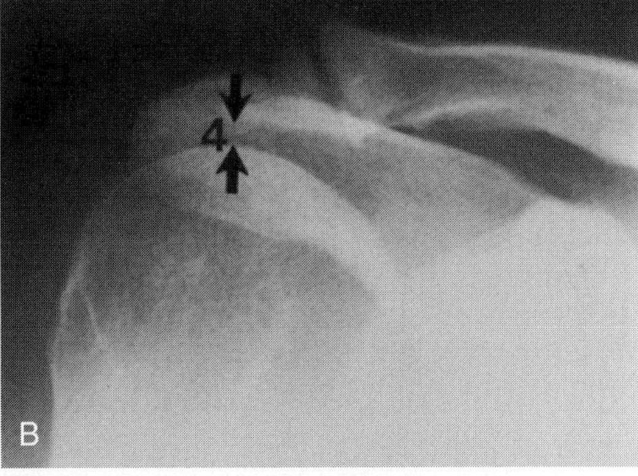

Figure 5-42 ■ A, Supraspinatus tear with fluid in the subacromial-subdeltoid bursa: coronal sonogram. A 69-year-old man presented with limited abduction of the shoulder. The transducer is positioned along the humerus, with the acromion (*ACR*) at the observer's right. The supraspinatus tendon is retracted and is not seen. Fluid within the subacromial-subdeltoid bursa (*small arrows*) occupies the space vacated by the supraspinatus tendon. The deltoid muscle covers the shoulder and originates from the acromion. Abbreviations: subcutaneous fat (*sc*), humerus (*HU*). **B,** Supraspinatus tear with fluid in the subacromial-subdeltoid bursa: conventional anteroposterior supine radiograph. Same patient as in **A.** The subacromial space is narrowed to 4 mm (*4*), and the acromioclavicular joint shows evidence of osteoarthritis. These findings are consistent with a complete supraspinatus tear.

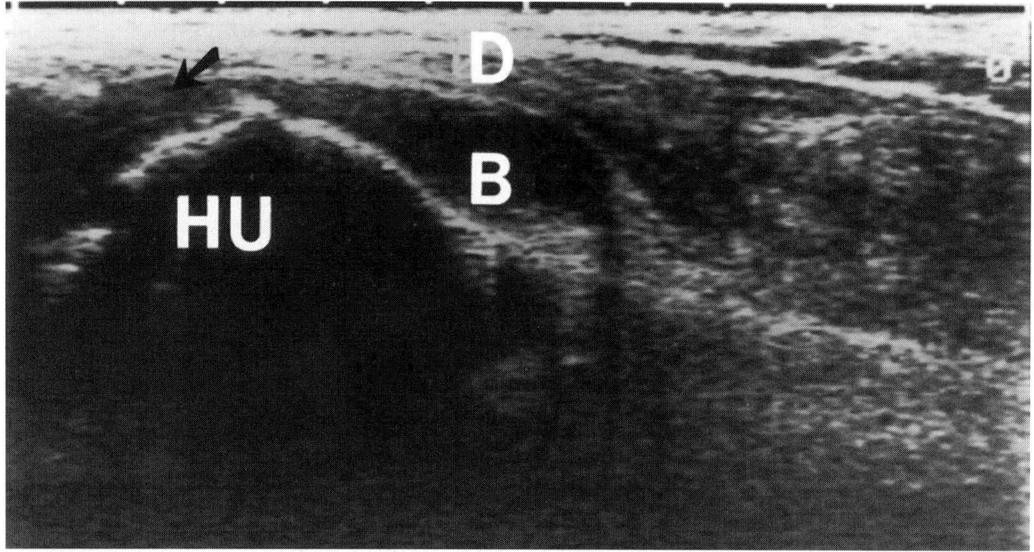

Figure 5-43 ■ Distention of the subacromial-subdeltoid bursa: coronal sonogram. The patient is a 45-year-old woman with a 2-year history of rheumatoid arthritis who presents with left shoulder pain. The position of the transducer is identical to that in Figure 5-42A. Proximal lies to the observer's left. A significantly distended subacromial-subdeltoid bursa (*B*) is noted, which is characteristic of rheumatoid arthritis. Aspiration is indicated for differentiation between chronic inflammatory disease and infection when the clinical picture is unclear. The bursa communicates with the joint space under the acromion (*curved arrow*). Abbreviations: deltoid (*D*), humerus (*HU*).

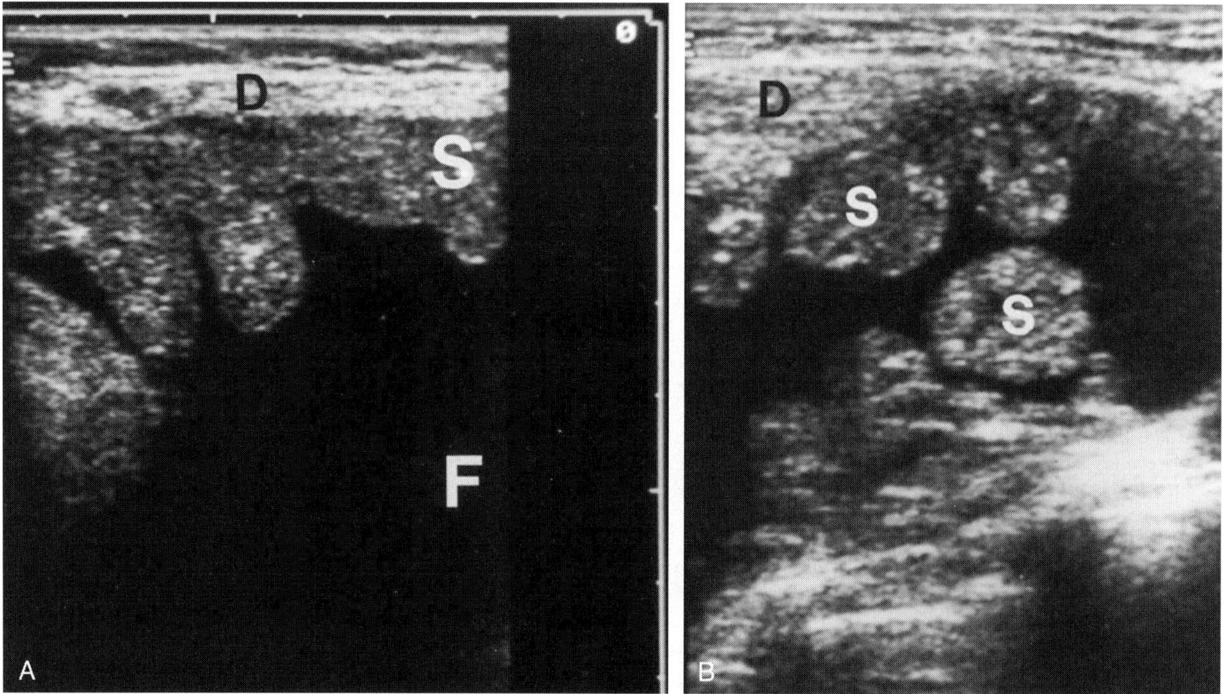

Figure 5-44 ■ **A,** Pannus in the subacromial-subdeltoid bursa: coronal sonogram. A 51-year-old woman with a 24-year history of rheumatoid arthritis who presents with palpable swelling and tenderness of the right shoulder. The position of the transducer is identical to that in Figure 5-43. The deltoid muscle (*D*) is atrophic. Distention of the subacromial-subdeltoid bursa is due to both fluid (*F*) and synovial proliferation (*S*). The hypertrophic synovial tissue has a polypoid appearance and is typically referred to as *pannus.* **B,** Pannus in the subacromial-subdeltoid bursa: transverse sonogram. Same patient as in **A.** The transducer is rotated 90 degrees, yielding a transverse image. Again noted is the polypoid appearance of the hypertrophic synovial tissue (*S*). The pannus is hypoechoic relative to the surrounding tissue and is surrounded by anechoic fluid. Abbreviation: deltoid (*D*).

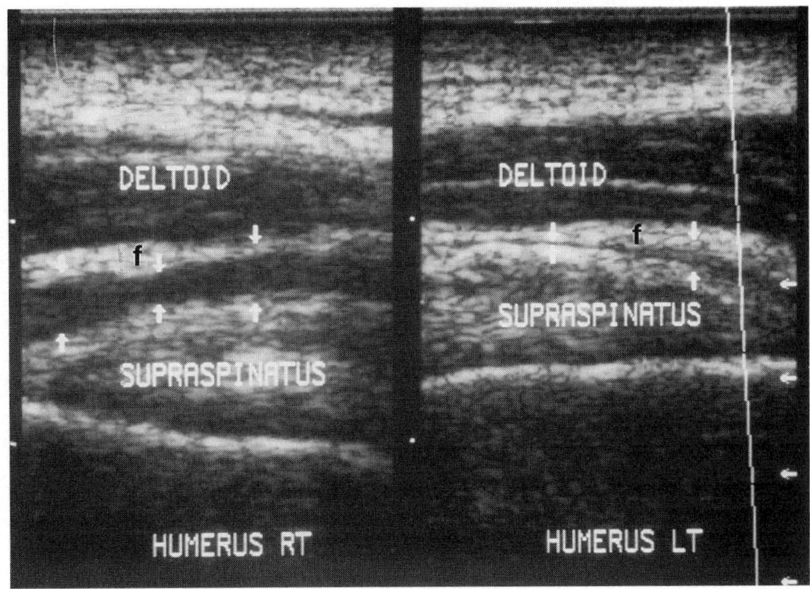

Figure 5-45 ■ Anatomy of the subacromial-subdeltoid bursa: split-screen coronal cuff sonography. This tennis player complains of pain in the right shoulder. The abnormal right shoulder (left image) shows a thickened right subacromial-subdeltoid bursa (*between the arrows*). Compare the symptomatic side with the normal left bursa (*between the arrows on the right image*). The hypoechoic bursal tissue of the affected shoulder is more than three times the thickness of normal synovial tissue. Volume increase of the bursa can involve the subacromial space and cause a clinical syndrome known as *impingement*. The hyperechoic tissue around the bursa represents the peribursal fat (*f*).

pumped into bursae during motion. Communicating bursae serve as potential reservoirs for joint effusions and thus minimize the deleterious effects of the effusion. The result is a cyst. Physiological studies indicate that a valvular mechanism is responsible for cyst development. Although the exact mechanism has not been elucidated, anatomical studies have demonstrated the pathways of communication with the joint space to be narrow channels between the ligaments and tendons (Jayson, 1981). Movement of the joint is thought to open and close the valve (Figs. 5-48 through 5-51). Pressure within the bursa is considerably higher than that within the joint space. Weight bearing on the joint will force fluid into the bursa against a pressure gradient while the valve is open (Jayson, 1981).

Sonography demonstrates a distended bursa containing hypoechoic or anechoic fluid. The definitive

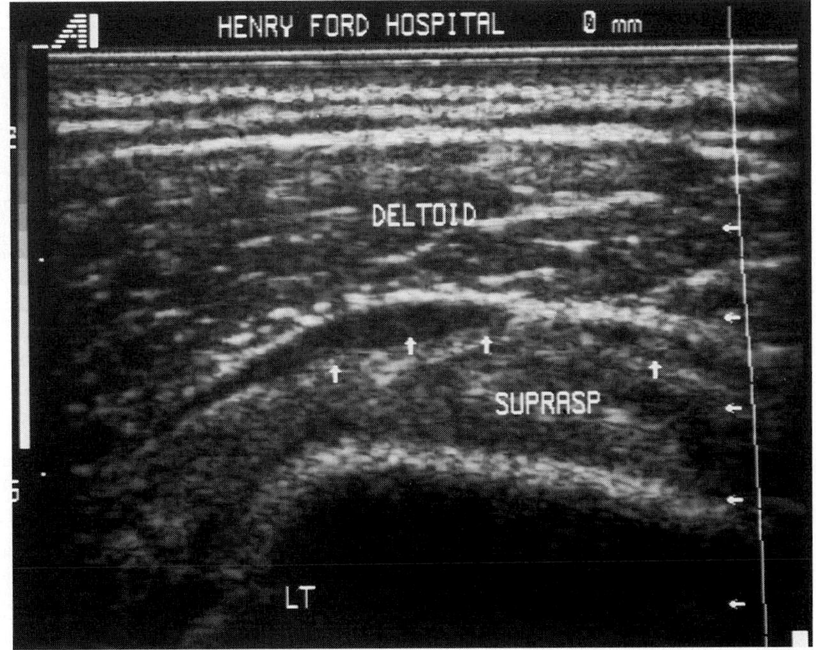

Figure 5-46 ■ Loculated fluid in impingement: transverse rotator cuff sonogram. Pain in this construction worker's shoulder is associated with excessive fluid in the subacromial-subdeltoid bursa. The fluid does not move around in the shoulder, as would be expected in acute synovitis. More fluid is seen in the anterior bursa (*three arrows*) compared with the bursa located more posteriorly (*one arrow*). That configuration did not change when pressure was applied with the transducer, indicating loculated fluid. This is relatively common in cases of chronic synovitis.

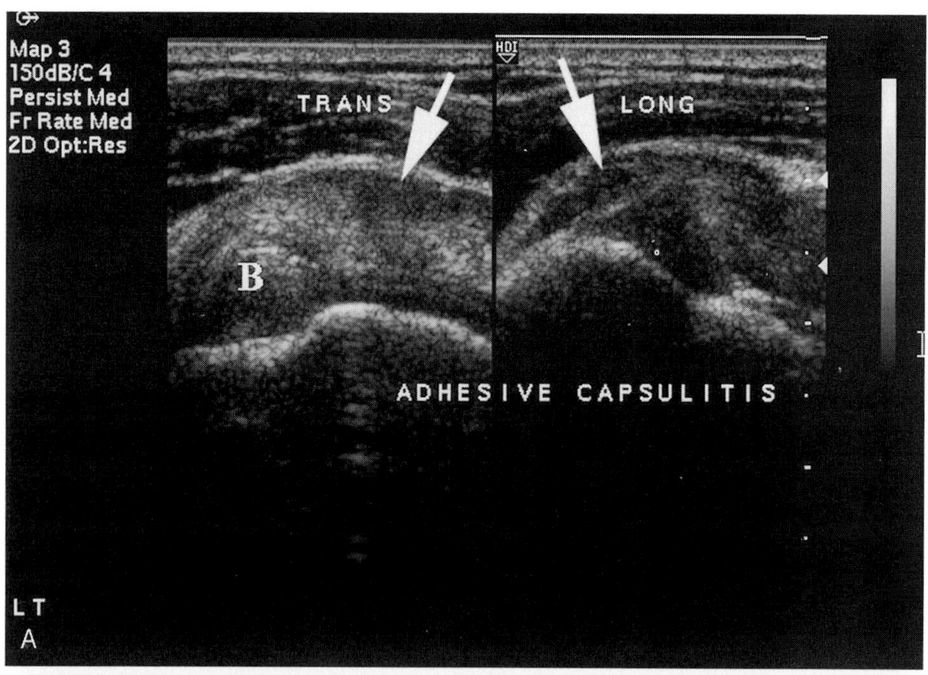

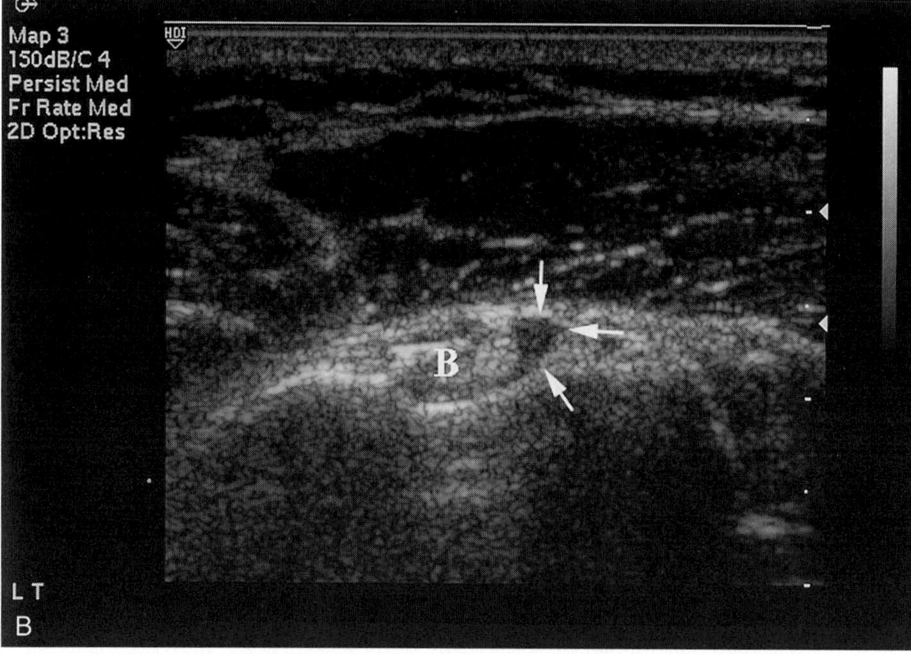

Figure 5–47 ■ **A,** Adhesive capsulitis: split-screen images of the rotator cuff. Pain in the left shoulder and inability to raise the arm brought this 38-year-old woman to the orthopedic clinic. Hypoechoic tissue (*arrows*) surrounds the long biceps tendon and the subdeltoid bursa in the affected shoulder. Histological examination of the tissues surrounding the rotator cuff of patients with adhesive capsulitis has revealed fibrosis. The fibrosis in this disease is similar to that in Dupuytren's disease. In addition, both diseases can occur together and in association with diabetes mellitus. Abbreviations: transverse view (*TRANS*), longitudinal view (*LONG*), long biceps tendon (*B*). **B,** Adhesive capsulitis: transverse sonogram through the distal long biceps tendon. Same patient as in **A.** A hypoechoic rim of tissue (*arrows*), probably thickened tendon sheath, surrounds the medial aspect of the long biceps tendon in most shoulders affected by adhesive capsulitis. The rotator cuff is typically intact. Abbreviation: long biceps tendon (*B*).

diagnosis can be made by identification of the slit-like channel connecting the bursa with the joint space. In an examination of the subdeltoid bursa, the communication with the joint space is a tear in the rotator cuff. Patients with rheumatoid arthritis have irregularity and thickening of the synovial lining of the bursa. Septic arthritis and other inflammatory processes have definite internal echos within the fluid and inhomogeneous filling of the bursa.

Baker's Cyst

Baker's cysts will be discussed as a separate entity because of the very frequent enlargement of the gastrocnemius-semimembranosus bursa. The popliteal cyst was first described by Adams (1840), who correctly identified the cyst as an enlarged bursa found medially in the popliteal fossa. Later, Baker described the lesion again and established the causal relationship between joint effusions and popliteal cysts (Baker, 1877).

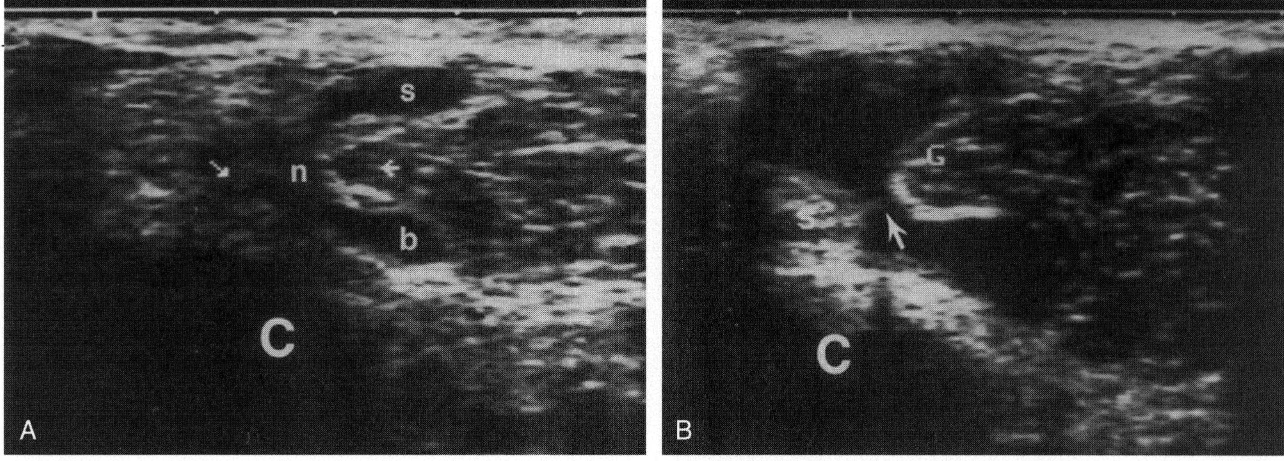

Figure 5–48 ■ **A,** Small Baker's cyst: transverse sonogram with the knee in slight flexion. The patient is a 39-year-old man with a medial meniscal tear. The transducer is positioned transversely over the medial aspect of the popliteal fossa just above the joint space. A Baker's cyst is divided into three anatomical parts: the base, the neck, and the superficial portion. Separating the joint capsule and the medial femoral condyle (*C*) from the medial gastrocnemius tendon (*horizontal arrow*) is the base (*b*) of a small Baker's cyst. The neck (*n*) of the Baker's cyst is a slit-like channel between the medial gastrocnemius tendon and the semimembranosus tendon (*oblique arrow*). Its superficial portion (*s*) extends posteriorly between the fascia and the medial gastrocnemius tendon. **B,** Same patient and transducer position as **A** but with the knee in extension. With the knee in extension, the neck of the bursa is narrowed (*arrow*), and a greater amount of fluid is seen in the superficial extent of the bursa. This supports the theory of a pump and valve mechanism in the formation of a Baker's cyst. Abbreviations: semimembranosus tendon (*S*), medial gastrocnemius tendon (*G*), medial femoral condyle (*C*).

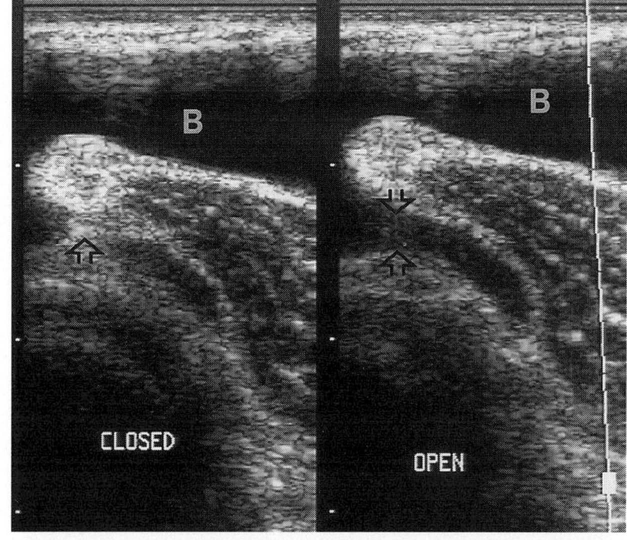

Figure 5–49 ■ Valve mechanism of Baker's cyst: transverse sonogram with split-screen tech-nique. A Baker's cyst (*B*) in a 49-year-old woman with a lateral meniscal tear. Firm pressure applied on the cyst by the transducer opens the valve to the joint space. The soft tissue valve consists of the apposition of two tendons: the medial gastrocnemius and the semimembranosus. The image on the left side of the split screen shows the two tendons in close contact (*open arrow*). The image on the right side demonstrates tendon separation with pressure applied (*two open arrows*). This tendon valve mechanism opens and closes during normal walking due to flexion and extension of the knee.

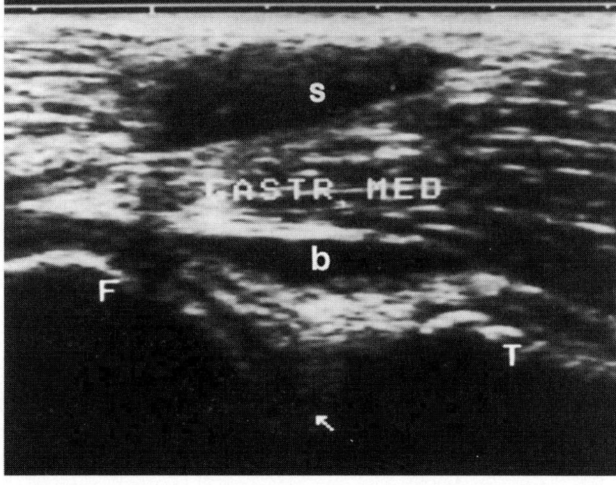

Figure 5–50 ■ Small Baker's cyst: longitudinal sonogram. Same patient as in Figure 5–48. In this image the transducer is oriented along the length of the medial gastrocnemius tendon. The medial gastrocnemius tendon is surrounded by the base (*b*) and superficial portion (*s*) of the Baker's cyst. In Baker's cysts that arise as a result of noninflammatory intra-articular disease, the fluid is uniformly anechoic. Clear fluid is obtained on aspiration of these joints. The synovial lining of these cysts is very smooth and regular. Deep to the base of the Baker's cyst lies the posterior extent of the joint capsule and the medial meniscus (*arrow*). Abbreviations: medial femoral condyle (*F*), proximal tibia (*T*).

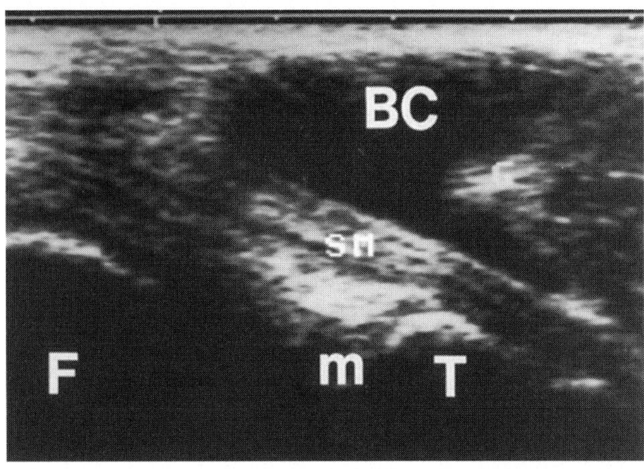

Figure 5–51 ■ Small Baker's cyst: longitudinal sonogram. Same patient as in Figure 5–48. The transducer is moved approximately 1 cm medial to that in Figure 5–50 to demonstrate the semimembranosus tendon (*SM*) in its long axis. Its insertion on the posterior aspect of the tibial epiphysis (*T*) is seen on the right. A small amount of joint fluid is present between the tendon and the posterior aspect of the medial meniscus (*m*). The neck of the bursa is located between the gastrocnemius tendon (*G*) and the semimembranosus tendon. The largest portion of the Baker's cyst is its superficial extent (*BC*).

The gastrocnemius-semimembranosus bursa is always found at the medial aspect of the popliteal fossa. Communication with the joint space of the knee develops after birth, probably during adolescence. Morphologically, the bursa is divided into three portions: the base, the superficial extent, and the neck (Canoso, 1981). Located between the joint capsule and the gastrocnemius tendon is the base of the bursa. Beneath the fascia is the superficial portion of the bursa. The neck of the bursa lies between the gastrocnemius and semimembranosus tendons, hence the name of this bursa (see Figs. 5–48 through 5–51). The slit-like channel of communication between the bursa and the joint space is closed during extension of the knee. This is accomplished by compression of the neck of the bursa between the medial femoral condyle and the gastrocnemius tendon. Flexion of the knee separates these structures and opens the channel (Canoso, 1981). Fluid enters the bursa due to a pressure gradient created between the joint space and the bursa. Foreign bodies are often observed within the lumen of the Baker cyst, another sign of the existence of a pressure gradient directed toward the bursa.

Two general categories of disease can result in bursal distention: pathology associated with increased intra-articular fluid and the inflammatory arthropathies. The diseases that result in increased intra-articular fluid have one common feature: they all result in irregularity of joint surfaces. Diseases included in this group are osteochondritis dissecans, osteochondral fractures, osteonecrosis, osteoarthritis, cartilage defects, meniscal lesions, and loose bodies. In these cases, fluid within the Baker's cyst is almost always anechoic (see Fig. 5–48).

Inflammatory arthropathies are characterized by increased fluid production and synovial proliferation within the joint and communicating bursae. Baker's cysts developing secondary to an inflammatory arthropathy tend to be much larger than those associated with other types of joint pathology (Fig. 5–52). Rheumatoid Baker's cysts characteristically have marked irregularity of the synovial lining, with numerous internal echos identified within the fluid (van Holsbeeck et al., 1988) (Fig 5–53). These large Baker's cysts can dissect the soft tissues in the legs in two different ways. The most common presentation is extension of the Baker's cyst dorsal to the gastrocnemius muscle in a subcutaneous location (Fig. 5–54). The other presentation, seen in rheumatoid Baker's cysts, is dissection of the fascial planes between the soleus and gastrocnemius muscles, extending between the muscles of the posterior compartment (Fig. 5–55). The pathogenesis of these differing presentations is easily understood. The gastrocnemius-semimembranosus bursa surrounds the medial gastrocnemius tendon (see Fig. 5–52). Swelling of the bursa can then extend ventral or dorsal to this tendon. The intermuscular extension is far less frequent, probably due to higher pressure within the muscle compartment in patients with normal muscle tonus.

Fibrin clots may also be seen as hyperreflective masses within a rheumatoid bursa (see Fig. 5–52). The largest of these rheumatoid Baker's cysts, filled with pannus, may rupture, resulting in changes within the surrounding fat and muscle (Figs. 5–56 and 5–57). These changes are due to inflammation secondary to enzymes found in the pathological bursal fluid. When they occur, the condition is often referred to as *pseudothrombophlebitis* because the clinical appearance of the leg is indistinguishable from that of acute thrombophlebitis (Jayson, 1981). Ultrasound will establish the correct diagnosis and is preferred over invasive studies such as contrast venography or arthrography. Noteworthy is that Baker's cysts remain in place after total knee arthroplasty (TKA). Loose bodies in these Baker's cysts

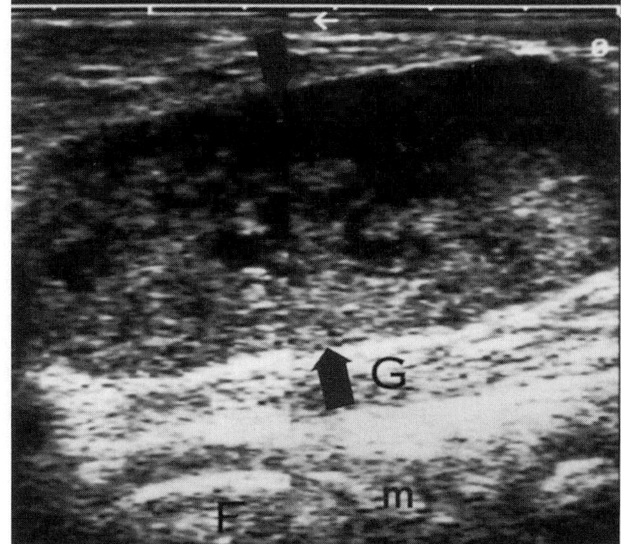

Figure 5–52 ■ Rheumatoid Baker's cyst: longitudinal sonogram. The patient is a 53-year-old man with a 10-year history of symmetrical arthritis involving the hands, feet, shoulders, and right knee. He was rheumatoid factor positive. At this time, he presented with increasing pain in the right calf. The position of the transducer is identical to that in Figure 5–50. No fluid is present in the base of the Baker's cyst between the medial gastrocnemius (*G*) and the meniscus (*m*). However, the superficial portion of the cyst is markedly distended with fluid (*large arrows*). Definite internal echos are identified moving within the fluid dependently. Synovial proliferation predominated along the anterior surface of the superficial extent of the bursa. Abbreviation: medial femur (*F*).

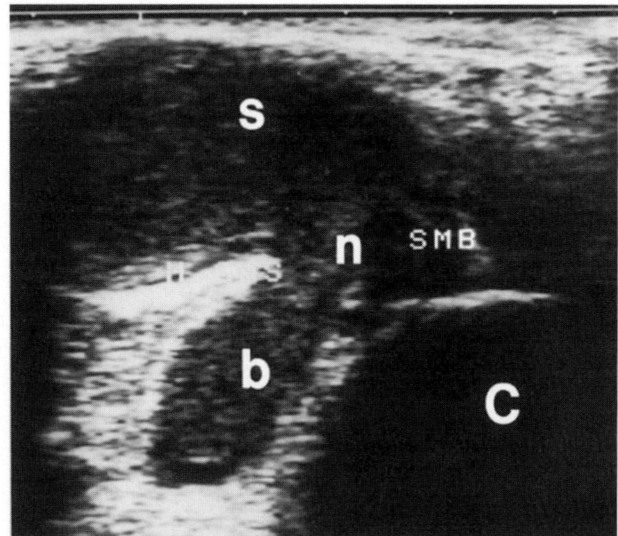

Figure 5–53 ■ Rheumatoid Baker's cyst: transverse sonogram. This 62-year-old woman presented with inflammatory-type pain in both knees. Swelling of the knees was greater on the left, with fullness in the left popliteal fossa. The patient was rheumatoid factor positive. Synovial biopsy results were consistent with chronic synovitis, consistent with rheumatoid arthritis. All portions of the Baker's cyst are markedly distended: base (*b*), neck (*n*), and superficial extent (*s*). The neck of the cyst is much wider than that seen in cases due to noninflammatory intra-articular disease. Wide separation of the medial gastrocnemius (*MGAS*) and semimembranosus tendons is observed. The synovial proliferation is seen diffusely as thickening of the walls, and debris is noted throughout. Abbreviations: medial femoral condyle (*C*), semimembranosus (*SMB*).

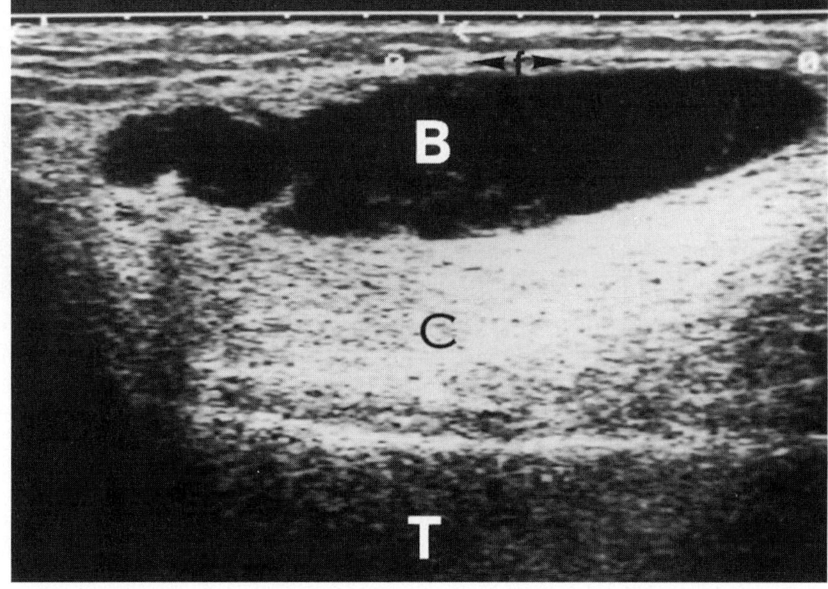

Figure 5–54 ■ Superficial extent of rheumatoid Baker's cyst: longitudinal sonogram. A 66-year-old woman with long-standing rheumatoid arthritis presented with pain and swelling of the right calf. This case demonstrates the location of dissection of the superficial portion of the rheumatoid Baker's cyst. It is the most frequent presentation of an enlarging rheumatoid Baker's cyst. The large superficial extent of this cyst (*B*) lies between the fascia (*f*) and calf muscles (*C*), displacing the muscles anteriorly. Rheumatoid Baker's cysts tend to be the largest, this one measuring more than 10 cm long. Again, irregularity of the synovial wall is noted. Abbreviation: tibia (*T*).

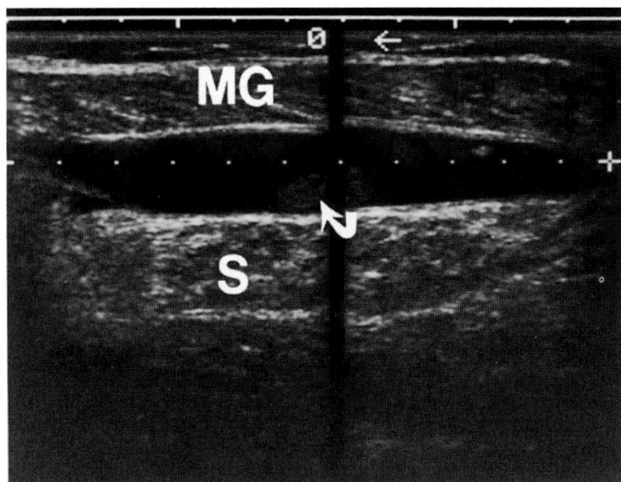

Figure 5-55 ■ Deep dissection of rheumatoid Baker's cyst: longitudinal sonogram. The patient is a 50-year-old man with polyarticular disease of 4 months' duration who presented with pain and swelling of the left leg. A 15-cm-long Baker's cyst extends into the calf deep to the medial gastrocnemius (*MG*) and superficial to the soleus (*S*). The bursa is filled with fluid and pannus (*curved arrow*), which is characteristic of rheumatoid disease.

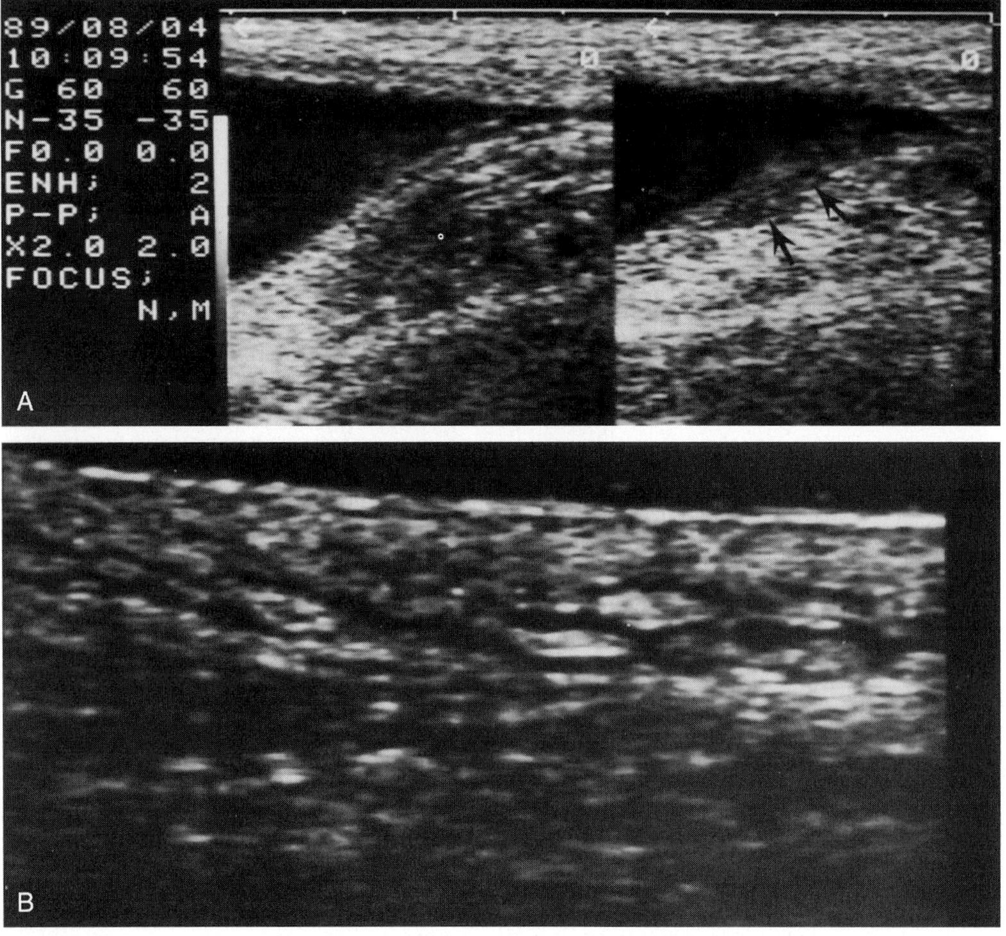

Figure 5-56 ■ **A,** Ruptured rheumatoid Baker's cyst: longitudinal sonogram. The calf of the right leg of this 46-year-old man was erythematous and edematous. The clinical presentation was consistent with deep venous thrombosis. A Baker's cyst that has ruptured is identified in the popliteal fossa. Note that the inferior border of the cyst is no longer rounded but instead is pointed. This is characteristic of a cyst that has ruptured. In the image on the right, pressure was applied with the transducer, and fluid was seen extravasating into the surrounding tissues (*arrows*). Sonographic examination for venous thrombosis and contrast venography were both normal. **B,** Ruptured rheumatoid Baker's cyst: longitudinal sonogram of the subcutaneous fat. Same patient as in **A.** A standoff pad was utilized. Fluid is identified surrounding the subcutaneous fat lobules, forming a reticular pattern. This is always seen in cases of ruptured Baker's cyst, but it may also be seen in deep venous thrombosis.

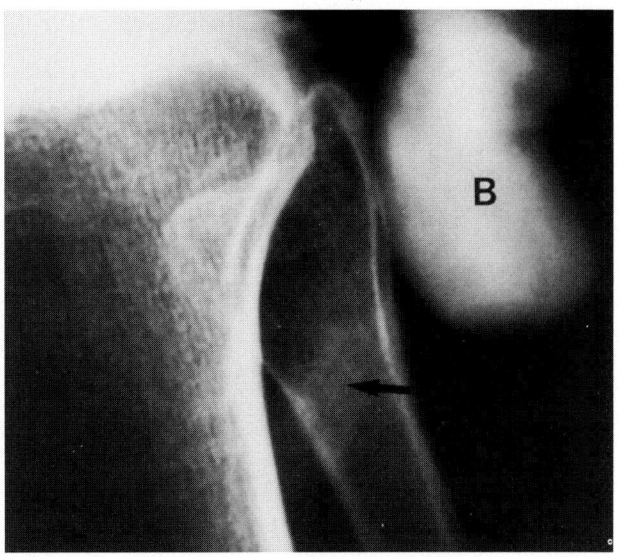

Figure 5–57 ■ Ruptured rheumatoid Baker's cyst: arthrography. Same patient as in Figure 5–45. Arthrography was performed to confirm the diagnosis. This image was obtained 45 minutes following injection of contrast material. Subtle leak of contrast material (*arrow*) is noted anterior and inferior to the Baker's cyst (*B*).

should not be mistaken for calcified soft tissue tumors. Pseudothrombophlebitis may even develop in patients after TKA. Synovial inflammation of the gastrocnemius-semimembranosus bursa can cause leg swelling in the postoperative patient. This is very important to keep in mind because the differential diagnosis of postoperative knee swelling includes more common complications, such as quadriceps tear, infection, and thrombophlebitis.

Studies comparing sonography with contrast arthrography in the diagnosis of Baker's cyst show the diagnostic accuracy to be equivalent (Resnick and Niwayama, 1988). In these patients, structural integrity of the joint cartilage is not an issue. Given the discomfort inherent in an invasive procedure, especially when the synovia are inflamed, ultrasound is the examination of choice. MRI is comparable in diagnostic accuracy and is noninvasive. However, the examination requires the patient to lie motionless for at least half an hour, far longer than the 5 to 10 minutes required to perform a careful ultrasound examination. This factor makes ultrasound the preferred examination, particularly in patients with crippling rheumatoid arthritis. Cost factors also favor ultrasound.

The differential diagnosis of a mass in the popliteal fossa includes popliteal artery aneurysm, varices, lymphocele, abscess, schwannoma, or other soft tissue tumors with cystic characteristics, as well as Baker's cyst (Scott et al., 1977). Absence of pulsa-

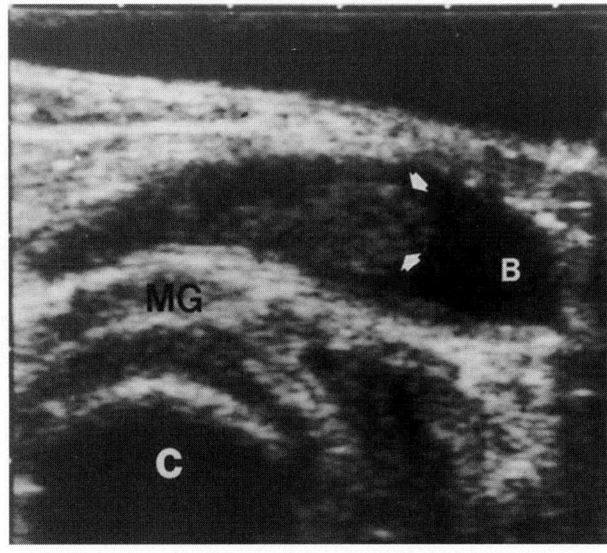

Figure 5–58 ■ Benign synovioma arising within Baker's cyst: longitudinal sonogram. A middle-aged man with a palpable mass in the popliteal fossa of the right knee. The transducer is aligned along the length of the medial gastrocnemius tendon (*MG*). A polypoid soft tissue mass (*small arrows*) is seen protruding into the Baker's cyst (*B*). Histological examination of the synovectomy specimen revealed a benign synovioma. Abbreviation: femoral condyle (*C*). (Courtesy of Dr. A. de Brabant, Milan, Italy)

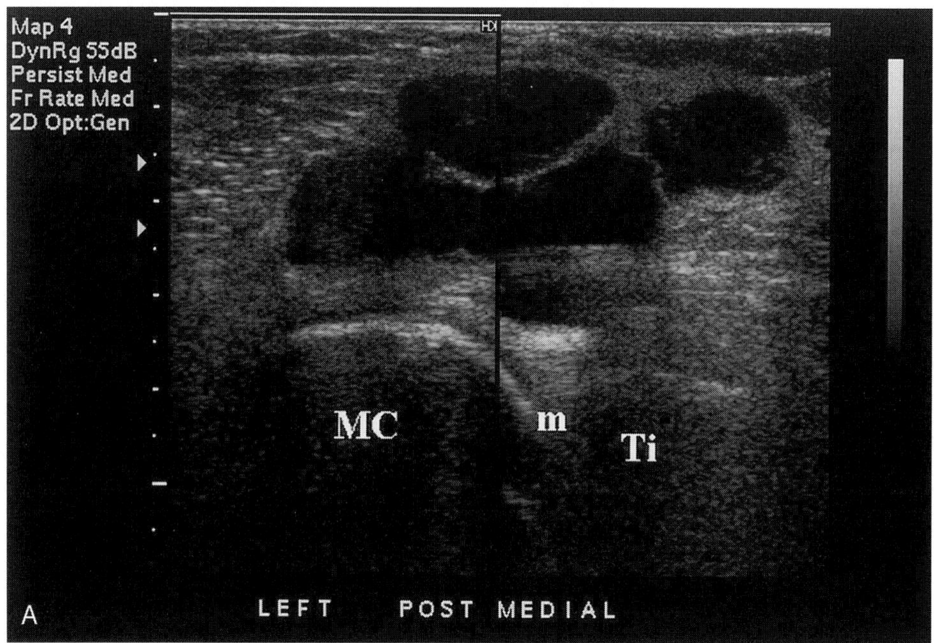

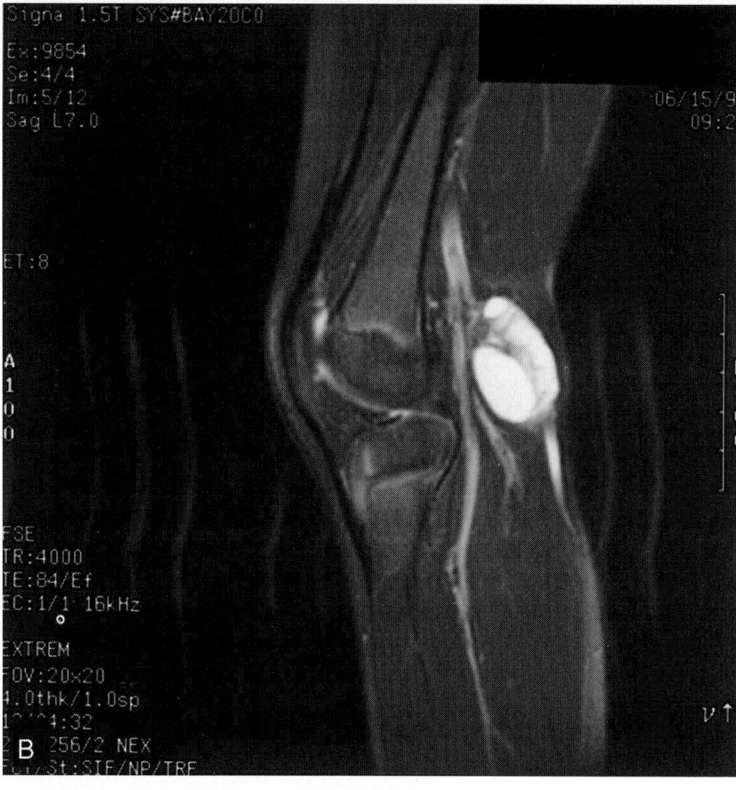

Figure 5-59 ■ **A,** Baker's cyst in a child: longitudinal sonogram through the medial popliteal space. A popliteal mass was detected clinically in this 10-year-old girl. The clinician noted that the mass seemed pulsatile and did not transilluminate as expected. The sonogram along the long axis of the Baker's cyst shows multiple septations within the mass. The location of the mass over the posterior horn of the medial meniscus (*m*) and over the medial gastrocnemius is typical of a popliteal cyst. Abbreviations: medial femoral condyle (*MC*), tibial plateau (*Ti*). **B,** Baker's cyst in a child: sagittal FSE T_2-weighted sequence with fat suppression. Baker's cysts in children are quite common lesions. These popliteal cysts are often very tense and rarely communicate with the joint space. Some lesions do not transilluminate; septations within these cysts may cause them to be opaque. This lesion pulsated due to its large size, high internal pressure, and close relationship to the popliteal artery laterally.

tion on gray scale imaging helps to exclude aneurysm. Conventional Doppler and color flow imaging will further exclude vascular pathology. The definitive diagnosis of Baker's cyst is made by identification of the channel of communication with the joint space adjacent to the medial femoral condyle. This is pathognomonic for Baker's cyst. Differentiation between Baker's cyst secondary to monoarticular rheumatoid arthritis and pigmented villonodular synovitis is based on clinical criteria. These entities are similar in their sonographic appearance (Fig. 5–58).

Traumatic Bursitis

In exceptional cases, a communicating bursa can become pathologically distended with fluid in the absence of articular disease. An example of this is the development of gastrocnemius-semimembranosus cysts in children. These cysts result from overload of the adjacent tendons. There is no evidence of ligamentous or meniscal disease. Local traumatic inflammation of the synovial lining of the bursa is the most likely etiology of this type of bursitis (Fig. 5–59).

Ultrasound examination in these cases reveals a distended bursa containing anechoic fluid. Communication with the joint is not detectable in children less than 10 years of age. The ligaments and menisci are normal.

Loose Body Entrapment

Communicating bursae such as the gastrocnemius-semimembranosus bursa have valvular connections with the adjacent joint, as described earlier. Fluid pumped into the bursa contains glycoproteins. As solute is reabsorbed from the bursa and new fluid is pumped in, the concentration of these glycoproteins progressively increases. The result is a collection of detritus within the bursa (Canoso, 1981). In addition, cartilage fragments may become trapped within the bursa (Fig. 5–60). Some of these loose bodies may calcify and become visible on conventional radiographs (Figs. 5–61 and 5–62). However, sonography is more sensitive, identifying both calcified and noncalcified loose bodies within the bursa as hyperreflective foci, with or without shadowing (Fig. 5–63). Baker's cysts containing loose bodies tend to be intermittently painful and tender to palpation. Synovial osteochondromatosis can occur in the synovium of a bursa. The calcifications tend to be smaller than calcific loose bodies. The diseased synovium is thickened, and calcifications appear adherent to the synovium (Pai and van Holsbeeck, 1995).

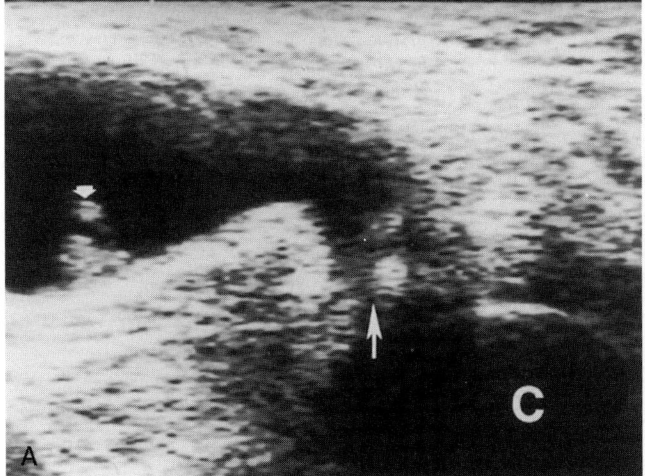

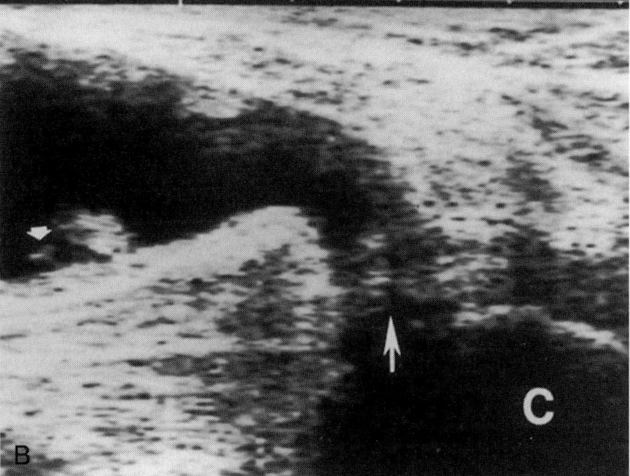

Figure 5–60 ▪ **A,** Meniscal fragments within a Baker's cyst: transverse sonogram. The patient is a 41-year-old man who sustained trauma to the left medial meniscus and presented with progressive swelling of the knee over the past 2 months. The transducer is positioned transversely over the medial aspect of the left popliteal fossa. Communication of the Baker's cyst with the joint space is demonstrated (*large arrow*). Several meniscal fragments (*small arrow*) are identified within the cyst. **B,** Pressure applied with the transducer demonstrated movement of the fragments within the cyst. Arthroscopy showed a medial meniscal tear and multiple meniscal fragments loose within the joint. Loose bodies are preferentially trapped within Baker's cysts. Abbreviation: medial femoral condyle (*C*).

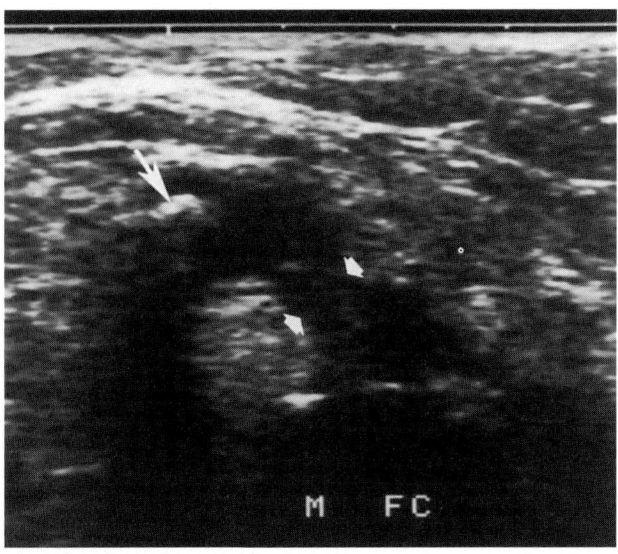

Figure 5–61 ■ Calcified loose body within Baker's cyst: transverse sonogram. A 50-year-old woman with pain and swelling in the right popliteal fossa. The position of the transducer is identical to that in Figure 5–49. A calcified loose body (*large arrow*) 8 mm in diameter is identified in the superficial portion of the bursa with prominent acoustic shadowing. The diameter of the loose body exceeds that of the neck of the Baker's cyst (*arrowheads*). This implies that it has increased in size since its entrapment within the cyst. Abbreviation: medial femoral condyle (*MFC*).

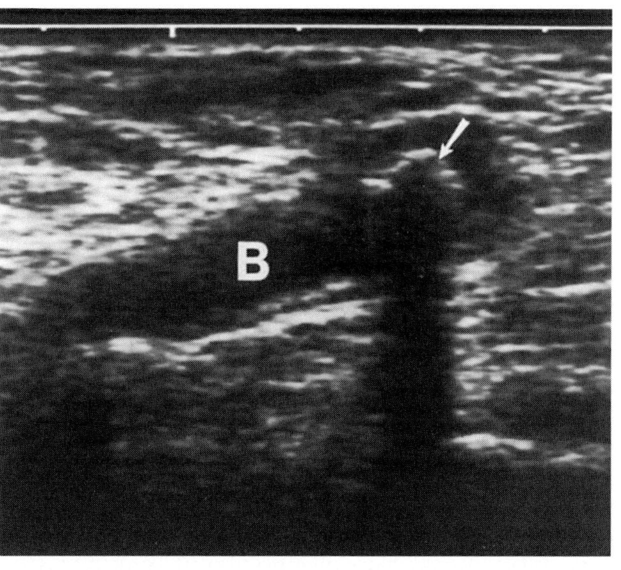

Figure 5–62 ■ Calcified loose body trapped within Baker's cyst: longitudinal sonogram. This calcified loose body (*arrow*) caused pain and swelling in the popliteal fossa of a 75-year-old woman. Note the prominent acoustic shadow. Abbreviation: Baker's cyst (*B*).

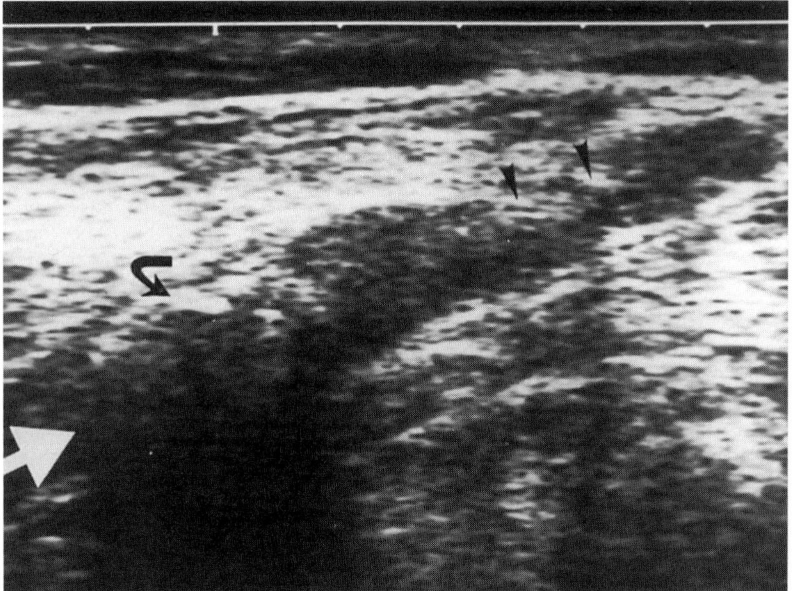

Figure 5–63 ■ Loose bodies trapped within Baker's cyst: longitudinal sonogram. The patient is a 69-year-old man with pain in the left popliteal fossa. Numerous echogenic foci fill an elongated Baker's cyst (*large white arrow*). Some of these foci demonstrate marked acoustic shadowing (*curved arrow*), whereas shadowing is more subtle with others (*arrowheads*). Only the largest of these loose bodies were evident on the conventional radiograph. Shadowing does not necessarily indicate calcification.

References

Adams R: Chronic rheumatic arthritis of the knee joint. *Dublin J Med Sci* 17:520–522, 1840.

Baker WM: On the formation of synovial cysts in the leg in connection with disease of the knee joint. *St Bartholomew's Hosp Rep* 13:245–261, 1877.

Baudrillard JC, et al: Synovial cysts of unusual location. Two cases and review of the literature. *J Radiol* 67:201–207, 1986.

Canoso JJ: Bursae, tendons and ligaments. *Clin Rheum Dis* 7:189–221, 1981.

Chandler SB: The iliopsoas bursa in man. *Anat Rec* 58:235–240, 1934.

Codman EA: The shoulder: *Rupture of the Supraspinatus Tendon and Other Lesions in or about the Subacromial Bursa.* Boston, Thomas Todd Co, Printers, 1931.

De Palma AF: *Surgery of the Shoulder.* Philadelphia, JB Lippincott Co, 1950.

Gardner DL: *Pathology of the Connective Tissue Diseases.* London, Edward Arnold, 1965.

Jayson MIV: Protective value of synovial cysts in rheumatoid knees. *Ann Rheum Dis* 31:179–182, 1981.

Lindgren PG, Willen R: Gastrocnemius-semimembranosus bursa and its relation to the knee joint. Anatomy and histology. *Acta Radiol* 18:497–512, 1977.

Newman JS, et al: Detection of soft-tissue hyperemia: Value of power Doppler sonography. *AJR* 163: 385–389, 1994.

Nicholas JA, Hershman EB: *The Lower Extremity and Spine in Sports Medicine.* St Louis, CV Mosby Co, 1986.

Pai VR, van Holsbeeck M: Synovial osteochondromatosis of the hip: Role of sonography. *JCU* 23:199, 1995.

Peterson L, Renström P: *Sports Injuries.* Chicago, Year Book Medical, 1986.

Rakofsky M: *Fractional Arthrography of the Shoulder.* Stuttgart, Gustav Fischer, 1987.

Resnick D, Niwayama G: *Diagnosis of Bone and Joint Disorders.* Philadelphia, WB Saunders Co, 1988.

Scott WW, et al: B-scan ultrasound in the diagnosis of popliteal aneurysms. *Surgery* 81:436, 1977.

van Holsbeeck M, et al: Staging and follow-up of rheumatoid arthritis of the knee. Comparison of sonography, thermography, and clinical assessment. *J Ultrasound Med* 7:561–566, 1988.

van Holsbeeck M, Introcaso J: Sonography of the postoperative shoulder. *AJR* 152:202, 1988.

van Holsbeeck M, Strouse PJ: Sonography of the shoulder: Evaluation of the subacromial-subdeltoid bursa. *AJR* 160:561–564, 1993.

Chapter 6
Sonography of Ligaments

Traumatic injuries of ligaments in the knee and ankle are quite common, most often seen in athletes participating in contact sports. Clinical examination is valuable only in cases of acute complete rupture, but it usually cannot be performed immediately following injury. Chronic ligamentous injury and meniscal tears associated with either acute or chronic trauma are poorly evaluated with clinical examination. Arthroscopy provides direct visualization of the cruciate ligaments and menisci, but extracapsular ligaments are not evaluated. Cruciate ligaments are often difficult to evaluate with arthrography, and like arthroscopy, arthrography examines only intra-articular structures. CT lacks sufficient contrast resolution to define ligamentous structures. In addition, its limitation to transverse axial imaging makes it inappropriate for evaluation of most ligaments. Ultrasound and MRI are the only diagnostic modalities well suited for examination of ligaments. Both of these imaging techniques provide multiplanar capability and demonstrate ligamentous anatomy well. The advantages of ultrasound over MRI are the short examination time, the ability to provide a dynamic examination, reasonable cost, and availability. These factors are most significant in the setting of acute injury. Ultrasound examinations are universally available to emergency room physicians, but considerable delay is encountered in scheduling MRI examinations. Often the prognosis depends on prompt initiation of therapy.

Examination Technique

In the examination of ligaments, high-frequency transducers are of the utmost importance. Linear arrays of 12, 10, 7.5, and 5 MHz are acceptable. The highest frequency available is preferred because ligaments are generally thin, superficially located structures. Low-frequency transducers, less than 5 MHz, are not acceptable for the examination of ligaments. Since ligaments are usually located quite superficially, a standoff pad may be required to image extra-articular ligaments. Intra-articular ligaments, such as the cruciates of the knee, are well demonstrated without a standoff. Careful attention must be paid to gain and time gain compensation (TGC) settings. Oversaturation of images will result in failure to identify ligaments. Ligaments are normally hyperreflective and will blend in with the strong echos produced by cortical bone when gain or TGC are set too high. Identification and examination of ligaments are made considerably easier if the transducer is always aligned along the length of the ligament to be examined. Transverse images are of little diagnostic value. As in other musculoskeletal ultrasound examinations, comparison with the contralateral extremity is often valuable.

Normal Sonographic Structure of Ligament

Many ligaments of the hand, wrist, shoulder, hip, knee, and ankle can be examined sonographically. These include the vincula tendineum, collateral ligaments of the phalanges, triangular fibrocartilage of the wrist, dorsal hood, collateral and annular ligaments of the elbow, coracoacromial ligament of the shoulder, iliofemoral ligament of the hip, collateral ligaments of the knee, and tibiofibular, fibulotalar and deltoid ligaments of the ankle. Ligaments are composed of dense, regular connective tissue similar to that of tendons. Their structure differs from that of tendons in that more interweaving of collagen fibers is observed in ligaments, giving them a less regular histological and sonographic appearance (Bloom and Fawcett, 1980). All of these liga-

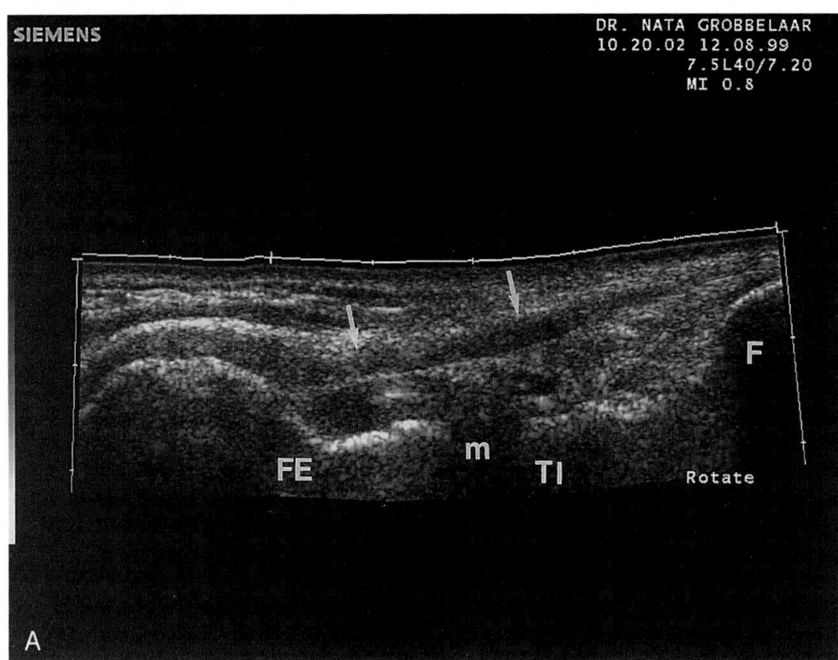

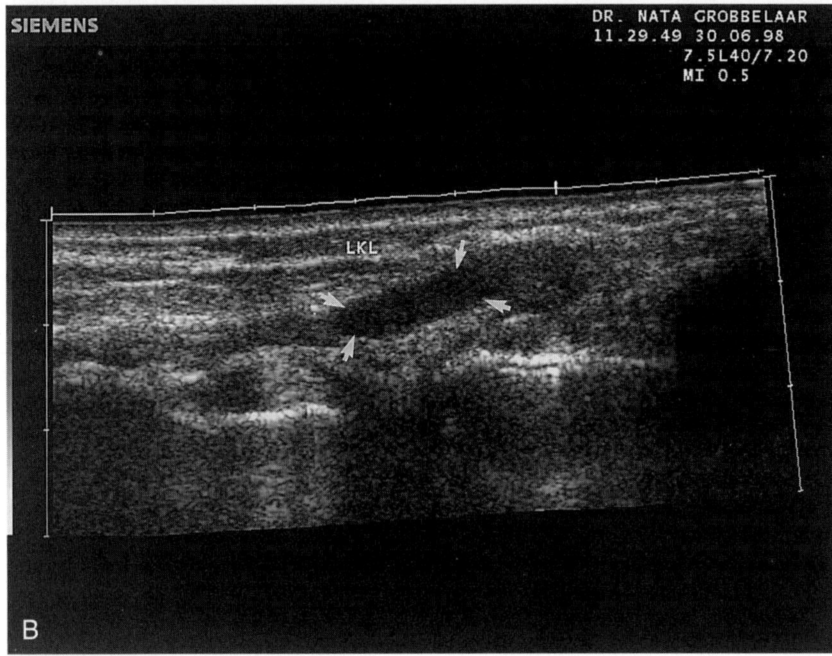

Figure 6-1 ■ **A,** Normal lateral collateral ligament: longitudinal sonogram with extended-field-of-view technique. A normal collateral ligament is identified in this 30-year-old physician. The transducer moves over the posterior lateral aspect of the knee and makes a compound image of the entire lateral collateral ligament (*arrows*). The inferior aspect lies to the observers right, with the caudal portion of the transducer over the fibular head (*F*). The biceps femoris tendon encircles the lateral ligament from the lateral side, appearing like a horseshoe on transverse images. This sometimes makes it difficult to distinguish these two as separate hyperechoic structures on longitudinal images. Abbreviations: distal femur (*FE*), lateral meniscus (*m*), proximal tibia (*TI*). (Courtesy of Dr. N. Grobbelaar, private practice, Pretoria, South Africa.) **B,** Abnormal lateral collateral ligament: longitudinal sonogram with extended-field-of-view technique. This young rugby player injured his knee through a rotational force. The player fell down with his foot firmly planted while another player hit him on the top of the knee. Ultrasound detects swelling and a hypoechoic defect (*between arrows*) in the lateral collateral ligament. Note the swelling through retraction proximal and distal to the defect. Surgery confirmed a complete tear of the lateral collateral ligament. Abbreviation: lateral collateral ligament (*LKL*). (Courtesy of Dr. N. Grobbelaar, private practice, Pretoria, South Africa.)

ments (Fig. 6-1), with the exception of the medial collateral ligament of the knee, appear as homogeneous, hyperechoic bands approximately 2 to 3 mm thick closely approximating the bony contours.

The medial collateral ligament (MCL) of the knee is a specialized structure and therefore requires a more detailed description. This ligament, also called the *tibial collateral ligament,* is a broad, flat structure approximately 9 cm long that extends from the medial femoral condyle to the medial aspect of the proximal tibia (Fig. 6-2). It is divided into superficial and deep components separated by a zone of loose areolar connective tissue (Fig. 6-3). The superficial component is a band of dense, regular connective tissue anchoring the medial femoral condyle to the proximal tibia. Many physicians consider the deep component to be composed of two smaller ligaments connecting the medial meniscus to the femur and tibia. These are referred to as the *meniscofemoral* and *meniscotibial ligaments.*

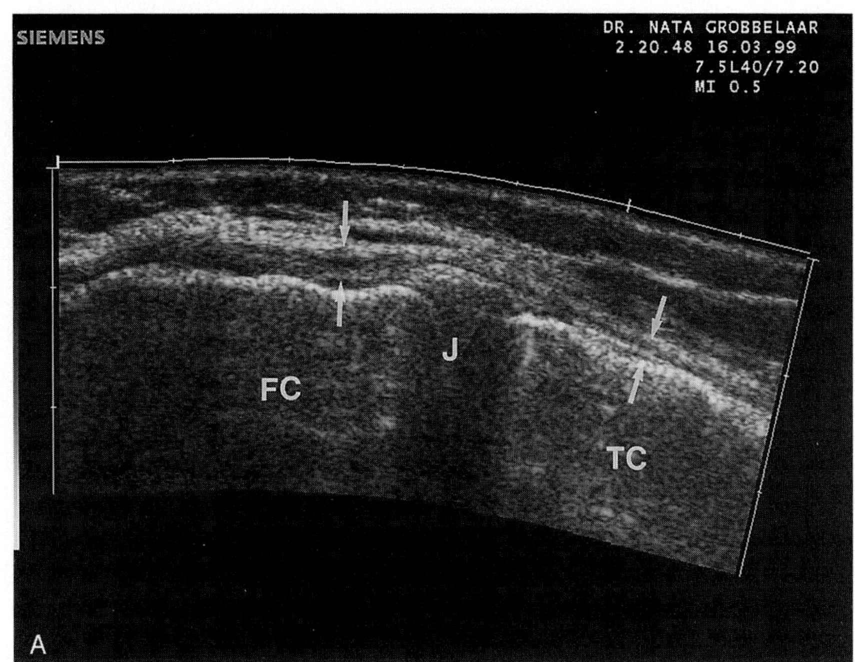

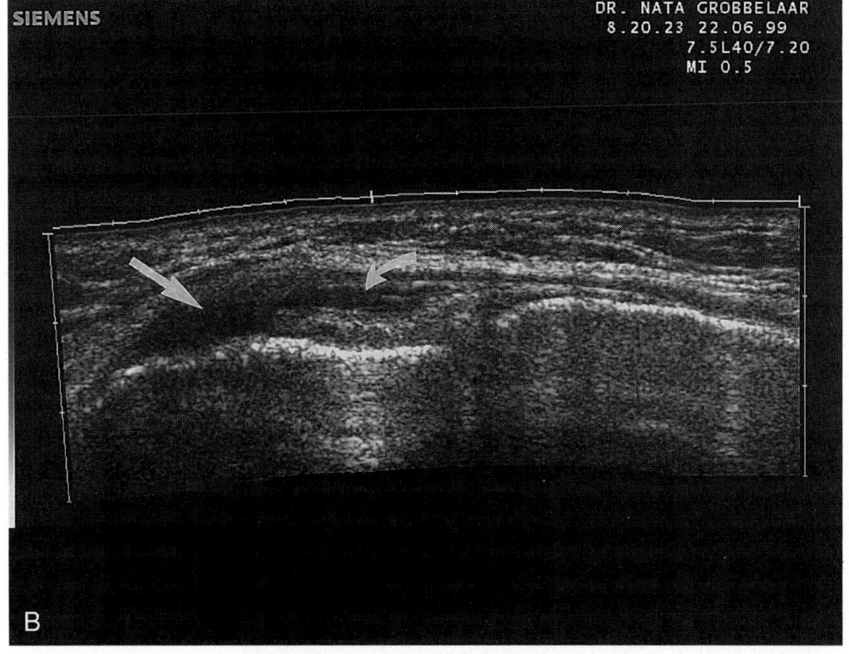

Figure 6-2 ■ **A,** Normal femoral and tibial insertion of the medial collateral ligament: extended field-of-view image in the coronal plane. This image of the knee of a 30-year-old man was obtained with the patient in lateral decubitus position and his leg extended. The normal medial collateral ligament can measure up to 9 cm in length. It originates from the most proximal aspect of the medial femoral condyle (*FC*), covers the joint space (*J*), and inserts on the medial tibial condyle (*TC*) several centimeters below the margin of the tibial plateau. The locations for measuring the thickness of the proximal and distal segments of the ligament are noted (*arrowheads*). The proximal segment is measured at the depth of the concavity of the medial femoral condyle. The distal segment is measured at a point halfway between the tibial plateau and the most distal extent of the ligament. Note the trilaminar structure of the MCL, best seen at the site of proximal measurement. (Courtesy of Dr. N. Grobbelaar, private practice, Pretoria, South Africa.) **B,** Abnormal femoral insertion of the medial collateral ligament: extended field-of-view image in the coronal plane. After a fall down some stairs, this 39-year-old man observed his knee swell up rapidly. Pain on the medial aspect of the knee corresponded to the origin of the MCL. The compound image of the MCL shows a tear (*straight arrow*) in the proximal portion of the ligament. Fluid leaks (*curved arrow*) in between the layers of the more distal ligament, which is still intact. Note the significant swelling of the proximal ligament at the site of maximal concavity of the medial femoral condyle, the location at which the ligament is typically measured. (Courtesy of Dr. N. Grobbelaar, private practice, Pretoria, South Africa.)

Ultrasound demonstrates the MCL as a trilaminar structure: two hyperechoic layers separated by a hypoechoic zone. The hyperreflective bands correspond directly to the superficial and deep dense connective tissue ligaments. Loose areolar connective tissue forms the hypoechoic band that separates the superficial and deep components. In some patients, a bursa is found within this hypoechoic zone of loose connective tissue (Anderson, 1983; Clemente, 1985). Figure 6-4 is a radiograph of a cadaver knee specimen. Barium sulfate was injected into the middle hypoechoic layer of the MCL. A specimen radiograph was then obtained, demonstrating that the barium was within the substance of the MCL (Figs. 6-4 and 6-5). Histological sections were then made of the MCL, which showed barium confined to the loose areolar connective tissue that separates the deep and superficial layers of the ligament.

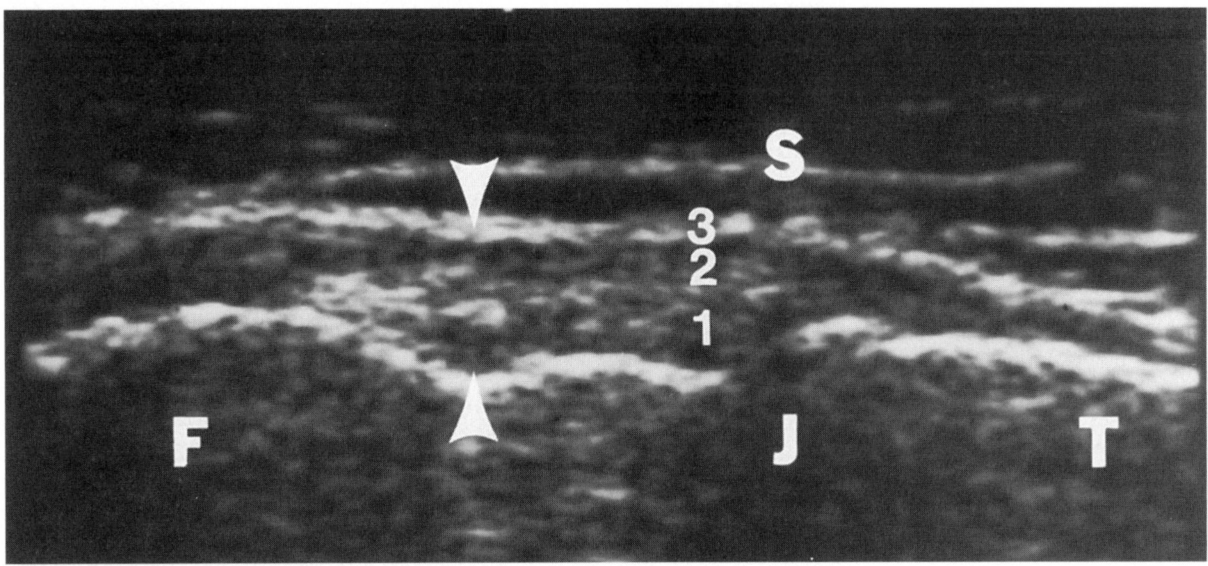

Figure 6-3 ■ Normal trilaminar structure of the MCL: coronal sonogram. This detailed image of the MCL better demonstrates the normal trilaminar structure of this ligament. The deep hyperechoic layer (*1*) is composed of the meniscofemoral and meniscotibial ligaments. Loose areolar connective tissue (*2*) separates the superficial and deep hyperechoic layers. Abbreviations and symbol: femur (*F*), joint space (*J*), superficial MCL (*3*), tibia (*T*), proximal measurement (*arrowheads*).

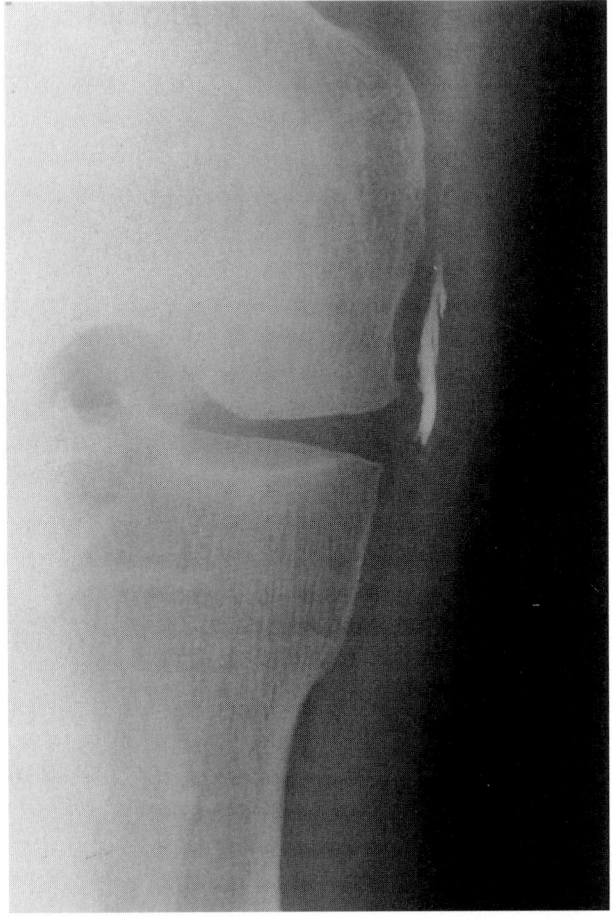

Figure 6-4 ■ MCL of an autopsy specimen: anteroposterior knee radiograph. It clearly demonstrates contrast material layering within an anatomically confined space after it had been injected into the layer indicated in Figure 6-3.

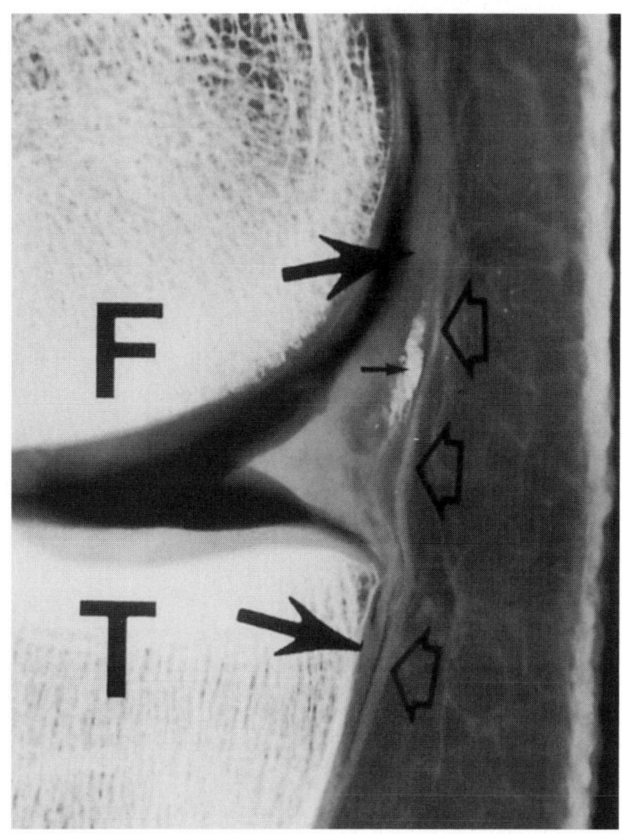

Figure 6–5 ■ MCL of an autopsy specimen: specimen radiograph. The knee in Figure 6–4 was then sectioned to yield 1-cm-thick coronal tissue specimens. A mammographic technique was used to obtain this specimen radiograph. Barium (*small arrow*) is identified layering within the MCL between the deep and superficial layers. The *large black arrows* indicate the meniscofemoral and meniscotibial ligaments, which stabilize the medial meniscus. Abbreviations and symbol: femur (*F*), tibia (*T*), superficial component of the MCL (*open arrows*).

Ligament Pathology

Intra-articular Ligaments

Ligaments are categorized by location: either intra-articular or extra-articular. This distinction is valuable in determining the best diagnostic approach. We have been successful in demonstrating tears of the intra-articular ligaments of the knee and wrist. Detection of tears of the cruciate ligaments or triangular fibrocartilage (Fig. 6–6) requires careful technique and some patience. In the knee, care must be taken to distinguish the ligament from intercondylar fat (Figs. 6–7 through 6–11). Approximately 60 degrees of flexion (Fig. 6–12) is required to obtain an adequate sonographic window on the anterior cruciate ligament. Clearly, in the acutely traumatized patient, this is rarely possible. Other investigators have experienced similar difficulties in imaging intra-articular ligaments using pulse-echo ultrasound (Laine et al., 1987; Richardson et al., 1988). A recent study focusing on the efficacy of ultrasound in the detection of acute cruciate ligament tears used a transverse approach over the origin of the anterior cruciate ligament (ACL). Sensitivity and specificity in detecting ACL tears were high. The course of the ligament is not well demonstrated, but hematoma resulting from ligament rupture can be shown with great accuracy (Ptasznik et al., 1995). Transmission ultrasound has shown promise in imaging intra-articular ligaments, but the equipment is not yet commercially available (Hentz et al., 1987). Therefore, we prefer to evaluate pathology of intra-articular ligaments with MRI at the present time.

Extra-articular Ligaments

Acute Ligament Injury

Clinical examination to detect complete ligament tears is quite reliable, but often the diagnosis is considerably delayed. Stress tests for the detection of joint laxity are used to identify ligament injury. Pain and swelling present at the time of injury make these tests inappropriate in the acute setting. Several weeks after injury, when pain and swelling have subsided, these tests may be administered and the diagnosis made. This delay is undesirable because surgical repair, if indicated, should be performed as soon as possible following injury to ensure the best possible result.

Ultrasound provides a reliable means of detecting acute ligament injury, both complete and partial tears. The simple, noninvasive nature of the exami-

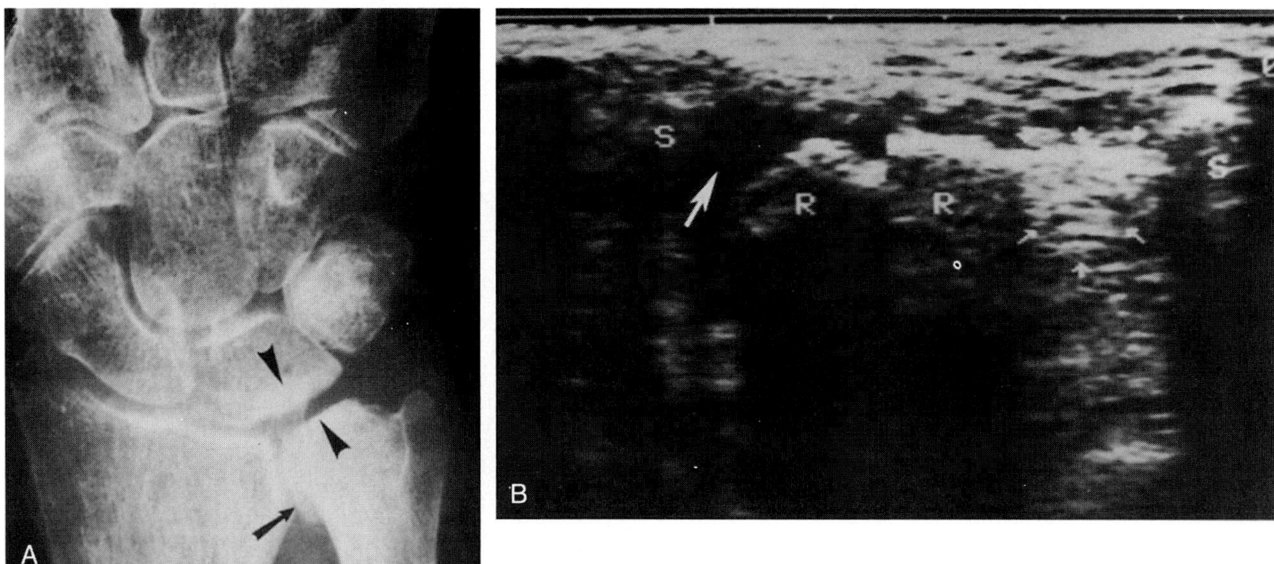

Figure 6-6 ■ **A,** Triangular fibrocartilage tear in the wrist: radiograph. The patient is a 62-year-old woman with pain in the ulnar side of the wrist during pronation and supination. Sclerosis (*arrowheads*) is demonstrated in the proximal lunate and distal ulna, indicative of abnormal motion. Osteophytic change and narrowing of the radioulnar joint (*arrow*) are also present. **B,** Triangular fibrocartilage tear in the wrist: transverse sonogram. Same patient as in **A.** The transducer is positioned over the volar aspect of the wrists, just distal to the ulnar head at the level of the ulnar styloid. Side-by-side comparison is provided in this split-screen image, with the asymptomatic left wrist at the observer's right. A normal triangular fibrocartilage (*arrows*) is identified between the radius (*R*) and ulnar styloid (*S*) of the left wrist. Complete absence of fibrocartilage is seen in the symptomatic right wrist (left image). Fluid (*white arrow*) fills the space previously occupied by the triangular fibrocartilage.

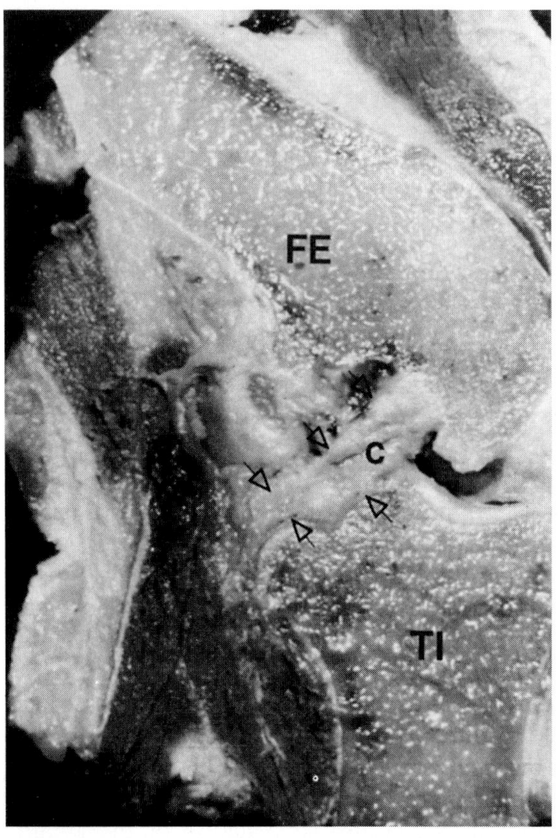

Figure 6-7 ■ Cadaver knee: longitudinal anatomical section through the posterior cruciate ligament (PCL). An oblique section was obtained through this cadaver specimen to bisect the PCL along its length. The PCL (*arrows*) travels obliquely and anteriorly from the most posterior aspect of the tibia to the medial femoral condyle (*FE*). Fat surrounds the ligament within the intercondylar fossa. Abbreviations: PCL (*C*), proximal tibia (*TI*).

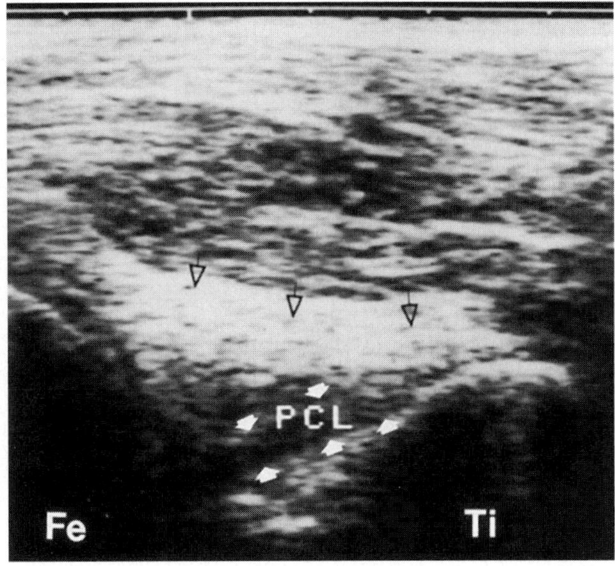

Figure 6-8 ■ Normal PCL: longitudinal sonogram. A normal PCL is seen in this 30-year-old man. The transducer is positioned over the popliteal fossa, with the cranial end obliqued slightly toward the medial. The PCL (*white arrows*) has a hypoechoic appearance relative to the surrounding fat. This is due in part to anisotropy. The *open arrows* indicate the normal posterior joint capsule, which appears markedly hyperechoic and curved anteriorly. Abbreviations: distal femur (*Fe*), proximal tibia (*Ti*).

nation and the short time required for examination make it ideal in the emergent setting. Patient selection must be based on a thorough clinical examination. Ultrasound is necessary in only a limited number of patients who present with equivocal clinical findings, especially when surgery is being considered (van Dijk et al., 1996). In cases of partial rupture, the involved area of the ligament appears markedly thickened and decreased in echogenicity. Complete ruptures are demonstrated as a discontinuity of the ligament, with the free ends separated by hematoma. The fluid occupying the gap will appear hypoechoic or anechoic, depending on how long after injury imaging is performed. In general, the diagnosis is most easily made when imaging occurs as soon after injury as possible. Some retraction of the ends of the ruptured ligament occurs, giving them a slightly rounded appearance.

In the ankle, the fibulocalcaneal and fibulotalar ligaments are most frequently involved. Two fibulotalar ligaments are present: anterior and posterior. The anterior fibulotalar ligament courses anteriorly and slightly inferiorly from the anterior aspect of the distal fibular epiphysis to insert on the lateral aspect of the talus. The posterior fibulotalar ligament is relatively short, running horizontally from the posterior aspect of the distal fibular epiphysis to the posterior talus. In 70% of ankle ligament ruptures, the anterior fibulotalar ligament (Figs. 6-13 and 6-14) is the only ligament involved. Combined rupture of the anterior fibulotalar and fibulocalcaneal ligaments is seen in 20% of cases (Peterson and Renstrom, 1986). The posterior fibulotalar ligament is rarely ruptured. The mechanism of injury to the ankle ligaments is nearly always supination and inward rotation of the foot.

A less common injury is sprain of the anterior tibiofibular ligament (Figs. 6-15 and 6-16). Pain in these sprains is localized above the lateral tibiotalar joint space. The injury occurs with external rotation

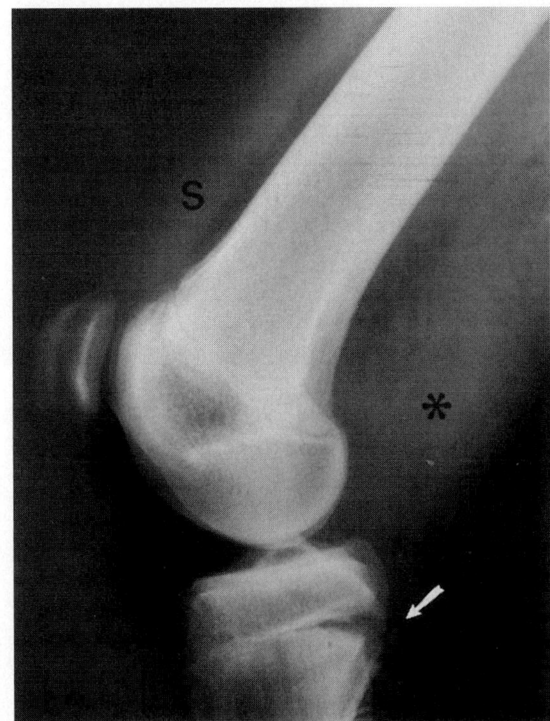

Figure 6-9 ■ Epiphysiolysis proximal tibia with associated PCL tear: lateral film of the knee. This 17-year-old boy felt a snap in his knee while hanging upside down with his foot caught in an elevator door. The tibial growth plate is markedly widened posteriorly, and an avulsed fragment of the tibial metaphysis is noted (*arrow*). Subcutaneous hemorrhage (*asterisk*) results in swelling of the soft tissues of the popliteal fossa. A distended suprapatellar bursa (*S*) is also well demonstrated.

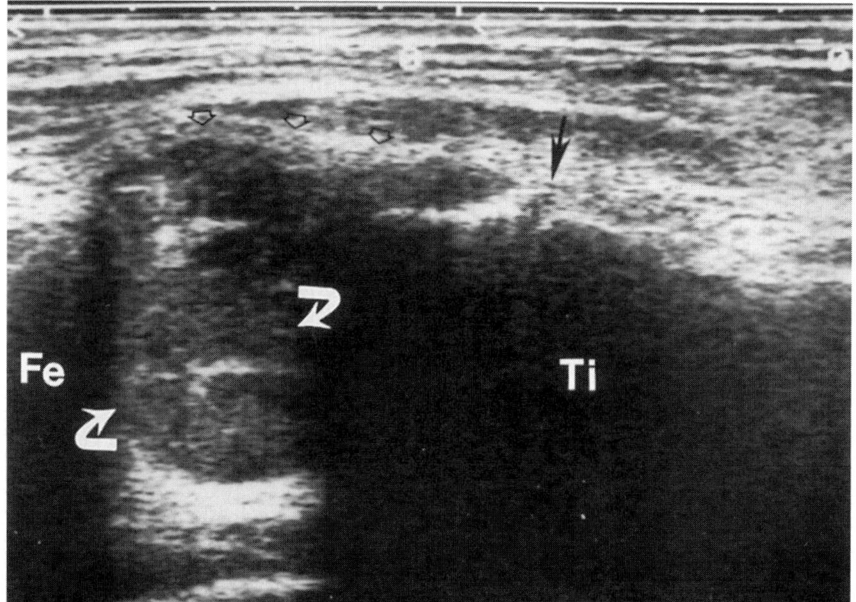

Figure 6-10 ■ Epiphysiolysis proximal tibia with associated PCL tear: longitudinal sonogram of the popliteal fossa. Same patient as in Figure 6-9. An ultrasound examination was requested to exclude vascular injury. The popliteal vessels were intact. Intercondylar hemorrhage is seen in the expected location of the PCL (*curved arrows*). The posterior joint capsule (*open arrows*) bows posteriorly, displaced by hemorrhage. At the level of the tibial growth plate, a small osseous fragment (*black arrow*) is identified. Abbreviations: distal femur (*Fe*), proximal tibia (*Ti*).

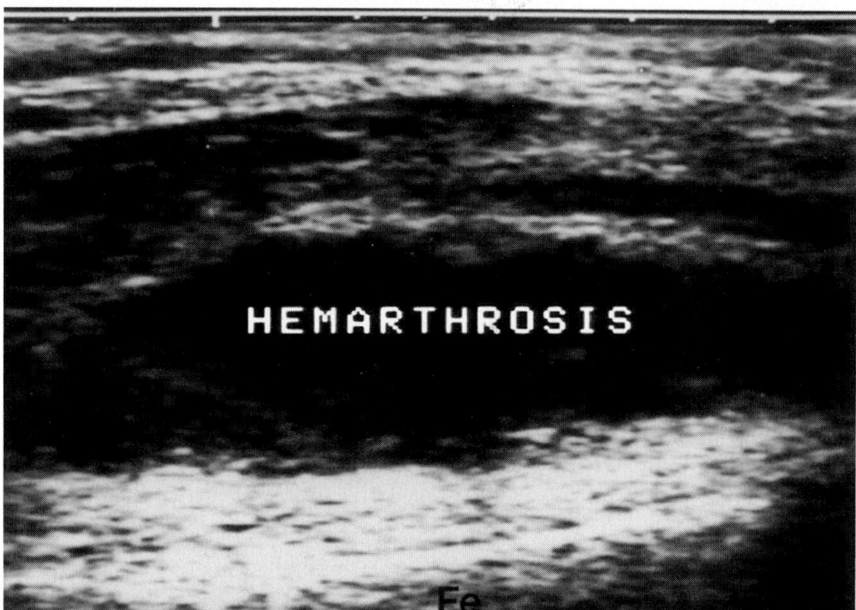

Figure 6-11 ■ Epiphysiolysis proximal tibia with associated PCL tear: longitudinal sonogram of the suprapatellar bursa. Same patient as in Figures 6-9 and 6-10. Significant intra-articular hemorrhage is seen within the suprapatellar bursa. This is a common finding in cruciate ligament tears.

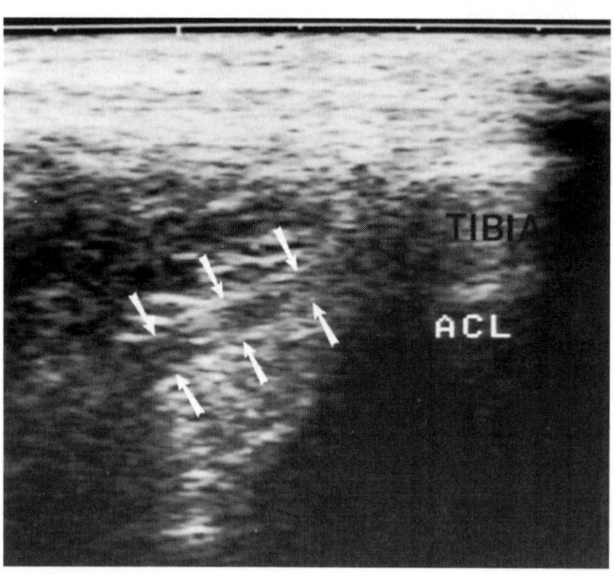

Figure 6-12 ■ Normal ACL: longitudinal sonogram. A normal ACL is seen in this asymptomatic 30-year-old man. The examination is performed with the knee in full flexion and the transducer positioned along the length of the ACL; the cranial end of the transducer is placed oblique to the lateral aspect. Like the PCL, the ACL (*arrows*) appears hypoechoic relative to the surrounding intercondylar fat.

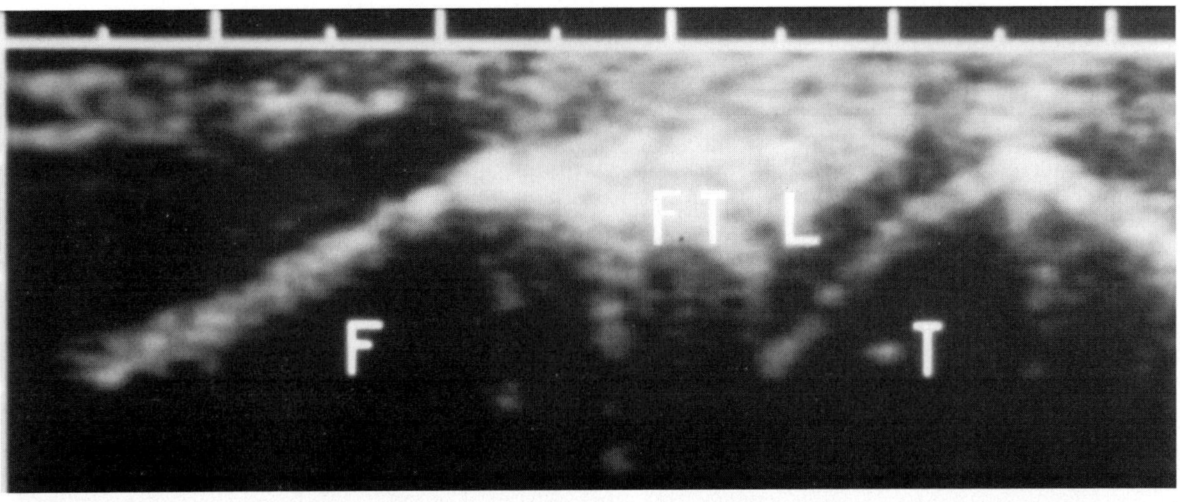

Figure 6-13 ■ Normal anterior fibulotalar ligament: oblique sonogram. Same person as in Figure 6-12. To examine the anterior fibulotalar ligament, the transducer is positioned over the lateral malleolus, angled 45 degrees anteriorly relative to the long axis of the fibula. The normal anterior fibulotalar ligament (*FTL*) is a hyperechoic band that connects the distal fibula (*F*) with the talus (*T*).

of the lower extremity on the ankle. *High ankle sprain* is the term used to describe a ligamentous injury of the tibiofibular ligament, which is difficult to diagnose by clinical exam or imaging modalities other than ultrasound (Bouffard et al., 1996). It most commonly occurs in American football players and results in prolonged disability (Box 6-1). Right-left comparison is necessary to make the diagnosis. Distraction at the syndesmosis is measured and compared with the normal side. An acutely disrupted ligament results in a cleft on transverse images over the lateral aspect of the lower tibia and fibula. Fluid in the tibiotalar joint may persist for prolonged periods of time. If associated with fracture, the lesion is called the *Maisonneuve injury* or *Dupuytren fracture*, depending on the site of the fibular fracture. The most common syndesmosis rupture is the anterior tear. The posterior tibiofibular ligament, the interosseous ligaments, and the interosseous membrane are more rarely injured. Therefore, most of these lesions are stable. However, recovery is prolonged, and the healing process may take months. These athletes are often incapacitated by pain. Taping is indicated to support the ankle in these circumstances, but this does little to alleviate the pain.

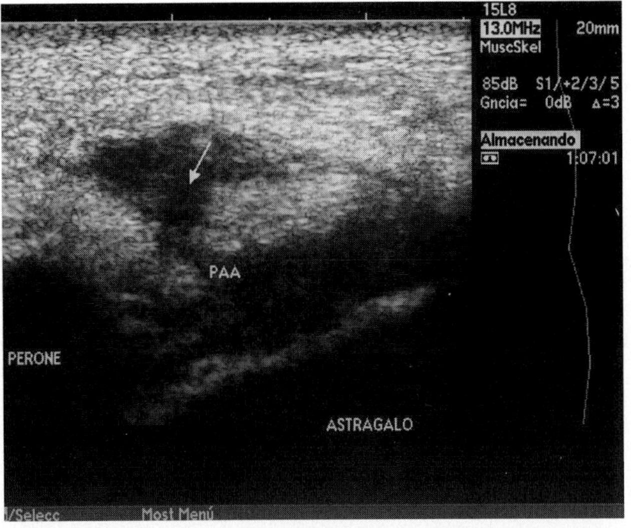

Figure 6-14 ■ Torn anterior fibulotalar ligament: oblique sonogram. This image was obtained only hours following inversion injury of the right ankle. The soft tissues are diffusely swollen, with hematoma separating the torn ends of the anterior fibulotalar ligament (*arrow*). Hematoma (*PAA*) is noted on the inside and outside of the joint capsule. Abbreviations: distal fibula (*PERONE*), talus (*ASTRAGALO*). (Courtesy of Dr. G. Rodriguez, Mount Sinai Hospital, Miami, Florida)

A separate distal fascicle of the anteroinferior tibiofibular ligament can exist as a normal variant. An inversion sprain can result in thickening of this ligament, and a chronic pain syndrome may develop. Abrasion of the articular cartilage and pain in the anterior ankle have been diagnosed as talar impingement. Granulation in the tibiofibular ligament can be confirmed sonographically prior to arthroscopic debridement (Fig. 6-17). Hypoechoic tissue is found at the inferior aspect of the syndesmosis and in the tibiotalar joint (Basset et al., 1990).

During the same examination in which integrity of the ligaments is evaluated, the peroneus tendons, Achilles tendon, and retrocalcaneal bursa should be examined for concurrent injury. In the remaining 9%

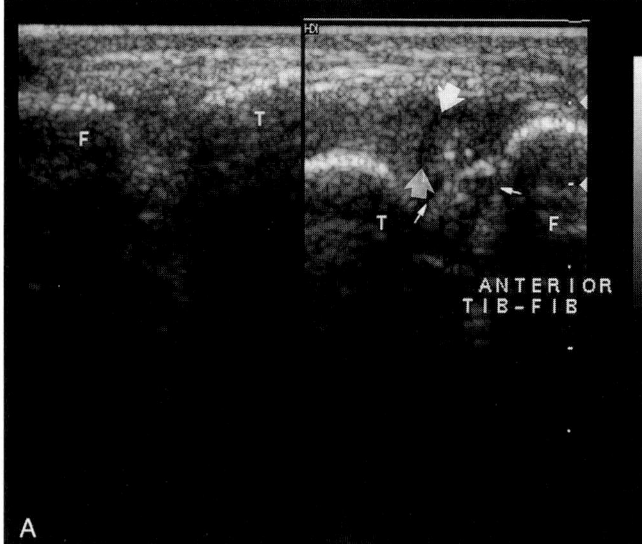

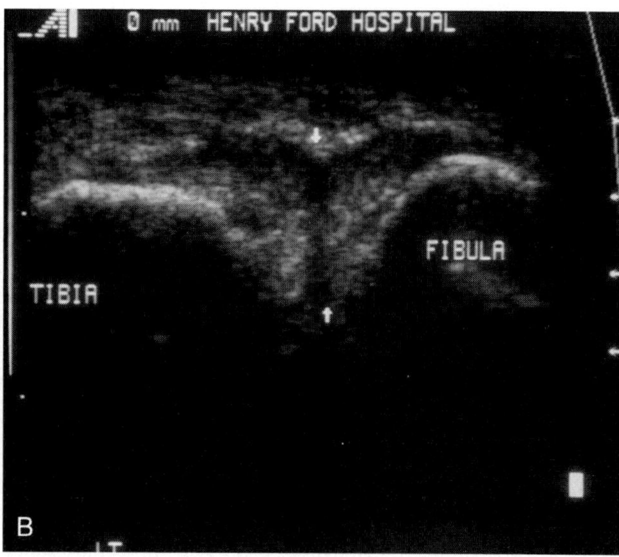

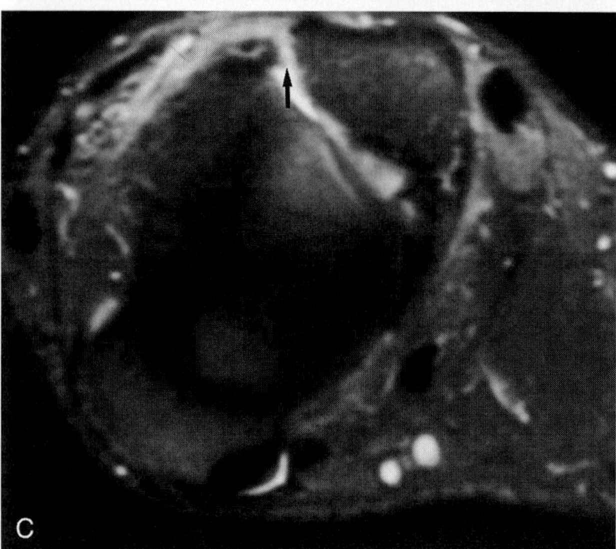

Figure 6–15 ■ **A,** Torn anterior tibiofibular ligament: transverse ultrasound scan of the anterior syndesmosis with split-screen comparison. While this 27-year-old professional football player was reaching for the ball, another player fell on his right calf. The injured player had to leave the field because of excruciating ankle pain. He was not able to bear weight at the time of the examination. The transducer was positioned above the tibiotalar joint, oriented transversely over the distal tibia and fibula. The left side of the split screen shows the normal relationship of the anterior distal tibiofibular joint. The disrupted right tibiofibular joint is shown on the right side. The distance between the tibia and fibula is wider (*small arrows*). A linear hypoechoic cleft disrupts the anterior tibiofibular ligament (*large arrows*). Abbreviations: tibia (*T*), fibula (*F*). **B,** Torn anterior tibiofibular ligament: follow-up transverse ultrasound scan of the anterior syndesmosis with split-screen comparison. Same patient and transducer position as in **A.** The patient's pain persisted, and he was not able to practice for the football games at all. A new ultrasound study was requested 3 weeks after the initial injury. The follow-up transverse ultrasound scan shows a syndesmosis rupture (*small arrows*), which is almost unchanged from the prior study. **C,** Torn anterior tibiofibular ligament: transverse T_2-weighted sequence of the syndesmosis. Same patient as in **A.** The fat-suppressed fast spin-echo images show complete disruption of the anterior tibiofibular ligament (*arrow*).

of acute ankle ligament ruptures, the deltoid ligament at the medial aspect of the ankle is involved. Pain and swelling over the medial aspect of the ankle may also be due to posterior tibial tendon rupture. This tendon is one of the principal stabilizers of the hind foot, and lesions of the posterior tibial tendon may mimic deltoid ligament injury. Surgical therapy is sometimes indicated in these cases, but the approach for these two types of lesions differs considerably. Ultrasound is extremely valuable in differentiating deltoid ligament injury from tendon injury, facilitating surgical planning.

Sonography is also valuable in the follow-up of healing ligament tears. Ligaments tend to heal quite slowly. The first evidence of restoration of ligament integrity is seen approximately 5 weeks following

Box 6–1
Indications for Ultrasound Examination of Ankle Ligaments

- Combined tear of the anterior fibulotalar and fibulocalcaneal ligaments (20% of acute tears)
- Injury of the anterior tibiofibular ligament (high ankle sprain)
- Granuloma of the distal fascicle of the anterior tibiofibular ligament
- Tear with extension through the superior peroneal retinaculum, resulting in peroneal tendon instability

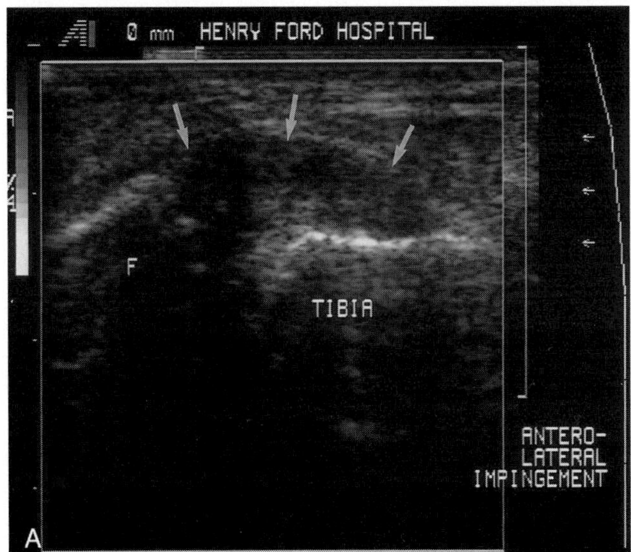

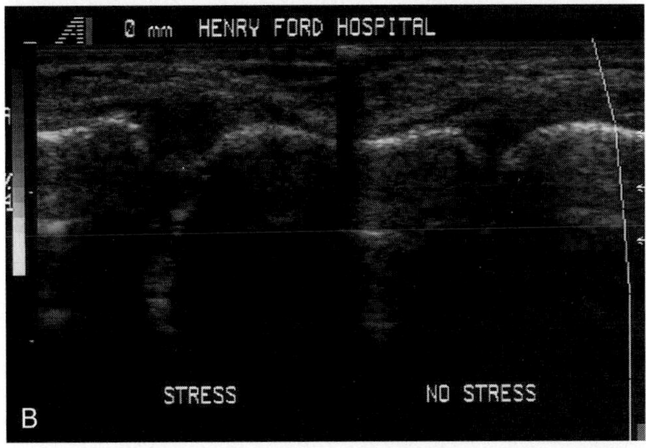

Figure 6–16 ■ **A,** Subacute tear of the anterior tibiofibular ligament: transverse sonogram. Persistent pain plagues this 50-year-old woman 2 months after she slipped while walking on ice. This transverse image of the anterior aspect of the syndesmosis demonstrates inhomogeneous swelling (*arrows*) in the expected location of the anterior tibiofibular ligament. Abbreviation: distal fibula (*F*). **B,** Subacute tear of the anterior tibiofibular ligament: sonographic stress test of the syndesmosis. Same patient as in A. The syndesmosis widens abnormally, with the foot brought into dorsiflexion (left side of the split screen). The tibiofibular joint returns to normal without stress (right side of the split screen).

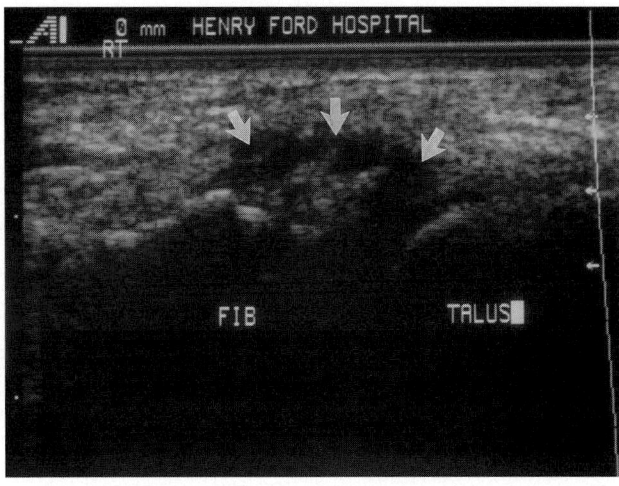

Figure 6–17 ■ Anterior tibiotalar impingement by granulation in the anteroinferior tibiofibular ligament: longitudinal sonogram. This obese 26-year-old man complains of chronic right ankle pain. The pain began over 1 year ago following an ankle inversion injury. The transducer is aligned along the long axis of the fibula. Mixed-echogenicity tissue (*arrows*) is identified at the lateral aspect of the tibiotalar joint between the fibula and the talus. Arthroscopic debridement removed a granuloma 1 cm in diameter. The anteroinferior band of the tibiofibular ligament, which was in continuity with the granuloma, appeared frayed and hypertrophied.

injury. Definite echos filling the gap in the ligament will be observed. After several months, the normal homogeneous, hyperechoic appearance of the ligament will be restored. Serial ultrasound examinations are valuable in helping to determine when normal activity may be resumed.

Injury to the collateral ligaments of the knee is quite common in athletes. Of these injuries, the MCL is most frequently involved. Complete rupture of the MCL is often accompanied by rupture of the ACL and tear of the medial meniscus (Hughston et al., 1976). The mechanism of injury is usually a blow to the lateral aspect of the knee, frequently in football and soccer (Peterson and Renstrom, 1986). An isolated MCL tear may also result from overaggressive arthroscopic surgery if the capsule is perforated.

The normal sonographic appearance of the MCL was described in detail earlier. Acute rupture (Figs. 6–18 through 6–23) of the MCL is identified as an interruption in the hyperechoic bands that form the ligament. Hypoechoic or anechoic fluid fills the gap, as seen in other ligament ruptures. Pressure applied with the transducer will displace fluid from the rupture site. The site of rupture most frequently observed is at the junction of the meniscofemoral and meniscotibial ligaments with the medial meniscus. This deep portion of the MCL is short and binds these structures tightly together. Therefore, traction applied to the ligament ruptures the deep portion first (Fig. 6–24) (Peterson and Renstrom, 1986). Hematoma may be confined to the hypoechoic layer if only the deep portion of the ligament is ruptured. If hematoma is present within the middle hypoechoic layer, a hemorrhagic bursitis is possible. Clearly, functional disability is most severe with rupture of both the superficial

Text continued on page 184

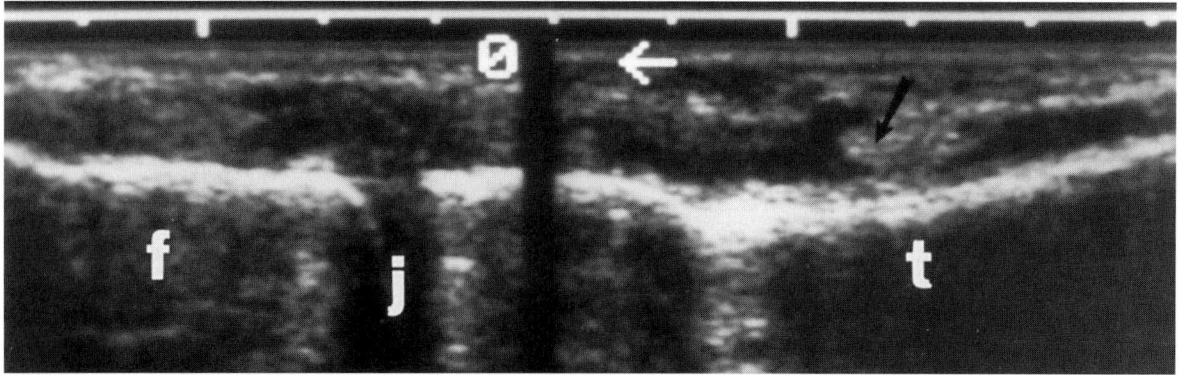

Figure 6–18 ▪ Acute rupture of the MCL: coronal sonogram. This 15-year-old hockey player was hit on the lateral aspect of the knee. He presented with pain and swelling over the medial aspect of the knee. A good physical examination could not be performed due to the severe pain and swelling; therefore, an ultrasound examination was performed. Hematoma replaces a large portion of the structure of the MCL. Only a small fragment of retracted ligament (*black arrow*) is seen distally. Abbreviations: distal femur (*f*), joint space (*j*), proximal tibia (*t*).

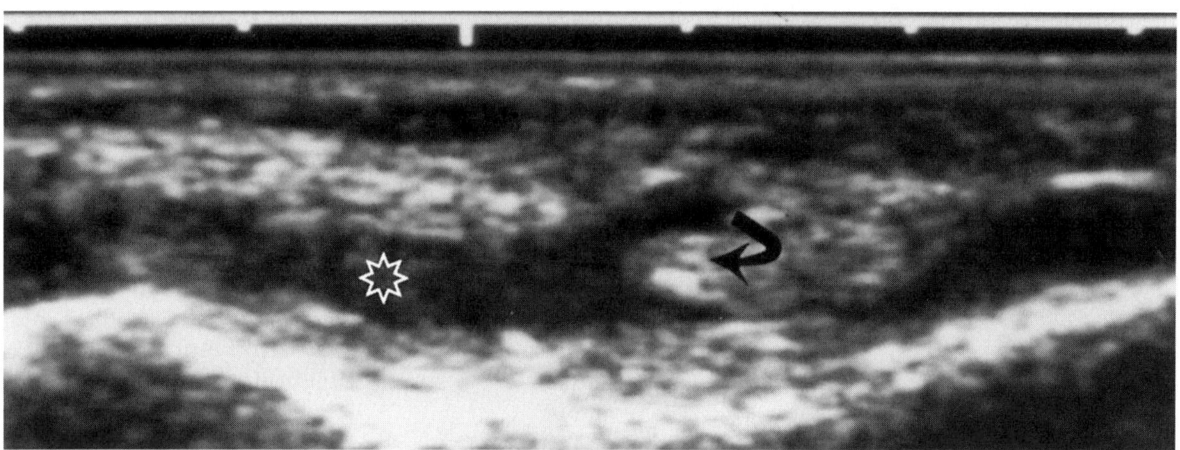

Figure 6–19 ▪ Acute rupture of the MCL: detail of the tibial MCL insertion. Same patient as in Figure 6–18. No normal ligament structure is identified. Hematoma (*asterisk*) surrounds a small, retracted fragment of the distal ligament (*curved arrow*). Two weeks after this examination, a physical examination was performed and revealed a grade III MCL tear. Results of the anterior drawer test were also positive, indicating ACL rupture. Results of a MacMurray test indicated a medial meniscal tear. This is a classic triad seen in acute MCL rupture.

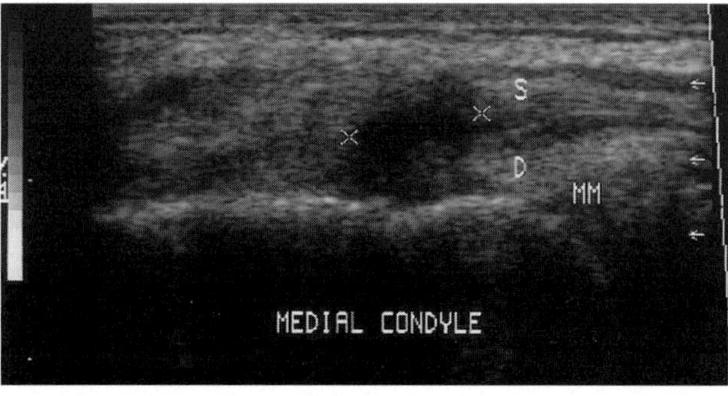

Figure 6–20 ▪ Proximal tear of the MCL: coronal sonogram along the medial knee. Five days ago, this 33-year-old firefighter injured his left knee on the job when falling with his foot caught in a crevice. The transducer is aligned along the medial collateral ligament. Both the superficial (*S*) and deep (*D*) layers of the MCL appear disrupted by hypoechoic hematoma (*between the calipers*).

Figure 6–21 ▪ Distal tear of the MCL: coronal sonogram along the medial knee. This 25-year-old hockey player received a blow to his knee while being checked against the boards. Tenderness was noted along the medial joint line. Focal disruption (*small arrow*) of the layered structure of the MCL is noted distal to the medial meniscus (*MM*).

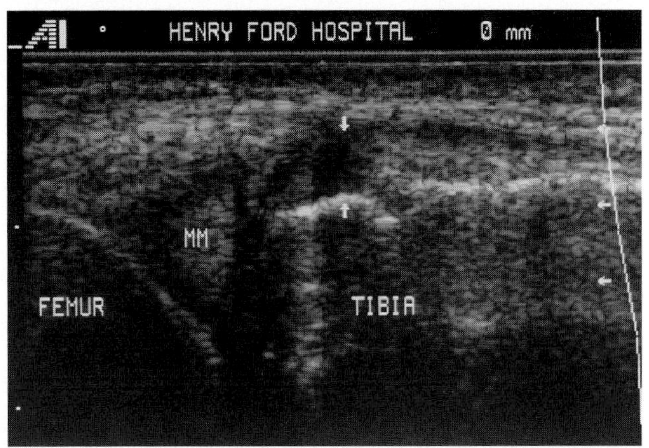

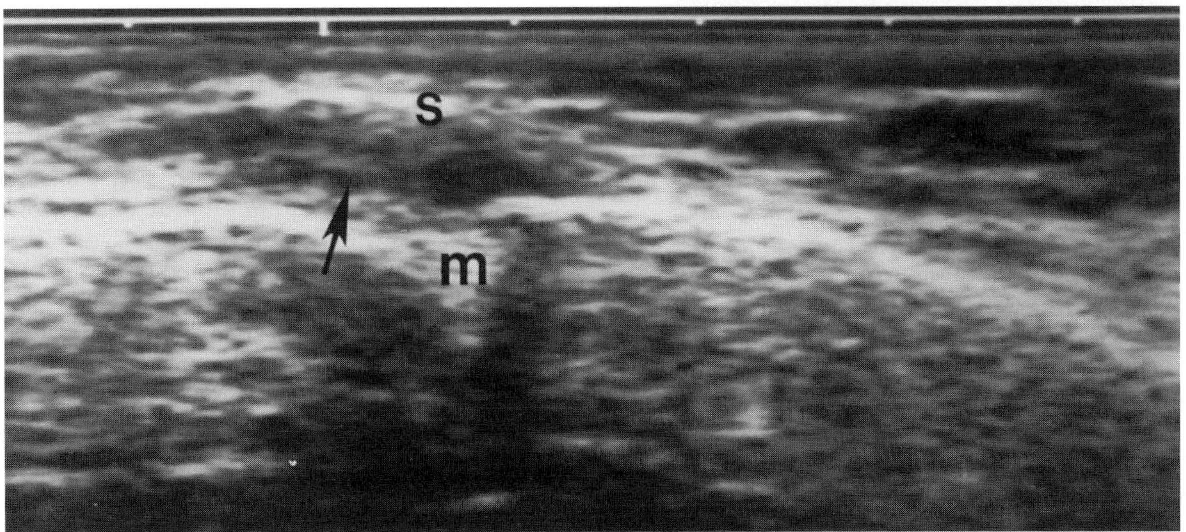

Figure 6–22 ▪ Partial MCL rupture: coronal sonogram. Three days ago, this 21-year-old soccer player was blocked while kicking. He presented with pain and swelling over the medial femoral condyle. This coronal sonogram demonstrates an intact superficial portion (*s*) of the MCL, which is displaced medially by a swollen, hypoechoic deep portion (*arrow*). This appearance is typical of partial rupture of the MCL. These lesions usually involve the proximal portion of the ligament to a greater extent than the distal portion and begin in the deep portion, involving only the superficial portion in more severe injuries. Abbreviation: normal medial meniscus (*m*).

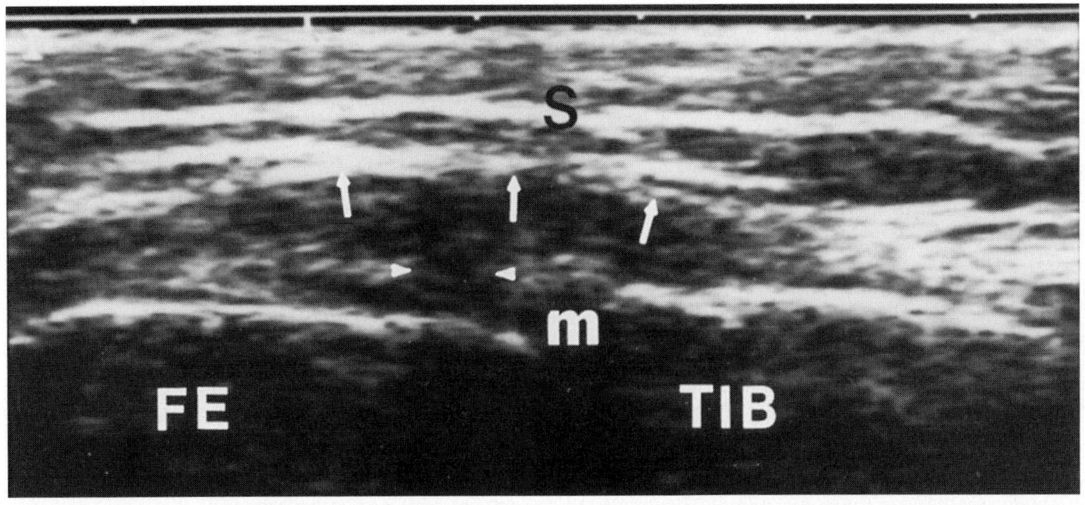

Figure 6–23 ▪ Partial MCL rupture: coronal sonogram. This pedestrian was hit on the lateral side of the knee while walking between two cars stopped in traffic. A gap is observed in the meniscofemoral ligament (*arrowheads*), and swelling of the tissues beneath the superficial portion of the ligament displaces it medially (*arrows*). Abbreviations: medial femoral condyle (*FE*), medial meniscus (*m*), proximal tibia (*TIB*), subcutaneous tissues (*S*).

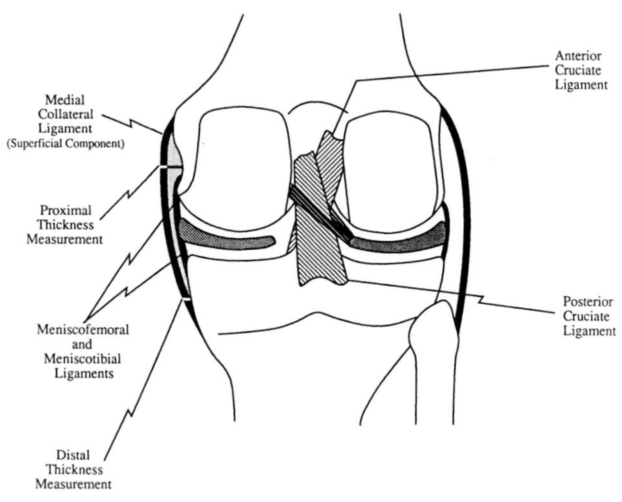

Figure 6–24 ■ Schematic diagram of ligaments of the knee. This posterior view of the knee demonstrates the trilaminar structure of the MCL. A hypoechoic zone of loose areolar connective tissue separates the hyperechoic superficial layer from the deep meniscofemoral and meniscotibial ligaments. Sites of standard measurement of the proximal and distal portions of the ligament are indicated. The proximal measurement is obtained at the point of greatest depth of the concavity in the medial femoral condyle. The distal portion of the ligament is measured at a point equidistant from the tibial plateau and the most distal extent of the ligament.

and deep components of the ligament. As stated earlier, pain and swelling limit clinical examination immediately following injury. Sonography will quickly make the diagnosis and accurately assess the extent of injury, allowing prompt institution of appropriate therapy.

Partial ruptures of the MCL will result in thickening of the ligament (see Fig. 6–22). Two standardized measurements of MCL thickness will help to detect subtle injury (see Fig. 6–24). Proximal and distal measurements of MCL thickness are obtained. The greatest depth of concavity of the medial surface of the femoral condyle is used as the proximal landmark for measurement. Normal thickness of the MCL at this point is 3.6 mm (S.D., 0.5 mm) (van Holsbeeck et al., 1988). This is often the most useful parameter because proximal swelling of the ligament is most frequently observed in MCL injury (van Holsbeeck et al., 1988).

The point at which the distal measurement of MCL thickness is obtained is determined by identifying a point equidistant from the tibial plateau and the most distal extent of the MCL. The thickness of the ligament at this point is normally 2.3 mm (S.D., 0.3 mm). Athletic conditioning without injury does not change the thickness or appearance of the ligament (van Holsbeeck et al., 1988). Acute changes in ligament thickness must be interpreted in light of which layer or layers are responsible. Thickening and decreased echogenicity of either the deep or superficial hyperechoic layers without an identifiable gap must be considered a partial rupture of the involved ligament. If the central hypoechoic portion of the MCL is thickened, the diagnosis of meniscal cyst must be considered. In these cases, the integrity of the deep hyperechoic portion of the MCL and the meniscus should be carefully examined. When the meniscofemoral ligament, meniscotibial

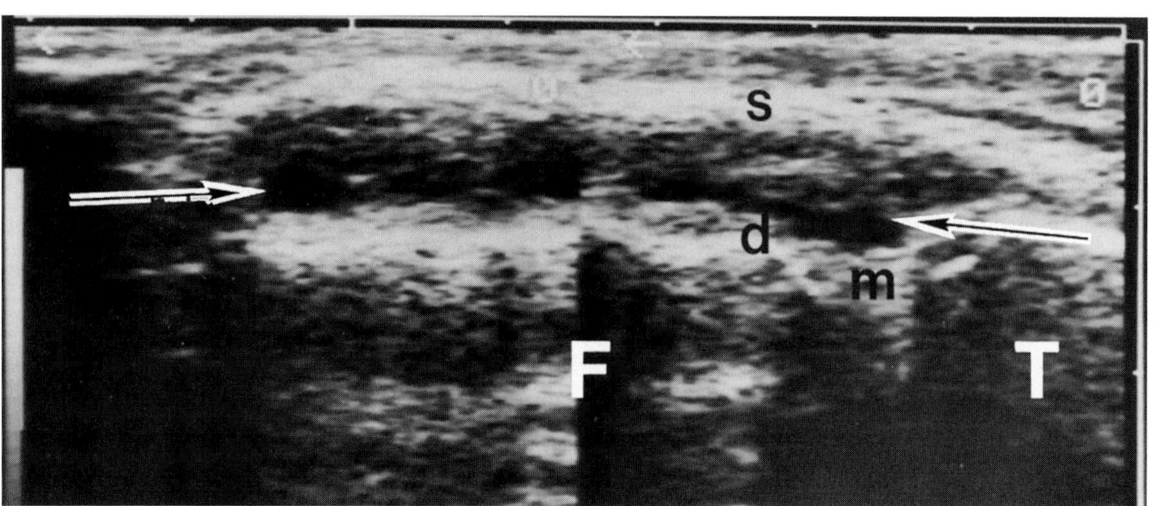

Figure 6–25 ■ Bursitis in the MCL: coronal sonogram. The patient is a 26-year-old man who was hit on the medial side of the knee during a judo match. Over the past 3 months, he continued to compete, with increasing pain and swelling over the medial aspect of the knee. A markedly hypoechoic fluid collection (*arrows*) separates the superficial (*s*) and deep (*d*) layers of the medial MCL. The medial meniscus (*m*) and dense connective tissue components of the ligament are intact. In a certain percentage of cases, a bursa separates the deep and superficial components of the ligament. Traumatic bursitis may then be seen in these patients. In this case, aspiration of the lesion for palliative reasons yielded clear bursal fluid. Abbreviations: distal femur (*F*), proximal tibia (*T*).

ligament, and meniscus are demonstrated to be intact, the presence of an enlarged bursa within the central portion of the ligament should be suspected (Fig. 6–25) (Lee and Yao, 1991). Follow-up examination after resolution of acute swelling may prove beneficial in these cases. It is important to assess the medial meniscus when the patient comes for a repeat study; the knee will then be easier to manipulate.

Ligaments are thickened capsular structures. Joint capsules between ligaments have a more delicate structure, and a tear in a capsule can be quite extensive and difficult to distinguish from a ligament tear. Rupture of the medial retinaculum of the knee is a typical example of a capsular tear. This retinaculum will tear when the patella dislocates laterally. The patella typically relocates spontaneously, and the pain at the medial knee is often interpreted as an MCL tear. Hemarthrosis and intra-articular damage to cartilage and subchondral bone are common in patients with a disruption of the medial retinaculum (Fig. 6–26).

Box 6–2
Ultrasound Examination of Difficult Clinical Conditions after Valgus Injuries

- Displaced UCL of the thumb (Stener lesion)
- Pain caused by stretch of the UCL of the elbow in baseball pitchers

Ulnar collateral ligaments (UCL) in the elbow and thumb have a lot in common with the MCL of the knee (Box 6–2). These ligaments also demonstrate a layered structure on sonography. Similar valgus injuries lead to rupture of these ligaments (Figs. 6–27 through 6–29). The lesions are often sports related, and reinjury is common. Chronic UCL injuries often require surgery (Fig. 6–28). The

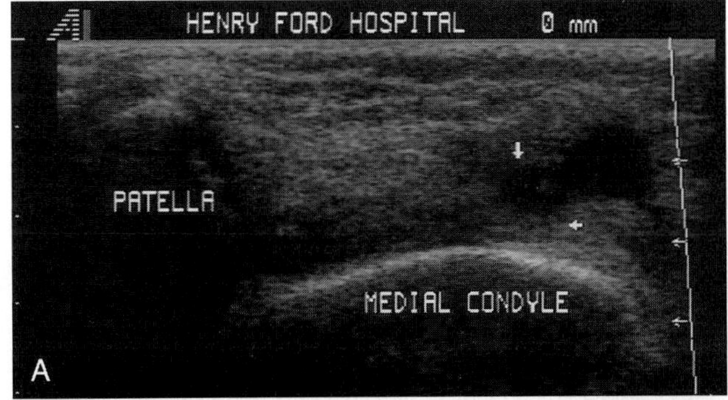

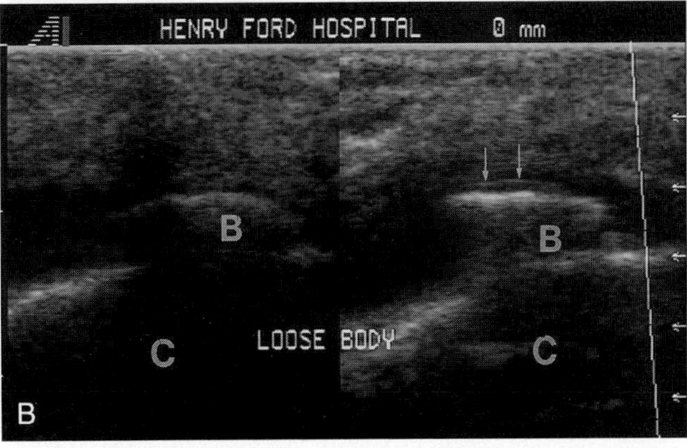

Figure 6–26 ▪ **A,** Acute tear of the medial retinaculum: transverse sonogram through the medial retinaculum. The right knee of this 22-year-old woman started swelling suddenly after a twisting injury. With the transducer placed transversely and medially to the patella, a defect was noted in the medial retinaculum (*arrows*). An active leak of fluid through this defect was observed during flexion/extension of the knee. **B,** Acute tear of the medial retinaculum: split-screen view over the medial suprapatellar recess. Same patient as in **A.** The image at the left side of the split screen shows the lateral recess with a loose body within the joint fluid. Notice how the position of the body (*B*) changes relative to that of the lateral femoral condyle (*C*) when the examiner's thumb and index finger apply side-to-side compression on the recess (at the right side of the split screen). The interface (*arrows*) between the hyaline cartilage, which covers the fragment of subchondral bone, and the joint fluid is visible only when fluid surrounds the loose body.

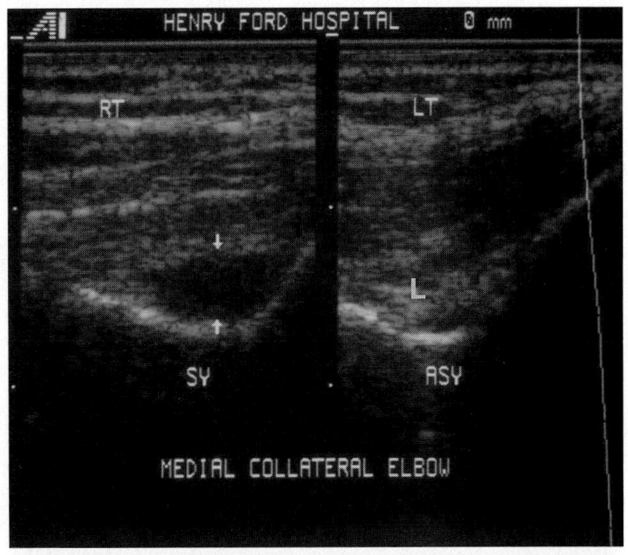

Figure 6–27 ▪ Acute tear of the UCL in the elbow: split-screen comparison of coronal images of the ulnar ligament in both elbows. While throwing a fastball, this professional baseball player experienced an acute sharp pain in the elbow. Now, 1 week after the injury, he is not able to play due to disabling pain. The left side of the split screen shows a fluid-filled defect (*between the arrows*) in the expected location of the UCL of the patient's right elbow. The right side of the screen shows the normal contralateral elbow with a normal anterior bundle (*L*) of the ligament. Abbreviations: symptomatic (*SY*), asymptomatic (*ASY*).

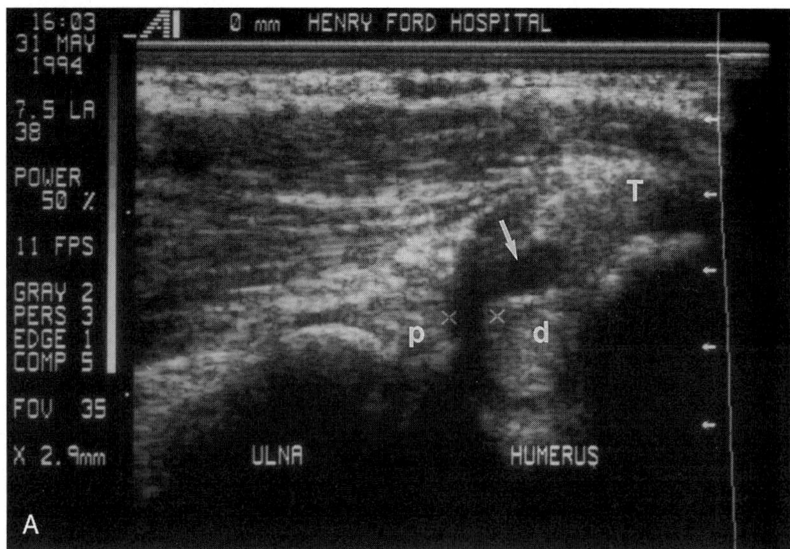

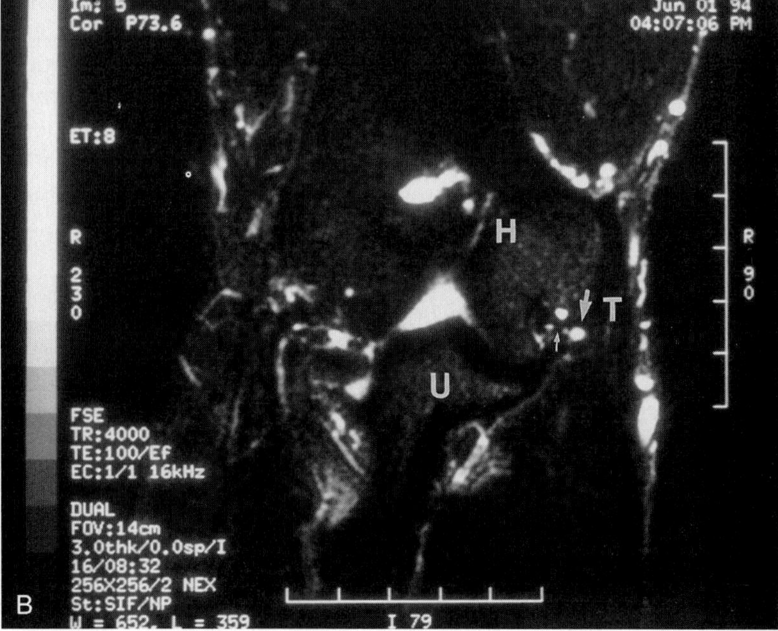

Figure 6–28 ■ **A,** UCL tear in the elbow: coronal sonogram. When pitching, this 30-year-old professional baseball player experiences medial elbow pain. The pain is at its maximum with valgus stress. The transducer is placed over the medial epicondyle of the humerus and over the proximal ulna, with its orientation along the fibers of the forearm flexors. Against convention, the orientation of the image shows proximal on the right and distal on the left. A fluid-filled defect (*cursors*) separates the proximal (*p*) and distal (*d*) stumps of the ruptured anterior bundle of the UCL. Joint fluid (*arrow*) leaks out beneath the origin of the flexor tendons (*T*). **B,** UCL tear in the elbow: coronal fast spin-echo T_2-weighted MRI image obtained with fat suppression. Same patient as in A. The small pocket of extra-articular fluid (*arrow*) is again noted deep to the origin of the flexor tendons (*T*). The fluid communicates with the joint through the small ligament tear, which was clearly visible on an ultrasound scan but barely perceptible (*small arrow*) on the MRI. The greater spatial resolution of the ultrasound examination relative to the MRI is often significant, as demonstrated here. Abbreviations: distal humerus (*H*), ulna (*U*).

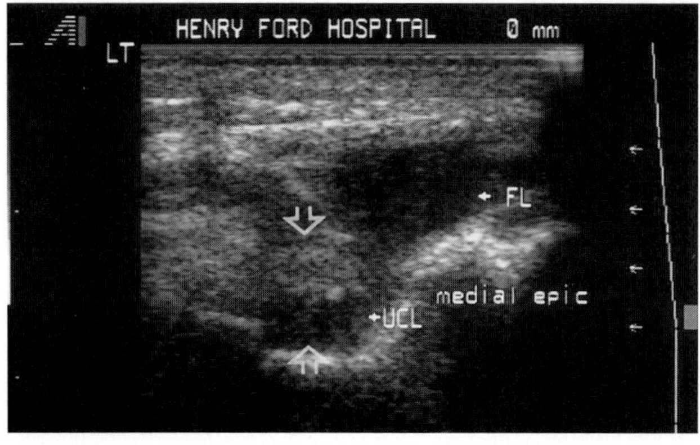

Figure 6–29 ■ Flexor tendon tear in the elbow: coronal sonogram. This 44-year-old woman felt a sharp pain in the elbow while playing softball. The clinical presentation was similar to that of the patients in Figures 6–27 and 6–28. The coronal sonogram, which has been oriented like the image in Figure 6–27, shows an anechoic defect in the injured common flexor tendon origin. The anterior bundle of the UCL (*between the open arrows*) of the right elbow is still intact.

ultrasound examination and the sonographic appearance of lesions at the base of the thumb are discussed in Chapter 16.

Treatment of ligament rupture varies, depending on the site of rupture and the extent of injury. Rapid diagnosis and assessment of the extent of injury are critical when the need for surgical repair is likely. The sooner the correct diagnosis is established and surgical repair is accomplished, the more favorable the outcome (Nicholas and Hershman, 1986). In cases with less extensive injury, splint, or cast immobilization for 5 to 6 weeks is the treatment most frequently employed (Hastings, 1980; Peterson and Renstrom, 1986). The direct and indirect consequences of immobilizing an athlete for 1.5 months are considerable. Therefore, establishing the definitive diagnosis with ultrasound is extremely important. The pathological changes in torn ligaments are slow to return to normal. In partial-thickness tears, the changes may be seen for 2 months and in full-thickness tears for up to 6 months (D'Erme, 1996).

Chronic Ligament Injury

The normal repair mechanisms of ligaments usually result in restitutio ad integrum when adequate therapy is instituted (Frank et al., 1983; Kannus, 1988; Laws and Walton, 1988). However, when clinical examination alone is used for diagnosis, some lesions pass undetected and go untreated (Hastings, 1986). Healing will then be considerably impaired in a manner similar to the formation of a pseudarthrosis following fracture. For this reason, we have chosen to refer to this lesion as *nonunion* of a ligament. We have identified two types of ligamentous nonunion, which have been confirmed at the time of surgery. The first is characterized by ligament interruption. Little or no reparative activity is evident. Sonography demonstrates the persistence of gaps or focal thinning of the ligament. This form of nonunion is observed in slightly less than 10% of cases (Fig. 6–30). One of the reasons this can occur is separation of the two torn ends of the ligament. The Stener lesion in the thumb is a typical example. A fascial layer separates the proximal and distal ends of the torn ligament.

In the majority of cases of ligamentous nonunion, a hypertrophic response (Fig. 6–31) with excessive formation of granulation tissue and mucoid degeneration is observed. The hypertrophic form of nonunion is a frequent complication of untreated partial ligament rupture. These chronic lesions are associated with pain and tenderness over the lesion. We have observed hypertrophic nonunion in sinus tarsi syndrome, chronic peroneal retinaculum rupture, and fibulotalar and deltoid ligament ruptures. Similar lesions are seen in the coracoacromial ligament in impingement syndrome of the shoulder, a common injury found in tennis players. Foci of granulation tissue in the plantar fascia of long-distance runners have also been identified sonographically. The pathogenesis of these lesions is most likely the same mechanism. The most common site of hypertrophic nonunion is the knee, particularly the MCL. Although it can be seen in football, basketball, and hockey players, it is characteristically

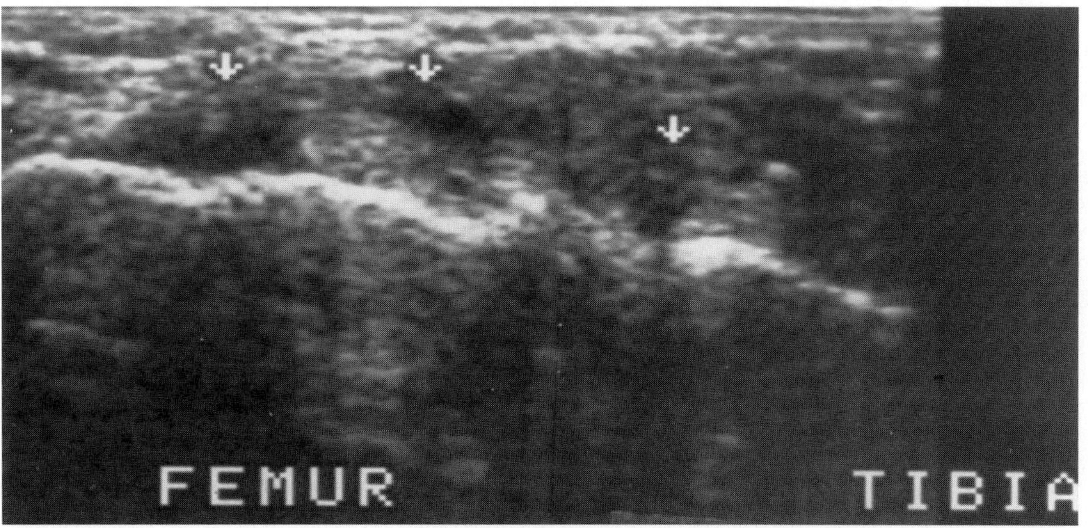

Figure 6–30 ▪ Chronic reinjury of the MCL: coronal sonogram. Six months ago, this 26-year-old man was hit by a car while cycling. At that time, he sustained a grade III tear of the MCL. Since then, he has reinjured the ligament twice. He presented with pain and swelling over the medial surface of the knee. The normal trilaminar structure of the ligament is no longer recognizable. It is markedly swollen, with three points of rupture (*arrows*) noted along the length of the ligament.

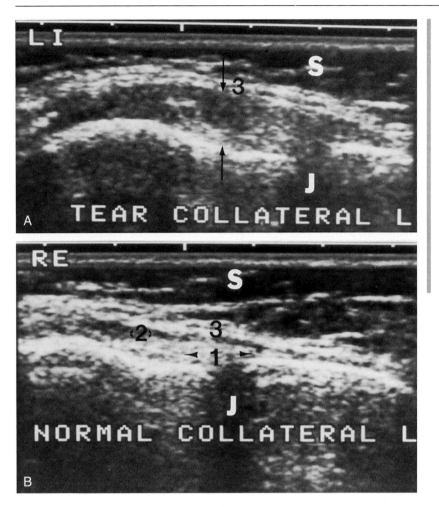

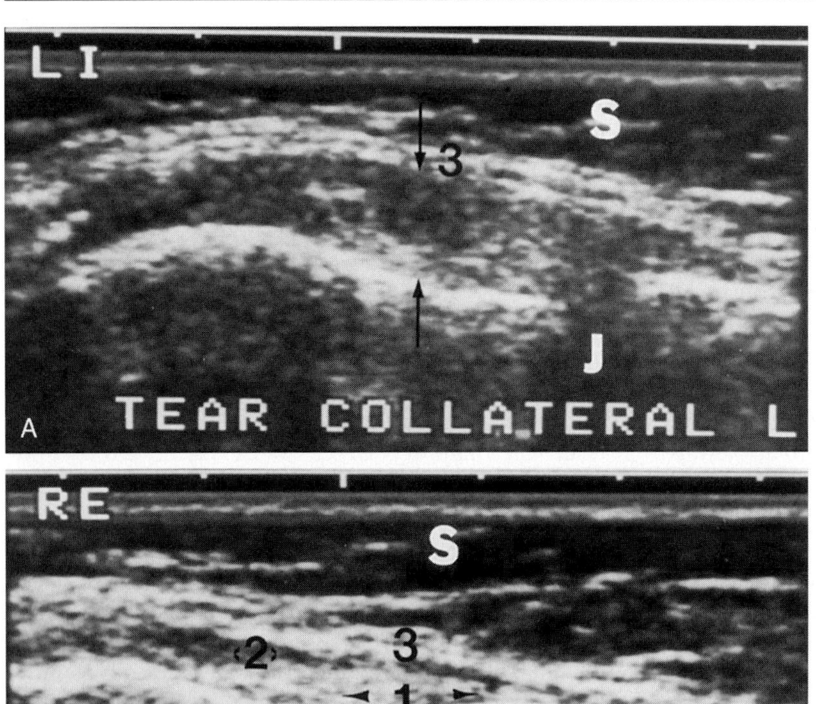

Figure 6–31 ■ Comparison of symptomatic and asymptomatic MCL: coronal sonogram. **A,** The patient is a 30-year-old soccer player who presented 5 months following a grade II rupture of the MCL. He continued to have pain, especially while kicking. The deep layer of the MCL is decreased in echogenicity and markedly swollen (*arrows*), displacing the superficial layer (*3*) medially. Abbreviations: joint space (*J*), subcutaneous tissues (*S*). **B,** The same patient as in **A,** asymptomatic knee. A normal trilaminar MCL is observed. The deep layer (*1*), composed of the meniscofemoral and meniscotibial ligaments, is intact. A normal hypoechoic layer of loose areolar connective tissue (*2*) separates the superficial layer (*3*) from the deep layer. Note that the proximal portion of the ligament is thicker than the distal portion. The mean thickness of a normal MCL is 3.6 mm (S.D., 0.5) at the proximal site and 2.3 mm (S.D., 0.3) at the distal site. Abbreviations: joint space (*J*), subcutaneous tissue (*S*).

found in soccer players. A soccer-style kicking motion applies a tremendous amount of valgus stress to the knee. The typical history is pain that is increased immediately before contact with the ball when kicking. This pain differs from that experienced with meniscal injury, which is characterized by an increase in pain immediately following contact with the ball (Nicholas and Hershman, 1986).

Hypertrophic ligamentous nonunion is easily recognized sonographically. A hypoechoic mass (Fig. 6–32) is identified within the highly echogenic

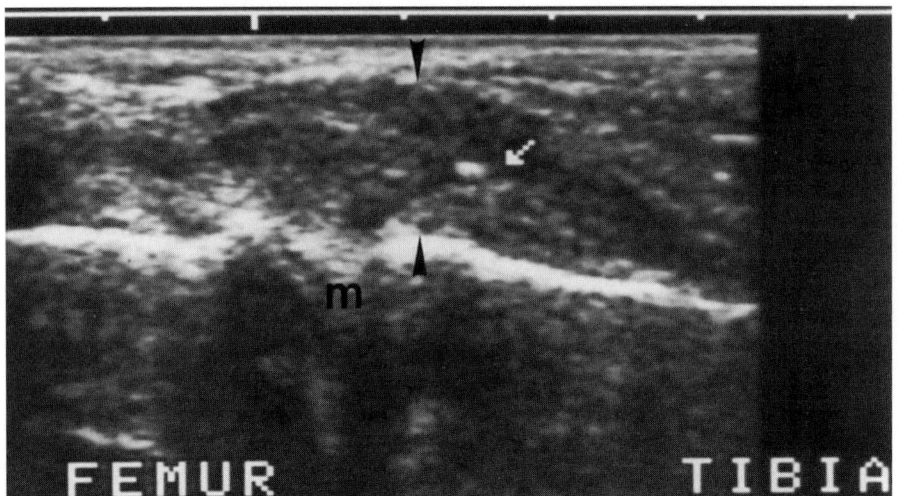

Figure 6–32 ■ Chronic calcified MCL lesion: coronal sonogram. A 19-year-old wrestler injured his right knee 5 months ago and continued to have pain. Global swelling of the MCL is noted, predominantly over the proximal tibia (*arrowheads*). A small calcification (*arrow*) is seen in the swollen middle portion of the ligament. These conditions are familiar to radiologists as Pellegrini-Stieda disease, but this understates the magnitude of the problem of chronic MCL injury. Calcifications are seen in only 14% of patients with chronic MCL injury. Abbreviation: medial meniscus (*m*).

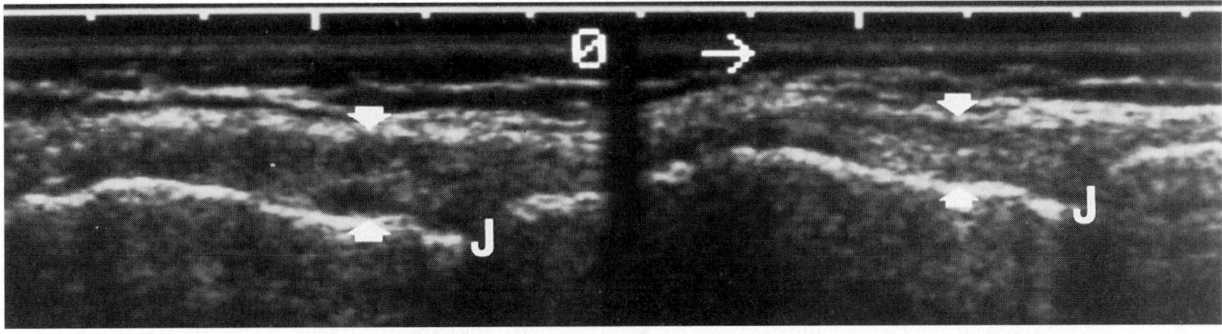

Figure 6–33 ■ Chronically painful MCL: coronal sonograms. One year ago, this farmer was hit on the lateral aspect of the left knee by an angry cow. He continued to have medial knee pain, especially when walking on irregular surfaces. The arthroscopic examination was normal. The symptomatic left MCL is on the left side in this split-screen image. The deep portion of the proximal ligament (*arrows*) is decreased in echogenicity and thickened compared with the asymptomatic right side. Abbreviation: joint space (*J*).

substance of the ligament. This is a striking finding since the normal ligament appears as a thin, hyperreflective band of tissue. Few internal reflections are observed within the hypoechoic soft tissue component of the lesion. As a result, they may initially be mistaken for meniscal cysts in the knee. However, when pressure is applied with the transducer, the hypoechoic material will respond like soft tissue. In a meniscal cyst, fluid beneath the transducer will be expressed when pressure is applied.

The sonographic picture of hypertrophic nonunion of the MCL is characterized by thickening and disruption of the normal trilaminar structure of the ligament (Fig. 6–33). In our experience, the thickening is more prominent in the proximal portion of the MCL (van Holsbeeck et al., 1988). This was observed in 91% of our patients. Calcium deposition in Pellegrini-Stieda disease is found in a similar distribution, suggesting that this is part of the same disease process (Ricklin et al., 1964; Peterson and Renstrom, 1986; Mink et al., 1987). Calcifications were observed sonographically in 14% of the patients in our series (Fig. 6–34 through 6–36). In all of our patients with hypertrophic nonunion, the capsular portion of the ligament was involved, whereas only one-third had involvement of both the superficial and deep components. This

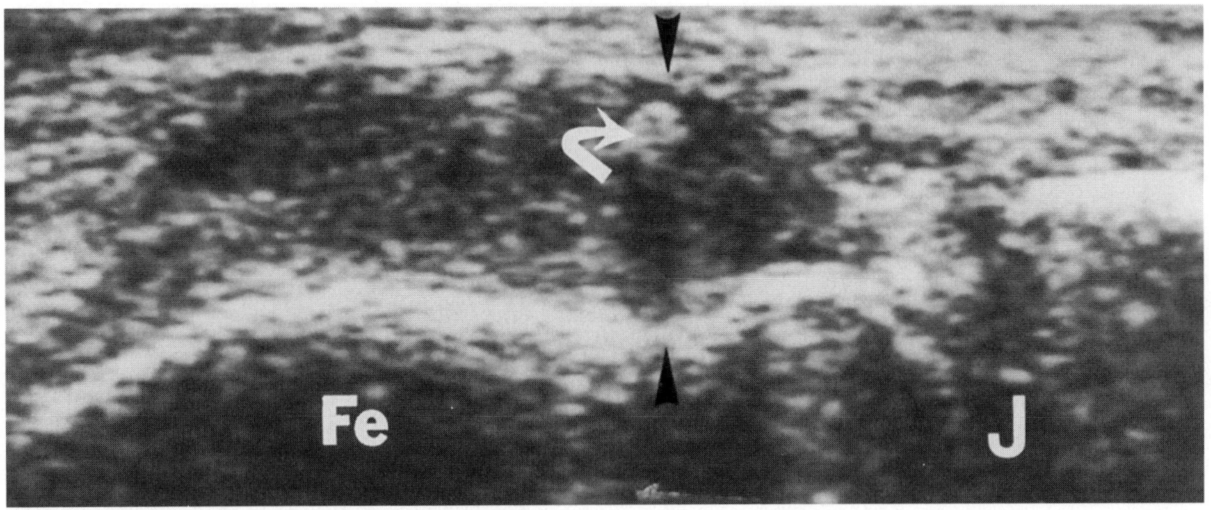

Figure 6–34 ■ Chronic MCL injury: coronal sonogram. At a routine physical examination prior to the conclusion of a trade to another team, this coronal image of the MCL in a 25-year-old football player demonstrates marked thickening (*arrowheads*) of the proximal ligament, with loss of the normal trilaminar structure in this region. A small calcification (*curved arrow*) with incomplete acoustic shadowing is also noted. Abbreviations: medial femoral condyle (*Fe*), joint space (*J*).

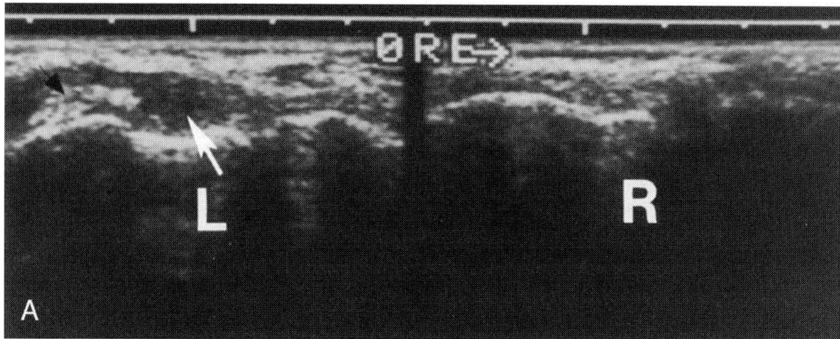

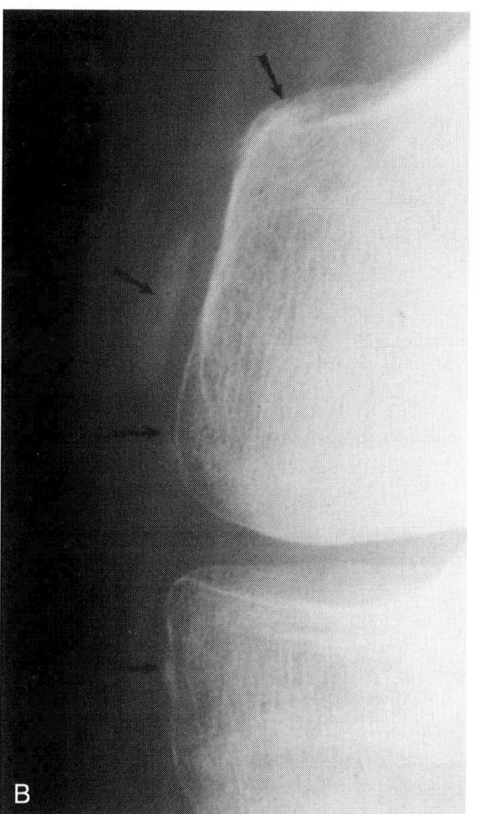

Figure 6–35 ■ **A,** Calcification in a chronic MCL lesion: coronal sonograms. The patient is a 19-year-old basketball player who injured his left knee three times in the past 6 months. He presented with persistent swelling and pain over the medial aspect of the left knee. The left MCL is markedly swollen and globally decreased in echogenicity (*white arrow*), with loss of the normal trilaminar structure. Echogenic calcifications (*black arrow*) are noted in several locations throughout the ligament. Abbreviations: symptomatic left knee (*L*), asymptomatic right knee (*R*). **B,** Calcification in a chronic MCL lesion: anteroposterior radiograph of the knee. Same patient as in **A.** Multiple foci of calcification and ossification (*arrows*) are noted within the substance and insertions of the ligament.

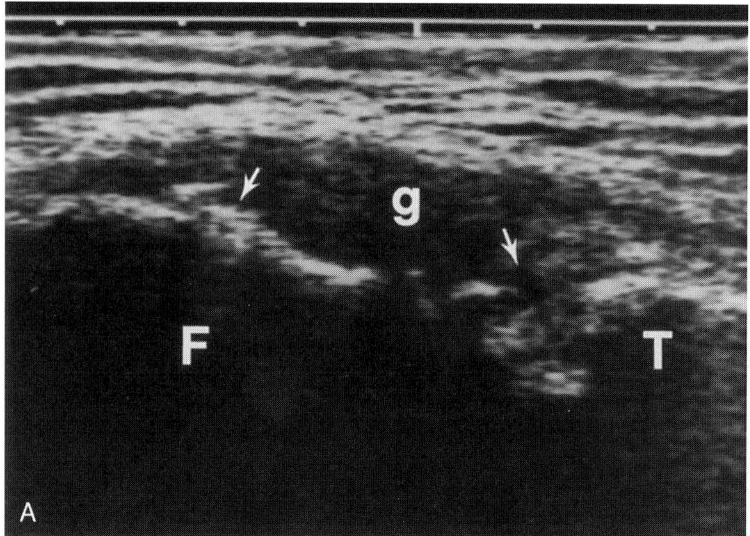

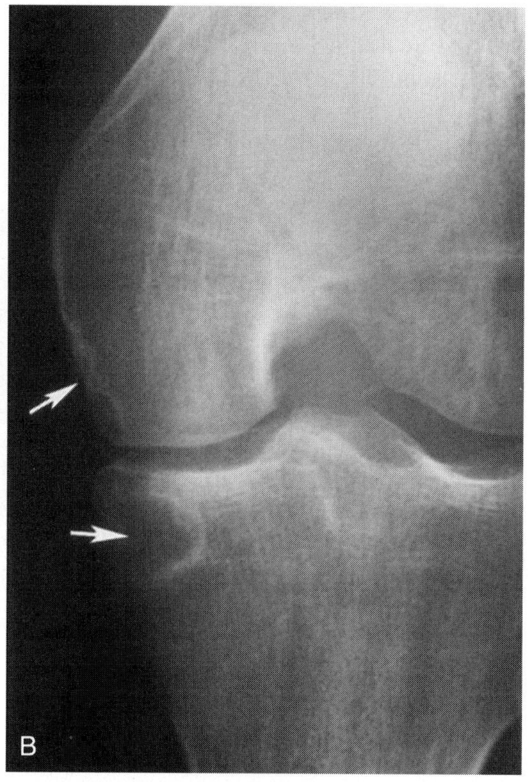

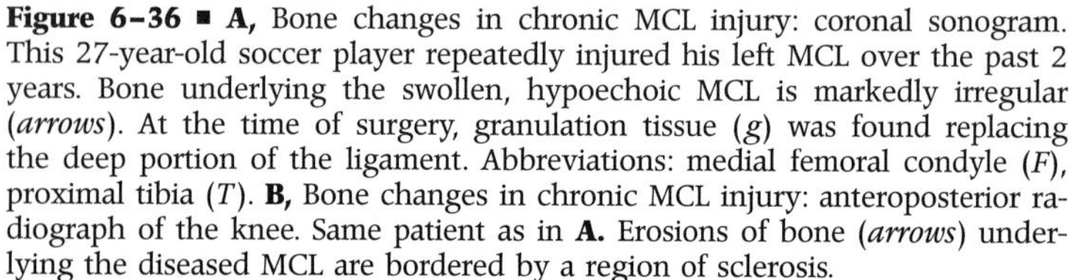

Figure 6–36 ■ **A,** Bone changes in chronic MCL injury: coronal sonogram. This 27-year-old soccer player repeatedly injured his left MCL over the past 2 years. Bone underlying the swollen, hypoechoic MCL is markedly irregular (*arrows*). At the time of surgery, granulation tissue (*g*) was found replacing the deep portion of the ligament. Abbreviations: medial femoral condyle (*F*), proximal tibia (*T*). **B,** Bone changes in chronic MCL injury: anteroposterior radiograph of the knee. Same patient as in **A.** Erosions of bone (*arrows*) underlying the diseased MCL are bordered by a region of sclerosis.

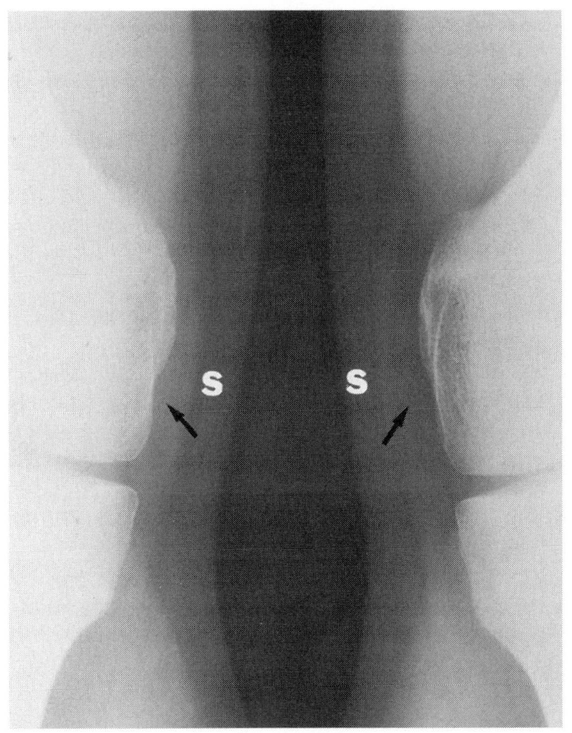

Figure 6–37 ■ Chronic MCL lesion: low-kilovoltage radiograph of the knees. Chronic MCL injury is poorly evaluated with radiographs. Calcifications are seen in only a small percentage of cases, and thickening of the ligament (*arrow*) is difficult to evaluate due to small variations in rotation. Abbreviation: subcutaneous tissue (*S*).

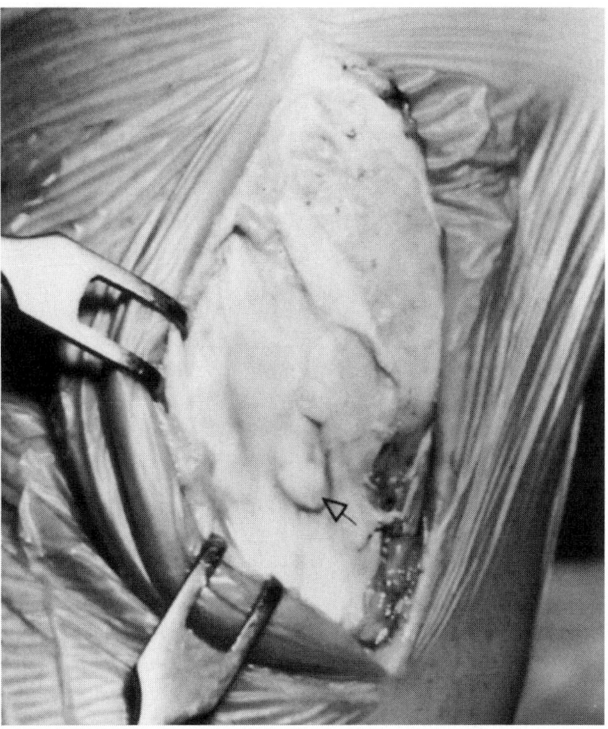

Figure 6–38 ■ Chronic MCL lesion: surgical findings. Foci of granulation tissue (*open arrow*) are often found in cases of chronic injury within the substance of the MCL at the time of surgery. Careful curettage and side-to-side suturing of the ligament margins usually result in good wound healing.

supports the hypothesis that tears of the MCL start in the deep component (Peterson and Renstrom, 1986; Mink et al., 1987).

Unfortunately, these lesions are frequently misdiagnosed without the assistance of ultrasound (Fig. 6–37). Arthroscopy is not valuable in the evaluation of these lesions. The arthroscopist can detect only indirect signs of these MCL lesions, such as "floating" of the medial meniscus (Mink et al., 1987). When arthroscopy is performed in these cases, it is often complicated by extravasation of large volumes of irrigation fluid. If unrecognized, this will result in a compartment syndrome with compression of the neurovascular bundle (Jackson and Dandy, 1976; Noyes et al., 1980; Casscells, 1984; Mink et al., 1987). In professional soccer players, 60% of patients with chronic medial knee pain and negative arthroscopy have hypertrophic nonunion of the MCL (van Holsbeeck et al., 1988). It is not unusual for these patients to present for sonographic examination after undergoing medial shelf resection with no relief of symptoms. Surgical repair of the hypertrophic MCL lesion with curettage of the granulation tissue and side-to-side suturing of the ligament margins provides relief of symptoms (Fig. 6–38). Normal healing occurs following proper immobilization. Histological examination of the surgical specimen reveals disruption of collagen fibers with foci of necrosis, vascular ingrowth, granulation tissue, and areas of mucoid degeneration (van Holsbeeck et al., 1988).

References

Anderson JE: *Grant's Atlas of Anatomy.* Baltimore, Williams & Wilkins Co, 1983.

Bassett FH, et al: Talar impingement by the anteroinferior tibiofibular ligament. A cause of chronic pain in the ankle after inversion sprain. *J Bone Joint Surg Am* 72(1):55–59, 1990.

Bloom W, Fawcett DW: *A Textbook of Histology,* ed 11, Philadelphia, WB Saunders Co, 1980.

Bouffard JA, Goitz HT, van Holsbeeck MT: Sonographic evaluation of high-ankle sprains, *Radiology* 201 (P): 399, 1996.

Casscells SW: *Arthroscopy: Diagnostic and Surgical Practice.* Philadelphia, Lea & Febiger, 1984.

Clemente CD: *Gray's Anatomy.* Philadelphia, Lea & Febiger, 1985.

D'Erme M: Le lesioni dei legamenti collaterali del collo del piede: diagnosi e follow-up con risonanza magnetica ed ecografia. *Radiol Med* 91:705–709, 1996.

Frank C, et al: Healing of the medial collateral ligament of the knee. *Acta Orthop Scand* 54:917–923, 1983.

Hastings DE: Knee ligament instability—a rational anatomical classification. *Clin Orthop* 208:104–107, 1986.

Hastings DE: The non-operative management of collateral ligament injuries of the knee joint. *Clin Orthop* 147: 22–28, 1980.

Hentz VR, Green PS, Arditi M: Imaging studies of the cadaver hand using transmission ultrasound. *Skeletal Radiol* 16:474–480, 1987.

Hergan K, Mittler C, Oser W: Ulnar collateral ligament: Differentiation of displaced and nondisplaced tears with US and MRI imaging. *Radiology* 194:65, 1995.

Hughston JC, et al: Classification of knee ligament instabilities. I: The medial compartment and the cruciate ligaments. *J Bone Joint Surg Am* 58:159–172, 1976.

Jackson RW, Dandy DJ: *Arthroscopy of the Knee.* New York, Grune & Stratton, 1976.

Kannus P: Long term results of conservatively treated medial collateral ligament injuries of the knee joint. *Clin Orthop* 226:103–111, 1988.

Laine HR, et al: Ultrasound in the evaluation of the knee and patellar regions. *J Ultrasound* 6:33–36, 1987.

Laws G, Walton M: Fibroblastic healing of grade II ligament injuries. Histological and mechanical studies in sheep. *J Bone Joint Surg Br* 70:390–396, 1988.

Lee JK, Yao L: Tibial collateral ligament bursa. *Radiology* 178:855, 1991.

Mink JH, Reicher MA, Crues JV III: *Magnetic Resonance Imaging of the Knee.* New York, Raven Press, 1987.

Nicholas JA, Hershman EB: *The Lower Extremity and Spine in Sports Medicine.* St Louis, CV Mosby Co, 1986.

Noyes FR, et al: Arthroscopy in acute traumatic hemarthrosis of the knee. *J Bone Joint Surg Am* 62:685–695, 1980.

O'Callaghan BI, Kohut G, Hoogewoud HM: Gamekeeper thumb: Identification of the Stener lesion with US. *Radiology* 192:477, 1994.

Peterson L, Renstrom P: *Sports Injuries.* Chicago, Year Book Medical, 1986.

Ptasznik R, et al: Value of sonography in the diagnosis of traumatic rupture of the anterior cruciate ligament of the knee. *AJR* 164:1461, 1995.

Richardson ML, et al: Ultrasonography of the knee. *Radiol Clin North Am* 26:63–75, 1988.

Ricklin P, Ruttiman A, Del Buono MS: *Meniscal Lesions: Practical Problems of Clinical Diagnosis, Arthrography and Therapy.* New York, Grune & Stratton, 1964.

van Dijk CN, et al: Diagnosis of ligament rupture of the ankle joint. Physical examination, arthrography, stress radiography and sonography compared in 160 patients after inversion trauma. *Acta Orthop Scand* 67(6): 566–570, 1996.

van Holsbeeck M, et al: Sonography of the medial collateral ligament [abstract]. *Radiology* 169(P):178, 1988.

Chapter 7 Pathophysiology and Patterns of Disease

Trauma is the most common etiological factor in diseases of the musculoskeletal system. Acute and chronic trauma can result in skeletal fractures, as well as muscle, tendon, and ligament rupture. The injury may result in either complete or partial disruption of the involved structure. Motor vehicle accidents and other forms of blunt trauma often result in extensive fractures and soft tissue injury. In contrast, occupational and sports-related injuries have a marked predominance of soft tissue injury. The rate at which force is applied and the magnitude of the force determine the type of injury that will result. If force is slowly applied, an avulsion fracture will probably result at the insertion of a ligament of tendon. When force is applied rapidly, the most common injury will be a midsubstance tear of the soft tissue structure involved (Nicholas and Hershman, 1986). Tears at the musculotendinous junction occur at a critical tension, which is proportional to the degree of stretch of the muscle. In an animal model, tears at the musculotendinous junction consistently occurred when the muscle was stretched to 125% of its resting length (Nicholas et al., 1986). Bones and muscles usually heal quite readily after acute injury. In contrast, tendons and ligaments tend to heal very slowly, if at all. In this chapter, we will look more closely at mechanisms of injury and healing in the musculoskeletal system. Osseous fractures have been examined extensively by many other authors and therefore will not be addressed in this chapter. Instead, we will focus more closely on soft tissue injury.

Muscle Rupture

The etiology of muscle rupture is straightforward. A cause-and-effect relationship between trauma and the muscle rupture can almost always be established. The patient often recalls the event resulting in acute pain and loss of function of the involved muscle. Muscle injury can result from either direct or indirect trauma. Indirect trauma is often experienced during athletic activity. Eccentric loading of a muscle that spans two joints is most commonly the mechanism of injury. Typical examples are rupture of the rectus femoris muscle in soccer players and of the medial gastrocnemius muscle in tennis players (Fig. 7–1). Professional soccer players commonly develop foot speed of approximately 120 mph when striking the ball, resulting in a ball velocity in excess of 60 mph. The forces placed on the quadriceps muscle during this motion leave little doubt as to the mechanism of injury. Adductor tears are also quite common in soccer players. Tears of the hamstrings are most commonly seen in athletes required to develop sudden bursts of speed, such as sprinters, soccer players, and baseball players.

Direct trauma is most commonly seen in accident victims but may also be seen in some athletes. Blunt trauma directly to a muscle results in a crush type of injury and rupture. The muscle may be compressed between an external object and a bone or between two external objects. Football players often experience these types of muscle injury when struck by another player's helmet.

Healing of these injuries most commonly results in the formation of a dense fibrous scar. However, myositis ossificans may develop in some cases, most commonly following direct crush injuries. The factors predisposing to the formation of myositis ossificans are not well established, but the presence of a large hematoma separating wound margins appears to favor its development. Imaging characteristics of muscle injury and patterns of healing are discussed in detail in Chapter 3. Therefore, this discussion will not be repeated here.

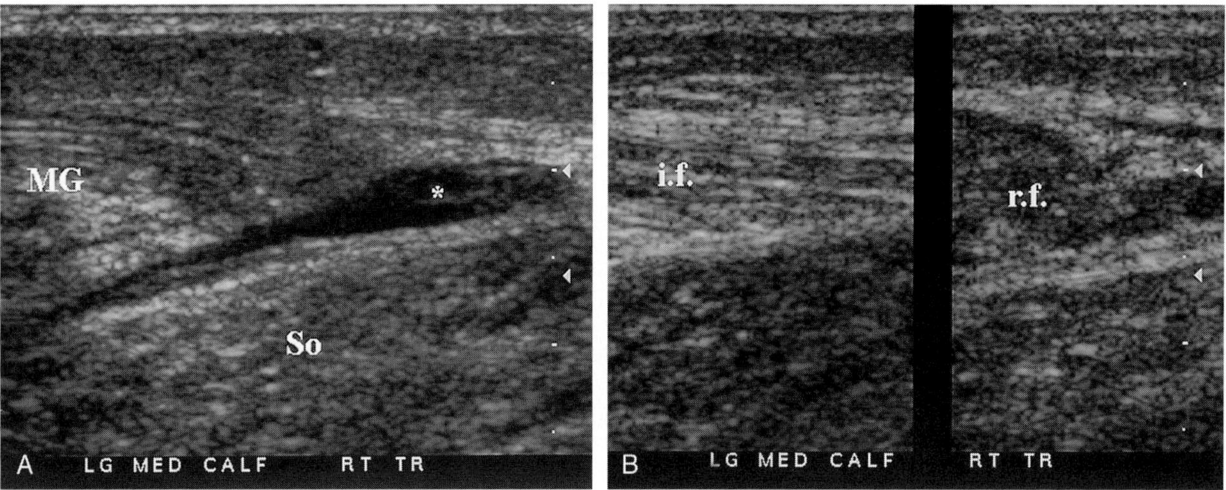

Figure 7–1 ■ **A**, Medial gastrocnemius tear: longitudinal sonogram. The patient is a 37-year-old tennis player who felt a sudden sharp pain in the right medial calf when rallying to the net. This image of the distal end of the medial gastrocnemius (*MG*) as it joins the aponeurosis with the soleus (*So*) demonstrates a muscle boundary lesion. Hematoma (*) separates the torn gastrocnemius from the underlying soleus. **B**, Medial gastrocnemius tear: split-screen examination through the left and right gastrocnemius muscles. Same patient as in **A**. The intact fibers of the left medial gastrocnemius (*i.f.*) contrast with the retracted fibers (*r.f.*) of the right medial gastrocnemius.

Tendon Rupture

Rupture of tendons may be the result of direct penetrating trauma or indirect trauma caused by excessive loading during physical activity. Sports-related injury is the leading cause of tendon injury and rupture. Tendon ruptures often occur at their point of attachment to bone. Sharpey's fibers, which anchor the tendon to bone, are the structures at risk. A typical example of this type of tendon injury is rupture of the distal biceps humeri tendon (Fig. 7–2). Rupture of the distal biceps humeri tendon is quite common, is difficult to diagnose clinically, and requires prompt surgical repair to restore function. This tendon rupture is easily diagnosed sonographically by imaging the radial tuberosity, which can be visualized only with the arm in pronation. Careful comparison with the asymptomatic side will allow accurate diagnosis of complete and partial tears. In full-thickness tears, the biceps humeri tendon retracts above the elbow and is identified over the brachialis muscle. The degree of tendon retraction is unusually large in these cases. Buckling of the tendon can cause refractile shadowing (Fig. 7–3).

The quadriceps and patellar tendons are also commonly injured by indirect trauma, which results in rupture at their anchor point onto bone. A slip and fall on ice or stairs is the most common mechanism of injury to the extensor complex of the knee (Figs. 7–4 through 7–7). Tears of the extensor

Text continued on page 198

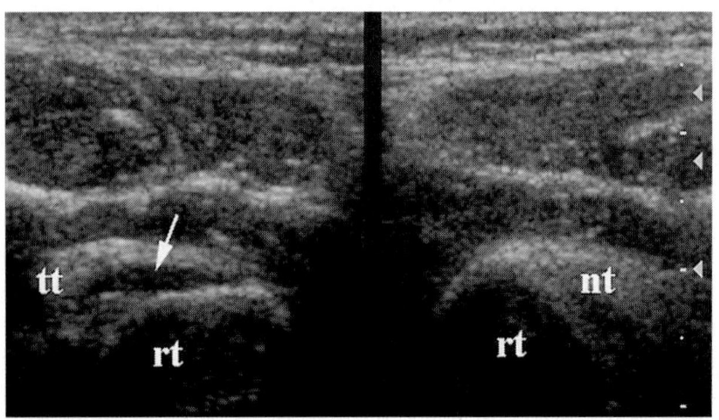

Figure 7–2 ■ Tear of the distal long biceps tendon: transverse sonogram. This 42-year-old construction worker experienced a pop in his left elbow while lifting a slab of concrete. The sonogram provides side-to-side comparison of the distal long biceps tendon at the insertion on the radial tuberosity (*rt*) with the forearm in pronation. On the left, a partial tear (*arrow*) is demonstrated in the symptomatic elbow. A normal tendon (*nt*) is shown on the right. Abbreviation: torn tendon (*tt*).

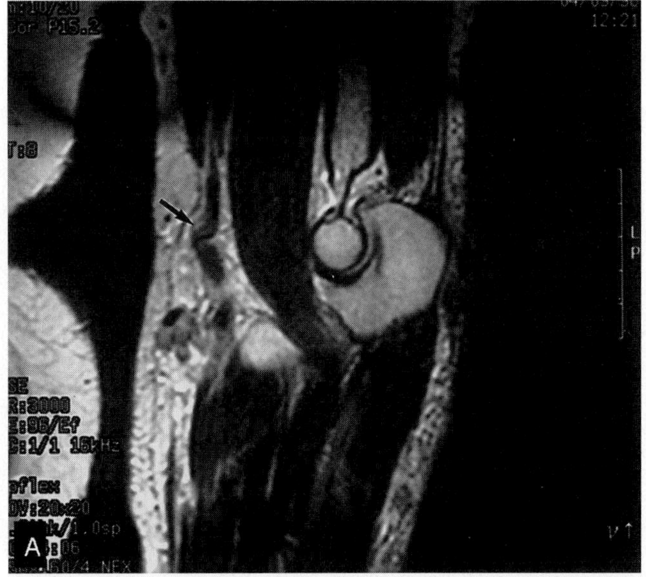

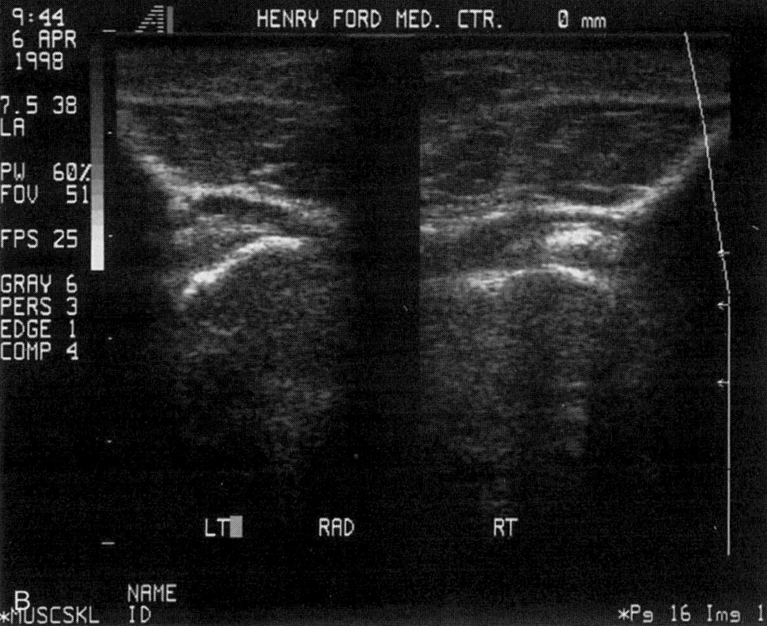

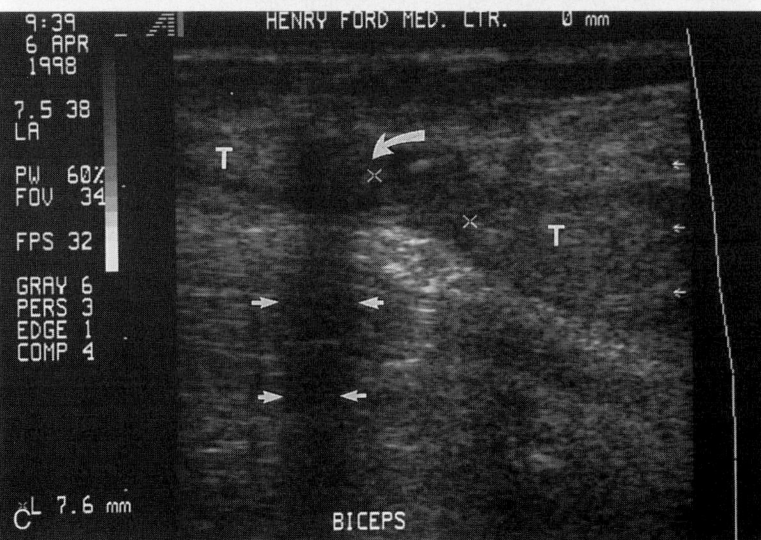

Figure 7–3 ■ **A**, Full-thickness tear of the distal biceps brachii: T_2-weighted sagittal image. A sudden onset of weakness in the elbow impairs this cardiologist's catheterization skills. The sagittal image through the affected left elbow shows the buckled and retracted tendon (*arrow*). **B**, Full-thickness tear of the distal biceps brachii: split-screen comparison of the biceps brachii tendon insertions. Same patient as in **A**. Transverse images were obtained with the arm pronated and with the transducer over the radial tuberosities (*RAD*). The left tendon insertion (*LT*) seems detached and surrounded with fluid. The right tendon insertion (*RT*) appears normal. **C**, Full-thickness tear of the distal biceps brachii: longitudinal image with the transducer in an antecubital position. Same patient as in **A**. Misinterpretation is common in this type of tear, which is caused by artifact induced by buckling of the retracted tendon (*T*). The transducer in this figure is aligned along the tendon, as displayed on the MRI image in **A**. The buckling causes refractile shadowing (*arrows*) and a false hypoechoic defect (*curved arrow*). The examiner was misled and was led to believe that the tendon was retracted proximal to the site of buckling (*between the calipers*).

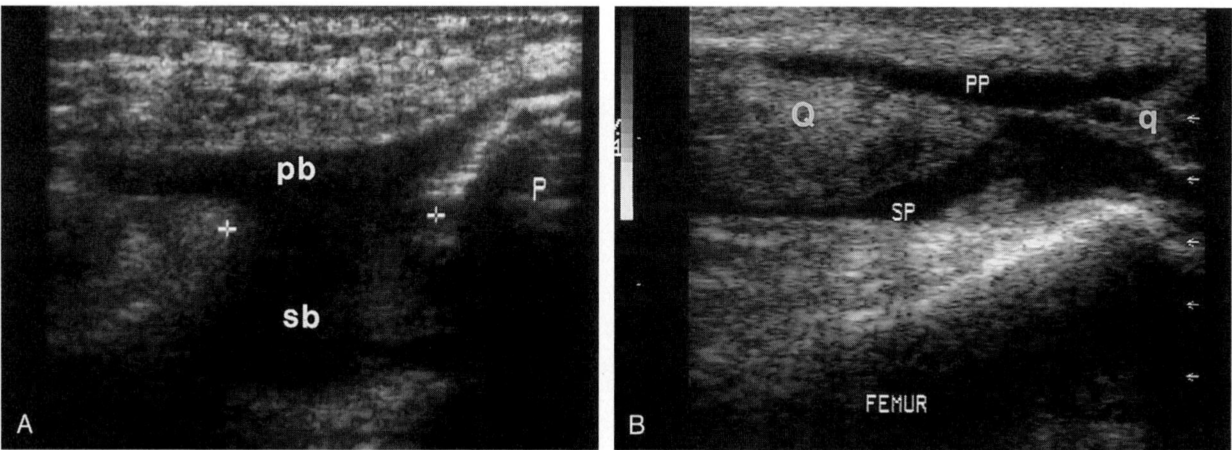

Figure 7–4 ■ **A**, Full-thickness quadriceps tendon tear: longitudinal sonogram. After slipping on a patch of ice, this 37-year-old male was unable to straighten his right leg. Significant ecchymosis and swelling surrounded the knee joint. A large discontinuity is present within the quadriceps tendon approximately 10 mm proximal to the patella (*P*). Note that there is now free communication between the suprapatellar (*sb*) and prepatellar (*pb*) bursae. This injury is similar to that sustained by President Clinton. **B**, Full-thickness quadriceps tendon tear: longitudinal sonogram. Fall similar to that in **A**. In this patient, there is communication between the prepatellar bursa (*PP*) and the suprapatellar bursa (*SP*) as well. The fluid leaks through a defect between the proximal (*Q*) and distal (*q*) retracted ends of the quadriceps tendon.

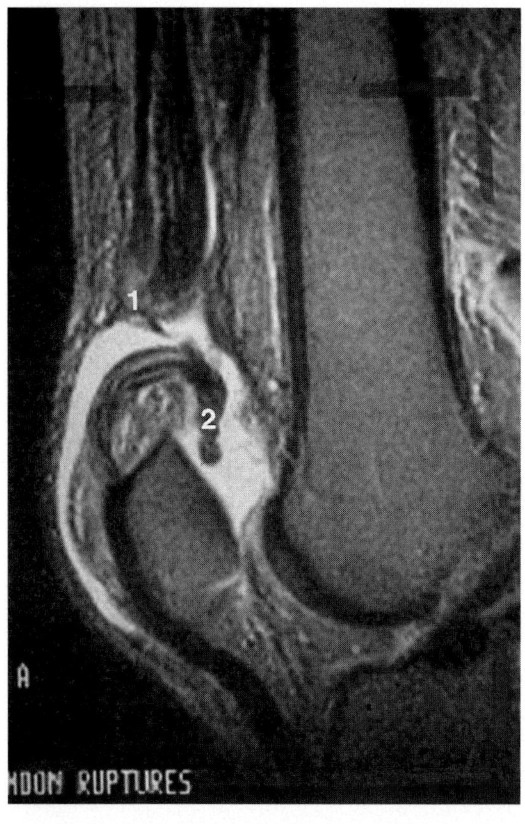

Figure 7–5 ■ Full-thickness quadriceps tendon tear: sagittal MRI (T_2 weighted). This T_2-weighted MRI of the knee depicts a similar injury to that shown in Figure 7–4. Again, the communication between the surrounding deep (suprapatellar) and superficial (prepatellar) bursae is clearly demonstrated. Note that the torn ends of the tendon curve away from each other. This curving causes refraction when imaged with ultrasound. Abbreviations: proximal quadriceps tendon (*1*), distal quadriceps tendon (*2*). (Courtesy of Jamshid Tehranzadeh, MD, VCI Medical Center)

Figure 7–6 ■ Full-thickness patellar tendon rupture: longitudinal sonogram. The patient is a 29-year-old male who felt a sudden sharp pain under his patella while jumping during a basketball game. This longitudinal image demonstrates disruption (*curved arrow*) of the tendon at the patellar apex. Calcifications (*small arrows*) within the tendon distal to the site of rupture indicate chronic tendon disease. Refraction artifact (*open arrows*) indicates the site of rupture.

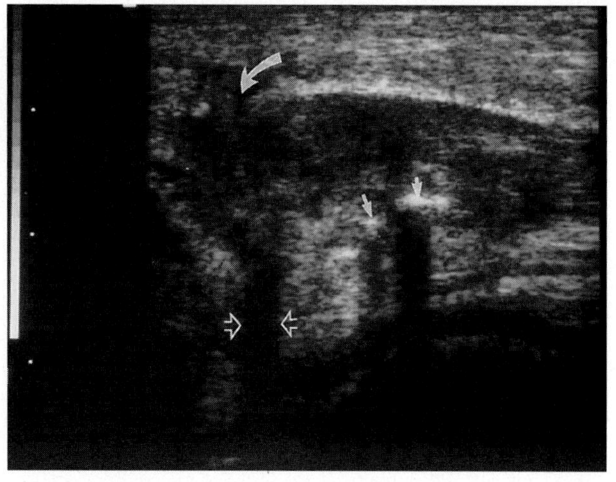

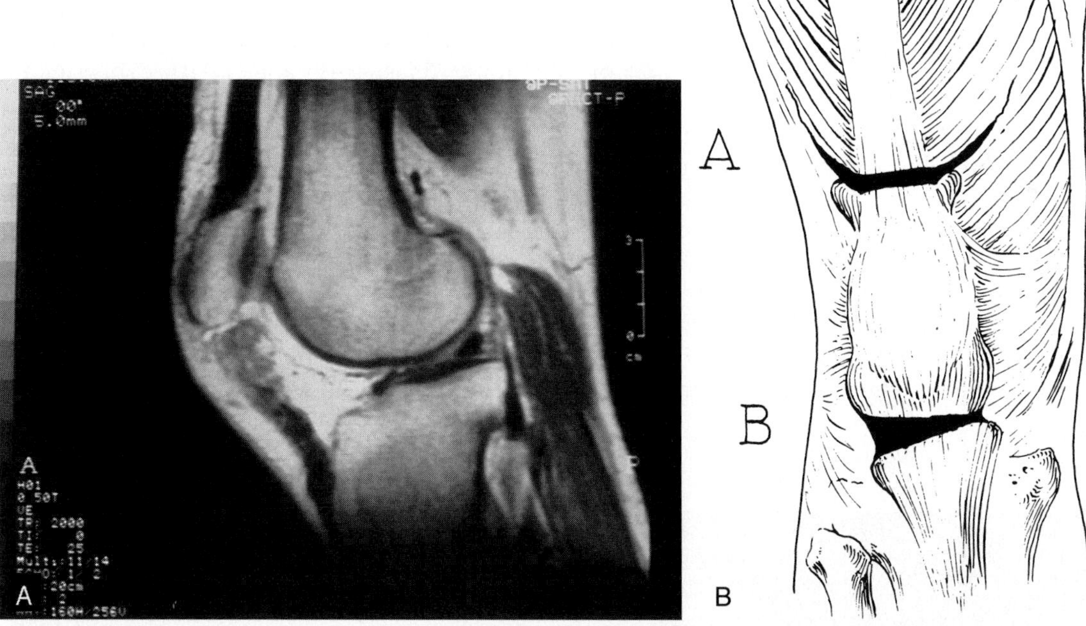

Figure 7–7 ■ **A**, Full-thickness patellar tendon rupture: sagittal MRI (T_2 weighted). A patellar tendon rupture identical to that shown in Figure 7–6 is shown on this sagittal MRI. Mild displacement of the patella and rotation is noted. A blunted configuration is seen on the torn end of the patellar tendon. This is probably the cause of refractile shadowing. The classic site of rupture is immediately beneath the patellar apex, as depicted in these two cases. **B**, Diagram of the ruptures of the extensor mechanism of the knee. Both quadriceps tears (*A*) and patellar tendon ruptures (*B*) occur most often around the bone surface of the patella. The tears frequently affect the distal quadriceps and the proximal patellar tendon, respectively. The black areas in the diagram represent the defects noted on the ultrasound image. The gap is typically filled with anechoic fluid. The torn ends of the tendon retract, and the fibers are often curled at the edges. (Courtesy of Jamshid Tehranzadeh, MD, VCI Medical Center)

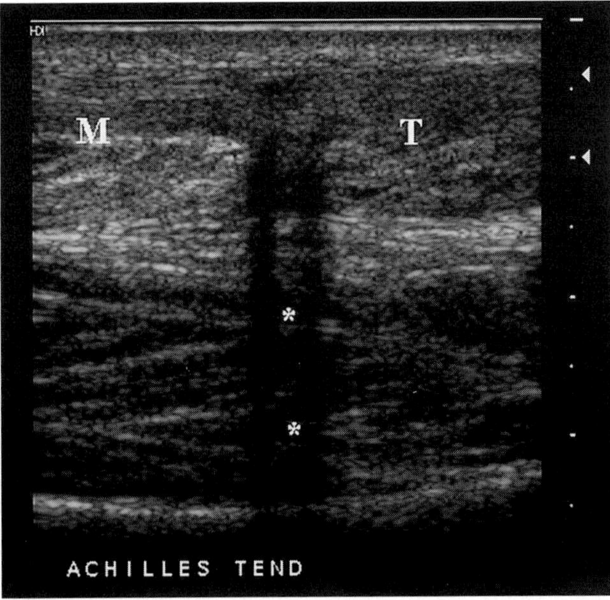

Figure 7–8 ▪ Musculotendinous tear of the Achilles tendon: longitudinal sonogram. A stabbing pain in the leg forced this 42-year-old soccer player to quit during the final game of league competition. The longitudinal sonogram shows a proximal tendon injury at the junction of the soleus muscle (*M*) and the Achilles tendon (*T*). The edges of the tear cause acoustic shadow because of refraction (*asterisk*).

tendons of the fingers, as well as both flexor and extensor tendons of the elbow, also commonly occur at their junction with bone. In the upper extremity, the forces involved may be as violent as that resulting in elbow dislocation or as minor as that experienced in finger hyperflexion. Factors predisposing to tendon rupture are increasing age, diabetes, hyperparathyroidism, inflammatory arthropathies, and enthesopathies. The most common inflammatory conditions resulting in soft tissue damage and tendon rupture are lupus erythematosus and rheumatoid arthritis.

Some tendons rupture more commonly at their musculotendinous junction (Fig. 7–8). Few tendons fail in their midsubstance. We have observed Achilles tendon ruptures in all three locations: the musculotendinous junction, the midsubstance and at the enthesis. In the Achilles tendon, the most common site of rupture is approximately 4–6 cm proximal to its insertion onto the calcaneus at the level of the tibiotalar joint. This unusual site of rupture has been attributed to the relative avascularity of the tendon in this region.

The peroneus tendons also exhibit a predisposition to rupture at an unusual site, the level of the distal lateral malleolus. A fragile retinaculum, the superior peroneal retinaculum, holds the peroneal tendons in place behind the posterior aspect of the lateral malleolus. Disruption of the retinaculum results in dislocation of the peroneal tendons. This subluxation is more likely to occur if the tendons are located in a shallow, bony groove behind the lateral malleolus or in cases with an abnormally rounded surface of the posterior fibula. Chronic tendon subluxation is perceived by patients as a click or snapping sensation in the posterior lateral aspect of the ankle (Figs. 7–9 and 7–10). This tendon instability results in pain, which can limit the patient's level of activity. The earliest signs of a pathophysiological reaction to peroneus tendon subluxation are thickening of the tendon sheath and increased fluid within the sheath. Chronic irritation of the tendons rubbing over the posterior bony crest of the fibula results in degeneration of the tendons. Flattening of the peroneus brevis tendon is the first sign of tendon degeneration (Fig. 7–10). Later, a longitudinal central split develops within the tendon

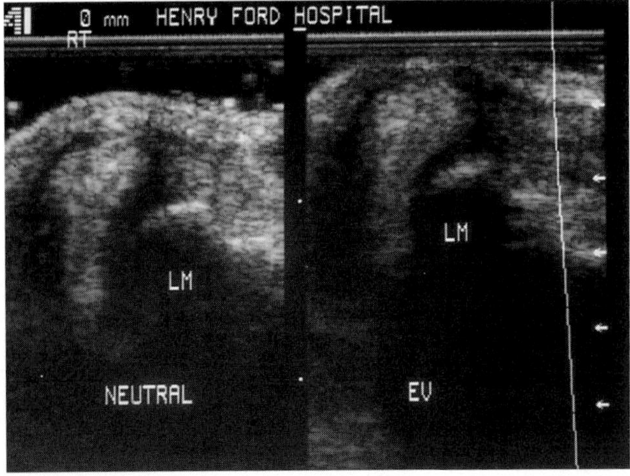

Figure 7–9 ▪ Peroneal tendon instability: transverse sonogram of the peroneal tendons with split-screen technique showing neutral and dorsiflexion-eversion. This young man injured his ankle 8 months ago. The pain and swelling were almost gone 4 weeks after the injury when he first noticed a twinge in his ankle while climbing stairs. Now he feels uncertain in his gait, and the pain that can occur at any time makes him apprehensive. He describes the discomfort as a sharp, stabbing ache associated with an audible click over his lateral malleolus. The image on the left was obtained with the transducer oriented transversely over the course of the tendons, with the ankle in neutral position. The image on the right shows the tendons when the ankle is dorsiflexed and everted. The tendons should be located behind the lateral malleolus (*LM*) or on the left side of the image. The abnormal tendons sublux laterally (toward the transducer) in the neutral position; the ankle dorsiflexion and eversion accentuate the abnormality. Abbreviation: dorsiflexion-eversion (*EV*).

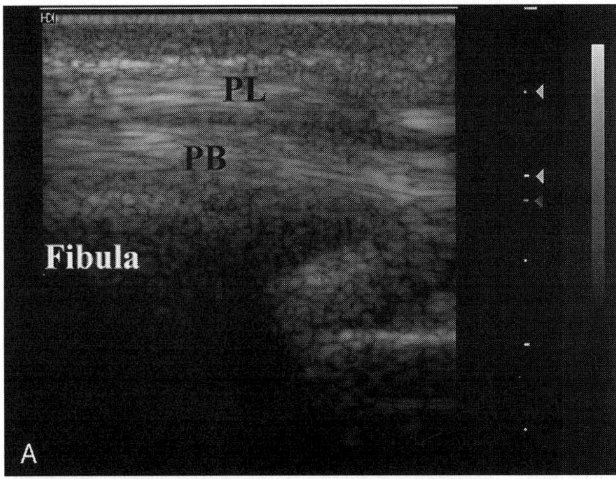

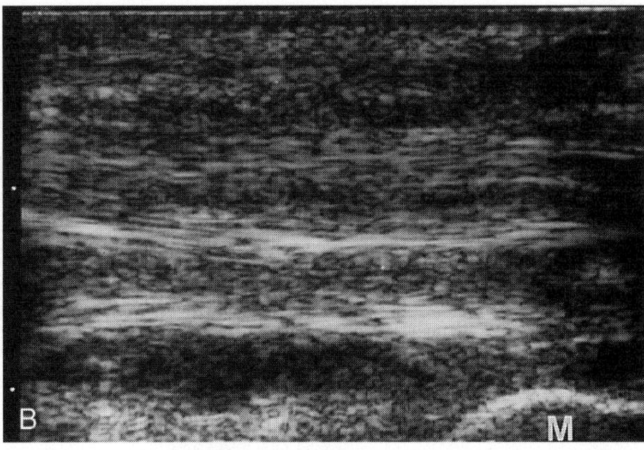

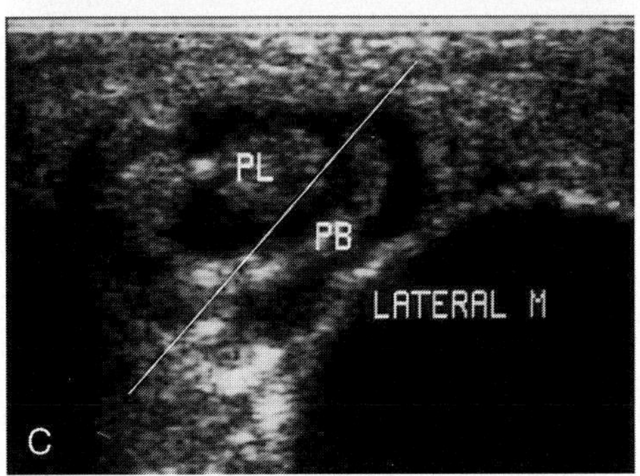

Figure 7-10 ■ **A,** Normal peroneal tendons: longitudinal sonogram. Scanning over the lateral aspect of the foot behind the fibula of a normal 27-year-old male yielded this image of the peroneal tendons. The peroneus longus (*PL*) is located superficially. The peroneus brevis (*PB*) lies deep to the peroneus longus, passing adjacent to the fibula. **B,** Longitudinal tear of the peroneus brevis: longitudinal sonogram. Eighteen months ago, this 31-year-old female suffered an injury of the right ankle and complains of persistent swelling. Several tendon layers are seen adjacent to the lateral maleolus, secondary to longitudinal fissuring of the peroneal tendons. A moderate amount of fluid is demonstrated within the tendon sheath. Abbreviation: lateral maleolus (*M*). **C,** Longitudinal tear of the peroneus brevis tendon: transverse sonogram. The transverse image explains the unusual layered appearance observed on the longitudinal scan (*B*). The torn peroneus brevis (*PB*) is hoof-shaped, and the tendon surrounds the peroneus longus (*PL*) in a semicircular fashion. Three layers will be identified if one scans the tendons longitudinally along the plane indicated by the thin white line. Partial volume averaging reinforces this type of artifact.

Figure 7-11 ■ **A,** Diagram of the longitudinal tear of the peroneus brevis. The most common tear of the peroneus brevis is depicted in this diagram. The wear and tear of the tendon caused by constant rubbing over the lateral malleolus in patients is hypothetical. **B,** Diagram of advanced peroneal tendon disease. Peroneus brevis and longus tears occur together in some patients. Both tendons appear flattened and split longitudinally. The pathology cannot be visualized longitudinally because the prominence of the fibula interferes with imaging. Transverse images show too many tendon bundles around the lateral malleolus.

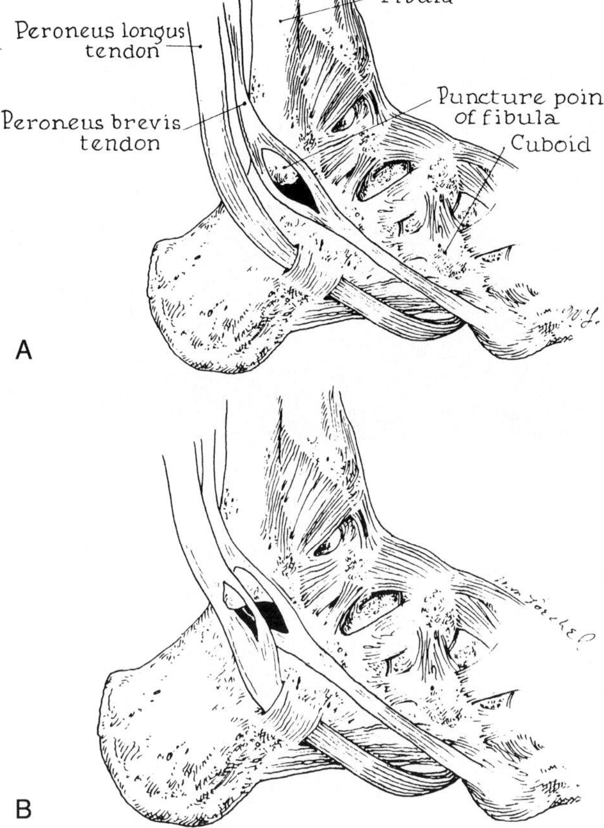

substance (Fig. 7–11). Similar changes in the peroneus longus tendon follow (Fig. 7–11). At this point, the sonographic picture may be somewhat confusing, giving the impression that four distinct tendons are present at the level of the distal fibula. The distal fibula may separate the torn peroneus tendons, protruding through the rent in a manner similar to that of a button passing through a buttonhole. In end-stage disease, complete rupture of the tendons occurs. However, an isolated transverse tear of the peroneus tendons is rare (see Fig. 4–22).

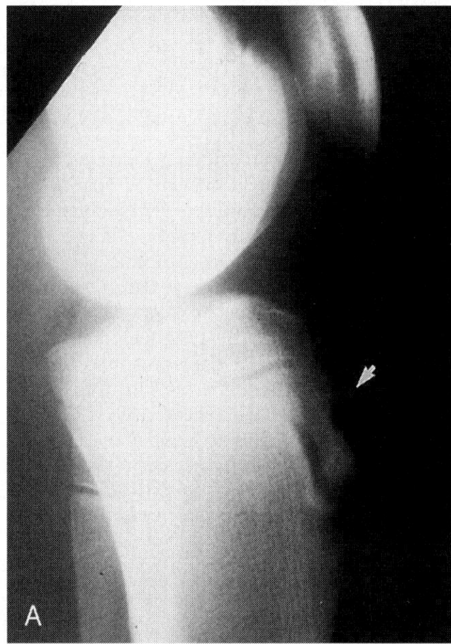

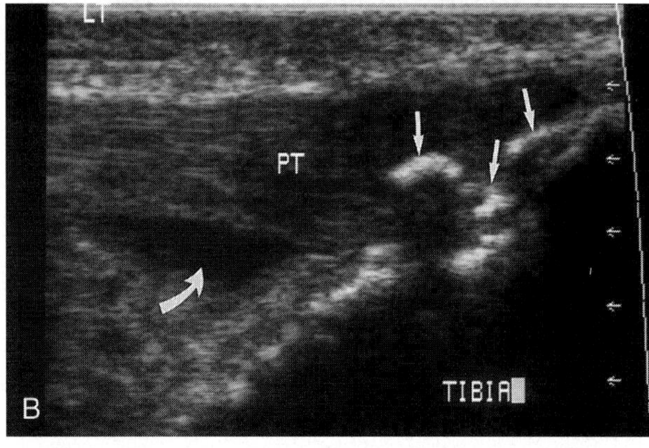

Figure 7–12 ■ **A**, Osgood-Schlatter disease: lateral knee radiograph. Because of painful swelling of the knee, this 15-year-old soccer player is not able to play competitively. The lateral radiograph demonstrates a small apophyseal fragment (*arrow*) in an abnormal proximal position. As in most radiographs, the soft tissues are not well shown. **B**, Osgood-Schlatter disease: longitudinal sonogram through the distal patellar tendon. Sonography of a knee with Osgood-Schlatter's disease shows small avulsions from the apophyseal cartilage (*arrows*). Those avulsions calcify, and they may grow as separate ossification centers. When the patient presents with acute pain, it is not unusual to see some swelling in the distal tendon (*PT*), and one can often observe fluid in the deep infrapatellar bursa (*curved arrow*).

Radiographic findings in tendon injury are few and usually nonspecific. These findings include focal soft tissue swelling, soft tissue atrophy, and small, bony avulsions. In some cases, soft tissue swelling may be absent in acute injury due to sparse vascularization of tendons and ligaments. Focal soft tissue atrophy is observed less frequently than soft tissue swelling and is also nonspecific with regard to the underlying pathology. Therefore, a more sensitive and specific imaging modality is required in the diagnosis of tendon rupture, such as ultrasound or MRI. Radiographs are accurate in diagnosing bony avulsions associated with tendon injury. Small flake-like osseous fragments identified on radiographs are good indicators of the site of tendon injury at the insertion of Sharpey's fibers, but they reveal little about the full extent of the injury (Rogers, 1992).

Tendon injuries in children and adolescents differ greatly from those seen in adults. The weak link in the musculoskeletal system of children and adolescents is the apophysis adjacent to its junction with a tendon (Fig. 7–12). Characteristic lesions are seen in Osgood-Schlatter disease and Sinding-Larssen-Johansson syndrome. Histologically, these lesions are microavulsions of the apophyseal cartilage (Ogdon, 1990) (Fig. 7–12). Ultrasound demonstrates a thickened, edematous tendon insertion and small fragments of cartilage avulsed from the apophysis. The avulsed cartilage fragments frequently appear hyperechoic relative to the normal apophyseal cartilage due to ossification occurring within the necrotic cartilage fragments (Fig. 7–12). Intratendinous lesions are extremely rare in children and adolescents. These are usually seen only in cases of direct penetrating trauma.

Tendon Degeneration

Tendon rupture may occur in association with little or no trauma. These tendon ruptures occur at sites of tendon degeneration, which significantly weaken the tendon. The best example of this type of tendon rupture involves the rotator cuff of the shoulder. The impingement theory has long been cited as the cause of the majority of rotator cuff tears (Neer, 1983). However, recent epidemiological and pathological evidence points to aging as the most important factor in the pathogenesis of rotator cuff tears (Ozaki et al., 1988; Fukuda et al., 1990; Matsen and Arntz, 1990; Milgrom et al., 1995). Our studies indicate that hand dominance and physical activity do not increase the incidence of rotator cuff tears. However, clinically symptomatic rotator cuff disease is more common on the dominant side. Also, the incidence of rotator cuff tears is equal in men and women (Milgrom et al., 1995), but men present more commonly with shoulder complaints related to rotator cuff disease. It is unclear whether the difference in the incidence of symptomatic rotator cuff lesions is related to differences in pain tolerance between men and women. Another explanation may be that women are more likely to reduce their level of activity when pain first develops, while men maintain a level of activity that results in progression of symptoms.

Many patients relate a cause-and-effect relationship between an event with minor trauma and the onset of their shoulder problems. The associated incidents vary from throwing a ball to falling on an outstretched arm or even playing a card game. These events may simply be the final event in a long series of minor traumatic events which result in tendon degeneration and progressive rotator cuff fiber failure. Matsen (1990) describes the process of chronic rotator cuff injury as an insidious process which goes unnoticed by the patient and has been referred to as *creeping tendon ruptures* (van Holsbeeck et al., 1998).

Box 7–1
Rotator Cuff Tendinopathy

- Begins as early as age 30
- Starts in the tendon (interstially, intratendinous, delamination)
- At age 60, 60% have tendon damage
- Often asymptomatic

Asymptomatic rotator cuff tears affect a large portion of the population, as many as 60% of individuals over 60 years of age (Box 7–1) (Milgrom et al., 1995). As people age, the rotator cuff becomes increasingly susceptible to rupture, and less force is required to result in tendon injury. Significant force is required to tear the rotator cuff of a 30-year-old individual, while relatively trivial force is needed to produce a tear in a 60-year-old. When a group of tendon fibers fail at the same time, the lesion becomes symptomatic, presenting as pain at rest exacerbated by extension, abduction, and external rotation. Acute extension of the tear may occur, associated with the sudden onset of substantial

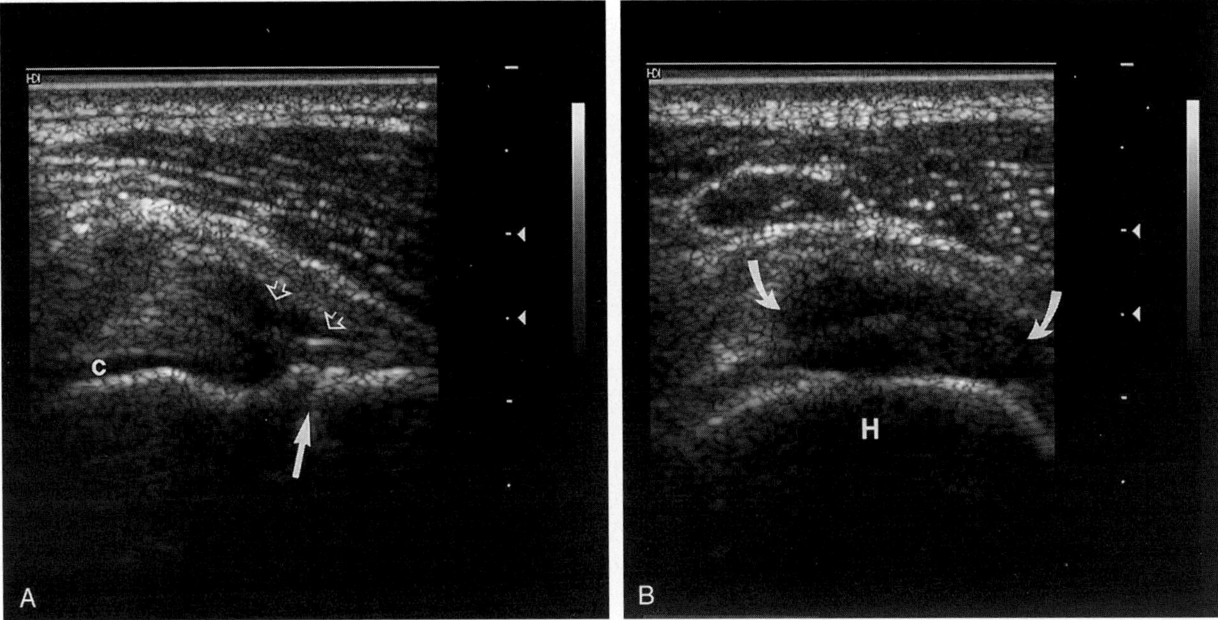

Figure 7–13 ▪ **A**, Partial-thickness rotator cuff tear: longitudinal sonogram. Several weeks of pain and weakness in the right shoulder caused this 42-year-old man to seek treatment. He was a recreational weight lifter. A lesion of mixed echogenicity (*open arrows*) is identified near the critical zone of the supraspinatus tendon 1 cm proximal to the most distal aspect of the tendon insertion. The cortical surface of the greater tuberosity is irregular (*arrow*). Abbreviation: cartilage of humeral head (*c*). **B**, Partial-thickness rotator cuff tear: transverse sonogram. Same patient as in **A**. The region of mixed echogenicity (*curved arrows*) is again noted in the supraspinatus tendon overlying the humeral head (*H*).

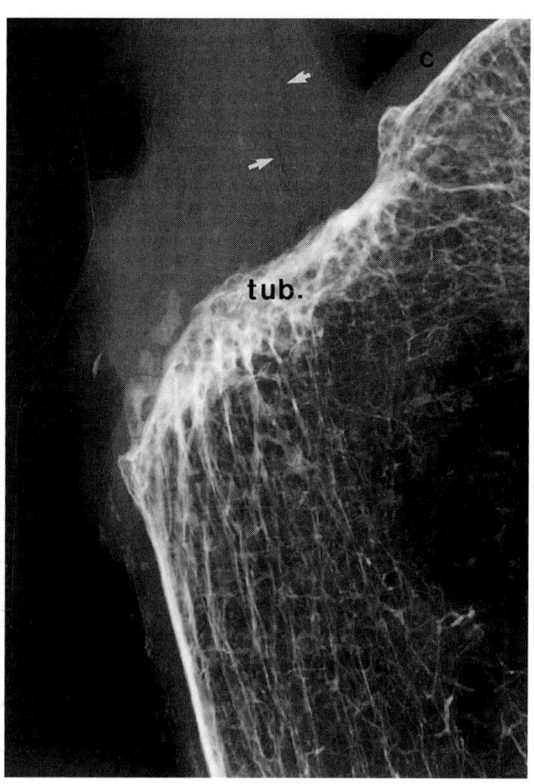

Figure 7-14 ■ Earliest signs of rotator cuff tear: microradiograph. A 5-mm-thick section obtained through the greater tuberosity of a cadaver specimen was radiographed using a 5-μm focal spot and high-detail film. This image demonstrates the earliest signs of rotator cuff tear, commonly referred to as *delamination* (*small arrows*) within the substance of the tendon. Note the bony irregularity of the enthesis at the greater tuberosity. Abbreviations: greater tuberosity (*tub*), humeral cartilage (*c*).

weakness in flexion, abduction, and external rotation. Although differences in the shape of the acromion, abnormalities of the acromioclavicular joint, and other factors may influence the susceptibility of the rotator cuff to tears, age-related deterioration appears to be the dominant factor (van Holsbeeck et al., 1998). Age-related tendon degeneration and loading factors are dominant in the determination of patterns of failure of the rotator cuff.

Tendon degeneration in the rotator cuff is a process which appears to begin at the age of 30 (Fig. 7-13). Postmortem studies have shown that this process begins interstitially (Fig. 7-14). It is unknown whether this process is reversible, and if so, at what point it becomes irreversible. References in the arthrography literature (Yamanaka, 1994) indicate that some partial tears may heal. In our experience with follow-up of both partial- and full-thickness tears, there is no significant potential for healing of these lesions. Inflammatory changes within the tendon adjacent to these tears may improve (Newman et al., 1994), but we have observed no decrease in the extent of the tears.

In both clinical and cadaver studies, we have observed two distinct patterns of partial-thickness rotator cuff tears (van Holsbeeck et al., 1995). The first type is a lesion of mixed echogenicity, with separate regions of decreased and increased echogenicity (Fig. 7-15). These lesions are typically identified along the articular (deep) surface of the tendon. A hyperechoic linear or curvilinear cleavage plane is outlined by a hypoechoic halo. This interface may relate to the retracted torn tendon fibers (Figs. 7-16 and 7-17).

The second type of partial rotator cuff tear is homogeneously hypoechoic or anechoic (Figs. 7-18 through 7-21). Typically, these tears are located either centrally within the tendon or along the bursal surface. The region of decreased echogenicity represents fluid in the majority of cases, but it may be due to myxoid degeneration.

Delamination within the critical zone of the rotator cuff is the most common pathological finding in autopsy studies (Codman, 1931, 1934). Sonographic evaluation of the critical zone is difficult due to anisotropy at the insertion of the supraspinatus tendon. The two thickest layers of the distal supraspinatus tendon (Clark and Harryman, 1992) are probably responsible for sonographic artifacts in the critical zone. One of these layers is highly anisotropic due to the regular longitudinal organization of the collagen fibers. The other layer does not demonstrate anisotropic properties. This

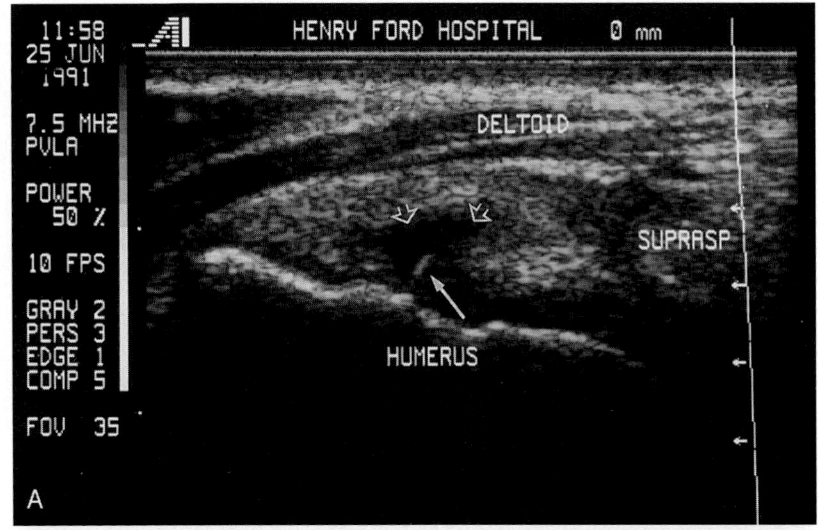

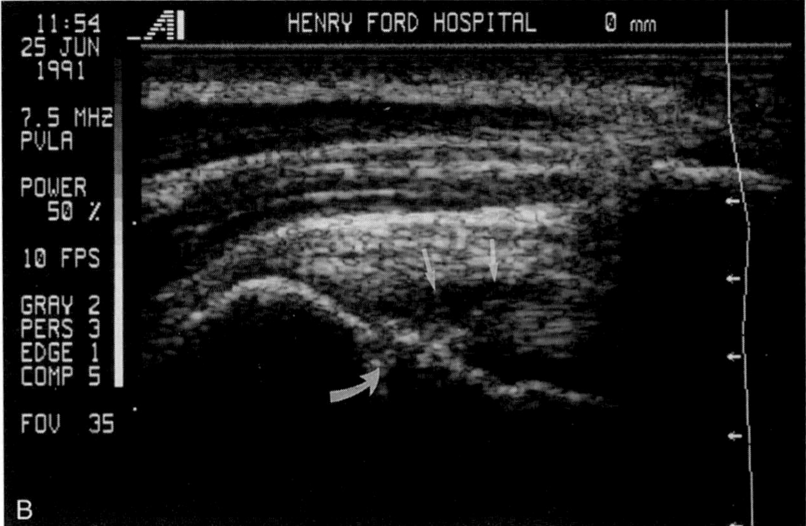

Figure 7–15 ■ **A**, Partial-thickness tear of the rotator cuff: longitudinal sonogram. This 49-year-old woman complains of unremitting shoulder pain for the past 5 weeks. The pain did not improve with physical therapy. A triangular region of decreased echogenicity (*open arrows*) is seen along the deep surface of the supraspinatus tendon at its insertion on the greater tuberosity. A curvilinear, highly echogenic focus (*arrow*) is noted centrally within this region. **B**, Partial-thickness tear of the rotator cuff: longitudinal sonogram. Same patient as in **A**. This image was obtained at a position 2 cm posterior to that shown in **A**. Delamination (*arrows*) is almost always associated with irregularity of the cortex of the tuberosity (*curved arrow*) at the tendon insertion.

great difference in imaging properties between the two layers is responsible for the difficulty in making a sonographic diagnosis of lesions in the critical zone. Often the interface between these two layers appears as a hyperechoic speckled pattern in normal patients (Fig. 7–22). As degeneration occurs, resulting in delamination, the retracted longitudinal fibers of the supraspinatus tendon result in a comma-shaped hyperechoic defect. The art of rotator cuff sonography requires the examiner to distinguish between artifact resulting from the normal interface of tendon layers and a true lesion caused by disruption of tendon fibers in the critical zone. An artifact will be transient, disappearing with angulation of the transducer. A true lesion will remain visible despite slight variation in the angle of incidence of the sound beam (Fig. 7–23). Calcifications appear as echogenic interfaces as well. However, they appear more round or spherical instead of the linear or stub-like interfaces of the partial-thickness tear (Fig. 7–24).

Secondary signs of rotator cuff pathology will also lead the examiner to the correct diagnosis. Synovitis (Middleton et al., 1986; Hollister at al., 1995) and degenerative changes in the cortical bone of the greater tuberosity (Wohlwend et al., 1998) are excellent indicators of associated rotator cuff pathology. Often synovitis is associated with fluid, which can extend into the bursa, joint space or biceps tendon sheath (Figs. 7–25 through 7–27). The hypoechoic thickening of the bursa is not always due to an effusion; synovial proliferation is sometimes difficult to differentiate (Fig. 7–28).

Degenerative bony changes occur along the surface of the greater tuberosity, which is left bare by the torn tendon fibers. These erosions may also be

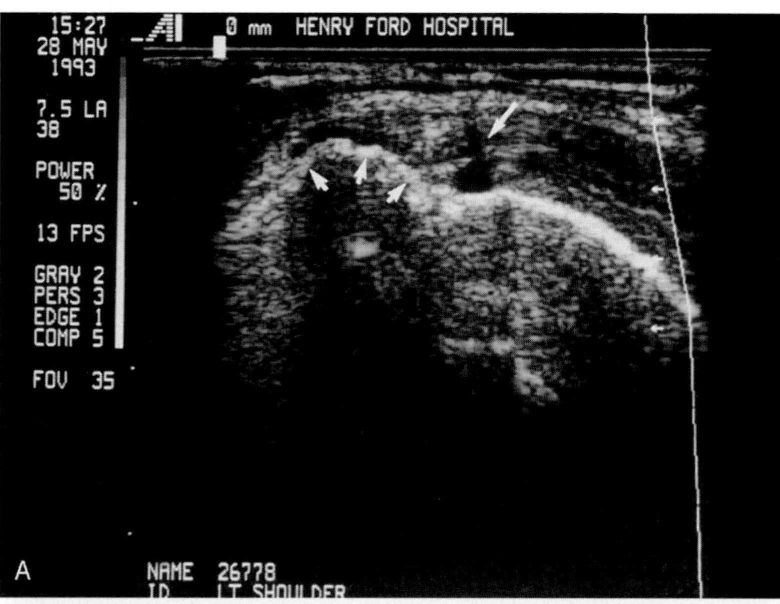

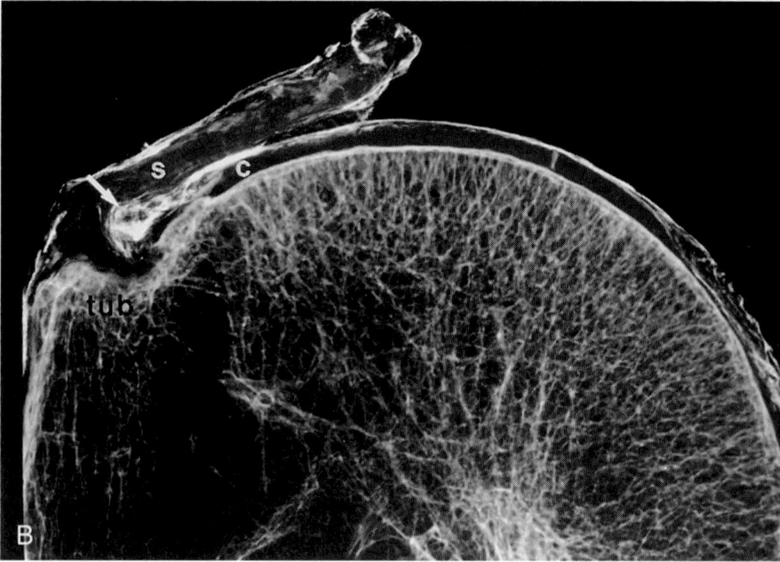

Figure 7–16 ■ **A**, Partial-thickness tear of the rotator cuff: longitudinal sonogram. A longitudinal image of the supraspinatus insertion of a cadaver specimen was obtained. Abnormal decreased echogenicity (*arrow*) is demonstrated surrounding a small triangular, echogenic focus in the critical zone of the tendon. The cortical surface of the tuberosity is irregular (*small arrows*). **B**, Partial-thickness tear of the rotator cuff: microradiograph. The specimen used to obtain the image in **A** was sectioned and radiographed after the surface of the tendon was coated with thin barium. Contrast material has penetrated into the pathological region of the tendon insertion (*white arrow*) shown on the ultrasound image. The triangular tendon fragment at the base of the lesion corresponds to the echogenic focus noted in the critical zone of the tendon. Note the irregular thinning of the cortical bone of the greater tuberosity (*tub*) and the adjacent articular cartilage (*c*) of the humeral head. Abbreviation: supraspinatus tendon (*s*).

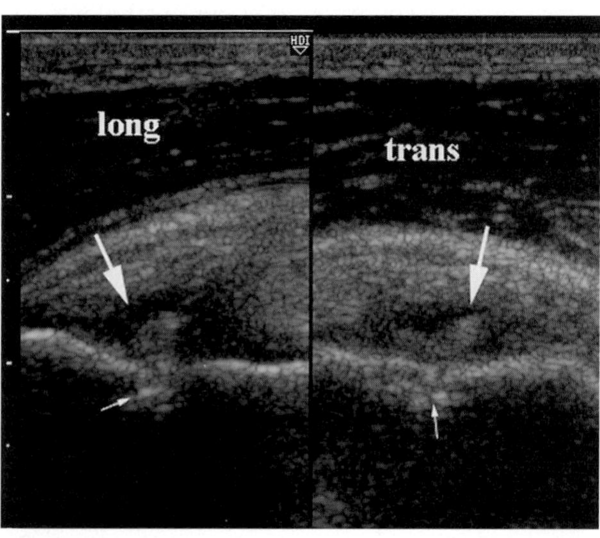

Figure 7–17 ■ The "stub" in partial-thickness rotator cuff tear: split-screen images over the anatomical neck of the proximal humerus. The hyperechoic focus in a lesion of mixed echogenicity is often stub-like and may well represent retracted fibers of torn tendon. If one is not sure whether the detected abnormality represents artifact or tear, one should try to show the lesion along different imaging planes. In this illustration, the images were obtained with the transducer positioned at almost 90 degree angles. Another helpful sign is the mirror bone change (*small arrows*) that is noted deep to the stub (*big arrows*).

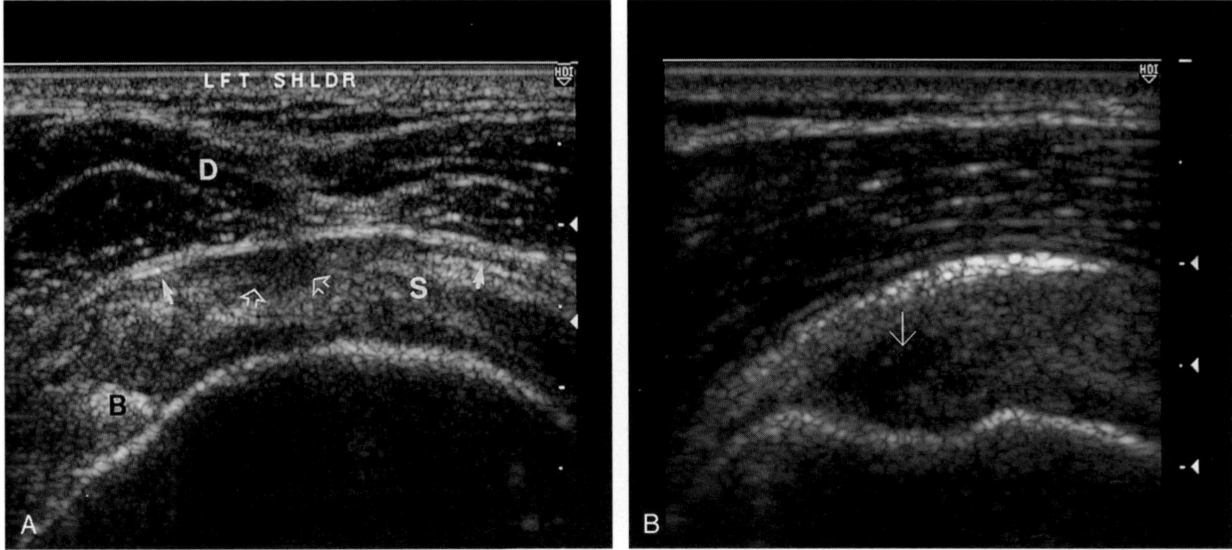

Figure 7–18 ■ **A**, Bursal surface partial-thickness rotator cuff tear: transverse sonogram. This 43-year-old tennis player cannot lift his left arm for serves or overhead shots. The bursal surface of the tendon appears hypoechoic and eroded (*open arrows*). Compare the region of the partial tear with the adjacent normal tendon surface (*arrows*). Abbreviations: intracapsular biceps tendon (*B*), deltoid (*D*), supraspinatus (*S*). **B**, Bursal surface partial-thickness rotator cuff tear: longitudinal sonogram. Same patient as in **A**. This longitudinal image shows the lesion (*arrow*), which continues to involve a deeper portion of the tendon.

seen along the anatomical neck of the humerus. Codman was the first to describe these bony changes observed in autopsy specimens (Codman, 1931, 1934) (Figs. 7–29 and 7–30). These findings were subsequently confirmed by other investigators using radiography (Golding, 1962), arthrography (Rakofski, 1987), and sonography (Patten et al., 1992; van Holsbeeck et al., 1995; Wohlwend et al., 1998). Our recent studies have confirmed the importance of identifying these secondary findings (Figs. 7–31 through 7–38). Bony changes are associated with both partial- and full-thickness tears of the rotator cuff, seen in as many as 70% of cases (Wohlwend et al., 1998). They are always identified at the site of the cuff lesion, and the size of the bony lesion corresponds very closely to the size of the rotator cuff tear. Both bone erosion and proliferation occur in combination at the site of the lesion. The degree to which each process occurs varies widely from one patient to another. In some, osteolysis will predominate; in others, bone proliferation will be the dominant reaction. This pattern of oste-

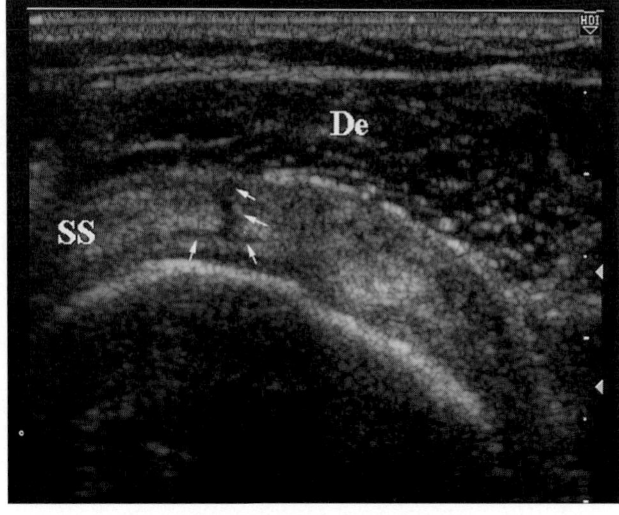

Figure 7–19 ■ Bursal surface tear and delamination: transverse sonogram. Frequently, one can observe partial-thickness tears which extend in two orthogonal planes. The tear within the tendon substance will often propagate parallel with the longitudinal fibers of the supraspinatus, as seen in this bursal side tear. The *small arrows* point at the tear and the associated delamination. Abbreviations: deltoid (*De*), supraspinatus (*SS*).

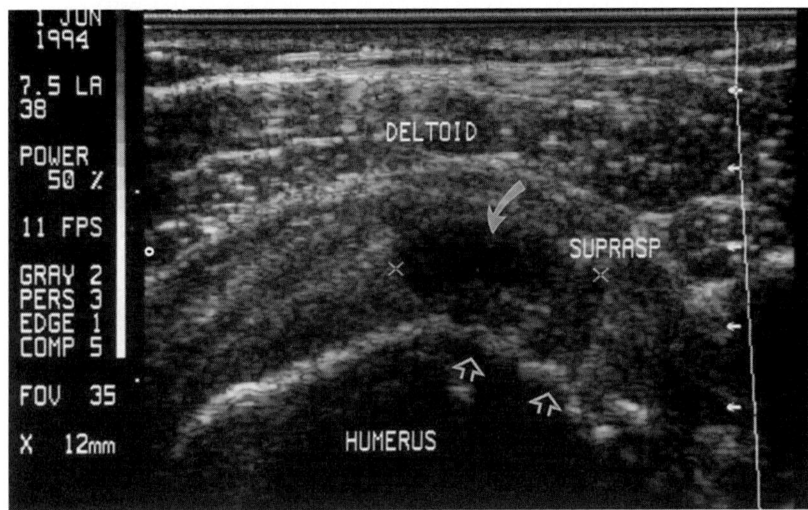

Figure 7–20 ■ Partial-thickness tear of the rotator cuff: transverse sonogram. Chronic right shoulder pain caused this 39-year-old male to seek treatment. He could not sleep due to the pain unless he supported his shoulder. A 12-mm lesion of mixed echogenicity is demonstrated in the deep portion of the supraspinatus tendon. An anechoic region (*curved arrow*) is noted. This appearance is not uncommon in partial tears. The region of irregularity of the cortical bone (*open arrows*) corresponds well with the size of the tendon lesion.

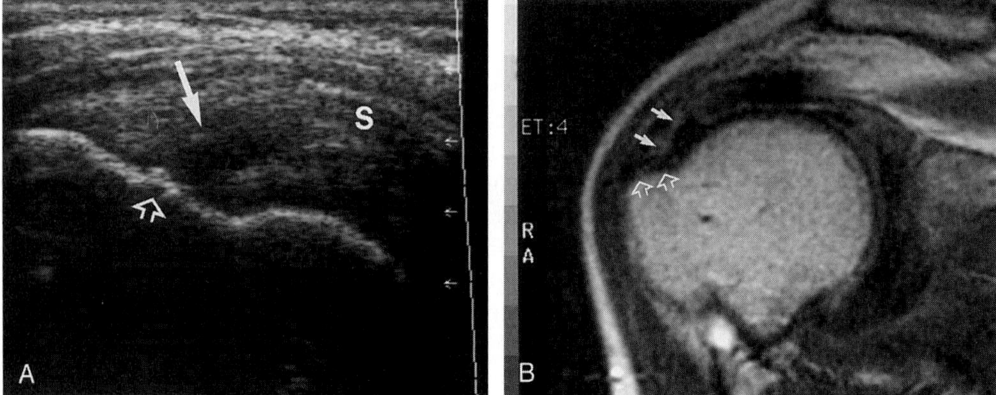

Figure 7–21 ■ **A**, Partial-thickness tear of the rotator cuff: longitudinal sonogram. Over the past 3 years, this 44-year-old female experienced intermittent pain in the right shoulder. It varied greatly in intensity, sometimes becoming quite severe. She worked as a clerk in a department store. The pain limited her activity at work. This longitudinal sonogram of the greater tuberosity region shows a hypoechoic lesion (*arrow*) along the supraspinatus tendon (*S*) insertion. Bony irregularity (*open arrow*) is again seen in association with the tendon lesion. **B**, Partial-thickness tear of the rotator cuff: coronal MR image (T_2 weighted). Same patient as in **A**. Orientation of this coronal fast spin-echo T_2-weighted MR image is identical to that of the sonogram shown in **A**. Inhomogeneous signal is seen in the critical zone of the tendon (*arrows*) corresponding to the region of partial tear demonstrated on the sonogram. On this MRI examination without the benefit of intra-articular gadolinium, it is almost impossible to distinguish between a partial tear and tendinosis. The lower spatial resolution of MRI also fails to demonstrate the cortical irregularity seen sonographically, which has been confirmed on gross pathological specimens. Symbol: greater tuberosity (*open arrows*).

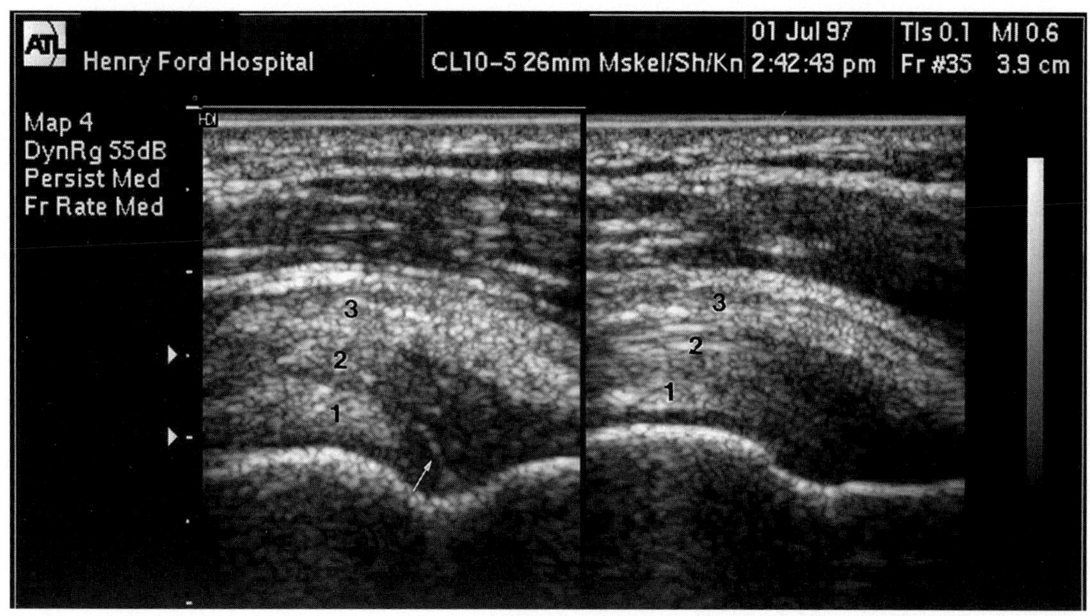

Figure 7–22 ■ Normal rotator cuff anisotropy: longitudinal sonograms. These two longitudinal images of the rotator cuff at the insertion onto the greater tuberosity were obtained with a 10-MHz transducer with differing degrees of angulation. A normal 32-year-old patient was imaged. Three layers are noted within the tendon. Detail of the internal tendon architecture varies, depending upon the angle of incidence of the sound beam. In the image on the right, greater detail of tendon fibers is seen in layer 2. The influence of anisotropy in layers 1 and 3 is less due to the variability of interwoven fibers in these layers. Orientation of the fibers in layer 2 is very consistent and parallel. Variation in transducer angulation results in changes in appearance of the hypoechoic zone near the tendon insertion. Interfaces between the tendon layers (*arrow*) appear as linear hyperechoic structures which vary upon angulation of the transducer. Key features which distinguish this from tendon pathology are the absence of bony irregularity and the variable appearance of the hypoechoic zone. An image of a true partial tear will not be dependent upon small changes in transducer angulation.

olysis and bone proliferation resembles that seen at fracture sites. Therefore, we feel that these lesions are posttraumatic. Neovascularity can be observed both histologically and sonographically in association with these lesions (Fig. 7–35). These vascular changes are similar to those observed at healing fracture sites and with Ilizarov bone-lengthening procedures.

Bony changes and their associated neovascularity are very helpful secondary signs of rotator cuff tears. Even the earliest partial-thickness tears are often associated with bony changes (see Figs. 7–13, 7–15, 7–20, and 7–38). Often this can be helpful in distinguishing artifact from true partial thickness tears.

Many full-thickness rotator cuff tears result from propagation of partial-thickness tears. These lesions are typically located in the critical zone of the supraspinatus tendon, about 1 cm proximal to the most lateral extent of the tendon insertion on the greater tuberosity (Figs. 7–39 through 7–41). Small full-thickness tears in the critical zone are referred to as *horizontal full-thickness tears*. They typically uncover the greater tuberosity and result in the bony irregularity discussed above (Fig. 7–42). These lesions are best visualized on longitudinal images (Fig. 7–43). It is helpful to observe the continuity of the bursal interface; discontinuity of this interface indicates the bursal extension of rotator cuff disease (Fig. 7–44). On transverse images, these lesions may be misdiagnosed as partial-thickness tears due to partial volume effects.

Longitudinal full-thickness rotator cuff tears extend along the length of the tendon and are observed less frequently than horizontal tears. Tears of this type more likely result from an acute traumatic injury. The proximal extent of the tear uncovers the articular cartilage of the humeral head. Differences in the acoustic properties between the fluid filling the tendon defect and the articular cartilage result in a sharp, highly echogenic interface. We refer to this as the *cartilage interface sign*, which is characteristic of large *longitudinal rotator cuff tears* (Figs. 7–45 through 7–48).

Patients with rotator cuff tears who do not undergo surgical repair describe their disease as a chronic process with recurrent exacerbations of their pain. At times their pain may be completely absent, a condition which patients often may attribute to either a steroid injection or physical therapy. Rarely, they experience spontaneous regression

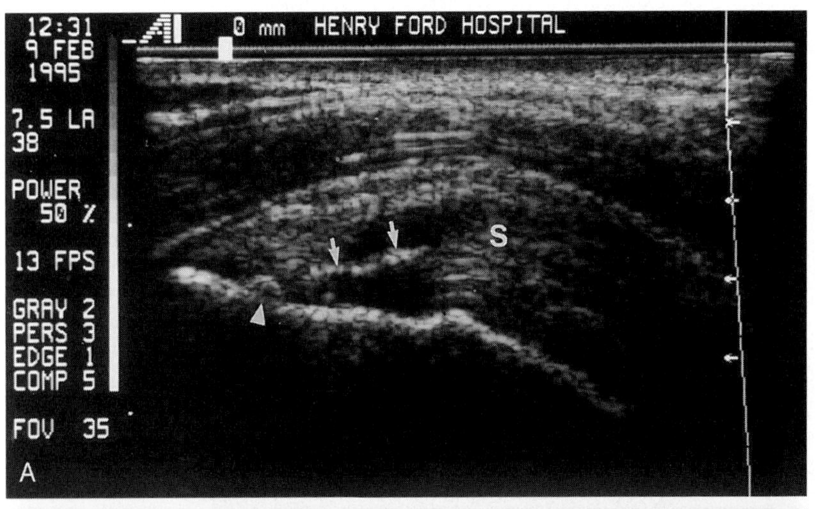

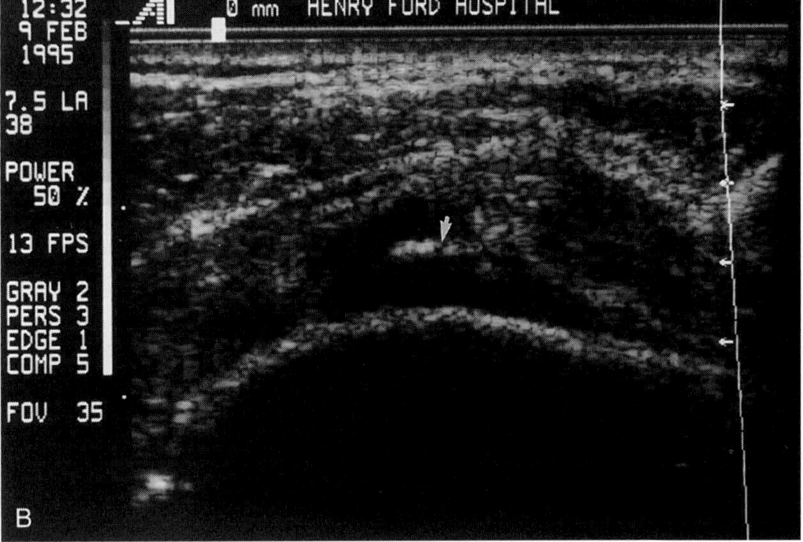

Figure 7–23 ■ **A**, Echogenic interface within the "critical zone": longitudinal sonogram. Radiographs and electromyographic studies were unremarkable in this 55-year-old male with localized tenderness over the deltoid insertion. A sharply defined echogenic line (*small arrows*) is outlined by a hypoechoic halo in the critical zone of the supraspinatus tendon (*S*), indicating the site of a partial thickness tear. Osseous irregularity (*arrowhead*). **B**, Echogenic interface within the critical zone: transverse sonogram. Same patient as in **A**. Again, a well-defined echogenic line (*arrow*) is surrounded by decreased echogenicity at the critical zone. The shape and size of the lesion did not change significantly with transducer realignment. This partial-thickness tear was confirmed at arthroscopy.

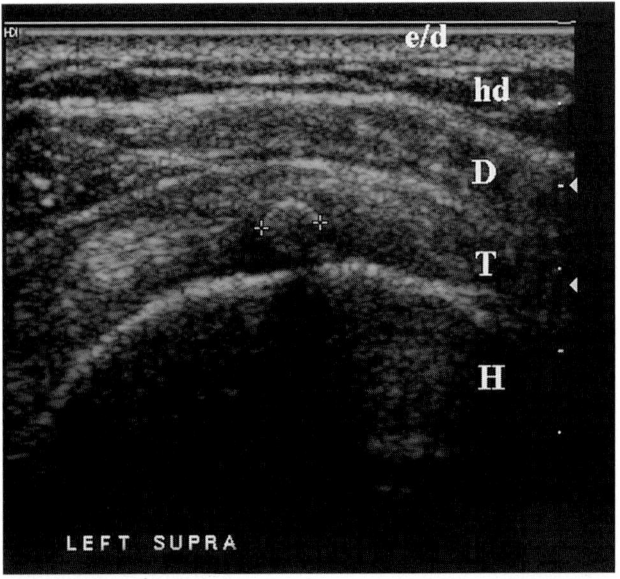

Figure 7–24 ■ Intratendinous calcification: transverse sonogram. A 48-year-old secretary presented with chronic left shoulder pain. A curvilinear hyperechoic line (*between the calipers*) with acoustic shadowing is seen within the deep portion of the supraspinatus tendon. The shape of the lesion and the presence of acoustic shadowing distinguish this calcification from a partial-thickness tear. However, regions of decreased echogenicity corresponding to tendon inflammation may surround these calcifications. This may make the definitive diagnosis more difficult, but the presence of acoustic shadowing leads to the correct diagnosis. Abbreviations: epidermis/dermis (*e/d*), hypoderm (*hd*), deltoid (*D*); supraspinatus tendon (*T*), humerus (*H*).

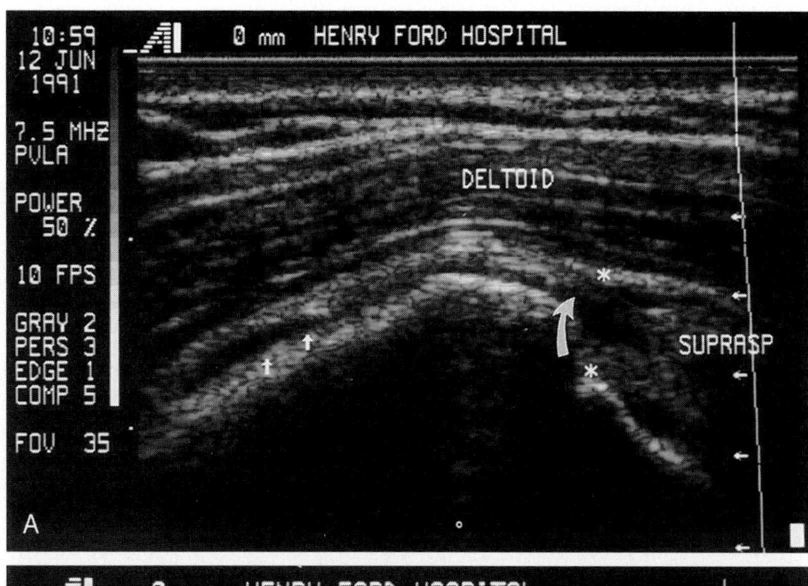

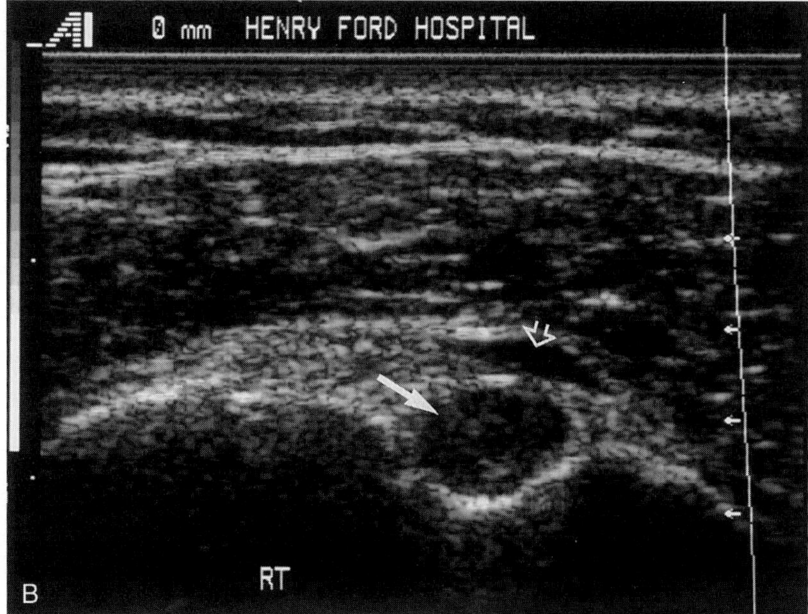

Figure 7–25 ■ **A**, Bursal fluid: longitudinal sonogram. After a fall on his outstretched arm, this 50-year-old man continues to complain of pain with movement of the shoulder. This longitudinal sonogram shows that the supraspinatus tendon is focally avulsed from the greater tuberosity. Hyperechoic peribursal fat (*) and the cortical surface of the greater tuberosity (*) are more closely approximated but are separated by a thin layer of anechoic fluid (*curved arrow*). Increased fluid (*arrows*) is also noted within the subacromial-subdeltoid bursa beyond the greater tuberosity. **B**, Bursal fluid: transverse sonogram. Same patient as in **A.** Increased fluid in the biceps tendon sheath (*arrow*) and in the bursal space (*open arrow*) is a common finding in rotator cuff disease. This fluid is in separate anatomical spaces, which closely approximate each other in this region anteriorly. When this combination of findings is observed, it is almost pathognomonic for a rotator cuff tear.

of symptoms, but complete remission of pain is very rare. In most cases the pain returns, often recurring in association with a seemingly insignificant trauma. Typically, patients with rotator cuff tears report that their pain is worse at night.

Many rotator cuff tears are completely asymptomatic, as demonstrated by a number of screening studies. It is not clear what factors determine which lesions will become painful. The size of the tear alone does not seem to be the factor determining if a pain syndrome results. Very large tears may remain asymptomatic, while small tears can cause disabling pain. A recent sonographic screening study of 100 volunteers discovered a high incidence of rotator cuff tears in pain-free shoulders (Milgrom et al., 1995). In addition, many of these patients had small effusions in either the biceps tendon sheath or the subacromial-subdeltoid bursa. Similar results have been reported in the MRI literature when normal shoulders were examined (Miniaci et al., 1995; Raven, 1995; Sher et al., 1995). This high incidence of rotator cuff tears has been confirmed in several cadaver studies (Keyes, 1933; Lindblom and Palmer, 1939; De Sèze et al., 1961). Therefore, the clinical significance of rotator cuff findings must be carefully evaluated in patients over the age of 50 years. In these cases, clinical judgment is the most important factor in distinguishing asymptomatic from symptomatic rotator cuff lesions. The sonographic identification of a rotator cuff tear should not stop the clinician from considering other possible causes of shoulder pain. In addition, the sono-

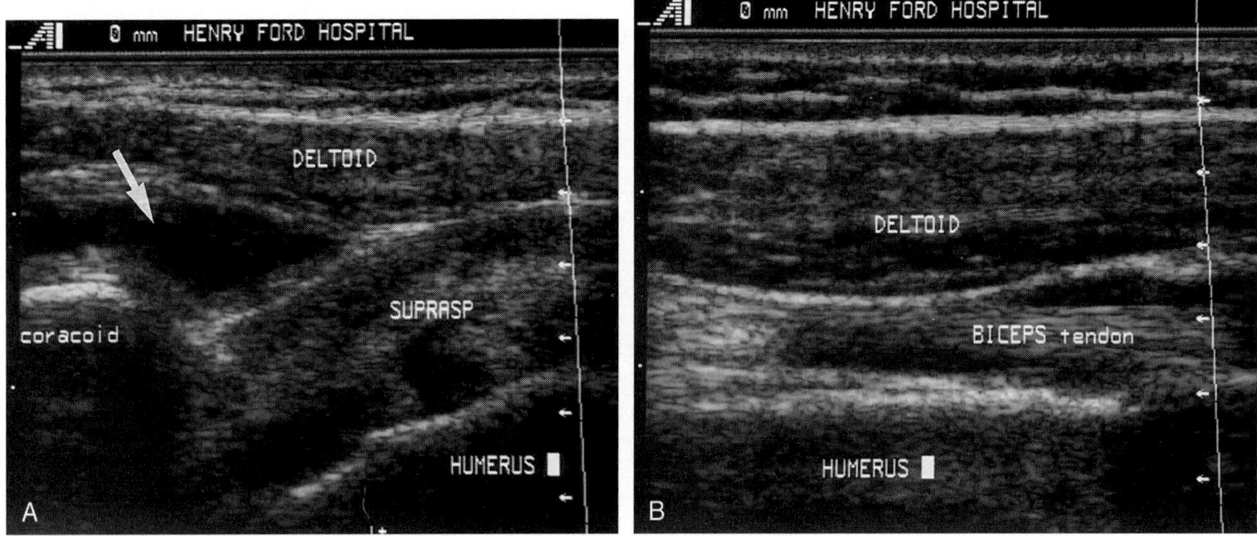

Figure 7–26 ■ **A**, Synovitis in rotator cuff disease: transverse sonogram. This 45-year-old male presented with constant intolerable pain in the left shoulder. A full-thickness rotator cuff tear was diagnosed sonographically. Fluid collecting in the subdeltoid bursa (*arrow*) may be seen as far medially as the coracoid process. **B**, Synovitis in rotator cuff disease: longitudinal sonogram. Same patient as in **A**. Fluid is seen in the tendon sheath of the long head of the biceps, both deep and superficial to the tendon. In over 50% of cases, fluid within the biceps tendon sheath is associated with a rotator cuff tear.

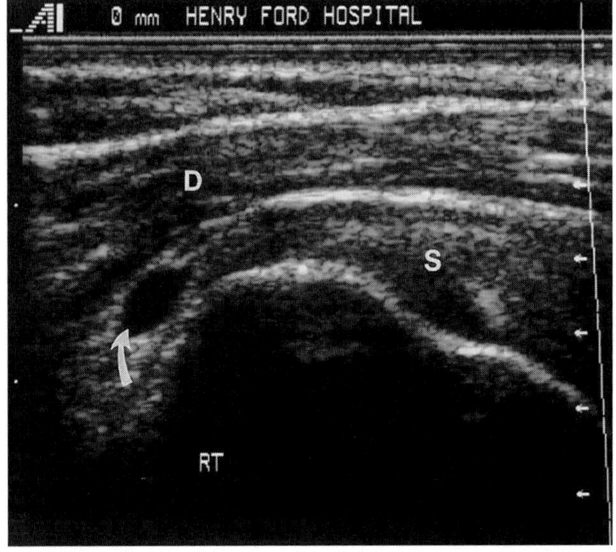

Figure 7–27 ■ Loculated fluid in the subacromial-subdeltoid bursa: longitudinal sonogram. A 53-year-old female presented with symptoms of impingement, but no rotator cuff tear was demonstrated sonographically. Anechoic fluid (*curved arrow*) is present within the subacromial-subdeltoid bursa. No change in the configuration of this fluid was observed with compression, appearing loculated. The presence of increased fluid within the bursa in the absence of a rotator cuff tear is rare. Abbreviations: deltoid (*D*), supraspinatus (*S*).

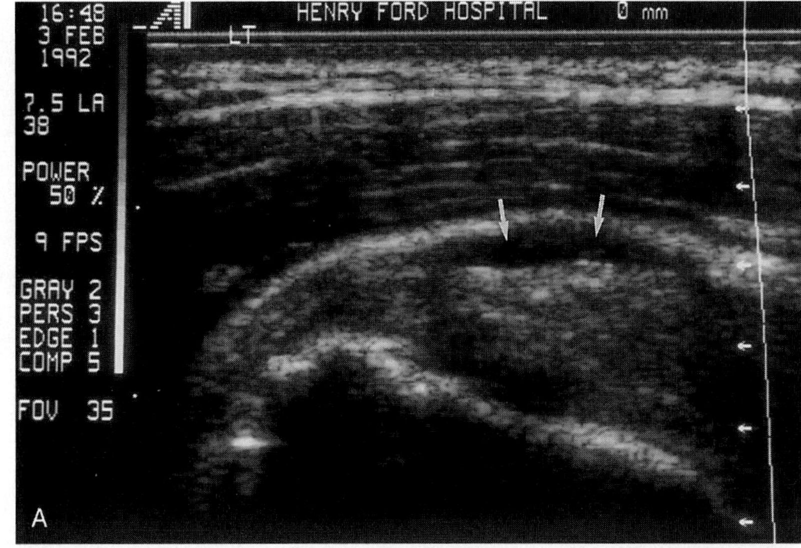

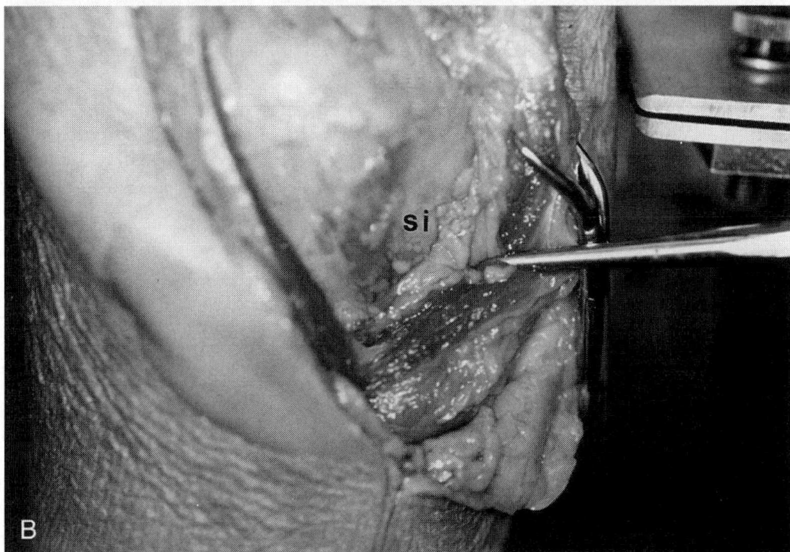

Figure 7–28 ■ **A**, Synovial thickening of the subacromial-subdeltoid bursa: longitudinal sonogram. A cadaveric shoulder specimen was scanned, demonstrating hypoechoic thickening (*arrows*) of the bursa. Pressure applied with the transducer did not deform this thickening. **B**, Synovial thickening of the subacromial-subdeltoid bursa: photograph of dissection. Dissection of the specimen to examine the subacromial-subdeltoid bursa was performed. Irregular synovial thickening (*si*) was observed on both superficial and deep walls of the bursa. "Rice bodies" within the bursa observed during surgical exploration of a joint are probably secondary to chronic irritation.

graphic examination should always be interpreted in conjunction with conventional radiographs. In an older patient population, it is not uncommon to discover evidence of osseous metastases, myeloma, or a Pancoast tumor on radiographic examination. Limited range of motion and pain on shoulder elevation can be due to a number of disease processes, of which rotator cuff disease is the most common. However, simultaneous occurrence of a full-thickness rotator cuff tear with a concurrent neoplasm involving or adjacent to the shoulder is not rare in our experience.

Patients with rotator cuff disease will usually consult their primary care physician or may present to the emergency room with a history of pain following acute trauma. In most cases, a radiograph will be obtained and is usually interpreted as normal. The patient will often be assured that nothing is wrong with the shoulder and will be sent home with a prescription for a nonsteroidal anti-inflammatory agent. It has been postulated that tendon fiber failure will continue, with recurrent episodes of pain associated with microtrauma (Matsen and Arntz, 1990). The patient is finally referred to an orthopedic surgeon after enduring pain for months or even years. At that point, the patient is so uncomfortable that he or she is willing to submit to invasive diagnostic studies such as arthrography, MR arthrography, and even arthroscopy. The cuff changes identified at this late stage are often full-

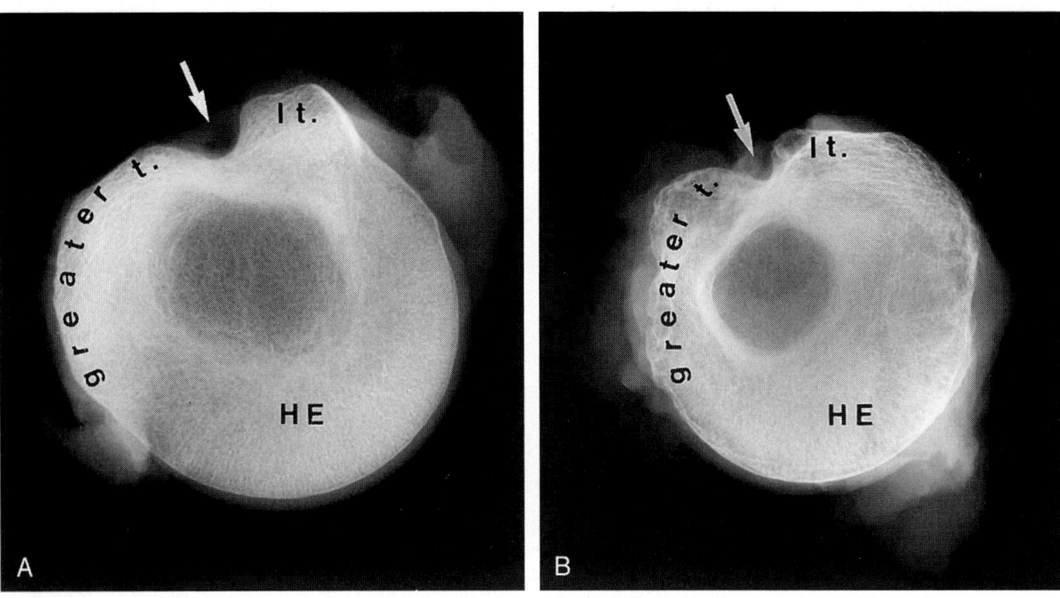

Figure 7-29 ■ **A**, Normal humeral head: axial radiograph. Smooth-flowing cortical contours are seen in this axial radiograph of a normal cadaveric humeral head. The rotator cuff in this specimen was normal. Abbreviations: lesser tuberosity (*lt.*), bicipital groove (*arrow*), humeral epiphysis (*HE*). **B**, Osseous degeneration associated with rotator cuff tears: axial radiograph. A large, complete supraspinatus tear was present in this cadaveric specimen. Note the marked cortical irregularity involving the greater tuberosity. Abbreviations: lesser tuberosity (*lt.*), bicipital groove (*arrow*), humeral epiphysis (*HE*).

thickness, and some are inoperable due to the extent of the tear. Clearly, there is a great need for noninvasive diagnostic imaging utilized earlier in the disease process. It is not usually necessary to perform more than one conventional radiographic examination of the shoulder prior to sonographic evaluation of the rotator cuff. The ultrasound examination may be performed on the patient's initial visit following radiography. This strategy would eliminate repetitive radiographic examinations and expedite the patient's therapy, resulting in significant cost savings.

Aging seems to be the strongest etiological factor in the degenerative process affecting the rotator cuff and the long head of the biceps tendon. Therefore, we choose the shoulder as a typical example of age-related tendon tears. Asymptomatic tendon tears are frequently observed in the shoulder, as discussed above, but asymptomatic tears are not observed elsewhere in the musculoskeletal system. Focal regions of tendon degeneration are commonly observed and frequently remain asymptomatic. We examined the tendons of 95 adolescents entering the athletic program at their school. Their mean age was 18 years, and the group was comprised of 52 males and 43 females. The quadriceps, patellar, and Achilles tendons were examined bilaterally, resulting in a total of 190 tendons of each type. Hypoechoic changes and swelling of the tendon was observed in seven patellar, two quadriceps, and two Achilles tendons. Two of the lesions had been symptomatic in the past but were asymptomatic at the time of the examination. These findings of tendon degeneration were not observed in a control group of 40 sedentary students with identical age profiles. We feel that in addition to age-related changes, repetitive stress will also result in degenerative tendinopathy, which is usually asymptomatic. These findings are supported by the work of other investigators (Khan et al., 1996, 1997). A recent study demonstrated that hypoechoic changes can precede symptoms or persist after resolution of symptoms in cases of patellar tendinosis. It is only speculation, but it appears likely that these subclinical lesions predispose tendons to subsequent rupture. This supposition is supported in part by the increased incidence of tendon rupture in patients who are more physically active.

Text continued on page 221

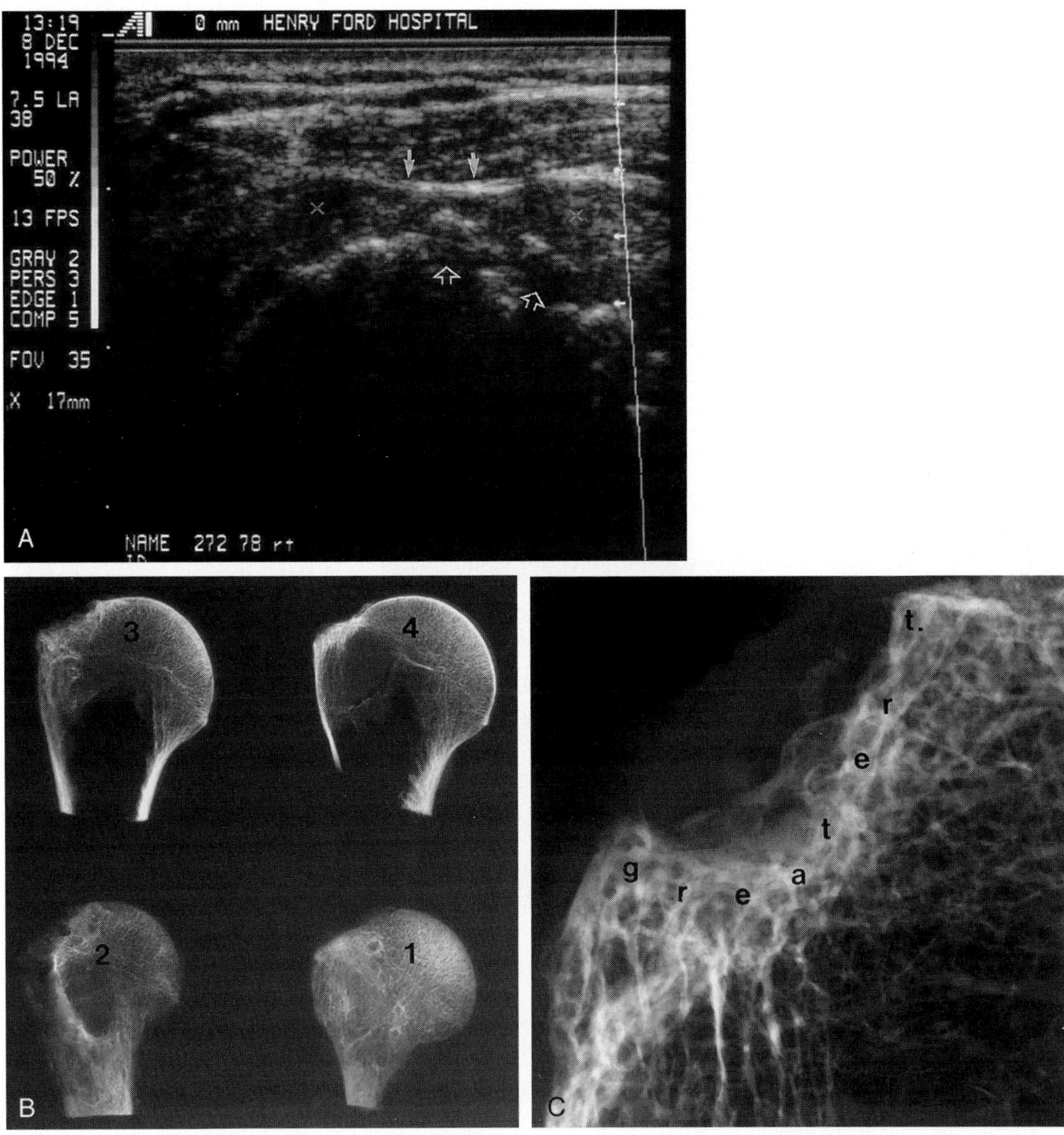

Figure 7-30 ■ **A**, Large full-thickness supraspinatus tear: transverse sonogram. Complete absence of the rotator cuff is seen, with a bony irregularity (*open arrows*) extending over the entire length of the tear. The width of the tear was measured at 17 mm (*calipers*). Note the displacement of the peribursal fat (*arrows*) and deltoid muscle into the defect created by the absent rotator cuff. **B**, Large full-thickness supraspinatus tear: section radiographs. The humeral head of the specimen imaged in **A** was sectioned coronally into four 1-cm-thick sections, and this radiograph was obtained. Section 1 is the most anterior segment containing the lesser tuberosity. The cortical surface of the lesser tuberosity is relatively smooth. The bicipital groove and the anterior third of the greater tuberosity are included in section 2. Marked cortical irregularity is present along the surface of the greater tuberosity and the anterior neck of the humerus. Section 3 contains the middle third of the greater tuberosity. Hypertrophic and erosive degenerative changes are seen in the cortex of the tuberosity. Section 4 contains the posterior third of the greater tuberosity, showing minimal cortical irregularity. **C**, Large full-thickness supraspinatus tear: microradiograph. A subsection of the greater tuberosity from section 3 in **B** was obtained and radiographed with magnification. The erosion and fragmentation of the greater tuberosity surface are better appreciated.

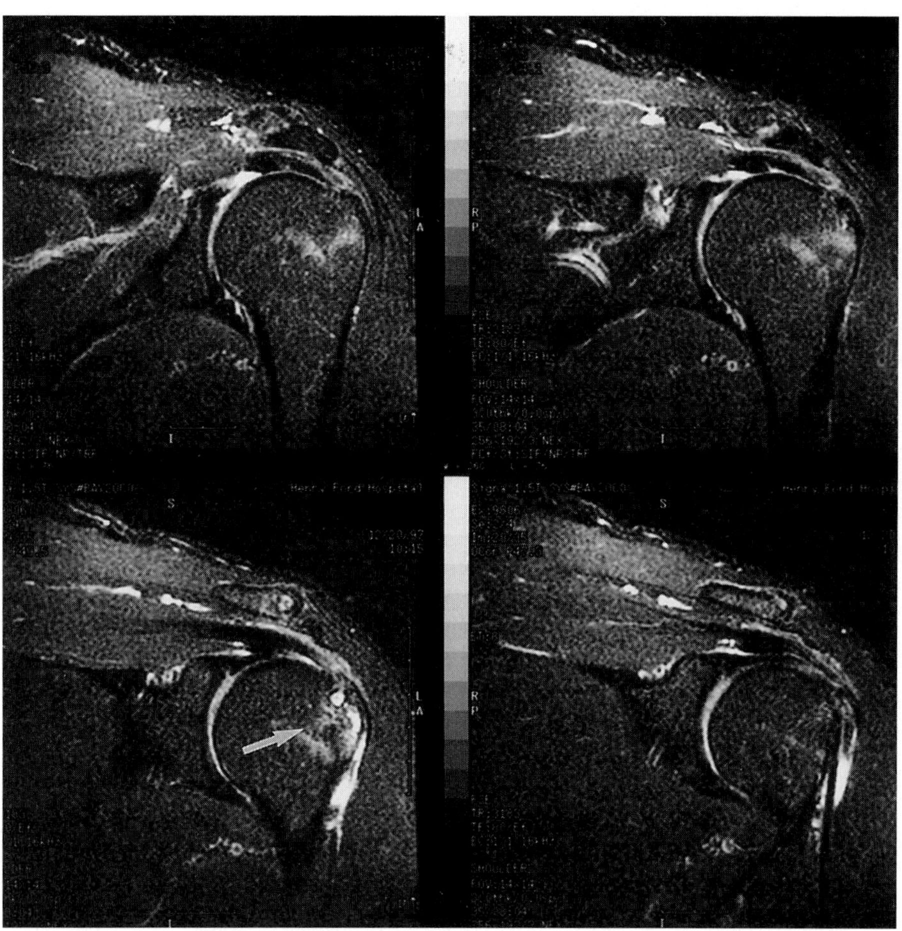

Figure 7–31 ■ Changes of the tuberosity surface and bone marrow: coronal MRI (T_2-weighted). It is rare to observe greater tuberosity changes on MRI studies. This patient has a full-thickness tear. The greater tuberosity bone surface and the bone marrow show abnormalities. The high signal intensity in the marrow is compatible with an inflammatory or a posttraumatic process as the cause for the change. Note that the malformation is most pronounced in the section deep to the biceps tendon groove (*arrow*).

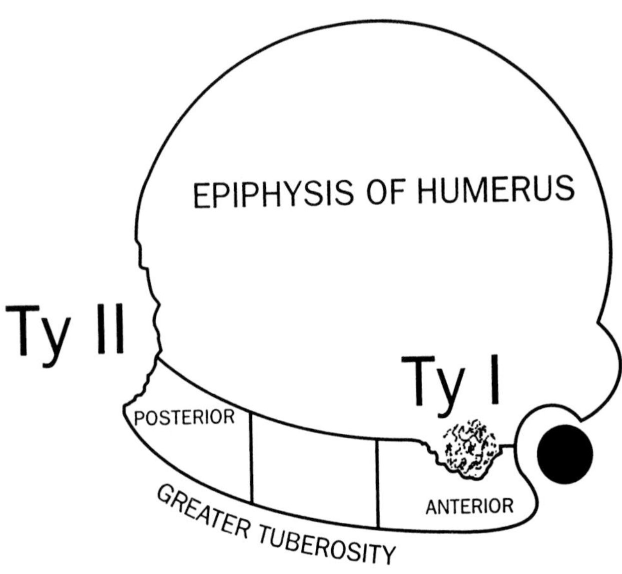

Figure 7–32 ■ Degenerative changes of the greater tuberosity: diagrammatic representation. In clinical practice, we observe two types of degenerative change involving the greater tuberosity. Type 1 changes involve the anterior aspect of the tuberosity and are almost always associated with partial- or full-thickness tears of the rotator cuff. Type 2 changes involve the posterior third of the greater tuberosity and the posterior surface of the anatomical neck of the humerus. The significance of the type 2 findings is not fully understood.

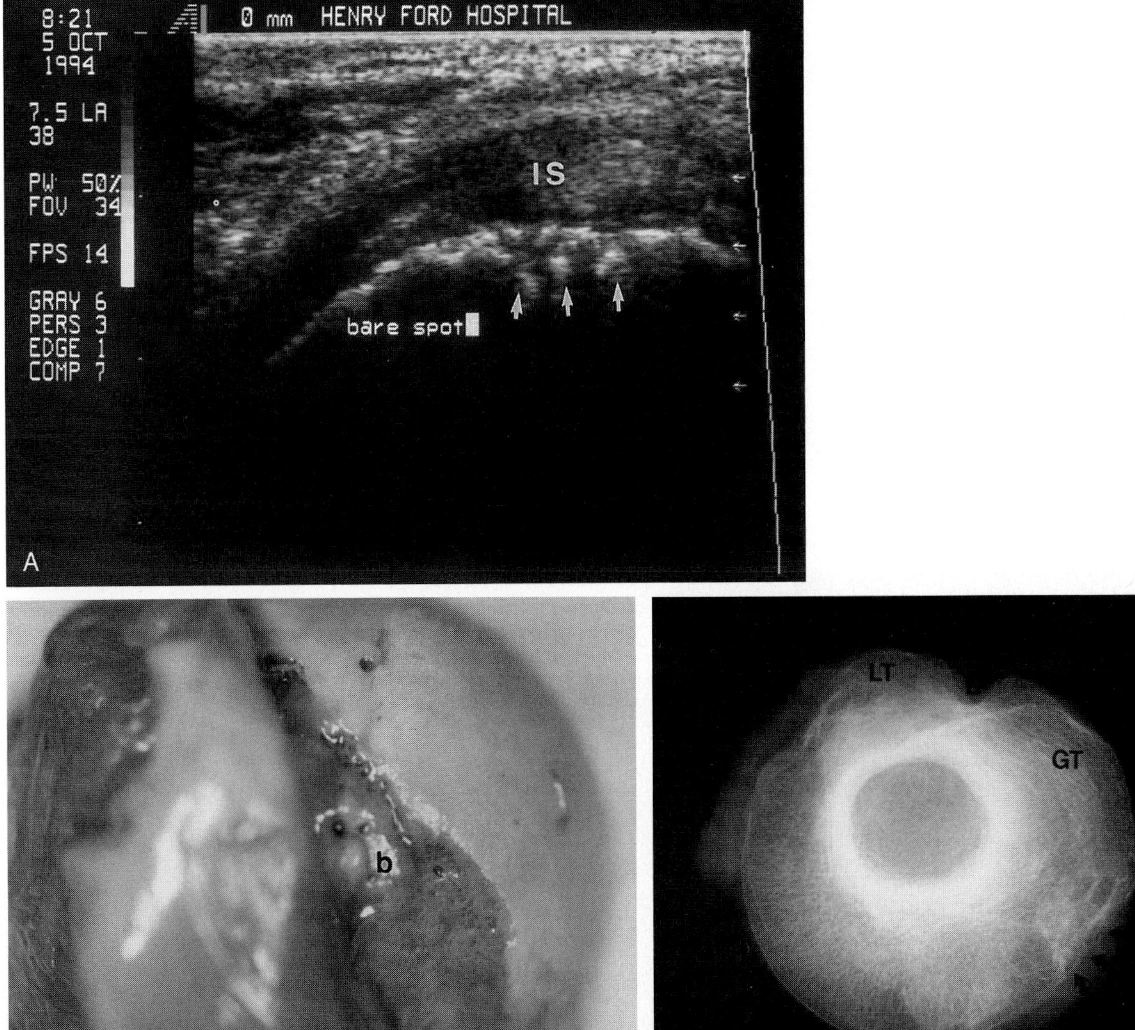

Figure 7–33 ■ **A**, Posterior greater tuberosity degenerative change: transverse sonogram. Pitting (*small arrows*) is observed along the posterior humeral neck in this image of a cadaver specimen deep to the infraspinatus tendon (*IS*). These changes are type 2 tuberosity changes. **B**, Posterior greater tuberosity degenerative change: specimen photograph. Same specimen shown in **A**. The cortical changes involving the posterior aspect of the greater tuberosity and anatomical neck lie in an area referred to as the *bare area* (*b*). This term was coined by arthroscopists because this region is often not covered by synovium. It often appears irregular. **C**, Posterior greater tuberosity degenerative change: specimen radiograph. An axial radiograph of this specimen was obtained. The bare area (*curved arrows*) is seen posteriorly as a segment of cortical irregularity distant from the anterior greater tuberosity (*GT*). Abbreviation: lesser tuberosity (*LT*).

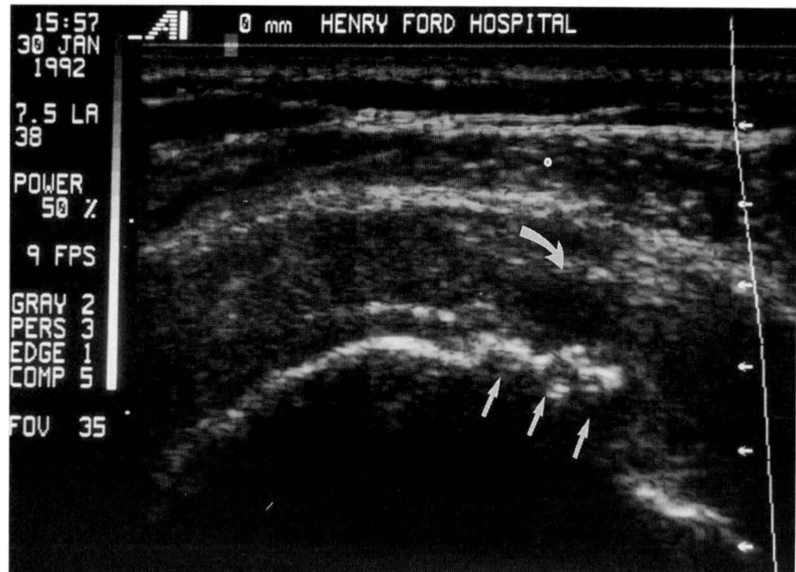

Figure 7–34 ■ Degenerative cortical changes: transverse sonogram. This 56-year-old female experienced increasing shoulder pain over the past month which was exacerbated by household work. A hypoechoic lesion (*curved arrow*) is demonstrated within the tendon of the rotator cuff superficial to a region of cortical irregularity (*arrows*). Cortical changes deep to a tendon abnormality reinforce the suspicion of a tear. A full-thickness tear of the rotator cuff was confirmed by arthroscopy.

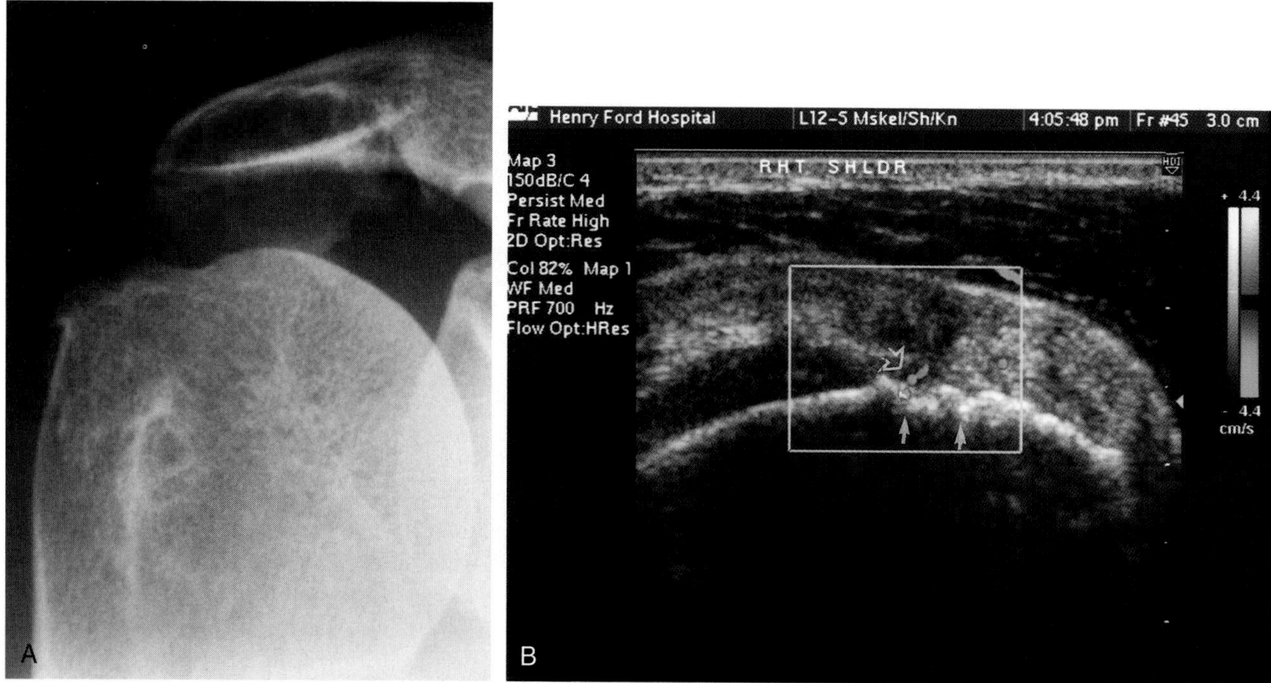

Figure 7–35 ■ **A**, Hypervascularity at site of tendon injury: anteroposterior radiograph. Degenerative changes of the cortex of the greater tuberosity are seen on this frontal radiograph of a 50-year-old automobile assembly line worker. He had experienced increasing pain during the repetitive lifting required in his job. Often these changes are overlooked when interpreting conventional radiographs of the shoulder. **B**, Hypervascularity at a site of tendon injury: transverse sonogram with power Doppler. A tendon lesion is present adjacent to the area of cortical irregularity (*arrows*). This region demonstrates increased vascularity, with bridging vessels (*arrowhead*) from the cortex to the diseased tendon.

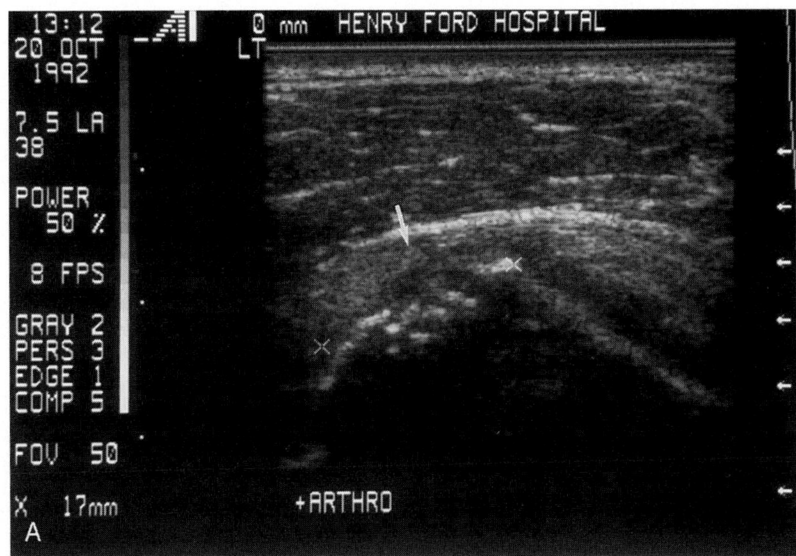

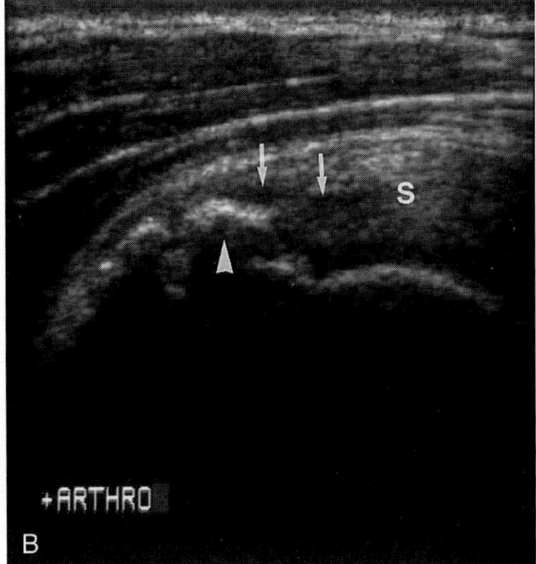

Figure 7–36 ■ **A**, Cortical changes associated with a full-thickness tear: transverse sonogram. After 5 months away from work due to disabling pain, this 43-year-old male presented for imaging evaluation of the left shoulder. He had to support the left shoulder carefully with pillows in order to sleep. Marked pitting of the cortical surface of the humerus (*x-x*) is present, associated with focal thinning of the tendon (*arrow*). **B**, Cortical changes associated with a full-thickness tear: longitudinal sonogram. Same patient as in **A**. This longitudinal image shows that the extent of the osseous irregularity (*arrowhead*) involves the full width of the tendon insertion. The tuberosity changes in **A** seem predominantly resorptive; in contrast, in this figure, they seem more proliferative instead. A hypoechoic cleft (*arrows*) separates the torn end of the tendon from the bone. Abbreviation: torn supraspinatos (*S*).

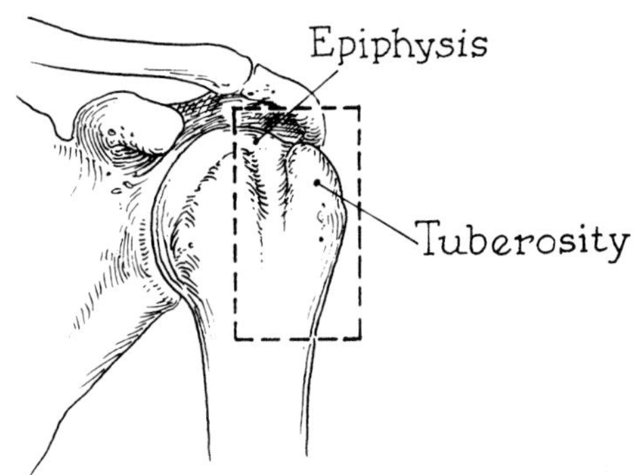

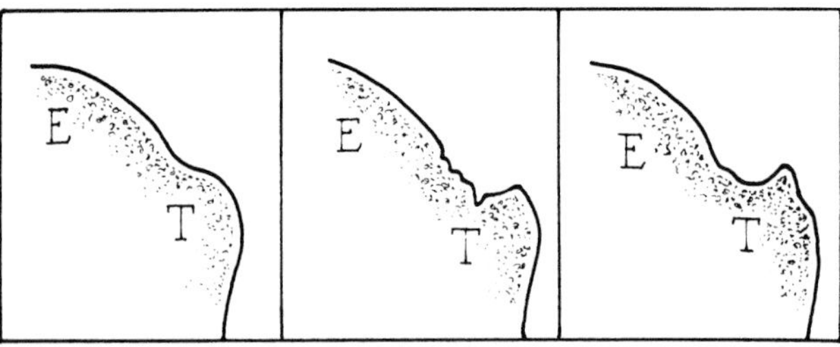

Figure 7-37 ■ Diagram of the contour of the normal and abnormal greater tuberosity. The degenerative bone changes observed in rotator cuff disease most frequently occur in the region indicated by the rectangle. The normal contour of the bone of the proximal humeral epiphysis (*E*) and greater tuberosity (*T*) is shown in the diagram at the bottom left. The two other diagrams depict common tuberosity changes in rotator cuff tendinopathy. The bone lesions can look like inflammatory erosions and can be predominantly destructive. However, the more typical lesions will have both areas of bone resorption and bone proliferation.

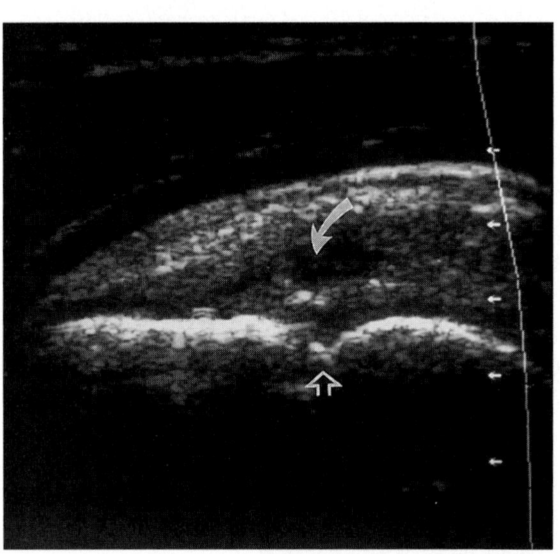

Figure 7-38 ■ Partial-thickness supraspinatus tendon tear: longitudinal sonogram. This 45-year-old radiological technologist experienced chronic shoulder pain when lifting patients. A small region of mixed echogenicity is noted in the deep portion of the supraspinatus tendon on this longitudinal image. The lesion (a "rim rent") is located directly over the anatomical neck of the humerus (*curved arrow*), as described by Codman (1934). The underlying cortical surface is irregular (*open arrow*).

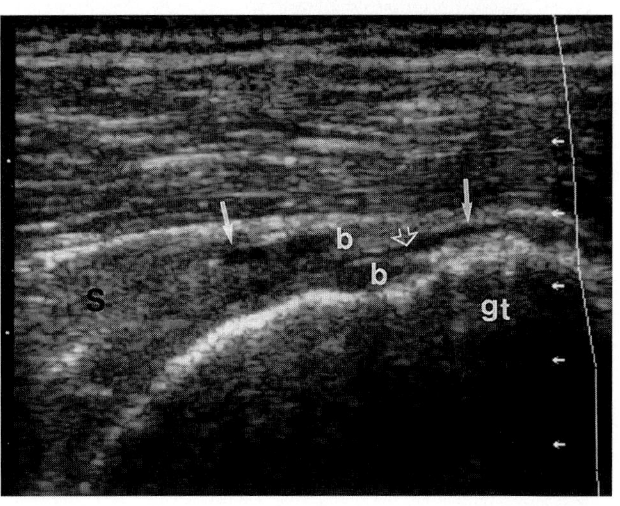

Figure 7-39 ■ Bursal thickening replacing tendon substance in a full-thickness tear: longitudinal sonogram. After a fall while shoveling snow, this 52-year-old female experienced severe pain and complete loss of shoulder elevation. She presented for imaging evaluation 4 months after her injury. Her clinical function had not improved with conservative management. The supraspinatus tendon (*S*) is retracted from its insertion (*arrows*) on the greater tuberosity (*gt*). Echogenic thickening of the bursal walls (*b*) fills the defect created by the torn supraspinatus tendon. Fluid within the bursal lumen (*open arrow*) is seen more closely approximating the surface of the greater tuberosity.

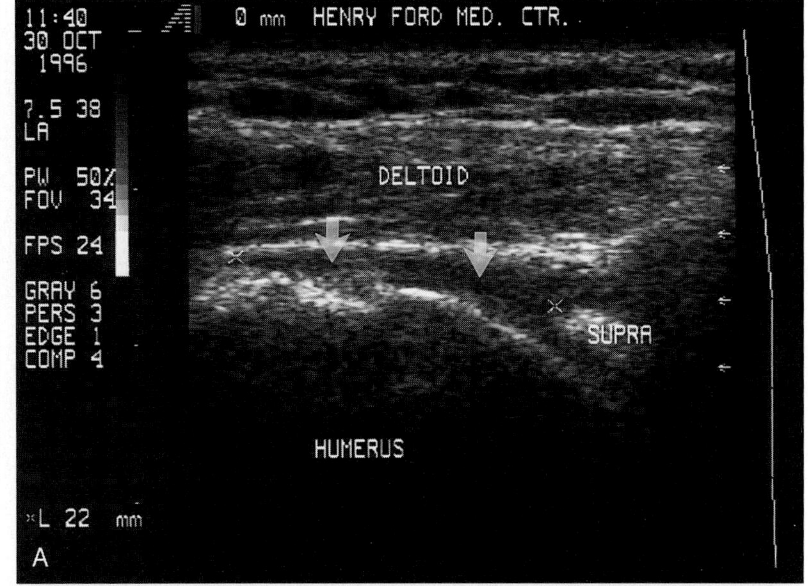

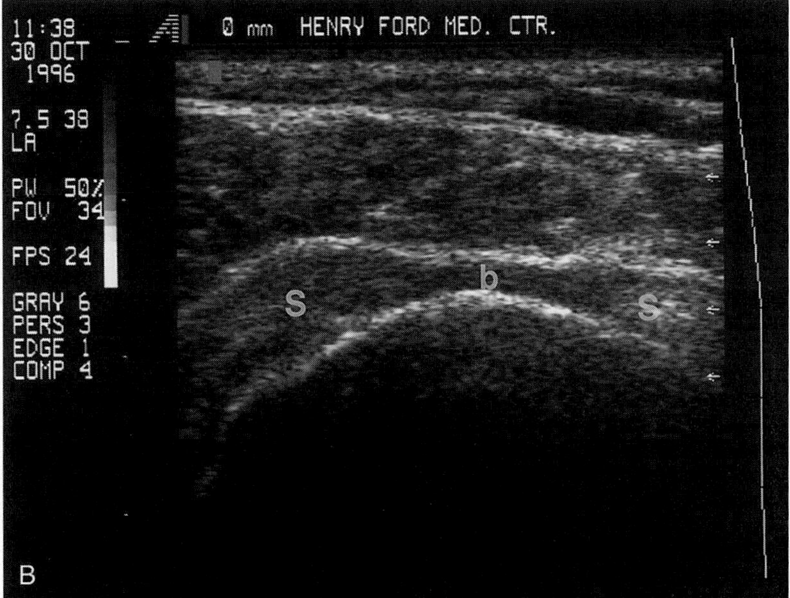

Figure 7-40 ■ **A**, Tendon retraction in a full-thickness tear: longitudinal sonogram. Five years ago, this 52-year-old male sustained a shoulder injury, with pain and minor limitation of shoulder range of motion. A prolonged rehabilitation program failed to improve his level of function. Shoulder pain limits his ability to play golf. He presents for preoperative evaluation prior to his retirement to Florida. The retracted stump of the supraspinatus tendon is seen over the humeral epiphysis. Retraction of the tendon is measured (*x-x*). Synovial thickening (*arrows*) of the bursal wall fills the retraction defect. This was demonstrated not to be fluid by compression applied with the transducer. **B**, Tendon retraction in a full-thickness tear: transverse sonogram. Same patient as in Figure **A**. The torn ends of the supraspinatus tendon (*S*) are separated by synovial thickening of the bursa wall (*b*).

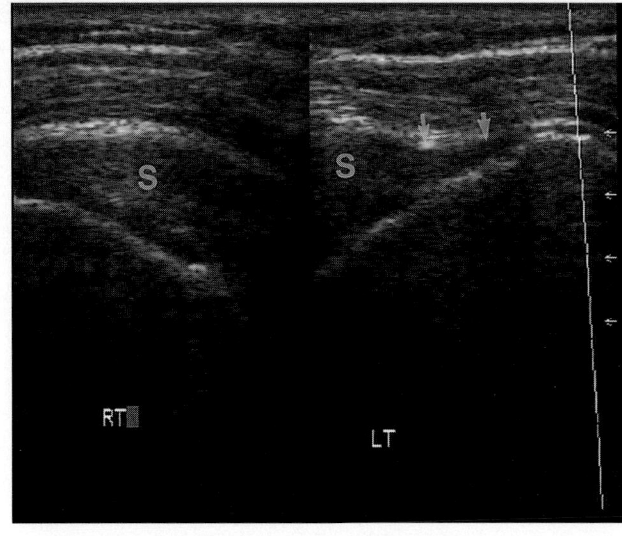

Figure 7-41 ■ Retracted supraspinatus tendon: longitudinal sonogram. Side-by-side comparison is shown in this split-frame longitudinal image of the supraspinatus tendons of a 56-year-old female with left shoulder pain. The pain developed while the patient was on crutches after bilateral total hip replacements. Retraction of the left (*LT*) supraspinatus tendon (*S*) has created a defect into which the subacromial-subdeltoid bursa and deltoid muscle have herniated. Hyperechoic peribursal fat (*arrows*) approximates the surface of the greater tuberosity. Normal anatomical relationships are demonstrated in the right (*RT*) shoulder.

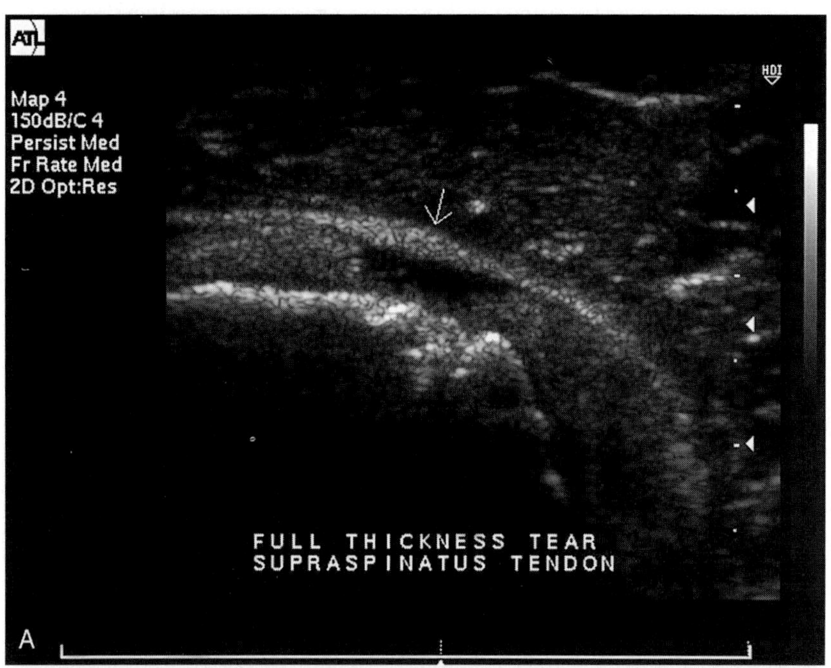

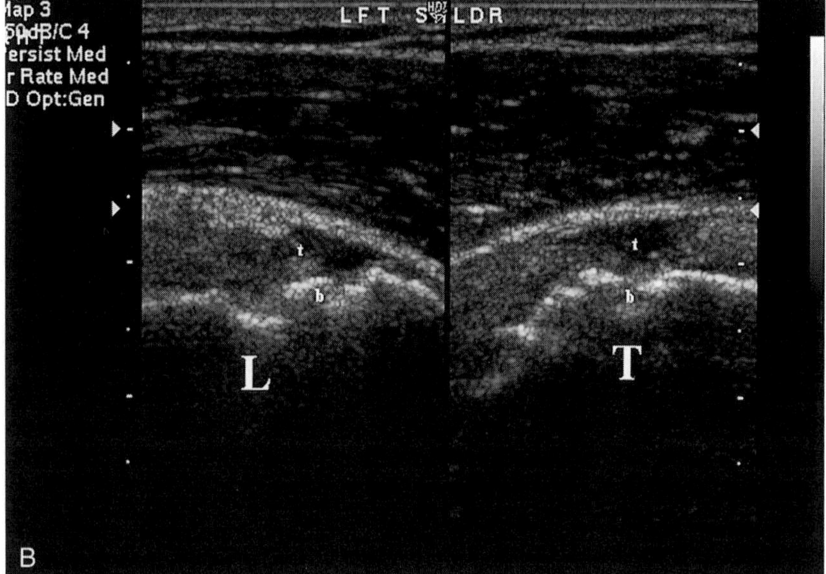

Figure 7–42 ■ **A**, Osseous irregularity associated with a full-thickness tear: transverse sonogram. A 48-year-old male presents with chronic throbbing pain of the left shoulder. A fluid-filled cleft (*arrow*) is demonstrated in the supraspinatus tendon. Cortical irregularity of the greater tuberosity deep to this lesion mirrors the dimension of the tear. **B**, Osseous irregularity associated with a full-thickness tear: split screen, longitudinal/transverse sonograms. Same patient as in **A**. These detailed, magnified images better demonstrate the degree of cortical irregularity associated with the tendon defect. Abbreviations: tendon tear (*t*), bone change (*b*), longitudinal image (*L*), transverse image (*T*).

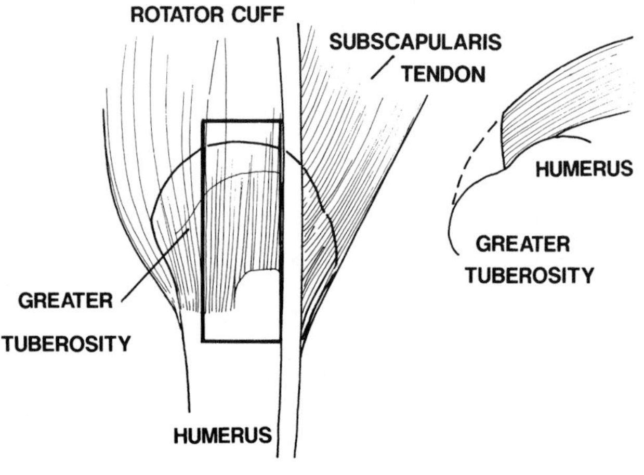

Figure 7–43 ■ Horizontal supraspinatus tears: diagrammatic representation. The diagram on the left demonstrates a horizontal tear from the surgeon's perspective. On the right, the corresponding anatomy is shown as it would be seen in a longitudinal sonographic image. The position of the transducer is shown by the rectangle in the image on the left. Horizontal tears comprise the vast majority of small rotator cuff tears.

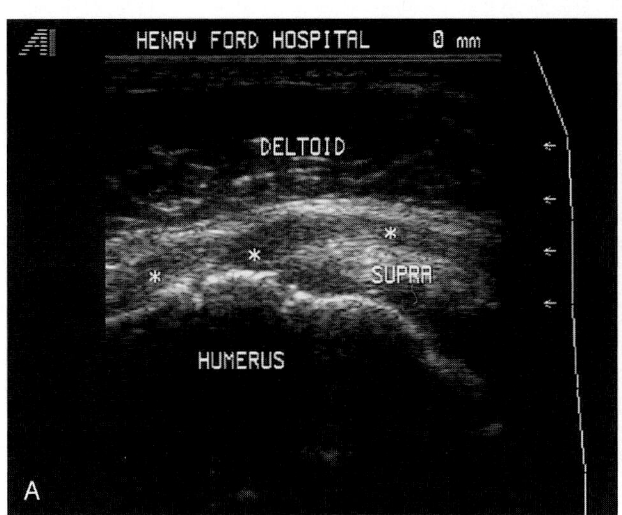

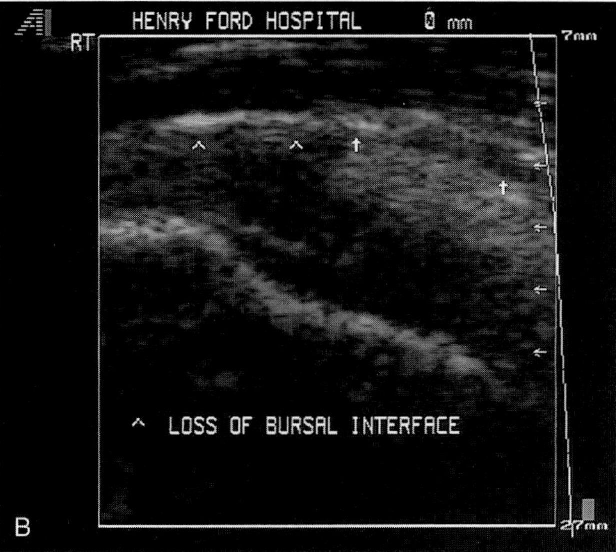

Figure 7–44 ■ **A**, Reactive bursal thickening: transverse sonogram. This 62-year-old female was treated conservatively for left shoulder pain. During the course of treatment, she received two intra-articular steroid injections. Marked thickening of the subacromial-subdeltoid bursa (*) fills the defect created by the full-thickness tear of the supraspinatus tendon. Note that the cortical irregularity of the greater tuberosity closely reflects the extent of the full-thickness tear. **B**, Reactive bursal thickening: longitudinal sonogram. Same patient as in **A**. The interface between the echogenic tendon and the bursa is clearly defined (*small arrows*). This allows accurate measurement of the extent of tendon retraction.

Tendinosis

In addition to the tendons of the rotator cuff, other tendons are affected by age related degenerative change (Figs. 7–49 through 7–52). The Achilles tendon is much more susceptible to rupture in a 40-year-old athlete than in a 20-year-old athlete. A significant difference is that tendinosis and rupture of the Achilles tendon have a higher correlation with the patient's level of physical activity than that seen in the rotator cuff. Acute traumatic tears of the Achilles tendon are less common when the tendon is normal. Acute tears usually extend through regions of tendinosis (Kannus and Jòzsa, 1991). We prefer the term *tendinosis*, rather than tendinitis because these lesions rarely contain inflammatory cells (Khan et al., 1996). Chronic overexertion in middle-aged athletes results in tendinosis and myx-

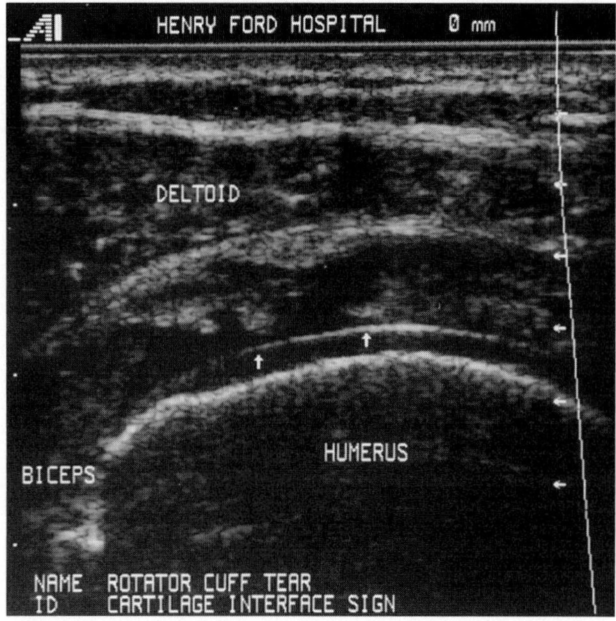

Figure 7–45 ■ Cartilage interface sign: transverse sonogram. After a fall on an outstretched arm, this 55-year-old male experienced severe shoulder pain. This transverse sonogram was obtained 1 week after his injury. Irregular tendon fragments are seen within an anechoic collection. A very echogenic line (*small arrows*) traces the surface of the articular cartilage of the humeral head. At surgery a full-thickness tear was found, which extended in the longitudinal axis of the tendon uncovering the humeral epiphysis.

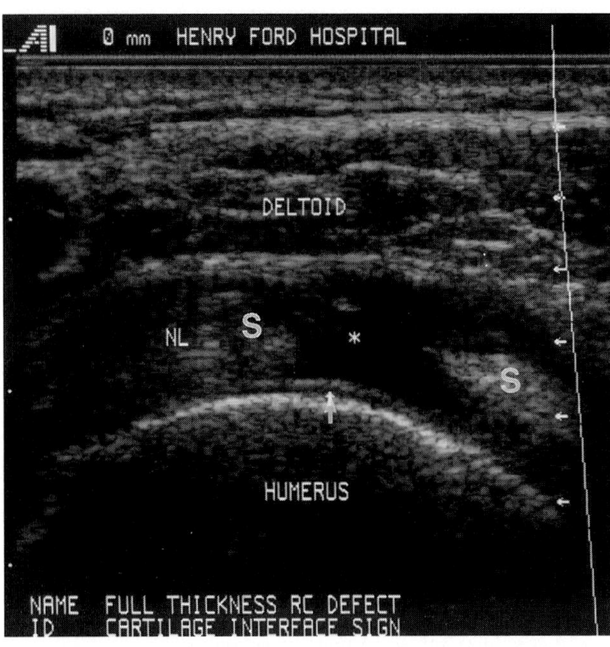

Figure 7–46 ■ Cartilage interface sign: transverse sonogram. This 29-year-old baseball player sustained a shoulder injury while sliding into home plate. An anechoic fluid collection (*) separates the torn ends of the supraspinatus tendon (*S*), creating a sonographic window to the cartilage surface (*small arrow*).

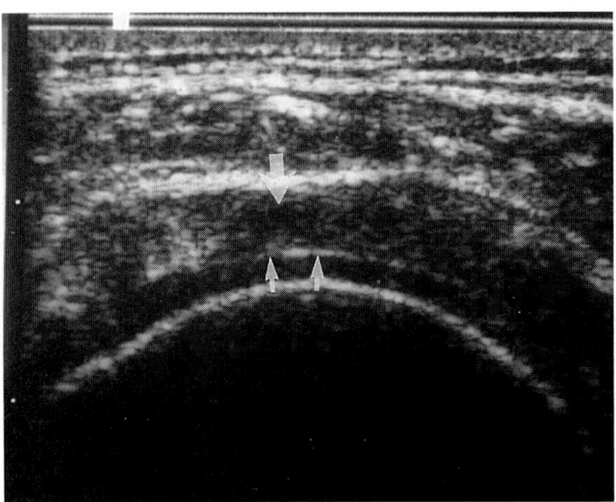

Figure 7–47 ■ Cartilage interface sign: transverse sonogram. The cartilage interface sign is most valuable when echogenic fluid fills the tendon defect. This transverse image illustrates the cartilage interface sign (*small arrows*) deep to a region of subtle abnormality within the supraspinatus tendon (*large arrow*). At surgery this proved to be a full-thickness tear 1 cm wide. The cartilage interface sign is the result of enhanced through-transmission associated with the fluid.

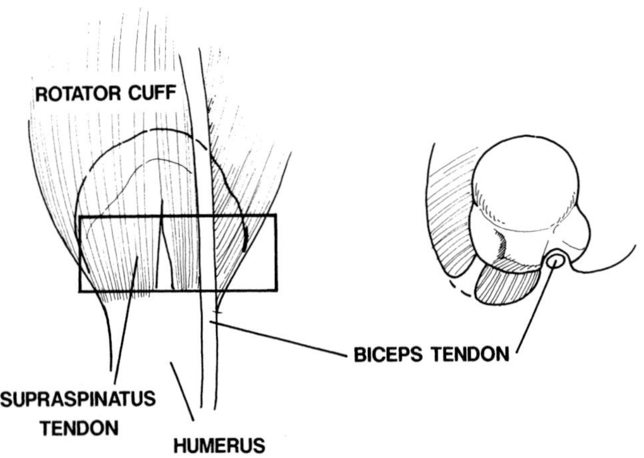

Figure 7–48 ■ Vertical supraspinatus tears: diagrammatic representation. Vertical tears are usually the result of acute traumatic injury. They are best visualized on transverse images. The cartilage interface sign is observed with vertical tears when they extend over the humeral epiphysis. Again, the diagram on the left depicts the surgeon's perspective, with the position of the transducer indicated by a rectangle. On the right is the diagrammatic representation of the corresponding ultrasound image.

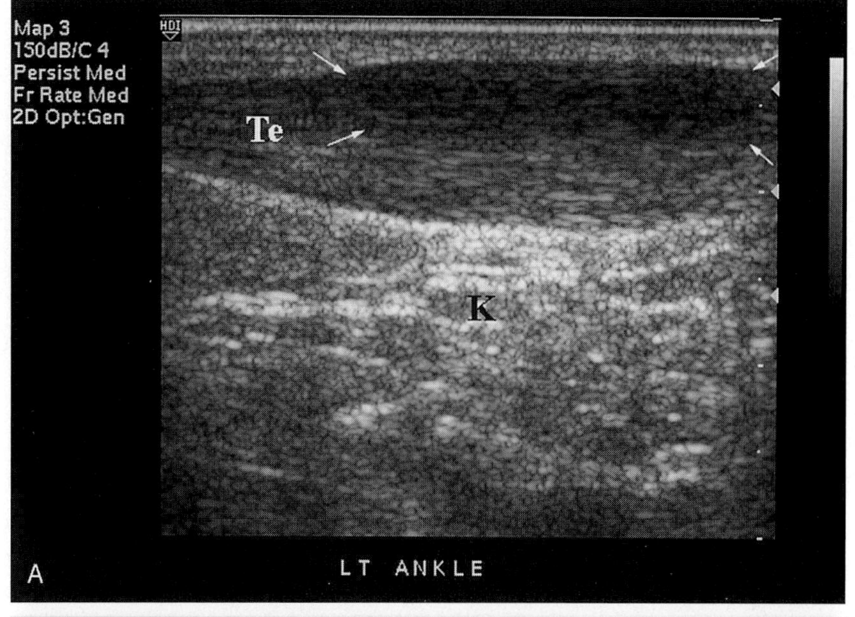

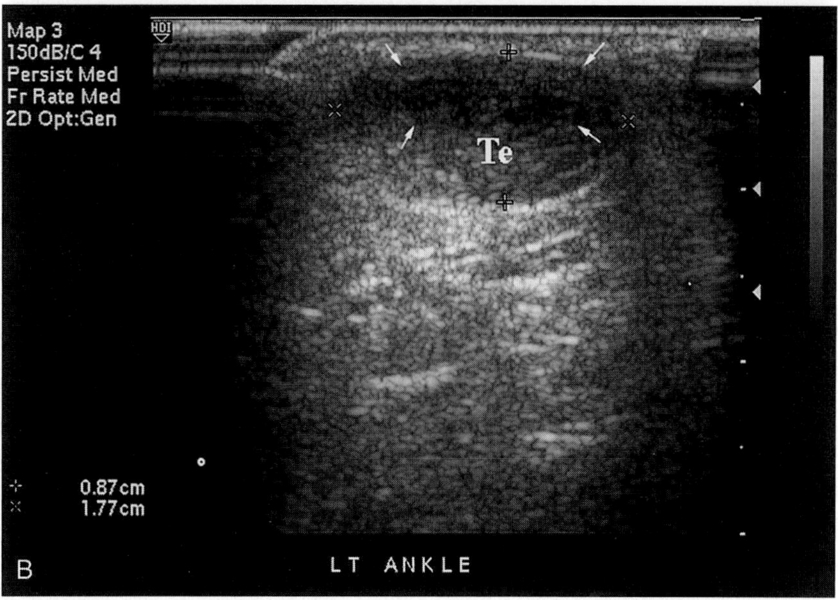

Figure 7-49 ■ **A**, Achilles tendinosis: longitudinal sonogram. The superficial portion of the Achilles tendon is markedly hypoechoic (*arrows*) in this 45-year-old jogger. The fibers involved are predominantly those contributed by the gastrocnemius. Marked diffuse thickening of the tendon, greater in the dorsal aspect, is also noted. The fibrillar pattern of the tendon is less apparent in the affected area, consistent with intratendinous degeneration. Abbreviations: Kager's fat pad (*K*); Achilles tendon (*Te*). **B**, Achilles tendinosis: transverse sonogram. Same patient as in **A**. Similar changes are seen in the transverse plane.

oid degeneration of the tendon (Martens et al., 1982; Khan et al., 1996). Some researchers have observed that all tendons which rupture spontaneously exhibit chronic disease histologically (Kannus and Jòzsa, 1991). They conclude that degenerative changes are relatively common in the general population. These lesions are commonly observed in individuals over 35 years of age and predispose the person to tendon rupture. Acute trauma is still the immediate cause of the tear, which occurs at the site of degeneration (Figs. 7-53 and 7-54). Kannus and Jòzsa detected hypoxic tendinopathy, mucoid degeneration, tendolipomatosis, and calcifying tendinopathy in 864 of 891 spontaneous tendon tears (Fig. 7-54). Similar findings have been observed in the tendons of race horses. Often ultrasound examination of a torn Achilles tendon will reveal areas of focal degeneration and calcification, which certainly predated the acute tear. Similarly, our examination of the contralateral Achilles tendon in these patients reveals significant tendon degeneration. In addition to tendinosis, corticosteroids predispose to full-thickness tendon tears.

Full-thickness tears in tendons which have their collagen fibers oriented along the long axis of the tendon demonstrate considerable retraction of the torn ends of the tendon. This is observed in the Achilles, posterior tibial (Fig. 7-55), quadriceps, patellar, biceps, and triceps tendons. The proximal portion of the tendon attached to viable muscle will

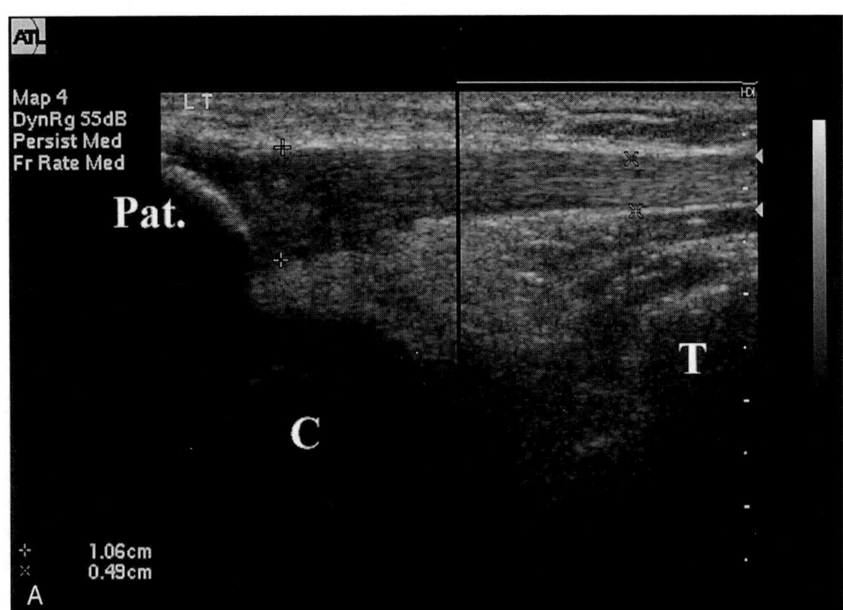

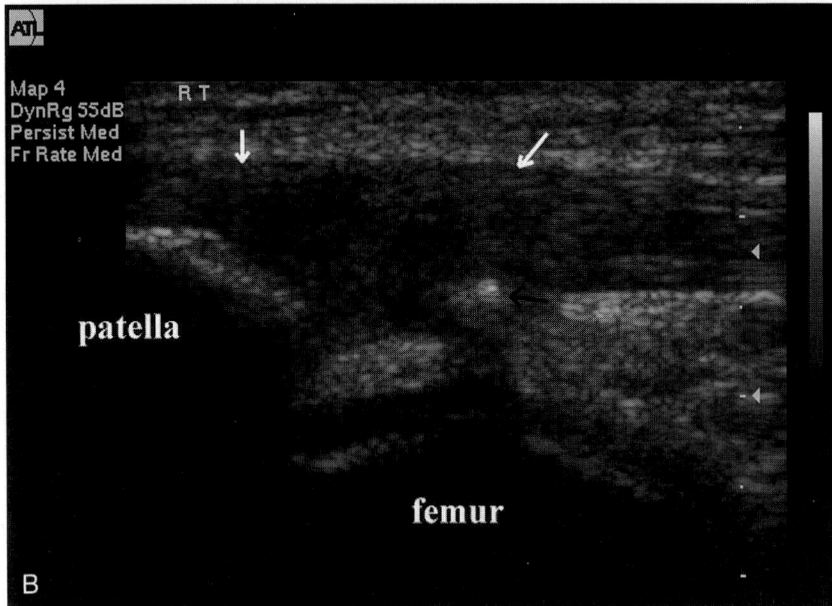

Figure 7-50 ■ **A**, Patellar tendinosis: longitudinal sonogram. Bilateral infrapatellar pain and swelling in this 32-year-old professional basketball player was refractory to conservative therapy. This longitudinal sonogram through the left patellar tendon demonstrates loss of the normal fibrillar pattern, decreased echogenicity of the tendon, and thickening (+) immediately below the patellar apex (*Pat.*). Abbreviations: femoral condyle (*C*), tibial plateau (*T*). **B,** Patellar tendinosis: longitudinal sonogram. Same patient as in **A.** A small calcification (*black arrow*) is seen within the deep portion of the tendon within a region of focal disruption. A more normal appearance of tendon architecture is noted more superficially (*white arrows*).

retract farther than the distal portion due to the intrinsic properties of the muscle (Fig. 7-56). Acoustic shadowing is present at the torn ends of the tendon. This artifact is probably due to refraction. The frayed ends of the tendon reflect the incident sound beam in all directions, with a very small percentage of the beam reflected back to the transducer. Refraction artifact may be seen in partial-thickness tears, but this is rare. Shadowing is seen in partial-thickness tears only when the tendon delaminates and a portion of the torn tendon folds back upon itself. Sometimes refraction artifact may be mistaken for shadowing due to calcification. These artifacts can coexist when tears occur through regions of tendinosis (Fig. 7-54). Recognition of refraction artifact in full-thickness tears is helpful in measuring the degree of retraction present at the rupture site, aiding the clinician in deciding if surgical repair is indicated (Fig. 7-54).

Chronic Overuse

Chronic overuse is a significant cause of tendon tears and other soft tissue injuries. Typical overuse

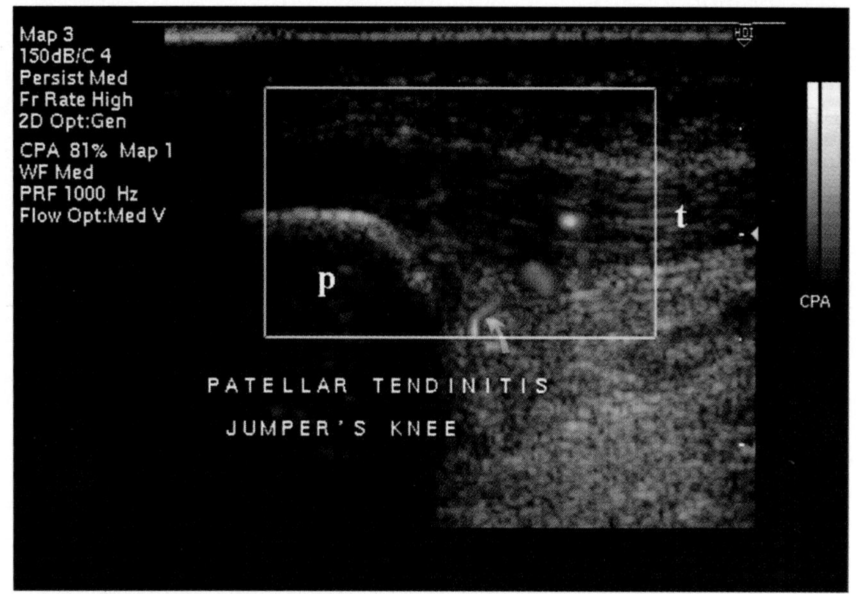

Figure 7–51 ■ Patellar tendinosis: power Doppler sonography. Classic changes of patellar tendinosis (generally referred to as *tendinitis*) are noted within the proximal portion of the patellar tendon of this 26-year-old soccer player. The hyperemia demonstrated here with power Doppler imaging is characteristic of the active painful phase of the disease. Feeding vessels (*curved arrow*) are typically observed entering from Hoffa's fat pad. Abbreviations: patellar tendon (*t*), patellar apex (*p*).

syndromes include posterior tibial tendon dysfunction in obese middle-aged females, jumper's knee in athletes, iliotibial band syndrome in runners, epicondylitis in the elbow (golf and tennis), de Quervain's tendinitis in the wrist, and plantar fasciitis in the foot (Kraushaar and Nirschl, 1999).

Posterior tibial tendon dysfunction in middle-aged women probably relates to foot pronation, which can be seen in association with valgus deformity of the knee and adipose tissue deposition along the medial aspect of the thighs. This chronic pronation results in elongation of the posterior tibial tendon. Edema and hyperemia within the substance of the tendon and effusion within the tendon sheath are the earliest signs observed sonographically (Fig. 7–57). Intrasubstance degeneration (Fig. 7–57), partial-thickness tears (Fig. 7–58), and full-thickness tears (Fig. 7–59) are seen in progressively more advanced disease. Kraushaar and Nirschl (1999) state that we should not use the term *tendinitis* for these conditions because they are not inflammatory per se. *Tendinosis* is a better term, as overuse is characterized by a fibroblastic and vascular response or by so-called angiofibroblastic degeneration. This book still uses both terms—tendinosis and tendinitis—as synonyms, thus conforming with standard clinical usage. Tears of the posterior tibial tendon are most frequently longitudinal and centered at the level of the medial malleolus (Fig. 7–60). Traumatic ankle injuries, such as fracture of the medial malleolus or ligamentous tear, often result in disruption of the flexor retinaculum. This allows anterior subluxation of the tendon (Fig. 7–61). The tendon moves out of the posterior tibial tendon groove, resulting in abrasion of the tendon along the anterior margin of this bony sulcus. The mechanism of injury is similar to that seen in subluxation of the peroneal tendons. Traumatic tears of the posterior tibial tendon can be quite variable in morphology. They may be longitudinal, transverse, L-shaped, or more complex in shape.

Rheumatoid arthritis affects the posterior tibial tendon through inflammation of the surrounding synovium. The tendon sheath demonstrates the classic findings of rheumatoid synovitis, and the tendon loses its normal fibrillar architecture. Tears are often full-thickness at the time of presentation. Onset of symptoms is rarely acute, and loss of function is indolent. Commonly, ultrasound examinations will reveal full-thickness tears which are irreparable due to the marked degree of retraction. Tendon grafts are often used to repair posttraumatic ruptures; however, in rheumatoid tears or other very-late-stage full-thickness tears, arthrodesis is the only therapeutic option. Triple arthrodesis is often used to treat the foot deformities resulting from posterior tibial tendon tears.

Of all the overuse syndromes, elbow tendinosis or tennis elbow is the best-known example. The origin of the extensor carpi radialis brevis is the primary site of this injury. In one-third of patients, the origin of the extensor digitorum communis is involved as well (Kraushaar and Nirschl, 1999). Histological studies combined with clinical data indicate that the changes are degenerative and occur when the tendon fails to heal properly after injury or

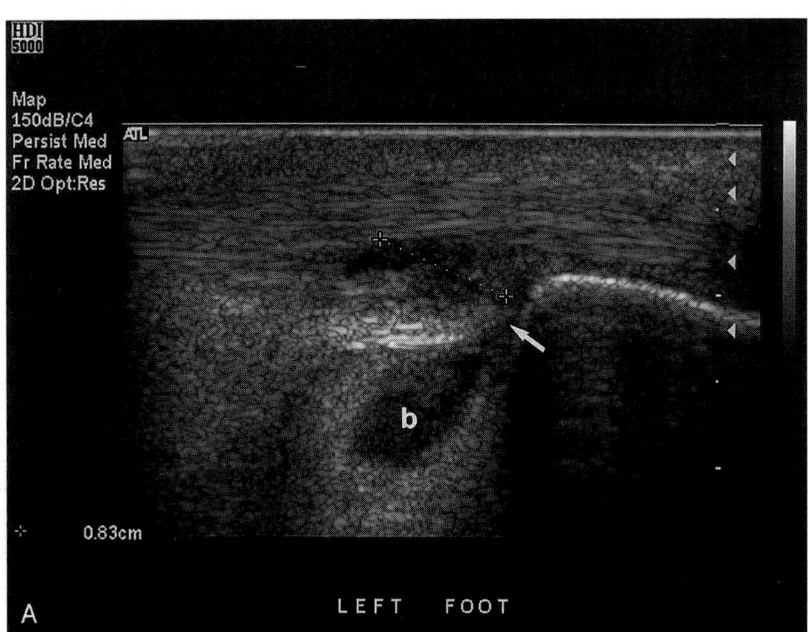

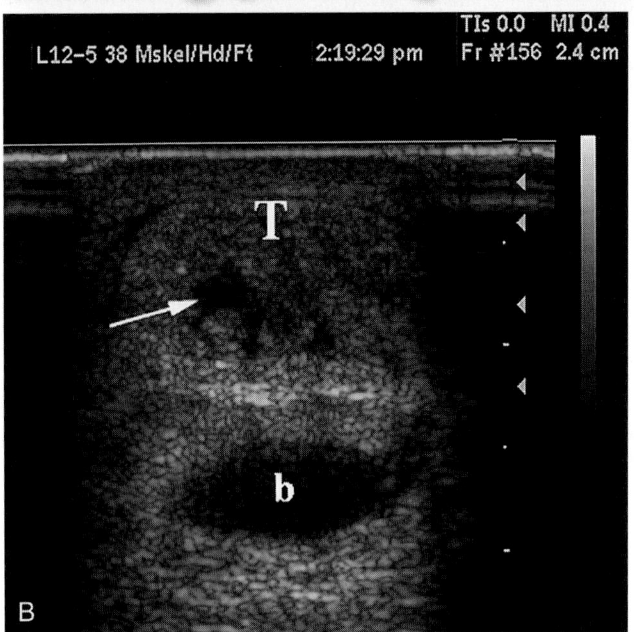

Figure 7-52 ■ **A**, Partial Achilles tendon rupture: longitudinal sonogram. Heel pain developed acutely in this middle-aged recreational athlete. This longitudinal image was obtained with the transducer over the enthesis of the Achilles tendon. An 8-mm-long focal disruption of the fibrillar pattern is noted in the anterior aspect of the tendon (*between the calipers*). Partial-thickness tears extend to the surface. This tear continues (*arrow*) into the synovial space of the retrocalcaneal bursa (*b*). **B**, Partial Achilles tendon rupture: transverse sonogram. Same patient as in **A**. The transverse image demonstrates the focal hypoechoic change (*arrow*) in the anterior aspect of the Achilles tendon (*T*). The adjacent retrocalcaneal bursa (*b*) is distended with fluid.

after repetitive microtrauma resulting from overuse (Kraushaar and Nirschl, 1999). The tendinosis infiltrate consists of active fibroblasts and vascular hyperplasia, unlike the infiltrate in inflammatory tendinitis, which is made up of lymphocytes and neutrophils. Proneness to this type of injury, which is observed in some patients, may be inherited. Patients with two or more clinical manifestations of the following conditions—bilateral tennis elbow, cubital tunnel syndrome, carpal tunnel syndrome, de Quervain tenosynovitis, trigger finger, or rotator cuff tendinosis—have been diagnosed as suffering from *mesenchymal syndrome* (Nirschl, 1969, 1988, 1992; Nirschl and Pettrone, 1979). This mesenchymal syndrome may relate to a potentially systemic abnormality of collagen cross-linkage (Kraushaar and Nirschl, 1999). Repair of tendons would then be impaired when the tolerable rate of stretch of tendon fibers has been exceeded. Tendons that develop microtears through overuse seem to tear through side-to-side dehiscence (Kraushaar and Nirschl, 1999). This may be why degenerative tears tend to be predominantly longitudinal. It has been shown that a net increase of more than 8% of the total length of a tendon results

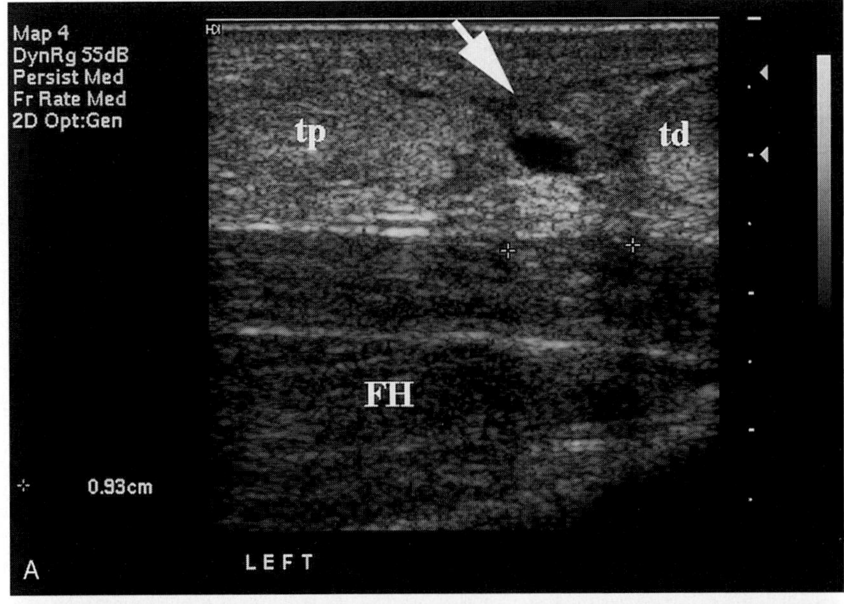

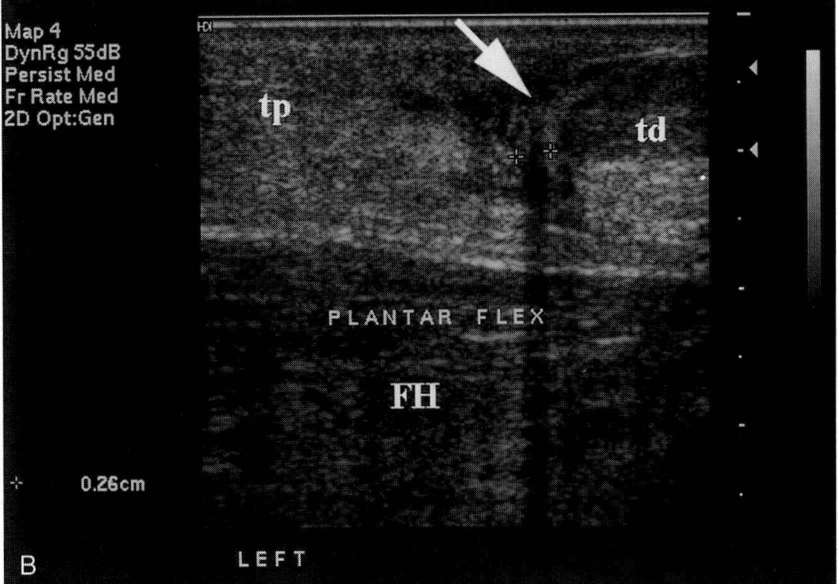

Figure 7-53 ■ **A**, Complete Achilles tendon rupture: longitudinal sonogram. This 38-year-old basketball player felt a sudden snap in his ankle, with loss of plantar flexion of his foot. A mixed-echogenicity collection (*arrow*) separates the torn ends of the tendon. Mild acoustic shadowing caused by refraction is observed at the tendon margins, indicating the degree of retraction. Abbreviations: proximal tendon (*tp*), distal tendon (*td*), flexor hallucis muscle (*FH*). **B**, Complete Achilles tendon rupture: longitudinal sonogram. Same patient as in **A**. The scan was repeated with the foot in plantar flexion, demonstrating good approximation of the proximal and distal ends of the torn tendon. The refractive shadowing (+) demonstrates a gap (*arrow*) of less than 3 mm. This is felt to be suitable for conservative treatment by casting in plantar flexion. Abbreviations: proximal tendon (*tp*), distal tendon (*td*), flexor hallucis muscle (*FH*).

in a tear (Jòzsa and Kannus, 1997). Complete tearing of the extensor origin in the elbow happens occasionally. It is often a relief to the patient who had been suffering from intolerable elbow pain up the time of the complete rupture.

Ligament Tears

Lateral and rotational forces applied to joints can result in ligament rupture. Ligament tears resulting from acute overload are typically seen in professional and amateur athletes. Abnormal valgus stress applied to the knee will result in rupture of the medial collateral ligament (MCL). A thumb caught in the strap of a ski pole will result in a gamekeeper's injury. Forceful throwing of a baseball can result in an ulnar collateral ligament (UCL) tear in the elbow. Healing of these ligaments can be impaired due to repetitive injury. A soccer player who continues to kick the ball with the medial side of his foot following MCL injury will certainly prevent the lesion from healing, and the injury will probably result in progression of disease. Other causes of impaired

Text continued on page 232

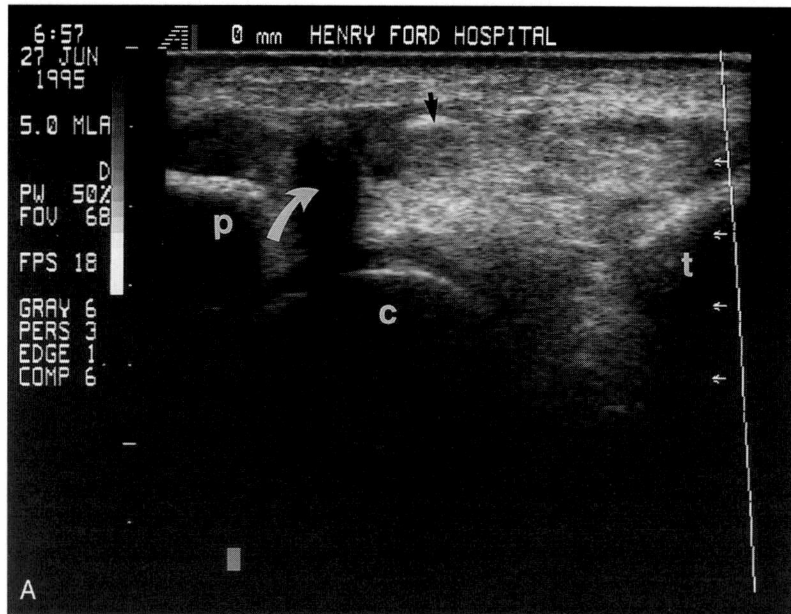

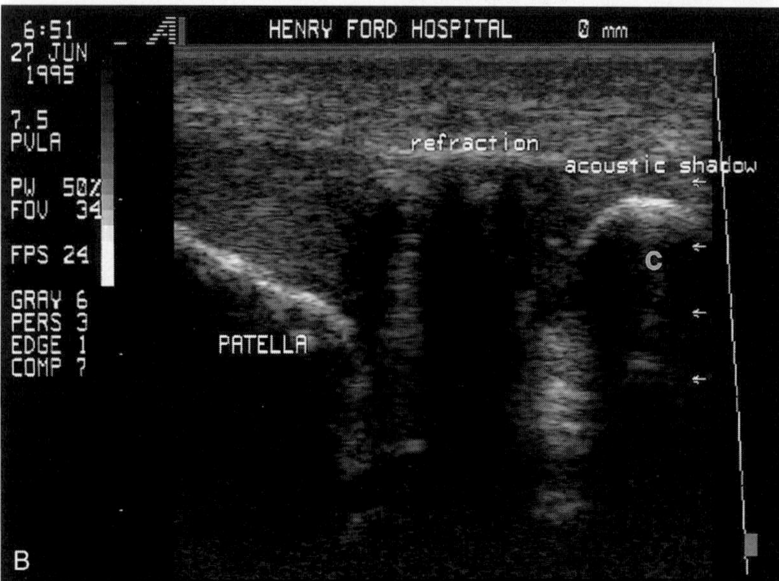

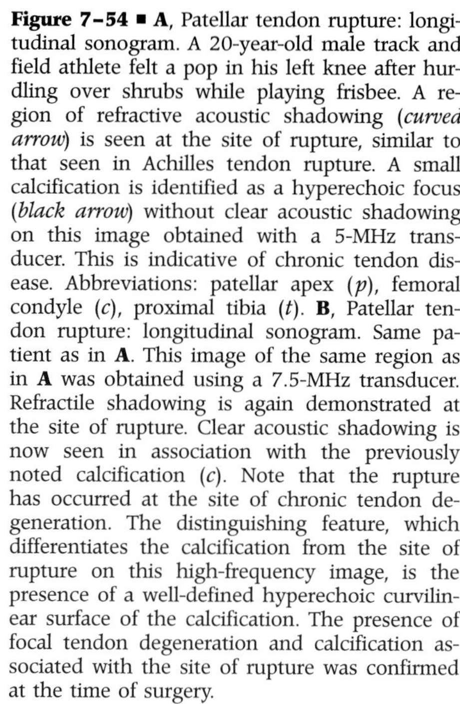
Figure 7–54 ■ **A**, Patellar tendon rupture: longitudinal sonogram. A 20-year-old male track and field athlete felt a pop in his left knee after hurdling over shrubs while playing frisbee. A region of refractive acoustic shadowing (*curved arrow*) is seen at the site of rupture, similar to that seen in Achilles tendon rupture. A small calcification is identified as a hyperechoic focus (*black arrow*) without clear acoustic shadowing on this image obtained with a 5-MHz transducer. This is indicative of chronic tendon disease. Abbreviations: patellar apex (*p*), femoral condyle (*c*), proximal tibia (*t*). **B**, Patellar tendon rupture: longitudinal sonogram. Same patient as in **A**. This image of the same region as in **A** was obtained using a 7.5-MHz transducer. Refractile shadowing is again demonstrated at the site of rupture. Clear acoustic shadowing is now seen in association with the previously noted calcification (*c*). Note that the rupture has occurred at the site of chronic tendon degeneration. The distinguishing feature, which differentiates the calcification from the site of rupture on this high-frequency image, is the presence of a well-defined hyperechoic curvilinear surface of the calcification. The presence of focal tendon degeneration and calcification associated with the site of rupture was confirmed at the time of surgery.

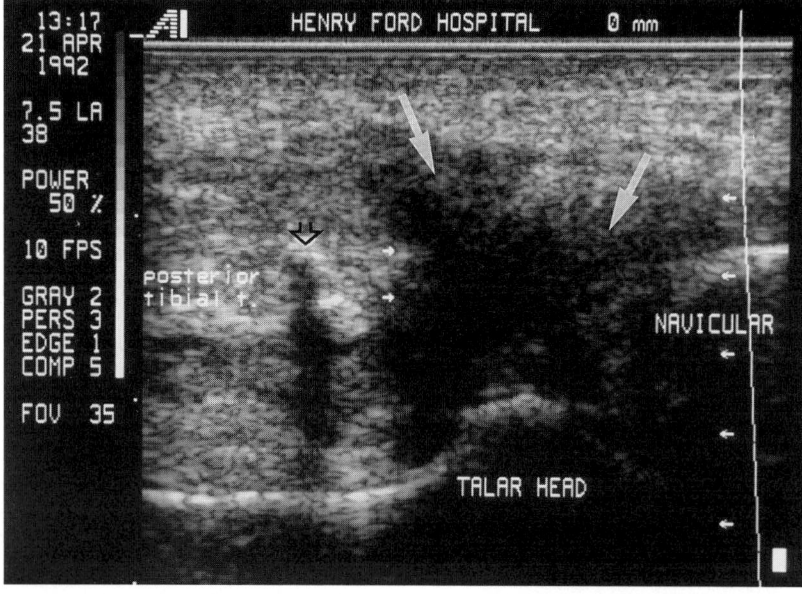

Figure 7–55 ■ Full-thickness tear of the posterior tibial tendon: longitudinal sonogram. After a missed attempt to kick the ball, which resulted in forceful eversion of the foot, this 30-year-old soccer player experienced severe pain and swelling over the medial aspect of the ankle. He also experienced nearly complete loss of ankle inversion. A hypoechoic fluid collection (hematoma, *large arrows*) separates the torn end of the posterior tibial tendon (*small arrows*) from its insertion on the navicular. A punctate calcification (*open arrow*) is present immediately proximal to the site of rupture.

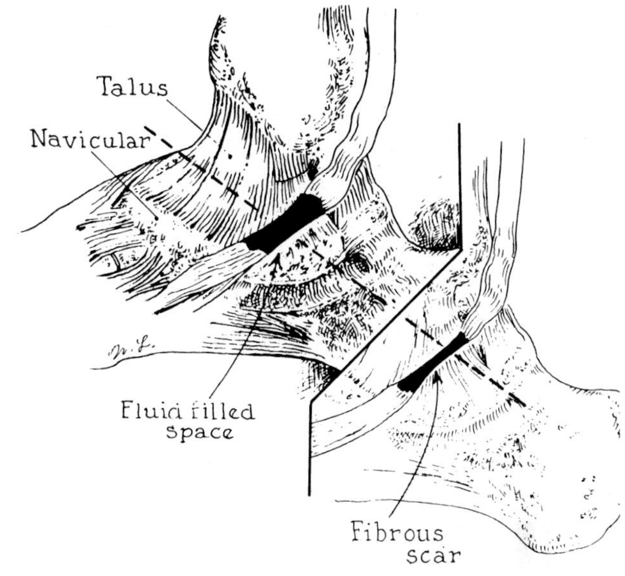

Figure 7–56 ■ Diagram of transverse tears of the posterior tibial tendon. Most transverse tears will be complete, and the defect caused by tear will fill in with anechoic fluid. The proximal disrupted tendon will often recoil significantly (*diagram*). Sometimes tears may fill with fibrous scar or a few longitudinal fibers of intact tendon may still show (*insert on right side of diagram*).

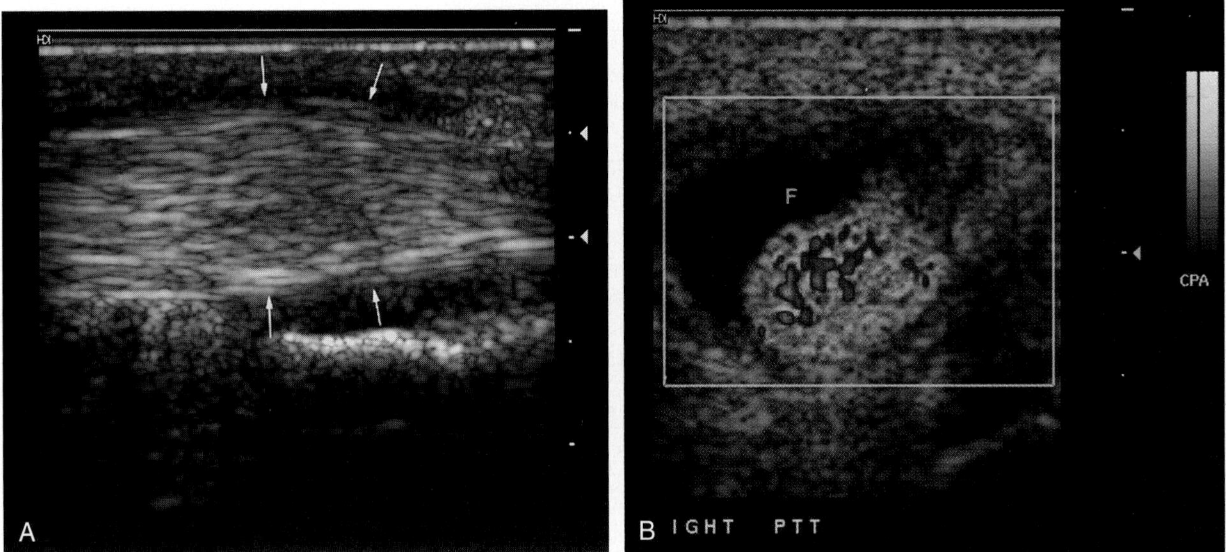

Figure 7–57 ■ **A**, Posterior tibial tendon overuse: longitudinal sonogram. An obese 52-year-old man visits the foot clinic because of chronic weakness in his right foot. Notes from the clinical exam describe a foot deformity characterized by foot pronation and heel valgus. The longitudinal sonogram of the posterior tibial tendon demonstrates segmental swelling of the tendon (*arrows*). The internal structure of the tendon is disorganized and hypoechoic. **B**, Posterior tibial tendon overuse: transverse sonogram with power Doppler sonography. Same patient as in **A**. The transverse image has been obtained with less pressure on the transducer. It is possible to show fluid (*F*) in the tendon sheath of the posterior tibial tendon using this technique. Hyperemia is also noted within the substance of the tendon.

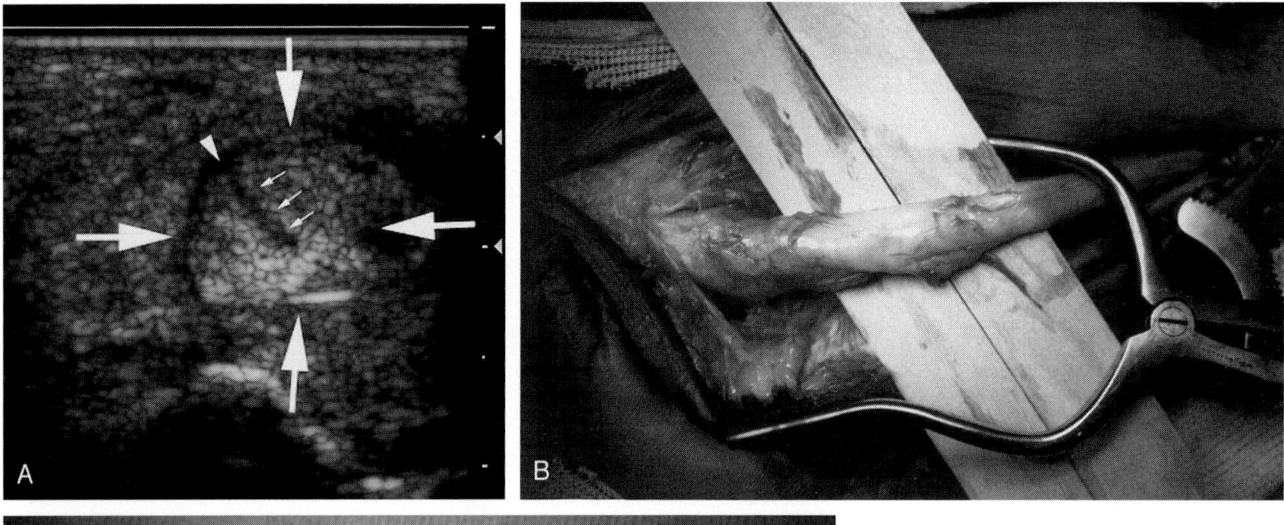

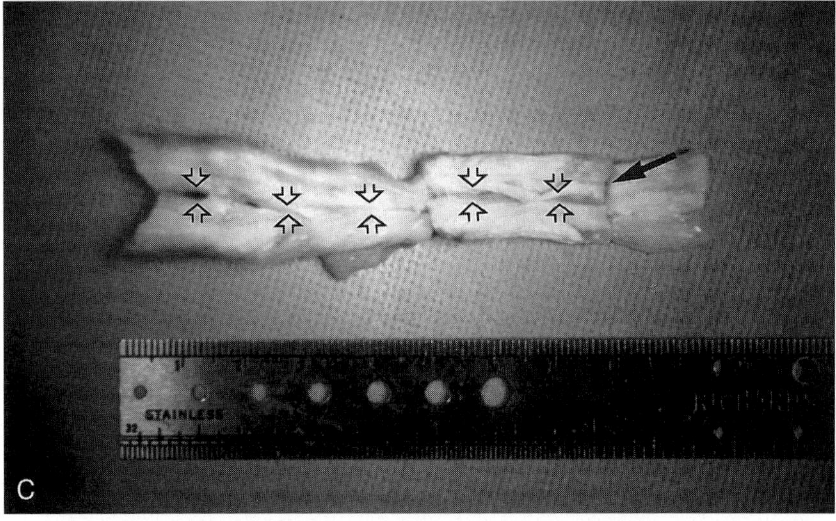

Figure 7–58 ■ **A**, Partial-thickness tear of the posterior tibial tendon: transverse sonogram. Pain and swelling around the medial ankle of this 56-year-old woman have been treated with a cast for a prolonged period of time. Ultrasound examination demonstrates a central hypoechoic cleft (*small arrows*) in the posterior tibial tendon (*large arrows*). As illustrated in this figure, the cleft extends to the surface in a very small segment of the tendon (*arrowhead*). **B**, Partial-thickness tear of the posterior tibial tendon: surgical exploration. Same patient as in **A**. Visual inspection of the tendon surface shows swelling and irregularity of the tendon. However, the partial tear demonstrated on ultrasound examination is not immediately visible on the tendon surface. **C**, Partial-thickness tear of the posterior tibial tendon: view of the bisected tendon. The resected specimen shows a longitudinal cleft (*open arrows*) within the tendon. The linear extension to the surface (*arrow*) corresponds to the abnormality demonstrated in **A**. Partial-thickness tears are characterized by surface extension. Treatment of this patient consisted of flexor digitorum transfer. The flexor digitorum was used as a graft to replace the diseased posterior tibial tendon.

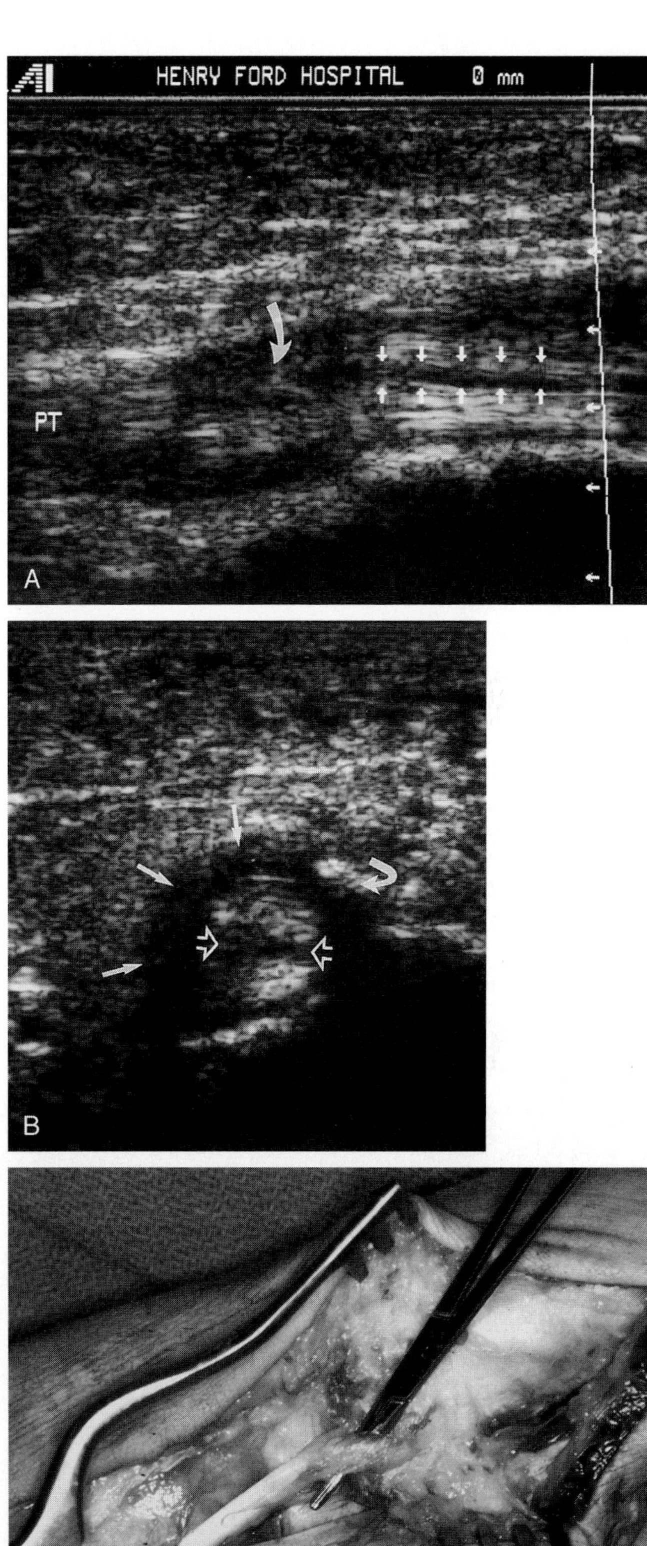

Figure 7–59 ■ **A**, Longitudinal tear of the posterior tibial tendon: longitudinal sonogram. This 45-year-old obese female experienced persistent pain at the medial aspect of the ankle following an ankle sprain several months ago. A longitudinal hypoechoic cleft (*arrows*) is present centrally within the posterior tibial tendon. A region of anisotropy and tendon degeneration (*curved arrow*) are noted more proximally within the tendon. Abbreviation: posterior tibial tendon (*PT*). **B**, Longitudinal tear of the posterior tibial tendon: transverse sonogram. Same patient as in **A**. Again, the longitudinal cleft (*open arrows*) is seen centrally within the posterior tibial tendon on this transverse image. A hypoechoic halo (*arrows*) is present within the tendon sheath, indicative of tenosynovitis. Degenerative spurring (*curved arrow*) of the anterior margin of the tibial groove is typical in patients with posterior tibial tendon pathology. **C**, Longitudinal tear of the posterior tibial tendon: surgical exploration. A surgical instrument is placed in the longitudinal tear of the posterior tibial tendon.

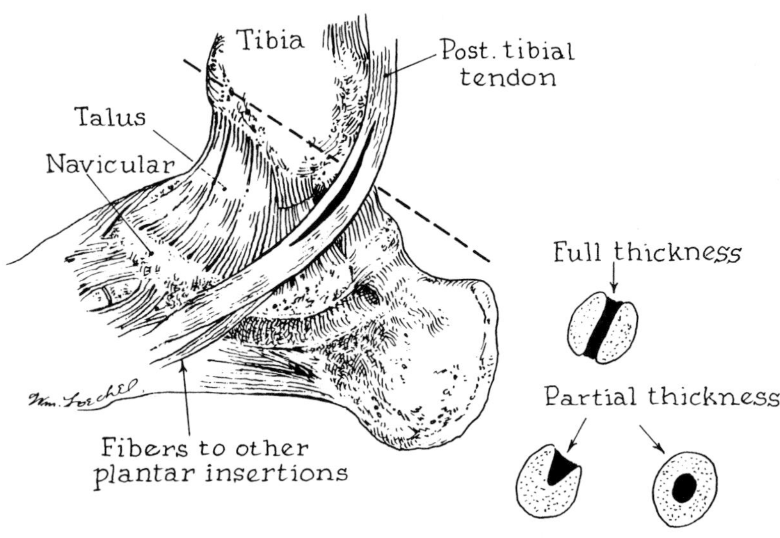

Figure 7–60 ■ Diagram of longitudinal tears of the posterior tibial tendon. Tears that follow the long axis of the tendon are typically referred to as *longitudinal tears*. Longitudinal tears are best seen on transverse images. The *hyphenated line* indicates the ultrasound scan plane. The images on the right illustrate different patterns of longitudinal tears. Partial-thickness tears that split the central fibers in the tendon cannot be observed during surgery. Only full-thickness longitudinal tears and partial thickness tears, which surface and extend into the synovial sheath covering the tendon, will be seen at surgery.

healing may relate to the degree of injury and anatomical features of the injury. The gamekeeper's injury is a good example. Valgus stress at the time of injury can be so forceful that the proximal UCL flips over the adductor fascia. This separates the proximal and distal ligament ends, preventing healing of this wound unless surgical apposition of the ligament ends is performed.

Ligamentous injuries can be associated with excessive shear forces or direct impact transmitted to the subchondral bone. These forces will result in osteochondritis dissecans, as well as chondral and osteochondral fractures. Osteochondral fracture involving the surface of the capitellum of the humerus in association with UCL tear in the elbow is a classic example. The valgus force which tears the UCL at the medial aspect of the elbow causes excessive pressure on the lateral column of the joint, resulting in impaction of the subchondral plate of the capitellum (Fig. 7–62).

Pulse-echo ultrasound is not the examination of choice for evaluation of intra-articular ligaments or joint cartilage. The role of ultrasound in the detection of joint pathology and investigation of internal

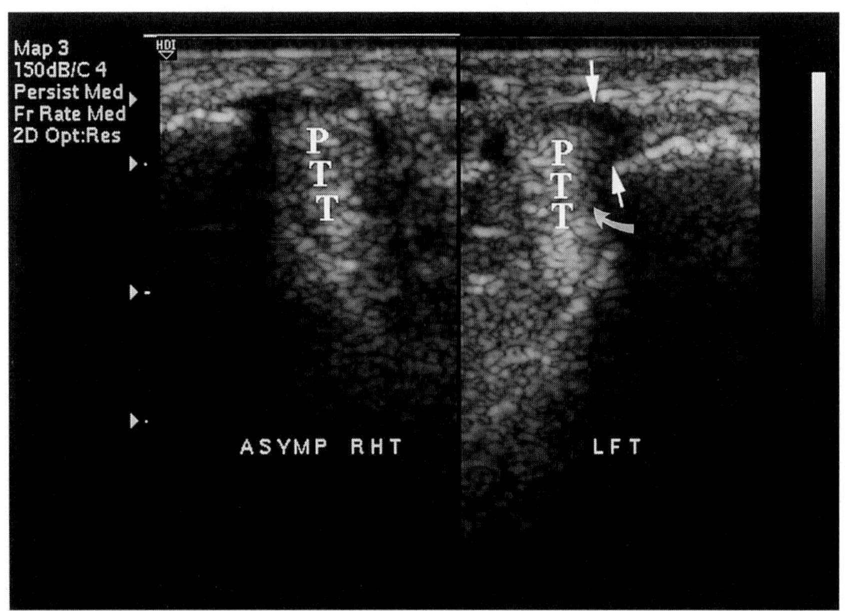

Figure 7–61 ■ Posterior tibial tendon subluxation: split-screen transverse sonograms. Medial ankle pain and swelling prompted this 54-year-old female to seek treatment. Posterior tibial tendon subluxation was observed with real-time imaging. These static images demonstrate mild medial subluxation of the left (*LFT*) posterior tibial tendon (*PTT*). The asymptomatic right (*RHT*) tendon is shown for comparison. A few millimeters of displacement of the symptomatic tendon relative to the medial malleolus is obvious (*big arrows*). Decreased echogenicity and erosion (*curved arrow*) of the tendon are noted at the point at which the tendon extends over the medial margin of the tibia.

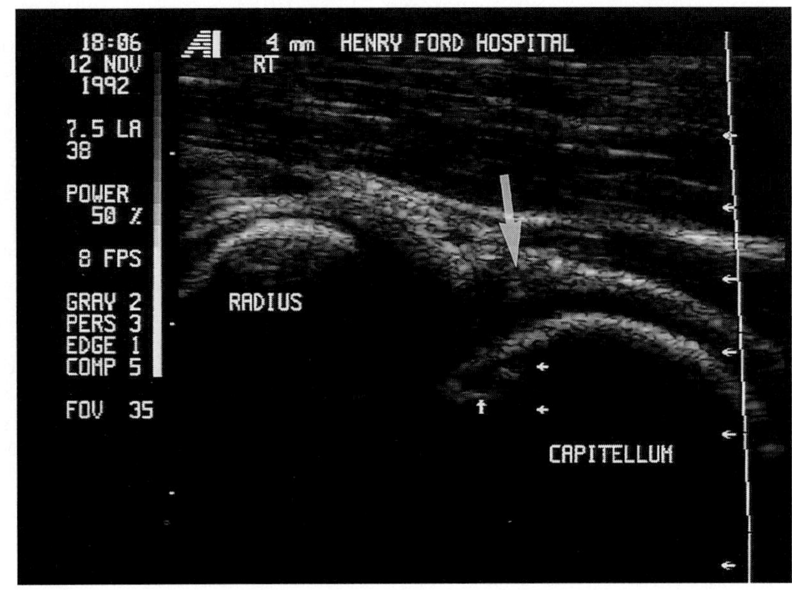

Figure 7-62 ■ Osteochondral injury of the capitellum humeri: sagittal sonogram. Months after rupturing the ulnar collateral ligament while throwing a baseball, this 15-year-old high-school student started complaining of pain on the lateral side of his elbow. The ultrasound transducer is aligned along the long axis of the extremity. An irregular subchondral lesion (*small arrows*) is noted in the capitellum. The cartilage over the capitellum demonstrates a cleft (*large arrow*). However, the fragment appeared stable, and the examiner's finger was not able to dislodge the fragment during the real-time examination. Panner's disease or osteochondral fractures of the capitellum are common in athletes with medial collateral ligament tears of the elbow. Abnormal valgus stress with traumatic impact on the lateral side of the elbow has been blamed for these lesions. In this sagittal image, distal is on the left and proximal on the right.

derangement will be discussed throughout the book where appropriate (see also Chapter 8).

References

Clark JM, Harryman DT: Tendons, ligaments, and capsule of the rotator cuff: Gross and microscopic anatomy. *J Bone Joint Surg* 74A(5):713–725, 1992.

Codman EA, Akerson IB: The pathology associated with rupture of the supraspinatus tendon. *Ann Surg* 93: 348–359, 1931.

Codman EA: *The Shoulder.* Boston, privately published, 1934.

De Sèze S, et al: Etudes sur l' épaule douloureuse. III. Etude anatomique de l' épaule sénile. *Rev Rhum* 28: 85–94, 1961.

Fukuda H, Hamada K, Yamanaka K: Pathology and pathogenesis of bursal-side rotator cuff tears viewed from histologic sections. *Clin Orthop* 254:75–80, 1990.

Golding FC: The shoulder—the forgotten joint. *Br J Radiol* 35:149–158, 1962.

Hollister MS, et al: Association of sonographically detected subacromial/subdeltoid bursal effusion and intraarticular fluid with rotator cuff tear. *AJR* 165:605–608, 1995.

Jòzsa LG, Kannus P (eds): Overuse injuries of tendons, in *Human Tendons: Anatomy, Physiology, and Pathology.* Champaign, IL, Human Kinetics, 1997, pp 164–253.

Kannus P, Jòzsa LG: Histopathological changes preceding spontaneous rupture of a tendon. *J Bone Joint Surg Am* 73(10):1507, 1991.

Keyes EL: Observations on rupture of the supraspinatus tendon. *Ann Surg* 97:849–856, 1933.

Khan KM, et al.: Patellar tendinosis: Findings at histopathologic examination, US, and MR imaging. *Radiology* 200:821–827, 1996.

Khan KM, et al: Patellar tendon sonography and jumper's knee in female basketball players: A longitudinal study. *Clin J Sport Med* 7(3):200–205, 1997.

Kraushaar BS, Nirschl RP: Tendinosis of the elbow: Clinical features and findings of histological, immunohistochemical and electron microscopy studies. *J Bone Joint Surg Am* 81(2):259–278, 1999.

Lindblom K, Palmer I: Ruptures of the tendon aponeurosis of the shoulder joint—the so called supraspinatus ruptures. *Acta Chir Scand* 82:133–142, 1939.

Martens M, et al: Patellar tendinitis: Pathology and results of treatment. *Acta Orthop Scand* 53:445–450, 1982.

Matsen FA, Arntz CT: Subacromial impingement. In: Rockwood CA and Matsen FA (eds): *The Shoulder.* Philadelphia, Saunders, 1990, pp 623–626.

Middleton WD, et al: Ultrasonic evaluation of the rotator cuff and biceps tendon. *J Bone Joint Surg Am* 68: 440–450, 1986.

Milgrom C, et al: Rotator cuff changes in asymptomatic adults. *J Bone Joint Surg* [*Br*] 77B:296–298, 1995.

Miniaci A, et al: Magnetic resonance imaging evaluation of the rotator cuff tendons in the asymptomatic shoulder. *Am J Sports Med* 23:142–145, 1995.

Neer CS: Impingement lesions. *Clin Orthop* 173:70–77, 1983.

Newman JS, et al: Detection of soft tissue hyperemia: Value of power Doppler sonography. *AJR* 163: 385–389, 1994.

Nicholas JA, Hershman EB: *The Lower Extremity and Spine in Sports Medicine.* St Louis, CV Mosby Co, 1986.

Nirschl RP: Mesenchymal syndrome. *Virginia Med Monthly* 96:659–662, 1969.

Nirschl RP: Prevention and treatment of elbow and shoulder injuries in the tennis player. *Clin Sports Med* 7: 289–308, 1988.

Nirschl RP: Elbow tendinosis/tennis elbow. *Clin Sports Med* 11:851–870, 1992.
Nirschl RP, Pettrone FA: Tennis elbow. The surgical treatment of lateral epicondylitis. *J Bone Joint Surg* 61A: 832–839, 1979.
Ogdon JS: *Skeletal Injury in the Child*, ed 2. Philadelphia, WB Saunders Co, 1990.
Ozaki J, et al: Tears of the rotator cuff of the shoulder associated with pathological changes in the acromion. *J Bone Joint Surg* 70A:1224–1230, 1988.
Patten RM, et al: Nondisplaced fractures of the greater tuberosity of the humerus: Sonographic detection. *Radiology* 182:201–204, 1992.
Rakofsky M: *Fractional Arthrography of the Shoulder*. Stuttgart, Gustav Fisher, 1987.
Raven PB: Asymptomatic tears of rotator cuff are commonplace. *Sports Med Dig* 17:11–12, 1995.
Rogers LF: *Radiology of Skeletal Trauma*, ed 2. New York, Churchill Livingstone, 1992.
Sher JS, et al: Abnormal findings on magnetic resonance images of asymptomatic shoulders. *J Bone Joint Surg* 77(A):10–15, 1995.
van Holsbeeck MT, et al: Ultrasound depiction of partial-thickness tear of the rotator cuff. *Radiology* 197: 443–446, 1995.
van Holsbeeck MT, et al: The rotator cuff, in Rumack, Wilson, Charboneau (eds): *Diagnostic Ultrasound*, Vol IV. St Louis, 1998: 26.
Wohlwend JR, et al: The association between irregular greater tuberosities and rotator cuff tears: A sonographic study. *AJR* 171:229–233, 1998.
Yamanaka K: Pathological study of the supraspinatus tendon. *J Jpn Orthop Assoc* 62:1121–1138, 1988.

Chapter 8
Sonography of Large Synovial Joints

Sonographic examination of large synovial joints is frequently requested because these joints are difficult to evaluate clinically. The shoulder, hip, and knee are deep-seated joints in which physical examination is limited. Ultrasound is dramatically changing our approach to the evaluation of joint disease. In Europe, ultrasound has already established its place as the primary means of evaluating periarticular disease of synovial joints. It is not limited by the size of the joint. Even the smallest interphalangeal joints can be examined sonographically. Currently in the United States, arthroscopy and MRI are the methods most frequently employed for evaluation of the knee. Arthroscopy is limited to the intra-articular structures. It permits the surgeon to examine the cartilage and perform corrective surgery in the same session. However, arthroscopy is an invasive technique not without risk to the patient. The risk of anesthesia and the possibility of damage to the periarticular soft tissues are not insignificant. MRI permits the radiologist to examine the subchondral bone and hyaline and fibrous cartilage, as well as the periarticular soft tissues. This is the information which is missing from a standard radiographic examination of a joint. However, the MRI examination is static, is relatively expensive, and cannot be performed without anesthesia in children.

The principal advantage of ultrasound over arthroscopy and MRI is its ability to examine the periarticular soft tissues with a more useful structural and anatomical detail. Many pain syndromes do not originate in bone or articular cartilage. Until now, these were presumptive clinical diagnoses. Sonography can be used to diagnose disease of the periarticular tissues with great sensitivity and specificity. It can detect tendinous, ligamentous, and muscular lesions. It can differentiate scar, granulation tissue, and complete and incomplete tears. Hemorrhagic and frictional bursitis can also be differentiated by their sonographic appearance. In addition, ultrasound is entirely noninvasive and requires no anesthesia or premedication.

Intra-articular disease can also be evaluated accurately using ultrasound. Ultrasound can quickly estimate the amount of intra-articular fluid. Changes in intra-articular fluid are easily detected, but this is a nonspecific finding seen in chondromalacia, osteoarthritis, rheumatoid arthritis, osteonecrosis, infection, intra-articular tumors, and chronic traumatic disease. In addition, ultrasound can identify synovial edema, hemarthrosis, and loose bodies within the joint. Cartilage and synovial thickness can be measured accurately, providing an excellent method to evaluate the effectiveness of treatment and the progression of disease (Aisen et al., 1984). Peripheral meniscal tears can also be detected, but in general, meniscal tears are better evaluated with MRI or arthroscopy.

In summary, ultrasound is a valuable tool in the diagnosis of both periarticular and intra-articular disease. It is the method of choice for evaluation of periarticular disease and the first step in the evaluation of intra-articular disease. If the intra-articular examination is normal, no further imaging studies are indicated. An abnormal sonographic examination is an indication for evaluation with MRI, arthrography, or arthroscopy.

Examination Technique

In the examination of superficially located joints, 5-, 7.5-, and 10-MHz transducers are utilized. These provide excellent spatial resolution in the evaluation of the joint capsule and synovia in elbows, hands, and feet. In the majority of patients, these transducers can also be used for examination of the shoulders, hips, and knees. However, in obese patients, it may be necessary to utilize a 3.5 MHz-transducer for these deep-seated joints. In these cases, sensitivity in

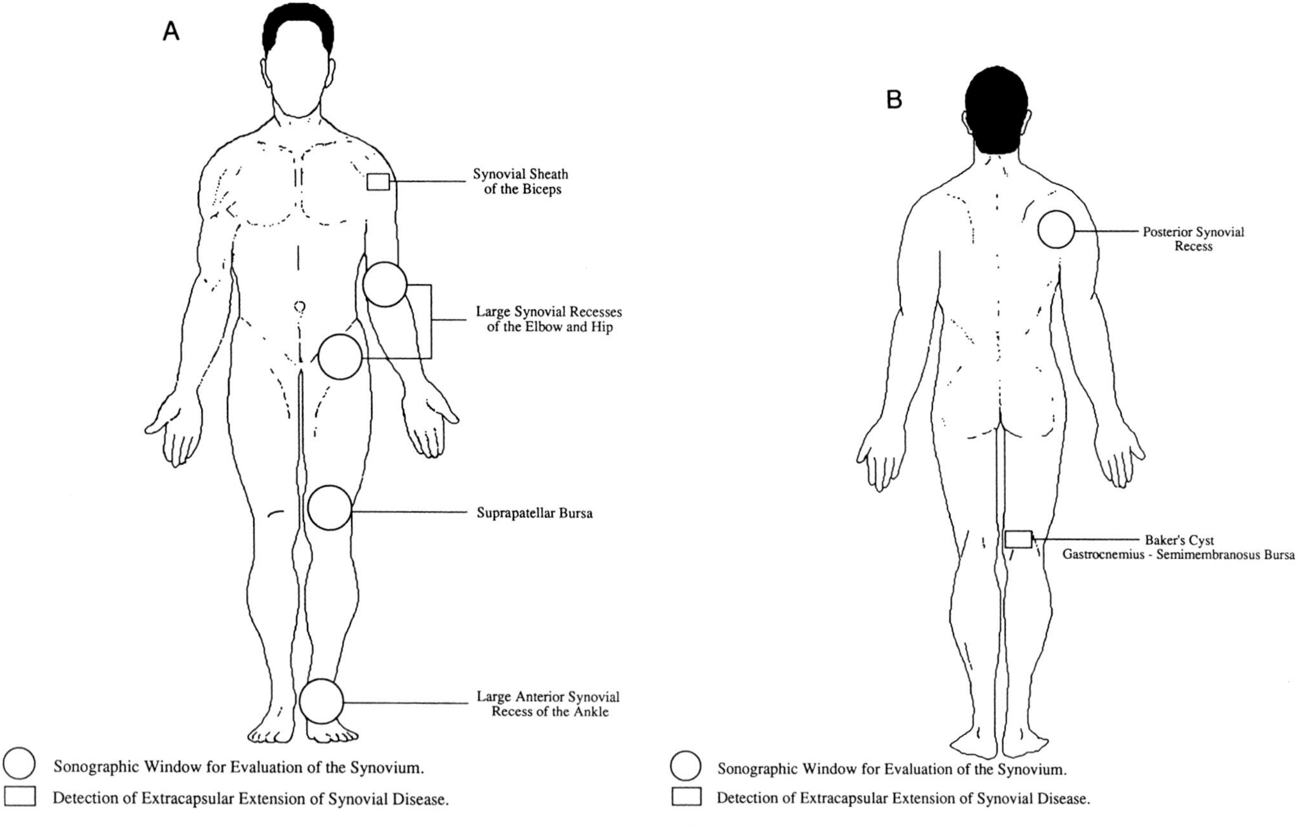

Figure 8–1 ▪ Sonographic windows for examination of the large synovial joints: anterior approach (**A**) and posterior approach (**B**).

detecting small lesions is decreased, but valuable information can still be obtained. When large synovial joints are scanned for intra-articular pathology and synovial disease, the examination is directed toward the largest synovial recesses of the joint not protected by bone. Flexion, extension, and internal or external rotation of the joint can further increase the field of view. Anteversion of the hip limits examination to the anterior approach. The shoulder joint is most accessible through the posterior synovial recess due to retroversion of the humeral head. Other approaches are restricted by bony protuberances. Figure 8–1 summarizes the recommended approaches to scanning the large synovial joints. In cases of extensive synovial disease, such as rheumatoid arthritis, the portal selected for scanning is not critical. Active rheumatoid disease of the shoulder enlarges the axillary and subcoracoid recesses, as well as the infraspinatus recess. Thus, the same diagnostic information can be obtained in rheumatoid patients regardless of which approach to the joint is selected. This is true for all large synovial joints with active disease. The progression of disease in the knee differs slightly from that in other joints. Early disease is best detected by examination of the suprapatellar recess, as shown in Figure 8–1A. However, chronic disease will enlarge the gastrocnemius-semimembranosus bursa, resulting in a Baker's cyst. Examination for Baker's cyst is performed using a posterior approach, scanning the medial aspect of the popliteal fossa.

Normal Sonographic Anatomy

In a normal joint, the bony contours are seen as hyperreflective lines with shadowing posteriorly. The epiphyseal growth plate is readily identified in children as a relatively hypoechoic band separating the epiphysis from the metaphysis. Cartilage covering the articular surfaces is depicted as a relatively hypoechoic, homogeneous stripe with smooth contours covering the epiphyses. The thickness of the articular cartilage is easily measured using the electronic calipers of the ultrasound unit. A minimal amount of fluid is normally found in the synovial recesses. The synovial leaves are separated by a fluid film approximately 2 to 3 mm thick (Figs. 8–2, through 8–4). Synovial tissue lining the joint is immeasurably thin, with smooth, regular contours

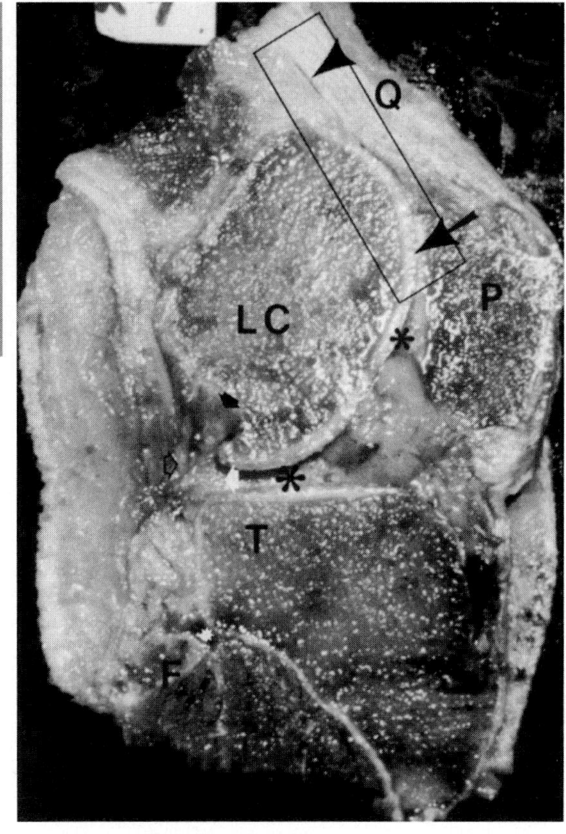

Figure 8–2 ▪ Sagittal anatomical section through the lateral compartment of the knee. The rectangular area indicates the region of greatest interest for routine examination of the knee. Deep to the quadriceps tendon (*Q*) lies the suprapatellar bursa (*black arrowhead*), which is an excellent indicator of intra-articular pathology. Normally, the walls of the suprapatellar bursa are extremely thin. Effusions, loose bodies, synovial edema, pannus, or tumor involvement change the volume and appearance of the bursa. Through the same sonographic window, we can image the cartilage of the femoral condyle (*large black arrow*). In the popliteal fossa, ultrasound can demonstrate the posterior joint capsule (*open black arrow*), the posterior cruciate ligament (*short black arrow*), and the meniscus (*white arrow*). Areas that are poorly visualized or not visualized include the cartilage of the patella, the tibial condyles, and the middle segment of the femoral condyles (*asterisk*). Abbreviations: lateral femoral condyle (*LC*), tibia (*T*), fibula (*F*), patella (*P*).

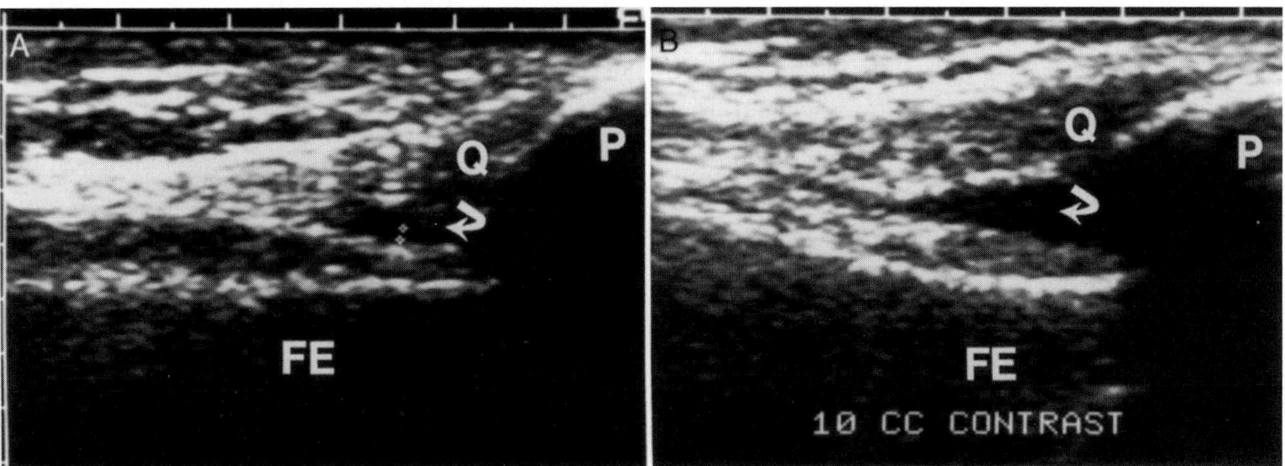

Figure 8–3 ▪ **A**, Normal suprapatellar bursa: longitudinal sonogram. The patient is a 20-year-old man with pain and tenderness inferior to the patella. Imaging was performed with the transducer oriented in the long axis of the quadriceps tendon using firm pressure. The inferior aspect of the transducer touches the middle of the basis patellae. A normal suprapatellar bursa (*curved arrow*) is approximately 1.5 to 3 cm long. It measures 2 to 3 mm in greatest thickness (compare to scale on top). Abbreviations: patella (*P*), femur (*Fe*), quadriceps (*Q*). **B**, Ten milliliters of contrast material was introduced for arthrography, which was normal. The anteroposterior diameter of the bursa (*curved arrow*) is increased by a factor of 5. Abbreviations: patella (*P*), femur (*Fe*), quadriceps (*Q*).

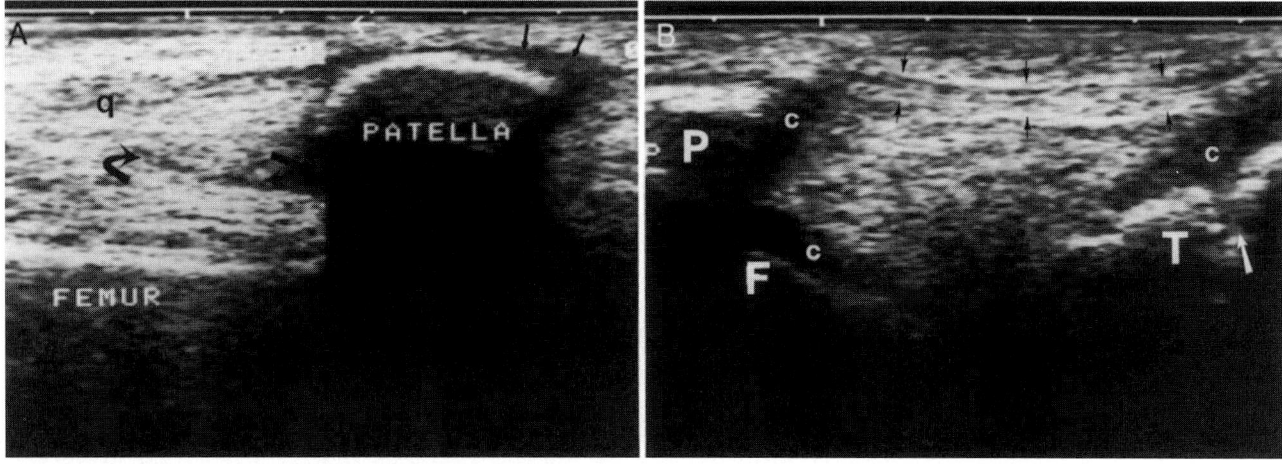

Figure 8–4 ■ **A**, Normal adolescent knee: longitudinal sonogram. A healthy 12-year-old boy. The knee is smaller, allowing visualization of the distal femur, patella, and proximal tibia on the same image. Deep to the quadriceps tendon (*q*), the suprapatellar bursa (*curved arrow*) extends 2 cm superior to the base of the patella. The anteroposterior dimension of the bursa is no more than 1 mm when firm pressure is applied with the transducer. Growth cartilage is still present around the apex of the patella (*arrows*). **B**, The transducer is moved inferiorly, now overlying the patellar tendon. A thick layer of cartilage (*c*) is noted covering the patellar apex (*P*), femoral condyle (*F*), and proximal tibia (*T*). The patellar tendon (*black arrows*) joins the patellar apex and the tibial tuberosity. A hypoechoic band (*white arrow*) in the proximal tibial represents the proximal growth plate.

(Fig. 8–5). Thin septae divide compartments within joints. These septae are called *plicae* when formed during embryological development (Figs. 8–6 and 8–7). Typically, the septae stand out clearly in an effusion. Plicae are hyperechoic relative to joint fluid; they appear thin, sheet-like, smooth and are no more than a few millimeters in thickness. A clearly identifiable hyperechoic line defines the joint capsule. In some joints, a significant layer of intracapsular fat separates the capsule and the synovium from each other. This is the case around the suprapatellar bursa in the knee and in the olecranon fossa in the elbow. Supporting ligaments demonstrate a lamellar appearance with alternating narrow hyperechoic and hypoechoic bands. Figures 8–8 through 8–11 illustrate the anatomy of the hips in children.

Sonography of Articular Pathology

Pathology of large synovial joints can be divided into those processes affecting the intra-articular structures and those involving the periarticular tissues. All structures lying within the synovial membrane, as well as the membrane itself, are considered intra-articular. Everything outside of the synovial membrane is considered periarticular.

Intra-articular Disease

Increased intra-articular fluid is a nonspecific finding indicative of joint pathology. It is seen in inflammatory processes, osteonecrosis, osteoarthritis, and tumors (Resnick and Niwayama, 1988; Gielen et al., 1990). A reactive synovitis, resulting in joint effusion, may be seen in cases of tumor adjacent to the joint. Despite the lack of specificity of this finding, joint effusion remains a valuable indicator of joint disease, and ultrasound is unquestionably the best means of detecting increased intra-articular fluid. Effusions as small as 1 mL are easily detected sonographically (Marchal et al., 1987). Sonography has proved to be more sensitive than blind aspiration of the joint (Adam et al., 1986; Peck, 1986; Marchal et al., 1987). A major advantage of ultrasound over other techniques, such as arthrography and MRI, in joint evaluation is that it not only detects fluid with great sensitivity, but it also guides aspiration of fluid with precision.

Transient Synovitis

Acute joint effusion in children is a difficult diagnostic problem for the clinician. Occurring in the hip, more than 95% of cases are the result of an idiopathic inflammatory process of the synovium. This process resolves spontaneously within 6 weeks

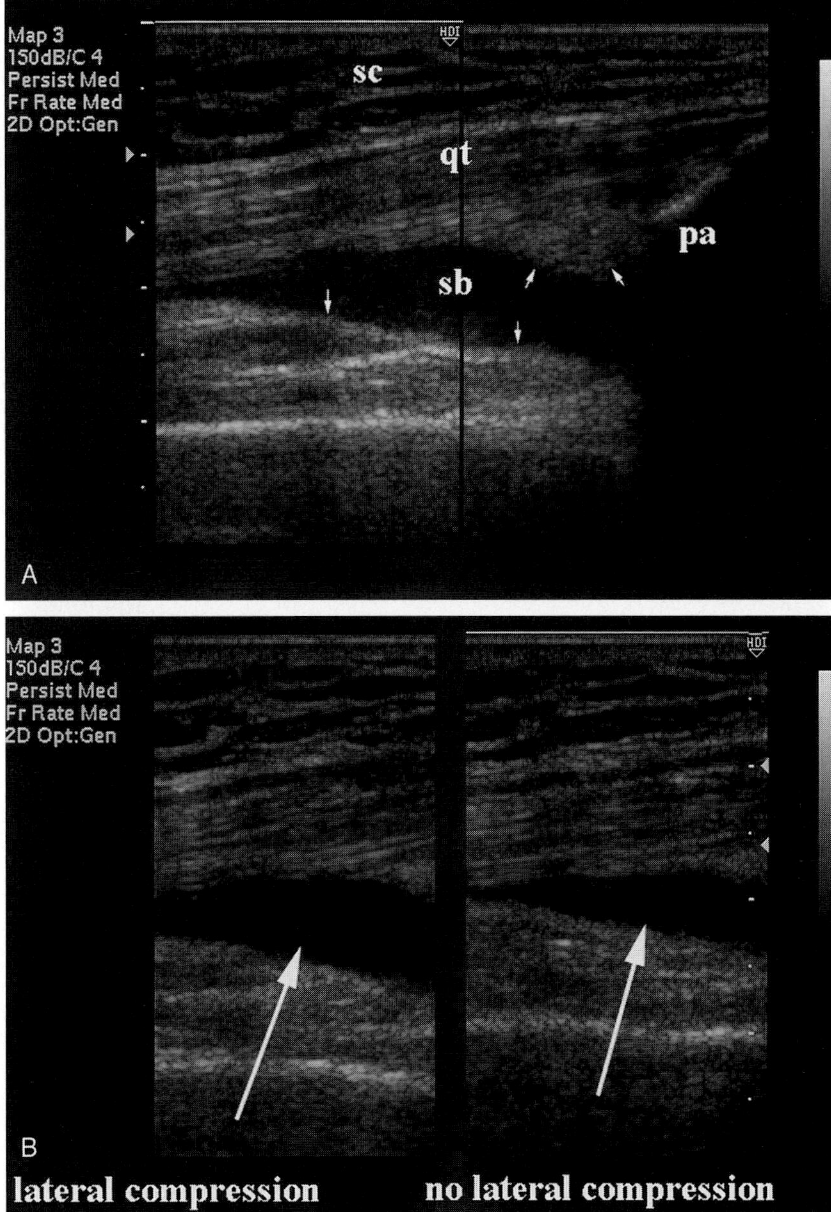

Figure 8–5 ■ **A**, Knee effusion: longitudinal image through the suprapatellar bursa. A knee joint effusion is present in this 36-year-old man with a meniscal tear. Anechoic fluid fills the suprapatellar bursa (*sb*). The transition between the effusion within the joint and the prefemoral and suprapatellar fat around the joint is abrupt (*arrows*). The normal synovial lining is imperceptible. Abbreviations: subcutaneous fat (*sc*), quadriceps tendon (*qt*), patella (*pa*). **B**, Knee effusion: longitudinal image through the suprapatellar bursa using split-screen technique. Same patient as in **A**. The image on the left side of the split screen shows the filling of the bursa (*arrow*) when the examiner's hand squeezes the medial and lateral recesses of the suprapatellar bursa. The image on the right side shows the bursa (*arrow*) without side compression. Quite often, reactive fluid in patients with meniscal tears will present as anechoic distention of the bursa. In acute effusions without inflammation, the thin synovial lining will be imperceptible.

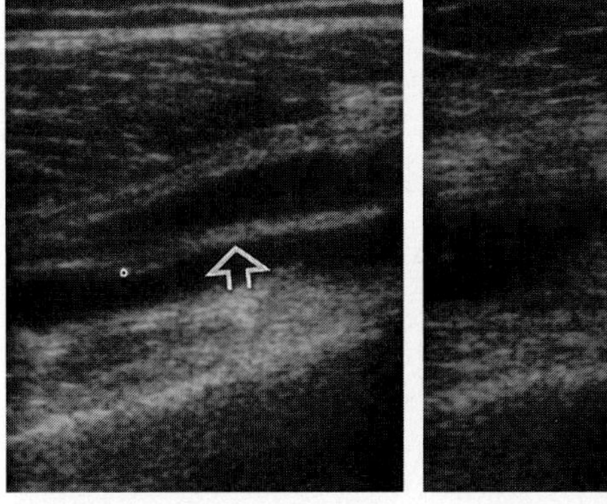

Figure 8–6 ■ Normal plicae: longitudinal images of the suprapatellar bursa using split-screen technique. Another patient with meniscal tear presents with knee effusion. A medial plica (*open arrow*) divides the suprapatellar bursa coronally on the left side of this split-screen image. This longitudinal image was obtained through the medial aspect of the bursa. An image through the midline of the knee is shown on the right side of the split screen. This image demonstrates the suprapatellar plica (*arrow*). The suprapatellar plica is present in over 95% of knees.

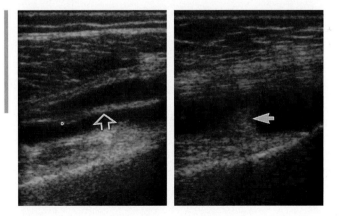

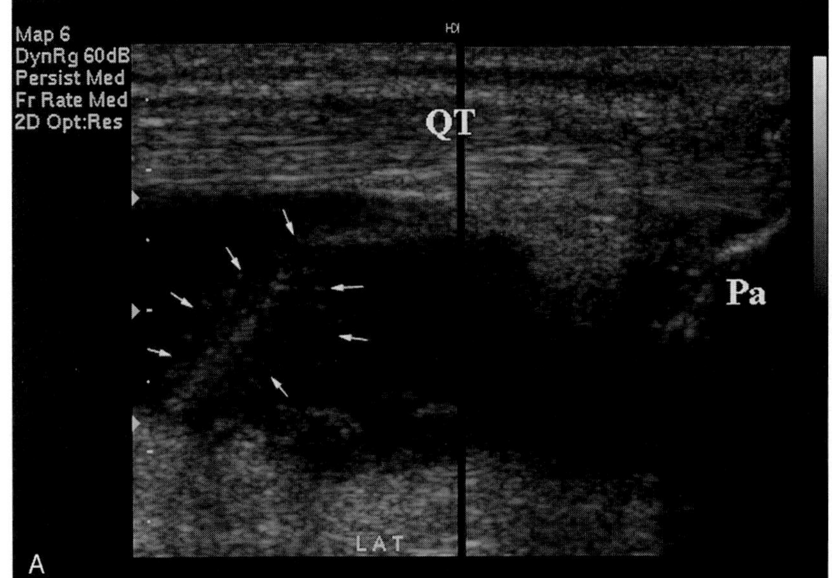

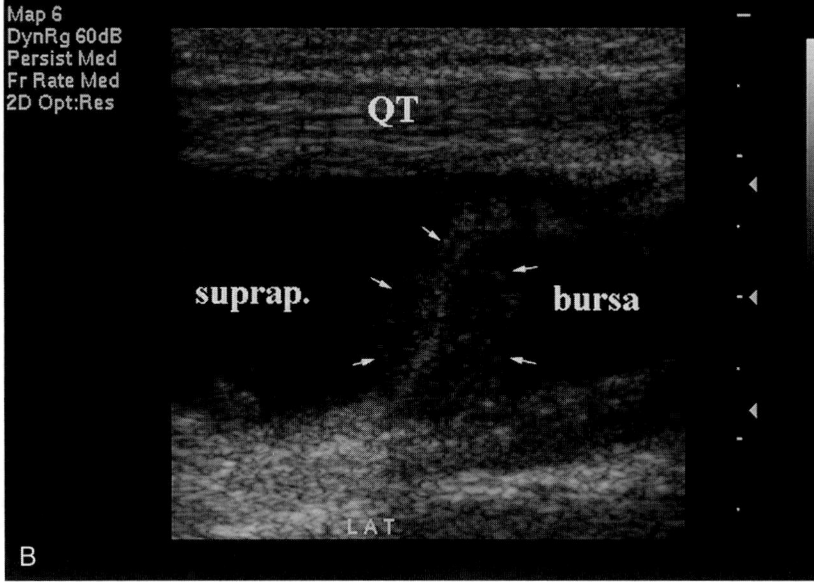

Figure 8–7 ■ **A**, Thickened suprapatellar plica: longitudinal sonogram through the suprapatellar bursa. Recurrent joint effusions plagued this 64-year-old man, who had osteoarthritis with several loose bodies in his knee. This sagittal image shows a thick suprapatellar plica (*arrows*). Abbreviations: patella (*Pa*), quadriceps tendon (*QT*). **B**, Thickened suprapatellar plica: longitudinal sonogram through the suprapatellar bursa. Same patient as in **A**. Detail of the thickened plica. Nodular tissue (*arrows*) surrounds the plica, which can still be recognized as a vague central hyperechoic line. The thickness of this septum exceeded 1 cm focally. Plicae can thicken in cases of chronic effusions and with inflammatory disease. Abbreviations: quadriceps tendon (*QT*).

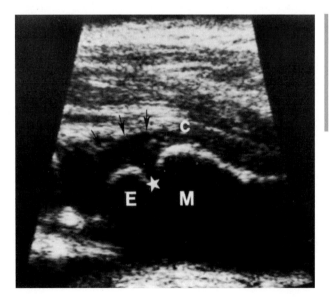

Figure 8–8 ■ Normal hip of a child: longitudinal sonogram. The patient is a normal 6-year-old boy. This image was obtained with the transducer aligned along the length of the femoral neck. Bony contours of the proximal femoral epiphysis (*E*) and metaphysis (*M*) are clearly demonstrated. The growth plate is identified as a hypoechoic band (*star*) distal to the femoral epiphysis. A hyperechoic band approximately 4 mm thick anterior to the femoral head represents the anterior joint capsule (*c*), also called the *iliofemoral ligament.* The epiphyseal cartilage is seen as a hypoechoic zone covering the femoral head (*arrows*).

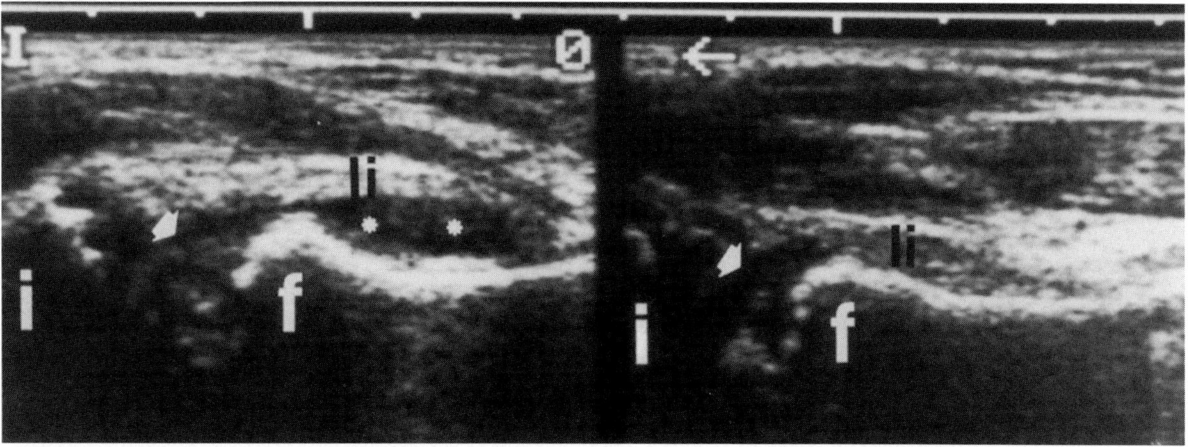

Figure 8–9 ■ Bilateral hips, unilateral effusion: longitudinal sonograms. The patient is an irritable 3-month-old boy who was not moving his left leg. The position of the transducer is identical to that in Figure 8–8. The anterior joint capsule is formed by the hyperechoic iliofemoral ligament (*li*) that connects the ilium and femur. Recognition of this structure is critical in making the diagnosis of hip effusion. A distance greater than 3 mm separating the iliofemoral ligament from the femoral cortex is diagnostic for an effusion. In this case, an effusion is identified in the left hip (*asterisk*) at the observer's left. The right hip, imaged for comparison, is normal. Epiphyseal cartilage (*white arrow*). Abbreviations: ilium (*i*), femur metaphysis (*f*).

without sequelae. Rarely, after repeated bouts of the disease, coxa magna may result. *Transient synovitis* is the preferred name for this disease because it clearly conveys the essential features of the disease. *Toxic synovitis* is a synonymous but less meaningful term.

In the past, the diagnosis of transient synovitis was one of exclusion. It was based on the clinical history and the finding of increased joint space of the hip medially, detected on conventional radiographs of the pelvis. The finding of joint space widening is valid only if the radiograph is an orthogonal projection. This severely limits the clinical value of this sign, with fewer than one-half of the cases (Marchal et al., 1987) of transient synovitis having joint space widening demonstrable on conventional radiographs. As a result, some clinicians

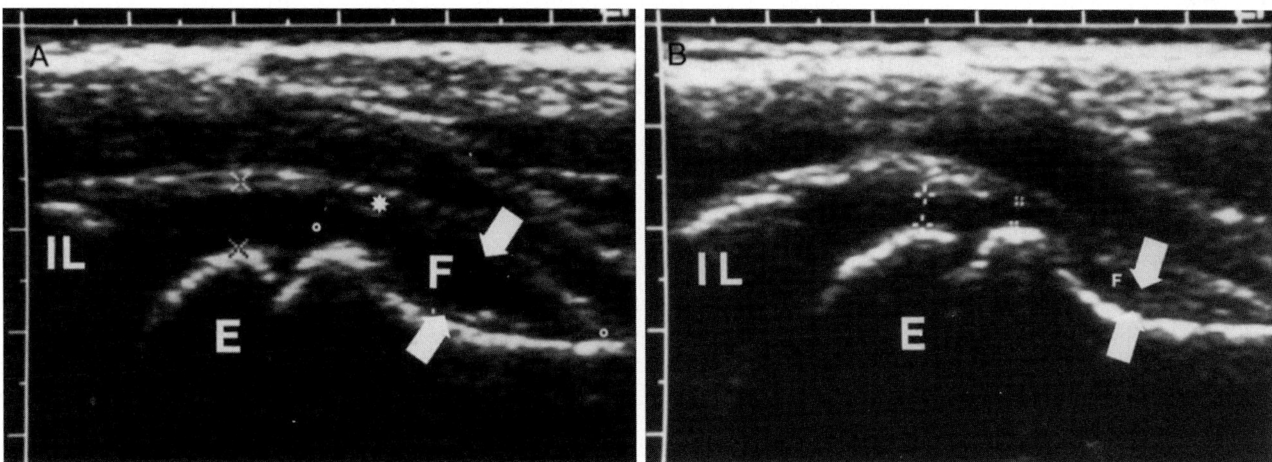

Figure 8–10 ■ **A**, Transient synovitis in a child: longitudinal sonogram. An 8-year-old girl who refused to bear weight on the left leg. The position of the transducer is identical to that in Figure 8–8. The capsule-to-cortex distance (*arrows*) is measured from the internal aspect of the iliofemoral ligament (*asterisk*) to the cortical surface at a point equidistant between the growth plate (*open circle*) and the insertion of the iliofemoral ligament on the femoral neck (*open circle*). In this case, the capsule-to-cortex distance is greater than 3 mm, indicative of joint effusion (*F*). A slightly thickened rim of capsule is seen covering the femoral neck. Abbreviations: femoral epiphysis (*E*), ilium (*IL*), epiphyseal cartilage (×). **B**, Transient synovitis: normal contralateral hip. Same patient as in **A**. The capsule-to-cortex distance is normal, 1 to 2 mm (*arrows*). A tiny fluid film (*F*) is noted between the iliofemoral ligament and the synovium. Abbreviations: ilium (*IL*), femoral epiphysis (*E*), epiphyseal cartilage (+).

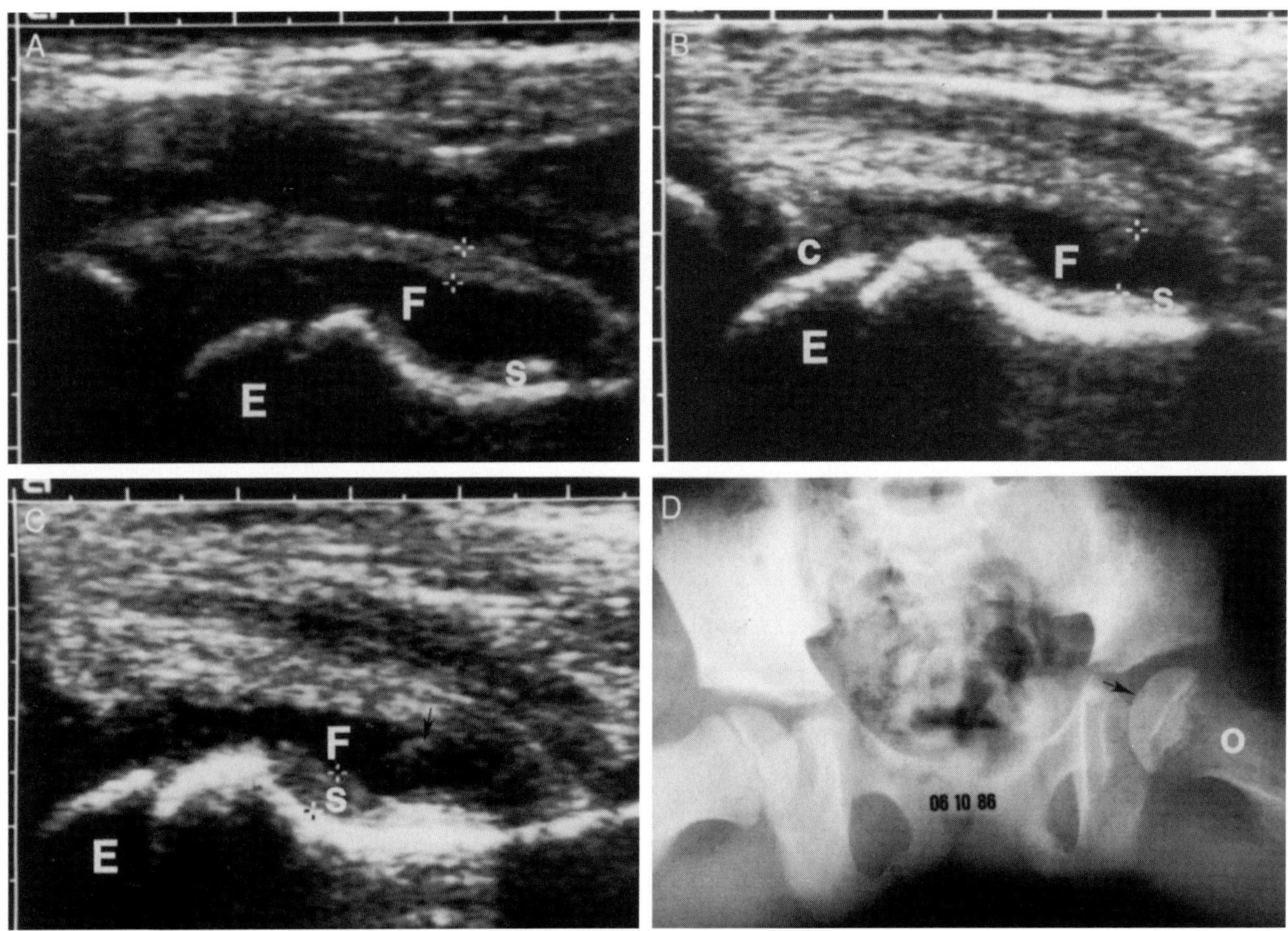

Figure 8-11 ■ **A,** Hip effusion in Legg-Calvé-Perthes disease: longitudinal sonogram. The patient is an 11-year-old boy with pain in the left leg over the past week. A large joint effusion (*F*) displaces the iliofemoral ligament (*between the cursors*) anteriorly, and a thin band of synovial tissue (*s*) and capsular tissue is identified around the femoral neck. Abbreviation: femoral epiphysis (*E*). **B,** Three weeks later, the amount of fluid is decreased (*between the cursors*), but an effusion is still present. The synovial-capsular tissue (*s*) around the femoral neck has increased in thickness. Abbreviations: cartilage (*c*), femoral epiphysis (*E*), fluid (*F*). **C,** Twelve weeks later, the femoral epiphysis (*E*) appears flatter. No change is observed in the quantity of intra-articular fluid (*F*). A further increase in synovial-capsular thickness (*cursors*) is noted, and the contour of the synovium has become quite irregular (*arrow*). **D,** Frog leg pelvic radiograph taken 12 weeks after the initial sonographic examination. The left femoral epiphysis is slightly flatter and more irregular than the right (*arrow*). The density of the left femoral epiphysis is increased relative to the osteoporotic femoral metaphysis (*open circle*), indicative of avascular necrosis.

have adopted unguided joint aspiration to confirm the diagnosis. In transient synovitis, serous or serosanguineous fluid is obtained (Vandeputte et al., 1971). However, unguided joint aspiration is not reliable unless performed by a clinician with considerable experience. Even when unguided joint aspiration is performed by experienced orthopedic surgeons, sonography has proved to be more sensitive in detecting joint effusion (Adam et al., 1986; Peck, 1986). Careful sonographic comparison with the asymptomatic side is mandatory. An effusion is detected by observing anterior displacement of the iliofemoral ligament by a fluid collection. Recent studies have shown separation of the anterior and posterior layers of the joint capsule by the effusion in transient synovitis (Robben et al., 1999). Asymmetry greater than 2 mm (see Figs. 8-9 and 8-10) or a capsule-to-bone distance greater than 3 mm is significant (Adam et al., 1986; Peck, 1986; Marchal et al., 1987; Dorr, 1988).

The differential diagnosis includes septic arthritis and Legg-Calvé-Perthes disease. Although these account for less than 4% of cases in our experience, they must be carefully considered in cases of acute hip pain with effusion in children. Ultrasound images in transient synovitis demonstrate a joint effusion composed of anechoic or markedly hypoechoic fluid. Effusions in septic arthritis are hypoechoic, with definite internal echos. Marked synovial irregularity and thickening of the joint capsule are also seen in septic arthritis (Dorr, 1988). In exceptional cases of septic arthritis, intra-articular gas bubbles may be identified as hyperechoic foci with "dirty" shadowing, indicative of infection with gas-producing organisms. Although the specificity of these findings is high, the decision to aspirate the joint to exclude infection must be based on clinical criteria. Several cases of early septic arthritis with anechoic fluid and minimal synovial changes have been reported (Marchal et al., 1987).

Sonographic characteristics of the joint effusions seen in transient synovitis and Legg-Calvé-Perthes disease are identical (Wingstrand, 1986; Marchal et al., 1987). Early diagnosis of Legg-Calvé-Perthes disease, before conventional radiographic findings are evident, is based on repeating the sonographic examination 6 weeks following the initial diagnosis of uncomplicated joint effusion. During this time, effusion resulting from transient synovitis will resolve. Persistence of a simple effusion is diagnostic of Legg-Calvé-Perthes disease. Cartilage edema, recognized as thickening of the cartilage, will also be seen in early stages of Legg-Calvé-Perthes disease. Later, flattening of the femoral head can be observed sonographically and on conventional radiographs (see Fig. 8-11). Small, loose bodies consisting of hyaline cartilage are not an unusual finding in the advanced cases of Legg-Calvé-Perthes disease.

Follow-up of Joint Effusions

In addition to suspected transient synovitis, sonographic follow-up examinations are extremely valuable in infectious and inflammatory arthritides: joint tuberculosis, septic joints, rheumatoid arthritis, psoriatic arthritis, and Reiter's disease. A decrease in the quantity of intra-articular fluid is the first sign of a positive response to therapy. The response can almost always be detected within 48 hours of initiation of treatment. Later, changes in the thickness of the synovia are seen (van Holsbeeck et al., 1988b). A more detailed discussion of the changes seen in rheumatoid arthritis is found in Chapter 11.

Septic Arthritis

Septic joint pathology is relatively rare in adults and much more common in children (Box 8-1). Immunocompromised patients, diabetics, drug addicts, and dialysis patients are at increased risk of septic arthritis. Blood-borne pathogens may directly seed to the synovial membrane or osteomyelitis may extend to involve a joint. The synovium is vulnerable because of the absence of a basement membrane protecting the highly vascular synovium (Middleton, 1993; Cimmino, 1997). Direct implantation of pathogens into a joint can occur with foreign body penetration of a joint or after placement of a joint prosthesis. Joint infection after intra-articular injection is a dreaded complication of local steroid treatment. Joint infections are most commonly due to a bacterial etiology, but the causes can also be fungal, mycobacterial, viral, or parasitic. Gram-positive cocci are the most common causative organism, with *Staphylococcus aureus* being the predominant organism. *S. aureus* is found in approximately 70% of adult pyarthroses. A quick Gram stain of hip fluid obtained by ultrasound-guided aspiration may confirm the diagnosis within an hour of admission. Definitive diagnosis requires culture of the synovial fluid. Amplification of DNA by the polymerase chain reaction (PCR) is a powerful technique which is gaining widespread use for diagnosis. PCR will aid in providing a rapid and accurate diagnosis of diseases such as Lyme arthritis and tuberculosis of joints.

Box 8-1
Facts to Remember When Scanning for Septic Arthritis

- Occurs in children, in immunocompromised adults, and in prosthetic joints
- 70% of pyarthroses are due to *Staphylococcus aureus*
- 75% of patients have a positive Gram stain (quickest test on fluid)
- 50% of patients have positive blood cultures
- 50% knee > 25% hip > 15% shoulder

Septic arthritis of the knee accounts for 40-50% of joint infections. Hip disease comprises 20-25% of cases, and shoulder disease accounts for 10-15%. These deep-seated joints are more difficult to evaluate clinically than the small joints in the hand and foot. Aspiration is often difficult because of the complex anatomy of these joints. Sonography can guide needles into narrow spaces between bone surfaces. Ultrasound-guided aspiration can avoid osteophytes and areas of capsular thickening. However, the main advantage of ultrasound is its ability to direct the needle into fluid collections, making "dry taps" a thing of the past. Some dry taps were attributable to technical failures, while others were due to the absence of a joint effusion. Joint swelling due to hypertrophic, inflamed synovium without effusion may account for some of these failures. A small, hypoechoic area surrounding the joint may be due to

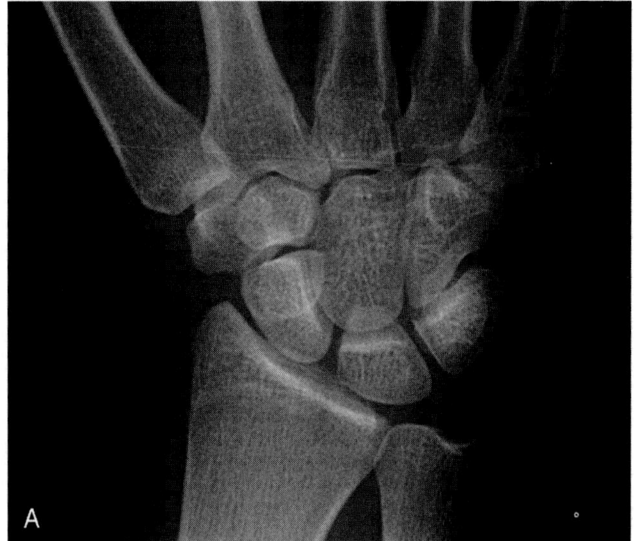

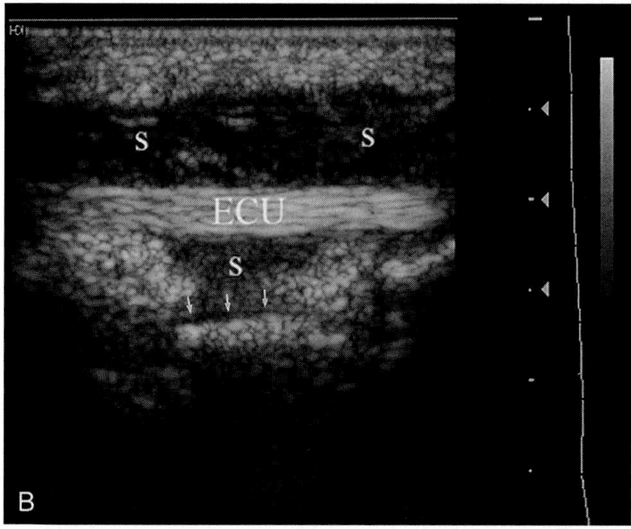

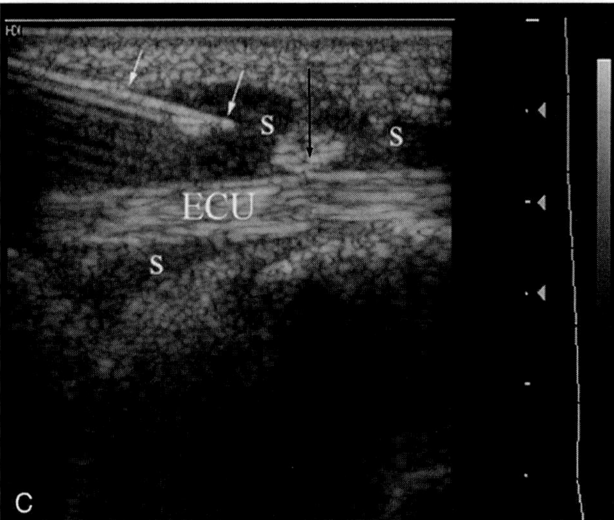

Figure 8-12 ▪ **A**, Gonococcal infection: radiograph of wrist. Wrist pain had been present for 5 days prior to hospital admission of this 17-year-old girl. She presented to the emergency department with fever, chills, and new pain in her left shoulder which had begun that day. Radiographs of the wrist are normal. **B**, Gonococcal infection: longitudinal sonogram over the dorsum of the wrist. Same patient as in **A**. Hypoechoic material is noted in a tendon sheath. No hyperemia is observed on the color Doppler study. Only the synovium (*s*) of the extensor carpi ulnaris (*ECU*) appears abnormal. The synovial space (*arrows*) of the carpus seems unaffected. **C**, Gonococcal infection: longitudinal ultrasound of the ECU tendon sheath during aspiration. Same patient as in **A**. A 19-gauge needle (*white arrows*) was introduced into the synovial sheath. Four milliliters of pus were aspirated. The sheath collapsed during aspiration (*black arrow*). The ultrasound study allowed us to sample the fluid selectively from the tendon sheath. The intercarpal joints were left untouched, and contamination of these joints was avoided. A blind aspiration may well have resulted in further spread of infection. Microscopic examination of a smear of joint fluid colored with Gram stain showed numerous polymorphonuclear leukocytes. Several cells were noted to have gram-negative, oval diplococci located intracellularly, a finding very suggestive of *Neisseria gonorrhoeae.* This positive result, which was obtained on the day of admission, facilitated treatment by more rapid administration of appropriate antibiotic therapy. Cervical cultures were positive for gonococcus despite the lack of urogenital symptoms.

synovitis rather than fluid. Power or color Doppler flow within this region must be used to substantiate synovial inflammation. The color flow in pannus typically appears as scattered color throughout abnormal tissue. Distinct from this, in infections, hyperemia demonstrated on color or power Doppler imaging will appear in the capsule or subsynovial layers around an infectious effusion (Breidahl et al., 1996). In some acute infections, however, there is often no demonstrable flow at all. Color flow in the center of an infected collection is typically absent, in contrast to the central color flow in pannus.

In most cases, fluid can be obtained under ultrasound guidance by advancing the needle through the thickened synovium. However, in patients who have large masses of synovium and little fluid, it may be necessary to utilize a core biopsy needle system. This method allows the operator to cut a piece of capsule and inflamed synovium. This technique facilitates the diagnosis of chronic infections, such as tuberculosis, fungal disease, and Lyme arthritis using tissue culture. Ultrasound adds accuracy to aspiration and biopsy of joints and eliminates potentially traumatic and unnecessary aspiration attempts in a normal joint.

In addition to detecting joint effusions, ultrasound can detect fluid collections outside of the joint, such as septic bursitis and soft tissue abscesses (Lombardi et al., 1992). Blind or fluoroscopi-

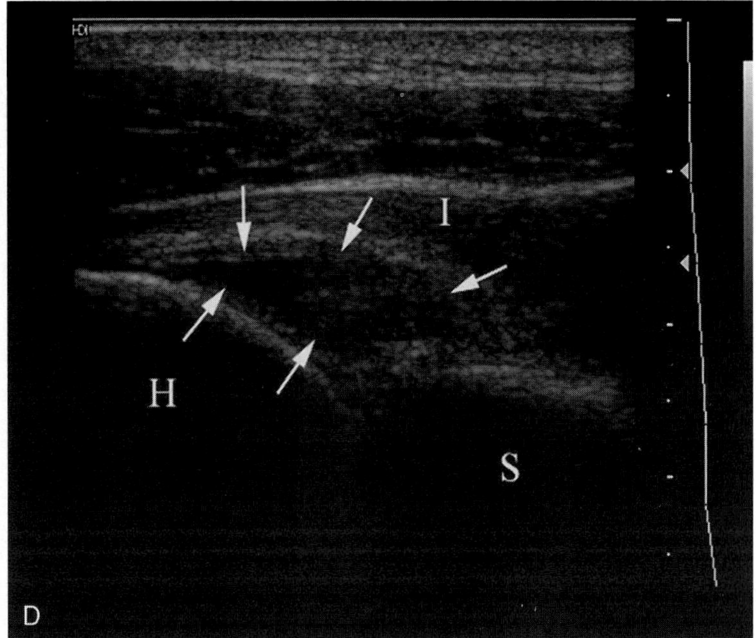

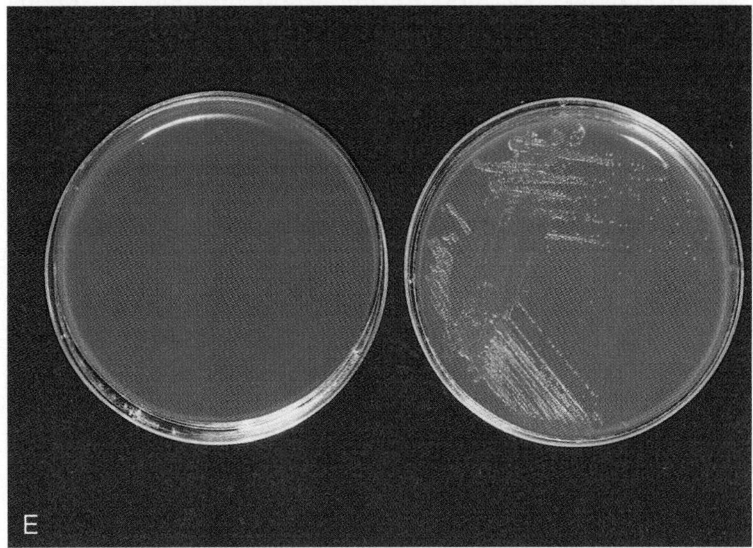

Figure 8–12 *Continued* ▪ **D**, Gonococcal infection: transverse ultrasound of the infraspinatus recess in the shoulder. Same patient as in **A**. Significant joint distention (*arrows*) was noted deep to the infraspinatus tendon (*I*). Maximal swelling was marked on the skin. A needle was then introduced, with its orientation perpendicular to the joint space between the posterior scapula (*S*) and the humeral head (*H*). Aspiration revealed clear serous fluid with low viscosity. The fluids of the wrist and shoulder were packaged separately. Laboratory exams that must be done on all fluid suspected of being infected include Gram stain, cell count, differential cell count, cultures, and sensitivity analysis. **E**, Gonococcal infection: cultures on Martin-Lewis agar. Same patient as in **A**. The examiner suspected gonococcal synovitis because of the patient's age, clinical history, and anecdotal experience of several prior aspirations of wrist joints which proved positive for this disease. Gonococci are difficult to culture; therefore, in view of the clinical suspicion, a Martin-Lewis agar was selected at the microbiology lab. Both the shoulder and wrist fluids were inoculated on this medium almost immediately after aspiration. The plates were then incubated in carbon dioxide for 24 hours at 37°C. The shoulder fluid spread over the petri dish on the left did not grow gonococcus. The wrist fluid in the dish on the right shows contiguous colonies of the typical small, hemispherical, transparent colonies of *N. gonorrhoeae.*

cally guided aspiration may transmit infected fluid from an infected extra-articular collection into a noninfected joint (Lombardi et al., 1992) (Fig. 8–12). Ultrasound will demonstrate where the fluid is and will allow targeted aspiration, without violation of the joint capsule.

Early signs of infection are pain and fever. Corticosteroid treatment and old age may mask infection because of their effect on body temperature regulation and the inflammatory response. Temperature then may be normal in patients with septic arthritis who are immunocompromised for any reason. Fifty percent of patients with a primary pyarthrosis have a positive blood culture (Golberg and Cohen, 1976).

Joint infection is characterized by an exudate of joint fluid. The exudate can be diagnosed sonographically by careful side-by-side comparison and measurement of the displacement of the capsule by the joint effusion. Animal studies have shown that an inflammatory exudate may be present within 3 hours after septic inoculation (Riegels-Nielsen et al., 1987). In over 600 joint aspirations, we have found only three cases in which the initial scan did not demonstrate increased joint fluid in patients who later proved to have a joint infection. Our recommendation is to repeat the ultrasound examination if fever and joint pain persist.

The effusion is typically hypoechoic relative to the surrounding soft tissues (Figs. 8–12 and 8–13). Most effusions contain a diffuse pattern of low-level echos (Fig. 8–14). Completely anechoic collections of infected joint fluid are rare. We have only observed these anechoic collections early in the course of infection. Hyperechoic effusions, however, are seen regularly (Fig. 8–15). In our experience, these hyperechoic effusions are observed more often in joints that are located superficially, like the tibiotalar and sternoclavicular joints. This appearance may confuse the inexperienced examiner. The collection can appear to be solid tissue on static examinations. During scanning, one will note fluctuation with swirling or layering within the fluid. The joint capsule and synovium are usually very hyperechoic in a septic joint. The size and echogenicity of an effusion may suggest an infectious or inflammatory etiology, but they are not pathognomonic. That is why we aspirate all fluid collections with symptoms or clinical settings that suggest infection. Hyperemia of the synovium seems to parallel the sensitivity of the joint upon puncture with the needle for diagnostic aspiration. Not all septic joints demonstrate synovial hyperemia. The duration of infection, the age of the patient, and the patient's immune status all influence the vascularity of the synovium.

When an effusion is detected, the depth from the skin surface is measured and a needle of appropriate length is selected. The transducer is positioned over the effusion, and an ink dot is placed on the skin at the midpoint of the ends of the transducer. The transducer is then repositioned orthogonal to the prior examination plane. The maximum joint effusion is marked once more, using the dots at the proximal and distal ends of the transducer. The dots are connected to form a + in both transverse and longitudinal orientations. The skin is prepared with Betadine and anesthetized with a 1% Lidocaine injection, provided that there are no contraindications, such as drug allergy. Scanning following aspiration can confirm complete aspiration and assess for any loculated fluid collections. Most

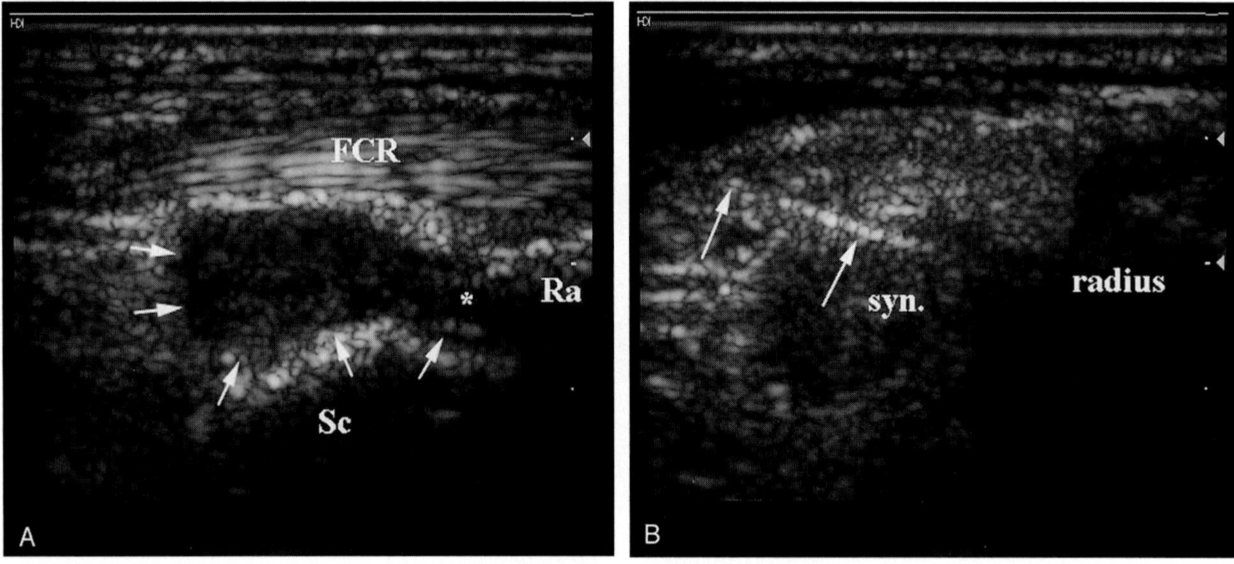

Figure 8–13 ■ **A**, Chlamydia infection: longitudinal ultrasound through the lateral aspect of the radiocarpal joint. On initial examination, pain and swelling in the wrist of this 19-year-old girl were judged to be of bony origin by the emergency room physician. The radiographs were negative, and the patient was referred for an ultrasound examination. Wrist joint swelling is noted with the transducer oriented over the lateral and volar aspect of the wrist. Hypoechoic swelling (*arrows*) in continuity with the radio-scaphoid joint (*) was interpreted as joint fluid, and aspiration was suggested. Power color Doppler did not show abnormal flow in this mass. Abbreviations: flexor carpi radialis (*FCR*), radius (*Ra*), scaphoid (*Sc*). **B**, *Chlamydia* infection: transverse ultrasound through the lateral aspect of the radiocarpal joint. Same patient as in **A**. Several attempts to aspirate fluid failed despite accurate localization of the needle within the hypoechoic mass. At the end of the study, saline was injected and reaspirated through the needle (*arrows*). The fluid from the joint washings tested positive for *Chlamydia trachomatis*. Subsequently, the smear from this young woman's cervix tested positive for *Chlamydia* as well. Abbreviation: synovium (*syn.*).

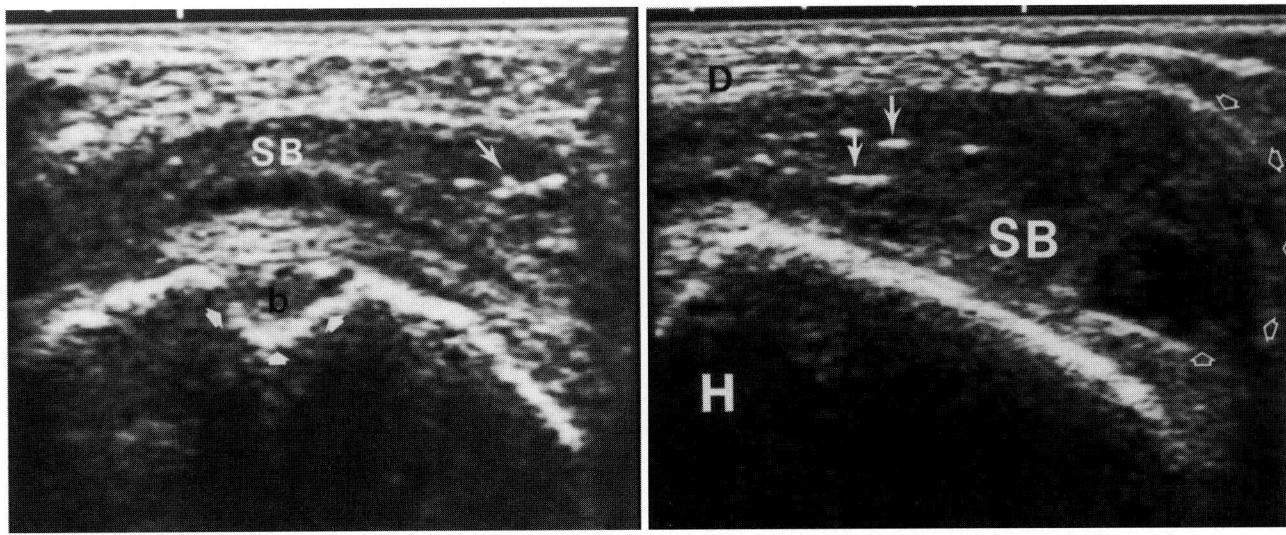

Figure 8–14 ■ **A**, Septic arthritis of the shoulder: transverse sonogram. This 65-year-old man initially presented with a history of right shoulder pain of 1 week's duration. He was treated by his family physician with intra-articular steroid injection. This relieved his symptoms temporarily, but he returned with increased pain and swelling 1 week later. He was afebrile, with minimal leukocytosis and an elevated erythrocyte sedimentation rate. The subacromial-subdeltoid bursa (*SB*) is filled with fluid that is only slightly less echogenic than the overlying deltoid muscle. Highly echogenic foci (*large arrow*) within the fluid collection are consistent with gas bubbles. A normal biceps tendon (*b*) is seen in the bicipital groove (*small arrows*). Blind aspiration of the joint was negative. Surgical drainage of the joint was performed based on the sonographic findings, and *Staphylococcus epidermidis* was cultured. **B**, Septic arthritis of the shoulder: coronal sonogram. Same patient as in **A**. A bulging subacromial-subdeltoid bursa (*SB*) is noted deep to the deltoid muscle (*D*). Note that the inferior extent of the bursa (*open arrows*) is larger than the superior aspect. A common error is to not identify the convex inferior margin of the distended bursa. Again noted are the echogenic gas bubbles (*large arrows*). Abbreviation: proximal humerus (*H*).

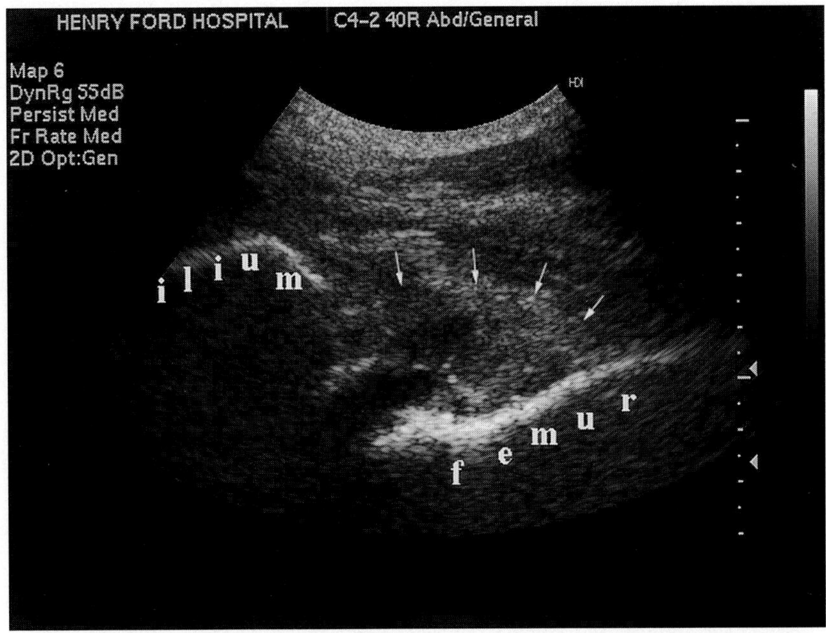

Figure 8–15 ■ Adult septic hip: longitudinal ultrasound. Chronic hip pain in this 43-year-old diabetic was suddenly exacerbated. Fever accompanied the increased pain, and the patient was referred for an emergent joint aspiration. The effusion is inhomogeneous but mainly hyperechoic relative to the surrounding soft tissues. The joint capsule bulges anteriorly (*arrows*). The femoral head has been partially destroyed. Hyperechoic specks of debris are noted anterior to the proximal femur. *Escherichia coli* grew from the cultured fluid.

infected fluid appears cloudy. A cell count of over 100,000 is almost pathognomonic for infection. Remember that the Gram stain is positive in 50–75% of patients with nongonococcal septic arthritis but in fewer than 25% of patients with *Neisseria gonorrhoeae.* Joint cultures are positive in 85% of nongonococcal infections but in only 25% of gonococcal infections.

Effusions in Trauma

Ultrasound is very helpful in distinguishing simple effusions from other types (Figs. 8–16 and 8–17). Hemarthrosis or lipohemarthrosis following intra-articular fracture, cruciate ligament tears, and meniscal tears, as well as dislocation can easily be identified. Free-floating blood clots or fat lobules are seen within the effusion (Fig. 8–18). These lobules are mobile and easily deformed when the examiner's hand or the transducer applies pressure. In many of these cases, aspiration of the joint is negative, probably due to obstruction of the needle lumen by clot or debris. Not all posttraumatic effusions consist of intra-articular hemorrhage. The fluid in the knee joint with meniscal tears is often anechoic. Knee flexion or compression of the lateral recess may move the fluid under the transducer. Both suprapatellar and medial patellar plicae may appear as normal variants of the suprapatellar bursa. The normal plicae are no more than a couple millimeters thick. Aspiration of these effusions yields serous fluid. Chronic posttraumatic effusions or inflammatory disease may cause thickening of the knee plicae, which may catch in the patellofemoral joint.

Synovial Edema and Pannus

Thickened, edematous synovia can be seen in inflammatory arthritides (Resnick and Niwayama, 1988), in amyloidosis (Gielen et al., 1990) with joint involvement (Fig. 8–19), and in tumoral involvement of the synovia (Resnick and Niwayama, 1988). Pigmented villonodular synovitis and synovial chondromatosis are two relatively common synovial tumors associated with synovial edema and thickening. Hypertrophic synovia are often hypoechoic, recognized as a dark band between surrounding muscle or fat (Cooperberg et al., 1978). Compression applied with the transducer affects the edematous synovia more than the adjacent muscle, tendons, ligaments, or fat. Therefore, compression is a helpful maneuver in identifying edematous synovial tissue (Fig. 8–20). A reliable and reproducible measurement of synovial thickness can be made only at maximal compression (van Holsbeeck et al., 1988b). All free fluid is then expelled from the region, and the measurement most closely reflects the true synovial thickness (Fig. 8–20).

Pannus is most commonly seen in cases of inflammatory arthritides, the classic example being rheumatoid arthritis. However, it can also be seen with chronic infections: tuberculosis, brucellosis, Lyme arthritis, and fungal infections. Additional information can be derived from increased blood flow in the synovium observed with color or power Doppler. Hyperemia is often present in patients with inflammatory and infectious synovitis (Fig. 8–21). Hyperemia has also been observed in pigmented villonodular synovitis, but it is rarely seen in osteoarticular amy-

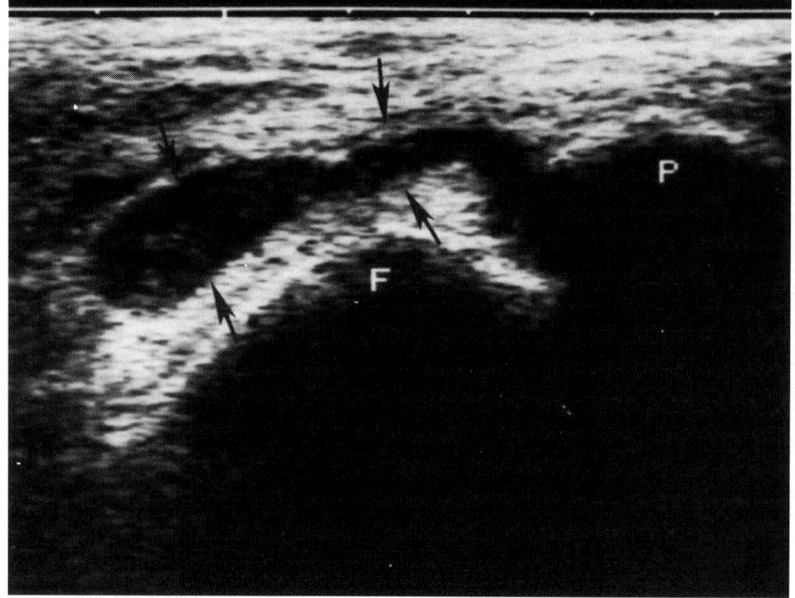

Figure 8–16 ■ Acute hemarthrosis of the knee: transverse sonogram. A 25-year-old man with trauma to the lateral aspect of the knee. Sonographic examination was performed about 10 hours following injury. The transducer is positioned transversely over the anterolateral aspect of the knee, approximately 2 cm above the joint space. The lateral joint recess (*arrows*) is filled with homogeneous, hypoechoic material. Aspiration of the joint was negative, presumably due to obstruction of the needle by clot. Arthroscopy performed 2 months later demonstrated a large bucket handle tear of the medial meniscus. Abbreviations: lateral femoral condyle (*F*), patella (*P*).

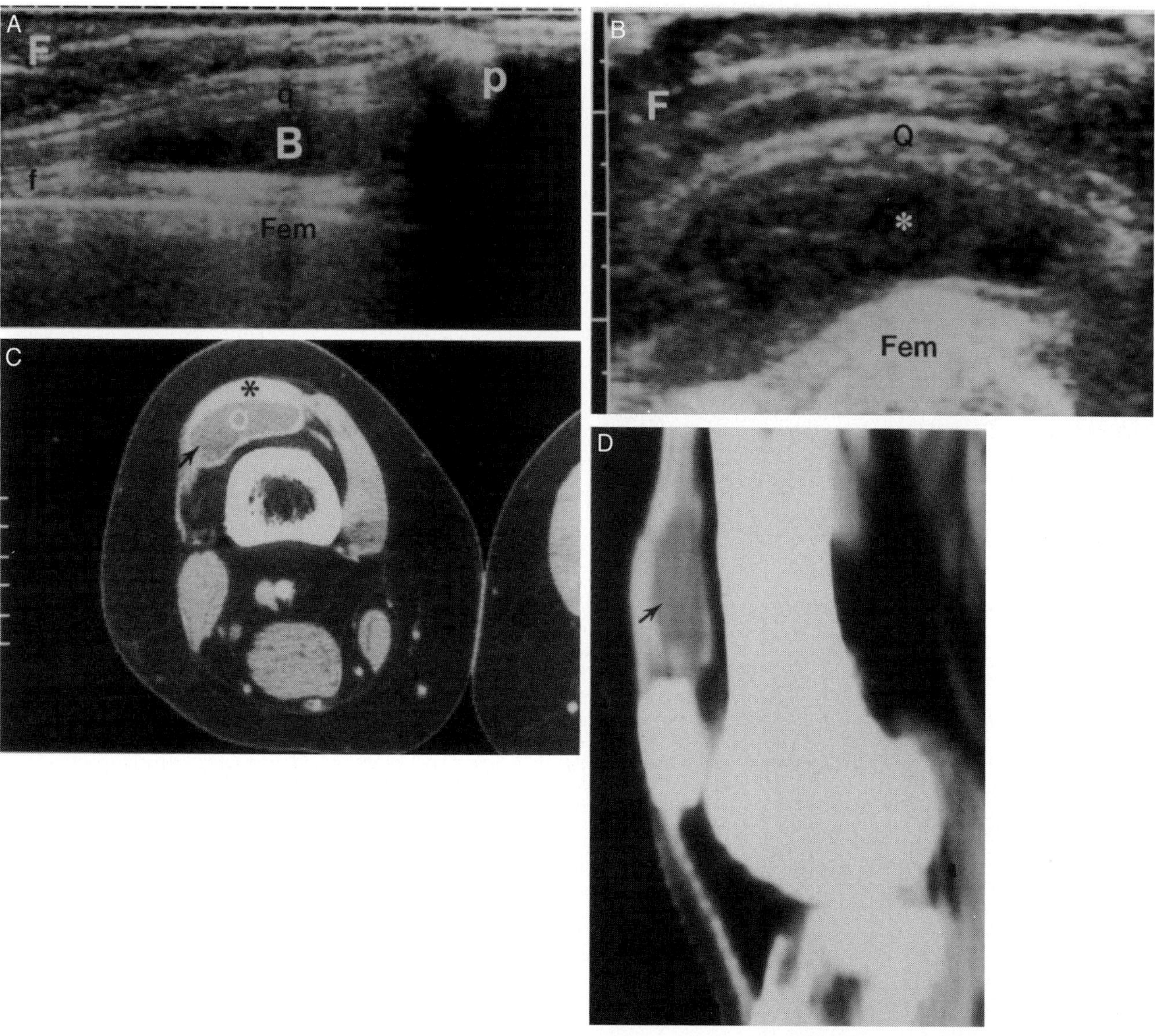

Figure 8–17 ■ **A**, Acute hemorrhagic bursitis: longitudinal sonogram. The patient is a 19-year-old female basketball player who received a blow to the knee during practice 3 days ago. Aspiration of the joint performed in the orthopedic surgeon's office yielded no fluid. The transducer is positioned at the superior aspect of the patella along the quadriceps tendon. A distended suprapatellar bursa (*B*) filled with hypoechoic fluid is noted deep to the quadriceps tendon (*q*). This homogeneous, hypoechoic fluid is consistent with recent hemorrhage. The fat (*f*) superior and deep to the bursa is hyperechoic, whereas the subcutaneous fat (*F*) is less echogenic. Hemorrhage in the knee is usually due to intra-articular fracture or to meniscal or cruciate tears. Hemorrhage localized to the bursa secondary to direct trauma, as in this case, is quite unusual. Abbreviations: femoral diaphysis (*Fem*), patella (*p*). **B**, Acute hemorrhagic bursitis: transverse sonogram. Same patient as in **A**. The transducer was rotated 90 degrees to yield a transverse image. The blood-filled suprapatellar bursa (*asterisk*) is again seen deep to the quadriceps tendon (*Q*). Abbreviations: subcutaneous fat (*F*), femur (*Fem*). **C** and **D**, Acute hemorrhagic bursitis: transverse and parasagittal CT. Same patient as in **A** and **B**. The distended, fluid-filled bursa (*arrows*) is demonstrated deep to the quadriceps tendon (*asterisk*). Density measurement of the fluid (*circle*) was 37 Hounsfield units. Note on the parasagittal image that the posterior joint capsule (*small arrow*) is not displaced.

loidosis, lipoma arborescens, and synovial osteochondromatosis. Villous synovial proliferation is often seen when pannus is present. Synechiae and fibrous adhesions within the synovial recesses are identified in later stages of disease. Fine particulate debris floating in the articular fluid may also be seen in rheumatoid joints. This is probably due to aggregation of fibrin within the inflammatory effusion, but it may also be seen following intra-articular corticosteroid administration (Worth et al., 1986). Infection does occur in rheumatoid joints, and aspiration is necessary to establish that diagnosis (Fig. 8–22).

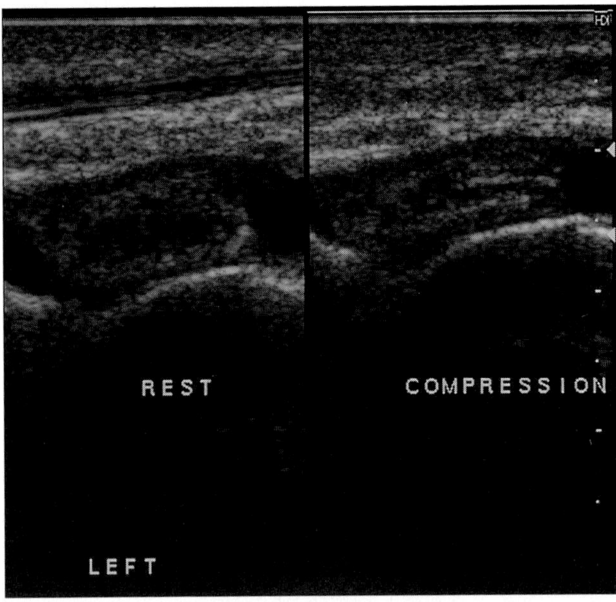

Figure 8–18 ■ Thrombus within the tibiotalar joint: longitudinal ultrasound with split-screen technique. The patient sustained an acute direct injury to the ankle joint. Longitudinal images through the anterior recess of the anterior tibiotalar joint demonstrate the lumen of that recess filled with thrombus. Pressure on the transducer deforms the thrombus, but the clot remains lodged in the recess, while some of the fluid has been expressed.

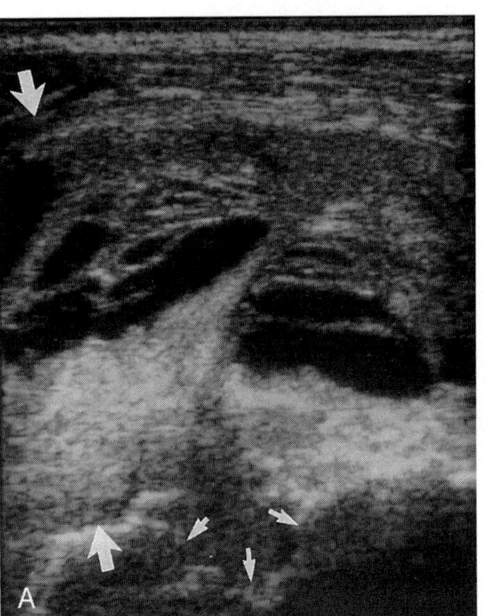

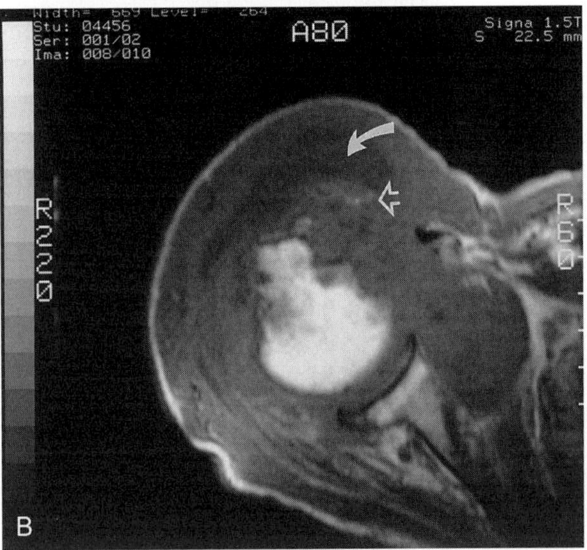

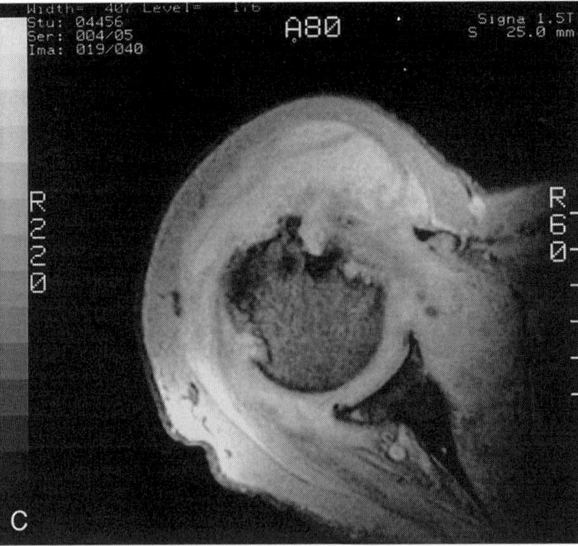

Figure 8–19 ■ **A**, Shoulder amyloidosis: transverse sonogram through the anterior subacromial-subdeltoid bursa. The subacromial-subdeltoid bursa of this renal dialysis patient demonstrates abnormal swelling and a layered structure of the bursal wall (*between the big arrows*). Fluid seems trapped in multiple compartments. The anatomical neck of the humerus is irregular, and punched-out defects deform its contour (*small arrows*). **B**, Shoulder amyloidosis: axial image through the glenohumeral joint using T_1 weighting. Same patient as in **A**. Low signal intensity fluid (*curved arrow*) and solid tissue of intermediate signal intensity (*open arrow*) are shown in the area which was imaged with ultrasound. Advanced destruction of the anatomical neck and greater tuberosity are also noted. **C**, Shoulder amyloidosis: axial image through the glenohumeral joint using gradient echo imaging. Same patient as in **A**. This pulse sequence demonstrates no hemosiderin. Therefore, pigmented villonodular synovitis is very unlikely. Unusual arthritic findings on this image include widening of the glenohumeral joint and deep, notch-like defects in the proximal humerus. Sediment within the bursal aspirate stained strongly with Congo red, indicating the presence of amyloid.

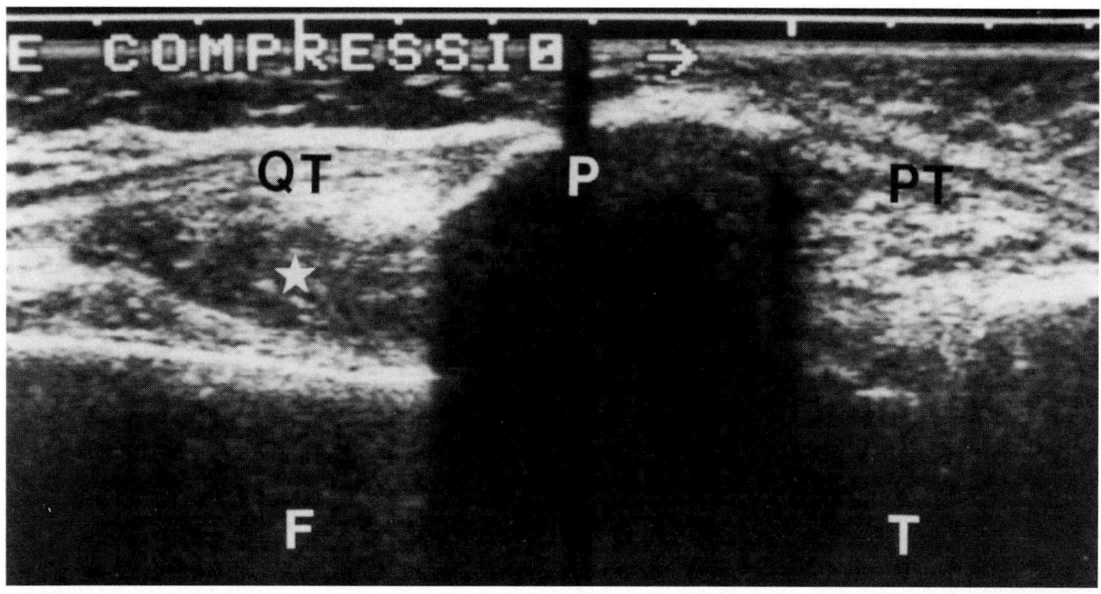

Figure 8–20 ▪ Rheumatoid arthritis of the knee: longitudinal sonogram with compression. A 58-year-old woman with a 16-year history of rheumatoid arthritis presented with new onset of pain in the right knee. The image is a sagittal view of the knee centered on the patella. Firm compression was applied with the transducer to express all of the fluid from the suprapatellar bursa. This allows reproducible measurement of the total synovial thickness (*TST*), the sum of the anterior and posterior walls of the suprapatellar bursa. In this case, the TST measures 1.7 cm, approximately eight to nine times greater than normal. The bursa is seen as a hypoechoic mass (*star*) deep to the quadriceps tendon. Pannus remains hypoechoic relative to the surrounding soft tissues despite firm compression to express joint fluid. Abbreviations: femur (*F*), quadriceps tendon (*QT*), patella (*P*), patellar tendon (*PT*), tibia (*T*).

Evaluation of synovial changes in large synovial joints is most easily performed at the suprapatellar recess of the knee, the anterior synovial recess of the hip, and the posterior synovial recess of the shoulder. All measurements of synovial thickness should be made with maximal compression applied by the transducer. This will yield the most accurate and reproducible measurements. Sonographic measurements of synovial thickness using this technique have been shown to be a reliable means of comparing the effectiveness of different therapies (Hammer et al., 1986; van Holsbeeck et al., 1988b).

Cartilage Pathology

Cartilage Structure

Articular cartilage is a gel of protein-polysaccharide complexes reinforced by a matrix of collagen fibers. The principal constituents of the polysaccharide portion are chondroitin and keratin sulfates, which are very hydrophilic (Sissons, 1987, in Taveras and Ferrucci, 1987). Chondrocytes are diffusely scattered throughout cartilage. The thickness of normal weight-bearing cartilage ranges from 1.2 to 1.9 mm (Aisen et al., 1984; Richardson et al., 1988). Cartilage of the growth plate differs principally in its arrangement of chondroblasts into regular pallisades of cells oriented in the long axis of the bone.

The sonographic appearance of articular cartilage is that of a thin, hypoechoic layer juxtaposed to the subchondral cortical bone. This hypoechoic appearance is probably a reflection of the homogeneous, hydrophilic structure of hyaline cartilage. Cartilage of the growth plate shares this homogeneous, hypoechoic appearance. Normal cartilage has sharp margins at both the articular and deep surfaces, making measurement of its thickness quite easy.

Fibrocartilage differs significantly from hyaline cartilage both histologically and sonographically. In fibrocartilage, the predominant component is collagen fibers, as the name implies. Densely packed bundles of collagen fibers are arranged in parallel. Cartilage cells that have differentiated from fibroblasts are scattered throughout this dense collagen matrix. In some cases, they are found in rows between the collagen bundles. A minute amount of ground substance surrounds these cells but is absent elsewhere (Bloom and Fawcett, 1975). This structure of tightly packed collagen with interspersed cartilage cells and minimal ground substance explains the hyperechoic appearance of fibrocartilage in ultrasound images. The menisci of the knee are composed of fibrocartilage and have a homogeneous, hyperechoic appearance. This is also true of the triangular fibro-

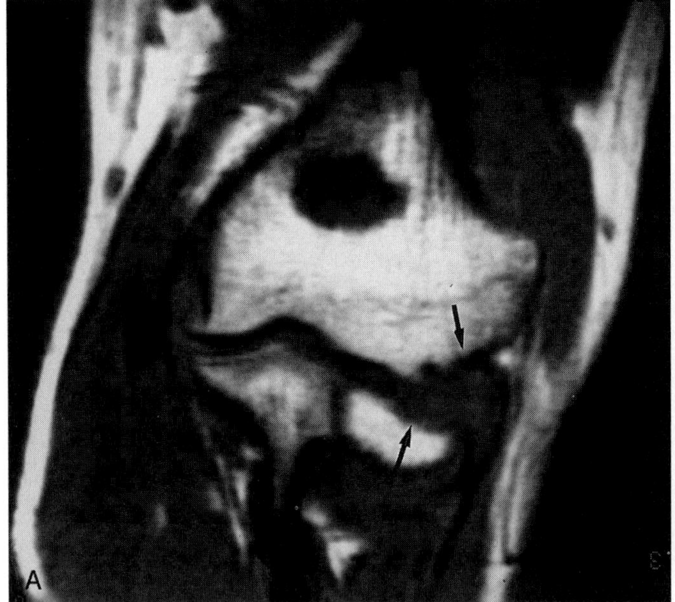

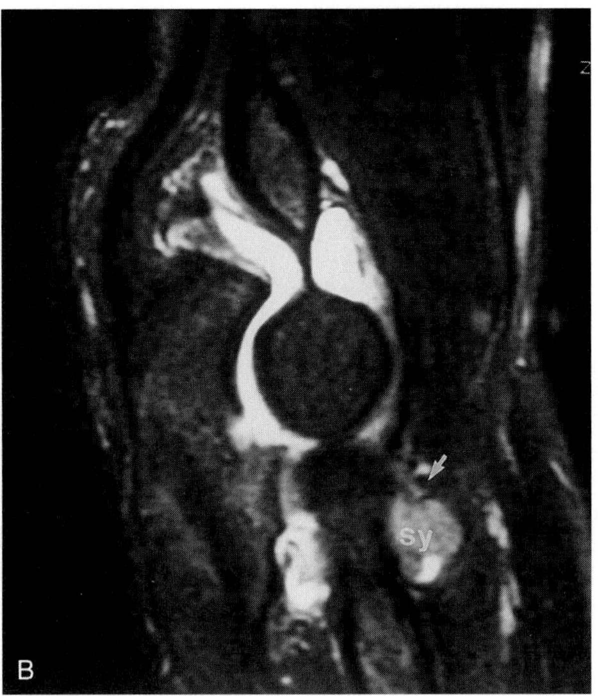

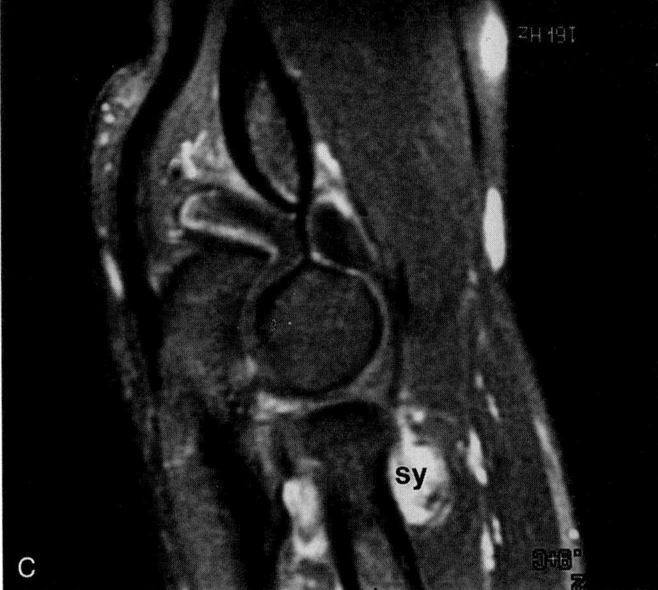

Figure 8–21 ■ **A**, Pannus in rheumatoid arthritis: coronal T_1-weighted MRI. Elbow swelling and pain in a patient with rheumatoid arthritis. This coronal T_1-weighted image demonstrates erosive changes in the capitellum and in the subchondral bone of the radial head (*arrows*). This sequence does not allow differentiation among joint fluid, joint capsule, synovium, ligaments, muscle. **B**, Pannus in rheumatoid arthritis: sagittal T_2-weighted MRI with fat suppression. Same patient as in **A**. Fluid fills the anterior and posterior recesses of the elbow joint. Note, however, the intermediate signal intensity of the synovium in the annular recess (*sy*). Symbol: annular ligament (*arrow*). **C**, Pannus in rheumatoid arthritis: sagittal T_1-weighted MRI with fat suppression after intravenous gadolinium administration. Same patient as in **A**. Fluid in the anterior and posterior recesses of the joint does not enhance, remaining dark. The hypertrophic synovial tissue (*sy*) or pannus in the annular recess enhances with gadolinium.

cartilage of the wrist and the menisci of the temporomandibular joints.

Cartilage Disease

Edema of cartilage is the earliest sign of pathological change. The normal cartilage margins become ill-defined, and the cartilage substance appears inhomogeneous (Aisen et al., 1984; Richardson et al., 1988). The thickness of the edematous cartilage increases slightly (Fig. 8–23). Comparison with the asymptomatic side is usually very helpful. Later, the surface of the involved cartilage will appear rough, and there will be measurable loss in thickness. This progression of disease can be seen in both inflammatory arthritis and osteoarthritis. The rate of disease progression and the response to therapeutic agents can be accurately monitored through serial sonographic examinations.

Chondral and osteochondral defects and osteochondritis dissecans can also be diagnosed sonographically (Selby et al., 1986) (Fig 8–24). Most commonly these are the sequelae of trauma, but they may also occur secondary to infarcts and epiphyseal osteonecrosis in older patients. Intra-articular fragments of cartilage may occur in these joints.

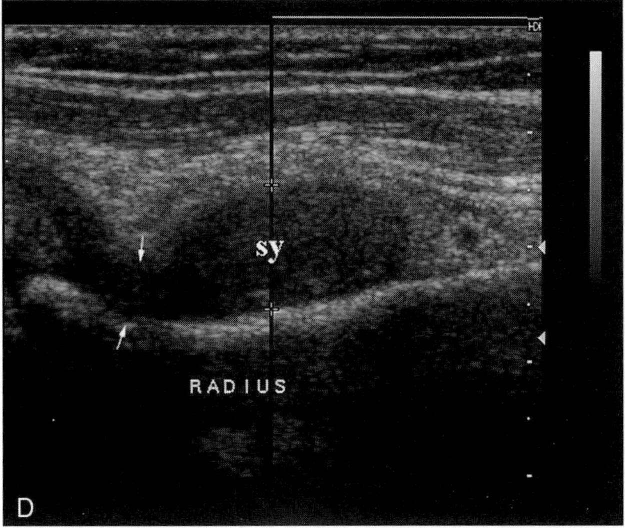

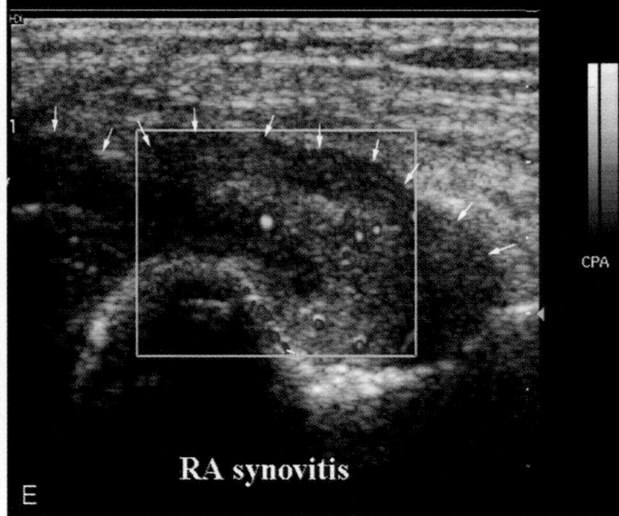

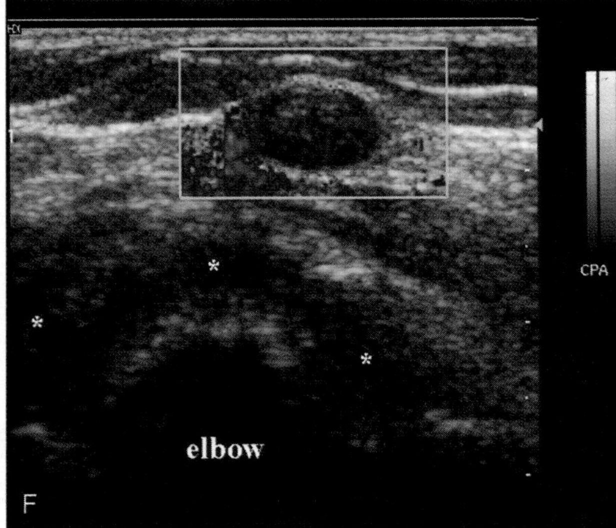

Figure 8-21 *Continued* ■ **D**, Pannus in rheumatoid arthritis: sagittal sonogram. Same patient as in **A**. The anterior aspect of the annular recess is distended by the hypertrophic synovium (*sy*). Compare this image with Figures 8-12 and 8-13. Notice that pannus cannot be distinguished from pus or synovial edema on gray scale imaging. The annular ligament causes concentric narrowing (*arrows*) at the proximal aspect of the recess. **E**, Pannus in rheumatoid arthritis: sagittal power Doppler ultrasound. Same patient as in **A**. Flow is demonstrated throughout the pannus (*arrows*). No flow is observed within the pus in Figure 8-12 or in the acute synovial edema in Figure 8-13. **F**, Rheumatoid nodule: longitudinal sonogram of the extensor surface of the elbow. Same patient as in **A**. Pannus is noted around the trochlea (*). In addition, a rheumatoid nodule (*insert*) is seen deep to the extensor fascia.

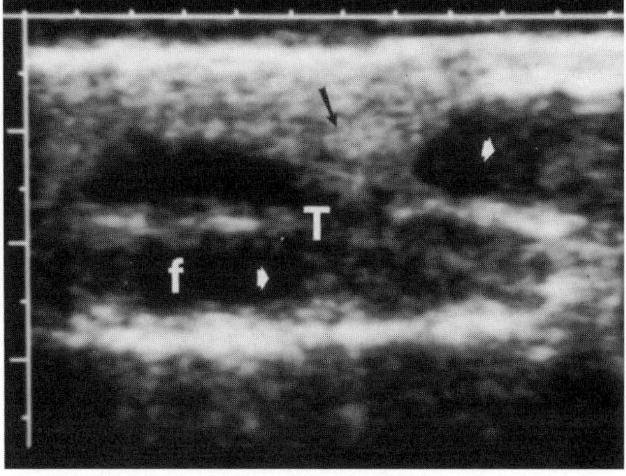

Figure 8-22 ■ Inflammatory distention of the biceps tendon sheath: longitudinal sonogram. A 62-year-old woman with rheumatoid arthritis for 12 years presented with pain, swelling, and fever after an intra-articular steroid injection in the right shoulder. The transducer is oriented along the long biceps tendon (*T*). Fluid within the synovial sheath (*f*) of the tendon displaces the tendon anteriorly. Compare this appearance with that of fluid within the subacromial-subdeltoid bursa shown in Figure 8-14B. Debris (*small arrows*) is noted within the fluid-filled sheath. Adhesions (*black arrow*) between the visceral and parietal synovia are also demonstrated. Aspiration of the fluid yielded frank pus, and *S. aureus* was cultured.

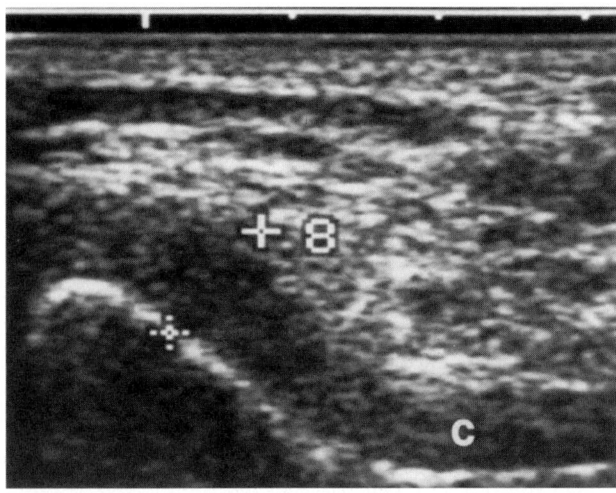

Figure 8–23 ■ Cartilage edema of the knee: transverse sonogram. This 66-year-old woman presented with a 6-year history of rheumatoid arthritis and 1 year of involvement of the right knee. The knee was flexed 90 degrees, and the transducer was placed transversely just above the patella. The hypoechoic articular cartilage (*c*) covering the femoral condyles measures approximately 8 mm thick, markedly thickened. The margins of the cartilage are indistinct, consistent with roughening of the articular surface.

These loose bodies calcify and become visible on conventional radiographs (Fig. 8–25). However, calcified and noncalcified loose bodies can be detected with ultrasound when there is increased intra-articular fluid (Frankel et al., 1998). Acoustic shadowing is frequently seen with loose intra-articular cartilage fragments, but it may be absent if little degenerative change has occurred in the cartilage (Fig. 8–26). Loose cartilage fragments that do not shadow are most commonly found following trauma in young, otherwise healthy patients. In the knee, loose bodies are preferentially trapped in Baker's cysts (Fig. 8–27). Therefore, examination of the popliteal fossa is mandatory in the evaluation of knees in which cartilage loss is observed. Loose bodies are not always surrounded by fluid. Detection of loose bodies in "dry joints" is often facilitated by the hypoechoic cartilage that surrounds the calcified portion of the intra-articular body (Fig. 8–28).

There are three cartilages in the body that can tear and form cysts as a consequence of these tears. Labral cysts occur around the shoulder, and hip and meniscal cysts occur around the knee. Trauma is the initial insult to the fibrous cartilage in these joints. Defects that extend from the joint through the joint capsule allow fluid to leak through the fibrous

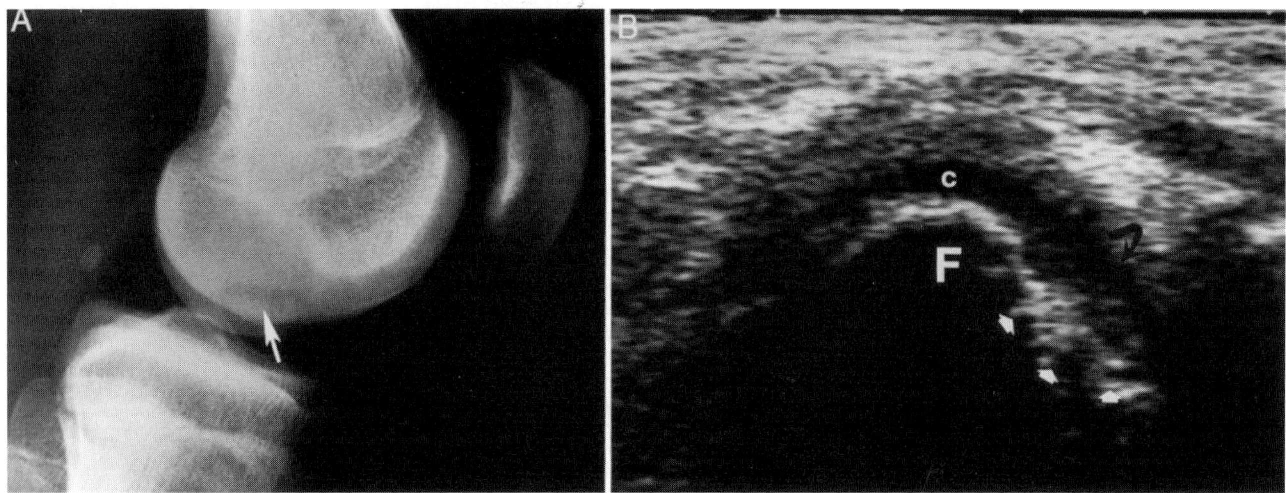

Figure 8–24 ■ **A**, Osteochondritis dissecans of the medial femoral condyle: lateral knee radiograph. An ovoid osseous fragment (*arrow*) is seen within a defect of the medial femoral condyle in this 13-year-old soccer player. **B**, Osteochondritis dissecans of the medial femoral condyle: longitudinal sonogram. Same patient as in **A**. The transducer is placed over the posteromedial aspect of the knee in full extension. The proximal aspect lies to the observer's left. Cartilage (*c* and *curved arrow*) overlying the osseous fragment (*small white arrows*) is intact. Abbreviation: medial femoral condyle (*F*).

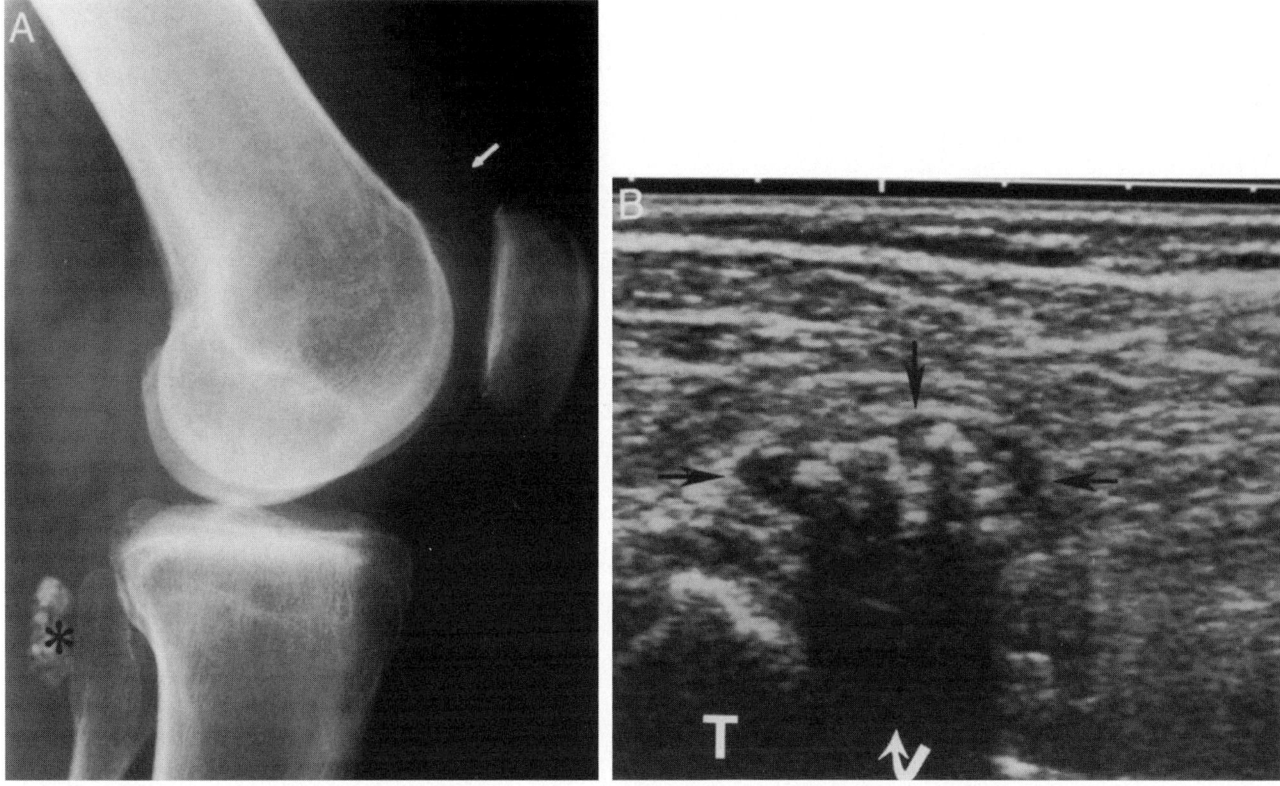

Figure 8–25 ■ **A**, Detection of loose bodies: lateral knee radiograph. This 55-year-old man presented with right knee pain. The radiograph demonstrates degenerative changes of the patellofemoral joint, and calcifications (*asterisk*) projected posterior to the fibular head. Enlarged suprapatellar bursa (*arrow*). **B**, Sonographic localization of loose bodies: longitudinal sonogram. Same patient as in **A**. This longitudinal sonogram was obtained at the medial aspect of the popliteal fossa, showing multiple calcifications with shadowing (*curved arrow*) within a small Baker cyst (*black arrows*). These were demonstrated as separate calcifications on real-time examination. Abbreviation: tibia (*T*).

cartilage and into the surrounding soft tissue structures, forming a cyst. Cysts around the shoulder (Figs. 8–29 through 8–31) cause the most dramatic clinical picture. These cysts have been called *suprascapular ganglia* because of the pressure they can exert on the suprascapular nerve. In addition to the pain and swelling they cause, these cysts are often associated with muscle atrophy. The most significant atrophy is noted in the infraspinatus muscle. Atrophy of the supraspinatus follows, with varying degrees of intensity. The muscle imbalance causes a subacromial pain which cannot be distinguished clinically from a rotator cuff tear. One should suspect this diagnosis in young patients, especially if they are weight lifters, volleyball players, or throwing athletes.

The workup of labral injuries usually requires MRI arthrography. These studies are expensive and invasive. Traumatic injuries of the superior and posterior labrum can be assessed with ultrasound in a number of cases (Figs. 8–32 and 8–33). New research indicates that ultrasound can also assist in the diagnosis of lesions of the anterior-inferior labrum; ultrasound is particularly useful if used immediately after a dislocation. The intra-articular hemorrhage from the dislocation improves the image and acts as a natural contrast medium.

Sonographic examination of the menisci of the knee has proved to be very valuable and is probably most useful in very young or very old patients because of difficulties encountered with MRI in these patient populations (Richardson et al., 1988; van Holsbeeck et al., 1988a). Posterior and peripheral meniscal tears are very well demonstrated using ultrasound. These are areas that are poorly evaluated with arthroscopy. Ultrasound examination is clearly indicated in patients with tenderness over the joint space, especially if the arthroscopic examination is normal. Small tears along the internal meniscal margin are easily missed

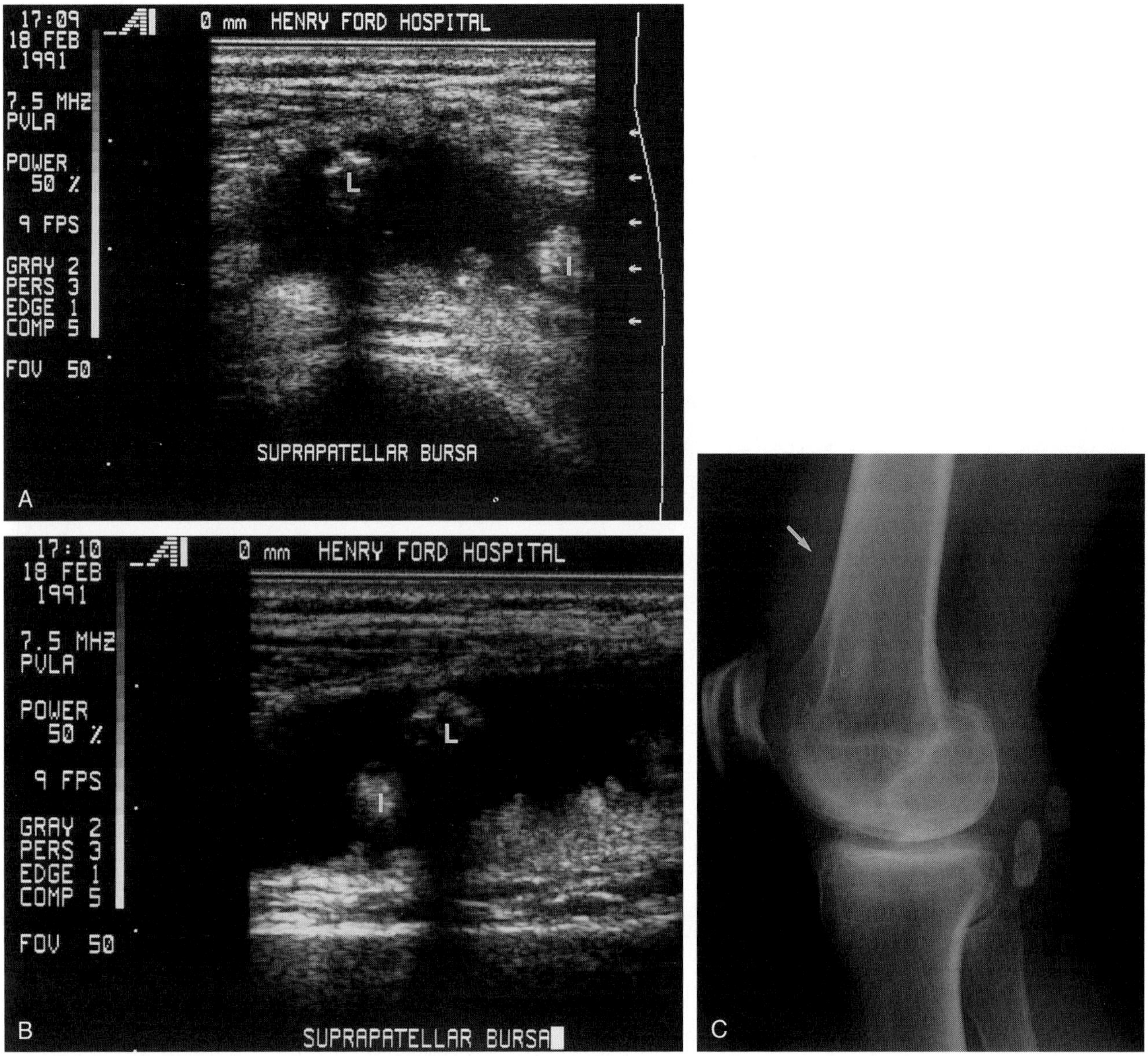

Figure 8–26 ■ **A**, Radiopaque and nonopaque loose bodies: transverse sonogram through the suprapatellar bursa. Intermittent locking of the knee was the chief complaint of this middle-aged man with posttraumatic arthritis of the knee. This transverse image of the suprapatellar bursa demonstrates two intraluminal loose bodies, which moved freely within the joint fluid. One loose body (*L*) casts a shadow, but the other body (*l*) is noted as a filling defect without a shadow. **B,** Radiopaque and nonopaque loose bodies: longitudinal sonogram through the suprapatellar bursa. Same patient as in **A**. The loose bodies have moved closer together on the current image. Again, one casts a shadow (*L*) and the other (*l*) does not. **C**, Radiopaque and nonopaque loose bodies: lateral knee radiograph. Same patient as in **A**. Two large, loose bodies are located within a Baker's cyst. These loose bodies project behind the femoral and tibial condyles. The suprapatellar bursa contains one vague calcification (*arrow*), which must represent the loose body with the accompanying acoustic shadow.

sonographically. Therefore, MRI remains the gold standard in the evaluation of meniscal tears. The high cost, frequent unavailability, and long examination time of MRI make ultrasound an essential first step in evaluation for meniscal tears.

Sonographic examination of the menisci of the knee is performed with the patient in the lateral decubitus position, with a cushion beneath the knee. The transducer is placed over the joint space in the long axis of the leg. Mild valgus stress is applied when the medial meniscus is examined. Varus stress is also applied for examination of the lateral

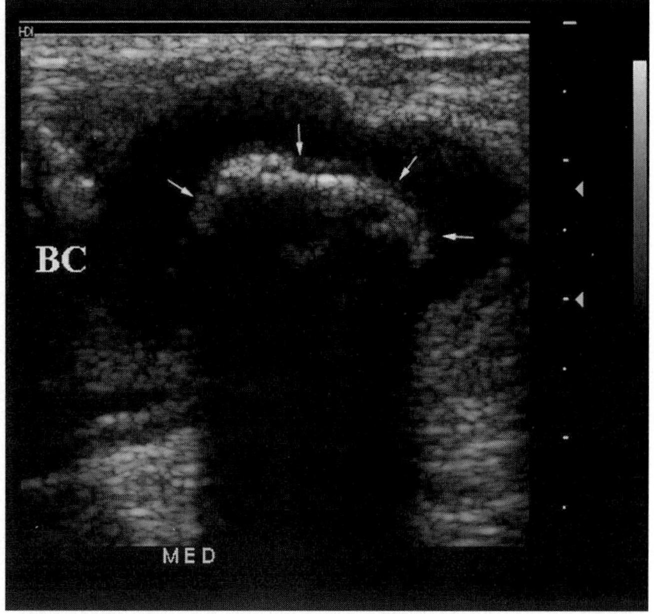

Figure 8–27 ■ Loose body in a fluid-filled Baker cyst: longitudinal ultrasound of the medial popliteal space. Loose body in an osteoarthritic knee. Most loose bodies are calcified and cast acoustic shadows. The surface of loose bodies is often irregular and covered by hypoechoic, noncalcified cartilage (*arrows*). Fluid within the synovial membrane facilitates the diagnosis. The examiner should try to squeeze the fluid into the recess which is suspected to hold the loose body. The diagnosis will be easily established when fluid surrounds the intraluminal structure. Abbreviation: Baker cyst (*BC*).

meniscus. Coronal imaging must be followed by transverse imaging. Once the meniscus is localized on coronal images, the transducer is rotated 90 degrees, parallel with the joint space. Examination of the menisci is most easily performed using an intraoperative fingertip linear array transducer. The meniscus is identified as a homogeneous, hyperechoic triangle situated between the hypoechoic layers of articular hyaline cartilage (Fig. 8–34). The posterior horns can be approached with a sector transducer through the popliteal space. Small amounts of synovial fluid may be seen in the recesses of the joint around the meniscus. Once the meniscus is localized in longitudinal images, axial images of the meniscus are obtained. Meniscal tears are identified as hypoechoic clefts or gaps within the hyperechoic fibrocartilage of the meniscus (Figs. 8–35 through 8–39). Richardson et al. (1988) have

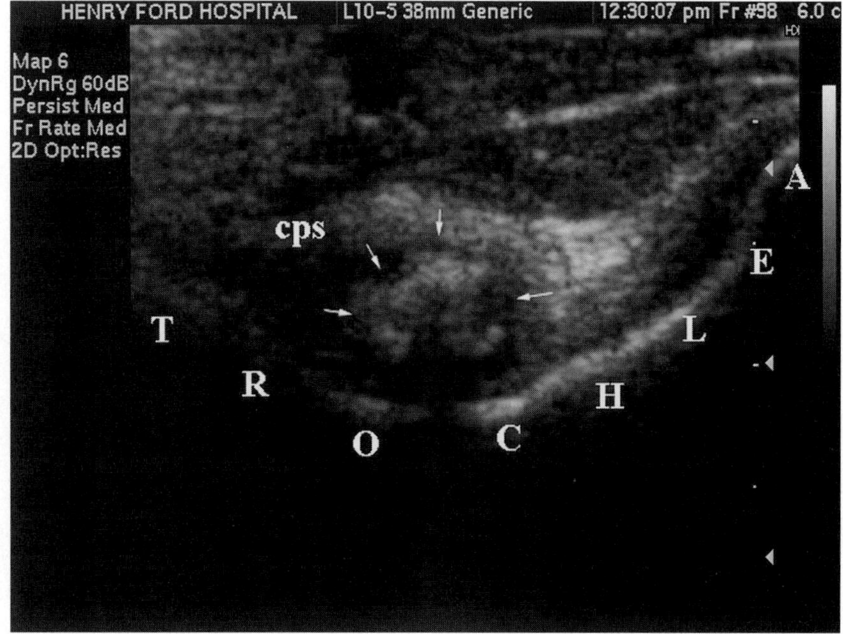

Figure 8–28 ■ Loose body in a "dry" olecranon fossa: transverse sonogram through the posterior elbow. This 38-year-old tennis player complained of posterior elbow pain. The clinician noted a significant extension deficit. The transducer has been positioned transversely over the distal humerus, at the junction of the posterior trochlea with the olecranon fossa just proximal. A loose body elevates the posterior joint capsule (*cps*). The core of the loose fragment exhibits the same echogenicity as the joint capsule and subchondral bone. A vague shadow is noted deep to the loose body. The only feature making this loose body stand out more clearly is its surface of hyaline cartilage. High-frequency transducers almost invariably show this cartilage as a thin, hypoechoic layer (*arrows*) covering the loose body. Without an intra-articular effusion, it is more difficult to detect loose bodies. The examiner must be very familiar with the normal joint anatomy and understand the histological architecture of loose bodies to detect the intra-articular cartilage fragments.

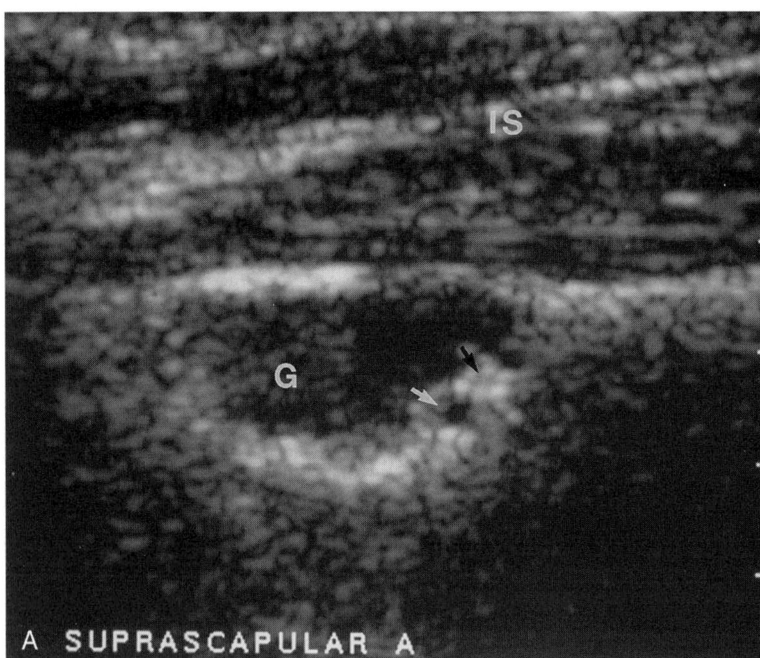

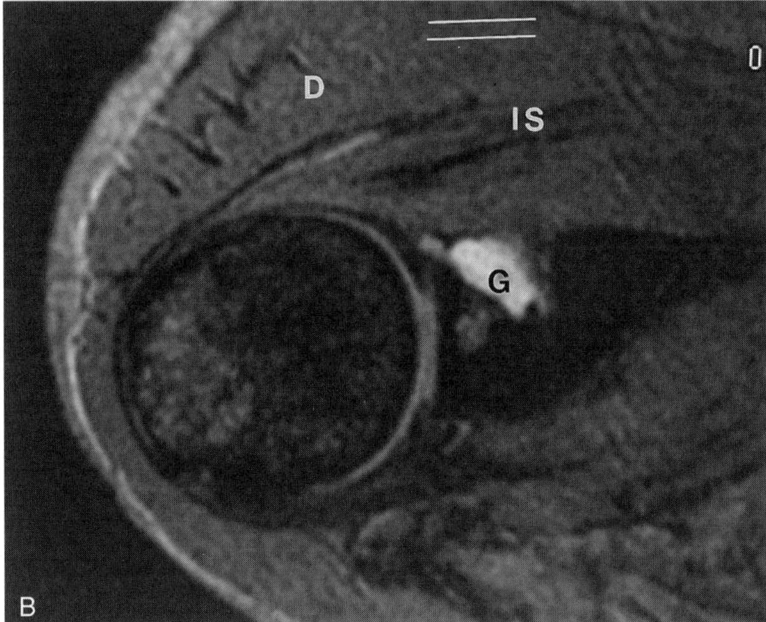

Figure 8-29 ■ **A**, Suprascapular ganglion found in the infraspinatus fossa: longitudinal ultrasound along the infraspinatus muscle and tendon. A young weight lifter complains of pain in the subacromial space. Muscle wasting is noted in both the supra- and infraspinatus fossae when compared with the asymptomatic left side. A hypoechoic ganglion (*G*) is noted deep to the infraspinatus muscle (*IS*). The suprascapular artery (*white arrow*) and nerve (*black arrow*) are compressed against the medial bony margin of the spinoglenoid notch. **B**, Suprascapular ganglion found in the infraspinatus fossa: axial gradient echo MRI. Same patient as in **A**. A ganglion (*G*) fills the spinoglenoid notch. Two white lines indicate the orientation of the transducer, which was used in **A**. Abbreviations: deltoid muscle (*D*), infraspinatus muscle and tendon (*IS*).

reported meniscal tears to be hyperechoic lesions. Their work was performed using cadaver specimens, and the hyperechoic appearance of the meniscal tears was probably the result of gas within the lesion. We have not observed hyperechoic meniscal tears in vivo. Joint fluid filling the gap in the torn meniscus results in a hypoechoic appearance.

Tears of the menisci are named according to their gross pathological appearance. A tear paralleling the internal border of the meniscus is called a *longitudinal tear*. If there is separation of the central portion of the meniscus along the margins of the tear, with the anterior and posterior aspects remaining attached to the peripheral meniscus, it is referred to as a *bucket handle tear*. *Radial tears* are oriented perpendicular to the peripheral margin of the meniscus. *Horizontal tears* extend from the superior or inferior surfaces of the meniscus to the periphery. Meniscal cysts are most frequently found in association with horizontal tears.

Text continued on page 263

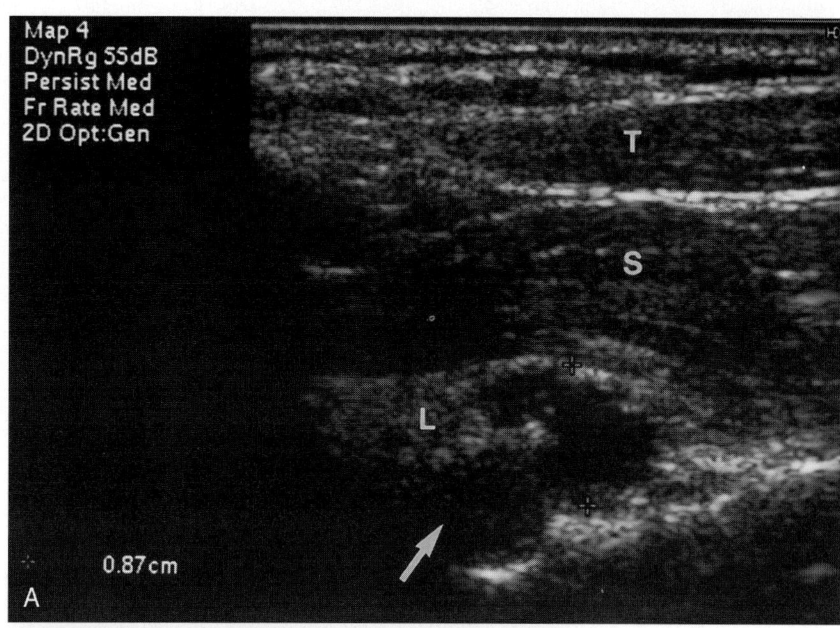

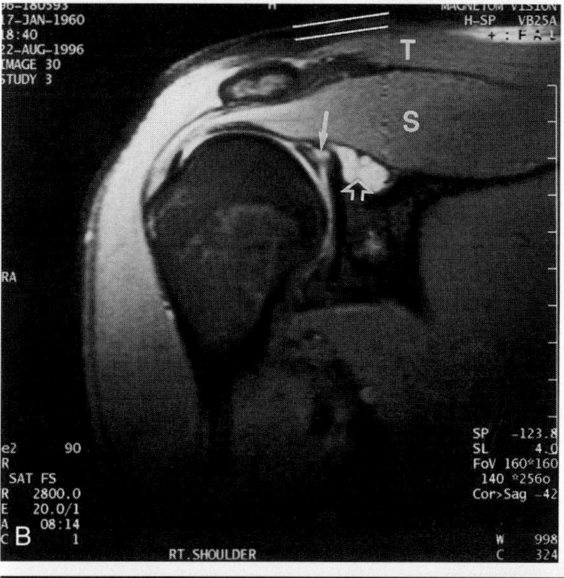

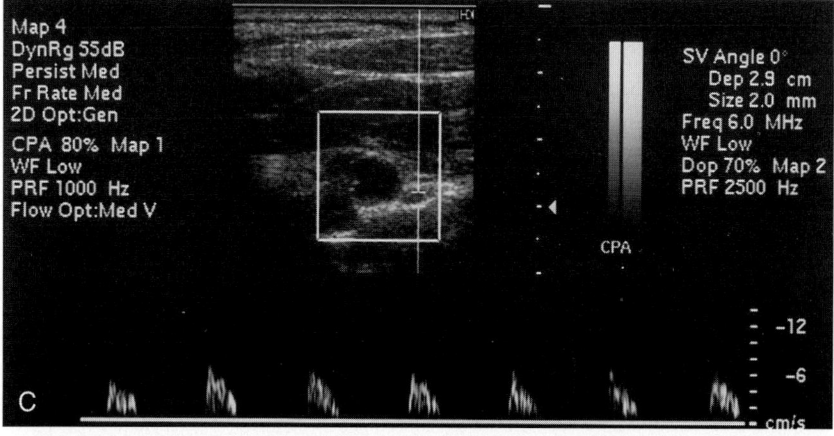

Figure 8–30 ■ **A**, Suprascapular ganglion found in the supraspinatus fossa: longitudinal sonogram along the supraspinatus muscle. Weakness in external rotation of the arm interferes with the game of this 36-year-old tennis player. A nagging pain in the arm, which wakes him at night, has been bothering him for weeks. A ganglion (*mass between the cursors*) is noted deep to the trapezius (*T*) and supraspinatus (*S*) musculature. The ganglion communicates (*arrow*) with the joint at the base of the labrum (*L*). **B**, Suprascapular ganglion found in the supraspinatus fossa: coronal proton density image with fat saturation. Same patient as in **A**. Smaller ganglia, like this one (*open arrow*), do not always extend as low as the infraspinatus fossa. These ganglia can be diagnosed by placing the transducer (*two white lines*) over the trapezius (*T*), aligned with the supraspinatus muscle and tendon (*S*). The tear (*arrow*) through the superior labrum is clearly visible on this image. **C**, Suprascapular ganglion found in the supraspinatus fossa: duplex Doppler sonography of the suprascapular artery. Same patient as in **A**. Normal arterial pulses are observed in the neurovascular bundle at the medial aspect of the ganglion. The MRI image in Figure 8–29B shows pulsation artifact from this artery along the medial margin of the mass as well.

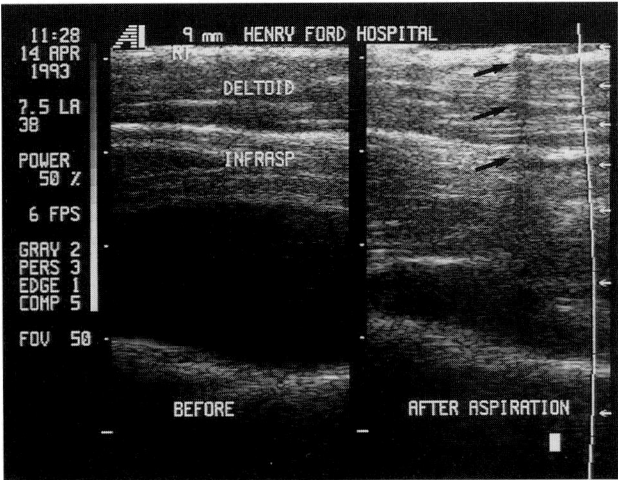

Figure 8–31 ■ Treatment of a suprascapular ganglion: split-screen technique with images aligned along the infraspinatus muscle. Impingement-like symptoms bother this physician, who is in his late thirties. He had been weight lifting on a regular basis prior to the onset of symptoms. A large ganglion is identified in both the supra- and infraspinatus fossae. Treatment options include surgical removal, arthroscopic debridement, and percutaneous aspiration. The patient-physician opted for the last procedure. The suprascapular nerve recovered, but three separate aspirations were required under ultrasound guidance. These images show the ganglion before (on left side of split screen) and after aspiration (on the right) of 8 cc of gelatinous fluid. The artifact (*arrows*) noted in the soft tissues superficial to the ganglion is caused by the metallic pellet used to mark the lesion on the skin.

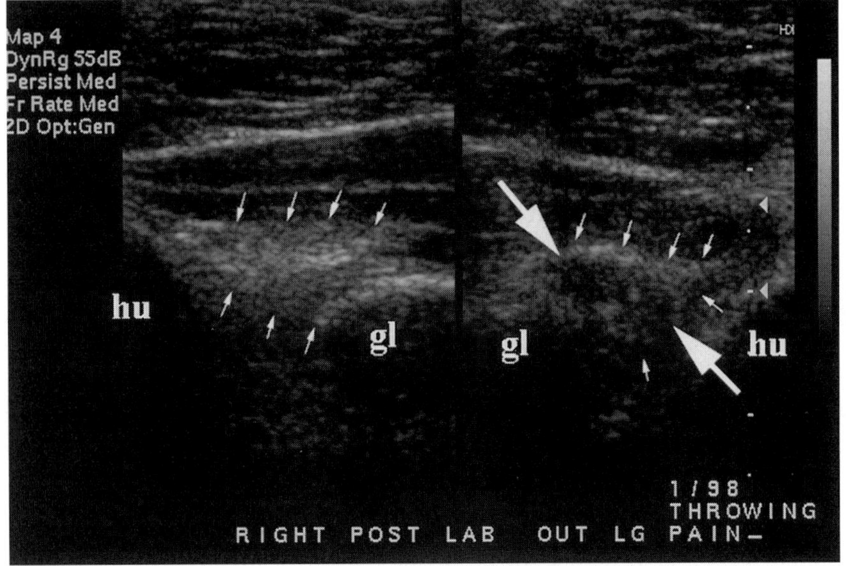

Figure 8–32 ■ Labral tear associated with a suprascapular ganglion: split-screen technique with images of the posterior labra. This 26-year-old man felt a snap in his shoulder while throwing a snowball. His shoulder felt unstable and weak for more than 3 months, and he experiences pain every time he lifts his arm. The normal left shoulder is noted on the left side of this split-screen image. The normal labrum appears hyperechoic and triangular in shape (*small arrows*). The abnormal labrum on the right side appears more hypoechoic, and a cleft (*large arrows*) interrupts its continuity. This patient also had a suprascapular ganglion medial to the tear. Abbreviations: humeral head (*hu*), glenoid (*gl*).

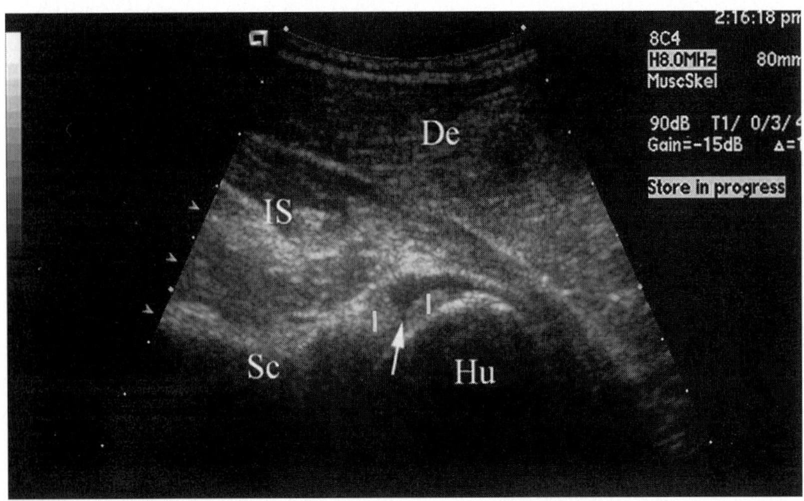

Figure 8–33 ■ Traumatic labral tear: oblique sonogram through the posterior shoulder and along the infraspinatus. A direct hit against the shoulder of this defensive lineman resulted in swelling and decreased range of motion of the joint. A labral tear (*arrow*) divides the labrum (*l*) into two pieces. An intra-articular effusion fills the infraspinatus recess and surrounds the torn labral pieces, serving as a natural contrast medium. Surgery confirmed a large tear. Abbreviations: deltoid muscle (*De*), infraspinatus muscle (*IS*), lateral scapula (*Sc*), humeral head (*Hu*).

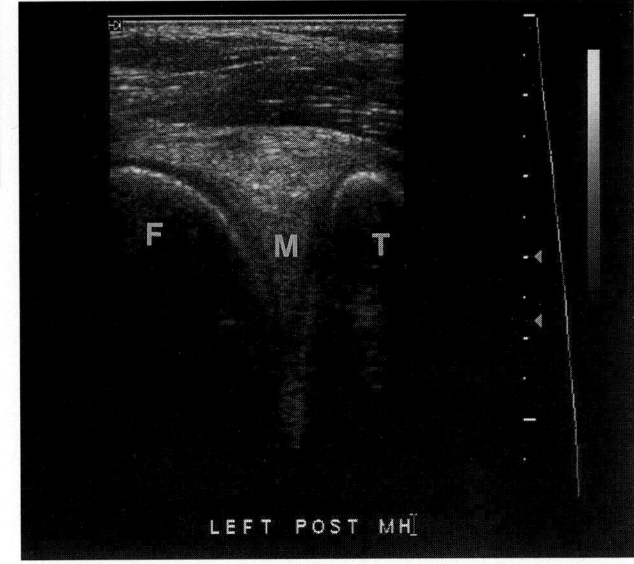

Figure 8–34 ▪ Normal medial meniscus: longitudinal sonogram. This image of the medial meniscus was obtained during a knee exam of one of our radiology fellows. It was obtained with the transducer placed longitudinally over the medial popliteal space of the right knee. The normal meniscus (*M*) is seen as a hyperechoic triangle between the femoral condyle (*F*) and the tibial condyle (*T*). Both condyles are covered by hyaline cartilage, which appears hypoechoic.

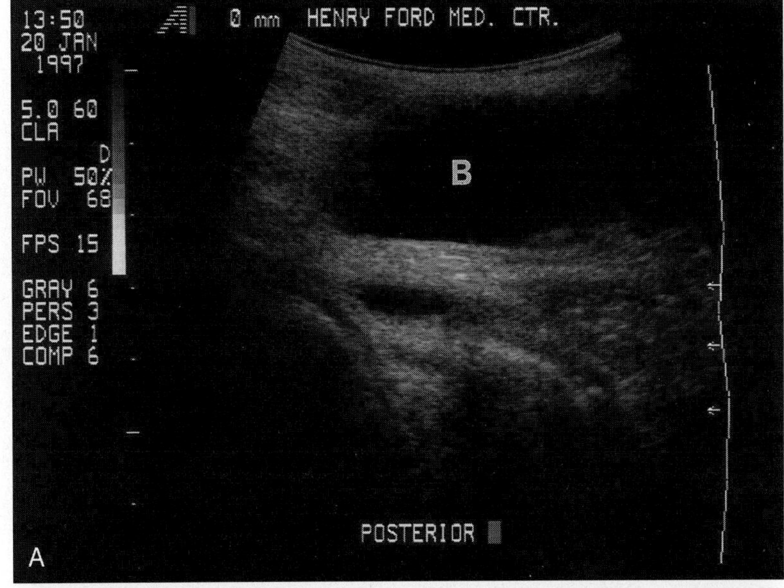

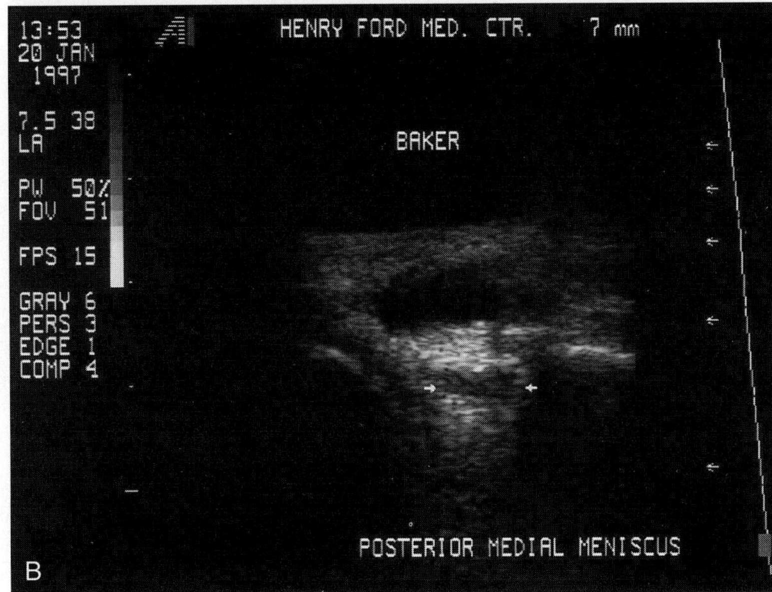

Figure 8–35 ▪ **A**, Abnormal medial meniscus: longitudinal sonogram. The patient is a young man who is about the same age as our radiology fellow in Figure 8–34. This athletic individual has a painful mass in the medial popliteal space. The anechoic mass in the medial aspect of the posterior knee represents a Baker cyst (*B*). **B**, Abnormal medial meniscus: longitudinal sonogram. Same patient as in **A**. Ultrasound image with a smaller depth of field. Popliteal cysts can be used as an acoustic window for evaluation of the posterior horn of the medial meniscus. A hypoechoic linear tear (*arrows*) is identified in the peripheral portion of the medial meniscus. This is a very common location for a traumatic tear of the meniscus.

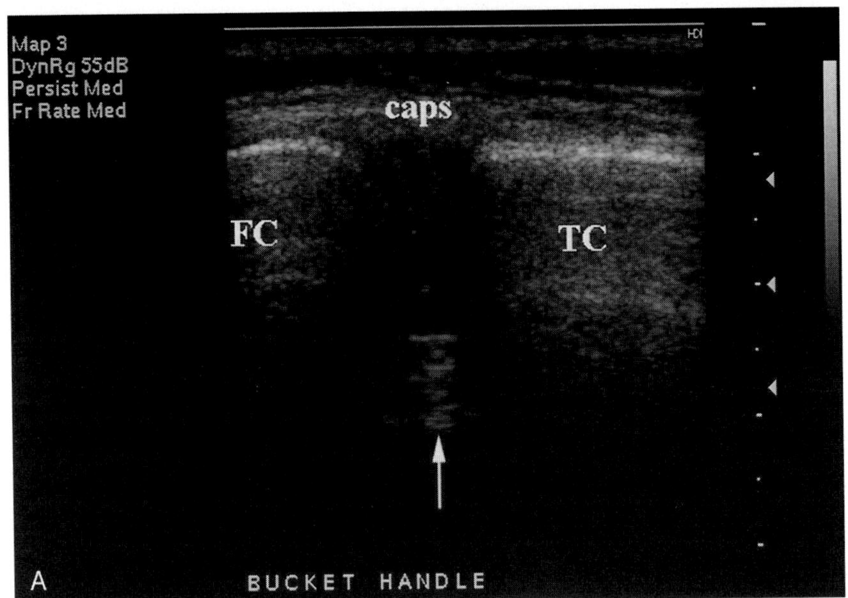

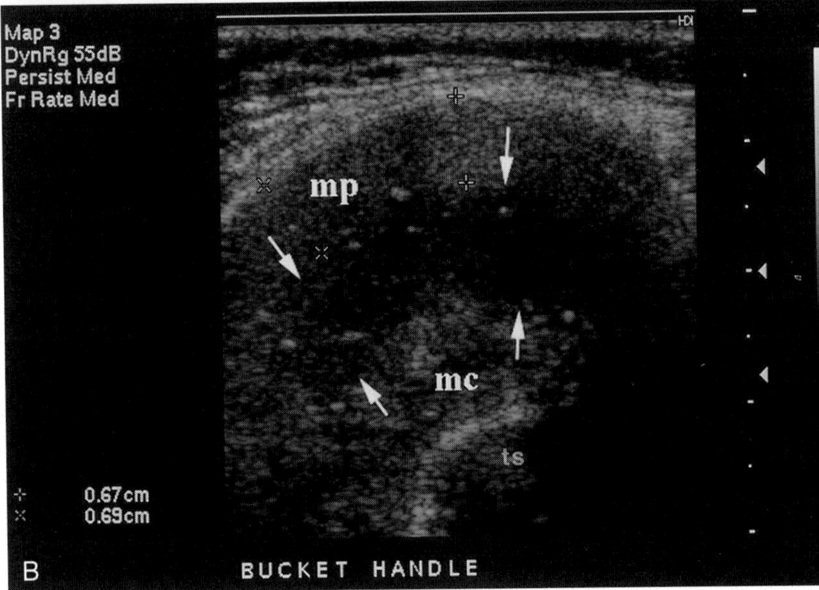

Figure 8–36 ■ **A**, Bucket handle tear of the medial meniscus: coronal sonogram. This patient experienced severe pain over the medial aspect of the knee and locking after injury during a soccer game. The position of the transducer is longitudinal, as in Figure 8–34, but now the transducer is over the medial side rather than over the posterior surface of the knee. A triangular fragment (*large arrow*) of the meniscus is separated from its peripheral attachment (*caps*) by fluid. Arthroscopy confirmed a bucket handle tear of the medial meniscus. Abbreviations: femoral condyle (*FC*), tibial condyle (*TC*). **B**, Bucket handle tear of the medial meniscus: transverse sonogram. Same patient as in **A**. The transducer is aligned transversely along the joint space. The anterior aspect lies to the left of the image. A cleft (*between the arrows*) is seen within the meniscus, indicative of a bucket handle tear. The torn central portion of the meniscus remains attached to the peripheral portion at the anterior and posterior extents of the meniscus. The peripheral fragment of meniscus (*mp*) measures no more than 7 mm. A normal meniscus measures over 1 cm. The central fragment of meniscus (*mc*) lies adjacent to the tibial spine (*ts*).

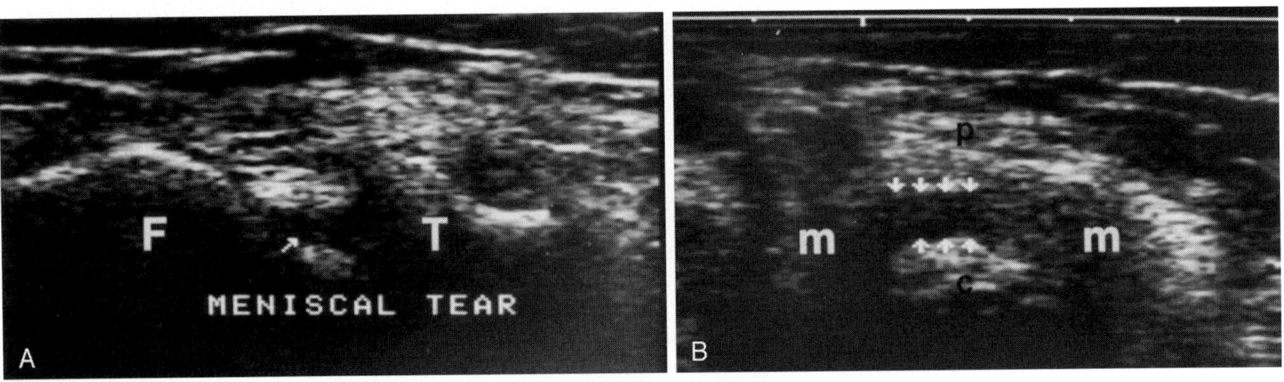

Figure 8–37 ■ **A**, Longitudinal meniscal tear: coronal sonogram. The patient is a 20-year-old football player with continued pain and swelling after being hit on the knee. A longitudinal meniscal tear is seen as a hypoechoic cleft (*arrow*) in the peripheral portion of the anterior medial meniscus. Abbreviations: femur (*F*), tibia (*T*). **B**, Longitudinal meniscal tear: transverse sonogram. Same patient as in **A**. The position of the transducer is identical to that in Figure 8–36B. The length of the meniscal tear (*arrows*) is demonstrated, dividing the meniscus (*m*) into peripheral (*p*) and central (*c*) fragments.

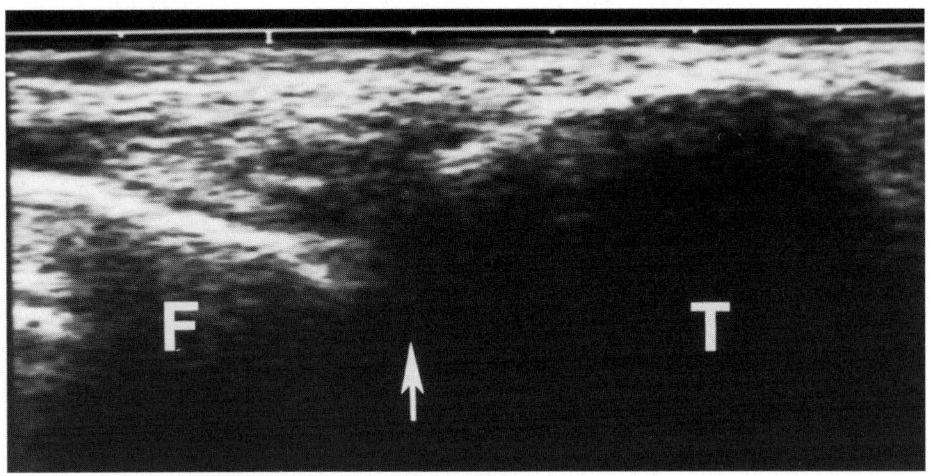

Figure 8–38 ■ Radial meniscal tear: coronal sonogram. This 52-year-old mechanic experienced severe pain on the medial side of the knee after standing up from a kneeling position. The image is obtained through the midportion of the medial meniscus. The normal triangular shape of the medial meniscus is not identified at the periphery of the joint space (*arrow*). When the medial meniscus is not identified on coronal images, lack of sufficient valgus stress must be considered as a possible cause. Abnormal echogenicity of the medial collateral ligament is also noted in this case, providing further evidence of injury. Abbreviations: femur (*F*), tibia (*T*).

Meniscal cysts are multiloculated collections of mucinous material associated with the meniscal margin (Figs. 8–40 and 8–41). The origin of these cysts is unknown but is probably related to trauma. Most meniscal cysts are associated with the lateral meniscus and communicate with the joint space through a horizontal meniscal tear (see Fig. 18–3) (Ferrer-Roca and Vilalta, 1980; Resnick and Niwayama, 1988). In theory, joint motion pumps intra-articular fluid through these tears, resulting in cyst development. However, medial meniscal cysts are usually isolated findings, rarely associated with meniscal tears. In these cases, primary myxoid degeneration of the meniscus is thought to be responsible for cyst formation (Resnick and Niwayama, 1988). Meniscal cysts were found in 7% of excised menisci.

A decade ago, the vast majority of meniscal cysts were diagnosed at surgery. Only the largest of these cysts were clinically palpable and were erroneously diagnosed as soft tissue tumors, pannus, pes anserinus tendinitis, or bursitis. Today, ultrasound is the most useful modality for the detection of meniscal cysts. Preoperative sonographic diagnosis of meniscal cysts has demonstrated these lesions to be more common than was previously suspected (Barrie, 1979; Ferrer-Roca and Vilalta, 1980).

Meniscal cysts are most frequently seen as hypoechoic cystic structures adjacent to the meniscus (see Fig. 8–41). Occasionally, they are anechoic. Reflectivity of the cyst contents is directly related to its viscosity. Loculations and meniscal fragments are frequently present within these cysts. Large meniscal cysts may erode bone under the margin of the

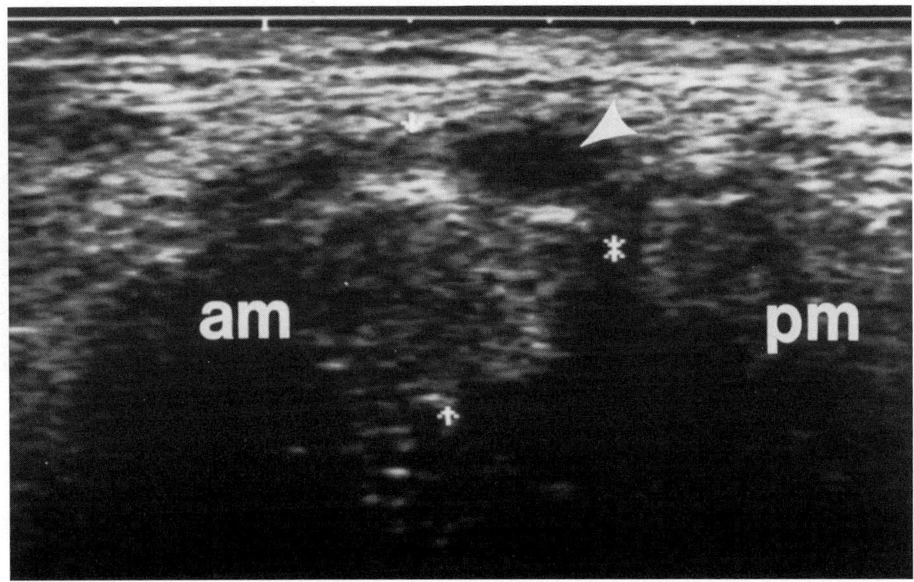

Figure 8–39 ■ Radial meniscal tear: transverse sonogram. Same patient as in Figure 8–38. The radial tear (*asterisk*) is confirmed in this plane of imaging. The tear separates the meniscus into anterior (*am*) and posterior (*pm*) fragments. *Arrows* indicate the normal dimension of the anterior meniscus. Fluid (*arrowhead*) is seen collecting between the medial collateral ligament and the peripheral margin of the meniscus.

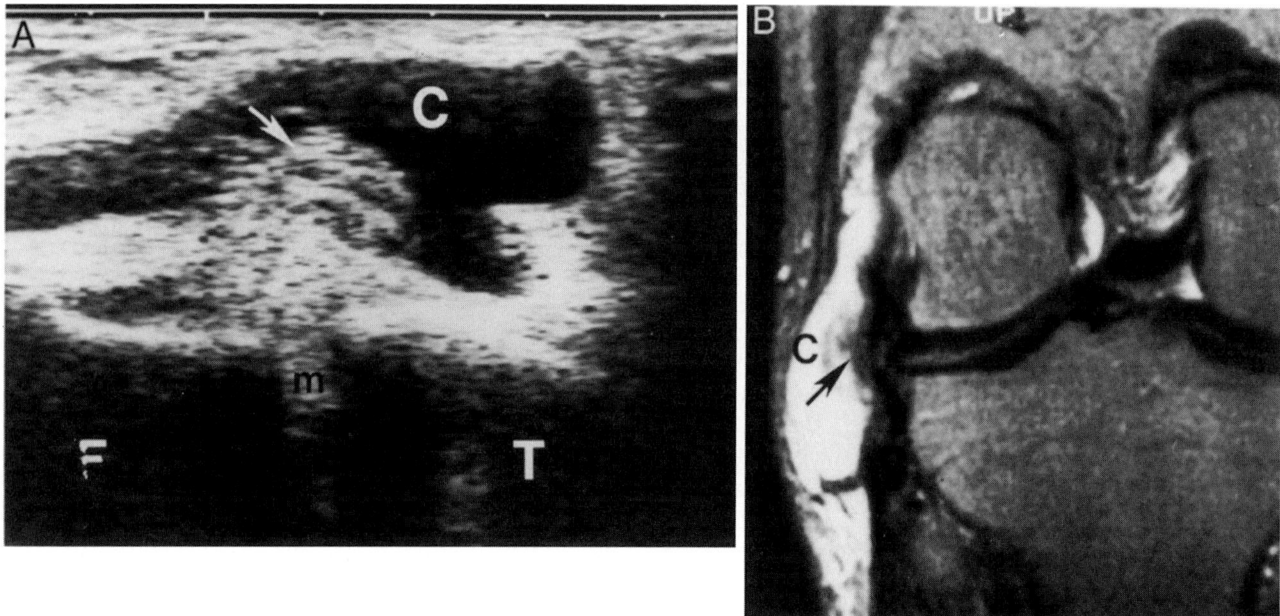

Figure 8–40 ■ Lateral meniscal cyst: coronal sonogram (**A**) and MRI (**B**). This 35-year-old man presented with pain and swelling over the posterolateral aspect of the knee. A cyst (C) surrounds the lateral meniscus (*m*). The lateral portion of the meniscus bulges into the cyst (*arrows*). These findings were confirmed with MRI and subsequently at surgery. Abbreviations: femur (*F*), tibia (*T*).

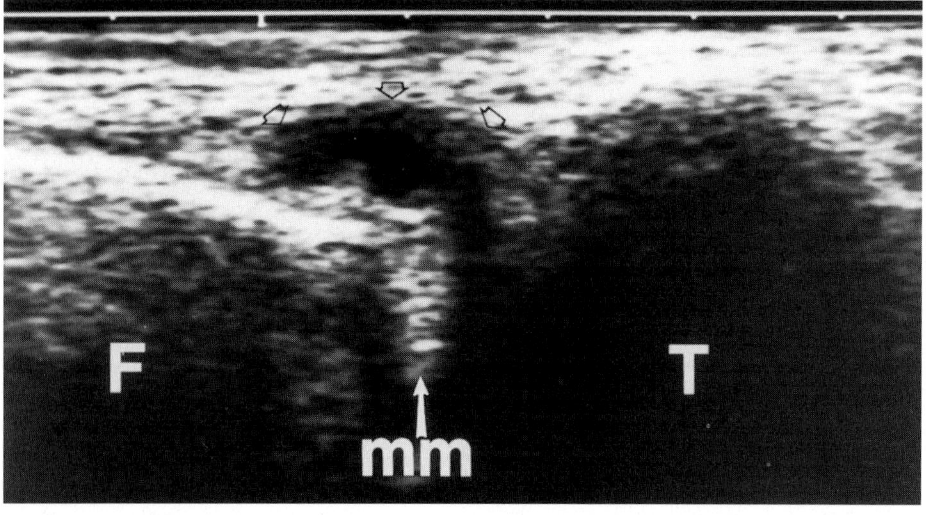

Figure 8–41 ■ Medial meniscal cyst: coronal sonogram. A small meniscal cyst (*open arrows*) associated with the medial meniscus (*mm*) is identified in this 55-year-old woman with chronic medial knee pain. This was an isolated finding; no tears were identified. Isolated meniscal cysts can be the sole cause of medial knee pain. Characteristically, meniscal cysts on the medial aspect of the knee are not associated with meniscal tears. However, lateral meniscal cysts are almost always associated with meniscal tears. Abbreviations: femur (*F*), tibia (*T*).

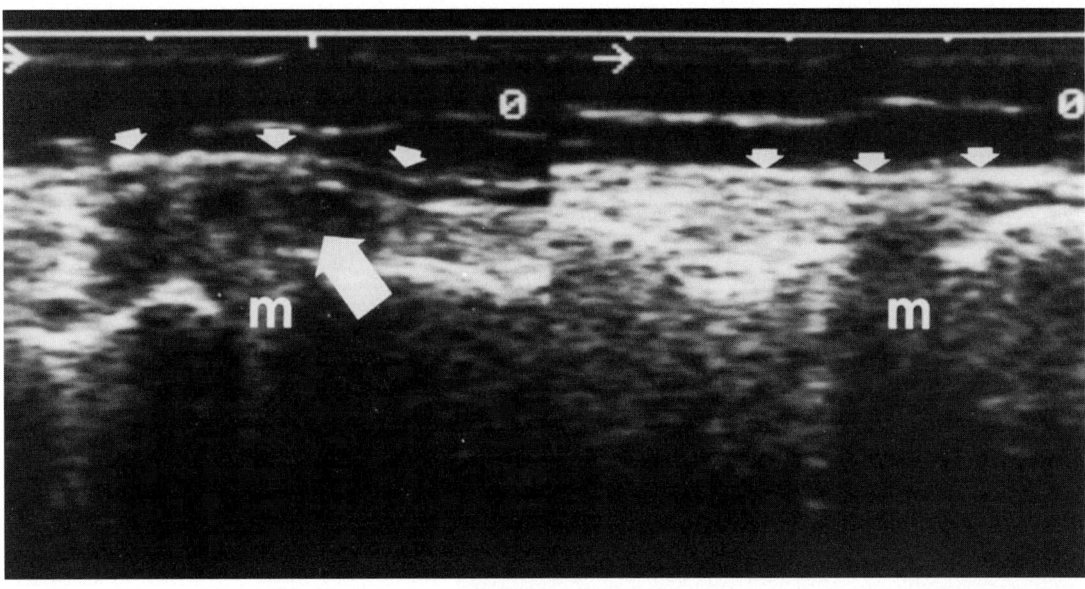

Figure 8–42 ■ Myxoid degeneration of the medial meniscus: coronal sonogram. This 50-year-old woman complained of pain over the medial aspect of the left knee. On the left side is the left medial meniscus; the right side shows the right medial meniscus for comparison. The left medial meniscus (*m*) bulges medially from the joint space (*arrow*) and elevates the medial collateral ligament (*small white arrows*). This small mass contains definite internal echos, unlike a meniscal cyst. Arthroscopy found the midsection of the meniscus to be enlarged and softened. Resection was performed, and histological analysis demonstrated myxoid degeneration.

tibial plateau, simulating an erosion of rheumatoid arthritis. Fluid within the cyst can be displaced from beneath the transducer when pressure is applied.

Degenerative changes of the menisci may be observed sonographically without associated meniscal cysts or tears. This is a frequent finding in the elderly. On sonographic images, the meniscus appears swollen and decreased in echogenicity (Fig. 8–42). The periphery of the meniscus bulges outward and is not compressible when pressure is applied with the transducer. Arthroscopy demonstrates swollen segments of the meniscus with myxoid degeneration. Good indications for meniscal sonography include clinical suspicion of meniscal cyst, acute meniscocapsular separations, the aging meniscus in patients over age 50, and discoid meniscus in children under 6 years of age (see Figs. 18–3, 18–4, 18–7, 18–8, 18–9, 18–11, and 18–12).

Loose Bodies

Intra-articular debris can be classified into four categories: (1) precipitation of fibrin, (2) degeneration of villi, (3) metaplasia of villi, and (4) desquamation of cartilage (Mori, 1979). Precipitation of fibrin is most frequently seen in cases of rheumatoid arthritis, but it may also occur in any chronic inflammatory process involving the synovia (e.g., tuberculosis) (Fig. 8–43) (Mori, 1979). In rheumatoid joints, the surfaces of the villi are covered with precipitated fibrin. These fibrin collections become dislodged and migrate to the synovial recesses of the joint. Sonography easily identifies them as hyperreflective foci floating in the synovial recesses (Fig. 8–44). This debris can be easily deformed by compression with the transducer (Worth et al., 1986).

Villi found in rheumatoid joints can undergo metaplasia, degeneration, and necrosis. Reduction in blood flow occurring with remission of an acute episode of inflammation will result in necrosis and shedding of the villi (Mori, 1979). Long, thin villi are most susceptible to this and therefore more likely to result in loose body formation. The sonographic appearance of these loose bodies is identical to that of fibrin clots. The presence of intact synovial villi and the clinical history will lead to the correct diagnosis (see Fig. 8–44). The joint recesses can be entirely filled with the synovial masses (Fig. 8–45).

Desquamation of articular cartilage can be a prominent feature of osteoarthritis, but it may also be seen in rheumatoid arthritis. Cartilage fragments can also be seen as loose bodies following intra-articular fracture or meniscal tear. Fragments of articular cartilage are often polygonal or thorn-like (Fig. 8–46). Like other loose bodies, they can be identified easily in the synovial recesses, but unlike

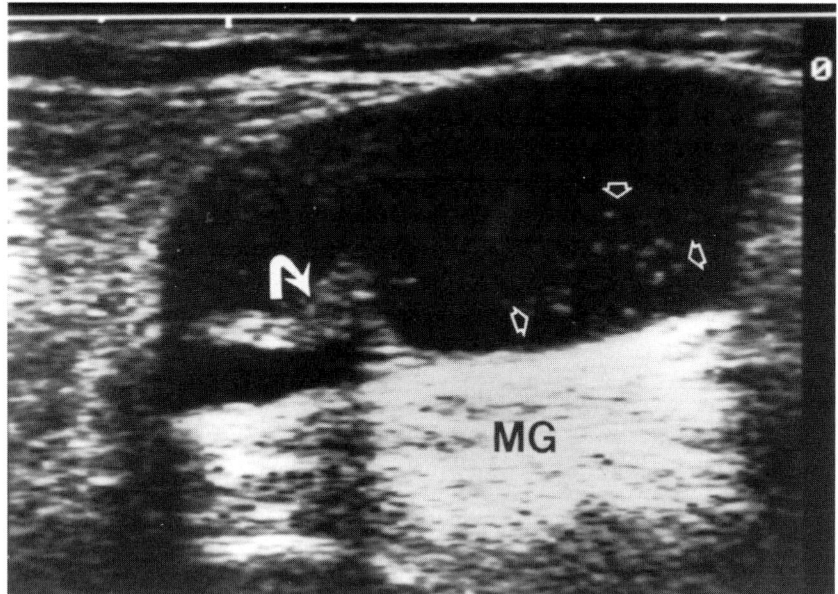

Figure 8–43 ■ Debris in rheumatoid Baker's cyst: longitudinal sonogram. This 50-year-old woman with long-standing rheumatoid arthritis was treated with an intra-articular injection of steroids the day before examination. Hyperechoic strands of tissue (*curved arrow*) are common in rheumatoid Baker's cysts. Echogenic debris is noted dependently in the Baker cyst (*open arrows*). This calcific debris is a frequent complication seen following the intra-articular injection of microcrystalline corticosteroid preparations. Abbreviation: medial gastrocnemius (*MG*).

fibrin clots and villi, they cannot be compressed. In addition, acoustic shadowing will be observed when calcification is present. Fibrinous or cellular material can be mistaken for cartilaginous material. Therefore, it is important to request the necessary clinical information before drawing conclusions from the ultrasound images.

In rheumatoid knees treated with intra-articular steroids, punctate echogenic material can be identified. These echogenic foci correspond to calcifications that frequently result from intra-articular injection of corticosteroids (see Figs. 8–43 and 8–47). Although easily identified on sonographic images, these calcifications are rarely visualized on conventional radiographs (Gilsanz and Bernstein, 1984).

Periarticular Disease

We define periarticular disease as those processes involving the tissues surrounding the joint, specifically extra-articular and extrasynovial tissues. Ultrasound

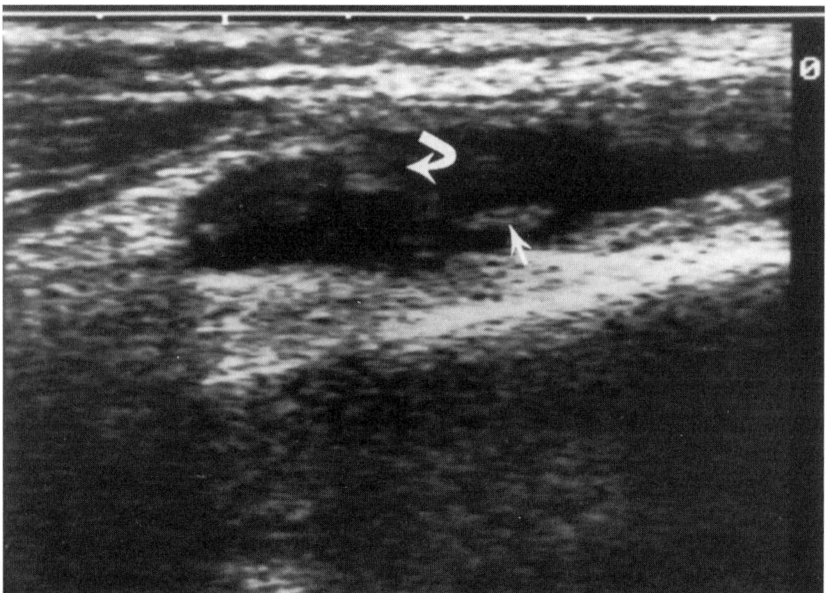

Figure 8–44 ■ Shedding of villi in rheumatoid arthritis: longitudinal sonogram. This patient is a 39-year-old woman with a 6-year history of rheumatoid arthritis and 6 months of knee involvement. She presented here with a flexion contracture of the right knee. This image is a longitudinal view of the suprapatellar bursa, which is distended with fluid. Irregular synovial proliferation is noted (*curved arrow*). Free-floating echogenic masses (*arrow*) are present within the bursa. Arthroscopy demonstrated these masses to be villi that had been shed from the synovial walls. Synovectomy with debridement of this debris was performed.

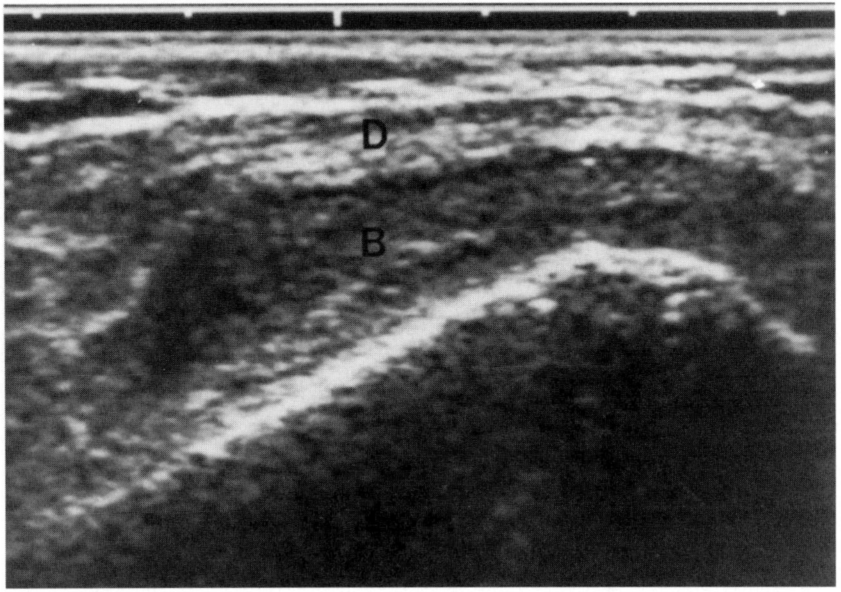

Figure 8–45 ▪ Rheumatoid shoulder disease: coronal sonogram. At the time of presentation, this 53-year-old woman with a 5-year history of rheumatoid arthritis complained of increasing right shoulder pain. The transducer is positioned in the coronal plane immediately inferior to the acromion. The acromion is just out of view to the observer's right. Hypoechoic material fills the subacromial-subdeltoid bursa (*B*). Ultrasound cannot always differentiate pannus from fibrinous debris. In this case, the sonographic appearance of the bursa explains why joint aspiration was negative despite prominent clinical swelling. Abbreviation: deltoid (*D*).

is clearly the most elegant technique for evaluation of this type of pathology. The FOV of arthroscopy is limited to the synovial cavity. This is also true of arthrography. In the past, clinicians had to rely entirely on clinical examination for the diagnosis of periarticular pathology. MRI can be helpful, but it is a static examination. Ultrasound is able to demonstrate periarticular anatomy under functional conditions, thus elucidating certain types of pathology. In addition, the high cost, lengthy examination, and frequent unavailability further limit the utility of MRI.

Tendon injuries, peritendinitis, bursitis, ligament tears, muscle tears, ruptures of the musculotendinous junction, and neurovascular lesions are all well evaluated using ultrasound. In other chapters of this volume, all of these lesions will be discussed in detail. At this point, we will confine our discussion to nerve and vascular lesions. Aneurysms, pseudoaneurysms, popliteal artery entrapment syndrome, adventitial cystic disease, venous thrombosis, and neuromas are abnormalities that may be encountered when large synovial joints are examined. Gray scale ultrasound with Doppler flow analysis is ideal for evaluation of vascular pathology. Peripheral nerves are also well evaluated using ultrasound.

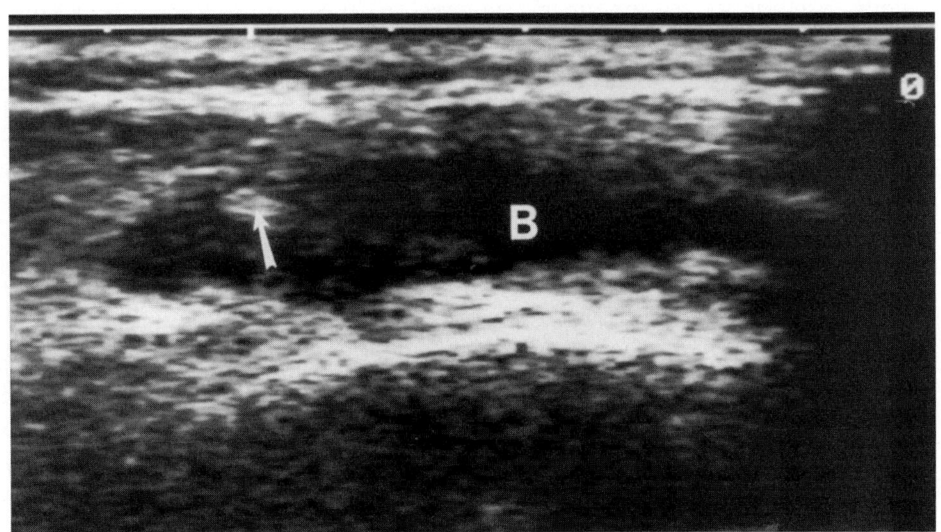

Figure 8–46 ▪ Meniscal fragment after meniscal surgery: longitudinal sonogram of the suprapatellar bursa. A meniscal fragment was lost in the joint during arthroscopic surgery on the left knee of this 37-year-old man. He presented with pain and locking of the knee. This longitudinal view of the suprapatellar bursa (*B*) demonstrates a hyperechoic meniscal fragment (*arrow*) within the lumen of the fluid-filled bursa. Manipulation by the examiner clearly showed this to be a free fragment.

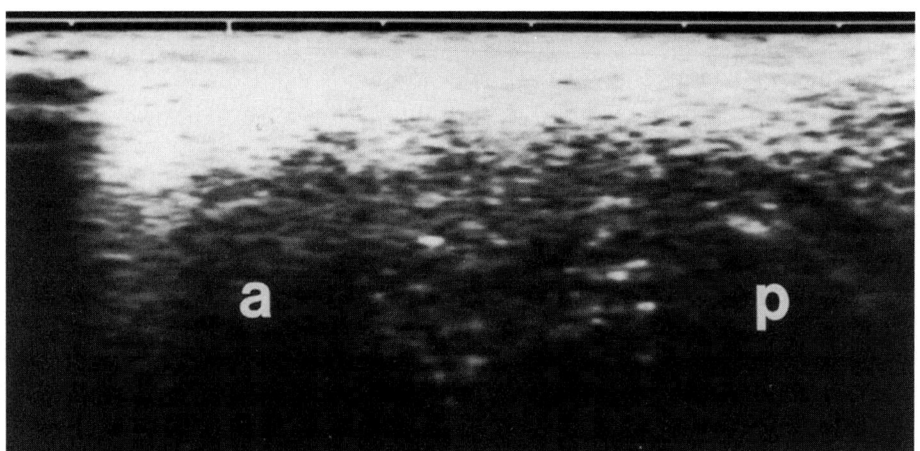

Figure 8–47 ▪ Steroid-related intra-articular debris: transverse sonogram of the lateral meniscus. The patient received an intra-articular injection of steroids 1 week prior to the examination. Throughout the meniscus, numerous tiny, highly echogenic foci are identified. These calcifications may also be observed on conventional radiographs. Abbreviations: anterior meniscus (*a*), posterior meniscus (*p*).

Aneurysms

Periarticular arterial aneurysms are most frequently seen adjacent to the hip and knee joints (Box 8–2). However, these vascular lesions may be identified adjacent to any joint. Congenital aneurysms are extremely rare. The vast majority are the result of atherosclerosis. Traumatic, mycotic, syphilitic, and poststenotic aneurysms are seen less frequently (Fig. 8–48). Aneurysms adjacent to joints resulting from atherosclerotic disease are found almost exclusively in the lower extremity (Fig. 8–49). Seventy percent of peripheral aneurysms are found in the popliteal artery. Fusiform aneurysms are most common in the common femoral arteries. These aneurysms are usually due to extension of an infrarenal abdominal aortic aneurysm that continues into the iliac and femoral vessels. Saccular aneurysms of the common femoral arteries generally occur at the site of anastomosis of prosthetic vascular grafts. Conversely, the majority of popliteal aneurysms are saccular. They usually present as asymptomatic masses in the popliteal fossa that are not pulsatile. Therefore, on clinical examination, they are difficult to distinguish from Baker's cyst (Fig. 8–50). These aneurysms usually contain a large amount of thrombus. As a result, there is a high risk of distal embolization of thrombus fragments. Surgical repair of these lesions is recommended for this reason. Rupture of these aneurysms is rare. Blood flow through these lesions is very slow, in some cases too slow to detect with color Doppler. Demonstrating continuity of the lesion with the superficial femoral artery leads to the correct diagnosis. In most cases, the distal superficial femoral artery is also ectatic. Popliteal aneurysms are frequently associated with other atherosclerotic aneurysms. Approximately 50% of cases are bilateral. Therefore, after the diagnosis of popliteal aneurysm is made, the popliteal fossa on the opposite side, the iliac regions, and the aorta should be examined.

Box 8–2
Popliteal Aneurysms

- 70% of peripheral aneurysms
- 50% are bilateral
- Difficult to detect (asymptomatic, hide in popliteal fat, not pulsatile)
- High risk—distal embolization

Poststenotic aneurysms are rare, usually found adjacent to the shoulder joint in the subclavian, axillary, and brachial arteries. They are frequently associated with cervical ribs or another type of thoracic outlet syndrome. Like popliteal aneurysms, they frequently result in distal embolization of fragments of luminal thrombus, requiring surgical intervention. These aneurysms are almost exclusively fusiform. The definitive diagnosis can be made sonographically with the demonstration of continuity with the brachial artery and the Doppler signal.

Aneurysms of the distal circulation are exceedingly rare and usually result from trauma or septic emboli. Traumatic aneurysms may occur anywhere in the circulation. They are pseudoaneurysms, with the flowing blood contained only by adventitia. As such, the risk of rupture is high, and surgical correction is indicated. Pseudoaneurysm located at a surgical anastomosis or a site of previous percutaneous entry of a catheter is a diagnosis that can be made with ultrasound noninvasively (McGahan and Goldberg, 1997). When pseudoaneurysms develop acutely after catheterization, they may be treated

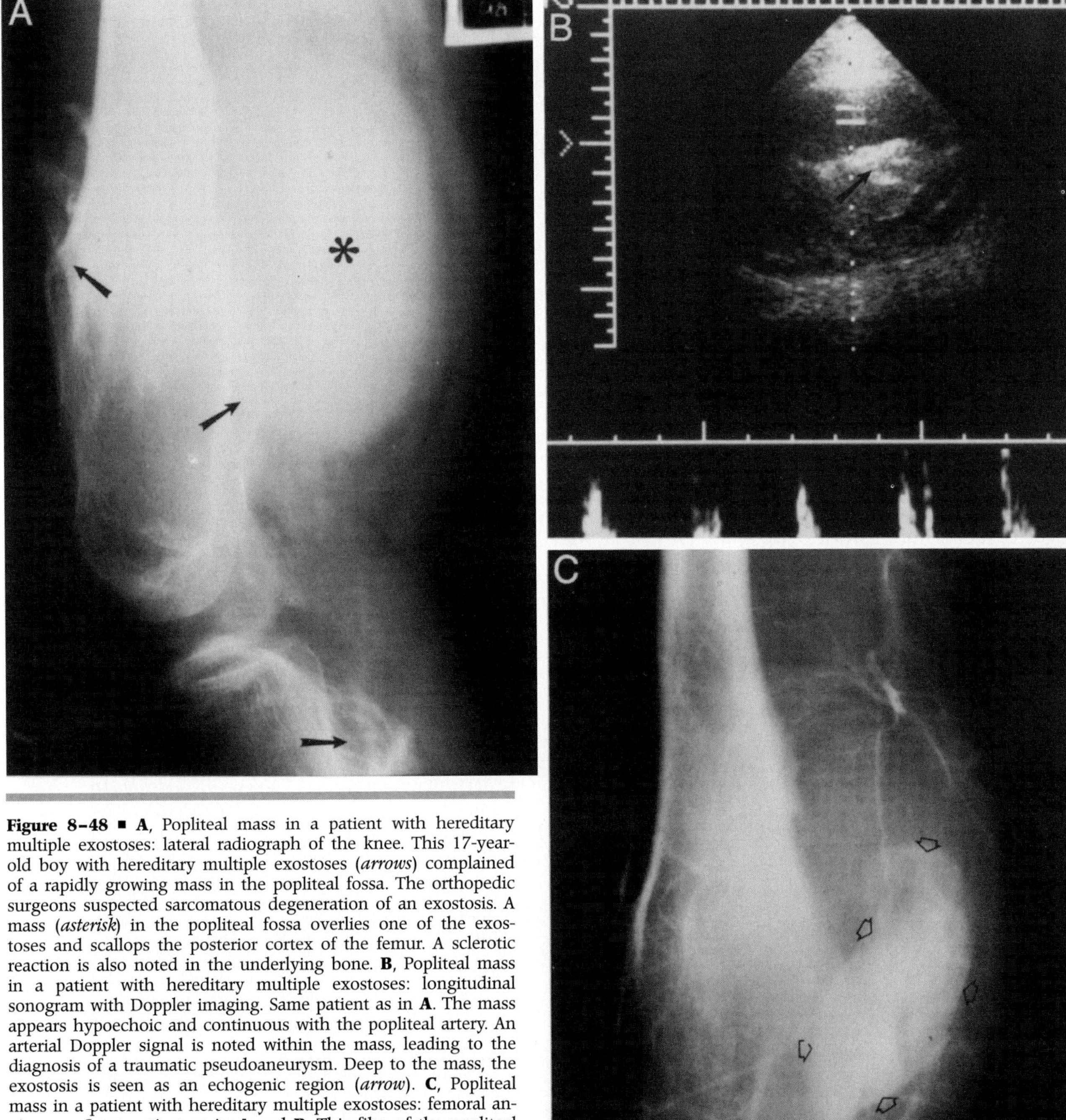

Figure 8–48 ■ **A**, Popliteal mass in a patient with hereditary multiple exostoses: lateral radiograph of the knee. This 17-year-old boy with hereditary multiple exostoses (*arrows*) complained of a rapidly growing mass in the popliteal fossa. The orthopedic surgeons suspected sarcomatous degeneration of an exostosis. A mass (*asterisk*) in the popliteal fossa overlies one of the exostoses and scallops the posterior cortex of the femur. A sclerotic reaction is also noted in the underlying bone. **B**, Popliteal mass in a patient with hereditary multiple exostoses: longitudinal sonogram with Doppler imaging. Same patient as in **A**. The mass appears hypoechoic and continuous with the popliteal artery. An arterial Doppler signal is noted within the mass, leading to the diagnosis of a traumatic pseudoaneurysm. Deep to the mass, the exostosis is seen as an echogenic region (*arrow*). **C**, Popliteal mass in a patient with hereditary multiple exostoses: femoral angiogram. Same patient as in **A** and **B**. This film of the popliteal region from the late arterial phase of a femoral angiogram demonstrates pooling of contrast material within the pseudoaneurysm (*open arrows*). The aneurysm was resected and a synthetic graft placed. Bone biopsy performed at the time of surgery demonstrated normal reactive bone.

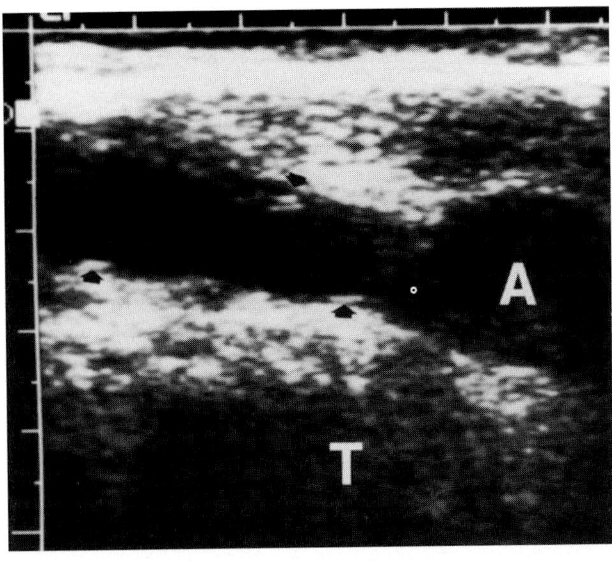

Figure 8–49 ■ Swelling of the left popliteal fossa: longitudinal sonogram. A mass was noted in the left popliteal fossa of this 62-year-old man during a routine physical examination. The clinical question was whether this mass was joint or vascular in origin. An ectatic popliteal artery with frank aneurysmal dilatation is demonstrated distally (*A*). Intimal calcifications are seen as hyperechoic lines (*arrows*). Abbreviation: proximal tibia (*T*).

with transcutaneous pressure applied with the surface of the transducer. Transcutaneous ablation of pseudoaneurysms with pressure applied on the transducer is successful in most cases if the patient is not systemically anticoagulated (Fellmeth et al., 1992).

Sonography does not have a role in the evaluation of acute penetrating trauma, but it is certainly indicated in more subtle forms of trauma. Color flow imaging can identify a free flap in vascular dissections. It is necessary to confirm the presence of the lesion by scanning transversely on the axis of the vessel. Velocity measurements can identify the true lumen of the dissection and determine whether both channels are patent (Bluth et al., 1989). Anechoic masses in the hand represent ganglia in the majority of cases. However, it is important to switch on

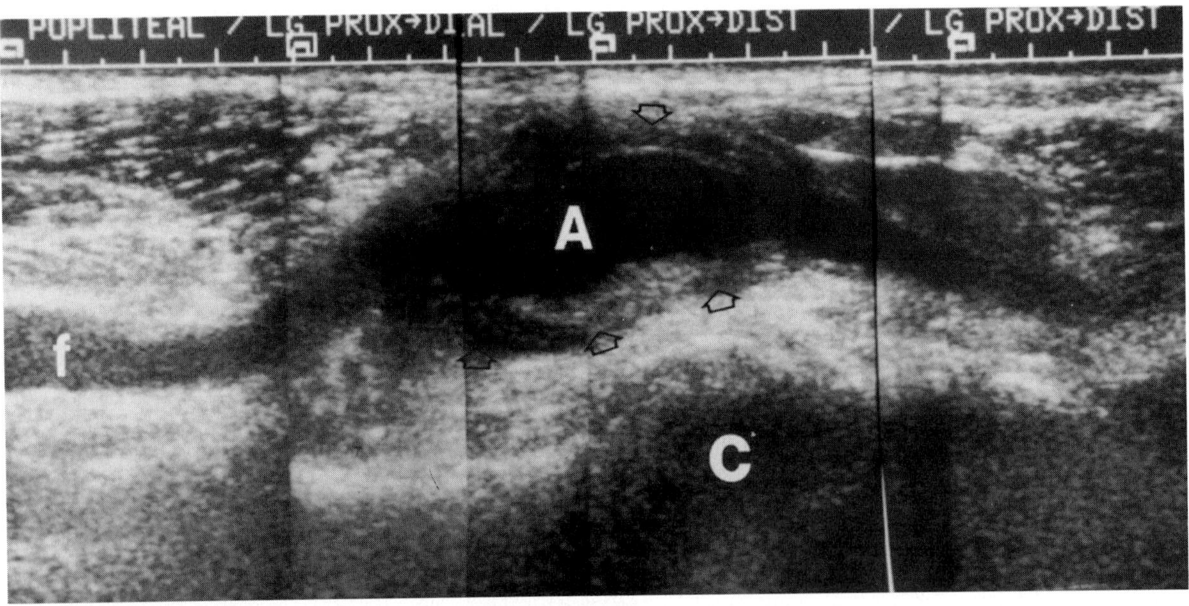

Figure 8–50 ■ Mass in the popliteal fossa: longitudinal sonogram. A mass in the right popliteal fossa of this 68-year-old man was thought to be a Baker cyst. The image displayed is a concatenation of serial longitudinal images obtained over a 16-cm length of the popliteal fossa. Aneurysmal dilatation (*A*) of the popliteal artery is noted to contain mural thrombus (*open arrows*). When an aneurysm of the popliteal fossa is discovered, the contralateral side, common femoral arteries, and abdominal aorta must be examined. This patient had aneurysmal dilatation of the opposite popliteal, bilateral common femoral, and bilateral iliac arteries and the infrarenal aorta. Abbreviations: junction of the superficial femoral artery and popliteal (*f*), lateral femoral condyle (*C*).

the Doppler or color Doppler to ensure that the lesion does not represent a pseudoaneurysm or arteriovenous fistula. Occasionally, arteriovenous fistulas result from penetrating trauma. If undiagnosed at the initial presentation, they can cause venous aneurysms secondary to increased flow. The lower extremity is a high-resistance system. If a high degree of diastolic flow is observed proximal to the site of injury, a fistula should be suspected.

Mycotic aneurysms are usually the result of bacterial endocarditis, but they may also occur from direct intra-arterial injection in drug abusers utilizing contaminated needles. Septic emboli lodge in the peripheral circulation, resulting in aneurysm formation, usually saccular. These lesions develop and expand rapidly, requiring timely, accurate diagnosis. Sonographically, these aneurysms have imaging characteristics identical to those of other aneurysms of the peripheral circulation. The diagnosis of mycotic aneurysm is based on clinical criteria.

Popliteal Entrapment Syndrome

Calf claudication in a young patient without other medical problems is probably due to popliteal artery entrapment syndrome. The normal course of the popliteal artery passes between the heads of the gastrocnemius muscle. Congenital malposition of the popliteal artery medial to or within the medial head of the gastrocnemius results in compression of the artery, which is greatest in extension. Initially this results only in decreased pedal pulses. However, this chronic irritation of the vessel results in intimal thickening and fibrosis. If it is undiagnosed, total occlusion of the vessel will occur. The severity of the claudication is dependent on the rate at which occlusion occurs and on the development of collateral flow. Diagnosis is based on identification of the popliteal artery within or medial to the medial head of the gastrocnemius muscle.

Cystic degeneration of the popliteal artery is another etiology of calf claudication. Narrowing of the popliteal artery in this condition is caused by compression from a mucoid cyst in the adventitia. It usually occurs in the middle third of the artery. Ultrasound is highly sensitive and specific in the identification of these cysts—perhaps more sensitive than arteriography if filming is performed in only the anteroposterior projection. Aspiration of the cyst under ultrasound guidance usually relieves the symptoms (Do et al., 1997). However, due to the possibility of recurrence, surgical therapy with synthetic graft placement may be desirable.

Venous Pathology

Sonography is playing an increasing role in the diagnosis and follow-up of deep venous thrombosis. Compression gray scale imaging and Doppler flow analysis are highly sensitive and specific for venous thrombosis (Fig. 8–51) (Lensing et al., 1989; Blebea et al., 1995; Sheiman and McArdle, 1995; Pezzullo et al., 1996). Examination of the popliteal fossa and hip should include evaluation of the patency and compressibility of the popliteal and femoral veins. The vein to be examined is localized in transverse images, and then the transducer is placed directly over the vessel, scanning its long axis. Pressure is applied with the transducer, and the response of the vessel is observed. If the lumen of the vein cannot be completely obliterated by compression, thrombus is present.

Nerve Lesions

Normal nerves appear as linear, fibrillar, hyperechoic structures in close proximity to vessels. Visualization of peripheral nerves depends strictly on the echogenicity of surrounding tissues (Martinoli et al., 1996). Nerve tissue is hyperechoic relative to muscle but slightly hypoechoic relative to tendons. Detection of nerves that course between muscle bellies is easy because of the sharp contrast between those anatomical structures. Distinctly more difficult is examination of nerves surrounded by hyperechoic connective tissue, such as the nerve in the cubital tunnel, nerves in elderly patients, nerves surrounded by scar, ligamentous fibrosis, and calcification. An experienced operator will enhance the examination significantly (Martinoli et al., 1996). Nerves can be followed along their course in the extremities from the axilla to the wrist in the arm and from the ischial spine to the ankle in the leg. Benign neural tumors are generally fusiform in shape and appear hypoechoic (Figs. 8–52 through 8–54). Neurilemmomas contain cystic spaces more often than neurofibromas (Box 8–3). The growth in those lesions is eccentric, in contrast to the central

Box 8–3
Cystic Masses in the Popliteal Fossa

- Baker's cysts (medial + joint communication)
- Aneurysms (midline or lateral)
- Neurilemmomas (lateral)
- Ganglia (midline/anywhere)
- Adventitial cystic disease of popliteal artery
- Caveat: cystic-appearing sarcomas (synovial sarcoma; myxoid liposarcoma, etc.)

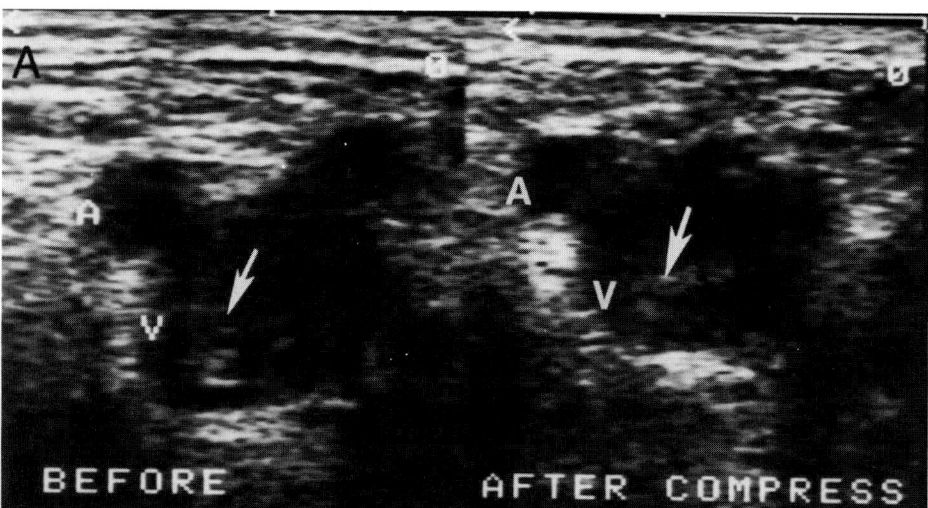

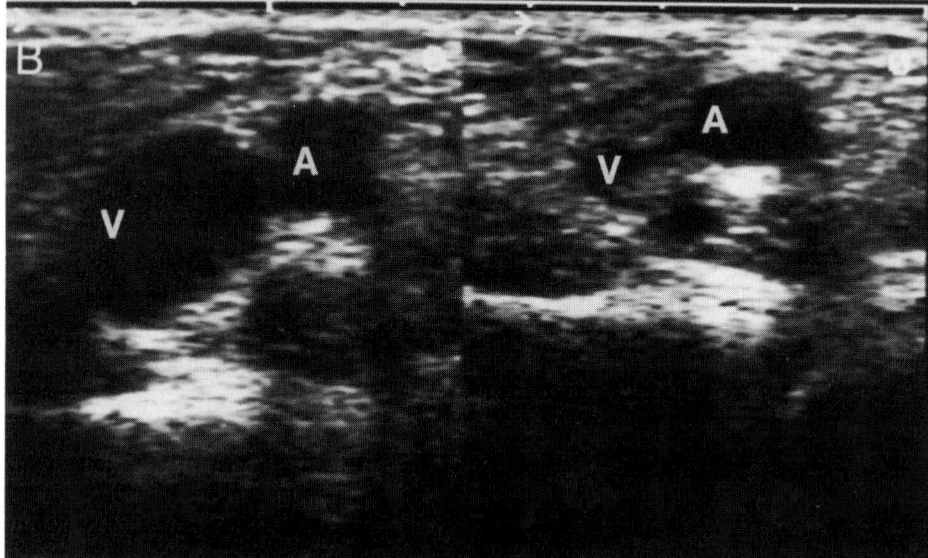

Figure 8-51 ■ **A**, Deep venous thrombosis of the lower leg: transverse sonograms. This 50-year-old woman presented to the emergency room with a 3-day history of erythema and swelling of the right lower extremity. She had a 10-year history of rheumatoid arthritis, and the clinical question was whether she had deep venous thrombosis or pseudothrombophlebitis. A compression study was performed of the common femoral vein (*V*) at the point of junction with the saphenous vein. Echogenic material (*arrow*) is noted within the vein. The dimension of the vein did not change when pressure was applied with the transducer. This is diagnostic of deep venous thrombosis. Abbreviation: femoral artery (*A*). **B**, Normal veins of the lower leg: transverse sonograms. Same patient and transducer position as in **A**, contralateral leg. The compression image is on the right. The common femoral vein is anechoic and fully compressible. This is the sonographic appearance of a normal vein. Abbreviations: common femoral artery (*A*), common femoral vein (*V*).

growth in neurofibromas. Sonography is a valuable first test when electromyography (EMG) indicates a peripheral nerve lesion. In addition, ultrasound can provide information about nerve processes in patients with distinct clinical symptoms even in the absence of EMG findings. Because nerve conduction tests reflect the status of the best-surviving nerve fibers, EMG can be negative in the presence of significant nerve disease. Nerve abnormalities can be studied following trauma or inflammation or with entrapment syndromes and tumors. Its ability to examine the entire extremity quickly provides another big advantage over MRI (see Chapter 16).

Recent investigations using 15-MHz transducers have shown that nerves appear to be composed of multiple hypoechoic, parallel, but discontinuous linear areas separated by hyperechoic bands. The hypoechoic areas are arranged in series, appearing well defined and elongated along the longitudinal axis of the nerve. Transverse sections show the hypoechoic areas to be rounded and embedded in a homogeneous, hyperechoic background (Martinoli et al., 1996). Histological correlation demonstrates the hypoechoic areas to be fascicles of neuronal fibers, whereas the hyperechoic background represents epineurium extending between the individual fascicles of nerve substance. Ultrasound has the ability to differentiate intraneural from extraneural lesions. This makes the technique valuable in identifying the etiology of peripheral neuropathies. Inflammatory swelling of nerves can be observed in Morton's neuromas (Redd et al., 1989) in the foot and in compressive neuropathies (Buchberger et al., 1992). Chronic trauma induces a lesion sonographically characterized by decreased echogenicity, probably edema, and loss of the normal fascicular pattern. These lesions are common and are often found in close proximity to joints. In some locations, nerve lesions may be

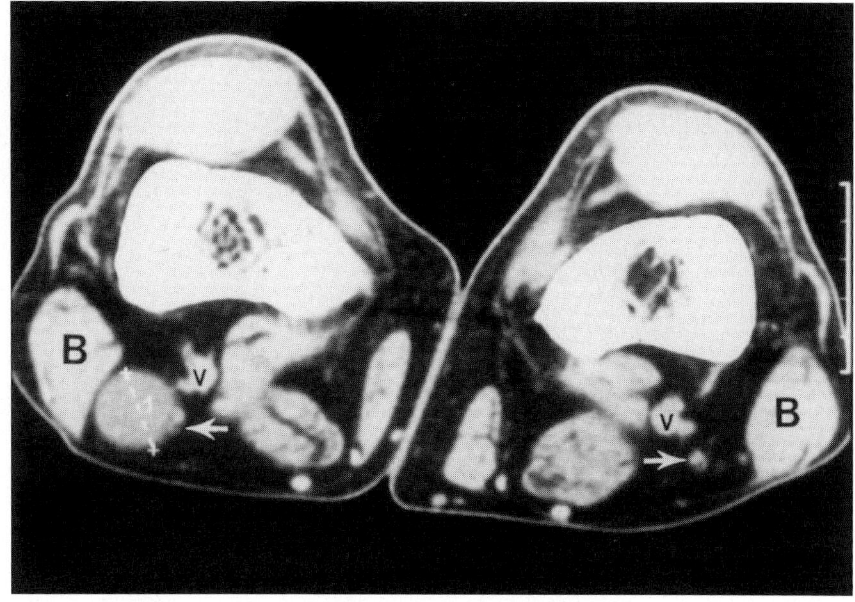

Figure 8–52 ■ Schwannoma in the right popliteal fossa: CT scan. Spinal CT was performed on this 30-year-old woman who presented with paresthesia of the right lower extremity. This examination was normal. CT of the lower extremities was performed following EMGs. A spherical mass 2.2 cm in diameter is seen arising from the lateral aspect of the tibial nerve (*arrow*). Abbreviations: biceps muscle (*B*), popliteal vein (*V*).

mistaken for a synovial or capsular process. Showing that the lesion is in continuity with a nerve is crucial in making the correct diagnosis (see Chapter 10).

Carpal tunnel is the best-known compressive neuropathy. However, a multitude of osteofibrous tunnels cause entrapment of nerves. Compression of the ulnar nerve has been observed sonographically in the cubital tunnel, the tibial nerve in the tarsal tunnel, and the superficial peroneal nerve under the fascia covering the peroneal compartment. The

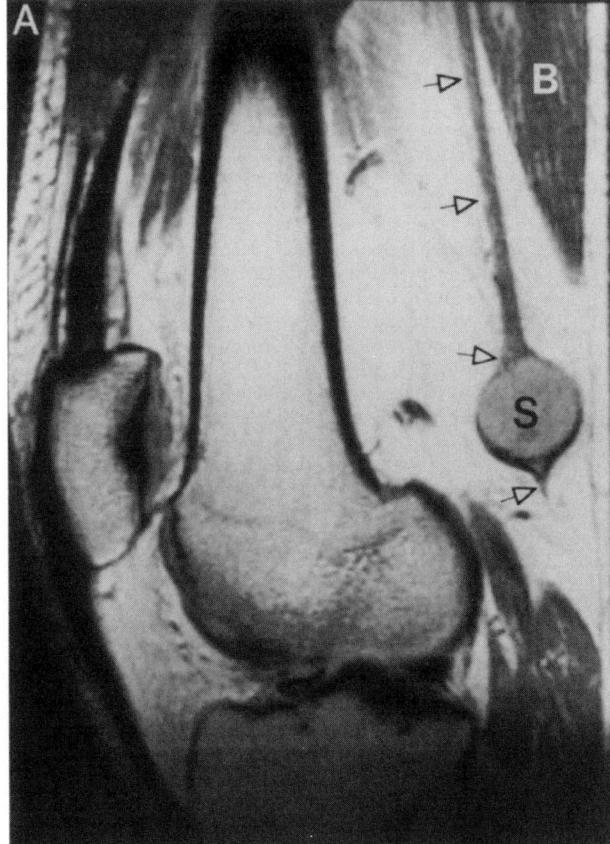

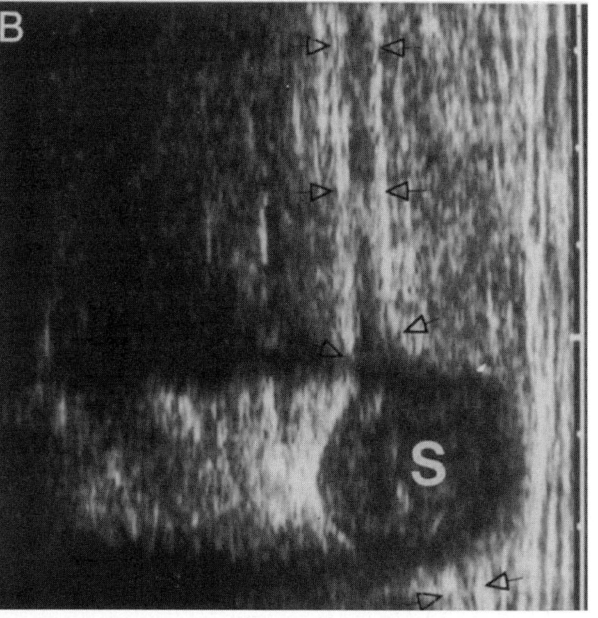

Figure 8–53 ■ **A**, Schwannoma in the popliteal fossa: sagittal T_1 MRI. Same patient as in Figure 8–52. A sagittal T_1-weighted spin-echo image demonstrates a mass continuous with the tibial nerve (*open arrows*) of slightly greater signal intensity. Abbreviations: biceps muscle (*B*), schwannoma (*S*). **B**, Schwannoma in the popliteal fossa: longitudinal sonogram. Same patient as in **A**. The image is oriented in the same manner as the MRI examination in **A**. Ultrasound demonstrates the schwannoma (*S*) continuous with the tibial nerve (*open arrows*). Note the increased through-transmission of sound deep to the lesion. This is a characteristic finding with schwannomas.

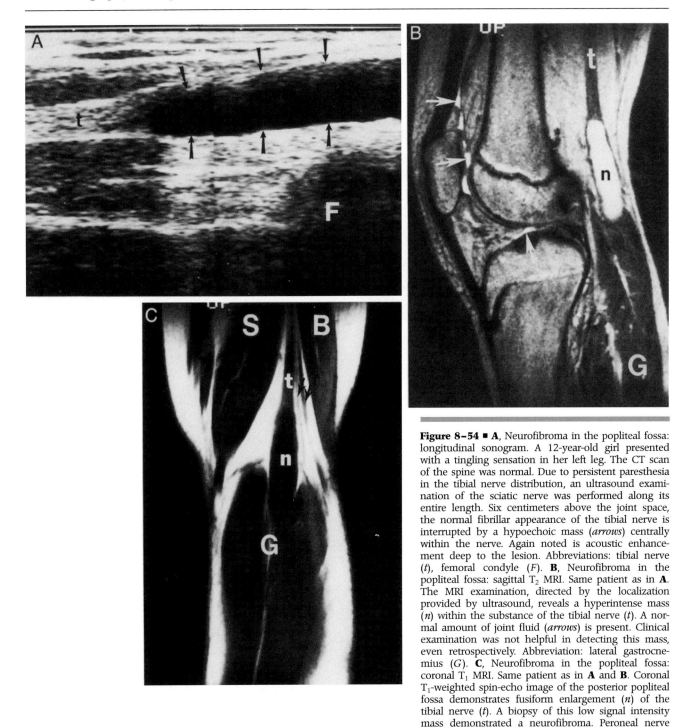

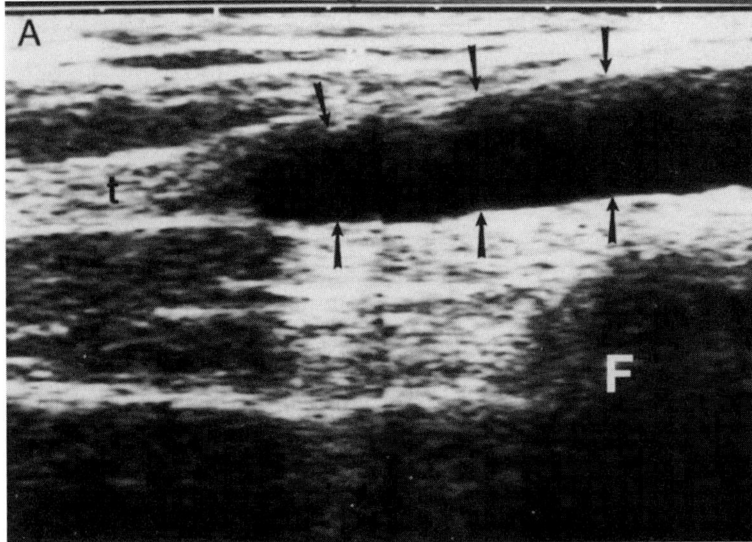

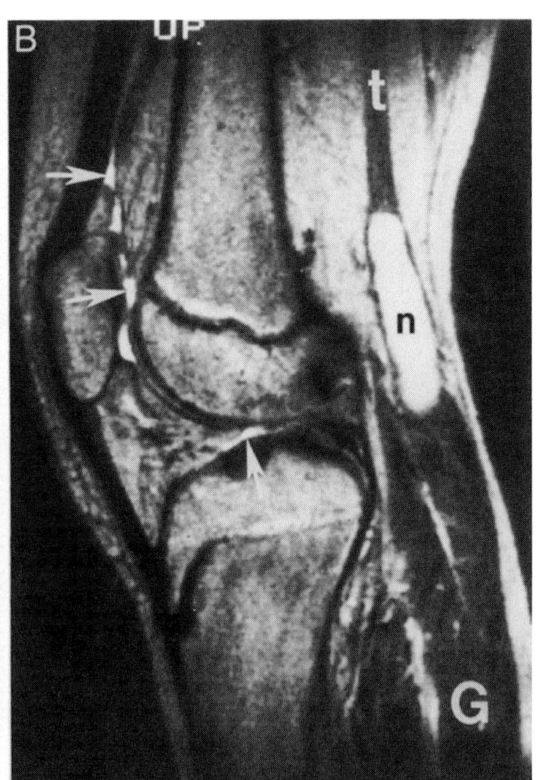

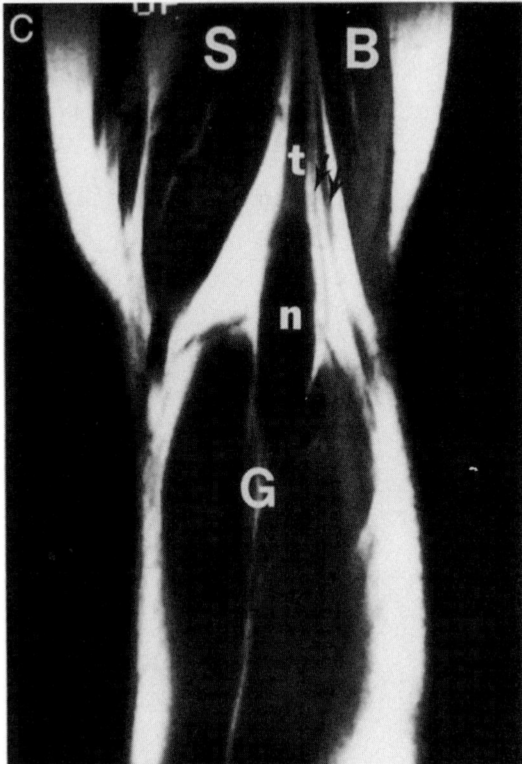

Figure 8–54 ■ **A**, Neurofibroma in the popliteal fossa: longitudinal sonogram. A 12-year-old girl presented with a tingling sensation in her left leg. The CT scan of the spine was normal. Due to persistent paresthesia in the tibial nerve distribution, an ultrasound examination of the sciatic nerve was performed along its entire length. Six centimeters above the joint space, the normal fibrillar appearance of the tibial nerve is interrupted by a hypoechoic mass (*arrows*) centrally within the nerve. Again noted is acoustic enhancement deep to the lesion. Abbreviations: tibial nerve (*t*), femoral condyle (*F*). **B**, Neurofibroma in the popliteal fossa: sagittal T_2 MRI. Same patient as in **A**. The MRI examination, directed by the localization provided by ultrasound, reveals a hyperintense mass (*n*) within the substance of the tibial nerve (*t*). A normal amount of joint fluid (*arrows*) is present. Clinical examination was not helpful in detecting this mass, even retrospectively. Abbreviation: lateral gastrocnemius (*G*). **C**, Neurofibroma in the popliteal fossa: coronal T_1 MRI. Same patient as in **A** and **B**. Coronal T_1-weighted spin-echo image of the posterior popliteal fossa demonstrates fusiform enlargement (*n*) of the tibial nerve (*t*). A biopsy of this low signal intensity mass demonstrated a neurofibroma. Peroneal nerve branches (*arrows*) look normal. Abbreviations: biceps muscle (*B*), gastrocnemius (*G*), semimembranosus (*S*).

typical compression neuropathy exhibits swelling proximal to the area of compression and flattening of the nerve within the narrow tunnel structure.

Morton's neuromas are not true neuromas, but fibrotic lesions induced by trauma. High-frequency ultrasound examination of Morton's neuromas in our patient population has shown a spectrum of disease. Edema and fusiform swelling of the interdigital nerve are the most common findings. In addition, lump-like masses, bursal thickening, hyperemia, thrombosed vessels, and callus have been found in association with the neural swelling. Others have observed swelling of a long segment of the nerve in rare diseases such as leprosy and intraneural ganglion cyst (Martinoli et al., 1996). Postsurgical or amputation neuromas can cause intense focal pain. Ultrasound is able to diagnose these lesions. They appear as hypoechoic masses with well-defined margins because of their fibrous capsule. Central hyperechoic changes are common; they have been attributed to fibrosis and calcification.

References

Adam R, et al: Arthrosonography of the irritable hip in childhood: A review of 1 year's experience. *Br J Radiol* 59:205–208, 1986.

Aisen AM, et al: Sonographic evaluation of the cartilage of the knee. *Radiology* 153:781–784, 1984.

Barrie HJ: The pathogenesis and significance of meniscal cysts. *J Bone Joint Surg Br* 61:184, 1979.

Blebea J, Strothman G, Fowl R: Bilateral lower-extremity US for deep venous thrombosis. *Radiology* 197:315, 1995.

Bloom W, Fawcett DW: *A Textbook of Histology*, ed 10. Philadelphia, WB Saunders Co, 1975.

Bluth EI, et al: Doppler color flow imaging of carotid artery dissection. *J Ultrasound Med* 8:149, 1989.

Breidahl WH, et al: Power Doppler sonography in the assessment of musculoskeletal fluid collections. *AJR* 166:1443–1446, 1996.

Buchberger W, et al: Carpal tunnel syndrome: Diagnosis with high-resolution sonography. *AJR* 159:793–798, 1992.

Cimmino MA: Recognition and management of bacterial arthritis. *Drugs* 54:50–60, 1997.

Cooperberg PL, et al: Gray scale ultrasound in the evaluation of rheumatoid arthritis of the knee. *Radiology* 126:759–763, 1978.

Do DD, et al: Adventitial cystic disease of the popliteal artery: Percutaneous US-guided aspiration. *Radiology* 203:743, 1997.

Dorr U: The painful hip joint. Diagnostic possibilities offered by sonography. *Fortschr Geb Röntgenstr Nuklearmed Erganzungsband* 148:487–491, 1988.

Fellmeth BD, et al: Repair of postcatheterization femoral pseudoaneurysm by color flow ultrasound guided compression. *Am Heart J* 123:547, 1992.

Ferrer-Roca O, Vilalta C: Lesions of the meniscus. II: Horizontal cleavages and lateral cysts. *Clin Orthop* 146:301, 1980.

Frankel DA, et al: Synovial joints: Evaluation of intraarticular bodies with ultrasound. *Radiology* 206:41–44, 1998.

Gielen JL, et al: Growing bone cysts in long-term hemodialysis. *Skeletal Radiol* 19:43–49, 1990.

Gilsanz V, Bernstein BH: Joint calcification following intraarticular corticosteroid therapy. *Radiology* 151: 647–649, 1984.

Goldberg DL, Cohen AS: Acute infectious arthritis. *Am J Med* 60:369–377, 1976.

Hammer M, et al: Sonography and NMR imaging in rheumatoid gonarthritis. *Scand J Rheumatol* 15: 157–164, 1986.

Lensing AWA, et al: Detection of deep-vein thrombosis by real-time B-mode ultrasonography. *N Engl J Med* 320:342–345, 1989.

Lombardi T, Sherman L, van Holsbeeck M: Sonographic detection of septic subdeltoid bursitis: A case report. *J Ultrasound Med* 11:159–160, 1992.

Marchal GJ, et al: Ultrasonography in transient synovitis of the hip in children. *Radiology* 162:825–828, 1987.

Martinoli C, et al: Ultrasonography of peripheral nerves. *J Peripheral Nerv Syst* 1(3):169–178, 1996.

McGahan JP, Goldberg BB: Diagnostic ultrasound. CD-ROM. Philadelphia, Lippincott-Raven, 1997.

Middleton DB: Infectious arthritis. *Prim Care* 20:943–953, 1993.

Mori Y: Debris observed by arthroscopy of the knee. *Orthop Clin North Am* 10:559–563, 1979.

Peck J: Ultrasound of the painful hip in children. *Br J Radiol* 59:205–208, 1986.

Pezzullo JA, Perkins AB, Cronan JJ: Symptomatic deep vein thrombosis: Diagnosis with limited compression ultrasound. *Radiology* 198:67, 1996.

Redd RA, et al: Morton neuroma: Sonographic evaluation. *Radiology* 171:415–417, 1989.

Resnick D, Niwayama G: *Diagnosis of Bone and Joint Disorders*, ed 2. Philadelphia, WB Saunders Co, 1988.

Richardson ML, et al: Ultrasonography of the knee. *Radiol Clin North Am* 26:63–75, 1988.

Riegels-Nielsen P, Frimodt-Moller N, Jensen JS: Rabbit model of septic arthritis. *Acta Orthop Scand* 58: 14–19, 1987.

Robben SGF, et al: Anterior joint capsule of the normal hip and in children with transient synovitis: US study with anatomic and histologic correlation. *Radiology* 210:499–507, 1999.

Selby B, et al: High resolution sonography of the menisci of the knee. *Invest Radiol* 21:332–335, 1986.

Sheiman RG, McArdle CR: Bilateral lower extremity US in the patient with unilateral symptoms of deep venous thrombosis: Assessment of need. *Radiology* 194:171, 1986.

Taveras JM, Ferrucci JT: Radiology: *Diagnosis—imaging—intervention*, Vol 5. Philadelphia, JB Lippincott, 1987, chap 1.

van Holsbeeck M, et al: Sonography of the medial collateral ligament [abstract]. *Radiology* 169:178, 1988a.

van Holsbeeck M, et al: Staging and follow-up of rheumatoid arthritis of the knee. Comparison of sonography, thermography, and clinical assessment. *J Ultrasound Med* 7:561–566, 1988b.

Vandeputte L, Mulier JC, Mulier F: Transient synovitis of the hip joint in children. *Acta Orthop Belg* 37: 186–193, 1971.

Wingstrand H: Transient synovitis of the hip in the child. *Acta Orthop Scand* 57(Suppl):45–46, 1986.

Worth WD, et al: Stellenwert der Arthrosonographie in die Beurteilung der Exsudativen und proliferativen Synovialitis. *Z Rheumatol* 45:263, 1986.

Chapter 9
Pediatric Musculoskeletal and Spinal Sonography

Michael A. DiPietro, M.D., and Theodore Harcke, M.D.

Applications for real-time sonography of the musculoskeletal system in children (Harcke et al., 1988) continue to grow and undergo refinement. This relates particularly to infancy, when radiography is of limited usefulness because it does not depict cartilage. Sonography clearly depicts the unossified hip, for example, and has thereby found widespread use in detecting developmental dysplasia of the hip in patients who are normal clinically. Its extreme sensitivity has increased our awareness of developmental maturation of the hip and of the possibility of monitoring minor abnormality with the intent of preventing overtreatment. Much of this chapter addresses DDH because there is widespread experience and considerable literature addressing ultrasound's role in this condition.

Other uses of sonography include distinguishing joint dislocations from displaced epiphyses (e.g., displaced Salter-Harris fractures), defining congenital skeletal anomalies, and delineating the extent of midline or near-midline soft tissue masses on the back with possible occult tethered spinal cord. There is growing interest in using ultrasound to detect inflammatory disease in joints and bones.

Developmental Dysplasia of the Hip

Background

The term *congenital dislocation of the hip* (*CDH*) was described as "an anomaly of the hip joint, present at birth, in which the head of the femur is, or may be, partially or completely dislocated from the acetabulum" (Dunn, 1969. p. 1037). The name was changed to *developmental dysplasia of the hip* (*DDH*) to better convey the scope of this condition, which has a range of abnormality and changes over time. DDH is regarded as a spectrum of instability: subluxable, subluxed, dislocatable, or dislocated hips with varying degrees of deformity (i.e., dysplasia) of the acetabulum. Cases of bilateral DDH which manifest variable severity from side to side further support the concept that this is a single but variable pathological entity.

DDH is perinatal, a late in utero alteration of a previously normally formed part, created by persistent gentle forces. There is another category of dislocation, teratological, in which the displacement occurs early in utero secondary to a problem such as myelodysplasia or arthrogryposis. In the teratological form, adaptive changes in the hips are advanced at birth and are usually obvious clinically and radiologically.

Both mechanical and physiological factors are implicated in DDH (Dunn, 1976b; Hensinger, 1979). The mechanical factor in deformation is constraint and compression of the fetus in utero. In utero spatial restriction of fetal leg movements can occur with oligohydramnios, first pregnancy (tight maternal uterine and abdominal muscles), and breech presentation (30–50% of DDH). Other deformations also caused by in utero constraint, such as sternocleidomastoid torticollis and metatarsus adductus, have an increased association with DDH. The physiological factor in DDH is laxity of the hip joint due to the influence of maternal hormones. This gender-related factor plays a role in the incidence of DDH and is thought to account for the 6:1 female: male ratio. Other genetic factors are also present since DDH is more likely to occur in infants who have a sibling or parent with DDH.

Near the time of birth, the joint capsule is elastic and stretched, resulting in a tendency for the femoral head to dislocate. However, the shape of the joint and the soft tissues are nearly normal, so that if the femoral head is kept in the acetabulum, the joint capsule will tighten and return to its normal configuration in a few weeks (Hensinger, 1979).

The dislocatable, unstable hip is treated by splinting with reliable, but not excessive, constraint until it can be held firmly by its own connective tissue, which had been stretched prior to birth. Ninety-six percent of DDH patients become radiologically and physiologically normal when they are treated early (Hensinger, 1979). When DDH is undetected and the hip is not reduced successfully, adaptive changes in the acetabulum (steep roof, pseudoacetabulum formation), femoral head (small, flattened, delayed ossification), ligaments, and muscles (contractures) occur; and with more deformity to reverse, obtaining a satisfactory reduction is difficult. Surgery is required in severe cases.

A clinical study, based on physical examination of 7,742 newborns, revealed an increased frequency of breech-delivered babies in the group with unstable or dislocated versus normal hips (17.3% vs. 4.4%) (Barlow, 1962). Of these newborns, 1.5% had dislocatable or dislocated hips soon after birth. However, 60% of those babies' hips became stable by 1 week and 90% by 2 months, with or without treatment. These patients also had normal 1-year follow-up physical examinations and radiographs, yielding a final DDH incidence of 0.15% of live births, similar to that reported in other series.

Most unstable newborn hips (80%) (Dunn, 1976b) resolve spontaneously, although this is unlikely after 2 months (Barlow, 1962). Adduction, extension, and immobility of the hips reduce the natural rate of resolution of dislocatable hips, whereas partial abduction and partial flexion encourage resolution. The possibility of spontaneous resolution creates controversy about early treatment of hips with minor instability and immaturity of the acetabulum (Berman and Klenerman, 1986). On the other hand, treatment, if eventually needed, is more difficult after 2 months of age due to the development of adductor muscle tightness. Barlow (1962) recommends treatment in the first week.

An autopsy study performed on babies who died during labor or soon after birth suggested that the crucial pathology of DDH is the labrum (Dunn, 1969, 1976a). Babies between 13 and 40 weeks' gestation with nonsubluxable hips showed little difference in general morphology over this wide gestational range. In those babies (27–44 weeks' gestation) with dislocatable hips, the cartilage labrum was shown to be everted and stretched posteriorly and superiorly to variable degrees. When dislocation was partial, the hip was restrained by the capsule and ligamentum teres, which, however, were stretched when instability and dislocation were worse. In addition, markedly unstable dislocated hips had the labrum inverted, the acetabulum shallow, and the femoral head small, pitted, discolored, and less spherical. The number of right and left abnormal hips was the same, although in clinical studies, left hip abnormality is more common. An incidence of 20% right and 25% bilateral DDH has been cited (Hensinger, 1979).

What constitutes DDH? Subluxable hips, dislocatable or dislocated hips, acetabular dysplasia with or without joint laxity, physiological immaturity of the acetabulum, and physiological laxity of the capsule in the newborn are all included in the condition. Since DDH is a treatable condition, and is treated with more success when intervention is begun early, attention has been given to early detection. Prior to the use of ultrasound, newborn screening was done by a clinical examination. One problem with evaluating the effect of screening and treating programs is the variability and indistinctness of the condition under study. "Distinctions between congenital dislocation, acetabular dysplasia, and normality are blurred in the mists of radiological images" (Catterall, 1984, p. 469). Reports concerning the management of DDH in infants less than 1 year of age seldom strictly define the criteria for diagnosis, yet DDH covers a broad spectrum between normality and severe dysplasia (Catterall, 1984).

The incidence of DDH in clinical screening programs is reported to be between 0.25% and 2% of live births, whereas before such programs existed it was 0.07% to 0.15% of live births (Place et al., 1978). The rate of late diagnosed cases was no different, and the apparent increase in the incidence of DDH could merely be a difference in classification, including many patients who might have recovered spontaneously without treatment (Place et al., 1978). A reportedly increased incidence from 0.15% (prescreen) to 0.18% (with screen) could have also been due to the detection of cases that formerly had gone unnoticed until adulthood (MacKenzie and Wilson, 1981). One might accept the high false-positive rate, with the risk of overtreatment, if the false-negative rate (DDH diagnosed late, missed in the newborn exam) dropped. Yet the reported incidence of late diagnosed (missed?) DDH was 0.078% of live births when all patients had newborn examinations (Place et al., 1978). The screening clinical examination that tests for increased joint laxity failed to prevent the occurrence of late DDH. With the advent of ultrasound, another method for screening became available. This will be discussed later in this chapter.

DDH is treated by splinting (holding) the hips in a flexed/abducted ("frog-leg") position. There are a variety of splints, some rigid and some permitting motion. A popular splint in the United States is the Pavlik harness, a dynamic splint that allows motion in a safe zone (MacEwen and Zembo, 1987). If one treats early, there is the possibility of needless and potentially dangerous overtreatment. However, if treatment is postponed until later, some cases might be missed or lost and treatment can be more difficult. Those who oppose immediate splinting cite the spontaneous resolution rate reported by Barlow (1962) together with the risk of iatrogenic avascular necrosis. The risk of avascular necrosis following splinting is 2.5% in one study (Saies et al., 1988). However, if extreme abduction is avoided during splinting, and if splinting is done early, before contracture, when little force is needed, the risk of avascular necrosis is minimized (Hansson et al., 1983; Tredwell and Davis, 1989).

For DDH cases that fail to respond to splinting and late detected cases, treatment is operative. The infant must undergo a closed reduction (under anesthesia) with casting. Open reduction is required if closed reduction is unsuccessful. Even when reduction is accomplished, further surgery may be required to provide an adequate acetabulum. A variety of iliac osteotomies are possible (MacEwen and Zembo, 1987).

Sonography

Historically, sonography developed along two lines. The initial pioneering work of Graf (1983) focused on acetabular morphology. Harcke (Harcke et al., 1984) began real-time scanning with a technique that mirrored the clinical examination and assessed stability as well as morphology.

Over the years, it has been established that real-time sonography can reliably assess three key features of the infant hip joint: (1) position: the relationship of the femoral head to the acetabulum; (2) stability: The change in position of the head in response to movement and stress—typically, this is modeled after the Barlow and Ortolani maneuvers and is referred to as *dynamic examination*; (3) morphology: the development of the bony and cartilaginous components of the acetabulum. Quantification of development has employed acetabular angles and coverage measurements that reflect the severity of dysplasia. As explained to parents, the hip joint is a ball in a socket, and we are checking for the position of the ball in the socket, the stability of the ball in the socket, and the shape of the socket and its coverage and containment of the ball.

In North America, most sonographers adopted a technique that incorporated both morphologic and dynamic assessment. The American College of Radiology (ACR) published a standard for examination of the infant hip. Simply stated, the ACR standard for assessment of the infant hip requires a check of the relationship of the femoral head to the acetabulum at rest and with stress (position and stability) and the development of the acetabular roof components (morphology) (American College of Radiology, 2000).

Technique

The hip has been studied from anterior and lateral approaches, with the lateral approach being more widely used. The lateral approach is emphasized in this chapter. A linear array transducer is recommended, with the highest frequency required in order to achieve adequate penetration. For newborn infants, the 7.5-MHz range is sufficient; as the infant reaches 3 months of age, a 5-MHz probe might be required. The electronically focused transducers allow wide latitude. Hip examination after 6 months of age generally shifts from ultrasound to radiography. If sonography in older infants is performed, the transducer frequency will change. From the lateral approach, two orthogonal planes, coronal and transverse, are used to confirm findings, as is common throughout sonography. Examination in both the coronal and transverse planes (with respect to the bony pelvis) can be performed while the hip position is changed and stress is applied. When using this method, one quickly realizes that the coronal images are similar to anteroposterior radiographs (Figs. 9–1 and 9–2), and transverse images are similar to cross-sectional images such as those provided by (CT) (Fig. 9–3) or MRI. However, since sono-

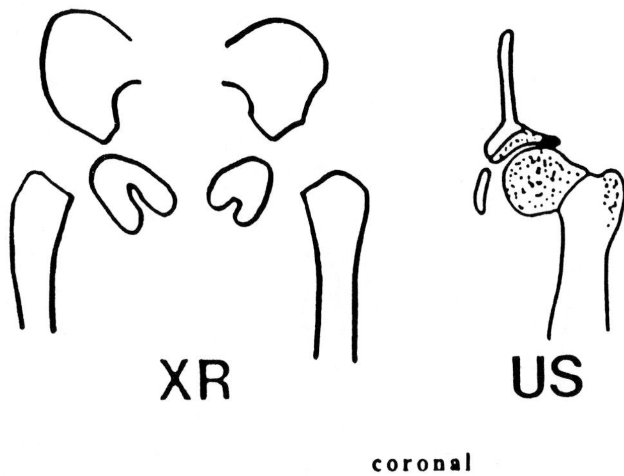

Figure 9–1 ▪ Schematic diagram of an anteroposterior hip radiograph (*XR*) and a coronal neutral sonogram (*US*).

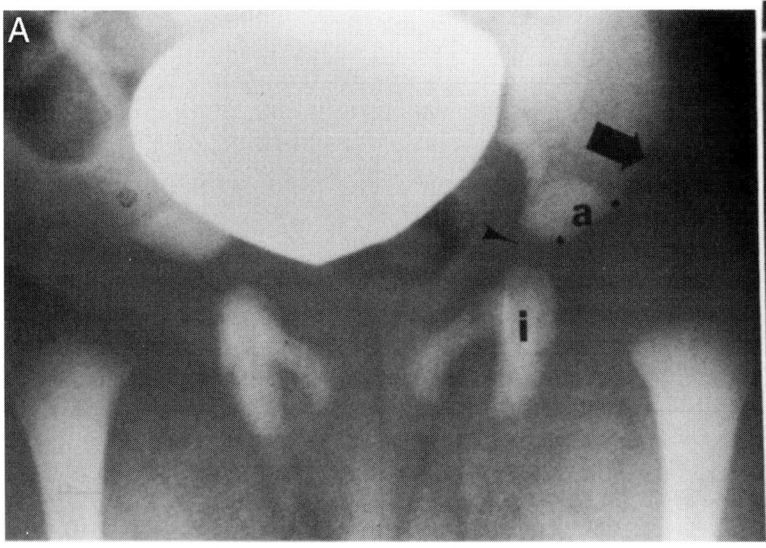

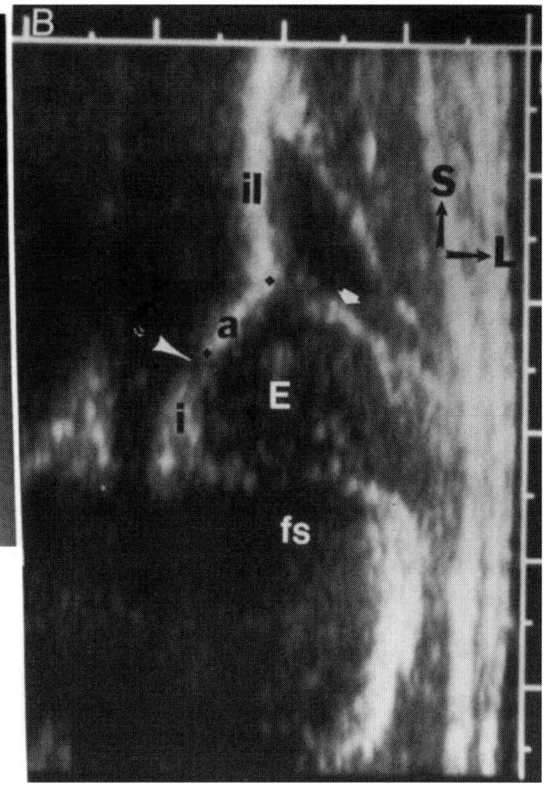

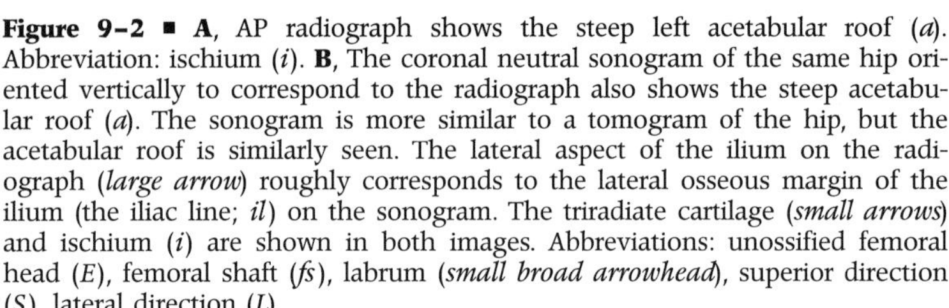

Figure 9–2 ■ **A**, AP radiograph shows the steep left acetabular roof (*a*). Abbreviation: ischium (*i*). **B**, The coronal neutral sonogram of the same hip oriented vertically to correspond to the radiograph also shows the steep acetabular roof (*a*). The sonogram is more similar to a tomogram of the hip, but the acetabular roof is similarly seen. The lateral aspect of the ilium on the radiograph (*large arrow*) roughly corresponds to the lateral osseous margin of the ilium (the iliac line; *il*) on the sonogram. The triradiate cartilage (*small arrows*) and ischium (*i*) are shown in both images. Abbreviations: unossified femoral head (*E*), femoral shaft (*fs*), labrum (*small broad arrowhead*), superior direction (*S*), lateral direction (*L*).

graphic images are displayed with the transducer surface at the top of the monitor, the orientation is lateral at the top, superior and anterior to the left of the viewing screen (Figs. 9–4 through 9–7).

It is important that the infant is relaxed for the examination. Feeding the infant just prior or during the examination is helpful. Performing the examination in a darkened room with the parent in contact with the infant is helpful. Older infants can be distracted with toys.

Complete examination of the hip incorporating coronal views in both anatomical (neutral) and flexed positions, together with transverse views in flexed and neutral positions, can be accomplished in 30 to 60 seconds by an experienced examiner. This assumes that the infant is relaxed and that the time re-

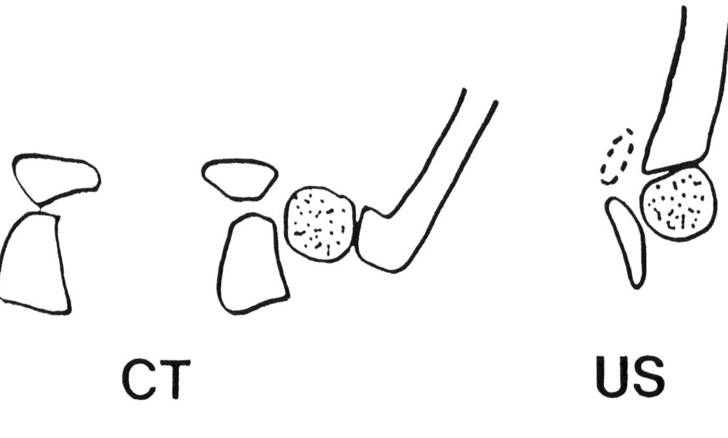

Figure 9–3 ■ Schematic diagram of a hip axial CT scan (*CT*) and a transverse flexion sonogram (*US*).

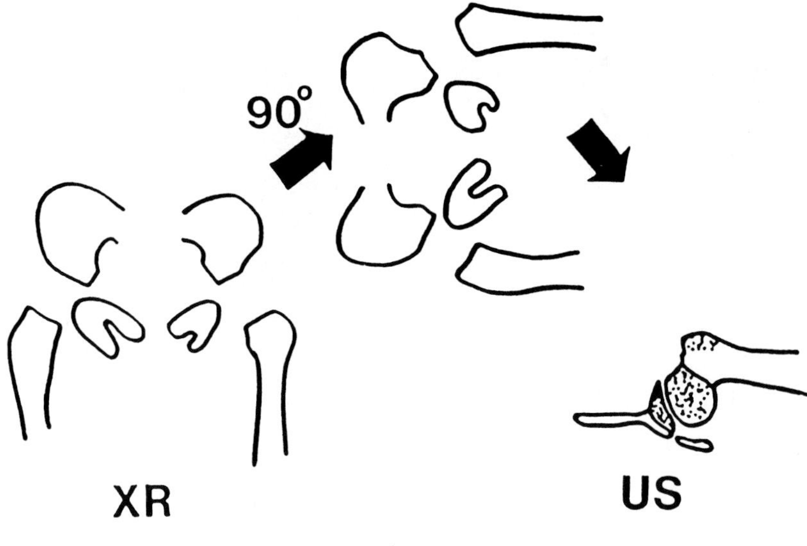

Figure 9–4 ▪ Schematic diagram of an AP hip radiograph (*XR*) rotated 90 degrees to match the coronal neutral sonogram (*US*) as it appears on the monitor.

quired to generate hard-copy images is not included. The total examination, including preparation and recording of images, can be done in 10 minutes.

In 1998, for the first time, the American Medical Association's *Manual of Common Procedures and Terminology* (*CPT-4*) included specific codes for examination of the infant hip (American Medical Association, 1998). Two levels of examination are recognized. A complete examination, which includes dynamic manipulation, is differentiated from a limited examination with one static view to assess morphology.

From the technical standpoint, there are some specific variations from routine sonographic scanning. With the infant in the supine position, the right hip is studied with the examiner holding the transducer in the left hand and the leg in the right hand. The opposite is true for examination of the left hip; here the transducer is in the right hand, and the left leg is maneuvered with the examiner's left hand. This "ambidextrous" scanning is required to perform a dynamic evaluation successfully. When the nondominant hand holds the transducer, it can be steadied by bracing the hand and arm on the

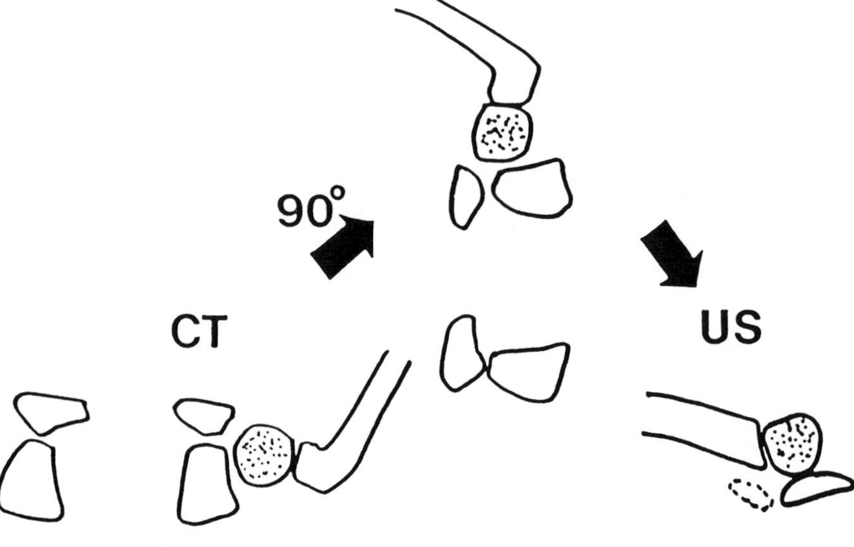

Figure 9–5 ▪ Schematic diagram of a hip axial CT scan (*CT*), rotated 90 degrees to match the transverse flexion sonogram (*US*) as it appears on the monitor.

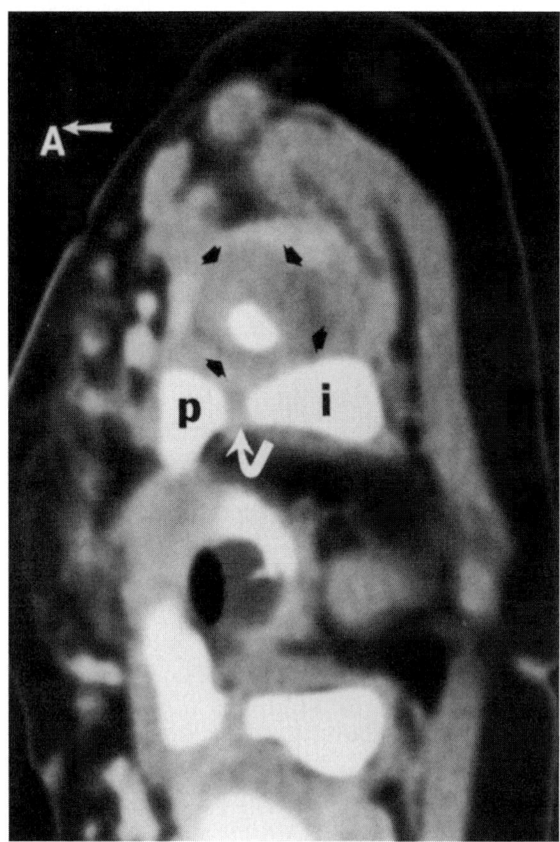

Figure 9–6 ■ CT scan of a pelvis rotated 90 degrees to correspond to the transverse sonographic view as it appears on the monitor. *Straight arrow* points anteriorly (*A*). The femoral head (*arrowheads*) with its ossified nucleus lies within the acetabulum. Abbreviations: pubis (*p*), ischium (*i*), triradiate cartilage (*curved arrow*).

bed. Alternatively, infants can be examined while on their side (decubitus position). In Europe this position is popular. It is a carryover from articulated-arm scanning of the late 1970s, and specific devices have been constructed to hold the baby in this position during hip scanning.

Hip sonography's significant advantage over radiography is its ability to distinguish cartilage from soft tissue. Cartilage is hypoechoic with respect to soft tissue; in the newborn, the proximal portion of the femur (femoral head and trochanter) is composed of cartilage. Within the cartilage, the vascular channels produce low-level specular echos. The femoral metaphysis and shaft, being osseous, produce bright-reflected echos. The immature acetabulum is composed of both cartilage and bone. It is formed by the ilium, ischium, and pubis, which meet to form the acetabulum or socket in a configuration referred to as the *triradiate cartilage*. Acetabular anatomy will then have hypoechoic cartilaginous components and echogenic bony components. The femoral head is maintained in the acetabulum by the hip capsule, which is echogenic and can be distinguished from the cartilage and overlying layers of muscle. When performing hip sonography, it is important to adjust the technical factors so that focal zones, echogenicity within the femoral head, and depth of field are optimal.

Coronal Anatomy and Pathology

A coronal view of the hip with the femur in neutral position was the projection advocated by Graf for assessing acetabular development. The hip is maintained in a physiologically neutral position; this represents about 20 degrees of flexion in the young infant. The transducer is maintained in the coronal plane with respect to the acetabulum. It is possible to obtain this view with the infant supine or in a lateral decubitus position. If the supine position is used, the transducer is held in the left hand when the right hip is examined and in the right hand for the left hip examination. If the lateral decubitus position is used, the infant is placed with the left side down for the right hip examination and with the right side down for the left hip examination. Graf (1984, 1987) has developed a device to maintain the infant in the lateral decubitus position. When this device is utilized, the transducer can be held with both hands on the lateral aspect of the hip.

In order to assess the hip joint in the coronal neutral view directly and consistently, it is mandatory to use a standard plane through the acetabulum (Fig. 9–8). The standard coronal plane is defined by three landmarks: (1) the iliac line or sonographic reflection from the lateral surface of the iliac bone proximal to the acetabulum; (2) the point where the iliac portion of the acetabulum transitions to the triradiate cartilage in the medial part of the acetabulum; and (3) the tip of the cartilage labrum as it extends from the acetabulum laterally over the femoral head to blend in with the hip capsule. In the correct plane, the iliac line is straight and is parallel to the margin of the image which represents the surface of the transducer. The transition point from the bony ilium to the triradiate cartilage is apparent because there is acoustic shadowing behind the bone and transmission of sound through the cartilage into the medial pelvic structures. The cartilage of the acetabulum extends laterally over the femoral head beyond the iliac line. Here, in the normal hip, it has a triangular configuration, with most of the labrum appearing hypo-

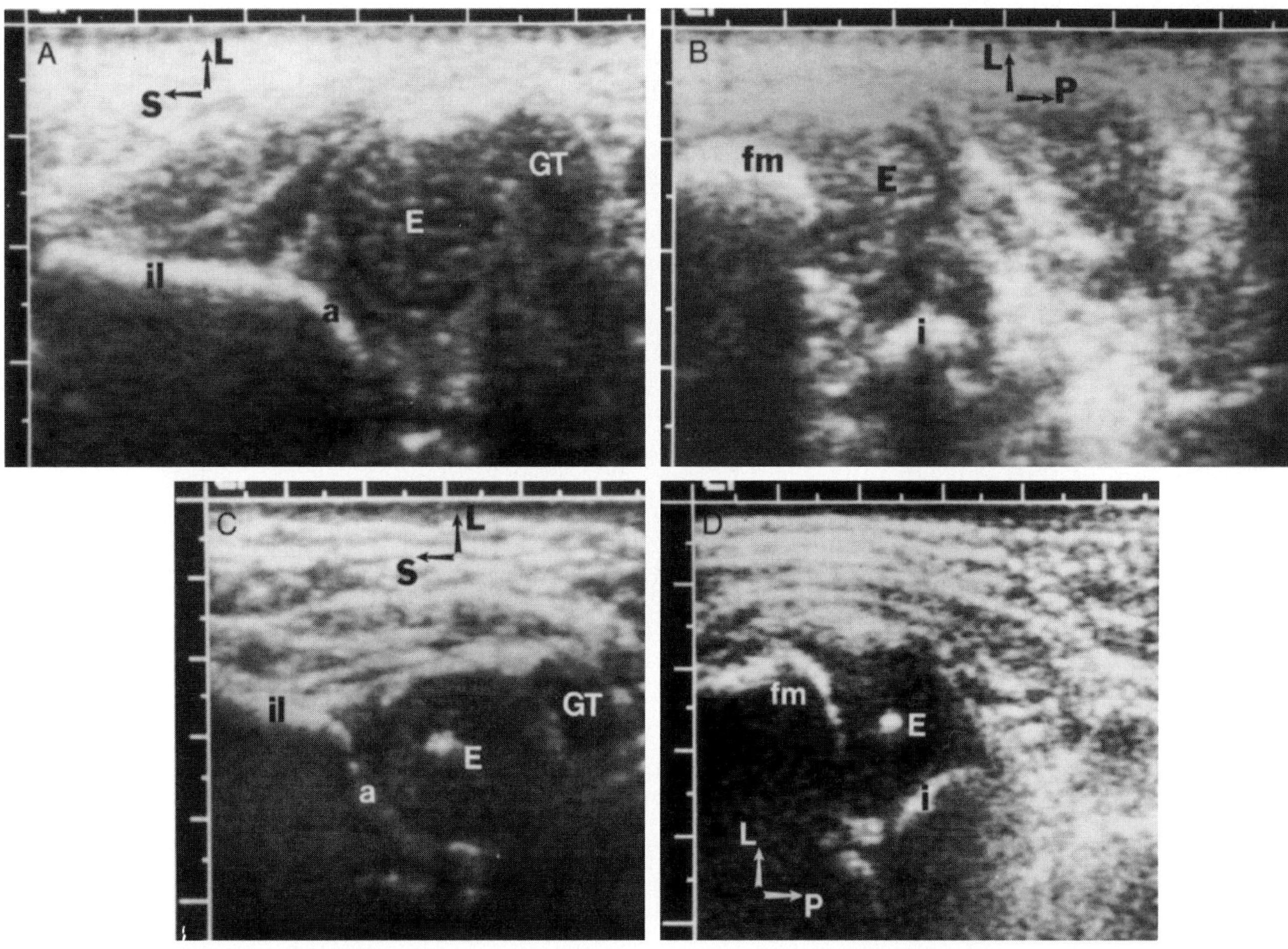

Figure 9–7 ■ **A** and **B**, Coronal and transverse views as seen on the monitor show a subluxed left hip at 3 days of age. Orientation arrows point laterally (*L*), superiorly (*S*), and posteriorly (*P*). The epiphysis (*E*) is displaced superiorly, laterally, and posteriorly. Abbreviations: ilium (*il*), acetabulum (*a*), femoral metaphysis (*fm*), ischium (*i*), greater trochanter (*GT*). **C** and **D**, Follow-up views at 4 months following stabilization in a Pavlik harness show normally positioned hips. Ossific nucleus of the femoral epiphysis (*E*) is seen.

echoic, like the femoral head. However, at the tip of the labrum, the cartilage becomes fibrous and exhibits increased echogenicity. It is the echogenic tip that constitutes the landmark.

The coronal neutral view is used principally to assess the development of the acetabulum. The inclination (steepness) of the acetabular roof can be measured on the sonogram by the alpha angle, as advocated by Graf (1984) (see Fig. 9–8). A second angle, the beta angle, was also incorporated into Graf's classification of dysplasia (Fig. 9–9). This labral measurement had a high degree of variation and has fallen out of favor. Measurement precision for the alpha angle is considered more reliable; however, variations ranging from 4.0 to 6.5 degrees are reported (Zieger and Schulz, 1986). Measuring acetabular angles and using these angles as a criterion for treatment has been proposed by Graf (Table 9–1). Not everyone has adopted this system because of variation. Measurement is considered optional in the standard examination, and it is possible to use a verbal description of the acetabulum that includes the appearance of the bony acetabular slope, the configuration of the lateral corner, and the appearance of the labrum.

A second technique for assessing acetabular development was described by Morin et al. (1985, 1999). Coverage of the femoral head by the bony acetabulum was determined from sonograms. The percentage of the diameter of the femoral head which was covered by the bony acetabulum in a normally seated hip was compared with the

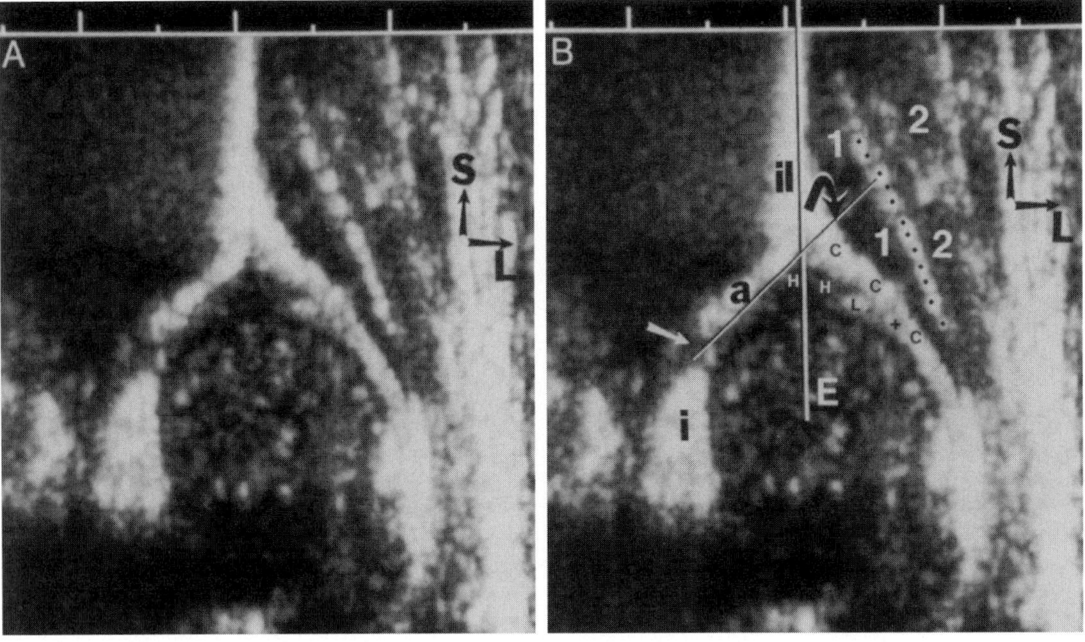

Figure 9–8 ▪ Coronal views of left hip displayed vertically both without (**A**) and with (**B**) labels. *Arrows* denote superior (*S*) and lateral (*L*). The unossified femoral head epiphysis (*E*) is well seated within the acetabulum beneath its ossified roof (*a*). The iliac line extended from the lateral iliac margin (*il*) shows the degree of femoral head coverage by its osseous acetabular roof. More laterally the femoral head is covered by the unossified roof, composed of hyaline cartilage (*H*), which will later ossify. Echogenic fibrocartilage at the lateral tip of the acetabular roof is the labrum (*L*). Ischium (*i*), triradiate cartilage (*straight arrow*), and joint capsule (*C*) are shown. Gluteus minimus (*1*) and gluteus medius (*2*) are separated by the intermuscular septum (*dots*). The Graf alpha angle (*curved arrow*), a measure of the steepness of the acetabular roof, is formed by the intersection of the iliac line (*il*) and a line along the osseous acetabular roof (*a*). The Graf beta angle (not shown), a measure of the superior deviation of the cartilaginous roof, would be drawn between the lateral aspect of the labrum (+) and the intersection of the iliac and osseous acetabular roof lines.

Table 9–1
Simplified Synopsis of Graf Sonographic Hip Types*

Type	Description	Alpha Angle (Degrees)	Beta Angle (Degrees)	Comment
I	Normal	*>60**		Should not dislocate in absence of a neuromuscular imbalance with altered biomechanics
IIa	Physiological immature *<3 mo.*	*50–59*		
IIb	Delayed ossification *>3 mo.*	50–59		
IIc	Very deficient bony acetabulum but femoral head still concentric	*43–49*	<77	At this stage beta angle becomes important
D	Femoral head *subluxed*	43–49	>77	Increased beta angle signifies an elevated, everted labrum and subluxation
III	*Dislocated*	<43	>77	
IV	*Severe* dysplasia/ dislocation	*Not measurable;* flat, shallow, bony acetabulum		*Labrum inverted; interposed* between femoral head and ilium

Adapted from Donaldson JS: Pediatric musculoskeletal US, in Poznanski AK, Kirkpatrick JA Jr (eds): *Diagnostic Categorical Course in Pediatric Radiology*. Oak Brook, Ill, Radiological Society of North America Publications, 1989, pp. 77–88; and Graf R: *Guide to Sonography of the Infant Hip*. New York, Thieme Medical Publishers, 1987.
*Distinguishing feature of each type is in italics.

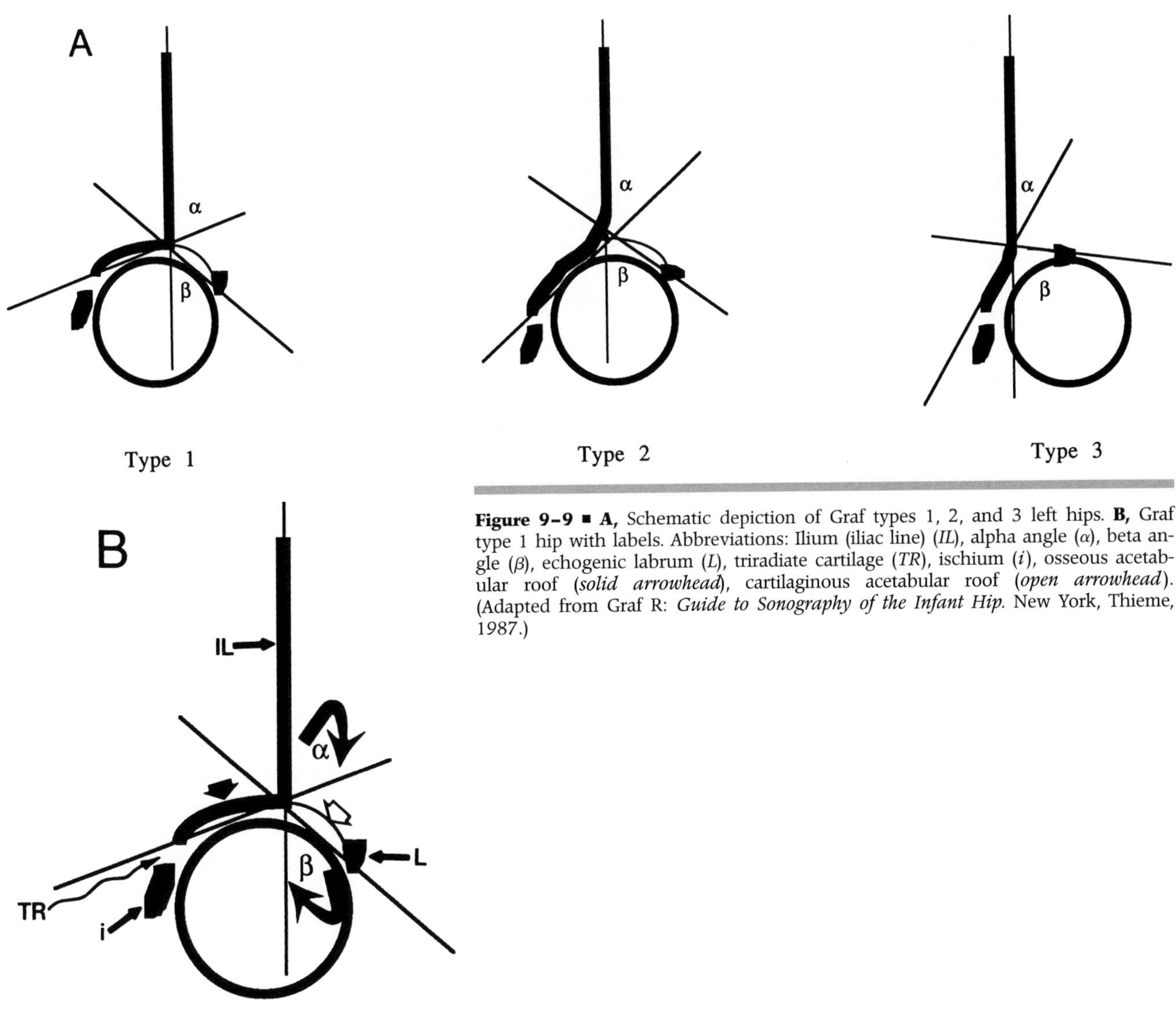

Figure 9-9 ▪ **A,** Schematic depiction of Graf types 1, 2, and 3 left hips. **B,** Graf type 1 hip with labels. Abbreviations: Ilium (iliac line) (*IL*), alpha angle (α), beta angle (β), echogenic labrum (*L*), triradiate cartilage (*TR*), ischium (*i*), osseous acetabular roof (*solid arrowhead*), cartilaginous acetabular roof (*open arrowhead*). (Adapted from Graf R: *Guide to Sonography of the Infant Hip.* New York, Thieme, 1987.)

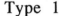

radiographic acetabular index. All hips with more than 58% of the femoral head covered by the bony acetabulum had normal radiographic measurements. Hips with less than 33% coverage had abnormal radiographic measurements with dysplastic acetabula. The percentages in between showed variable correlation. Some examiners utilize this coverage concept in assessing acetabular development (Terjesen et al., 1996).

In the coronal neutral view, dysplasia is manifested by other findings in addition to the inclination of the bony acetabulum. Displacement of the femoral head from the acetabulum is lateral, superior, or posterior, depending upon the severity of the dysplasia. The labrum also becomes deformed and fibrous when the femoral head is displaced. The hyaline cartilage changes to fibrocartilage, and the deformed labrum may be interposed between the femoral head and the acetabulum, preventing reduction (Fig. 9–10).

Coronal images of the hip can also be obtained with the hip flexed to 90 degrees. The transducer is oriented in the same plane as the coronal neutral view. The landmarks of the acetabulum are as found with the coronal neutral view; the major change is the absence of the femoral metaphyseal landmarks in the imaging plane (Fig. 9–11). Locating the standard plane with its key landmarks is also mandatory in the coronal flexion view. In the coronal flexion view, the hip can be dynamically examined.

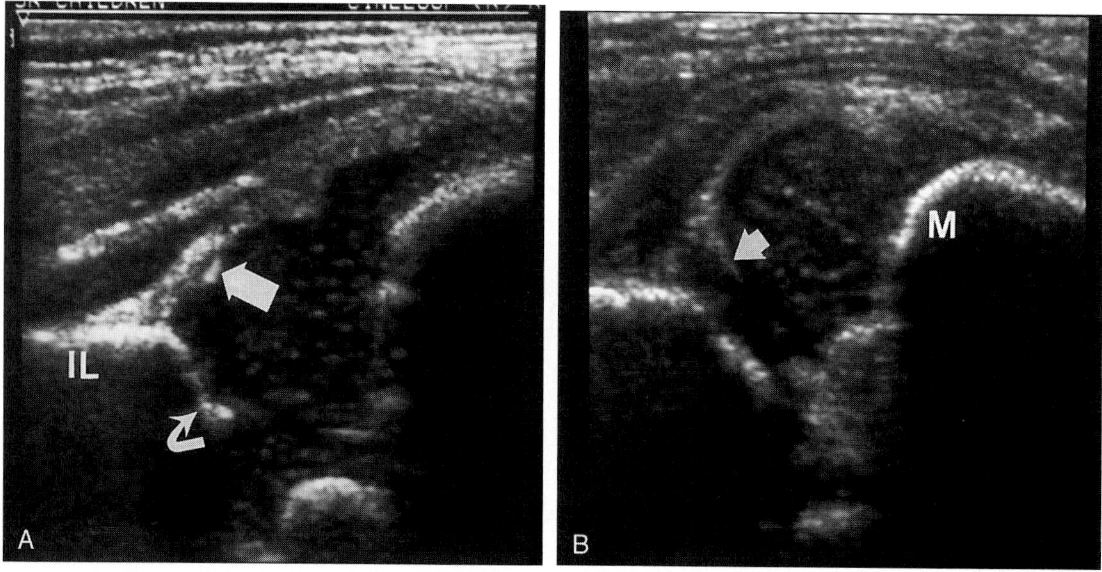

Figure 9-10 ■ Coronal/neutral views. **A,** Sonogram of normal hip. Note the bony acetabulum (*curved arrow*), the tip of the labrum (*straight arrow*), and the straight iliac line (*IL*). **B,** Sonogram of abnormal hip shows displacement of the femoral head laterally, with deformity of the labrum (*arrow*). Note the metaphysis (*M*).

Abduction and adduction of the femoral head enable the detection of instability and the assessment of femoral head/acetabular relationships with changes in position. Examining the hip in the coronal flexion view is analogous to the Barlow and Ortolani tests used clinically. During the examination, the sonographer moves the transducer in an anteroposterior direction so that the entire hip joint is evaluated. Anterior to the femoral head, the lateral curvilinear margin of the bony shaft of the flexed femur is encountered. Posteriorly, the back edge of the acetabulum can be visualized, with the

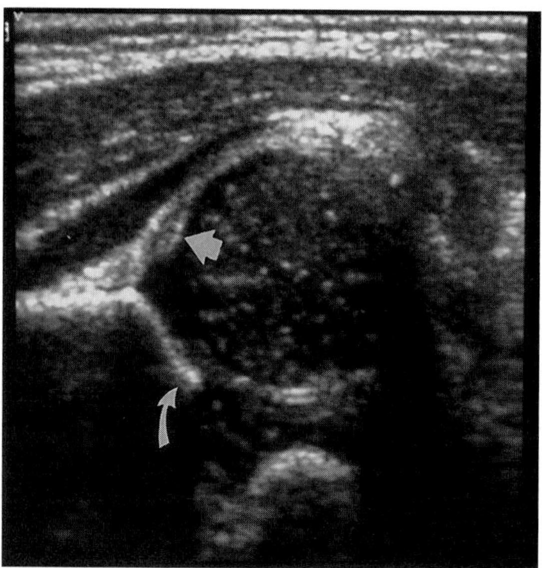

Figure 9-11 ■ Coronal/flexion view. The transducer is in the coronal plane, with the femur flexed to 90 degrees. Sonogram of normal hip shows the sonolucent femoral head resting against bony acetabulum (*curved arrow*). Note the fibrocartilaginous tip of the labrum (*straight arrow*).

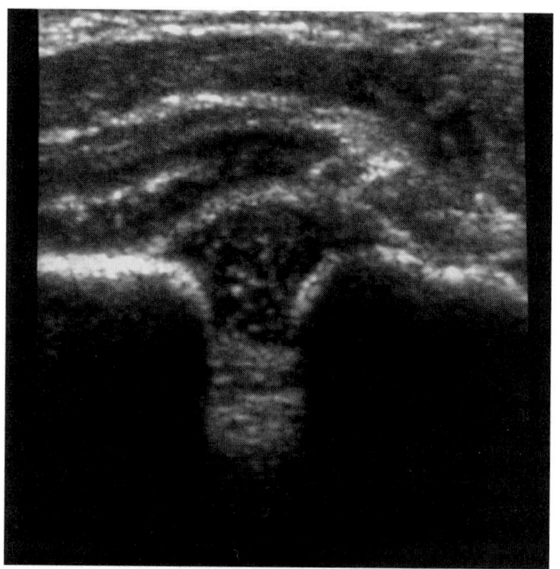

Figure 9-12 ■ Coronal/flexion view of the posterior acetabular lip. The normal view shows the posterior ray of the triradiate cartilage with none of the femoral head in this plane.

posterior lip of the triradiate cartilage becoming a critical landmark (Fig. 9–12). When the femoral head is normally positioned, the relationship of the head to the acetabulum is constant. This relationship does not change with adduction/abduction. Posterior stress is applied using a push/pull or piston movement with the hip flexed and the femur adducted. This is analogous to the Barlow maneuver, and its purpose is to demonstrate instability of the femoral head. Instability can vary from mild capsular laxity to complete dislocation. It is important that the infant is relaxed when this maneuver is performed. In a stable hip, the relationships at the posterior lip of the acetabulum are maintained without change when a gentle push in the posterior direction is applied. The sonographic image over the posterior lip reveals no portion of the femoral head entering that viewing plane during the maneuver.

With subluxation, the femoral head displaces laterally and/or posteriorly when the femoral head is in the flexed position. Soft tissue echos are seen between the medial aspect of the femoral head and the bony reflection from the medial acetabulum (Fig. 9–13A). In dislocation, the femoral head is positioned posteriorly and/or superiorly (Fig. 9–13B). With posterior dislocation, the femoral head appears in the plane of the posterior lip of the triradiate cartilage (Fig. 9–13C). In superior dislocations, the femoral head rests against the iliac bone. With an unstable hip, relationships can be determined and

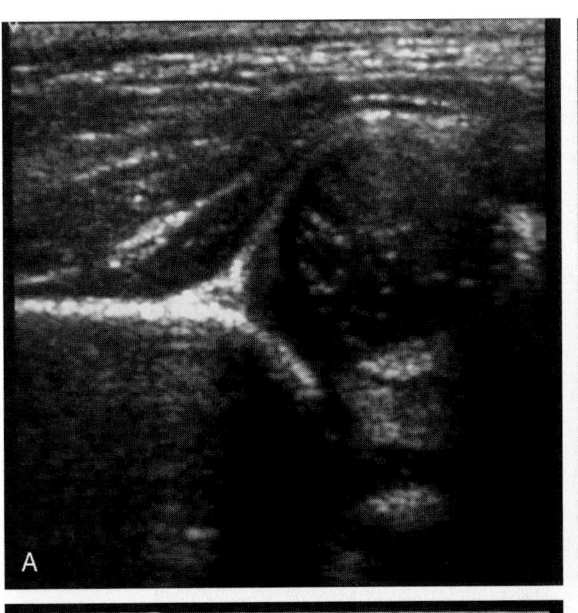

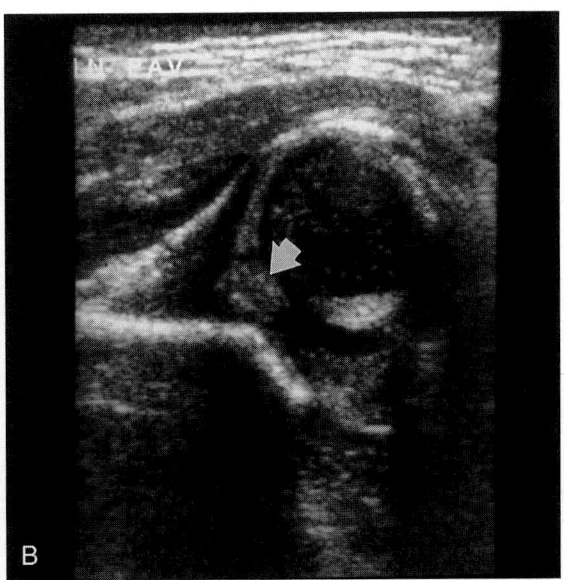

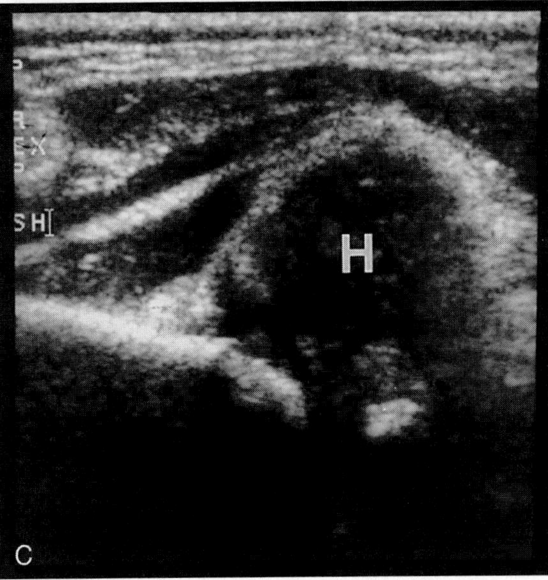

Figure 9–13 ▪ Coronal/flexion views, abnormal. The transducer is in the coronal plane, with the femur flexed to 90 degrees. **A**, Sonogram of subluxated hip shows the femoral head in contact with the superior lateral acetabular cartilage. The bony acetabulum is steeply angled. **B**, Sonogram of dislocated hip shows displacement of the sonolucent femoral head laterally and superiorly, with deformity and increased echogenicity of labrum (*arrow*). **C**, Posterior acetabular lip. The posteriorly displaced femoral head (*H*) appears over the triradiate cartilage.

instability which is not detected clinically becomes readily apparent.

Transverse Anatomy and Pathology

Common sonographic practice is to examine anatomy in orthogonal planes. This principle has been incorporated into sonographic assessment of the infant hip. The standard examination calls for evaluation in the transverse or axial plane with the hip flexed. In this orientation, it is possible to assess stability; this view is not used to determine the configuration of the bony acetabulum.

The transverse flexion examination is performed with the hip flexed at 90 degrees (similar to the coronal flexion view), and the transducer is maintained in the axial plane with respect to the body and pelvis (see Figs. 9–5 and 9–6). In practice, the transducer is positioned posterolaterally over the hip joint; to facilitate this placement, it is helpful to rotate the infant into an anterior oblique position. It is convenient to place a rolled towel under the back in order to maintain the infant's orientation comfortably. Anteriorly, the bony shaft of the metaphysis of the femur gives bright-reflected echos adjacent to the sonolucent femoral head. Bony echos from the acetabulum are seen posterior to the femoral head. In a normal hip, this produces a U configuration (Fig. 9–14A). The femur is adducted and abducted in order to check for instability. In the adducted position, posterior stress is applied. The U configuration changes to more of a V

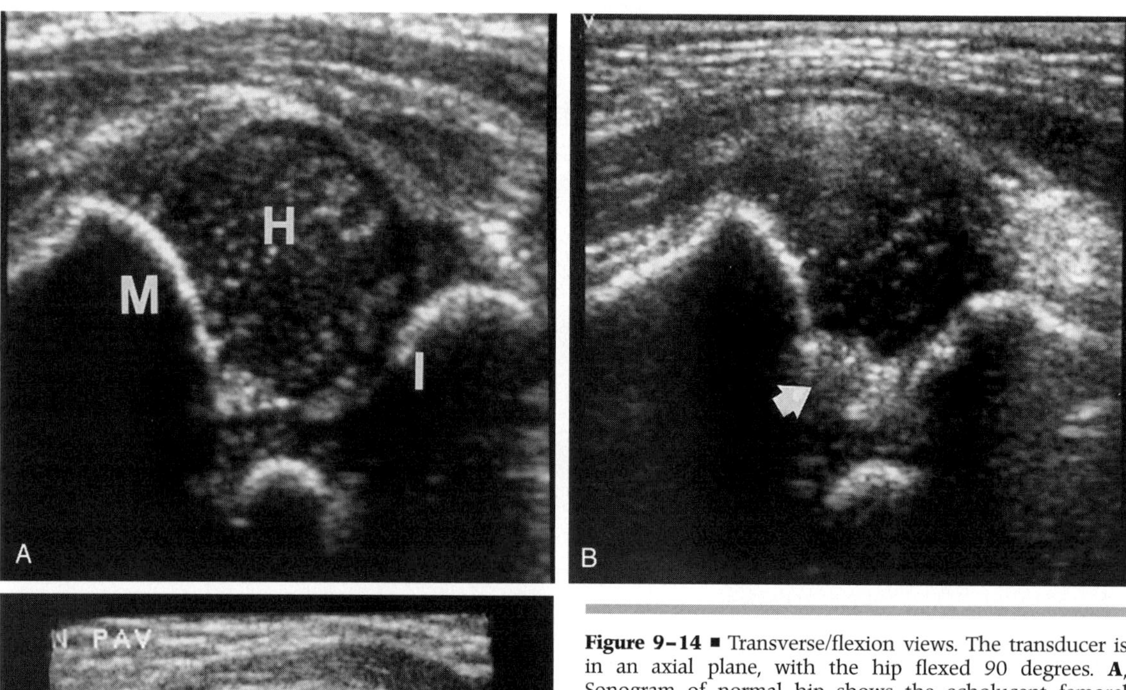

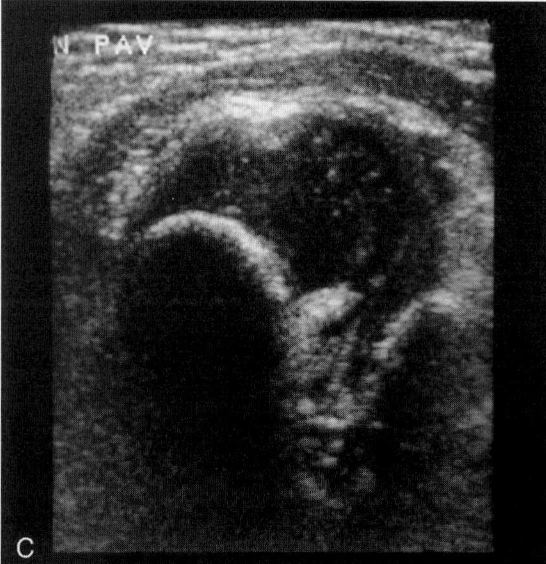

Figure 9–14 ▪ Transverse/flexion views. The transducer is in an axial plane, with the hip flexed 90 degrees. **A**, Sonogram of normal hip shows the echolucent femoral head (*H*) surrounded by the metaphysis (*M*) anteriorly and the ischium (*I*) posteriorly, forming a U around the femoral head. **B**, The subluxated hip is displaced laterally but remains in contact with the ischium. Echogenic tissue is in the acetabulum medially (*arrow*). **C**, Sonogram of dislocated hip shows a sonolucent femoral head displaced posterolaterally. The U configuration of the normal metaphysis and ischium is not seen.

orientation. When the hip is subluxated, the femoral head is displaced laterally in relation to the acetabulum but remains in contact with the ischial bone. Subluxation becomes dislocation when the head moves laterally or posterolaterally from the acetabulum (Fig. 9–14B).

In frank dislocation, the femoral head is positioned laterally, posteriorly, or superiorly. The U relationship cannot be obtained (Fig. 9–14C). A dislocated hip can be tested for reducibility by pulling the hip forward and abducting the flexed femur (the Ortolani maneuver). This abduction/adduction stress test defines the degree of instability. Subluxated hips can be classified as dislocatable or not dislocatable, and dislocated hips can be assessed for reducibility. Some dislocated hips are partially reducible but promptly redislocate when released. More severe dislocations are irreducible.

The transverse view can also be obtained when the hip is in physiologically neutral position (the position for the coronal neutral view). The transducer is directed horizontally into the acetabulum. The plane of interest is one that passes through the femoral head into the acetabulum at the center of the triradiate cartilage. In the normal hip, the sonolucent femoral head is positioned against the bony acetabulum; the midpoint of the head is centered at the back edge of the triradiate cartilage. The echos from the pelvic bones are found medially. The anterior echo is shorter in length and comes from the pubis; the longer posterior echo is produced by the ischium (Fig. 9–15A). If an ossific nucleus is present, one must angle the plane of the transducer above or below the nucleus to identify the triradiate cartilage. Acoustic shadowing by the ossification center must not be mistaken for the triradiate cartilage gap.

When a hip is subluxated, the transverse neutral view shows soft tissue echos between the femoral head and the acetabulum. The head is in contact with the posterior part of the acetabulum; the width and configuration of the gap depend on the degree of displacement. There is thicker cartilage over the pubic component of the acetabulum; this should not be mistaken for displacement of the femoral head. In dislocation, the head has no contact with the acetabulum (Fig. 9–15B). Most dislocations are posterior and superior. Because the dislocated femoral head may migrate superiorly, it is possible that the bony shaft of the femur will obscure the acetabulum. The presence of gross dislocation is manifested by failure to identify the triradiate cartilage where the round femoral head is located.

Clinical Applications

Sonography of the hip of the newborn infant can be used in two general situations: diagnostic assessment

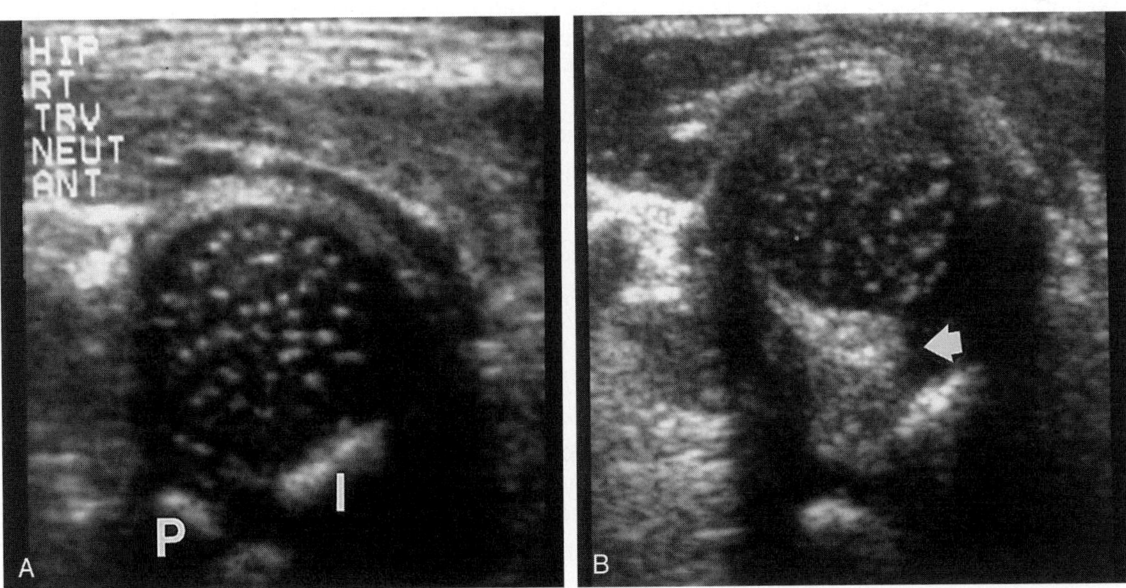

Figure 9–15 ▪ Transverse/neutral views. The transducer is perpendicular to the neutral femoral head in the axial plane of the acetabulum, as in Figure 9–14, except that the hip is not flexed. **A**, Sonogram of normal hip shows a sonolucent femoral head centered over the triradiate cartilage, with the pubis (*P*) anteriorly and ischium (*I*) posteriorly. **B**, Sonogram of dislocated hip shows a sonolucent femoral head displaced posterolaterally with a gap between the pubis and femoral head (*arrow*).

and management assessment. In most cases, referral for a diagnostic assessment is based upon a questionable or abnormal physical examination or on an increased risk of DDH. Routine use of ultrasound for mass screening has been done in some areas, but it is not a universally accepted concept and will be discussed separately. An assessment for management is performed on an infant who has been identified as having DDH and is undergoing observation or treatment. There are slight alterations in the way the sonogram is performed in these two types of assessments. However, the information desired concerns position, stability, and acetabular development in both cases.

Diagnostic assessment should include a complete examination, as proposed by the standard. This should include a dynamic or stress component. Sonography has been found to be highly specific and sensitive in comparison with clinical and radiographic evaluations (Clarke et al., 1985; Berman and Klenerman, 1986; Tonnis et al., 1990). In virtually every report of the accuracy of hip sonography, abnormal hips have been identified when the clinical and/or radiographic examination has been normal. DDH is a spectrum of pathology which ranges from mild laxity to irreducible dislocation. Acetabular dysplasia can exist with instability and can be found in a stable hip as well. With appropriate training and experience, the false-positive and false-negative rates for sonography should be in the 1–2% range. Clinically apparent dislocations have not been missed, and sonography has detected dislocations which were missed clinically (Ortolani negative). The few false-positive and false-negative sonographic results have involved cases of subluxation. Subluxation encompasses a range of capsular laxity and displacement, and the degree to which this is present is to some extent subjective. An accurate examination requires that the patient be relaxed and the examiner experienced in determining the amount of stress to apply to the hip. The false-negative examination is almost always due to lack of relaxation, which precludes obtaining optimal stress views, or to other technical difficulties related to the size of the patient and the development of femoral head ossification. Acetabular anatomy is obscured by an enlarging body habitus and increasing ossification in late infancy (Fig. 9–16). False-positive ultrasound cases are almost always the result of failure to employ correct technique, in particular the selection of correct transducer positioning. The acetabular roof can be falsely made to appear steeper than it really is. One value of a multiview examination is the opportunity to confirm sonographic findings in more than one plane. While a two-view exam meets the standard, a four-view exam provides more confidence, particularly when the sonographer is less experienced. Another rare but real potential pitfall is in the child with hip contracture or arthrogryposis. The fixed posture of the hip obscures the acetabulum, and the unossified greater trochanter can be mistaken for a dislocated, unossified femoral head.

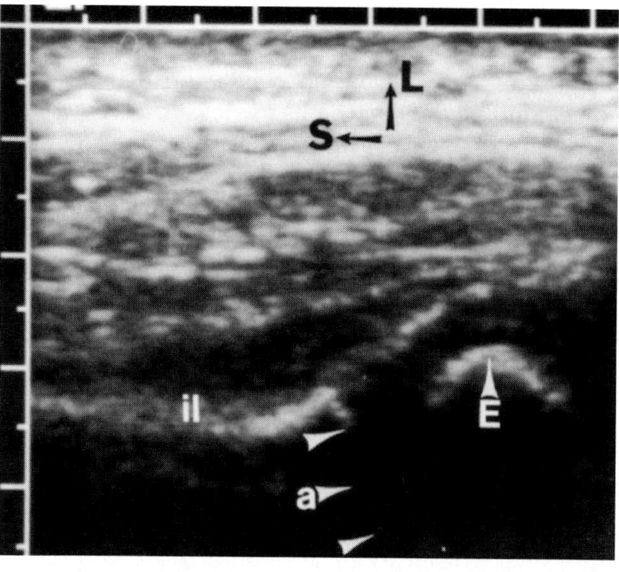

Figure 9–16 ■ Coronal view in a 15-month-old infant. Ossification and body habitus impairs visualization of the acetabulum (*a*). A large femoral head ossification (*E*) and the iliac line (*il*) are seen. Abbreviations: superior direction (*S*), lateral direction (*L*).

In examining infants for DDH, it is important to recognize that the natural history of this condition is that most infants improve spontaneously with time and do not require treatment. At present, we cannot distinguish those who will improve spontaneously from the few who will not. It has become popular to try to divide DDH into two categories of hip pathology: "neonatal, essentially sonographic DDH" and "true DDH" (Bialik et al., 1999). Very mild, clinically undetectable disease was recognized by Graf (1984), who defined it as a type IIA hip, and also by Harcke and Grissom (1990), who described mild subluxation and recognized physiological laxity with stress as a normal variant at less than 4 weeks of age. The concept of DDH as ranging in severity, with the potential to resolve spontaneously, has implications for both diagnostic and management protocols. We have learned that when capsular laxity and/or mild bony acetabular immaturity is seen in infants under 4 weeks of age, observation without treatment is reasonable and cost effective. A repeat sonographic examination at 4 to 6 weeks of age can confirm normalcy, and unnecessary treatment is therefore avoided.

As sonography became recognized as a more sensitive test for DDH than the clinical examination, mass screening for DDH was instituted in several areas of Europe. It became apparent that the initial newborn screening programs were leading to overtreatment (Szoke et al., 1988; Tonnis et al., 1990). An alternative to mass screening of all newborns was to screen a smaller segment of the population known to be at increased risk for DDH. In England, Boeree and Clarke (1994) studied risk factor–based screening. This did not eliminate all late cases in the population. In Norway, Rosendahl et al. (1994) tested three screening models: clinical screening, selective ultrasound screening, and universal ultrasound screening. While she found a slight difference in the number of late cases, with universal ultrasound screening producing the fewest, the differences in the groups were not statistically significant (Rosendahl et al., 1994). This continues to remain a controversial issue because conflicting data continue to arise. A study by Marks et al. (1994) in Conventry, England, reported that a program of universal ultrasound screening eliminated all late cases in that region. On the other hand, an epidemiological examination by Hernandez et al. (1994) of data from the literature using a decision analysis algorithm concluded that universal sonographic hip screening was not justified.

The implications of current literature for practice recommendations vary in different areas of the world. This variation is due in part to the size of countries and the healthcare systems which exist. In the United States, with a large and diverse population coupled with a complex system of health insurance, universal ultrasound screening has not been recommended by organizations such as the American Academy of Pediatrics (AAP). Current guidelines for practicing pediatricians, based on evidence-based literature and expert opinion, do not advocate routine sonographic screening of newborns (Harcke, 1995). Repeated clinical examination by the pediatrician is the cornerstone of the AAP guideline. The examiner must understand that Barlow/Ortolani-positive hips tighten, either in or out of the joint, and become normal between 2 weeks and 2 months of age. In the abnormal hip, the Ortolani "clunk" disappears and is replaced by limited hip abduction as the key clinical sign of DDH. The orthopedic surgeon, confirmatory clinical examination, and ultrasound and x-ray studies are secondary resources for the pediatrician. These are incorporated into an algorithm which takes into consideration that, while gaining wide acceptance, expert hip sonography is not available to all pediatricians. The selective ultrasound screening algorithms focus on a smaller segment of the population known to be at increased risk for DDH. Clarke and colleagues (Boeree and Clarke, 1994) proposed ultrasound for infants with an abnormal physical examination, positive family history, breech delivery, foot deformity such as clubfoot, or torticollis. This scheme will require about 10% of all newborns to undergo an ultrasound study. It should be recognized that the timing of the sonogram is critical. When the physical exam is abnormal shortly after birth, we suggest that ultrasound be done at 1 to 2 weeks of age. This allows hip instability to resolve on its own. Newborns with a risk factor for DDH and a normal clinical exam can be checked at 4 to 6 weeks. This avoids multiple exams in cases of transient instability and acetabular immaturity.

In infants diagnosed with DDH, sonography can be used to monitor hip position and acetabular development. This helps the orthopedic surgeon determine if, when, and how to institute treatment. It is now proposed that sonography be used routinely to follow borderline cases, particularly in very young infants, before a commitment is made to a treatment regimen (Bialik et al., 1999).

When the decision to treat is made, most of the devices used permit evaluation of the hip while it is held in flexion and abduction. The Pavlik harness, a dynamic splint commonly employed in many areas of the world for treatment of DDH, permits easy sonographic examination without its removal (Harcke et al., 1988). Hip sonography can be repeated frequently, without the need for radiographs or cross-sectional imaging. The harness permits dynamic examination, and real-time sonography provides three-dimensional information; continuing instability and posterior displacement are easily detected. Conversely, the examination can determine when stability has been achieved, and the use of the harness can then be discontinued (Grissom et al., 1988; Polaneur et al., 1990). Avascular necrosis of the femoral head is a complication of treating DDH in flexion abduction splints. Femoral head vascularity can be assessed by power Doppler to verify that the hip position is safe during treatment.

The Pavlik harness is not always successful, and rigid splinting or casting is another treatment alternative. Harding et al. (1997) recommended that dislocated hips treated with the Pavlik harness be followed weekly to establish improvement. If a dislocated hip does not reduce within 3 weeks, the harness should be abandoned in favor of traction and closed reduction.

When rigid splints or casting are utilized, ultrasound has been employed. Removing a plug from the cast over the posterior lateral aspect of the hip enabled an evaluation using standard views (Boal and Schwentker, 1985; Harcke et al., 1988).

Although this was successful, the examination is difficult and there was a question of compromising the reduction by removing the plaster plug. Consequently, we no longer do sonography of infants in rigid casts. A limited CT scan is utilized, with the localizer image enabling selection of one or two slices that document the hip position (Hernandez, 1984; Stanton and Capecci, 1992). MRI offers another alternative and produces no ionizing radiation; its high cost and the necessity for sedation are disadvantages. In rigid splints and casts that leave the anterior hip and groin exposed, an alternative sonographic view such as the one proposed by Dahlstrom et al. (1986) can be considered.

Epiphyseal Alignment

Unossified epiphyses are invisible on plain radiographs. However, as already shown when evaluating the hip for DDH, the cartilaginous epiphyses are well demonstrated sonographically. Radiographic malalignment of the humeral shaft with the glenoid or with the radius or ulna following a difficult, traumatic delivery may indicate a neonatal shoulder or elbow dislocation, respectively. However, since the epiphyses are radiolucent, their positions are unknown. The pediatric physis is relatively weak compared to the ligaments and tendons. Hence, fracture along the physeal plate with separation of the epiphysis from its metaphysis occurs as a result of trauma to the pediatric extremity. Neonatal extremity trauma resulting from a difficult delivery is a pertinent clinical scenario. Distinguishing between dislocation of the entire bone from a joint (e.g., shoulder or elbow), including its unossified epiphysis and diaphysis, and a displaced Salter-Harris fracture of the epiphysis (i.e., slipped epiphysis) is often impossible on plain radiographs of neonates and young infants. The latter condition should be

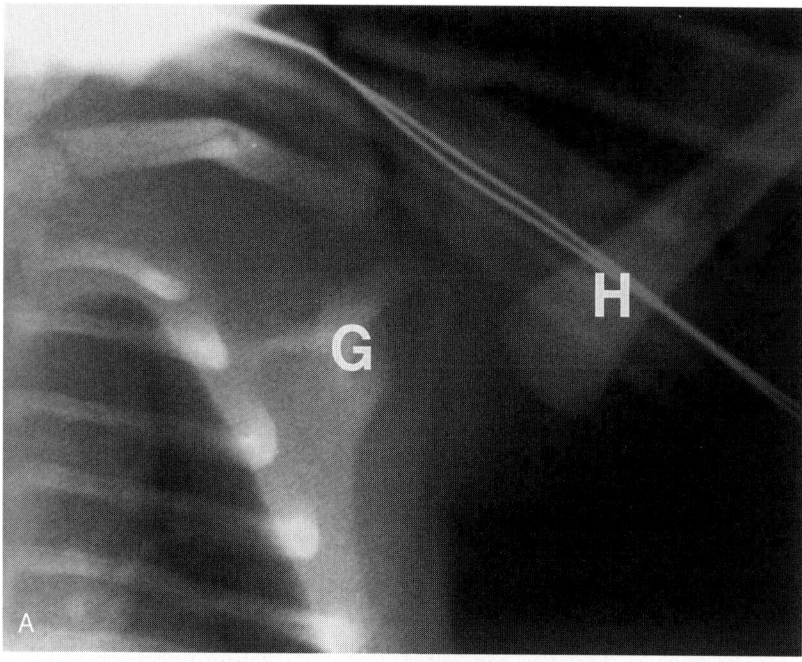

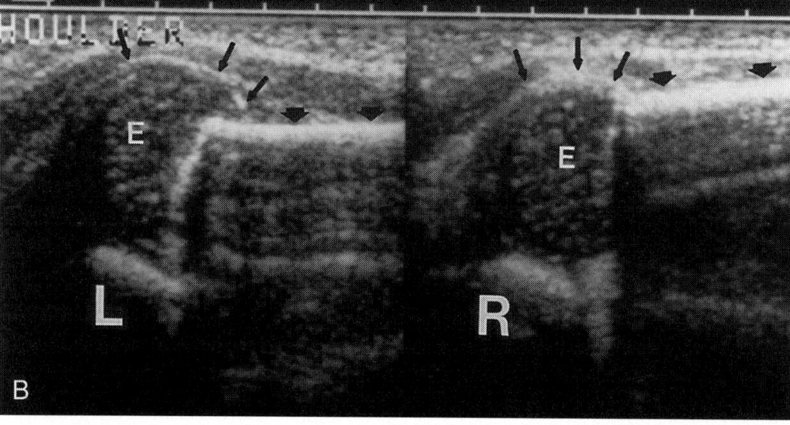

Figure 9-17 ■ Salter-Harris I fracture dislocation of the left proximal humerus. **A,** AP radiograph of the left shoulder. The left humeral head is not ossified. The humeral shaft (*H*) does not align with the glenoid (*G*). **B,** Longitudinal sonograms of the left (*L*) and right (*R*) proximal humeri displayed on a split-screen format. The epiphysis (*E*) of the left humerus (*arrows*) has slipped off the humeral shaft (*arrowheads*), indicative of a Salter-Harris 1 fracture. The normal alignment of the right proximal humeral (*R*) epiphysis (*E, arrows*) and shaft (*arrowheads*) is shown for comparison.

suspected in this age group. Formerly, arthrography was required to outline the epiphysis and to show its relationship to the joint and the shaft (White et al., 1987). Sonography can now answer the question (Zieger et al., 1987a; Broker and Burbach, 1990). A slipped proximal humeral epiphysis is usually well demonstrated in the coronal plane from a lateral approach (Fig. 9–17). Confirmatory transverse views and, when appropriate, gentle internal and external rotation of the humerus can be helpful. Sonography should be performed from multiple projections, with careful attention to orientation. Being present during scanning and noting the position of the transducer on the extremity is always helpful. Comparison with the normal opposite extremity, similarly positioned, can be helpful.

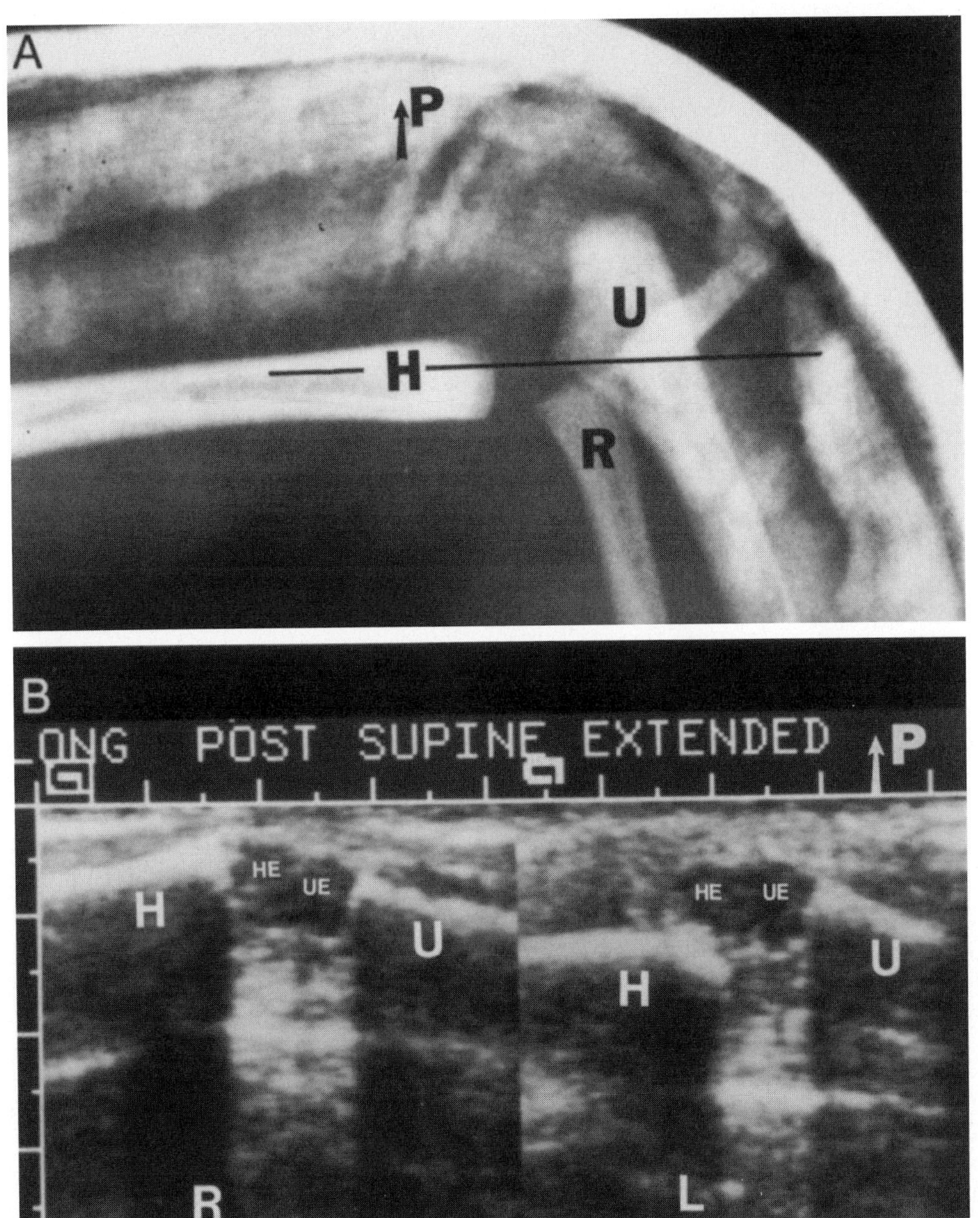

Figure 9–18 ▪ **A,** Lateral radiograph of this newborn's left elbow in a posterior splint (*P*) shows obvious elbow malalignment. The *arrow* points posteriorly. The radius (*R*) and ulna (*U*) are posterior to the humerus (*H*). Status of the unossified elbow epiphyses is unknown from the radiograph. **B,** Sagittal views of both elbows were obtained from their posterior aspects and are shown on the split screen in a projection matching that of the radiograph. The right hypoechoic distal humeral (*HE*) and proximal ulnar (*UE*) epiphyses (note the through-transmission) are normally aligned with their shafts. The left distal humeral epiphysis is separated from its shaft but remains aligned with the ulna, indicating that this is a displaced Salter-Harris 1 fracture through the distal humeral physis rather than an elbow dislocation.

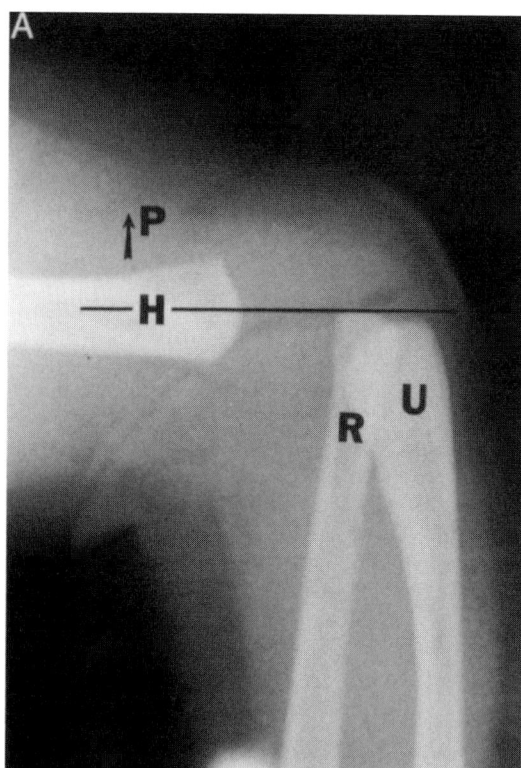

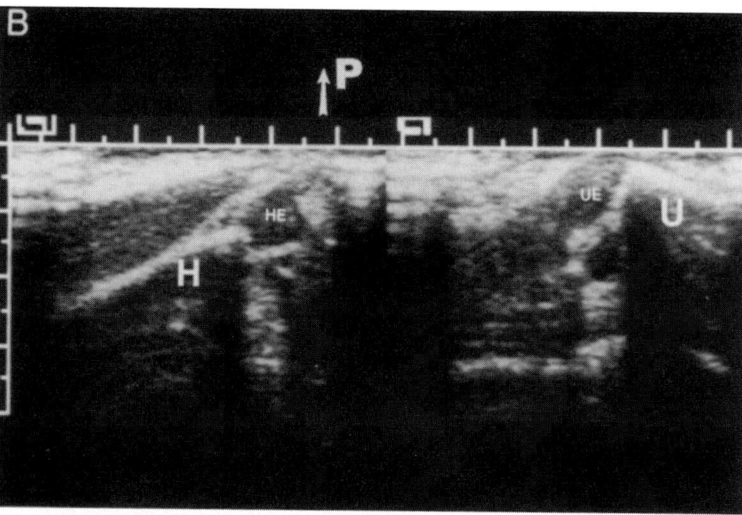

Figure 9–19 ▪ **A**, The lateral view of the elbow shows posterior displacement (*P*) of the radius (*R*) and ulna (*U*) with respect to the humerus (*H*), as in Figure 9–18. **B**, The similar posterior longitudinal sonogram of the elbow shows that the epiphyses (*HE, UE*) remain aligned with their respective shafts, although not with each other, indicating a true elbow dislocation. The humerus and ulna were in different anatomical planes and therefore could not be displayed together on the same sonogram.

Displaced distal humeral condylar fracture (Fig. 9–18) was distinguished from congenital elbow dislocation (Larsen syndrome) (Fig. 9–19) in two neonates using a posterior (i.e., sagittal) approach. Although the plain radiographs were similar in these examples, the sonograms showed the different relationships of the unossified epiphyses and their shafts, distinguishing displaced epiphysis (see Fig. 9–18) from dislocated elbow (see Fig. 9–19). Longitudinal imaging from the medial and lateral aspects of the elbow provides coronal views which, when used with transverse views, are helpful in examining older children with fractures involving incompletely ossified elbows and displaced cartilaginous ossification centers or fragments (Barr and Babcock, 1991; Markowitz et al., 1992). Two cases of congenital

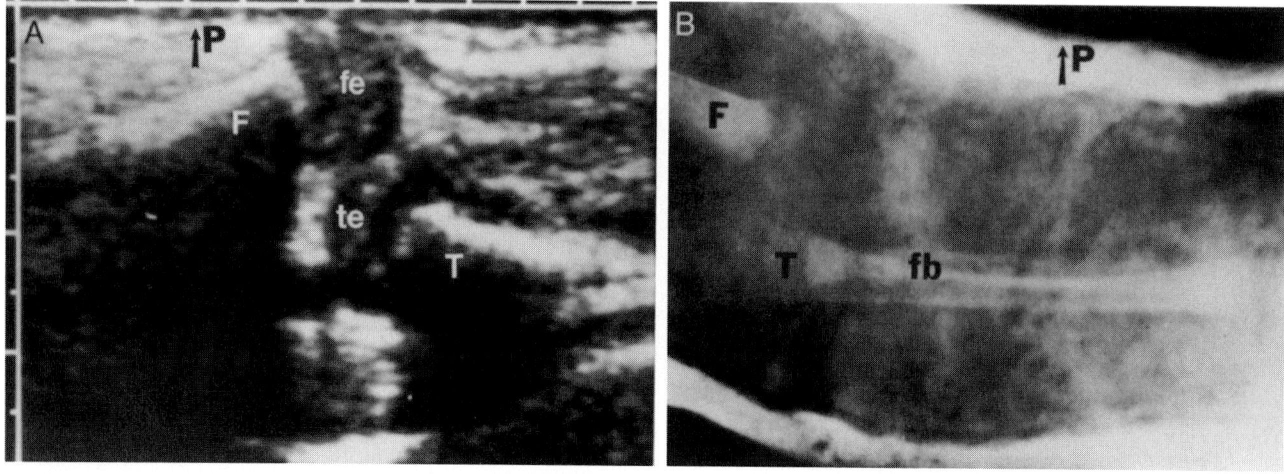

Figure 9–20 ▪ **A**, Longitudinal sonogram obtained from the posterior aspect (*P*) of the knee and in the same orientation as the plain radiograph shows that the unossified distal femoral epiphysis (*fe*) and proximal tibial epiphysis (*te*) remain with their respective shafts, indicating a true dislocation. Abbreviations: femur (*F*), tibia (*T*). **B**, The lateral radiograph obtained through a plaster cast shows a dislocated knee in this neonate. The *arrow* points posteriorly (*P*). The tibia (*T*) and fibula (*fb*) are displaced anteriorly with respect to the femur (*F*).

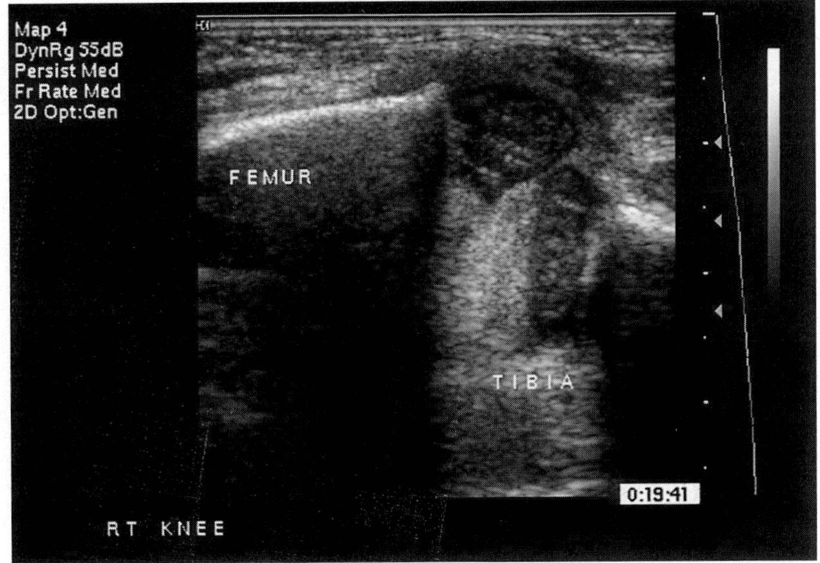

Figure 9–21 ■ Longitudinal sonogram from the anterior aspect of the knee in a neonate with Larsen syndrome and congenital dislocation. (Courtesy of Marnix van Holsbeeck, M.D., Henry Ford Hospital, Detroit)

knee dislocation show distal femoral and proximal tibial epiphyses which are displaced from each other but still aligned to their respective shafts (Figs. 9–20 and 9–21).

Slipped capital femoral epiphysis (SCFE), a cause of hip pain in older children, is actually a Salter-Harris 1 fracture. Epiphyseal displacement can be noted on sonography (Dorr et al., 1988), but the diagnosis is usually made on plain radiography. The most likely scenario is its incidental detection in the older child who is undergoing hip sonography for a suspected joint effusion (vide infra). Plain radiography, not sonography, is the indicated study when SCFE is suspected. Sonographic visualization of the epiphysis at this age is limited. Anterior scanning across the physis and along the proximal femoral neck, as for an effusion, shows the posteromedial displacement of the epiphysis. Another cause of hip pain, Legg-Calvé-Perthes disease, usually occurs in a younger child than SCFE but might also be detected during scanning a painful hip for effusion (Suzuki et al., 1987; Dorr et al., 1988). After the initial ischemic phase, irregular, fragmented ossification and flattening of the femoral head are present. Synovitis, lateral extrusion of the femoral head, and femoral head reconstitution were noted in one series of cases (Wirth et al., 1992). An effusion can occur as part of either SCFE or early Legg-Calvé-Perthes disease (Suzuki et al., 1987; Dorr et al., 1988; Wirth et al., 1992).

Extremity Deformities

Sonography has been used to measure lower extremity rotational deformities, femoral anteversion, and tibial torsion (Joseph et al., 1987; Terjesen and Anda, 1987; Harcke et al., 1988). It use is not widespread, and measurement techniques vary. However, both rotational deformities are assessed easily and reproducibly with CT (Hernandez et al., 1981; Hernandez, 1983). Sonographic depiction of unossified bone can be used in other deformities and malformations such as tibial hemimelia, proximal focal femoral deficiency (PFFD), congenital deficiency of the femur (Grissom and Harcke, 1994), clubfoot, and vertical talus. In vertical talus, sonography shows the alignment of the unossified navicular with the talus (Fig. 9–22) (Schlesinger et al., 1989). Difficulty arises in establishing reliable and reproducible measurements in congenital clubfoot deformity. Although cartilaginous tarsals are visible, their oval and elliptical contours and alignment vary with the position and movement of the foot.

Inflammation and Infection

To look for an effusion, the hip joint is scanned from an anterior (ventral) approach in both longitudinal and transverse planes. Fluid tends to accumulate anterior to the femoral neck in the inferior, caudal recess of the joint (Figs. 9–23 and 9–24). One scans in the sagittal plane over the extended hip and rotates the transducer slightly to be parallel with the long axis of the femoral neck. External rotation of the hip will bring the medial, most inferior recess of the joint space into the scanning plane, facilitating the detection of small effusions.

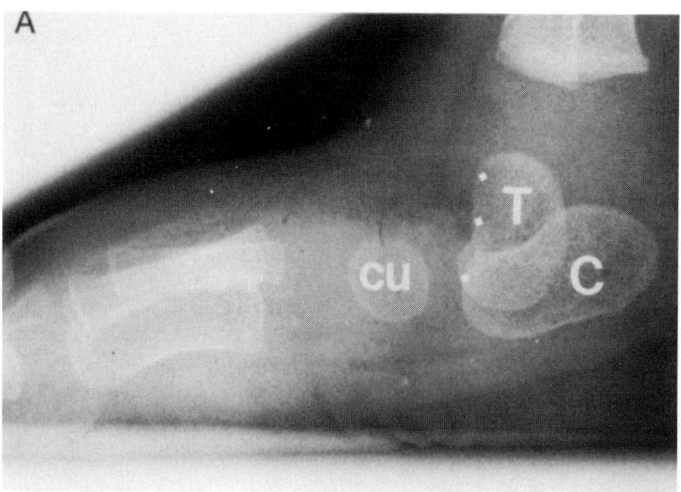

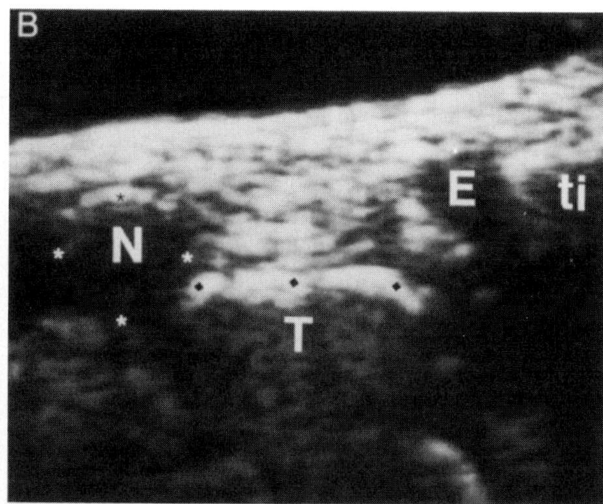

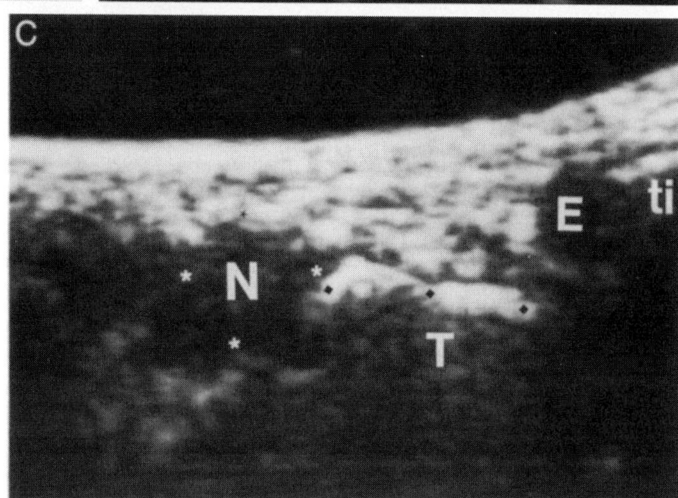

Figure 9–22 ■ **A**, Lateral radiograph of the foot and ankle in a 7-month-old infant with vertical talus. Abbreviations: talus (*T*), calcaneus (*C*), cuboid (*cu*). **B**, Sagittal sonogram obtained from the dorsum of the foot over the talus and navicular demonstrates the dorsal displacement of the unossified navicular (*N*) relative to the talus. The dorsal aspect of the talus is marked with *three dots* for orientation. **C**, Comparison view of the normal foot shows normal alignment of the unossified navicular with the talus. Abbreviations: unossified distal tibial epiphysis (*E*), ossified distal tibia (*ti*). (From Schlesinger AE, Deeney VFX, Caskey PF: *Pediatr Radiol* 20:134–135, 1989. Used with permission.)

Effusions as small as 1 ml can be detected (Marchal et al., 1987). Three criteria have been used to detect hip effusion:

1. An absolute measurement where the anterior joint capsule is displaced 3 mm or more anterior to the femoral neck at a point halfway between the physis and the caudal insertion of the joint capsule on the femoral neck.
2. Distention of the joint capsule 2 mm more than the asymptomatic, presumably normal side. It is important, therefore, that the scanning planes and positions of the hips (i.e., extension, rotation) be identical.
3. Simple observation of the shape of the joint capsule. It is normally concave anteriorly, parallel to the curvature of the femoral neck. If it is convex anteriorly, this indicates bulging of the joint capsule, which in most cases is due to an effusion.

The anterior bulge of the joint capsule is best seen with the hip extended. When the hip is flexed, the fluid is redistributed, the anterior aspect of the joint capsule is less distended, and the effusion is less apparent (Marchal et al., 1987). An irritable hip may be flexed and difficult to extend. The anterior joint capsule consists of an anterior and a posterior layer of fibrous tissue. The anterior layer is normally slightly thicker and more echogenic than the posterior layer (Robben et al., 1999). Distinguishing septic arthritis from sterile effusion (i.e., transient synovitis) on the basis of sonography remains difficult in many cases, even when power color Doppler is used. Increased echogenicity of the fluid and a thick articular capsule (more than 2 mm) may suggest septic arthritis (Zieger et al., 1987b; Dorr et al., 1988). No measurable thickening of either layer of the anterior joint capsule occurs with transient synovitis (Robben et al., 1999). However, plain radiographic and sonographic findings do not reliably differentiate infected from sterile hip effusions (Miralles et al., 1989; Zawin et al., 1993). Septic effusions can show increased capsular blood flow on power Doppler scans (Fig. 9–25), but this finding

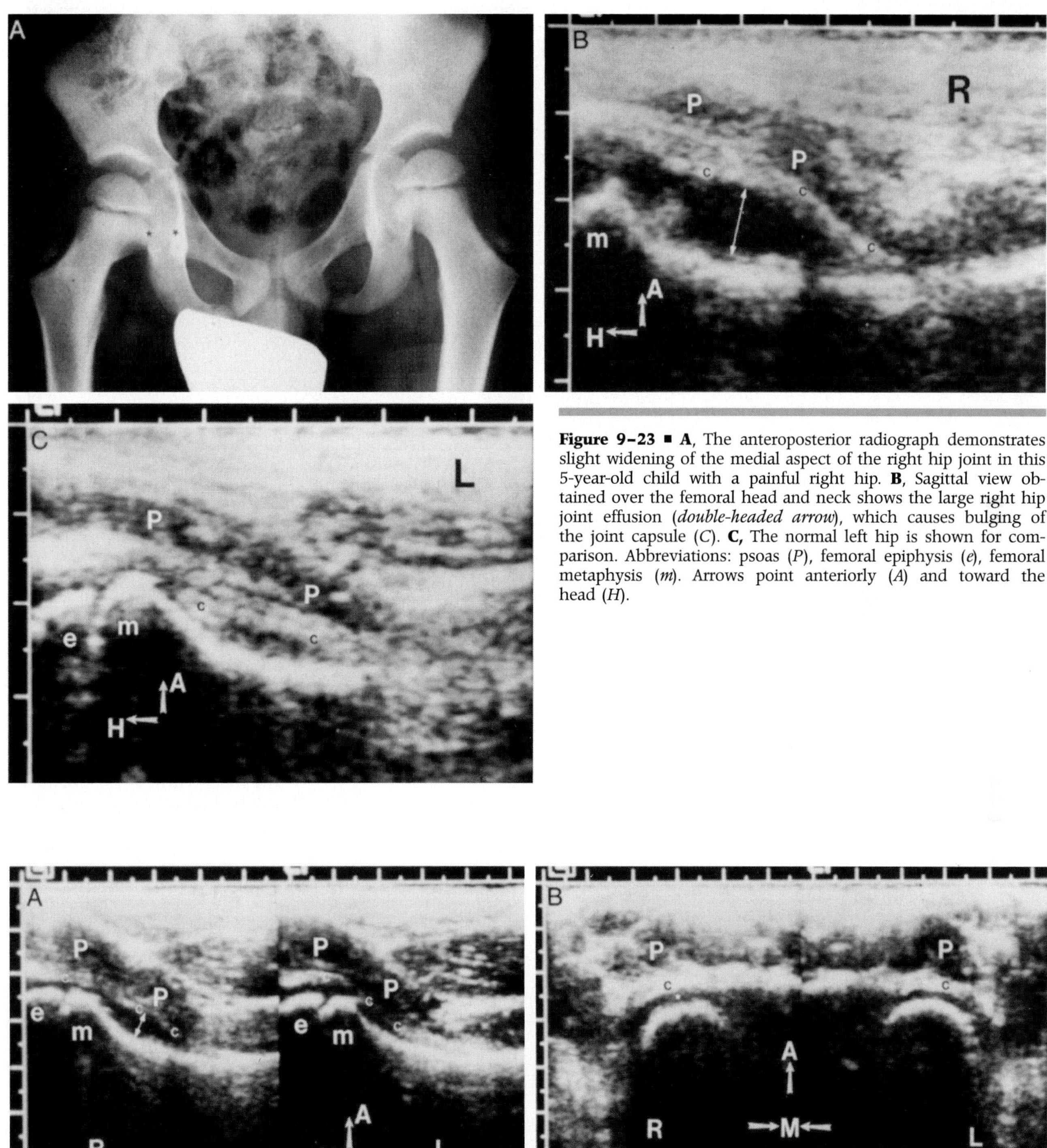

Figure 9–23 ■ **A**, The anteroposterior radiograph demonstrates slight widening of the medial aspect of the right hip joint in this 5-year-old child with a painful right hip. **B**, Sagittal view obtained over the femoral head and neck shows the large right hip joint effusion (*double-headed arrow*), which causes bulging of the joint capsule (*C*). **C,** The normal left hip is shown for comparison. Abbreviations: psoas (*P*), femoral epiphysis (*e*), femoral metaphysis (*m*). Arrows point anteriorly (*A*) and toward the head (*H*).

Figure 9–24 ■ Sagittal (**A**) and transverse (**B**) views of both hips viewed on split screens demonstrate a small right hip effusion (*double-headed arrow* on the sagittal view and *star* on the transverse view). One milliliter of clear fluid was aspirated. *Arrows* point anteriorly (*A*), superiorly (*S*), and medially (*M*). Abbreviations: joint capsule (*C*), psoas (*P*), femoral epiphysis (*e*), femoral metaphysis (*m*), right (*R*), left (*L*).

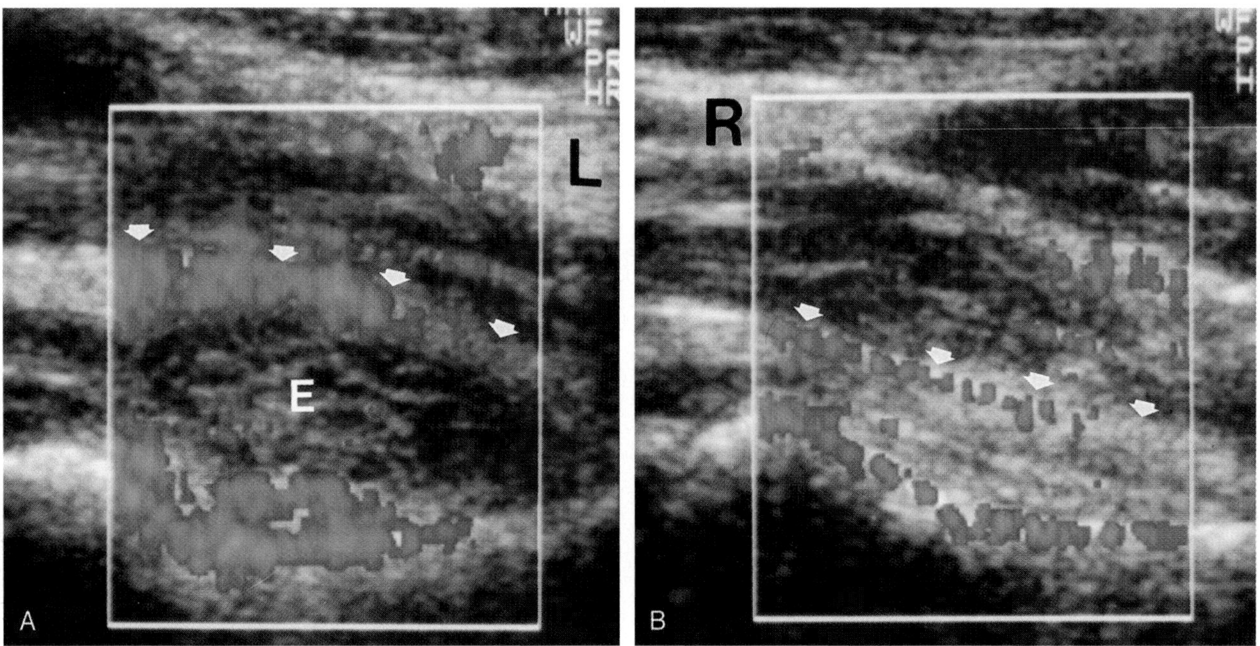

Figure 9–25 ■ Power Doppler scan of septic arthritis of the left hip joint. Sagittal anterior views of the left (**A**) and comparison normal right (**B**) hip joints show the left joint effusion (*E*) with internal echoes and an increased power Doppler signal of its bulging joint capsule (*arrowheads*). The capsule of the normal right hip is not bulging, and its power Doppler signal serves as a normal comparative baseline. The power Doppler settings were identical for both hips. (Reprinted with permission from Strouse PJ, DiPietro MA, Adler RS. Pediatric hip effusions: Evaluation with power Doppler sonography. *Radiology* 206:731–735, 1998.)

was not sensitive enough to preclude the need to aspirate the hip when the power Doppler study was negative (Strouse et al., 1998). Sensitivity below 100% was also substantiated in an animal model (Strouse et al., 1999). Sonography can also detect effusions in other joints (Fig. 9–26).

Osteomyelitis can present sonographically with a small focal fluid collection adjacent to bone (Abiri et al., 1989). Subperiosteal fluid (pus) can be detected (Fig. 9–27). Sonography has been used to evaluate and follow children with osteomyelitis (Abernethy et al., 1993; Wright et al., 1995; Riebel et al., 1996). Color Doppler sonography can show increased flow in and around the infected perios-

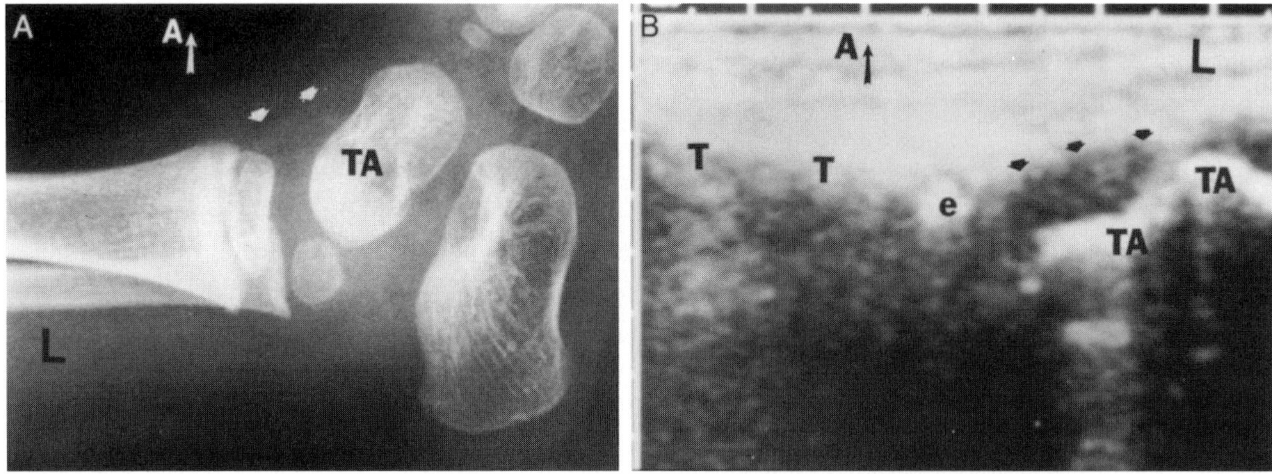

Figure 9–26 ■ **A**, Lateral radiograph of the left ankle oriented to match the sonogram (*arrow* points anteriorly, *A*). Note the ankle joint fullness (*arrowheads*) anterior to the talus (*TA*). **B**, The sagittal sonogram shows the joint effusion anterior to the talus. Abbreviations: distal tibial shaft (*T*), distal tibial epiphysis (*e*). *Arrow* points anteriorly.

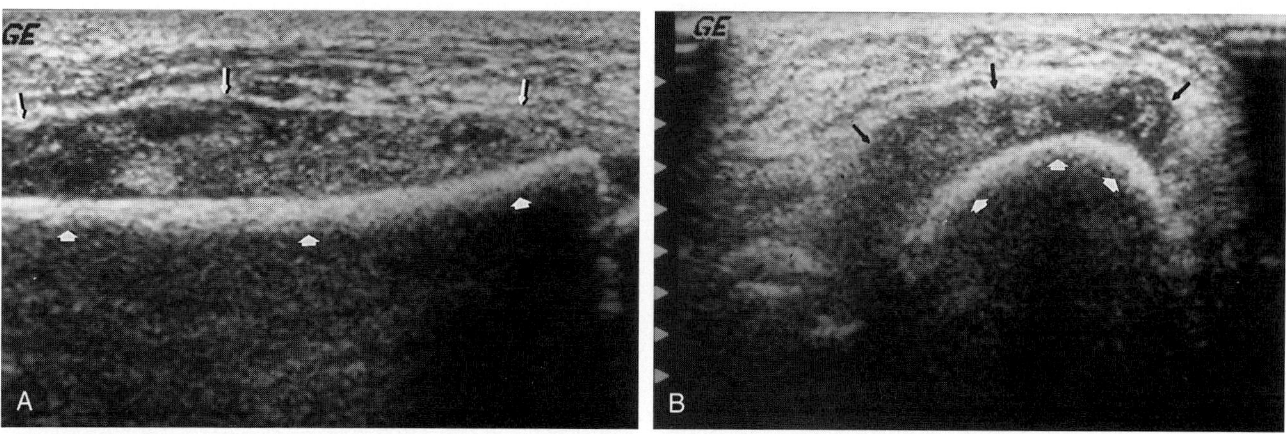

Figure 9–27 ■ Sagittal (**A**) and transverse (**B**) views of subperiosteal complex fluid (*arrows*) along the distal fibular shaft (*arrowheads*).

teum in children with advanced acute osteomyelitis (Chao et al., 1999).

Occult fractures have been detected (Graif et al., 1988) on sonography. In one example, hip sonography was requested to exclude effusion in a 2-month-old girl who would not move her leg. The hip study was negative, but sonography along the rest of the leg discovered a metaphyseal corner (Salter-Harris 2) fracture of the distal tibia, which was confirmed by radiography and was later shown to be due to child abuse (Fig. 9–28).

Fibromatosis Colli

This soft tissue "mass" is specific to pediatrics. It is the palpable, firm bulge in the central portion of a sternocleidomastoid muscle in a young infant presenting with torticollis (Kraus et al., 1986). The baby's head is often characteristically turned, as would be expected with unilateral sternocleidomastoid shortening or contraction. The ipsilateral ear is toward the ipsilateral shoulder, and the chin is toward the contralateral side. Scanning along the long axis of the sternocleidomastoid muscle shows the characteristic bulge of the muscle compared to the normal side (Fig. 9–29). It often responds to physical therapy.

The Spinal Canal

Sonography of the pediatric spinal canal is most commonly performed in the infant to look for an

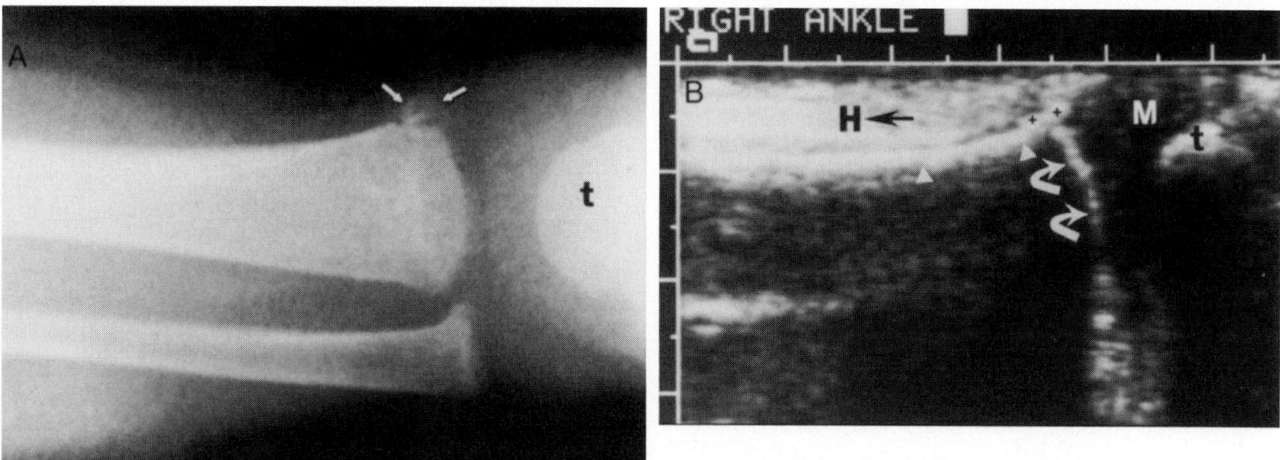

Figure 9–28 ■ **A**, AP radiograph showing a medial distal tibial metaphyseal corner fracture (*arrows*). **B**, Coronal sonogram oriented similarly shows the corner fracture (++) which led to the confirmatory radiograph. Abbreviations: unossified medial malleolus (*M*), talus (*t*), distal tibial metaphysis (*curved arrows*), distal medial tibial shaft (*arrowheads*). The *arrow* points to the patient's head (*H*).

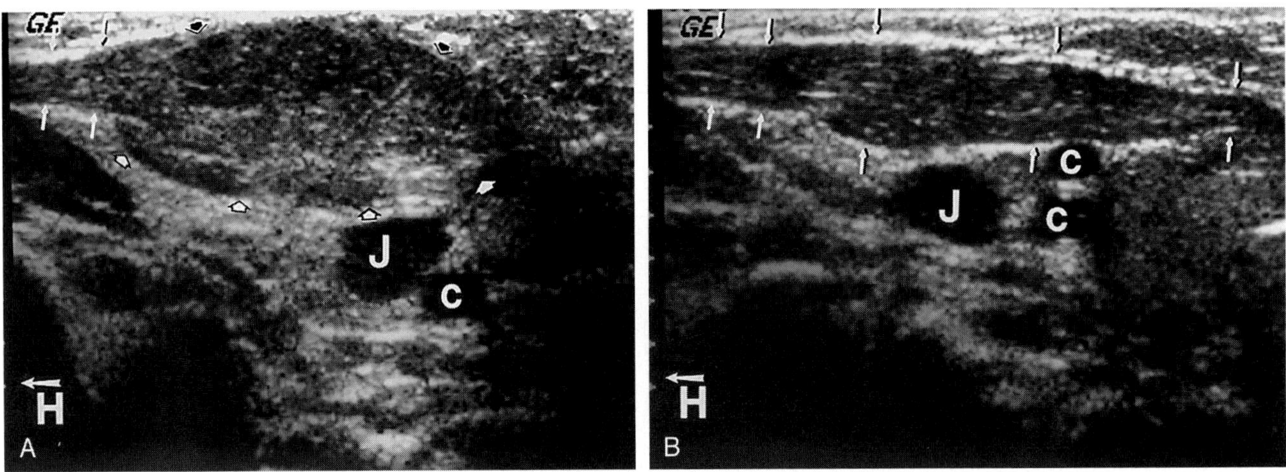

Figure 9–29 ■ Fibromatosis colli in a young infant. Sagittal views of the (**A**) left side of the neck, with a firm, palpable mass, and a comparison view of the (**B**) normal right side of the neck. The sternocleidomastoid muscle (*arrows*) has a normal appearance and contour on the right. It has a very thickened central portion (*arrowheads*) on the left which blends with normal-appearing muscle superiorly (*arrows*). The *large arrow* points toward the head (*H*). Jugular (*J*) and carotid (*c*) vessels are medial to the sternocleidomastoid muscles.

occult tethered spinal cord. Although its use is limited in the older child, it can often determine the level of the conus medullaris (DiPietro, 1998; DiPietro and Garver, 1998). Sonography can be used to assess a mass on the back which is better characterized in terms of its location (tissue plane) and extent than its histology. The echotexture and margins of the mass are noted, but this aspect of the evaluation is limited. When the mass is near the midline, its relationship to the spinal canal should be determined (Figs. 9–30 through 9–32). Although spinal sonography is performed predominantly to

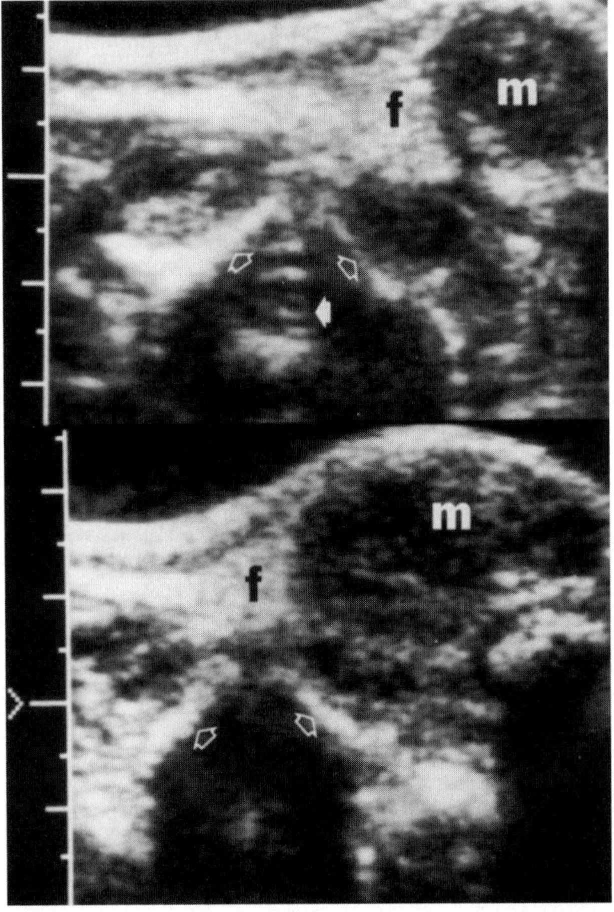

Figure 9–30 ■ Transverse sonograms obtained over the upper back of a 5-day-old infant demonstrate a 6 by 3 cm lobulated mass which is medial to the right scapula. The mass (*m*) is within subcutaneous fat (*f*) but superficial to paraspinal muscles, with no invasion of the spinal canal. Surgical pathological diagnosis was hemangiopericytoma. The thoracic lamina (*open arrowheads*) and spinal cord (*solid arrowhead*) are noted.

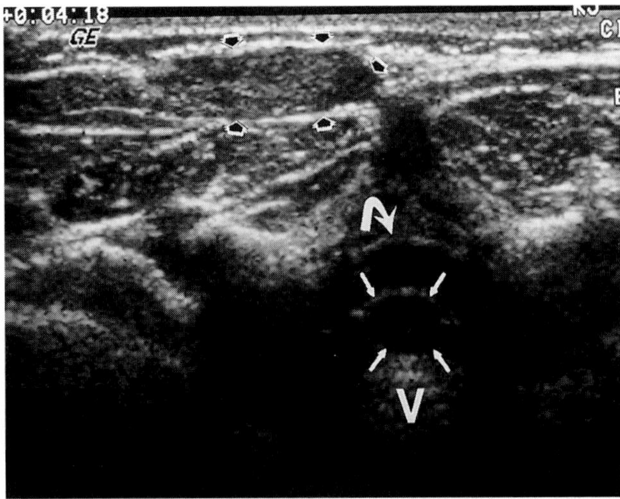

Figure 9–31 ■ Transverse view of a palpable subcutaneous mass (*arrowheads*) on the upper left lumbar area, remote from the spinal canal. Abbreviations: spinal canal dorsal dura (*curved arrow*), spinal cord (*straight arrows*), vertebral body (*V*).

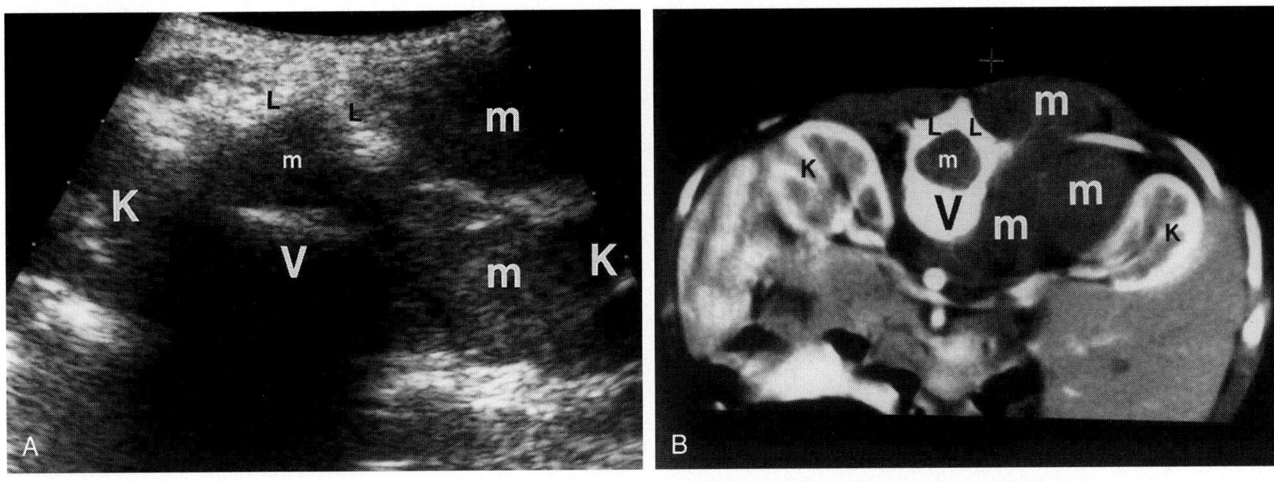

Figure 9–32 ■ **A**, transverse sonogram (courtesy of Sue Kaste, M.D., St. Jude's Hospital, Memphis) and **B**, correlative CT scan show a palpable right paraspinal mass (*m*) extending into the spinal canal and displacing the ipsilateral right kidney (*K*). Abbreviations: vertebral body (*V*), laminae (*L*).

evaluate the spinal canal, spinal cord, and cauda equina, a vertebral anomaly is sometimes detected (Fig. 9–33).

Technique and Normal Anatomy

The spinal canal is examined from the back. The child is usually prone, with sufficient flexion produced by a pillow, towel, or blanket roll under the child to separate the posterior vertebral elements and thereby provide an acoustic window into the spinal canal. Care must be taken not to hyperflex a small baby and compromise respiration. The child can also be studied in the decubitus posture or while sitting or being held by a parent. These alternative positions will work as long as spine flexion is adequate. We prefer using a linear array transducer at the highest frequency allowing adequate

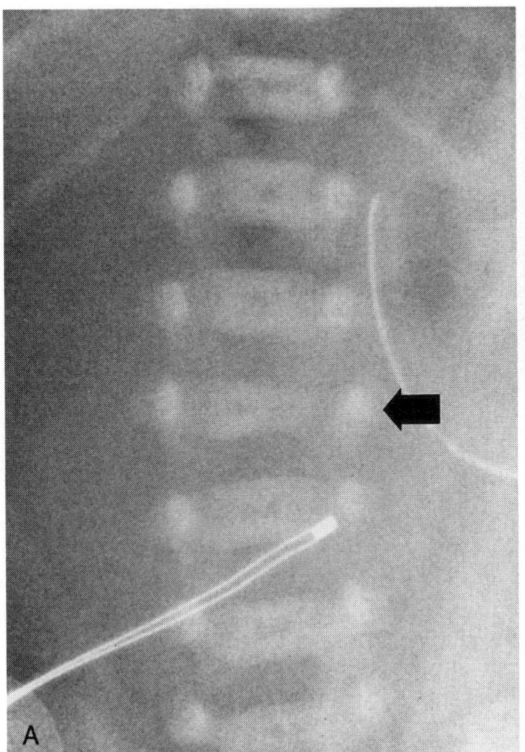

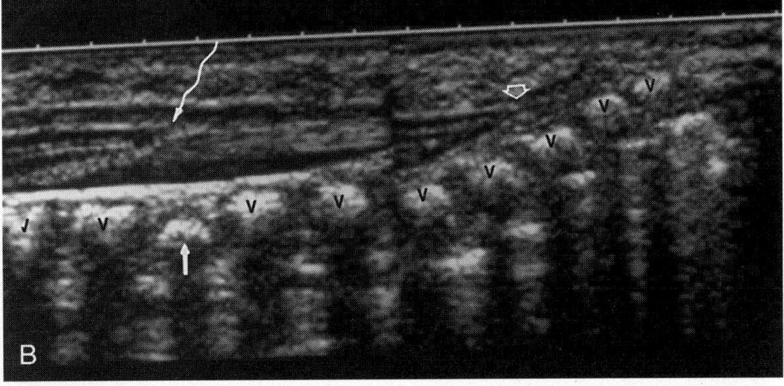

Figure 9–33 ■ Hypoplastic vertebral body. **A**, Frontal radiograph of the lumbar spine shows the hypoplastic left portion of a midlumbar vertebral body (*arrow*). **B**, Split-screen composite longitudinal sonogram of the lumbosacral spine shows vertebral bodies (*v*) and the single midlumbar hypoplastic body (*straight arrow*). The *wavy arrow* denotes the tip of the conus medullaris, and the open arrowhead denotes the caudal end of the thecal sac, both normal. (Reprinted with permission from DiPietro MA, Garver KA. Sonography of the neonatal spinal canal. In Haller JO (ed), *Textbook of Neonatal Ultrasound*. New York, Parthenon Publishing Group, 1998.)

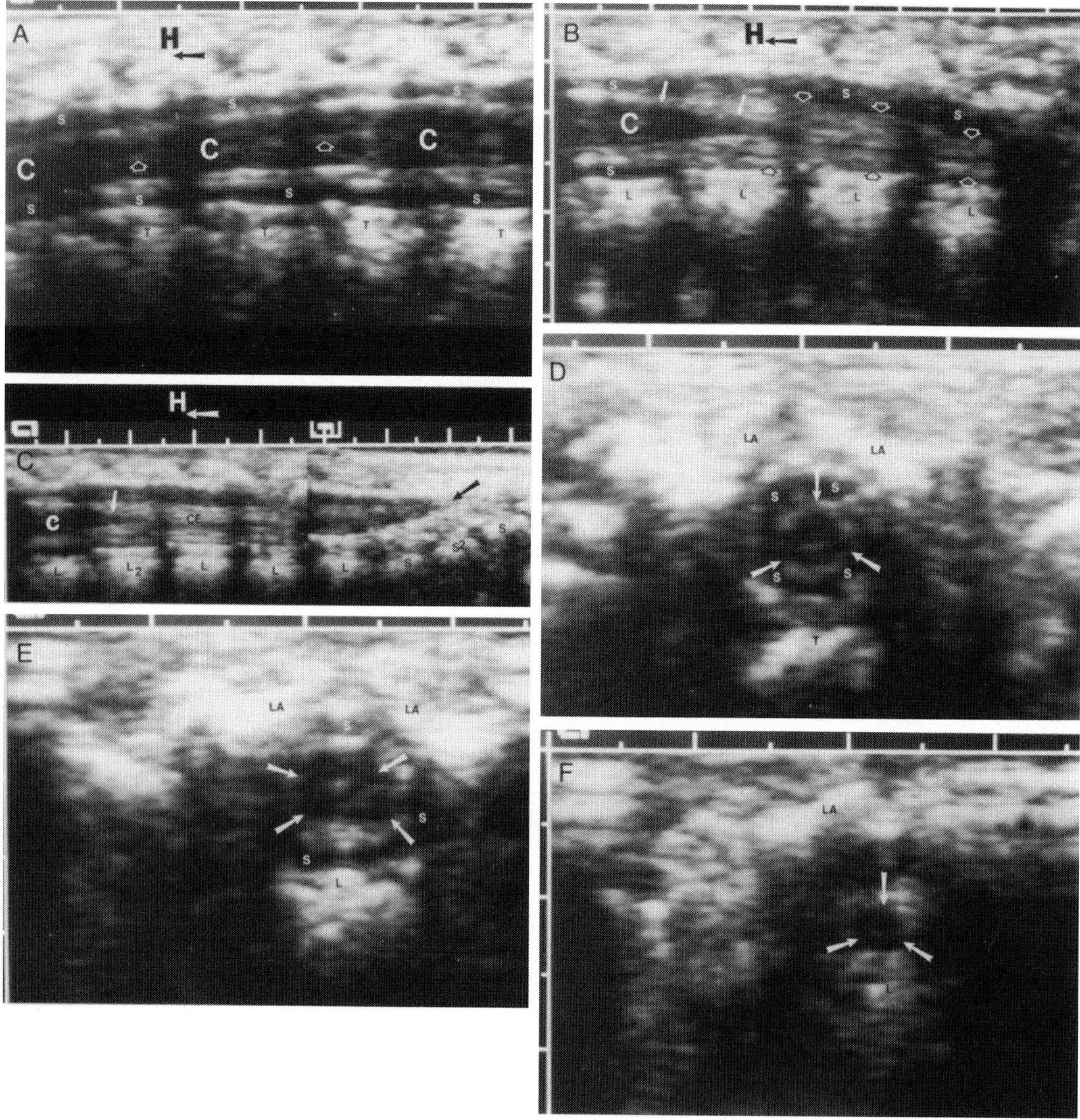

Figure 9-34 ■ **A-C**, Intraspinal sonogram of a normal 5-week-old infant. Sagittal views are oriented with the patient's head toward the viewer's left. **A**, The hypoechoic middle to lower thoracic and lumbar spinal cord (*C*) is shown with the echogenic central echo complex (*open arrowhead*). **B**, The distal portion of the cord tapers (*white arrows*), forming the conus medullaris. Longitudinal echogenic nerve roots (*open arrowheads, CE*) extend through the remainder of the spinal canal as the cauda equina. **C**, The split screen enables one to depict accurately most of the lumbosacral canal in one picture. The caudal extent of the thecal sac (*black arrow*) usually corresponds to S2. The *arrow* points toward the head (*H*). Abbreviations: subarachnoid space (*white S*), thoracic vertebra (*T*), lumbar vertebra (*L*), sacral segments (*black S*). **D-H**, Transverse views of the spinal canal at various levels. **D** and **E**, The hypoechoic spinal cord is outlined (*straight arrows*). In **E**, the spinal cord is thickest at the high lumbar level. **F** and **G**, In the upper lumbar canal, the cord (*arrows*) tapers at the conus medullaris (*open arrowheads*), surrounded by echogenic nerve roots forming the cauda equina (*CE*).

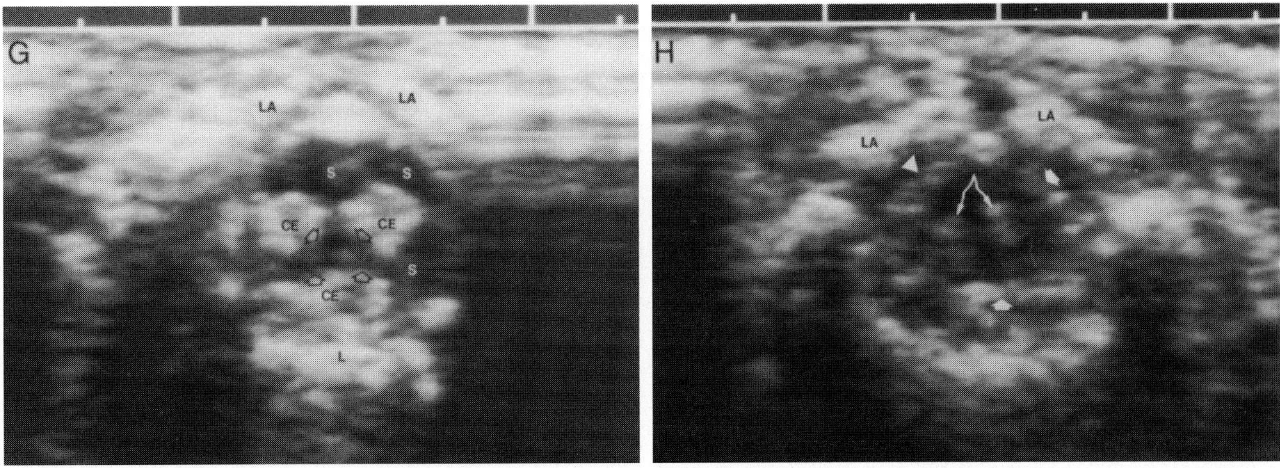

Figure 9–34 *Continued* ■ **H**, The cauda equina extends into the lower lumbosacral canal, appearing as echogenic clusters (*wavy arrows*). Abbreviations: thoracic vertebra (*T*), lumbar vertebra (*L*), lamina (*LA*), subarachnoid space (*S*), the margins of the low lumbar canal (*closed arrowheads*).

penetration, which can be up to 13 MHz. We also use a curved transducer for better contact in longitudinal views at the craniocervical junction and at the margin of a protuding mass or meningocele with the skin surface. Scanning is performed in the longitudinal (sagittal) and transverse (axial) planes along the spine (Fig. 9–34). Posterior spinal ossification is incomplete in neonates and young infants, allowing a panoramic sonographic view of the spinal canal. A broad view is also obtained by making a composite picture, with the split-screen function available on many units (Fig. 9–35A).

Scanning in the sagittal plane along the length of the canal (Fig. 9–35) shows the hypoechoic cord within the canal surrounded by cerebrospinal fluid (CSF) containing echogenic nerve roots. A longitudinal echogenic line down the center of the cord is referred to as the *central echo complex*. It is very close to the central canal and was shown on a sonographic histoanatomical study to be the interface between the myelinated ventral white commissure of the cord and the dorsal extent of its ventral median fissure (Nelson, Sedler et al., 1989). The tip of the conus medullaris is identified by its taper in the upper lumbar canal (Fig. 9–35C). The caudal end of the thecal sac containing CSF is usually at S2 (Koroshetz and Taveras, 1986).

It sometimes helps novice scanners to start scanning sagitally over the sacrum, which is identified by its stair-like appearance (Fig. 9–35E), to identify the spinal canal, and to follow the canal cephalad. Transverse views of the cord (Fig. 9–36) show the central echo complex as an echogenic dot in the central portion or slightly ventral to the center of the hypoechoic cord (Fig. 9–36C). Dura mater lines the canal (Fig. 9–36D), and echogenic roots of the cauda equina surround the cord. In addition to nerve roots at approximately the 10, 2, 4, and 8 o'clock positions, as noted on transverse views of the cord (Figs. 9–36D,E), horizontal echogenic dentate ligaments are seen at the 3 and 9 o'clock positions (Figs. 9–36A,B). The size and shape of the spinal cord vary with its vertebral level (Gusnard et al., 1986; Kawahara et al., 1987). The cord diameter is less at the midthoracic than at the thoracolumbar junction and cervical levels. Cauda equina surrounds the conus (Fig. 9–36E) and separates into right and left nerve clusters as it descends in the lumbar canal (Figs. 9–36F,G). One can mistake an echogenic cluster of nerves for an echogenic intracanalicular mass when viewing a single static image. However, during real-time scanning, it is easy to note that the cauda equina consists of many small echos (i.e., nerve roots) which oscillate and undulate within the CSF. The orientation of dorsal and ventral roots of the cauda equina can have a spider-like appearance at the tip of the conus (Fig. 9–37A). It can superficially resemble and be mistaken for diastematomyelia on a static image (Fig. 9–37B), but this should also not be a problem during real-time scanning.

Midline artery and lateral veins are seen in the ventral portion of the spinal canal on color Doppler scans (Figs. 9–38 and 9–39). Sagittal views of the tip of the sacrum show the hypoechoic, unossified coccyx. Newer-generation high-frequency transducers allow delineation of the separate coccygeal centers (Fig. 9–40). Spinous processes have an inverted U

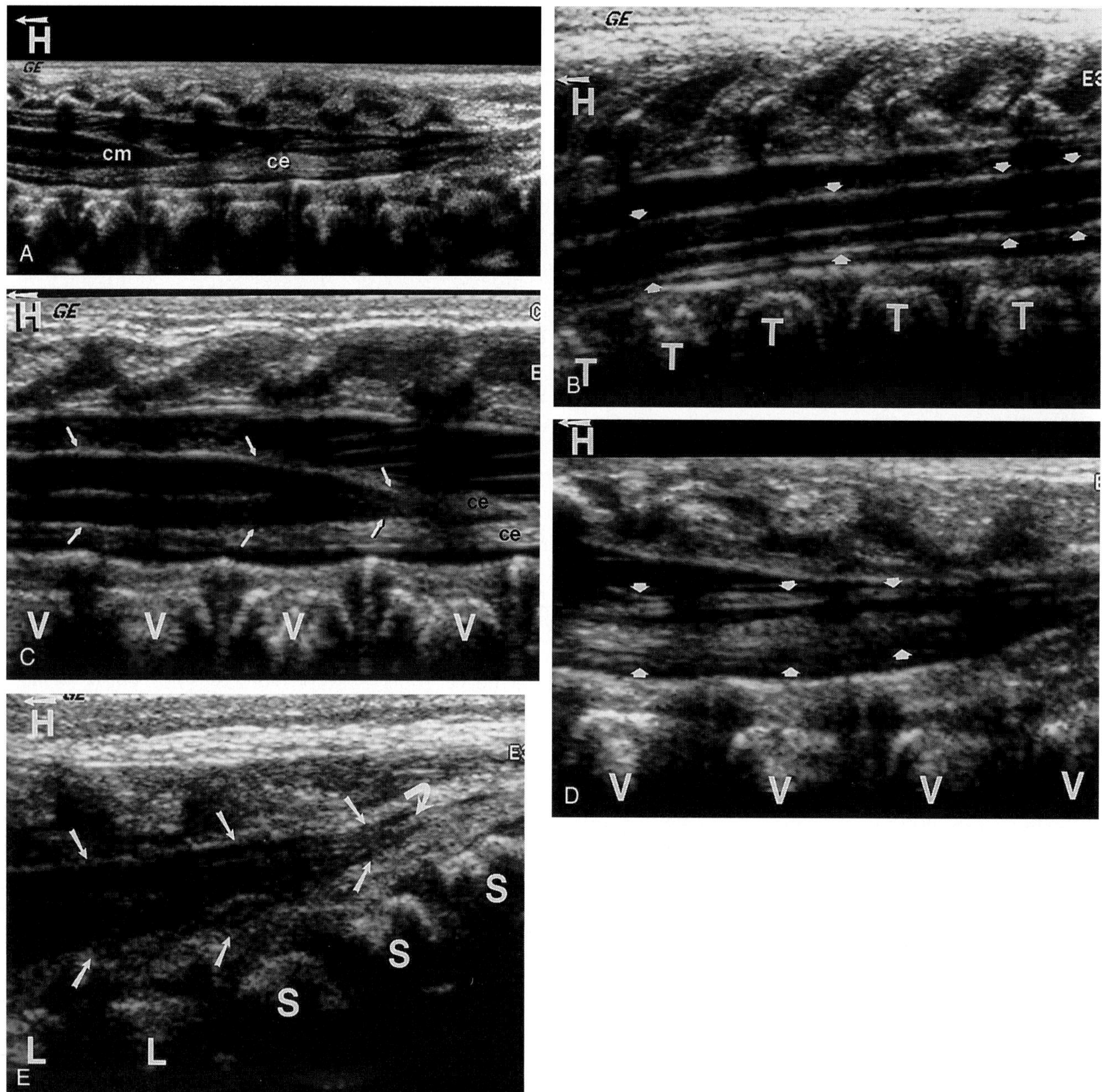

Figure 9–35 ■ Sagittal views of the neonatal spinal canal. **A**, Composite split screen showing a panoramic view of the entire lumbar canal. Abbreviations: conus medullaris (*cm*), cauda equina (*ce*). **B**, Detailed view of the midportion of the thoracic spinal canal showing the cord (*arrowheads*), which is more ventral superiorly, toward the upper thoracic canal. Abbreviations: thoracic vertebra (*T*). The *arrow* points toward the head (*H*). **C**, Detailed view of the upper lumbar cord and conus medullaris (*arrows*). Abbreviations: vertebral bodies (*V*), cauda equina (*ce*). **D**, Detailed view of the cauda equina (*arrowheads*) within the low lumbar and upper sacral canal. Abbreviation:vertebral bodies (*V*). **E**, detailed view of the lumbosacral junction and thecal sac (*straight arrows*), which tapers at its caudal end (*curved arrow*) at S2–S3. Abbreviations: lumbar vertebral bodies (*L*), sacral vertebral bodies (*S*).

appearance on sagittal images (Fig. 9–41), which in premature neonates are cartilaginous in the midline. More laterally, one sees lamina which resemble overlapping roof tiles (Fig. 9–42). Advanced ossification of the posterior spinal elements limits visualization of the spinal canal in the older child. Visualization is more segmental due to acoustic shadowing from the ossified posterior elements. However, if the child is properly positioned (i.e., flexed) and is not obese, the low thoracic and lumbosacral spinal canal can be seen well enough to identify and locate the conus medullaris (Figs. 9–43 and 9–44).

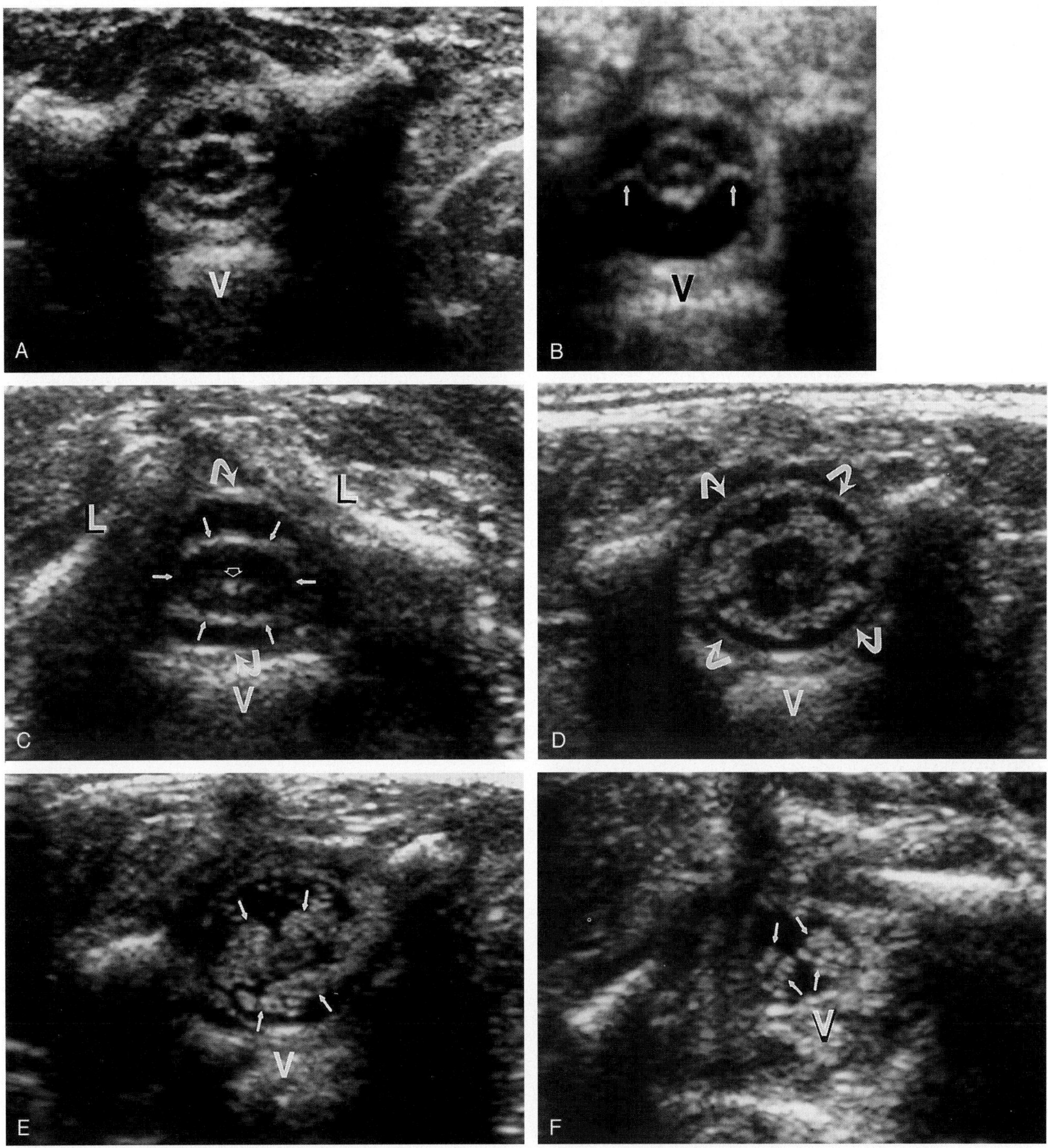

Figure 9–36 ■ Transverse views of the neonatal spinal canal. **A**, Midthoracic cord. Echogenic nerve roots at the 2, 4, 8, and 10 o'clock positions. Horizontal dentate ligaments at the 3 and 9 o'clock positions. Abbreviation: vertebral body (*V*). **B**, Midthoracic cord with dentate ligaments (*arrows*) at the 3 and 9 o'clock positions. Abbreviation: vertebral body (*V*). (Reprinted with permission from DiPietro MA, Garver KA. Sonography of the neonatal spinal canal. In Haller JO (ed), *Textbook of Neonatal Ultrasound.* New York, Parthenon Publishing Group, 1998.) **C**, Cord (*straight arrows*) at the thoracolumbar junction with the cord's central echo complex (*open arrowhead*) and dura (*curved arrows*). Abbreviations: vertebral body (*V*), vertebral laminae (*L*). **D**, Upper lumbar cord surrounded by nerve roots. Dura (*curved arrows*) lines the spinal canal. Abbreviation: vertebral body (*V*). **E**, Nerve roots (*arrows*) surround the conus medullaris in the upper lumbar canal. Abbreviation: vertebral body (*V*). **F**, Nerve roots of the cauda equina (*arrows*) forming right and left clusters in the middle and low lumbar canal. Abbreviation: vertebral body (*V*).

Figure continued on following page

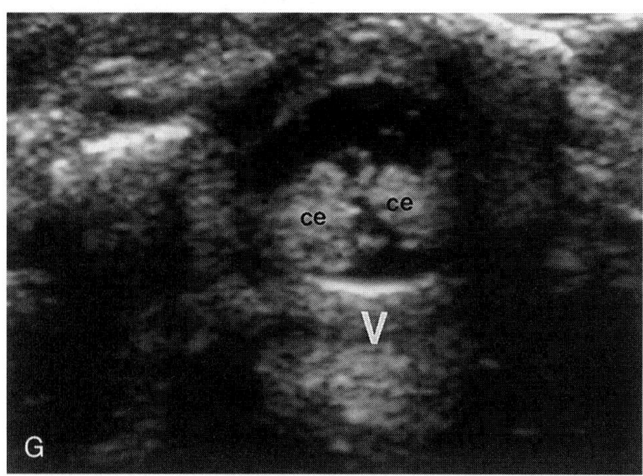

Figure 9–36 *Continued* ■ **G**, Cauda equina (*ce*) as right and left clusters of nerve roots in the middle and low lumbar canal. Abbreviation: vertebral body (*V*).

Spinal sonography in the older child had been performed with 5-MHz transducers, but newer equipment with improved penetration now allows it to be performed at higher frequencies (Fig. 9–45). It is sometimes helpful to use an interlaminar approach by moving the transducer slightly off midline and aiming it medially toward the canal between the shadowing lamina. The tip of the conus per se might not be seen, but its location can be inferred if the cord is seen at one vertebral level and only cauda equina is seen at the adjacent level. Information obtained from spine sonography in the older child is limited. One can often determine the level of the conus and whether or not it is oscillating (vide infra), but that information may adequately address the extent of the clinical question. Spinal canal sonography rivals MRI in the neonate (Rohrschneider, Forsting, et al., 1996), but there is no question that as the child grows, anatomical detail on MRI exceeds that on sonography. However, since sonography is easily performed and often more readily available, in experienced hands it may suffice, depending on the clinical situation and the question to be answered.

The tip of the conus medullaris can be located in neonates (Hill and Gibson, 1995) and often beyond infancy (DiPietro, 1993). The level of the tip of the conus medullaris is normally at or cephalad to vertebral body L2, although it can extend to the superior aspect of L3 (DiPietro, 1993). The conus levels varied little with age. However, a study which included premature infants showed a few conus tips extending to L3–L4 (Wolf et al., 1992). The vertebral level of the conus tip can be determined in several ways. One can simply note the level by looking at the patient's back while scanning. A high lumbar position is normal, and a low lumbosacral position is abnormal. Vertebral levels can be counted sonographically using the lowest rib bearing vertebra (Fig. 9–46) or the lumbosacral (L5–S1) junction recognized by its angle similar to a lateral radiograph (Beek et al., 1994) (see Figs. 9–34C and 9–35E). When looking for the lowest rib sonographically, one must scan far enough laterally (i.e., over the kidneys) so that lumbar trans-

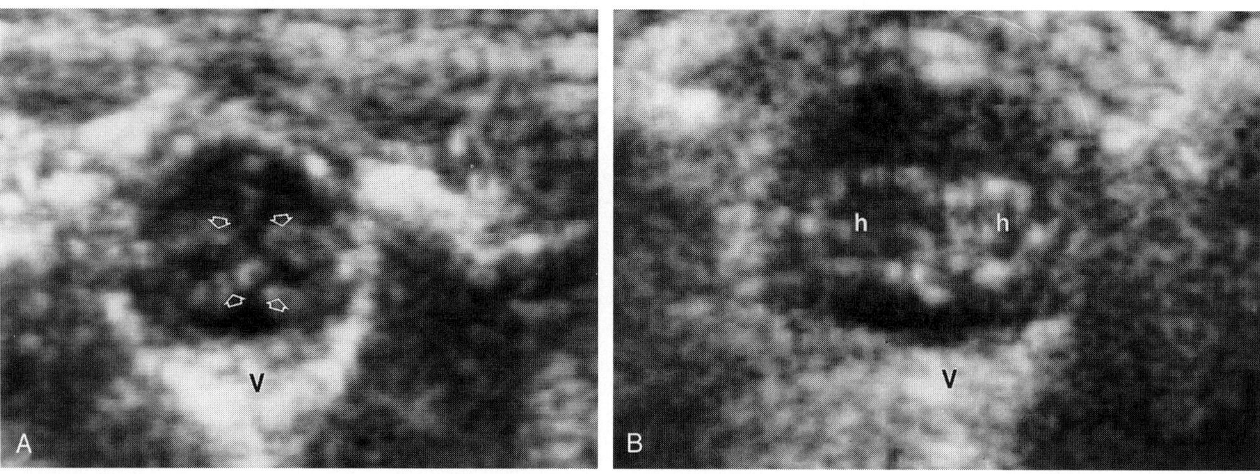

Figure 9–37 ■ **A**, Transverse view of the dorsal and ventral nerve roots (*arrowheads*) at the cauda equina, not to be mistaken for diastematomyelia (*see* **B**). Abbreviation: vertebral body (*V*). **B**, Transverse view of the right and left hemicords (*h*) in diastematomyelia. Abbreviation: vertebral body (*V*). (Reprinted with permission from DiPietro MA. The pediatric spinal canal. In Rumack CM, Wilson SR, Charboneau JW (eds), *Diagnostic Ultrasound,* ed 2. New York, Mosby, 1998.)

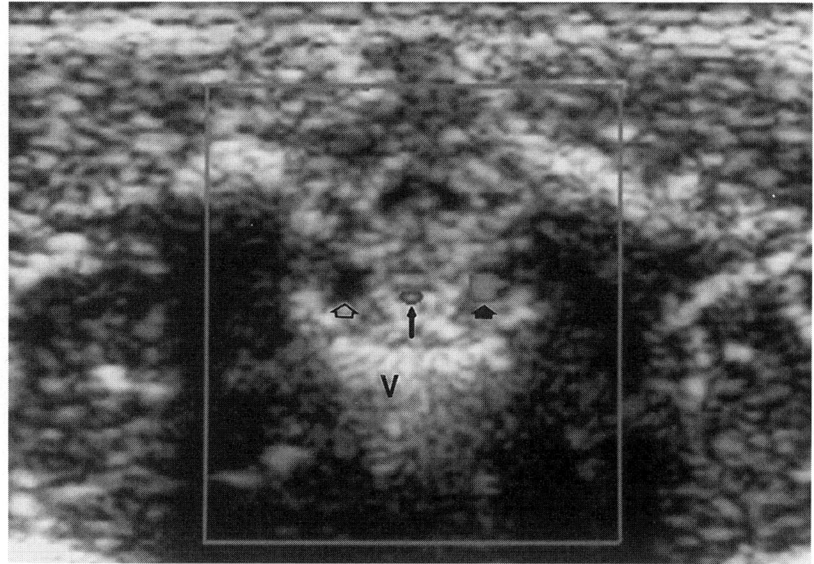

Figure 9–38 ■ Normal color flow Doppler imaging (filmed in black and white) at the conus medullaris. Bilateral ventral epidural veins (*arrowheads*) without (*open arrowhead*) and with (*solid arrowhead*) flow signal. The central flow signal (*straight arrow*) is in the anterior spinal artery. Abbreviation: vertebral body (*V*). (Reprinted with permission from DiPietro MA. The pediatric spinal canal. In Rumack CM, Wilson SR, Charboneau JW (eds), *Diagnostic Ultrasound,* ed 2. New York, Mosby, 1998.)

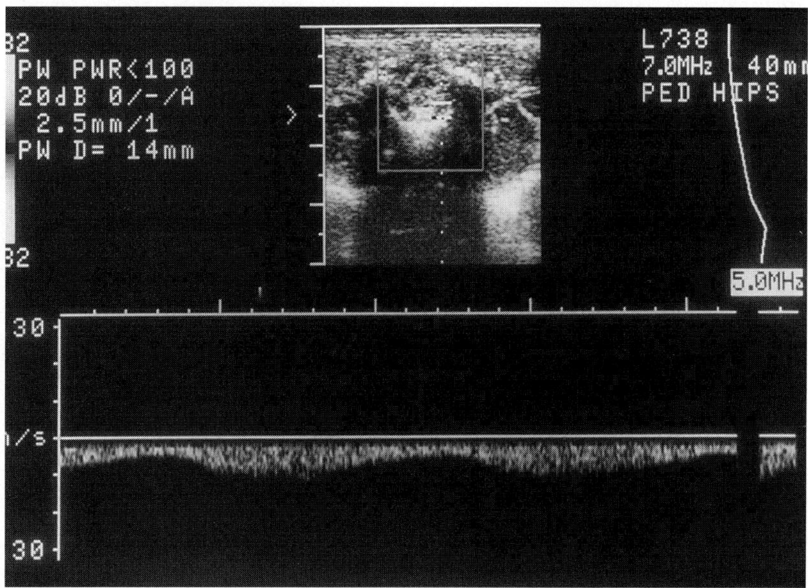

Figure 9–39 ■ Doppler waveform from the right epidural vein at the level of the conus.

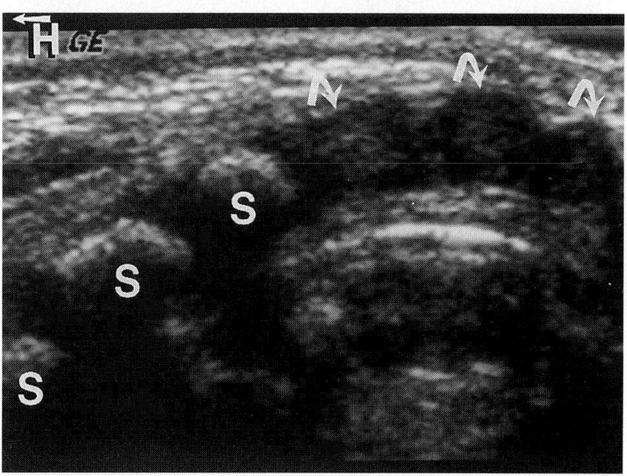

Figure 9–40 ■ Sagittal 13 MHz view of the neonatal sacrum showing ossified sacral vertebral bodies (*S*) and unossified coccygeal segments (*curved arrows*).

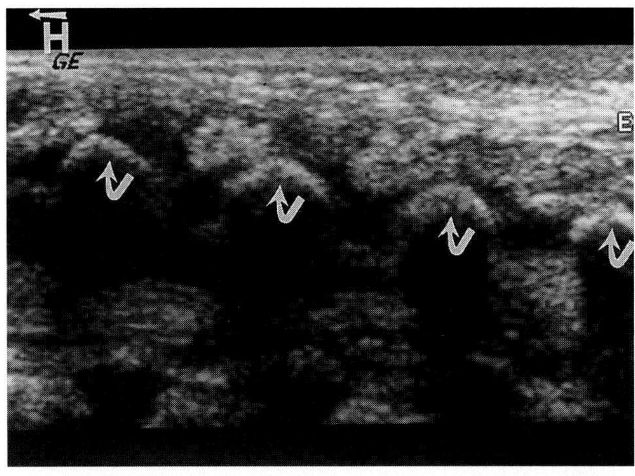

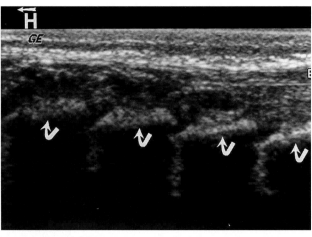

Figure 9–41 ■ Sagittal view of spinous processes (*curved arrows*).

Figure 9–42 ■ Sagittal view of laminae (*curved arrows*).

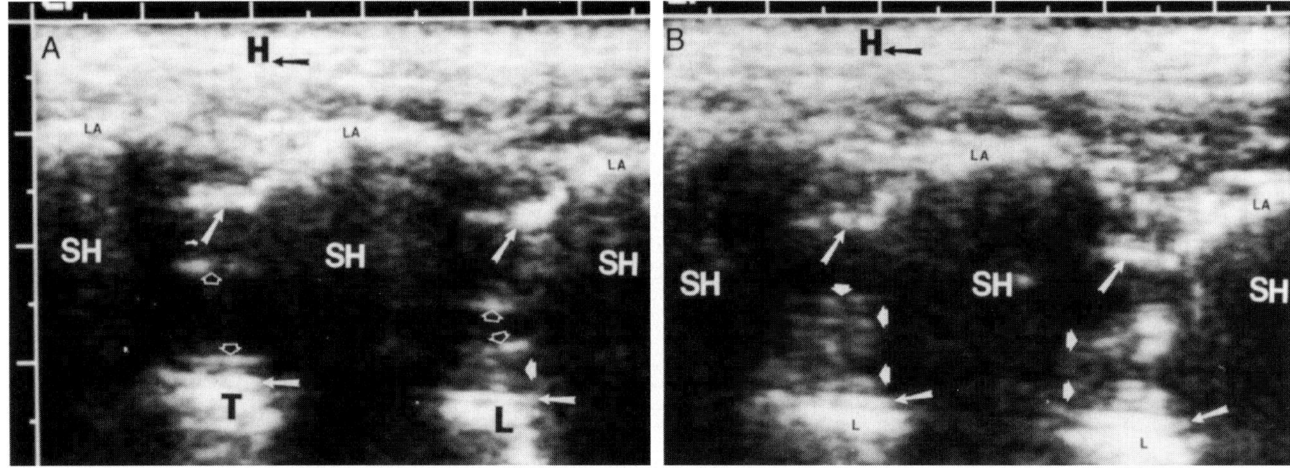

Figure 9–43 ■ Sagittal views of the low thoracic to midlumbar spinal canal in a 9-year-old child. **A**, Normal tapering of the spinal cord (*open arrowheads*) indicating the position of the conus medullaris at the thoracolumbar junction. **B**, At the next sequential caudal levels, the cord is no longer seen. Only echogenic strands of the cauda equina (*closed arrowheads*) are visible. Abbreviations: laminae (*LA*) with shadowing (*SH*), dura (*arrows*), thoracic vertebrae (*T*), lumbar vertebrae (*L*).

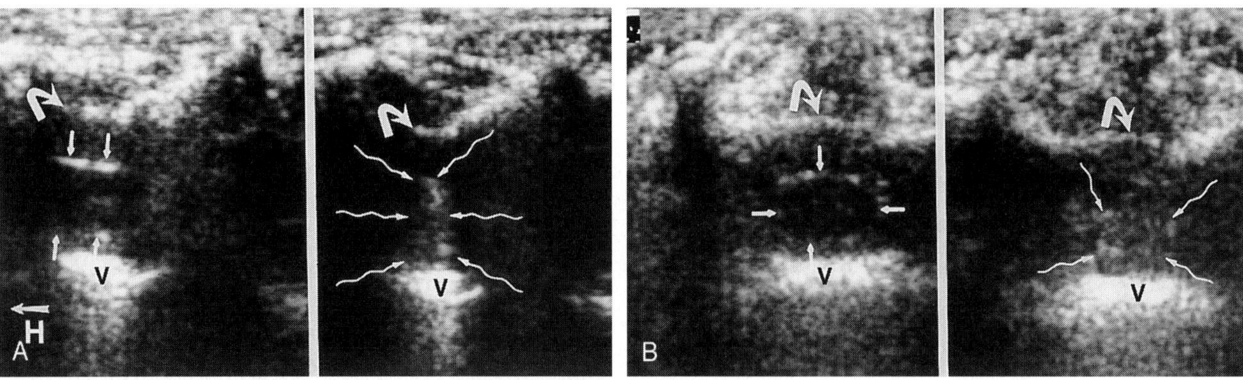

Figure 9–44 ■ Normal conus in a 9-year-old child. **A**, Sagittal views. **B**, Transverse views. Consecutive levels displayed on split screens show the cord (*straight arrows*) in the high lumbar canal, but the next lower vertebral level (*the right frames of the split screens*) show only the cauda equina (*wavy arrows*). Abbreviations: dorsal dura (*curved arrows*), vertebral bodies (*V*). (Reprinted with permission from DiPietro MA. The pediatric spinal canal. In Rumack CM, Wilson SR, Charboneau JW (eds), *Diagnostic Ultrasound,* ed 2. New York, Mosby, 1998.)

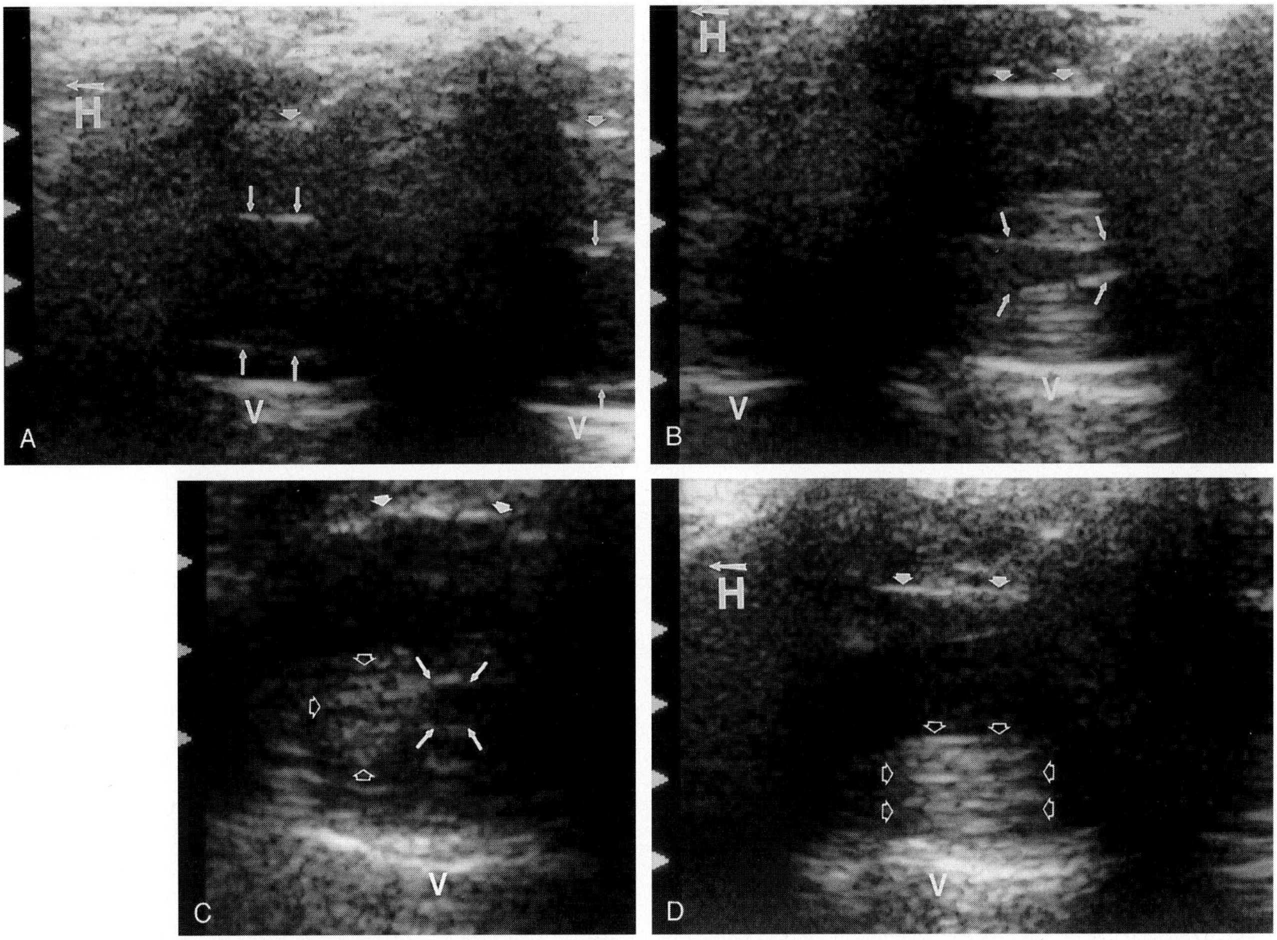

Figure 9–45 ■ Normal cord, conus, and cauda equina at 9 MHz in a 7-year-old child. **A**, Sagittal low thoracic upper lumbar cord. Abbreviations: spinal cord (*arrows*), dorsal dura (*arrowheads*), vertebral bodies (*V*). **B**, Sagittal conus (*arrows*) with surrounding echogenic cauda equina. Abbreviations: dorsal dura (*arrowheads*), vertebral bodies (*V*). **C**, Transverse conus (*arrows*) and adjacent cauda equina (*open arrowheads*). Abbreviations: dorsal dura (*solid arrowheads*), vertebral body (*V*). **D**, Sagittal cauda equina (*open arrowheads*). Abbreviations: dorsal dura (*solid arrowheads*), vertebral body (*V*).

verse processes are not mistaken for ribs. One can count cephalad from the sacrum, noting that the neonatal coccyx is cartilaginous (Beek et al., 1994) (Fig. 9–47) and that the caudal tip of the thecal sac often corresponds to S2 (Koroshetz and Taveras, 1986) (see Figs. 9–34C and 9–35E). Since landmarks can vary (e.g., a patient might have 11 or 13 ribs), a questionable conus position somewhere in the midlumbar region may warrant careful marking of the position of the conus tip on the skin with a radiopaque marker and then obtaining a radiograph to verify the level.

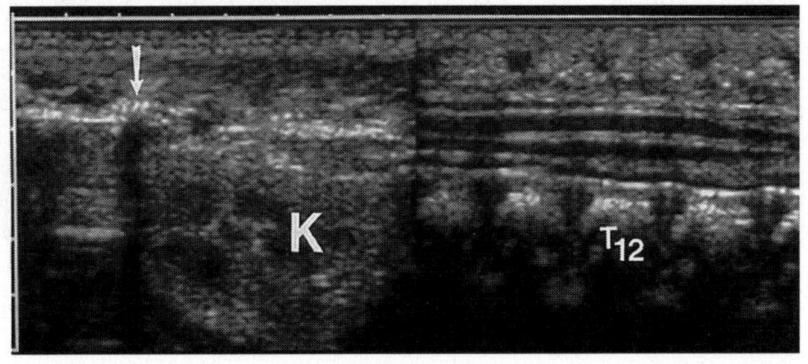

Figure 9–46 ■ Longitudinal split screen showing a method of estimating vertebral levels. The left frame identifies the lowest rib (*arrow*) over the kidney (*K*). The rib is followed back to the spine sonographically to presumably identify T_{12}, as noted in the right frame. (Reprinted with permission from DiPietro MA, Garver KA. Sonography of the neonatal spinal canal. In Haller JO (ed), *Textbook of Neonatal Ultrasound*. New York, Parthenon Publishing Group, 1998.)

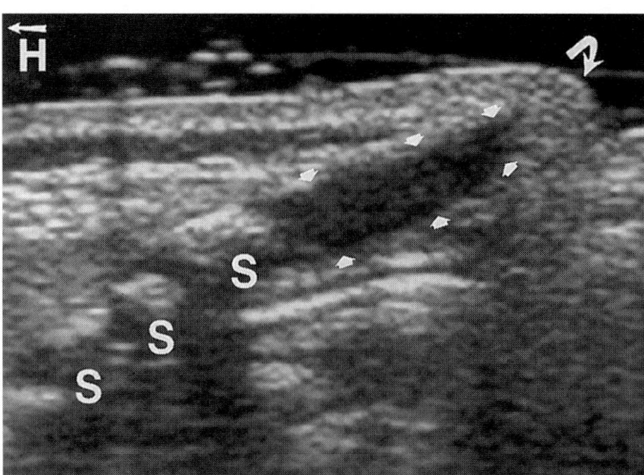

Figure 9–47 ■ Sagittal view of the unossified neonatal coccyx (*arrowheads*). The coccygeal tip causes a slight protrusion (*curved arrow*) of the skin in this case. Abbreviation: ossified sacral elements (*S*).

The hypoechoic coccyx should not be mistaken for a pilonidal cyst when scanning a baby with a low sacrococcygeal cutaneous dimple. This should be less of a problem with the use of newer high-frequency transducers which clearly show the cartilaginous nature of distinct individual coccygeal segments (see Fig. 9–40). Occasionally a pilonidal cyst (Fig. 9–48) or a sinus tract (Fig. 9–49) is detected. A tiny hairline tract could be missed, and the caretakers of a child with a deep cutaneous dimple are advised to see their clinical physician if the dimple ever exudes fluid or looks inflamed.

The Tethered Spinal Cord

Pediatric spinal canal sonography is requested most commonly to detect an occult tethered spinal cord which is suspected because of a midline (or near-midline) cutaneous abnormality on the back such as hemangioma (Albright et al., 1989), dermal sinus, dimple, skin tag, hairy patch, aplasia cutis (Higginbottom et al., 1980), or subcutaneous lipoma. These lesions can be stigmata of an underlying tethered cord which can be asymptomatic, especially in early infancy (Powell et al., 1975; Hall et al., 1981; Kriss and Desai, 1998). The tethered cord is a pathological fixation of the spinal cord in an abnormal caudal location, so that the cord suffers mechanical stretching, distortion and ischemia with daily activities, growth and development (Reigel, 1983). Neurologic deficits include reflex changes, sensory and motor loss, weakness, and sphincter problems. The child may be neurologically intact at birth but develops progressive deficits with growth spurts

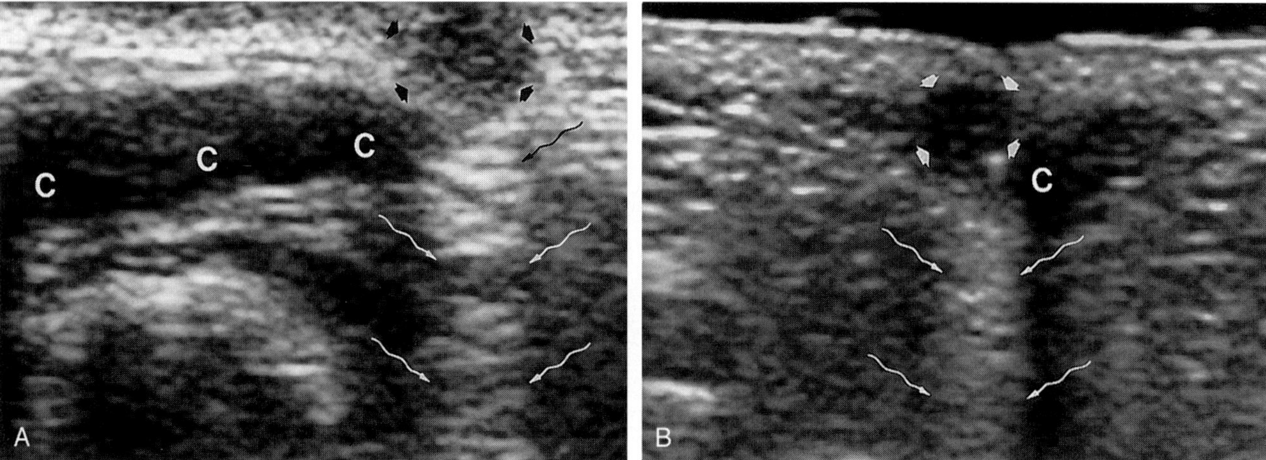

Figure 9–48 ■ Small subcutaneous pilonidal cyst (*arrowheads*) with through-transmission (*wavy arrows*) adjacent to unossified coccyx (*C*). **A,** Sagittal view. **B,** Transverse view.

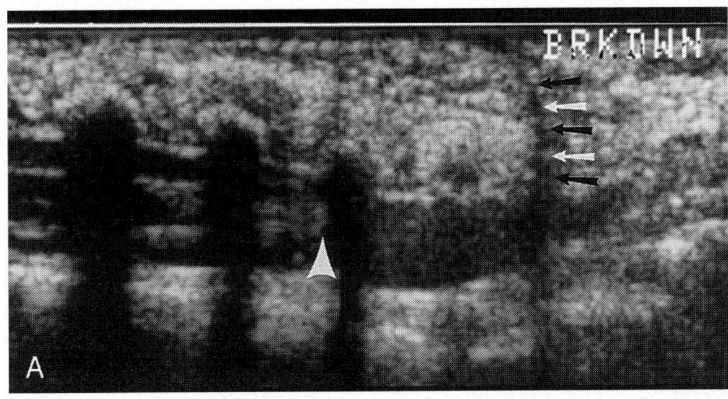

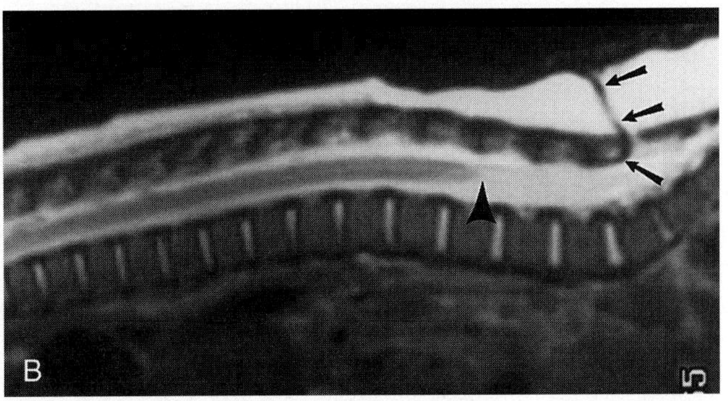

Figure 9-49 ▪ Dermal sinus (*arrows*) at the lumbosacral junction extending to the spinal canal. Abbreviation: conus tip (*arrowhead*). **A**, Sagittal sonogram. **B**, Sagittal MRI scan. (Reprinted with permission from DiPietro MA, Garver KA. Sonography of the neonatal spinal canal. In Haller JO (ed), *Textbook of Neonatal Ultrasound.* New York, Parthenon Publishing Group, 1998.)

(Hoffman et al., 1985) which include abnormal gait or lower-extremity deformity (Anderson, 1975; Lhowe et al., 1987). Progressive neurological impairment results from stretching of the cord as the child grows. It is generally thought that early detection of a tethered cord is important so that it can be released early, before neurological deficit progresses with growth of the child (Till, 1968; Hall et al., 1981; Fone et al., 1997). However, questions regarding the need to untether the cords of asymptomatic and neurologically intact children have been raised (Bodensteiner, 1995; Pierre-Kahn et al., 1997).

Spinal sonography is requested most commonly for the child with a sacral cutaneous dimple. Dimples are common findings and were present in 1.4% of a series of 1997 consecutive newborns. In addition, there were 1.2% "presumed sinuses" in this study, which predated the availability of sonography (Powell et al., 1975). The very caudal, shallow, central cutaneous pit which is visible only after the buttocks have been separated and which has no other additional cutaneous stigmata is unlikely to have an underlying occult tethered cord (Radkowski et al., 1990; Gibson et al., 1995; Kriss and Desai, 1998). However, it should be very caudal, very shallow, not eccentric, and without an asymmetric skin fold or any other abnormality (M.A. Radkowski, personal communication, 1999).

Appearance and Causes of Tethered Cord

The tethered cord is usually recognized by its extension into the low lumbar or sacral canal (Fig. 9-50). Cords can be tethered by lipoma (can be associated with lipomyeloschisis or lipomyelomeningocele), fibrolipoma, thick or tight filum terminale, diastematomyelia, meningocele, myelomeningocele (or myeloschisis), or a combination of these (Reigel, 1983; Gusnard et al., 1986; Naidich et al., 1986; Raghavendra et al., 1988; Zieger et al., 1988; Nelson et al., 1989; Glasier et al., 1990; Kaffenberger et al., 1992; Korsvik and Keller, 1992; Kriss et al., 1995a; Kriss et al., 1996; DiPietro, 1998; DiPietro and Garver, 1998; Kriss and Desai, 1998). Myelomeningoele and myeloschisis are open (i.e., not skin-covered) forms of spinal dysraphism referred to as *spina bifida aperta.* The others are skin-covered and are associated with occult tethering of the spinal cord. When associated with dysraphism they are referred to as *spina bifida occulta.* Subcutaneous lipomas over the lower back are highly suspect for an associated occult tethered cord. The lipoma often extends into the canal through focal midline defects in dura, bone, muscle, and fascia, attaches to the cord, and tethers it (Fig. 9-51). The types of intraspinal lipomas vary with respect to their sites of insertion in the spinal canal, attaching to meninges, cord, conus, filum terminale, or a combination of these. Many terms are used in reference to intraspinal lipomas, sometimes interchangeably. The subarachnoid space and cord bulge through the spina bifida into subcutaneous tissues, forming a *lipomyelomeningocele.* If the meninges do not bulge and the cord remains intracanalicular, it is a *lipomyelocele. Leptomyelolipoma* refers to a lipoma with a subcutaneous component and a large direct interface with the cord (Emery and Lendon, 1969; Chapman, 1982). *Lipomyeloschisis,* as the three roots comprising the word

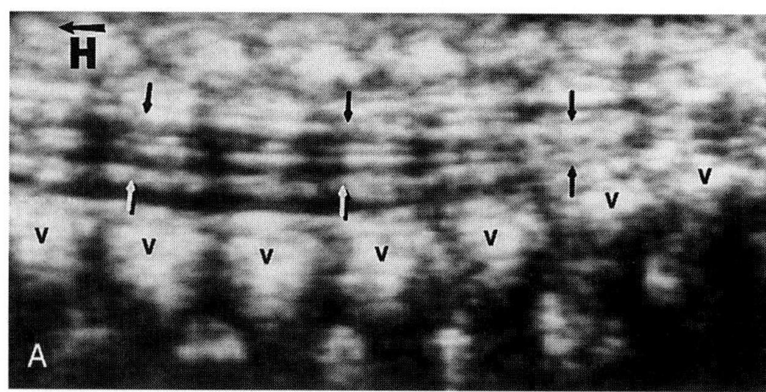

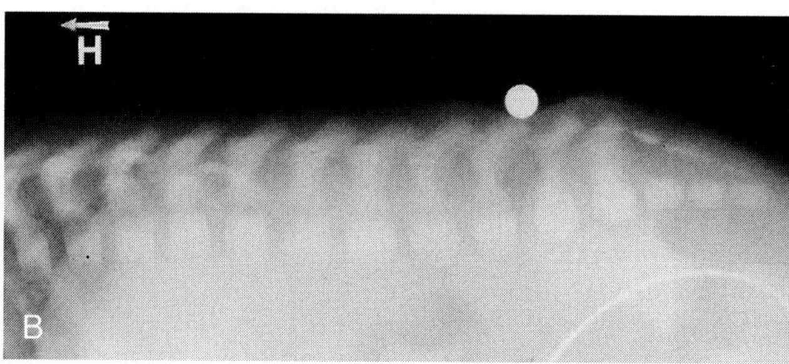

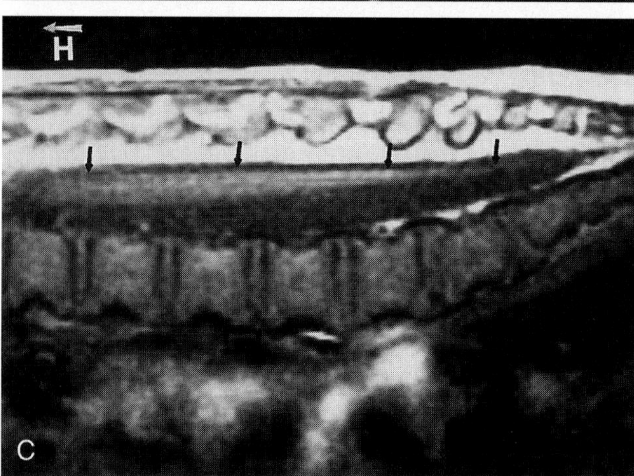

Figure 9–50 ■ **A**, Sagittal sonogram of the lumbosacral canal shows the spinal cord (*arrows*) extending to the sacral canal in a neonate with imperforate anus. Abbreviation: vertebral bodies (*V*). **B**, Lateral radiograph of the same neonate's lumbosacral spine shows the marker at the low level of the conus, as determined on sonography and the wide sacral canal. **C**, Sagittal MRI scan in the same baby confirming the tethered spinal cord (*arrows*). (Reprinted with permission from DiPietro MA. The pediatric spinal canal. In Rumack CM, Wilson SR, Charboneau JW (eds), *Diagnostic Ultrasound,* ed 2. New York, Mosby, 1998.)

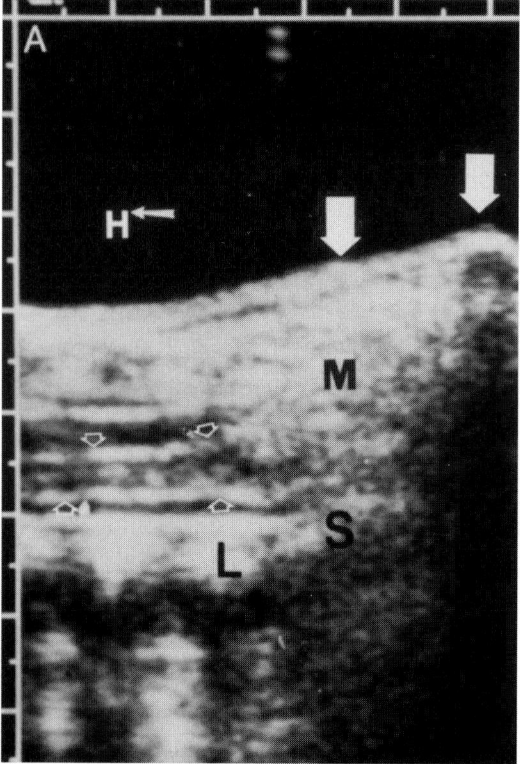

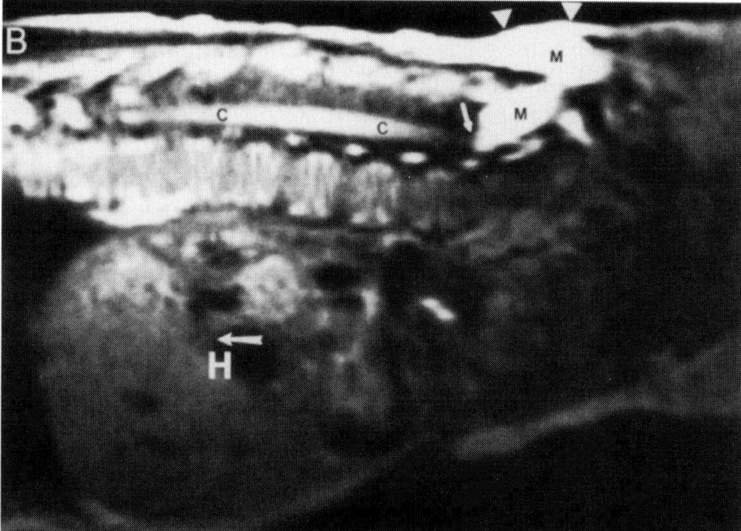

Figure 9–51 ■ **A**, Sagittal sonogram. **B**, Sagittal MRI scan. Eight-week-old infant with an intraspinal lipoma and a tethered spinal cord. The spinal cord (*C and open arrowheads*) is seen extending to the lumbosacral (*L, S*) junction, where it is connected to a large, echogenic fatty mass (*M*), which extends into the subcutaneous soft tissues and causes a visible bump (*solid arrowheads*) on the patient's back.

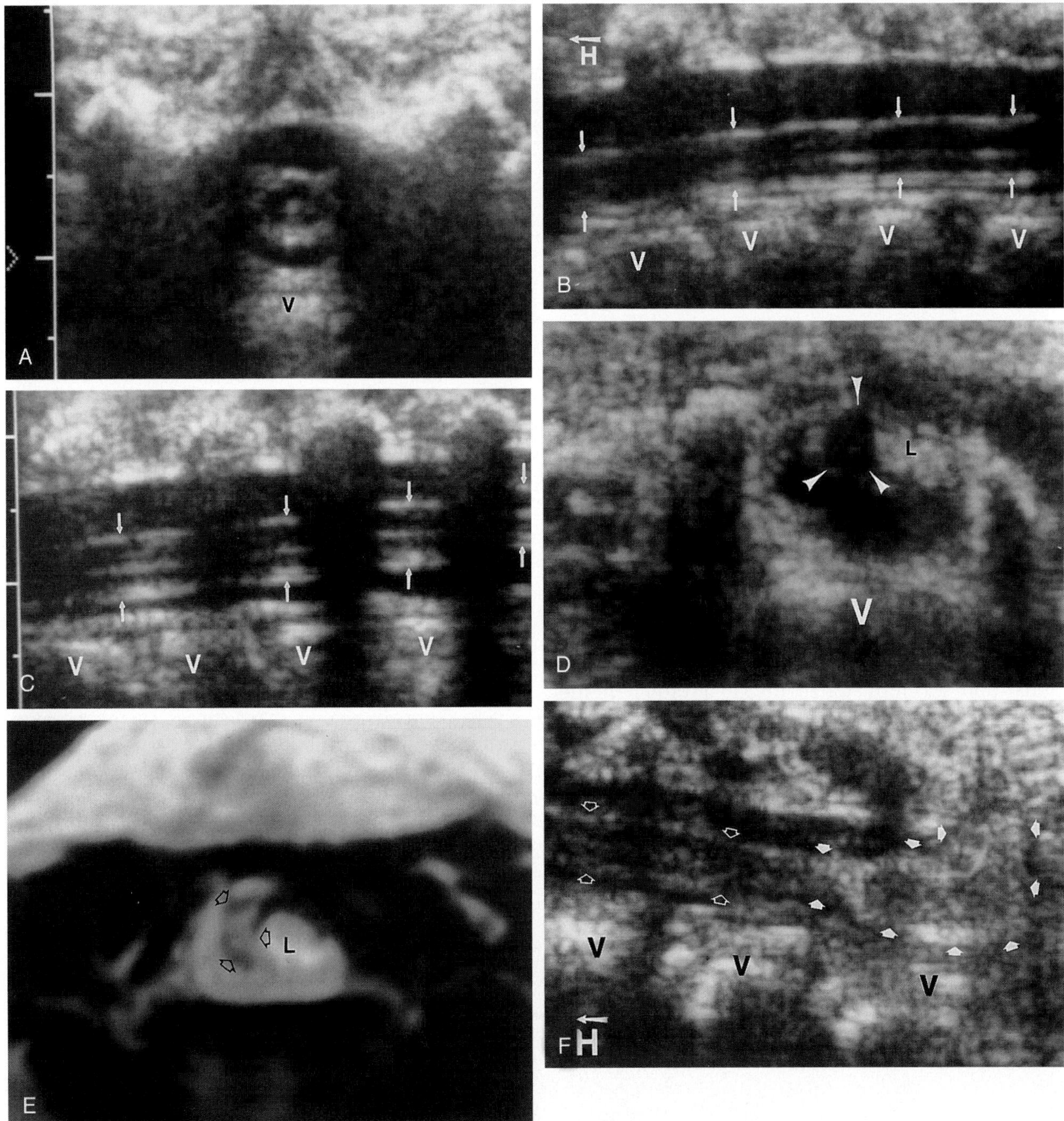

Figure 9–52 ■ Spinal cord tethered by a lipoma in the low lumbar canal. **A**, Transverse sonogram of the midlumbar cord, cephalad to the tethering. Abbreviation: vertebral body (*V*). **B**, Longitudinal sonogram of the lower thoracic–upper lumbar cord (*arrows*) cephalad to the tethering. Abbreviation: vertebral bodies (*V*). **C**, Longitudinal sonogram of the midlumbar cord (*arrows*), cephalad to the tethering. The tethered cord extends dorsally as well as caudally. Abbreviation: vertebral bodies (*V*). **D**, Transverse sonogram of the low lumbar canal showing the cord (*arrowheads*) tethered dorsally and caudally by an intracanalicular lipoma (*L*) to the right of the cord. Abbreviation: vertebral body (*V*). **E**, Transverse MRI of the low lumbar canal, as in (*D*). The cord (*arrowheads*) is tethered dorsally and caudally by the intracanalicular lipoma (*L*) on its right. **F**, Sagittal sonogram of the lumbosacral canal showing the cord (*open arrowheads*) tethered in the low lumbar canal by the lipoma (*solid arrowheads*). Abbreviation: vertebral bodies (*V*).

Figure continued on following page

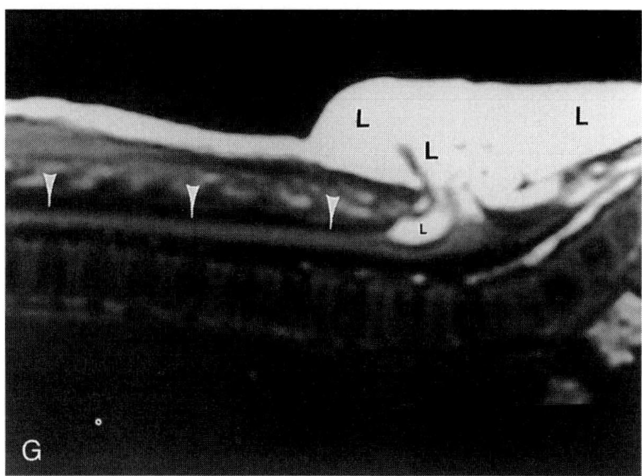

Figure 9-52 *Continued* ■ **G**, Sagittal MRI scan of the lumbosacral canal, as in (**F**). The cord (*arrowheads*) is tethered at the lumbosacral junction by the lipoma (*L*), which extends from the subcutaneous tissues into the spinal canal. (Reprinted with permission from DiPietro MA, Garver KA. Sonography of the neonatal spinal canal. In Haller JO (ed), *Textbook of Neonatal Ultrasound*. New York, Parthenon Publishing Group, 1998.)

indicate, refers to dorsal dysraphism and lipoma attached to the dorsal aspect of the partially cleft cord (Naidich et al., 1983). These entities are not mutually exclusive. Leptomyelolipoma and lipomyeloschisis include intradural lipoma, lipomyelocele, and lipomyelomeningocele, depending on the position of the meninges and cord. Myelomeningocele is an entirely different malformation from lipomyelomeningocele, with different embryology and pathological anatomy. It will be discussed separately (vide infra).

The caudal aspect of the cord is tethered in a caudal and eccentric (often dorsal) position in the spinal canal (Figs. 9-52 and 9-53). In addition, normal brisk spinal cord oscillations are often absent or damped in the region of the tether. In regard to normal spinal cord oscillation, brisk dorsoventral oscillations of the cord and cauda equina are normally evident during real-time scanning after 1 or 2 months of age. These oscillations occur at the heart rate. They might be seen in the neonatal period, but they are not always apparent. Some slower cord motion may be seen as the neonate moves, breathes, or cries. The brisk oscillation of the cord can be documented on M-mode sonography (Zieger and Dorr, 1988; Schumacher et al., 1992). Loss of or diminished oscillation near the level of tethering occurs often but not always. Oscillation usually remains brisk distant from the tether and is progressively damped as one scans closer to the point of tethering, often as the cord is assuming a more eccentric position within the canal. However,

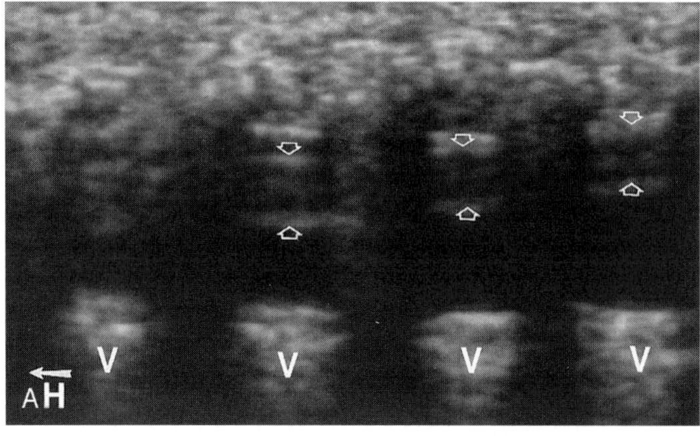

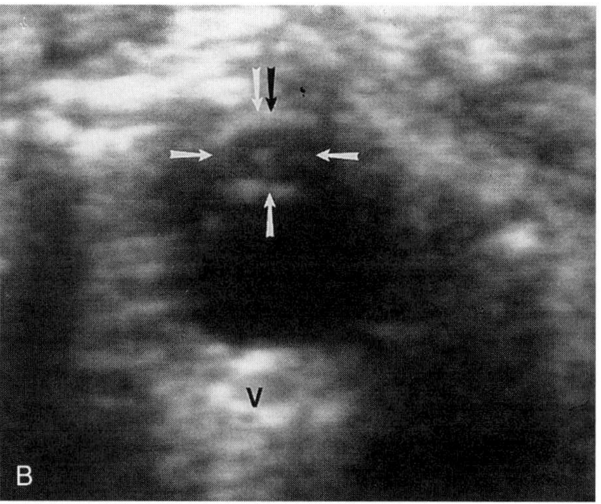

Figure 9-53 ■ **A**, Longitudinal sonogram of the low lumbar canal. The tethered cord (*arrowheads*) is too dorsal and caudal. Abbreviation: vertebral bodies (*V*). **B**, Transverse sonogram of the low lumbar canal, as in (**A**). The dorsal position of the tethered cord (*arrows*) is striking. Abbreviation: vertebral body (*V*). (Reprinted with permission from DiPietro MA. The pediatric spinal canal. In Rumack CM, Wilson SR, Charboneau JW (eds), *Diagnostic Ultrasound*, ed 2. New York, Mosby, 1998.)

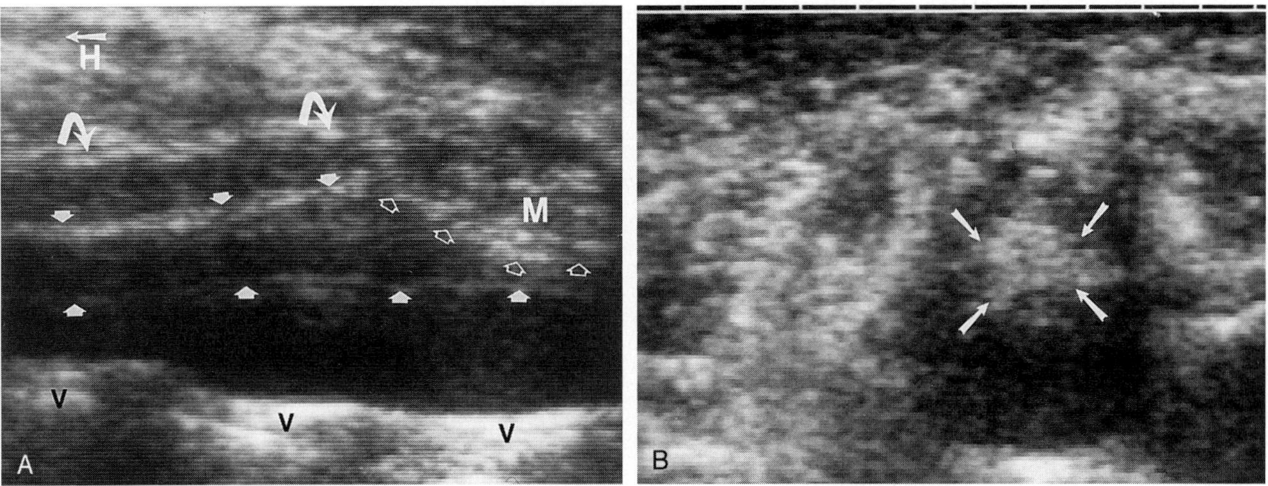

Figure 9–54 ■ Repaired lipomyelomeningocele in a 3-year-old girl. **A**, Longitudinal sonogram shows some residual lipoma (*M*) and the cord–lipoma interface (*open arrowheads*) on the cord's (*solid arrowheads*) dorsal surface. *Curved arrows* denote the dorsal dura. Abbreviation: vertebral body (*V*). **B**, Transverse sonogram shows a residual echogenic lipoma (*arrows*). (Reprinted with permission from DiPietro MA. The pediatric spinal canal. In Rumack CM, Wilson SR, Charboneau JW (eds), *Diagnostic Ultrasound,* ed 2. New York, Mosby, 1998.)

oscillation may be normal in the young (i.e. smaller) child with an obviously tethered cord. Oscillation will probably diminish as the child grows if the tethered cord is not released.

The lipoma–cord interface can be intimate with lipomatous infiltration of the cord, rendering complete resection of the lipoma from the cord difficult and hazardous. Resection is limited to that necessary to untether the cord safely (Hoffman et al., 1985). Understandably, some residual lipoma will be noted on postoperative scanning (Fig. 9–54), although the cord should be less eccentric within the canal and should oscillate more freely than it did preoperatively.

Diastematomyelia (Fig. 9–37B) with focal sagittal splitting of the cord, conus, or filum terminale is a cause of tethered cord which can occur alone or in conjunction with other tethering lesions, such as myelomeningocele. The septum splitting the cord can be osseous, fibrous, or cartilaginous, and the vertebral column is almost always abnormal (Naidich et al., 1986). Associated spina bifida provides an acoustic window; on the other hand, intersegmental laminar fusion, which is also common with diastematomyelia, impedes visualization (Naidich et al., 1986).

Associated Caudal Malformations

Malformations including imperforate anus (anorectal atresia), cloacal exstrophy, and caudal regression have an increased incidence of occult tethered cord and are therefore routinely screened (Tunnell et al., 1987; Karrer et al., 1988; Appignani et al., 1994; Nievelstein et al., 1994; Beek et al., 1995; Tsakayannis et al., 1995; Long et al., 1996). Although in one series the incidence of tethered cord was greatest in patients with high imperforate anus (44%), it was also substantial in patients with low imperforate anus (27%). Fifty-two percent of those tethered cords were asymptomatic, and 26% had no vertebral anomaly (Long et al., 1996). Therefore, we perform screening spinal sonography on all babies with imperforate anus, regardless of its level or the spine radiographic findings. Sacral anomalies, including crescentic or scimitar-shaped sacra, can occur with or without imperforate anus. These patients and patients with an increased interpediculate distance in the spine are screened for occult tethered cord (Yates et al., 1983). Children with the Currarino triad of ectopic, stenotic, or imperforate anus, crescentic sacrum, and a presacral mass (anterior meningocele, teratoma, or enteric cyst) have also been reported to have tethered cord and intradural lipoma (Currarino et al., 1981; Kirks et al., 1984; Gudinchet et al., 1997).

Normal Variants and Hydromyelia

The central echo complex in the lower neonatal cord and conus often appears as a pair of dots and a pair of lines in the transverse and longitudinal views, respectively (Fig. 9–55). This is a common normal finding and should not be mistaken for

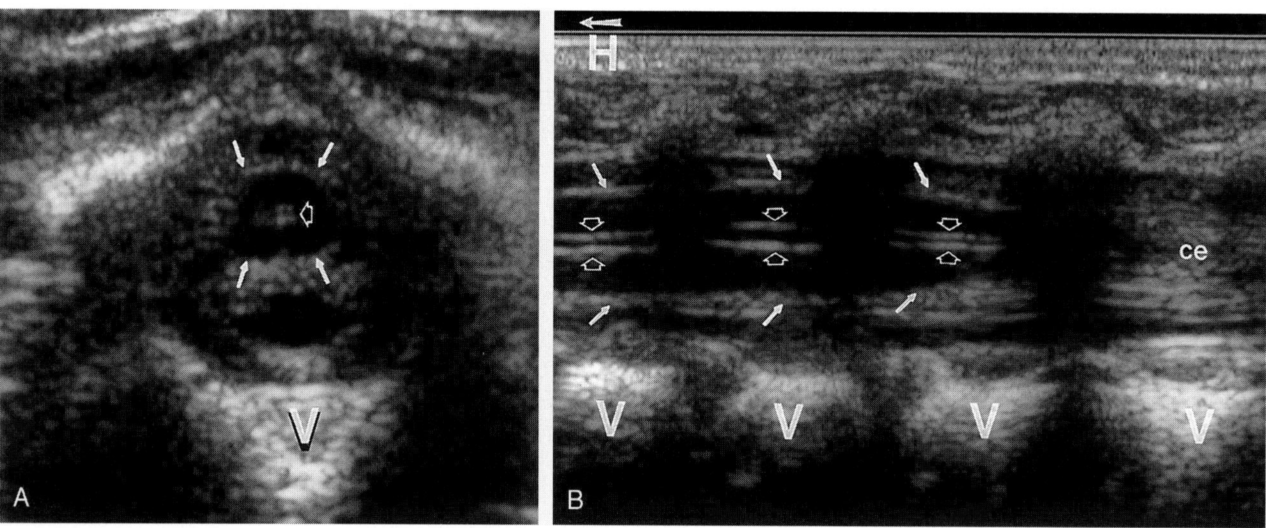

Figure 9-55 ■ **A**, Transverse sonogram and **B**, longitudinal sonogram of the low thoracic- upper lumbar cord (*arrows*) in a neonate. The central echo complex appears as two lines (*open arrowheads*). Abbreviations: vertebral bodies (*V*), cauda equina (*ce*).

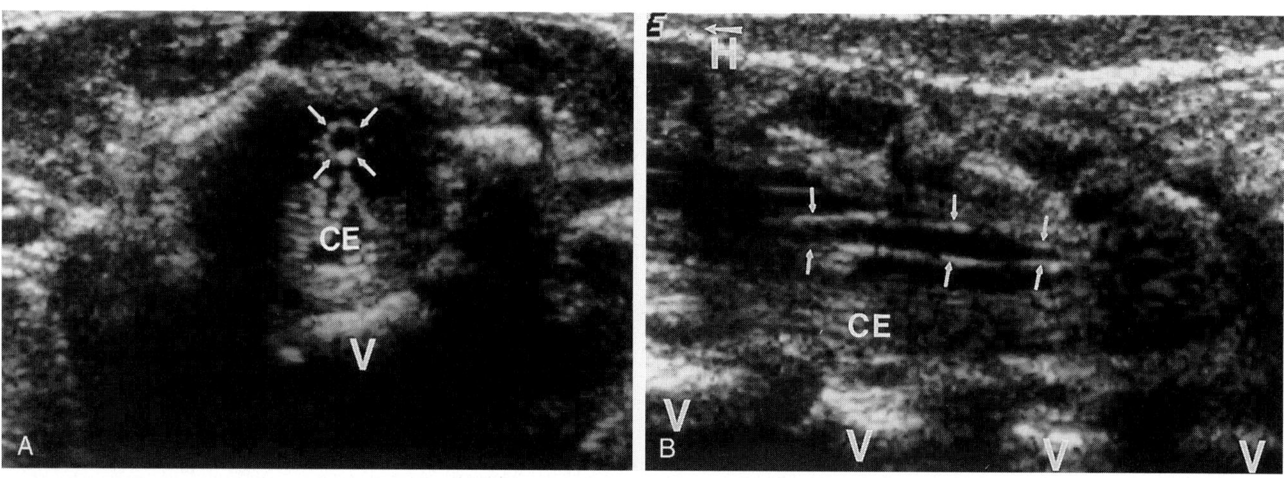

Figure 9-56 ■ **A**, Transverse sonogram and **B**, longitudinal sonogram of the filum terminale (*arrows*), which is mildly distended with fluid (a "filar cyst"). Abbreviations: cauda equina (*CE*), vertebral bodies (*V*).

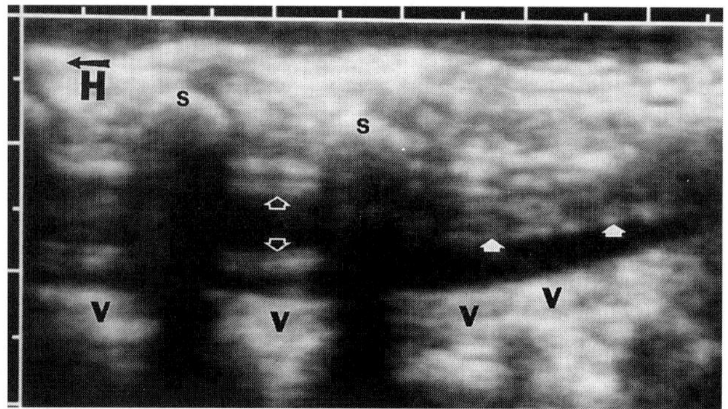

Figure 9-57 ■ Longitudinal sonogram of a 3-month-old boy with a repaired myelomeningocele, with cord extending into the sacral canal. The most caudal portion of the cord (*solid arrowheads*) is thin and echogenic. The low lumbar cord has marked hydromyelia (*open arrowheads*). Abbreviations: vertebral bodies (*V*), spinous processes with shadowing (*S*). (Reprinted with permission from DiPietro MA. The pediatric spinal canal. In Rumack CM, Wilson SR, Charboneau JW (eds), *Diagnostic Ultrasound*, ed 2. New York, Mosby, 1998.)

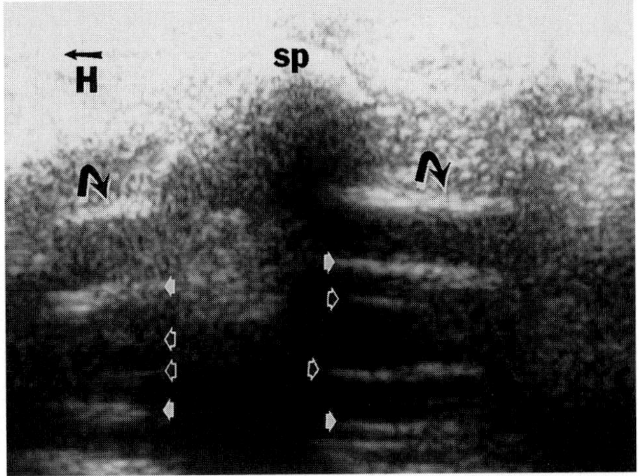

Figure 9–58 ■ Longitudinal sonogram showing hydromyelia of the low thoracic cord. Abbreviations: dilated central canal (*open arrowheads*), dorsal and ventral margins of the cord (*solid arrowheads*), dorsal aspect of spinal canal (*curved arrows*), spinous process with shadowing (*sp*).

hydromyelia. Sometimes there is a more prominent focal dilatation of the central canal in the lower cord and conus, a persistent terminal ventricle, which is an insignificant anatomical variant (Coleman et al., 1995; Kriss et al., 1995b; Rypens et al., 1995). It is an embryological remnant, a result of incomplete regression of the caudal neural tube formed from the caudal cell mass between gestational weeks 4 and 7. The caudal cell mass regresses to form the conus and the filum terminale. It therefore seems possible that the small filar cyst which is sometimes seen within an otherwise normal filum terminale is also a

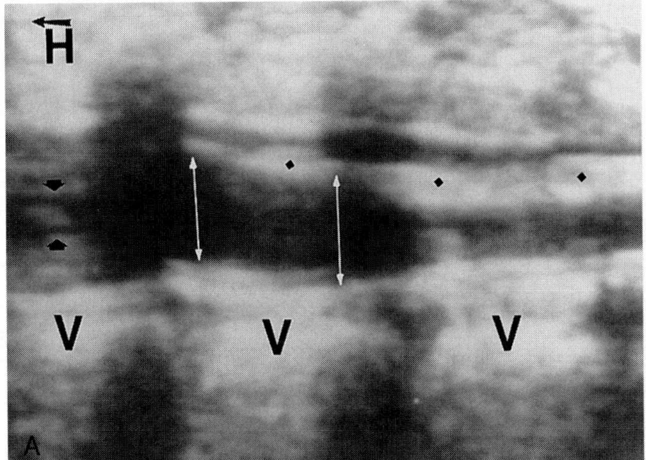

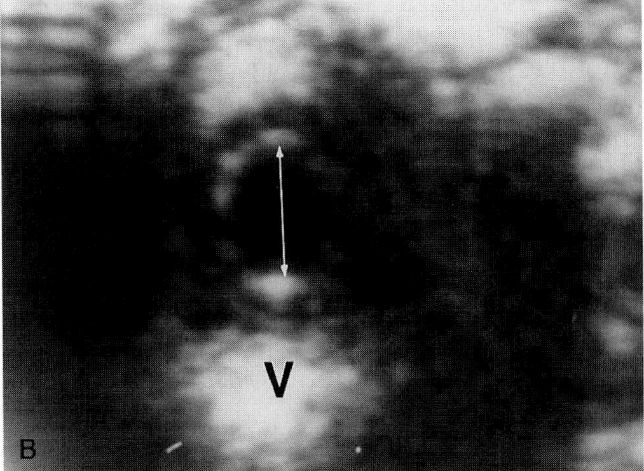

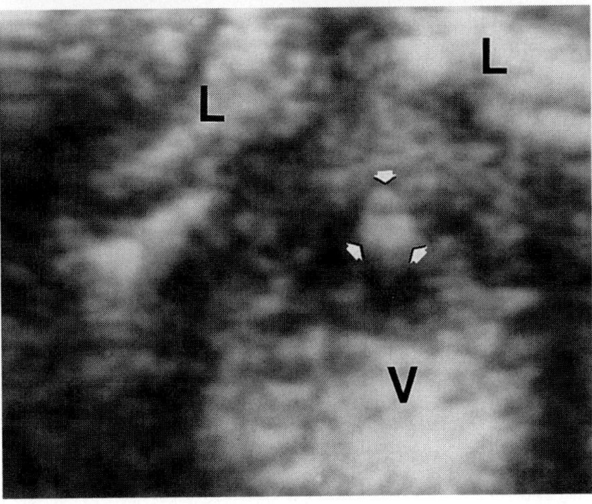

Figure 9–59 ■ **A**, Longitudinal sonogram of a large filar cyst (*double-headed arrows*) caudal to the spinal cord (*arrowheads*) and a thick filum terminale (*black diamonds*) more caudally. Abbreviation: vertebral bodies (*V*). **B**, Transverse sonogram of the large filar cyst (*double-headed arrow*). Abbreviation: vertebral body (*V*). **C**, Transverse sonogram more caudally through the thick filum terminale (*arrowheads*). Abbreviations: vertebral body (*V*), laminae (*L*). (Reprinted with permission from DiPietro MA, Garver KA. Sonography of the neonatal spinal canal. In Haller JO (ed), *Textbook of Neonatal Ultrasound*. New York, Parthenon Publishing Group, 1998.)

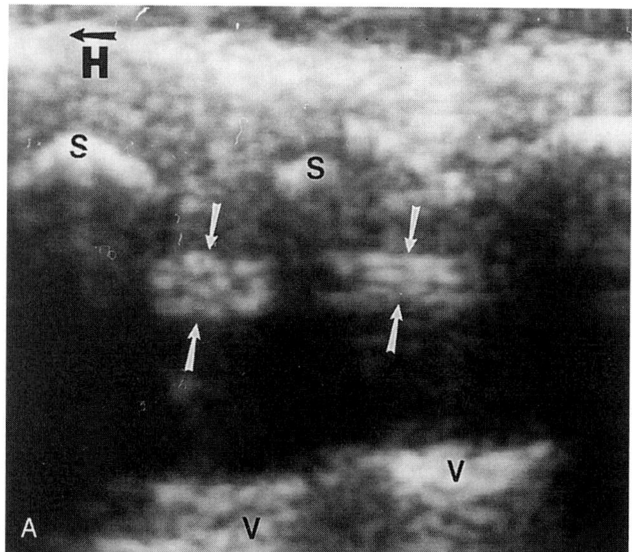

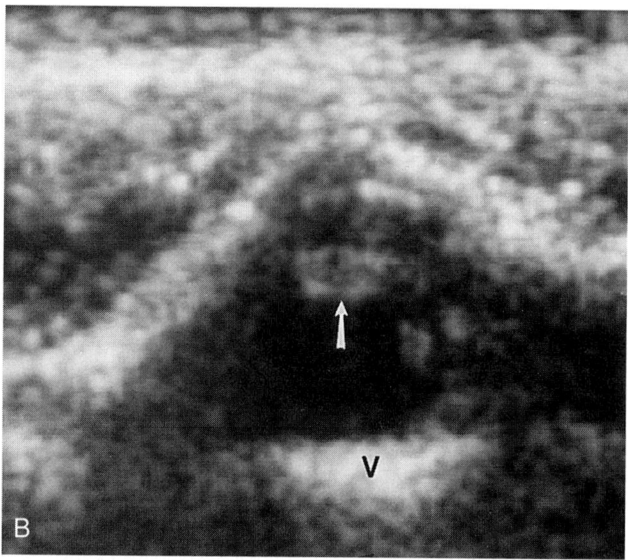

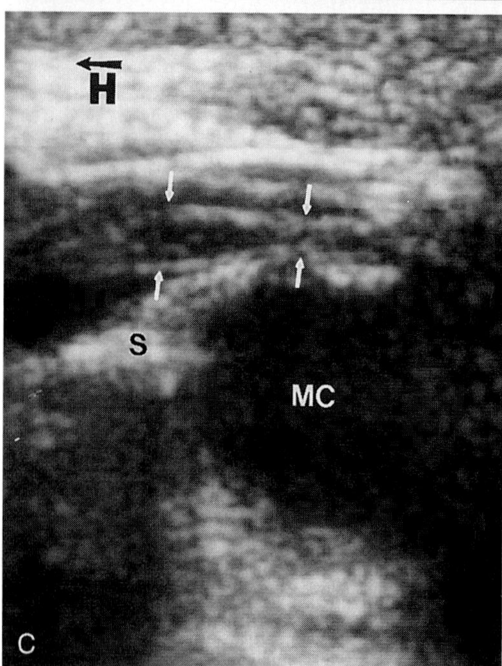

Figure 9-60 ■ **A**, Longitudinal sonogram of a thick filum terminale (*arrows*) in the sacral canal of a 6-year-old girl with a tethered cord. Abbreviations: vertebral bodies (*V*), spinous processes (*S*). **B**, Transverse sonogram through the thick filum terminale (*arrow*). Abbreviation: vertebral body (*V*). **C**, Longitudinal sonogram more caudally in the sacrum (*S*) showing the thick filum terminale (*arrows*) attached to an anterior meningocele (*MC*). (Reprinted with permission from DiPietro MA. The pediatric spinal canal. In Rumack CM, Wilson SR, Charboneau JW (eds), *Diagnostic Ultrasound,* ed 2. New York, Mosby, 1998.)

persistent terminal ventricle but within the caudal cell mass which regressed to form the filum terminale (Fig. 9-56). Another consideration is that it is a "thin arachnoid pseudocyst" (Rypens et al., 1995).

Tethered cords are associated with more extensive terminal syringohydromyelia (Fig. 9-57) (Iskandar et al., 1994). Hydromyelia can be noted on sonography (Fig. 9-58), but unless the patient is a neonate or young infant, its extent will be best seen on MRI.

Meningocele and Myelomeningocele

A cord can be tethered by a thick filum terminale (Fig. 9-59) which can exist alone or can accompany other malformations (Fig. 9-60). Meningoceles can be anterior (Fig. 9-60), posterior (Fig. 9-61), or even lateral. Meningoceles are usually considered to be empty sacs (see Fig. 9-60), but they can contain lace-like strands of "filmy arachnoid trabeculae" (Fig. 9-62) (Naidich and McLone, 1986). Dorsal bands of atretic neurovascular or fibrous tissue can even tether the cord in cases of meningocele or atretic (sacless) meningocele (i.e., meningocele manque) (Kaffenberger et al., 1992; Kriss et al., 1996). In contrast to meningocele, tubulation of the spinal cord is incomplete in myelomeningocele or myeloschisis. The role of sonography in these neonates is predominantly to evaluate the remainder of the cord for an additional lesion, such as diastematomyelia,

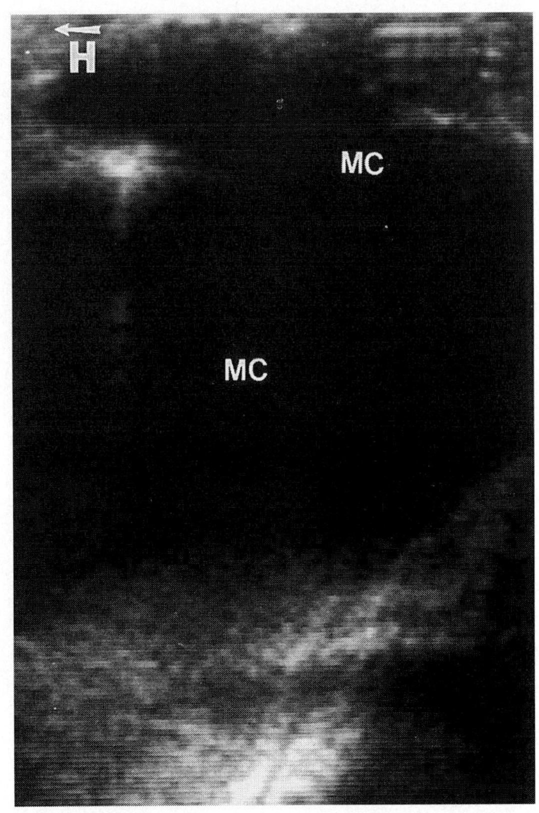

Figure 9-61 ■ Longitudinal sonogram of a lumbar meningocele (*MC*) showing the empty sac. (Reprinted with permission from DiPietro MA. The pediatric spinal canal. In Rumack CM, Wilson SR, Charboneau JW (eds), *Diagnostic Ultrasound,* ed 2. New York, Mosby, 1998.)

hydromyelia, lipoma, or thick filum terminale (Emery and Lendon, 1969; Glasier et al., 1990). Scanning of the open lesion per se is usually not essential or recommended unless it is done with the approval of the neurosurgeon and with a protective plastic drape on the lesion. Use enough coupling gel on the drape, do not let it touch the lesion, and apply no pressure to the lesion. One sees the cord entering the defect where the nontubulated portion of the cord forms the neural placode with its nerve roots extending through the sac (Fig. 9-63). Retethering of the cord following repair of myelomeningocele, also known as *secondary tethering,* can occur at any time (Nelson et al., 1988). The

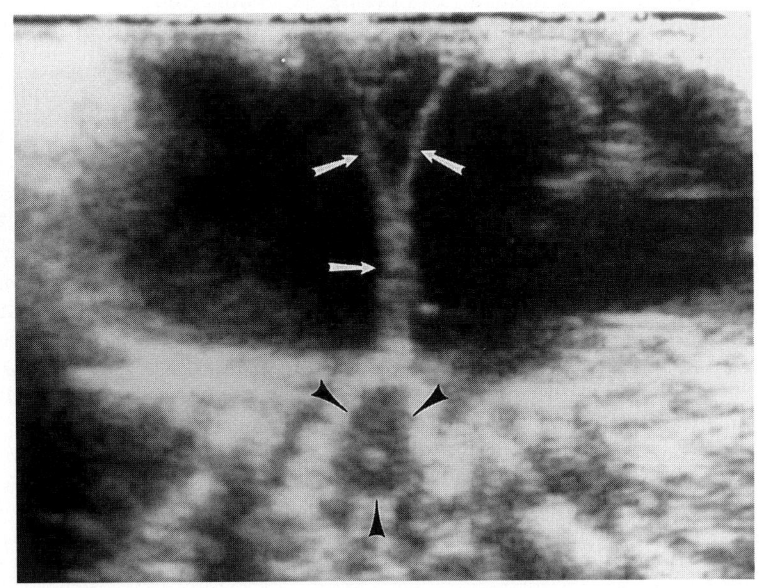

Figure 9-62 ■ Transverse sonogram of the lumbar cord (*black arrowheads*) at the level of an unrepaired meningocele in a newborn. The spinal cord lies entirely within the spinal canal. In this example, the cord's shape is distorted dorsally by strands of lace-like pia-arachnoid (*white arrows*) which extend dorsally into the meningocele. (Reprinted with permission from DiPietro MA, Garver KA. Sonography of the neonatal spinal canal. In Haller JO (ed), *Textbook of Neonatal Ultrasound.* New York, Parthenon Publishing Group, 1998.)

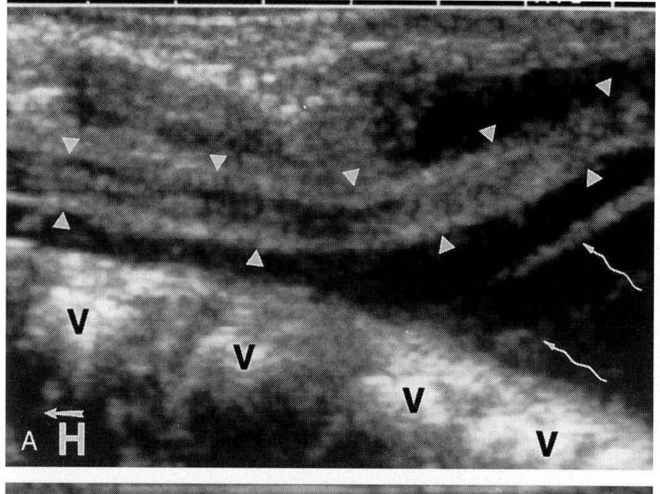

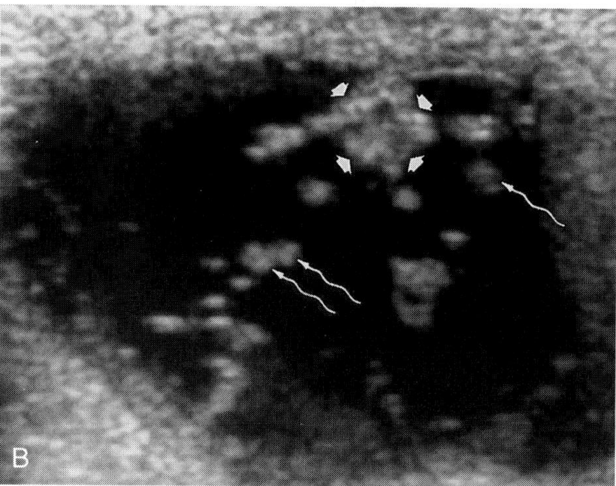

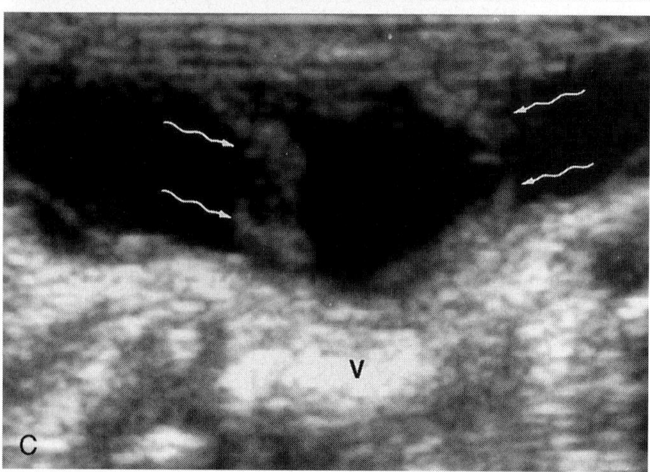

Figure 9–63 ■ **A**, Longitudinal sonogram of a newborn's unrepaired myelomeningocele. The spinal cord (*arrowheads*) is abnormally hyperechoic where it extends into the sac. Nerve roots (*wavy arrows*) extend ventrally and cephalad from the neural placode (not shown), in the dorsal aspect of the sac. Abbreviation: vertebral bodies (*V*). **B**, Transverse sonogram showing the caudal hyperechoic cord (*arrowheads*) dorsal within the myelomeningocele sac, with multiple nerve roots (*wavy arrows; only three are labeled*). **C**, Transverse sonogram showing nerve roots (*wavy arrows*) extending ventrally from the neural placode, which is in the dorsal caudal aspect of the sac. Abbreviation: vertebral body (*V*). (Reprinted with permission from DiPietro MA, Garver KA. Sonography of the neonatal spinal canal. In Haller JO (ed), *Textbook of Neonatal Ultrasound*. New York, Parthenon Publishing Group, 1998.)

cord position usually remains caudal, so that sign is not useful on MRI. Selective sonography may be requested to look for cord oscillation close to the repair site. The value of the presence or absence of caudal cord oscillation in evaluating secondary tethering is not definitely established.

References

Abernethy LJ, Lee YC, Cole WG: Ultrasound localization of subperiosteal abscesses in children with late-acute osteomyelitis. *J Pediatr Orthop* 13:766–768, 1993.

Abiri MM, Kirpekar M, Ablow RC: Osteomyelitis: Detection with US. *Radiology* 172:509–511, 1989.

Albright AL, Gartner JC, Wiener ES: Lumbar cutaneous hemangiomas as indicators of tethered spinal cords. *Pediatrics* 83:977–980, 1989.

American College of Radiology: ACR Appropriateness Criteria™ 2000. *Radiology* (supp) 215(S):819–827, 2000.

American Medical Association: *Current Procedural Technology (CPT)*. Chicago, American Medical Association, 1998.

Anderson FM: Occult spinal dysraphism: A series of 73 cases. *Pediatrics* 55:826–835, 1975.

Appignani BA, Jaramillo D, Barnes PD, et al: Dysraphic myelodysplasias associated with urogenital and anorectal anomalies: Prevalence and types seen with MR imaging. *AJR* 163:1199–1203, 1994.

Barlow TG: Early diagnosis and treatment of congenital dislocation of the hip. *J Bone Joint Surg [Br]* 44:292–301, 1962.

Barr L, Babcock DS: Sonography of the normal elbow. *AJR* 157:793–798, 1991.

Beek FJA, Bax KMA, Mali WPTM: Sonography of the coccyx in newborns and infants. *J Ultrasound Med* 13:629–634, 1994.

Beek FJA, Boemers TML, Witkamp TD, et al: Spine evaluation in children with anorectal malformations. *Pediat Radiol* 25:S28–S32, 1995.

Beek FJA, Van Leeuwen MS, Bax NMA, et al: A method for sonographic counting of the lower vertebral bodies in newborns and infants. *Am J Neuroradiol* 15:445–449, 1994.

Berman L, Klenerman L: Ultrasound screening for hip abnormalities: Preliminary findings in 1001 neonates. *Br Med J* 293:719–722, 1986.

Bialik V, Bialik GM, Blazer S, et al: Developmental dysplasia of the hip: A new approach to incidence. *Pediatrics* 103:93–99, 1999.

Boal DKB, Schwentker EP: The infant hip: Assessment of real-time ultrasound. *Radiology* 157:667–672, 1985.

Bodensteiner J: Standard of care: The blind leading the blind? [editorial]. *Clin Pediatr* 34:655–656, 1995.

Boeree NR, Clarke NMP: Ultrasound imaging and secondary screening for congenital dislocation of the hip. *J Bone Joint Surg* 76B:525–533, 1994.

Broker FHL, Burbach T: Ultrasonic diagnosis of separation of the proximal humeral epiphysis in the newborn. *J Bone Joint Surg [Am]* 72:187–191, 1990.

Catterall A: What is congenital dislocation of the hip [editorial]. *J Bone Joint Surg [Br]* 66:469–470, 1984.

Chao H-C, Lin S-J, Huang Y-C, et al: Color Doppler ultrasonographic evaluation of osteomyelitis in children. *J Ultrasound Med* 18:729–734, 1999.

Chapman PH: Congenital intraspinal lipomas: Anatomic considerations and surgical treatment. *Child's Brain* 9: 37–47, 1982.

Clarke NMP, Harcke HT, McHugh P, et al: Real-time ultrasound in the diagnosis of congenital dislocation and dysplasia of the hip. *J Bone Joint Surg [Br]* 67: 406–412, 1985.

Coleman LT, Zimmerman RA, Rorke LB: Ventriculus terminalis of the conus medullaris: MR findings in children. *Am J Neuroradiology* 16:1421–1426, 1995.

Currarino G, Coln D, Votteler T: Triad of anorectal, sacral, and presacral anomalies. *AJR* 137:395–398, 1981.

Dahlstrom H, Oberg L, Friberg S: Sonography in congenital dislocation of the hip. *Acta Orthop Scand* 57: 402–406, 1986.

DiPietro MA: The conus medullaris: Normal US findings throughout childhood. *Radiology* 188:149–153, 1993.

DiPietro MA: The pediatric spinal canal. In Rumack CM, Wilson SR, and Charboneau JW (eds), *Diagnostic Ultrasound,* ed 2. Chicago, Mosby-Year Book, 1998, pp 1589–1615.

DiPietro MA, Garver KA: Sonography of the neonatal spinal canal. In Haller JO (ed), *Textbook of Neonatal Ultrasound.* New York, Parthenon, 1998, pp 147–163.

Dorr U, Zieger M, Hauke H: Ultrasonography of the painful hip: Prospective studies in 204 patients. *Pediatr Radiol* 19:36–40, 1988.

Dunn PM: Congenital dislocation of the hip (CDH): Necropsy studies at birth. *Proc R Soc Med* 62:1035–1037, 1969.

Dunn PM: The anatomy and pathology of congenital dislocation of the hip. *Clin Orthop* 199:23–27, 1976a.

Dunn PM: Perinatal observations on the etiology of congenital dislocation of the hip. *Clin Orthop* 119:11–22, 1976b.

Emery JL, Lendon RG: Lipomas of the cauda equina and other fatty tumours related to neurospinal dysraphism. *Dev Med Child Neurol* Suppl 20(Suppl): 62–70, 1969.

Fone PD, Vapnek JM, Litwiller SE, et al: Urodynamic findings in the tethered spinal cord syndrome: Does surgical release improve bladder function? *J Urol* 157: 604–609, 1997.

Gibson PJ, Britton J, Hall DM, et al: Lumbosacral skin markers and identification of occult spinal dysraphism in neonates. *Acta Paediatr* 84:208–209, 1995.

Glasier CM, Chadduck WM, Leithiser RE Jr, et al: Screening spinal ultrasound in newborns with neural tube defects. *J Ultrasound Med* 9:339–343, 1990.

Glasier CM, Seibert JJ, Williamson SL, et al.: High resolution ultrasound characterization of soft tissue masses in children. *Pediatr Radiol* 17:233–237, 1987.

Graf R: New possibilities for the diagnosis of congenital hip joint dislocation by ultrasonography. *J Pediatr Orthop* 3:354–359, 1983.

Graf R: Fundamentals of sonographic diagnosis of infant hip dysplasia. *J Pediatr Orthop* 4:735–740, 1984.

Graf R: Guide to *Sonography of the Infant Hip.* New York, Thieme, 1987.

Graif M, Stahl-Kent V, Ben-Ami T, et al: Sonographic detection of occult bone fractures. *Pediatr Radiol* 18: 383–385, 1988.

Grissom LE, Harcke HT: Sonography in congenital deficiency of the femur. *J Pediatr Orthop* 14:29–33, 1994.

Grissom LE, Harcke HT, Kumar SJ, et al: Ultrasound evaluation of hip position in the Pavlik harness. *J Ultrasound Med* 7:1–6, 1988.

Gudinchet F, Maeder P, Laurent T, et al: Magnetic resonance detection of myelodysplasia in children with Currarino triad. *Pediatr Radiol* 27:903–907, 1997.

Gusnard DA, Naidich TP, Yousefzadeh DK, et al: Ultrasonic anatomy of the normal neonatal and infant spine: Correlation with cryomicrotome sections and CT. *Neuroradiology* 28:493–511, 1986.

Hall DE, Udvarhelyi GB, Altman J: Lumbosacral skin lesions as markers of occult spinal dysraphism. *JAMA* 246:2606–2608, 1981.

Hansson G, Nachemson A, Palmen K: Screening of children with congenital dislocation of the hip joint on the maternity wards in Sweden. *J Pediatr Orthop* 3: 271–279, 1983.

Harcke HT: The role of ultrasound in diagnosis and management of developmental dysplasia of the hip. *Pediatr Radiol* 25:225–227, 1995.

Harcke HT, Clarke NMP, Lee MS, et al: Examination of the infant hip with real-time ultrasonography. *J Ultrasound Med* 3:131–137, 1984.

Harcke HT, Grissom LE: Performing dynamic sonography of the infant hip. *AJR* 155:837–844, 1990.

Harcke HT, Grissom LE, Finkelstein MS: Evaluation of the musculoskeletal system with sonography. *AJR* 150: 1253–1261, 1988.

Harding MG, Harcke HT, Bowen JR, et al: Management of dislocated hips with Pavlik harness treatment and ultrasound monitoring. *J Pediatr Orthop* 17:189–198, 1997.

Hensinger RN: Congenital dislocation of the hip. *Clin Symp* 31(1):1–31, 1979.

Hernandez RJ: Evaluation of congenital hip dysplasia and tibial torsion by computed tomography. *J Comput Tomogr* 7:101–108, 1983.

Hernandez RJ: Concentric reduction of the dislocated hip. Computed-tomographic evaluation. *Radiology* 150: 266–268, 1984.

Hernandez RJ, Cornell RG, Hensinger RN: Ultrasound diagnosis of neonatal congenital dislocation of the hip. A decision analysis assessment. *J Bone Joint Surg* 76B: 539–543, 1994.

Hernandez RJ, Tachdjian MO, Poznanski AK, et al: CT determination of femoral torsion. *AJR* 137:97–101, 1981.

Higginbottom MC, Jones KL, James HE, et al: Aplasia cutis congenita: A cutaneous marker of occult spinal dysraphism. *J Pediatr* 96:687–689, 1980.

Hill CA, Gibson PJ: Ultrasound determination of the normal location of the conus medullaris in neonates. *Am J Neuroradiol* 16:469–472, 1995.

Hoffman HJ, Taecholarn C, Hendrick EB, et al.: Management of lipomyelomeningoceles: Experience at the Hospital for Sick Children, Toronto. *J Neurosurg* 62:1–8, 1985.

Iskandar BJ, Oakes WJ, McLaughlin C, et al: Terminal syringohydromyelia and occult spinal dysraphism. *J Neurosurg* 81:513–519, 1994.

Joseph B, Carver RA, Bell MJ, et al: Measurement of tibial torsion by ultrasound. *J Pediatr Orthop* 7:317–323, 1987.

Kaffenberger DA, Heinz ER, Oakes JW, et al: Meningocele manque: Radiologic findings with clinical correlation. *Am J Neuroradiol* 13:1083–1088, 1992.

Karrer FM, Flannery AM, Nelson MD Jr, et al: Anorectal malformations: Evaluation of associated spinal dysraphic syndromes. *J Pediatr Surg* 23:45–48, 1988.

Kawahara H, Andou Y, Takashima S, et al: Normal development of the spinal cord in neonates and infants seen on ultrasonography. *Neuroradiology* 29:50–52, 1987.

Kirks DR, Merten DF, Filston HC, et al: The Currarino triad: Complex of anorectal malformation, sacral bony abnormality, and presacral mass. *Pediatr Radiol* 14: 220–225, 1984.

Koroshetz AM, Taveras JM: Anatomy of the vertebrae and spinal cord. In Taveras JM (ed): *Radiology: Diagnosis-Imaging-Intervention.* Philadelphia, JB Lippincott Co, 1986, p 5.

Korsvik HE, Keller MS: Sonography of occult dysraphism in neonates and infants with MR imaging correlation. *RadioGraphics* 12:297–306, 1992.

Kraus R, Han BK, Babcock DS, et al: Sonography of neck masses in children. *AJR* 146:609–613, 1986.

Kriss VM, Desai NS: Occult spinal dysraphism in neonates: Assessment of high-risk cutaneous stigmata on sonography. *AJR* 171:1687–1692, 1998.

Kriss VM, Kriss TC, Warf BC: Dorsal tethering bands of the meningocele manque: Sonographic findings. *AJR* 167:1293–1294, 1996.

Kriss VM, Kriss TC, Babcock DSS: The ventriculus terminalis of the spinal cord in the neonate: A normal variant on sonography. *AJR* 165:1491–1493, 1995b.

Kriss VM, Kriss TC, Desai NS, et al: Occult spinal dysraphism in the infant. Clinical and sonographic review. *Clin Pediatr* 34:650–654, 1995a.

Lhowe D, Ehrlich MG, Chapman PH, et al: Congenital intraspinal lipomas: Clinical presentation and response to treatment. *J Pediatr Orthop* 7:531–537, 1987.

Long FR, Hunter JV, Mahboubi S, et al: Tethered cord and associated vertebral anomalies in children and infants with imperforate anus: Evaluation with MR imaging and plain radiography. *Radiology* 200:377–382, 1996.

MacEwen GD, Zembo MM: Current trends in the treatment of congenital dislocation of the hip. *Orthopedics* 10:1663–1669, 1987.

MacKenzie WG, Wilson JG: Problems encountered in the early diagnosis and management of congenital dislocation of the hip. *J Bone Joint Surg [Br]* 63:38–42, 1981.

Marchal GJ, Van Holsbeeck MT, Raes M, et al: Transient synovitis of the hip in children: Role of US. *Radiology* 162:825–828, 1987.

Markowitz RI, Davidson RS, Harty MP, et al: Sonography of the elbow in infants and children. *AJR* 159: 829–833, 1992.

Marks DS, Clegg J, Al-Chalabi AN: Routine ultrasound screening for neonatal hip instability. Can it abolish late-presenting congenital dislocation of the hip? *J Bone Joint Surg* 76B:534–538, 1994.

Miller F, Liang Y, Merlo M, et al: Measuring anteversion and femoral neck shaft angle in cerebral palsy. *Dev Med Child Neurol* 39:113–118, 1997.

Miralles M, Gonzalez G, Pulpeiro JR, et al: Sonography of the painful hip in children: 500 consecutive cases. *AJR* 152:579–582, 1989.

Morin C, Harcke HT, MacEwen GD: The infant hip: Real-time US assessment of acetabular development. *Radiology* 157:673–677, 1985.

Morin C, Zouaoui S, Delvalle-Fayada A, et al: Ultrasound assessment of the acetabulum in the infant hip. *Acta Orthop Belg* 65:261–265, 1999.

Naidich TP, McLone DG: Congenital pathology of the spine and spinal cord. In Taveras JM (ed): *Radiology: Diagnosis-Imaging-Intervention.* Philadelphia, JB Lippincott Co, 1986, p 18.

Naidich TP, McLone DG, Mutluer S: A new understanding of dorsal dysraphism with lipoma (lipomyeloschisis): Radiologic evaluation and surgical correction. *AJR* 140:1065–1078, 1983.

Naidich TP, Radkowski MA, Britton J: Real-time sonographic display of caudal spinal anomalies. *Neuroradiology* 28:512–527, 1986.

Nelson MD Jr, Bracchi M, Naidich TP, et al: The natural history of repaired myelomeningocele. *RadioGraphics* 8:695–706, 1988.

Nelson MD Jr, Sedler JA, Gilles FH: Spinal cord central echo complex: Histoanatomic correlation. *Radiology* 170:479–481, 1989.

Nelson MD Jr, Segall HD, Gwinn JL: Sonography in newborns with cutaneous manifestations of spinal abnormalities. *Am Fam Physician* 40:198–203, 1989.

Nievelstein RAJ, Valk J, Smit LME, et al: MR of the caudal regression syndrome: Embryologic implications. *Am J Neuroradiol* 15:1021–1029, 1994.

Pierre-Kahn A, Zerah M, Renier D, et al: Congenital lumbosacral lipomas. Child's *Nerv Syst* 13:298–334, 1997.

Place MJ, Parkin DM, Fitton JM: Effectiveness of neonatal screening for congenital dislocation of the hip. *Lancet* 2:249–251, 1978.

Polaneur PA, Harcke HT, Bowen JR: Effective use of ultrasound in the management of congenital dislocation and/or dysplasia of the hip (DDH). *Clin Orthop* 252: 176–181, 1990.

Powell KR, Cherry JD, Hougen TJ, et al: A prospective search for congenital dermal abnormalities of the craniospinal axis. *J Pediatr* 87:744–750, 1975.

Radkowski MA, Byrd SE, McLone DG: Unpublished data. 1990 Clinical and sonographic correlation of sacrococcygeal dimples. Presented at the 33rd annual meeting of the Society for Pediatric Radiology, April 19–22, 1990.

Raghavendra BN, Epstein FJ, Pinto RS, et al: Sonographic diagnosis of diastematomyelia. *J Ultrasound Med* 7:111–113, 1988.

Reigel DH: Tethered spinal cord. *Concepts Pediatr Neurosurg* 4:142–164, 1983.

Riebel TW, Nasir R, Nazarenko O: The value of sonography in the detection of osteomyelitis. *Pediatr Radiol* 26: 291–297, 1996.

Robben SGF, Lequin MH, Diepstraten AFM, et al: Anterior joint capsule of the normal hip and in children with transient synovitis: US study with anatomic and histologic correlation. *Radiology* 210:499–507, 1999.

Rohrschneider WK, Forsting M, Darge K, et al: Diagnostic value of spinal US: Comparative study with MR in pediatric patients. *Radiology* 200:383–388, 1996.

Rohrschneider WK, Fuchs G, Troger J: Ultrasonographic evaluation of the anterior recess of the hip: A prospective study of 166 asymptomatic children. *Pediatr Radiol* 26:629–634, 1996.

Rosendahl K, Markestad T, Lie RT: Ultrasound screening for developmental dysplasia of the hip in the neonate: The effect of treatment rate and prevalence of late cases. *Pediatrics* 94:47–52, 1994.

Rypens F, Avni EF, Matos C, et al: Atypical and equivocal sonographic features of the spinal cord in neonates. *Pediatr Radiol* 25:429–432, 1995.

Sahin F, Selcuki M, Ecin N, et al: Level of conus medullaris in term and preterm neonates. *Arch Dis Child* 77: F67–F69, 1997.

Saies AD, Foster BK, Lequesne GW: The value of a new ultrasound stress test in assessment and treatment of clinically detected hip instability. *J Pediatr Orthop* 8:436–441, 1988.

Schlesinger AE, Deeney VFX, Caskey PF: Sonography of the nonossified tarsal navicular cartilage in an infant with congenital vertical talus. *Pediatr Radiol* 20: 134–135, 1989.

Schumacher R, Kroll B, Schwarz M, et al: M-mode sonography of the caudal spinal cord in patients with meningomyelocele: Work in progress. *Radiology* 184: 263–265, 1992.

Stanton RP, Capecci R: Computed tomography for the early evaluation of developmental dysplasia of the hip. *J Pediatr Orthop* 12:727–730, 1992.

Strouse PJ, DiPietro MA, Adler RS: Pediatric hip effusions: Evaluation with power Doppler sonography. *Radiology* 206:731–735, 1998.

Strouse PJ, DiPietro MA, Teo E-L HJ, et al: Power Doppler evaluation of joint effusions: Investigation in a rabbit model. *Pediatr Radiol* 29:617–623, 1999.

Suzuki S, Awaya G, Okada Y, et al: Examination by ultrasound of Legg-Calve-Perthes disease. *Clin Orthop* 220: 130–136, 1987.

Szoke N, Kuhl L, Hendrichs J: Ultrasound examination in the diagnosis of congenital hip dysplasia of newborns. *J Pediatr Orthop* 8:12–16, 1988.

Terjesen T, Anda S: Femoral anteversion in children measured by ultrasound. *Acta Orthop Scand* 58:403–407, 1987.

Terjesen T, Holen KJ, Tegnander A: Hip abnormalities detected by ultrasound in clinically normal newborn infants. *J Bone Joint Surg* 78B:636–640, 1996.

Till K: Spinal dysraphism: A study of congenital malformations of the back. *Dev Med Child Neurol* 10:470–477, 1968.

Tonnis D, Storch K, Ulbrich H: Results of newborn screening for CDH with and without sonography and correlation of risk factors. *J Pediatr Orthop* 10:145–152, 1990.

Tredwell SJ, Davis LA: Prospective study of congenital dislocation of the hip. *J Pediatr Orthop* 9:386–390, 1989.

Tsakayannis DE, Shamberger RC: Association of imperforate anus with occult spinal dysraphism. *J Pediatr Surg* 30:1010–1012, 1995.

Tunell WP, Austin JC, Barnes PD, et al: Neuroradiologic evaluation of sacral abnormalities in imperforate anus complex. *J Pediatr Surg* 22:58–61, 1987.

White SJ, Blane CE, DiPietro MA, et al: Arthrography in evaluation of birth injuries of the shoulder. *J Can Assoc Radiol* 38:113–115, 1987.

Wirth T, LeQuesne GW, Paterson DC: Ultrasonography in Legg-Calve-Perthes disease. *Pediatr Radiol* 22:498–504, 1992.

Wright NB, Abbot GT, Carty HM: Ultrasound in children with osteomyelitis. *Clin Radiol* 50:623–627, 1995.

Wolf S, Schneble F, Troger J: The conus medullaris: Time of ascendence to normal level. *Pediat Radiol* 22: 590–592, 1992.

Yates VD, Wilroy RS, Whitington GL, et al: Anterior sacral defects: An autosomal dominantly inherited condition. *J Pediatr* 102:239–242, 1983.

Zawin JK, Hoffer FA, Rand FF, et al: Joint effusion in children with an irritable hip: US diagnosis and aspiration. *Radiology* 187:459–463, 1993.

Zieger MM, Dorr U, Ultrasonography of hip joint effusions. *Skeletal Radiol* 16:607–611, 1987b.

Zieger M, Dorr U: Pediatric spinal sonography. Part I: Anatomy and examination technique. *Pediatr Radiol* 18:9–13, 1988.

Zieger M, Dorr U, Schulz RD: Sonography of slipped humeral epiphysis due to birth injury. *Pediatr Radiol* 17:425–426, 1987a.

Zieger MM, Dorr U, Schulz RD: Pediatric spinal sonography. Part II: Malformations and mass lesions. *Pediatr Radiol* 18:105–111, 1988.

Zieger M, Schulz RD: Method and results of ultrasound in hip studies. *Ann Radiol (Paris)* 29:383–386, 1986.

Chapter 10 Sonography of the Dermis, Hypodermis, Periosteum, and Bone

Epidermis, Dermis, and Hypodermis

The epidermis and dermis combined are referred to as the *corium* or, more commonly, as the *skin*. Stratified squamous epithelium forms the epidermis, which is usually on the order of 100 μm thick. Highly cornified regions of the skin are the exception. Epidermis of the palms of the hands and soles of the feet may be up to 2 mm thick. The dermis is the primary supporting structure of the skin, containing vessels, nerves, lymphatics, glands, hair follicles, and a thick network of collagen fibers (Bloom and Fawcett, 1980). It typically measures 1 to 3 mm thick. The subcutaneous tissue, the hypodermis, consists of loose connective tissue and fat cells (Fig. 10–1). The thickness of the hypodermis varies greatly, depending on the region of the body and the body habitus of the patient. Blood vessels and nerves traverse the hypodermis on their way to the dermis. The high-frequency transducers (12, 10, 7.5, and 5 MHz) currently available are capable of distinguishing the skin from the hypodermis. A standoff pad is required for this examination. The skin appears as a uniform, hyperechoic layer of variable thickness, as described earlier. A distinction between epidermis and dermis cannot be made on the basis of sonographic images. Hypodermis has a much less echogenic appearance, containing some linear and curvilinear echogenic septa. These echogenic septa correspond to the fibrous interconnections supporting the hypodermis (Fig. 10–1) (Vincent, 1988). Closely associated with this network of fibers are blood vessels, nerves, and lymphatics (Fig. 10–2).

Pathology of the skin is well evaluated by clinical examination, and biopsy is easily performed. Ultrasound currently has no role in clinical evaluation of lesions confined to the skin, but it may someday be of value in the follow-up of systemic diseases affecting the skin, such as scleroderma. A current research application is measurement of the thickness of the corium following full-thickness burns (Fig. 10–3).

Ultra-high-frequency examination of the subcutaneous tissues has shown potential in staging of malignant melanoma and in identification of occult spread of tumor (Fig. 10–4) (Fornage and Lorigan, 1989; Fornage et al., 1993; Nazarian et al., 1996; Lassau et al., 1997; Tregnaghi et al., 1997). Some very small or soft tumors may not be palpable, but they can be easily detected sonographically due to their vascularity. This is true of melanoma (Fig. 10–4), glomus tumors, hemangiomas, and endometriomas (Fig. 10–5). Glomus tumors are among the most painful lesions of the soft tissues. These tumors made up of glomus cells have been diagnosed with both gray-scale and color Doppler; they are typically round, hypoechoic, and extremely vascular. The lesions may be only a couple of millimeters in diameter and often hide under the nail plate or in the pulp at the distal end of the fingers (Fornage, 1988a; Fornage and Rifkin, 1988).

Ultrasound's ability to distinguish the skin from the hypodermis and underlying muscle also makes it valuable in anthropomorphic studies. Measurement of the subcutaneous fat layer is easily performed using sonography and is more reproducible than other methods. This parameter is applied in several formulas to calculate lean body mass, a valuable indicator of the level of conditioning in athletes (Fried, 1986; Chiba et al., 1989).

Lesions of the subcutaneous tissues are well evaluated with sonography. Edema in the hypodermis results in markedly increased echogenicity (Figs. 10–6 and 10–7) (Vincent, 1988). The sonographic appearance of edema in the hypodermis is the inverse of that normally seen. Fibrous septa now

Text continued on page 329

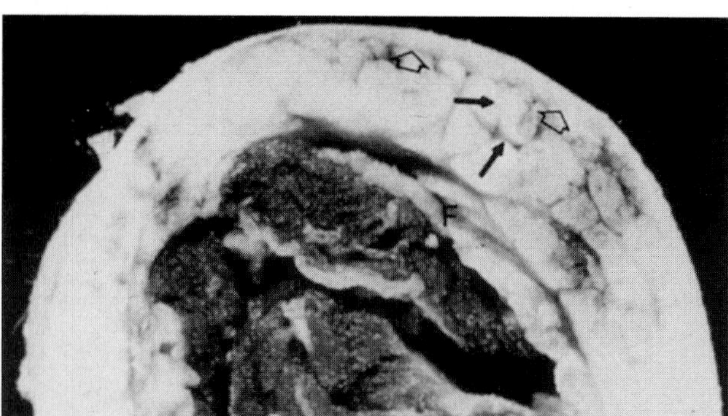

Figure 10-1 ■ Subcutaneous fat: transverse anatomical section. A loose fibrous connective tissue network (*black arrows*) provides a structural matrix for the subcutaneous fat. This connective tissue network anchors the skin (*open arrows*) to the underlying fascia (*F*) while allowing a moderate degree of motion between the layers.

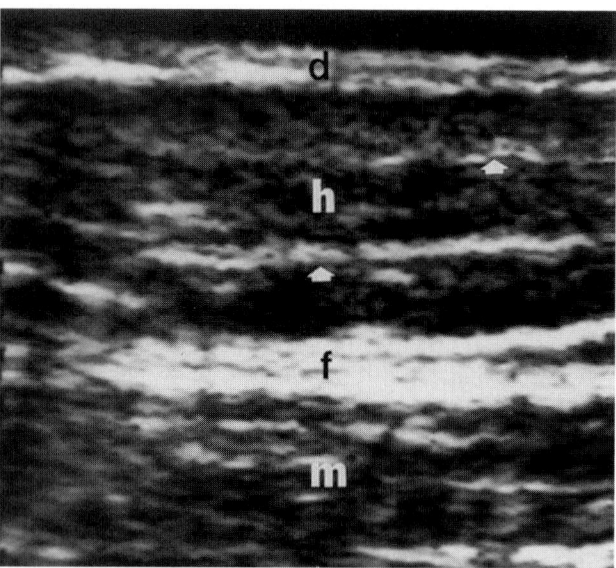

Figure 10-2 ■ Normal skin and subcutaneous tissues: longitudinal sonogram of the thigh. This longitudinal image obtained of a moderately obese 25-year-old man demonstrates the epidermis and dermis as a single hyperechoic layer (*d*). Its thickness varies considerably, depending on the location. Subcutaneous fat appears hypoechoic relative to the collagen-rich dermis. The subcutaneous fat appears less echogenic as the ratio of fat to lean body mass increases. Fibrous septa (*arrows*) within this layer are hyperreflective relative to the fat lobules. The septa contain vessels and nerves. As they become more widely separated by larger fat lobules, echogenicity of the fat decreases. Abbreviations: hypodermis/subcutaneous fat (*h*), fascia (*f*), muscle (*m*).

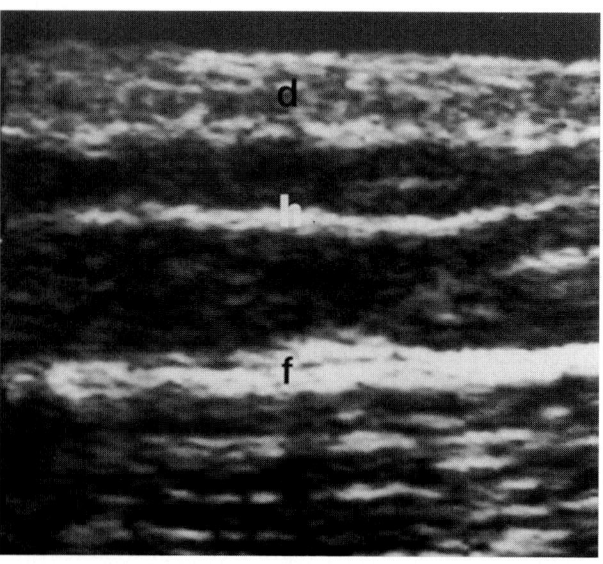

Figure 10-3 ■ Skin changes following a burn wound: longitudinal sonogram. A 20-year-old man 3 months following a large second-degree burn of the anterior thigh. The position of the transducer is identical to that in Figure 10-2. Fibrous scarring of the dermis (*d*) results in marked thickening of this hyperechoic layer. In this case, it is increased in thickness approximately fourfold. The degree of scarring is a function of the depth of the burn, complication of healing by infection, and genetic factors. Abbreviations: hypodermis (*h*), fascia (*f*).

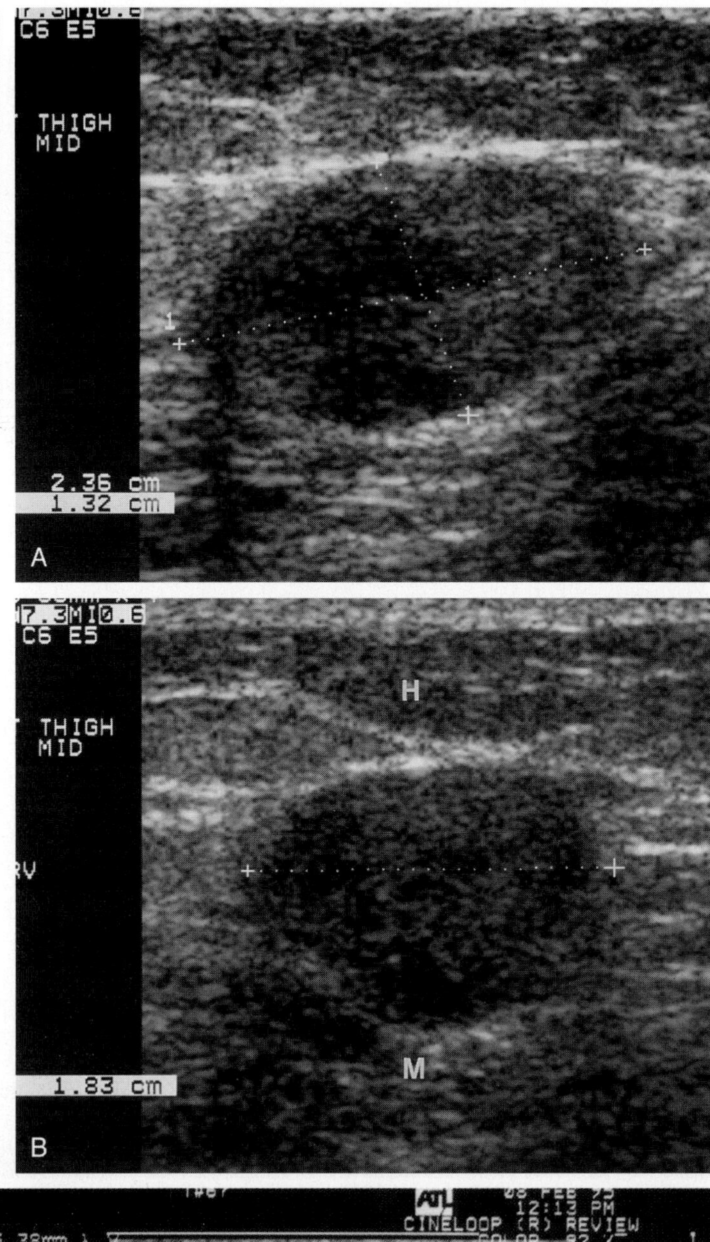

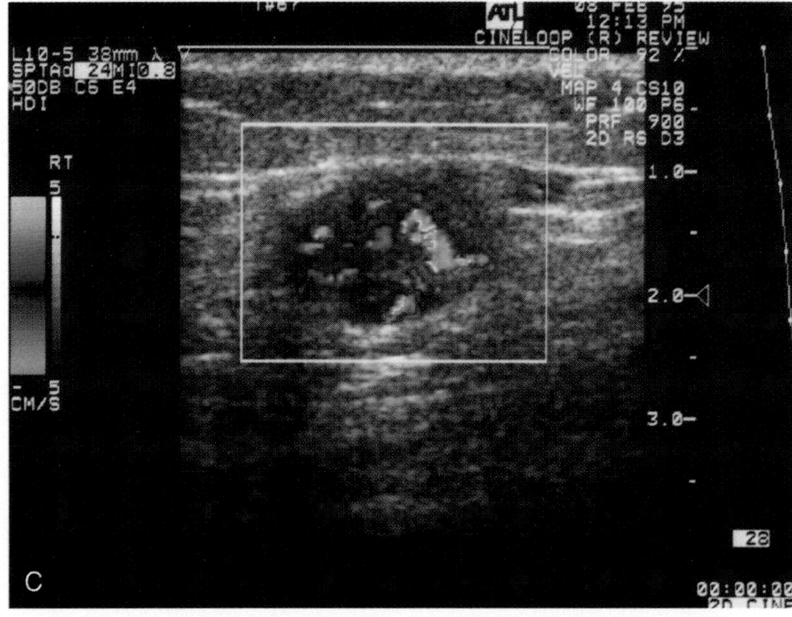

Figure 10–4 ■ **A,** Melanoma spreading in the hypodermis: longitudinal ultrasound. This 70-year-old man had a melanoma resected from his right lower extremity. The screening ultrasound scan detects a hypoechoic lesion deep in the hypodermis of his right thigh. The lesion was not clinically palpable. **B,** Melanoma spreading in the hypodermis: transverse ultrasound. Same patient as in **A.** The lesion appears homogeneous, hypoechoic, and well circumscribed. The soft tissue nodule is located deep in the hypodermis (*H*), and a mass effect on the underlying muscle (*M*) is obvious. **C,** Melanoma spreading in the hypodermis: color Doppler ultrasound. Same patient as in **A.** The color Doppler images show hyperemia throughout the lesion. The lesion was excised under ultrasound guidance. Subsequently, the patient developed lung metastases and died 6 months after this examination. (Courtesy of L. Nazarian, MD, Thomas Jefferson University Hospital.)

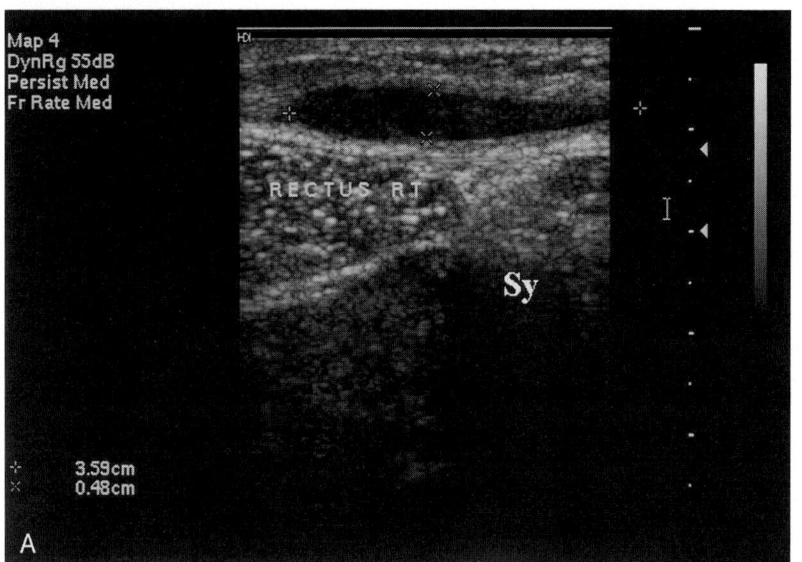

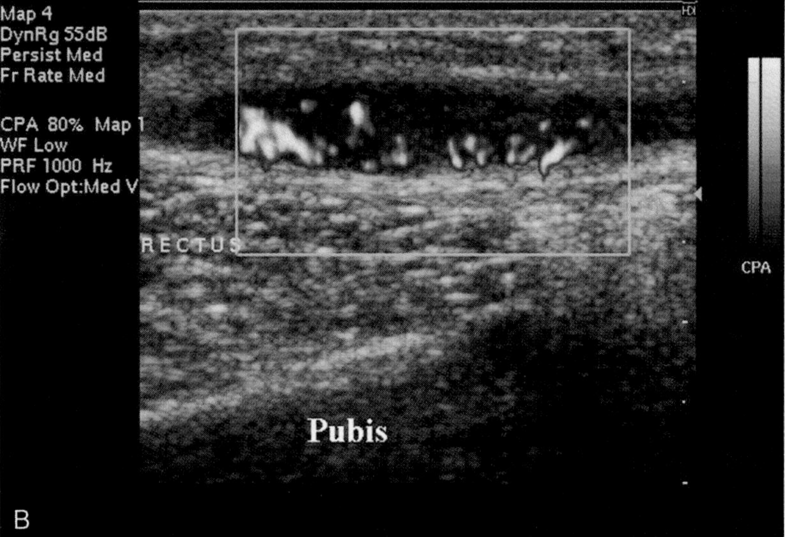

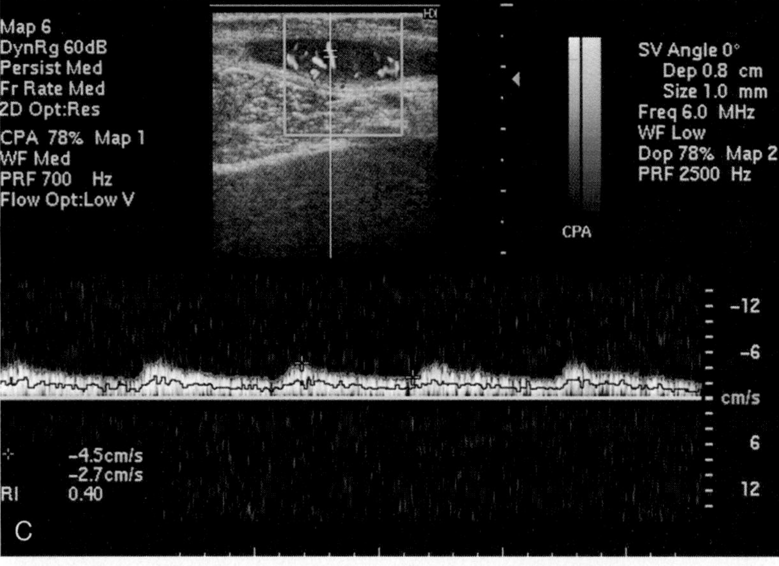

Figure 10–5 ■ **A,** Endometrioma of anterior abdominal wall: transverse sonogram. CT, MRI, and routine abdominal ultrasound examinations performed for this 38-year-old female with midline anterior abdominal wall pain were negative. She complained of swelling in the region, which was not clinically palpable. This high-frequency transverse ultrasound image of the anterior abdominal wall revealed a hypoechoic mass (*x-x*) anterior to the rectus muscles adjacent to the symphysis (*Sy*). **B,** Endo-metrioma of anterior abdominal wall: Transverse sonogram with power Doppler. Same patient as in **A.** Power Doppler demonstrated that this mass is highly vascular. The patient was questioned more carefully, revealing a history of prior cesarean section and varying discomfort associated with menses. This led to the correct diagnosis of endometrioma, which was confirmed at surgery. **C,** Endometrioma of anterior abdominal wall: transverse sonogram with duplex Doppler. Same patient as in **A.** A low-resistance waveform is confirmed with duplex Doppler.

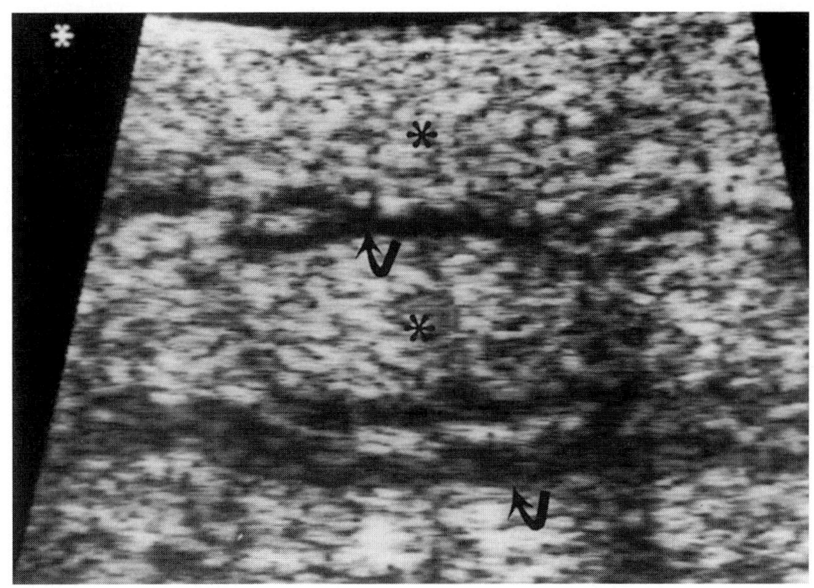

Figure 10–6 ■ Marked edema of the hypodermis: longitudinal sonogram of the thigh. This 42-year-old woman presented with deep venous thrombosis of the right leg. The transducer is positioned over the posterior thigh just above the popliteal fossa. Compare this image with the normal appearance of the hypodermis shown in Figure 10–2. The dermis can no longer be distinguished from the hypodermis. A complete reversal in the echogenicity of structures within the hypodermis is observed. The fibrous septa (*curved arrows*) containing distended lymphatics appear hypoechoic relative to the markedly echogenic fat lobules (*asterisks*). Increased reflectivity of the fat lobules may be attributed to microscopic fat–fluid interfaces resulting from edema.

appear hypoechoic relative to the surrounding echogenic fat. This is probably due to minute fat–fluid interfaces, which result from excess interstitial fluid. Echogenicity of the septa may, in fact, be slightly decreased due to distended lymphatics.

Generalized edema of the subcutaneous tissues is seen in cellulitis, panniculitis, lymphedema, venous insufficiency, subcutaneous hemorrhage (Fig. 10–8), and ruptured Baker's cyst (Fig. 10–9). The diffuse swelling seen in lymphedema involves the hypodermis and muscles equally (Yeh and Rabinowitz, 1982). Edema seen in thrombophlebitis tends to be greater in muscles, which appear hypoechoic. Cellulitis can have a nodular tumor-like appearance in intravenous (IV) drug abusers. However, in other patients with cellulitis, a gradual transition from abnormal to normal will be observed (Gitschlag et al., 1982; Yeh and Rabinowitz, 1982; Sandler et al., 1984). Subcutaneous abscess is visualized as a hypoechoic fluid collection bounded by increased echogenicity of the surrounding soft tissues. Debris is commonly identified within the fluid. Foreign bodies are often the inciting agents responsible for subcutaneous abscess. When wooden fragments are trapped within the subcutaneous tissues, the ensuing inflammatory reaction will decompose the piece

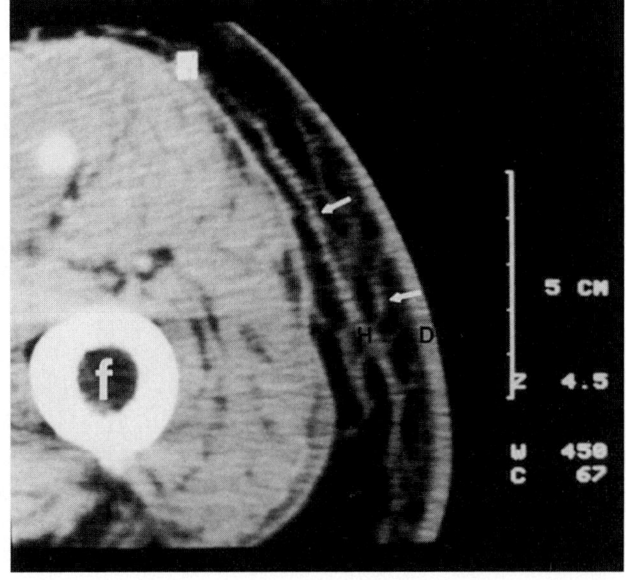

Figure 10–7 ■ Edema of the hypodermis: CT of the thigh. Marked edema of the hypodermis (*H*) is seen in this patient with a mycotic aneurysm of the femoral artery. Thickened septa (*arrows*) are seen throughout the subcutaneous fat. Normally, these septa are almost imperceptible. Note that the thickest septa run parallel to the skin (*D*) and fascia. Abbreviation: femur (*f*).

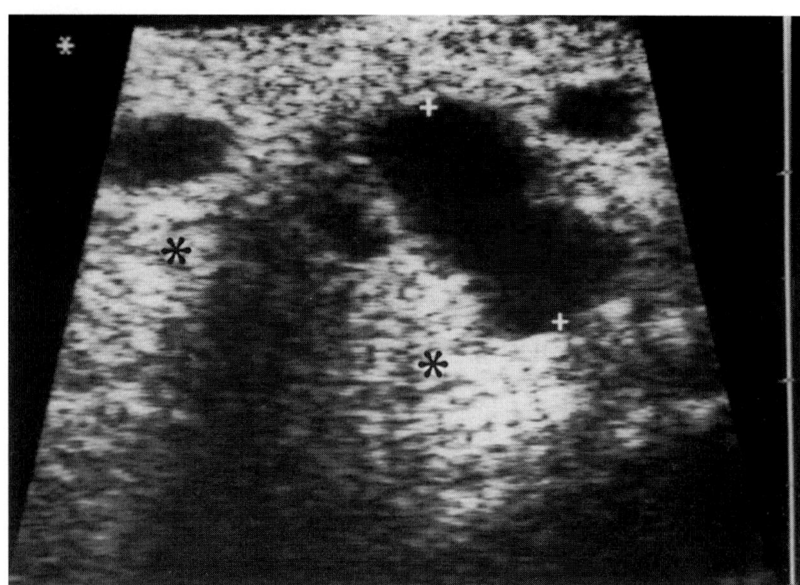

Figure 10-8 ■ Subcutaneous hemorrhage: transverse sonogram. The patient is a 28-year-old volleyball player who was kicked in the thigh during a match. He presented with redness and induration of the anterior thigh. This transverse image of the upper thigh demonstrates multiple hypoechoic fluid collections indicative of hematoma (between calipers). The surrounding fat appears markedly hyperechoic (*asterisks*). No septa are identified, probably due to rupture.

of wood. The echogenic wood splinter becomes progressively less echogenic until it finally disappears within the inflammatory collection. Some foreign bodies are not the result of accident but are surgically introduced. Vascular grafts (Fig. 10–10) and orthopedic implants may serve as a nidus for infection. Regardless of the cause, sonography is a valuable tool in the diagnosis of inflammatory lesions of the hypodermis. Trauma can also affect the subcutaneous tissues. Hematomas can present as anechoic or hypoechoic collections, sometimes demonstrating fluid-fluid levels. It is quite common to see a fluid accumulation persist in the deep layers of the subcutis when bruises are followed up sonographically. These seromas have been observed long after trauma in patients with significant contusions of the pelvis and hips, as well as in patients following extensive pelvic surgery. Seromas are most commonly seen in individuals with extensive subcutaneous fat in the thighs and hips. Ultrasound images have shown fragments of fat floating within the seroma, which may be responsible for de-

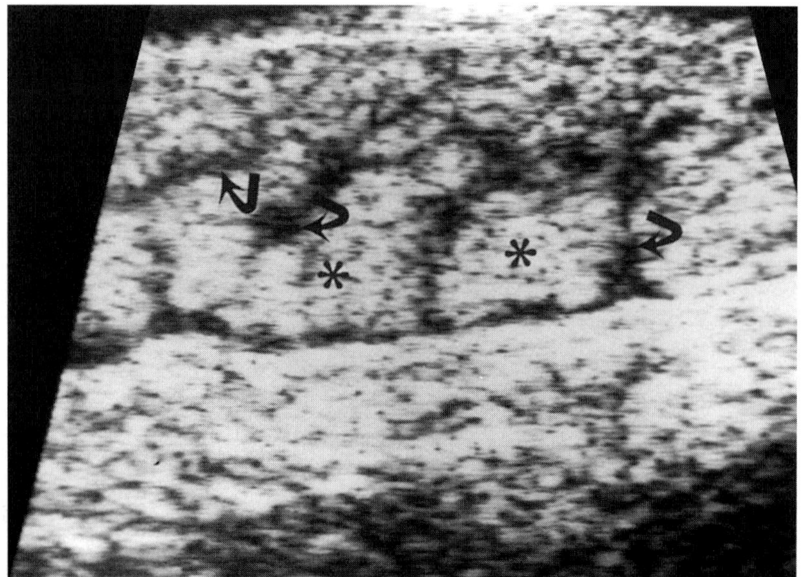

Figure 10-9 ■ Edema of the hypodermis: longitudinal sonogram of the posterior calf. In this patient with recently diagnosed rheumatoid disease, marked edema of the hypodermis is noted following rupture of a Baker's cyst. Again, reversal of the normal echo texture of the hypodermis is noted. Fat lobules (*asterisks*) appear markedly hyperechoic, and the connective tissue septa (*curved arrows*) are hypoechoic. In the calf, septa running perpendicular to the fascia and skin are more prominent. This appearance of the edematous hypodermis is always seen in cases of ruptured Baker's cyst.

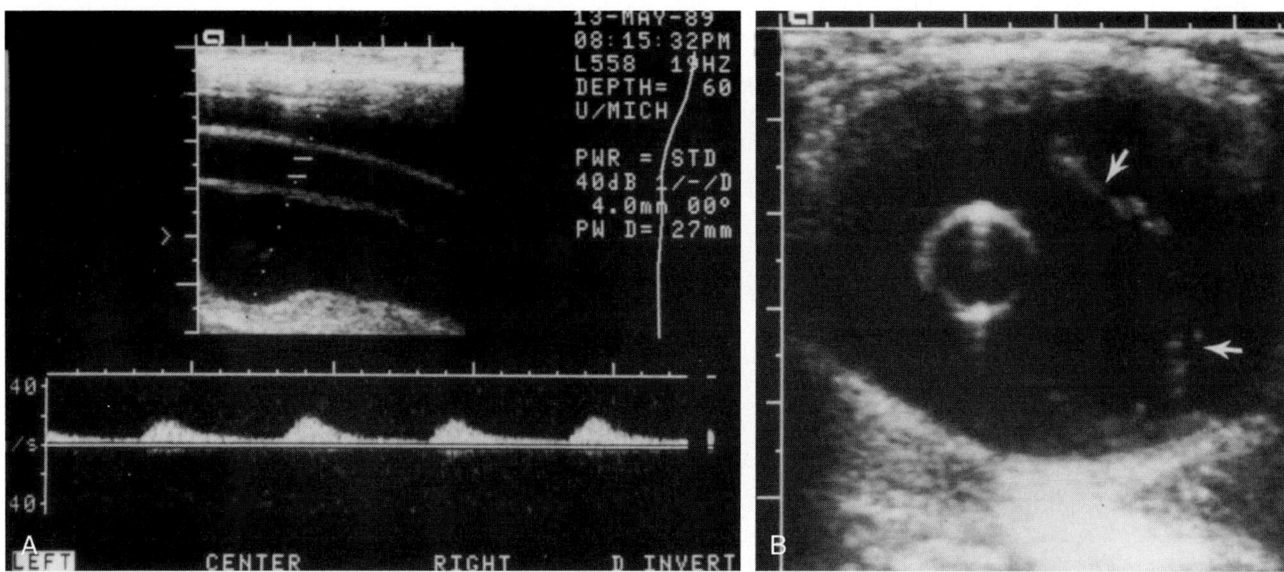

Figure 10–10 ■ **A,** Extra-anatomical bypass graft infection: longitudinal sonogram. This 64-year-old man with bilateral axillary-femoral bypass grafts presented with systemic sepsis and induration over the right graft. A large fluid collection is noted surrounding the graft, which is demonstrated to be patent by Doppler ultrasound. The surrounding subcutaneous fat is diffusely increased in echogenicity, and debris is seen floating within the collection. **B,** Extra-anatomical bypass graft infection: transverse sonogram. Same patient as in **A.** Once again, clumps of debris (*arrows*) are identified within this inflammatory collection. Aspiration was performed under ultrasound guidance, and cultures yielded *Streptococcus viridans.* Note the reverberation artifact off of the anterior and posterior walls of this Gore-Tex graft.

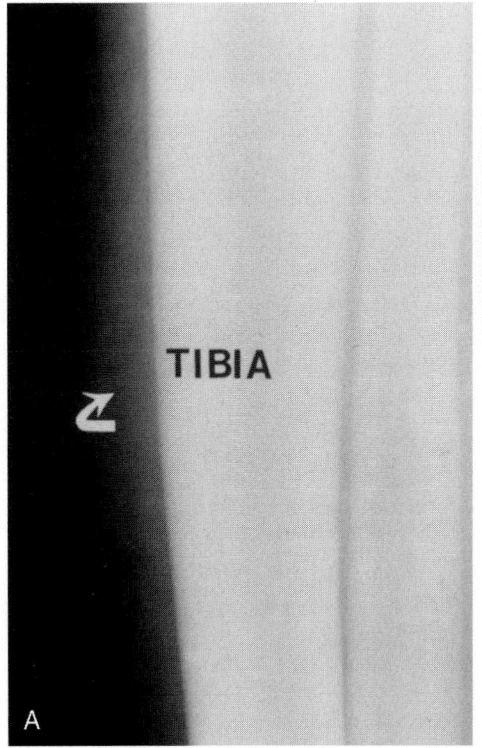

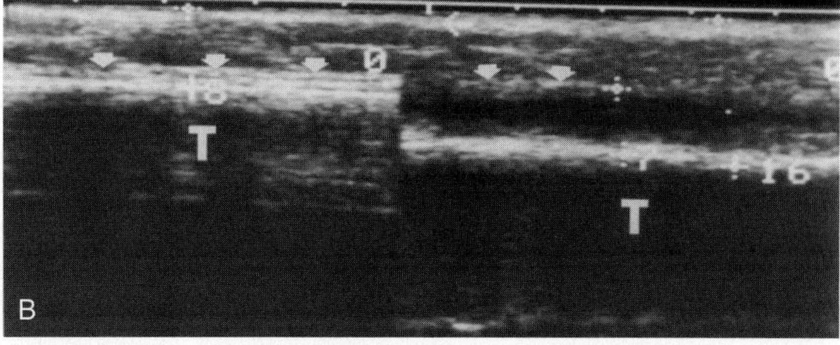

Figure 10–11 ■ **A,** Acute osteomyelitis: lateral radiograph. A 25-year-old diabetic man who presented with 2 days of fever and pain over the midtibia. No osseous changes are present. Some edema (*curved arrow*) of the soft tissues overlying the tibia is noted. **B,** Acute osteomyelitis: longitudinal sonogram of the anterior tibia. Same patient as in **A.** The transducer is positioned over the anteromedial surface of the tibia. Side-to-side comparison is provided in this split-screen image, with the asymptomatic left tibia on the left. A normal relationship of the hyperechoic fascia/periosteum (*arrows*) to the tibial cortex is seen on the left. A hypoechoic fluid collection elevates the fascia/periosteum off of the tibial cortex on the right. Soft tissue overlying the right tibia is twice as thick as the normal left side. Abbreviation: tibia (T).

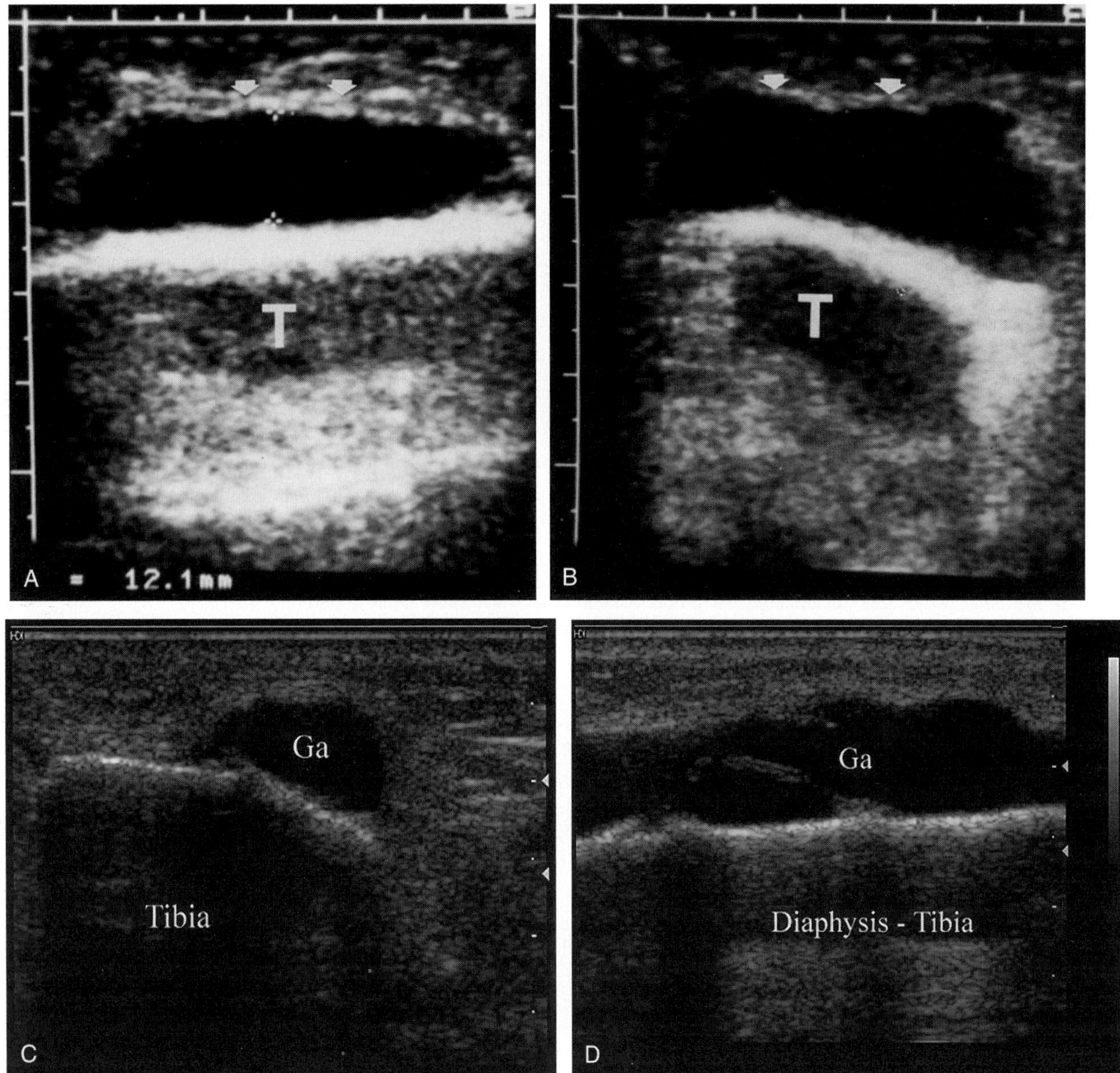

Figure 10–12 ■ **A,** Subperiosteal hematoma: longitudinal sonogram. This 22-year-old soccer player received a blow to the anterior tibia. He presented with continued pain and swelling 5 days after injury. The transducer is positioned over the midtibia along its length. Anechoic hematoma elevates the periosteum (*arrows*). Abbreviation: tibia (*T*). **B,** Subperiosteal hematoma: transverse sonogram. Same patient as in **A.** The hematoma that elevates the periosteum (*arrows*) tracks along the anteromedial cortex of the tibia (*T*). **C,** Focal swelling and pain over the anterolateral surface of the tibia plagues this active 38-year-old man in his daily activity. The lesion limits him in his athletic endeavors. An accumulation of anechoic material shows over the tibial surface and forms a very focal mass (*Ga*). The underlying tibial cortex appears slightly irregular. **D,** Same patient as in **C.** The long-axis view of this anechoic mass shows an elongated lesion with multiloculated structure displaying increased through-transmission.

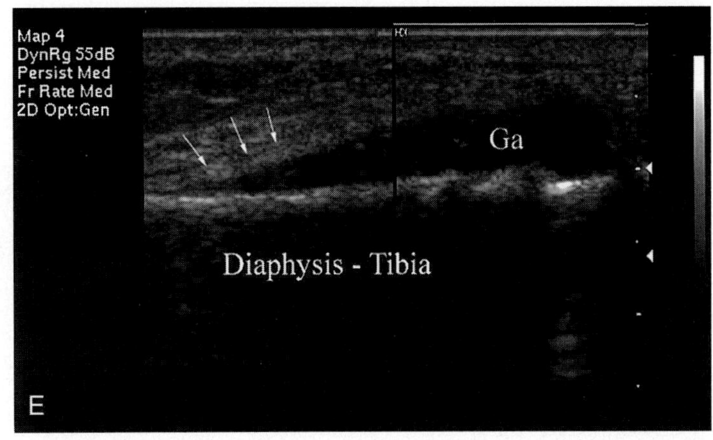

Figure 10–12 *Continued* ■ **E,** Same patient as in **C.** With the 12-MHz transducer over the proximal aspect of the lesion, one can discern the smooth transition between the normal periosteum and the elevated periosteum. Note the irregularity of the tibial bone surface. The hyperechoic periosteum (*arrows*) can be distinguished at the edge of the lesion. Aspiration of the ganglion (*Ga*) yielded gelatinous material. Pathology confirmed myxoid ground substance in the fluid. Subperiosteal ganglia, unlike subperiosteal hematoma and pus, cause a more focal bulging of the bone's periosteal envelope, as illustrated in **C.**

layed organization of the blood clot and healing. Ultrasound can assist in draining these collections. Drainage tends to relieve pain and often accelerates healing (see Chapter 14).

Periosteum

Thickening of the periosteum is a nonspecific finding seen in trauma, fracture, osteotomy, infection, tumor, Paget's disease, venous stasis, hypertrophic pulmonary osteoarthropathy, metabolic diseases, and endocrinopathies (Resnick and Niwayama, 1988). Sonography will clearly demonstrate periosteal thickening, but in the majority of cases, conventional radiography is the best method to survey the periosteum. Two specific exceptions to this statement are the diagnosis of osteomyelitis and stress fracture. In these cases, ultrasound is superior in the detection of a periosteal reaction, well before mineralization becomes evident on radiography.

Acute osteomyelitis is recognized on sonographic images by elevation of the periosteum by a hypoechoic layer of purulent material (Fig. 10–11) (Abiri et al., 1988). Stripping of the periosteum from the surface of the bone by fluid is more common in children than in adults. An explanation for this may be that the periosteum is more loosely attached to the bone in children. This appearance is identical to that of subperiosteal hemorrhage or subperiosteal ganglion, but the clinical history will usually clinch the diagnosis (Fig. 10–12). The absence of soft tissue between the fluid and cortical bone helps to differentiate osteomyelitis from other fluid collections (Abiri et al., 1988). The diagnosis of acute osteomyelitis by ultrasound, with aspiration and culture of the offending organism, often expedites initiation of appropriate therapy (Figs. 10–13 and 10–14). Results of the ultrasound examination are usually positive 24 hours following the onset of fever in cases of osteomyelitis. Results of radionuclide scintigraphy using technetium 99m-methylene diphosphonate become positive after approximately 48 to 72 hours. Gallium-67 scintigraphy takes up to 72 hours just to obtain adequate images, thus delaying the diagnosis by up to 5 days. Radiographic changes indicative of osteomyelitis may not become evident for 1 week or more.

In chronic osteomyelitis, sonography is not only valuable in making the diagnosis, but can also be used to assess involvement of the adjacent soft tissues and guide placement of a percutaneous drainage catheter (van Sonnenberg et al., 1987). Unlike acute osteomyelitis, changes in the surrounding soft tissues are often observed in chronic osteomyelitis. Soft tissue abscess related to chronic osteomyelitis is identified as a hypoechoic or anechoic fluid collection. These collections are noted to extend around the bony contours in more than 70% of cases (van Sonnenberg et al., 1987) (Fig. 10–15).

After sonographic localization of the abscess, a needle can be placed into the collection under sonographic guidance. A percutaneous drainage catheter is then placed using the Seldinger technique. The collection is aspirated dry, and the cavity is irrigated with sterile saline until the fluid returned is clear. It is of the utmost importance that the patient be given IV antibiotics immediately prior to placement of a percutaneous drainage catheter because this procedure will result in bacteremia. This approach is very efficient because diagnosis and therapy are accomplished in the same session (van Sonnenberg et al., 1987). Further imaging studies, such as CT, MRI, or radionuclide scintigraphy, are not necessary in cases of chronic osteomyelitis with a periosteal fluid collection. Ultrasound will make the diagnosis and assist with aspiration and drainage. Obtaining a sample of the fluid is of the

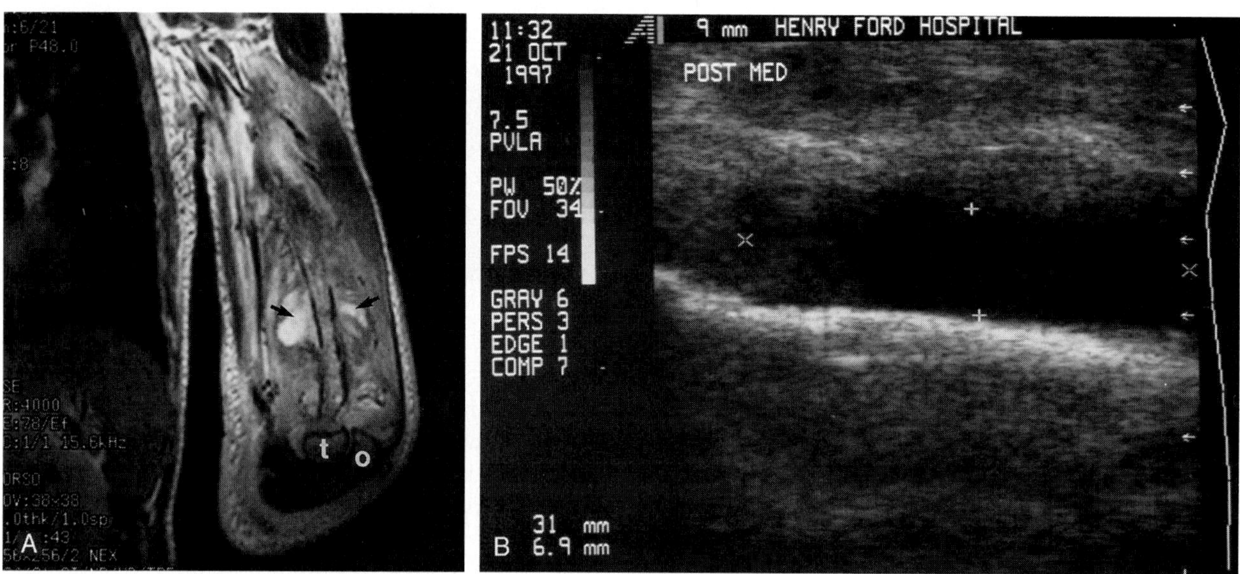

Figure 10-13 ■ **A,** Acute osteomyelitis of the humerus: sagittal T_2-weighted MRI. This 43-year-old male intravenous drug abuser presented with fever, pain, and swelling of his left arm. Abnormally increased signal is present within the marrow of the left humerus, as well as within the surrounding soft tissues (*arrows*). Abbreviations: olecranon (*o*), trochlea (*t*). **B,** Acute osteomyelitis of the humerus: longitudinal sonogram. Same patient as in **A.** The transducer is aligned along the long axis of the humeral diaphysis at the posterior medial aspect. The largest subperiosteal fluid collection (+) was identified in this region. Ultrasound-guided fluid aspiration yielded 10 cc of purulent material. *Staphylococcus aureus* was identified as the causative organism in cultures.

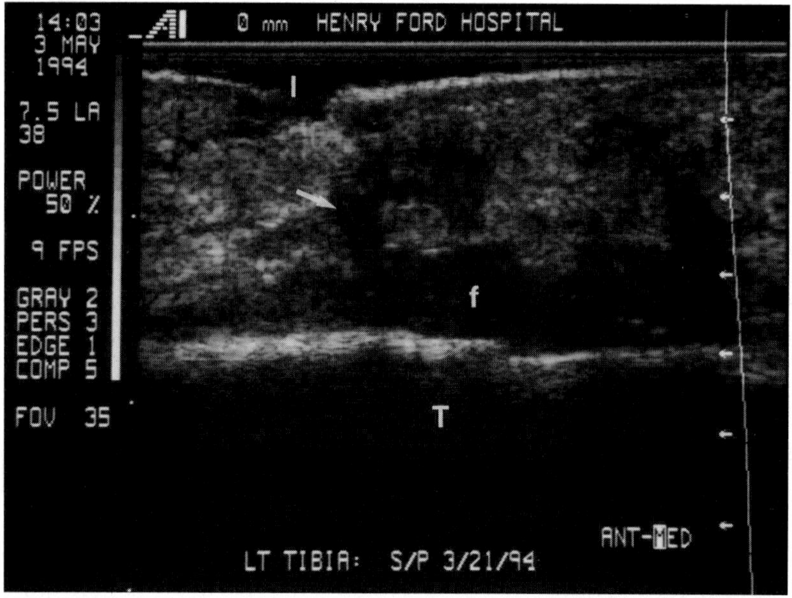

Figure 10-14 ■ Acute posttraumatic osteomyelitis of the tibia: longitudinal sonogram. Six weeks ago, this 45-year-old male sustained a grade I open tibial fracture in a motor vehicle accident. He was initially treated with a nonreamed intramedullary nail. He now presents without fever but with increasing swelling over the tibia. This longitudinal sonogram reveals a parosteal fluid (*f*) collection at the fracture site, which is highly unusual 6 weeks following injury. A skin laceration (*l*) is seen in continuity (*arrow*) with the fluid collection, but no drainage was present clinically. The fluid was aspirated under ultrasound guidance, which yielded purulent material containing *S. aureus.* Abbreviation: tibia (*T*).

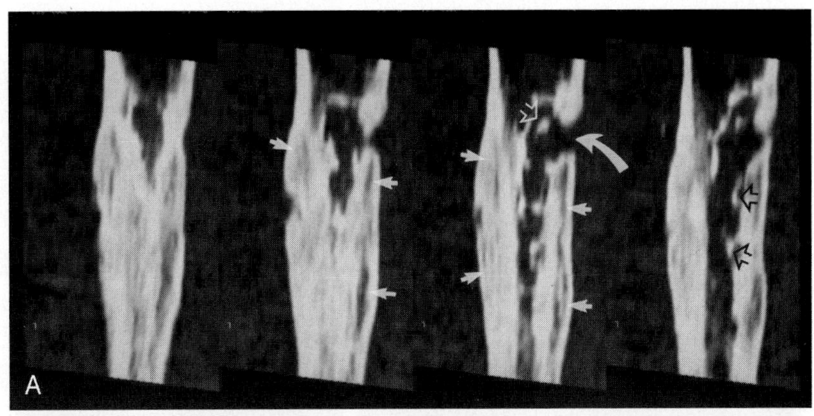

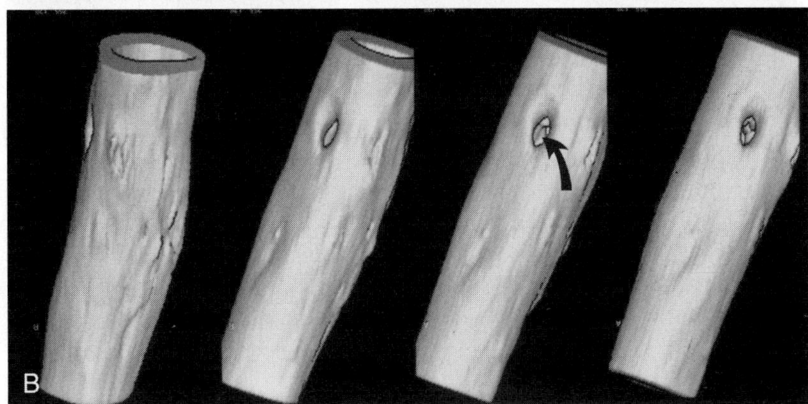

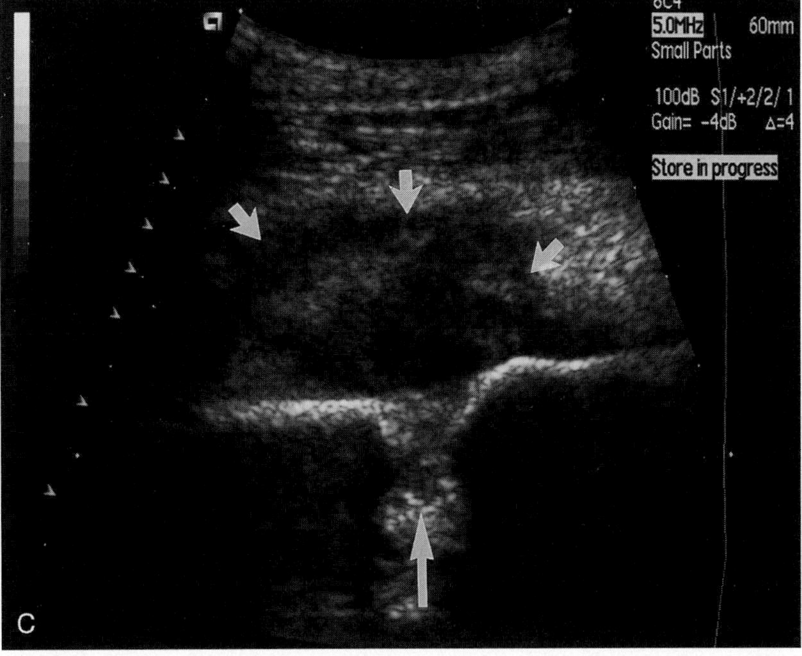

Figure 10–15 ■ **A,** Chronic osteomyelitis of the femur: sagittal CT reconstruction. These sagittal reconstructions created from axial CT images demonstrate classic changes of chronic osteomyelitis in this 35-year-old male, who suffered an open femur fracture at age 20. He now presents with recent onset of thigh pain. The involucrum (*small arrows*) is seen as a mantle of new bone surrounding the femoral diaphysis. Multiple sequestra (*open arrows*) are noted within the medullary space. The cloaca (*curved arrow*) is seen at the posterior border of the femur. However, noncontrast CT is unable to identify parosteal fluid collections, making it unsuitable for guiding aspiration for cultures. **B,** Chronic osteomyelitis of the femur: three-dimensional CT surface reconstruction. Same patient as in **A.** The extent of the cloaca (*curved arrow*) is better defined. **C,** Chronic osteomyelitis of the femur: longitudinal sonogram. Same patient as in **A**. A heterogeneous collection of fluid and granulation tissue (*short arrows*) is seen surrounding the opening of the cloaca (*long arrow*). Localization of the fluid collection facilitates aspiration and culture. (Courtesy of B. van Holsbeeck, MD, P. Lefere, MD, and L. van den Daelen, MD, Stedelijk Ziekenhuis, Roeselare, Belgium.)

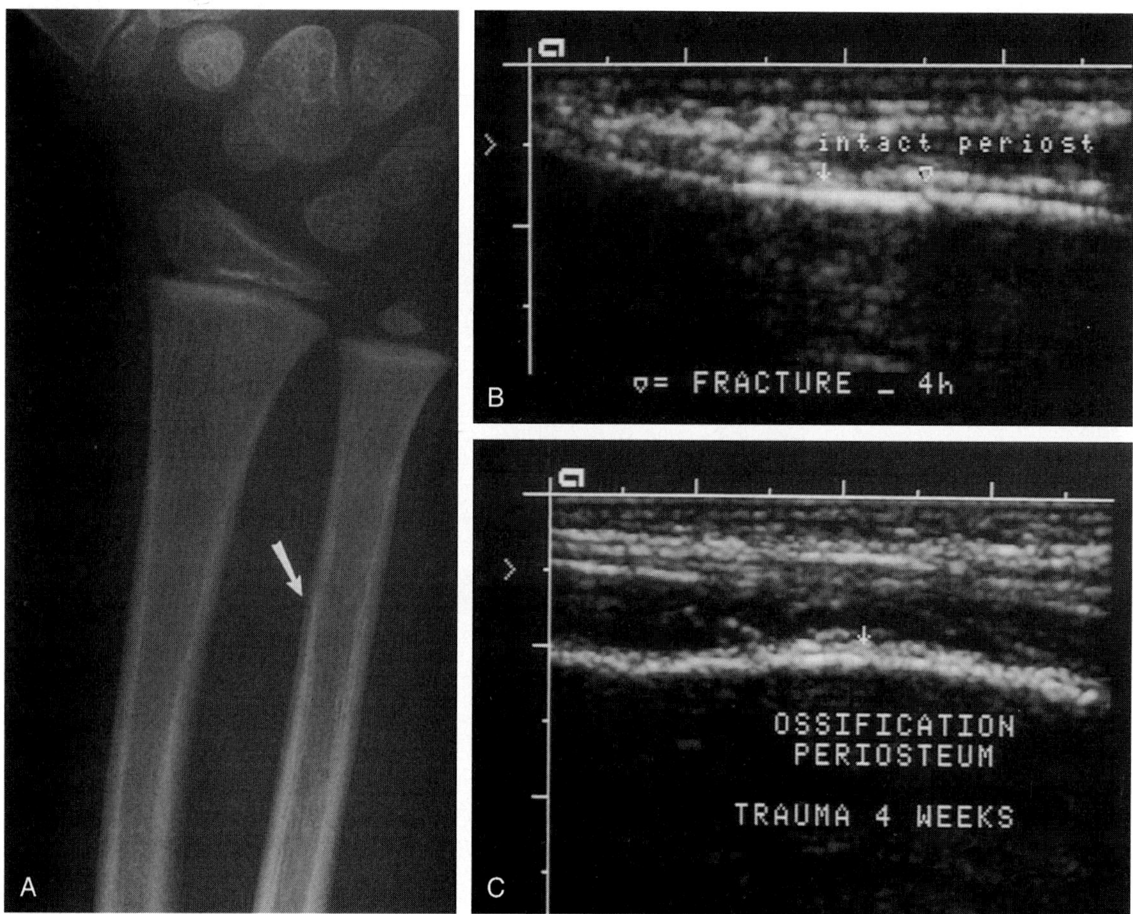

Figure 10–16 ■ **A,** Acute hairline fracture of the ulna: anteroposterior radiograph. A minute cortical discontinuity (*arrow*) is noted in the distal ulna of this 7-year-old boy following a playground injury. **B,** Acute hairline fracture of the ulna: longitudinal sonogram. Same patient as in **A** 4 hours after trauma. The transducer is placed over the distal ulna along its length. Hematoma slightly elevates the ulnar periosteum (*arrow*) adjacent to the site of cortical discontinuity (*arrowhead*). **C,** Four and a half weeks after injury, the cortical discontinuity is no longer recognized, and a periosteal reaction (*arrow*) is observed as a homogeneous, hyperechoic layer overlying the cortex.

utmost importance in planning further treatment. MRI will be needed in the evaluation of diabetic feet and in the diagnosis of long bone osteomyelitis when periosteal fluid is absent (Craig et al., 1997).

The periosteal reaction seen in other disease processes differs slightly from that seen in osteomyelitis. A very thin, hyperechoic line defines the soft tissue–periosteal interface. The thickened periosteum appears less echogenic, measuring several millimeters thick. These findings have been most helpful in the diagnosis of stress fractures and hairline fractures (Fig. 10–16). Stress fractures are most frequently seen in the lower extremities of runners. The clinical symptoms of pain related to exercise, associated with local tenderness, are rather nonspecific. Ultrasound will make the diagnosis by identifying focal periosteal thickening in the symptomatic region (Fig. 10–17). The examination can be performed at the time of the patient's initial presentation, weeks before radiographic changes are apparent. At the same time, other soft tissue lesions can be excluded as the source of pain (Fig. 10–18).

The differential diagnosis of periosteal thickening in the tibia includes the fascial thickening seen in shin splints. Fascial thickening in shin splints will be limited to the site of attachment of the fascia cruris. The ability to differentiate these two entities is one of the principal advantages of ultrasound over radionuclide scintigraphy in the diagnosis of stress fractures.

Other areas in which sonographic evaluation of the periosteum has proved of value include the demonstration of a favorable response during Ilizarov bone lengthening and follow-up of Paget's

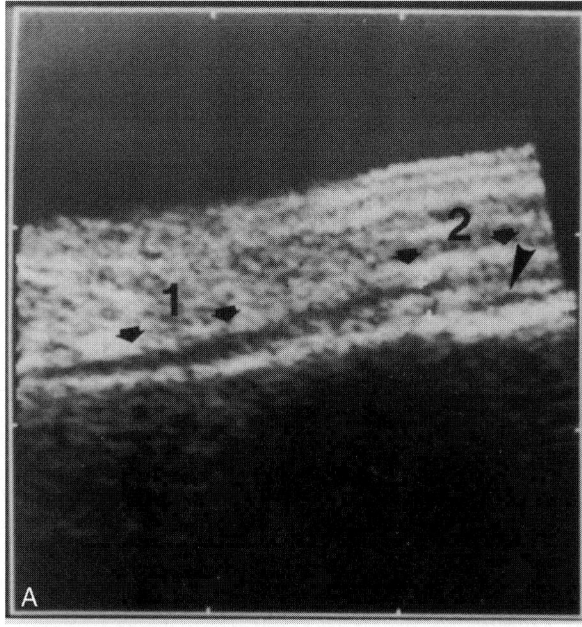

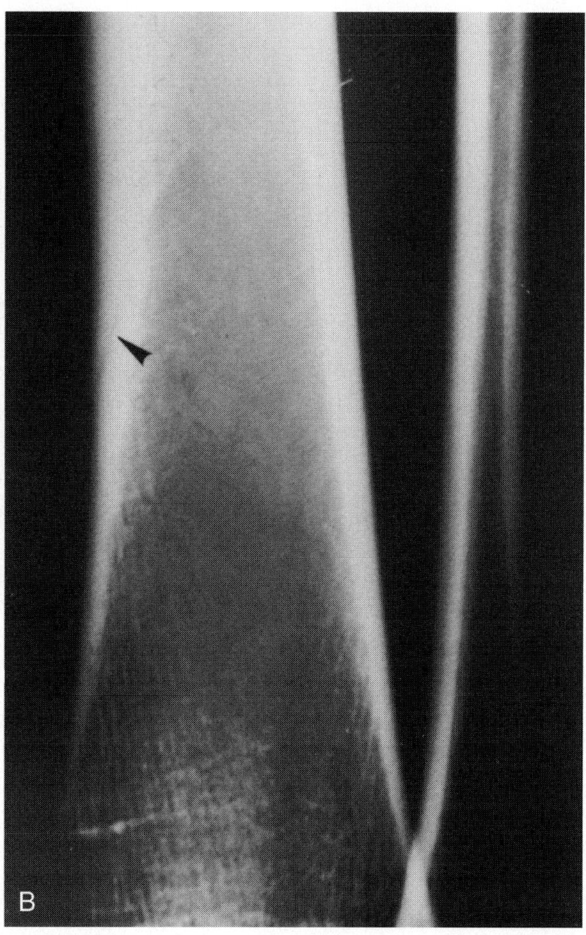

Figure 10–17 ■ **A,** Stress fracture distal tibia: longitudinal sonogram. A 19-year-old woman who attempted to run in a marathon with little prior training. She experienced persistent pain over the distal tibia and presented 5 days after the race for evaluation. Convertional radiographs were normal. Sonography was performed because of the strong suspicion of stress fracture. The transducer was positioned over the point of maximal tenderness along the medial aspect of the distal tibia. Periosteal thickening (*arrows*) and a reaction (*arrowhead*) are observed, more prominent distally. The number *1* indicates the edge of the periosteal reaction, and the number *2* indicates the center. **B,** Stress fracture distal tibia: anteroposterior radiograph. Same patient as in **A** 8 days after injury. A tiny cortical discontinuity (*arrowhead*) is identified in the medial cortex of the distal tibia in the region of abnormality observed with ultrasound. This was not evident on the prior radiographic examination. Stress fractures in the tibia are usually oblique, making differentiation from vascular canals difficult.

disease. Evaluation of periosteal thickening of the tibia (Fig. 10–19) in Paget's disease has been shown to be an indicator of disease activity (Maldague and Malghem, 1987). The evaluation of the Ilizarov bone lengthening technique is discussed in Chapter 9.

Bone

The bone–soft tissue interface is highly reflective, seen as a bright line with acoustic shadowing deep to the interface. The inability to image the medullary cavity of bone using pulse-echo ultrasound has led to the misconception that it is not well suited for the evaluation of bone. However, the high reflectivity of cortical bone and the tomographic nature of ultrasound imaging make it ideal for evaluation of bony contours (Figs. 10–20 and 10–21). In all musculoskeletal ultrasound examinations, the identification of grooves, fossae, tuberosities, trochanters, and epicondyles guides the study. For example, we distinguish the subscapularis and supraspinatus tendons of the rotator cuff by identification of the bicipital groove. Pathological changes in the bony contours are equally well recognized. Marginal erosions and synovial inclusions found in rheumatoid disease are more easily seen sonographically than with conventional radiography (van Holsbeeck et al., 1988). These findings may assist in early diagnosis of inflammatory arthritis. Ultrasound has also proved valuable in the detection of Hill-Sachs lesions (Graf and Schuler, 1988). These post-traumatic defects are often hard to visualize on conventional radiographs. The large number of

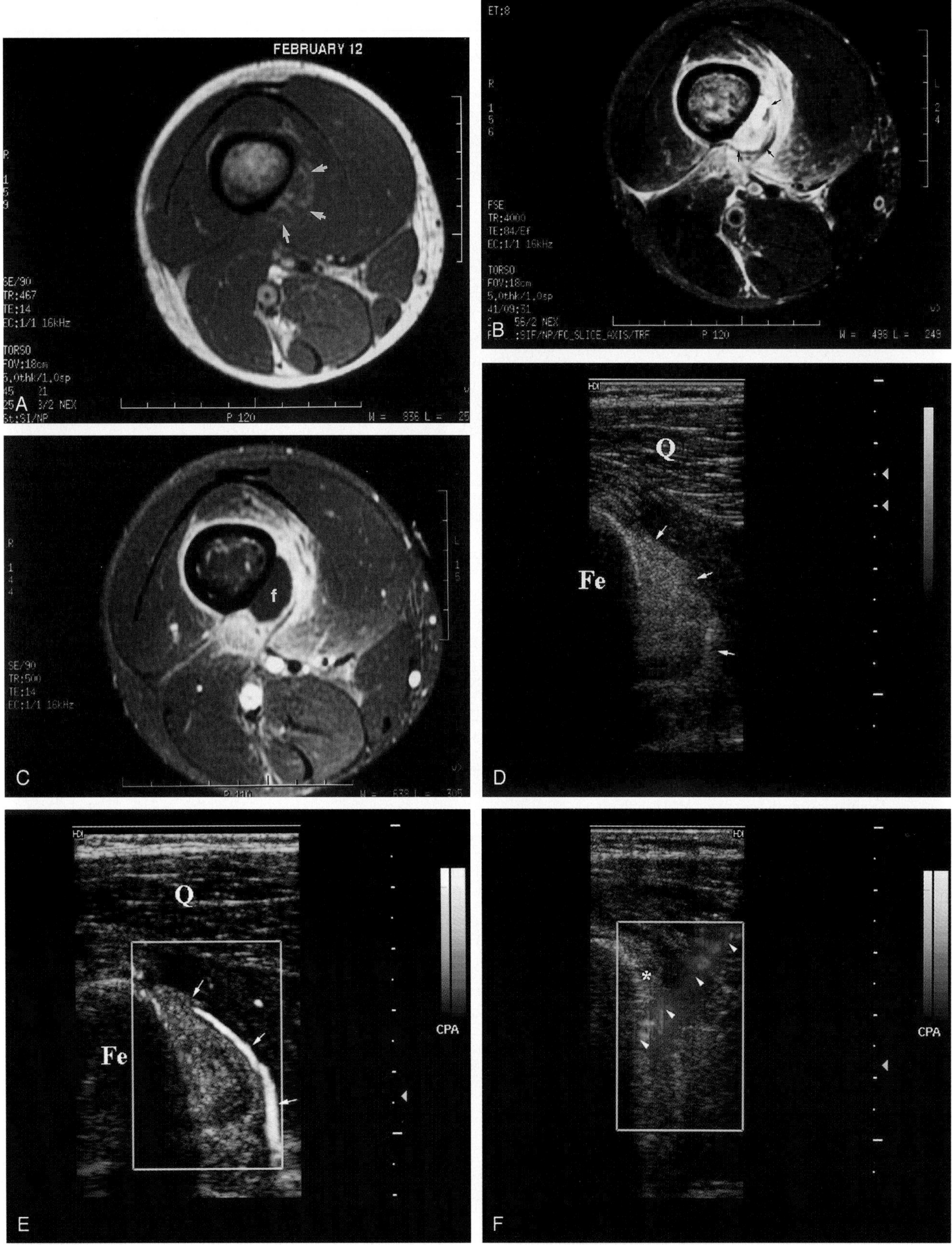

Figure 10–18 ■ *See legend on opposite page*

Figure 10–18 ▪ A, Subperiosteal hemorrhage: axial T_1-weighted MRI. A 26-year-old male with sickle cell disease presented with intense pain in the right thigh. The MRI examination revealed a parosteal mass (*arrows*) of mixed signal intensity associated with the posteromedial aspect of the femur. Anteroposterior, lateral, and oblique radiographs of the femur were negative. **B,** Subperiosteal hemorrhage: axial fast spin echo T_2-weighted fat saturation MRI. Same patient as in **A.** Fluid and edema are noted in and deep to the vastus medialis. Some edema was also noted within the bone marrow. On this sequence the mass is seen elevating the periosteum (*arrows*). **C,** Subperiosteal hemorrhage: axial T_1-weighted fat saturation MRI post-gadolinium infusion. Same patient as in **A.** There is intense enhancement of the periosteum and surrounding muscle. The mass does not enhance, consistent with the presence of fluid (*f*). **D,** Subperiosteal hemorrhage: transverse sonogram. Same patient as in **A**. The subperiosteal mass (*arrows*) demonstrated on MRI appears hyperechoic, consistent with either hemorrhage or pus. Abbreviations: quadriceps muscle (*Q*), femur (*Fe*). **E,** Subperiosteal hemorrhage: transverse sonogram with power Doppler. Same patient as in **A.** Hyperemia is seen in cortical vessels and periosteum (*arrows*), but no flow is demonstrated within the mass. Abbreviations: quadriceps muscle (*Q*), femur (*Fe*). **F,** Subperiosteal hemorrhage: transverse sonogram with power Doppler. Same patient as in **A.** Ultrasound guidance was utilized for aspiration of the mass. The needle is clearly demonstrated using power Doppler, with minimal motion of the needle (*arrowheads*). The periosteum (*asterisk*) has now collapsed.

special projections advocated for radiographic visualization of these lesions indicates the difficulty of this problem. Angulated internal rotation views, Hermodsson's tangential projection, and Stryker's, Didiee, and West Point views are all helpful (Resnick and Niwayama, 1988). However, they are often difficult to obtain and interpret. Ultrasound will quickly and clearly demonstrate the contours of the entire circumference of the humeral head. Hill-Sachs deformity is recognized as a defect in the cortical contour of the posterolateral surface of the humeral head. The lesion is the result of anterior shoulder dislocation, with the humeral head impacting on the anteroinferior aspect of the glenoid. The typical patient is a young, active adult. Identification of Hill-Sachs lesions is important because it indicates a

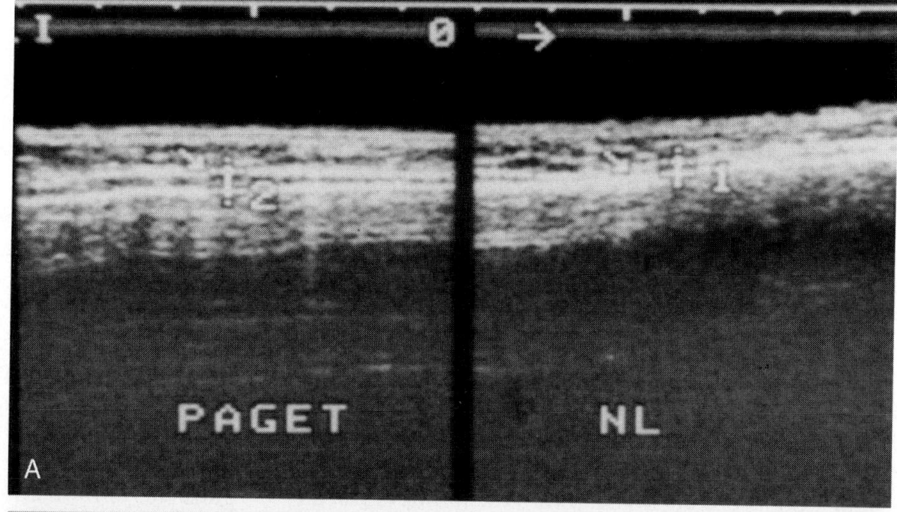

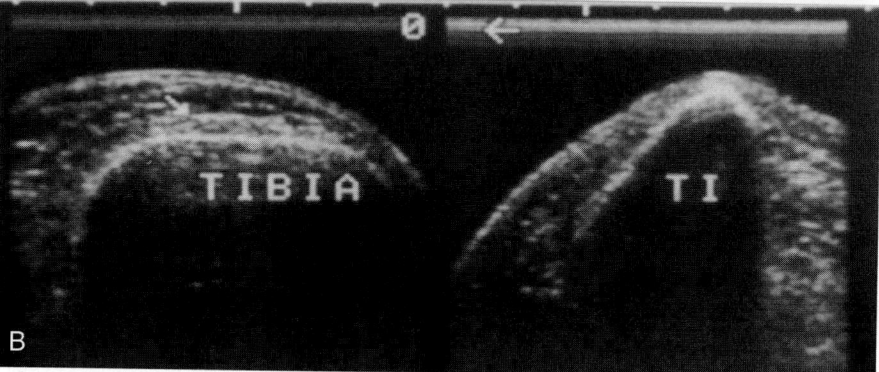

Figure 10–19 ▪ A, Periosteal thickening in Paget's disease: longitudinal sonogram of the tibia. The patient is a 70-year-old man with Paget's disease involving the right tibia. Side-by-side comparison is provided with these longitudinal images of the midshaft of the tibia. Periosteum of the involved tibia is twice as thick as that on the normal side. **B,** Periosteal thickening in Paget's disease: transverse sonogram of the tibia. Same patient as in **A.** These transverse images were obtained at the same level as the longitudinal images. A normal inverted V shape of the tibia (*TI*) is seen on the right. On the left, the tibia affected by Paget's disease is grossly deformed and surrounded by a markedly thickened periosteum (*arrow*).

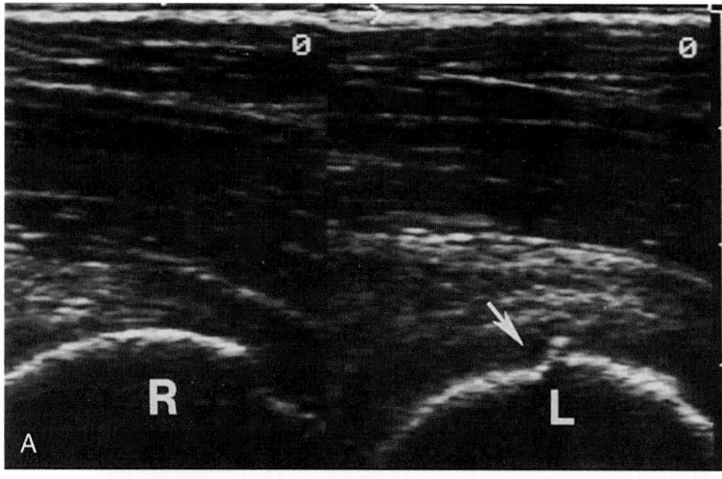

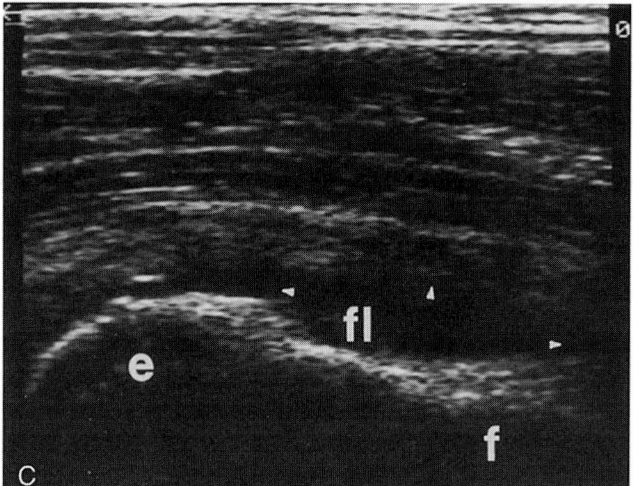

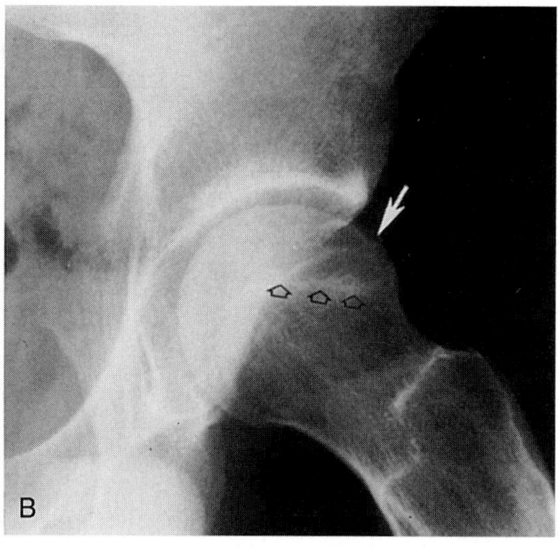

Figure 10–20 ■ **A,** Subchondral fracture with hip effusion: longitudinal sonogram. An alcoholic with left hip pain. The transducer is positioned parasagittal over the femoral head; side-by-side comparison is provided. A smooth contour of the right femoral is noted with normal articular cartilage. A cortical step-off (*arrow*) is seen on the left femoral head, and the articular cartilage is markedly thickened. Subchondral fracture is most often seen in osteonecrosis and is generally accepted as the cause of pain in these patients. Abbreviations: right femoral head (*R*), left femoral head (*L*). **B,** Subchondral fracture with hip effusion: frog leg radiograph. Same patient as in **A.** Anteroposterior radiographs were normal. A band of sclerosis (*open arrows*) in the femoral head is indicative of osteonecrosis. Overlying the region of osteonecrosis is a segment of cortical irregularity (*white arrow*). **C,** Subchondral fracture with hip effusion: longitudinal sonogram. Same patient as in **A** and **B.** The transducer is aligned over the left femoral neck (*f*). An anechoic fluid collection (*fl*) elevates the anterior joint capsule (*arrowheads*). Effusions are commonly found in cases of osteonecrosis. The irregular epiphysis (*e*) is again noted.

predisposition for recurrent luxation. In addition to evaluation of the sequelae of dislocation, ultrasound can be valuable in demonstrating subluxations at joints that are difficult to evaluate radiographically (Fig. 10–22). One example is the symphysis pubis (Fig. 10–23). Disruption of the pubic symphysis is a relatively common injury in soccer players due to the torsional stress induced while forcefully kicking. The ensuing pelvic pain is usually investigated with an anteroposterior radiograph, which is invariably unremarkable. Real-time sonographic examination quickly and easily demonstrates the abnormal movement. Similarly, subluxation can be noted sonographically at the acromioclavicular, radioulnar and tibiofibular joints. Some of those subluxations may be intermittent or difficult to diagnose secondary to problems with radiographic projection. Ultrasound can diagnose dislocations with great ease because it can evaluate the relationships of structures in real time. Comparison with the uninjured side can also be obtained quite easily. Stress can be applied to demonstrate instability, if this is clinically suspected.

Fractures that are occult on conventional radiographs can often be detected with sonography (Figs. 10–24 through 10–26). Unsuspected fracture findings are quite common in shoulder examinations. Impingement in the subacromial space may be due to subacute fractures of the greater tuberosity. Greater tuberosity fractures often go unnoticed radiographically if they are only minimally displaced. Callus formation then contributes to narrowing of the subacromial space, and the patient presents with symptoms of a torn rotator cuff. Often the patient presents with an exacerbation of symptoms weeks after the injury, when callus

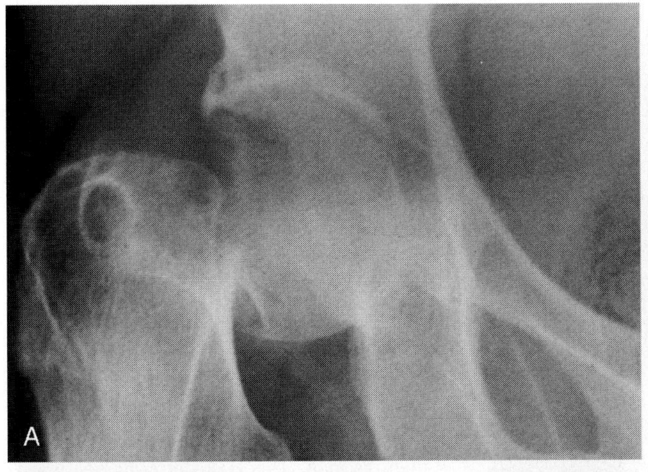

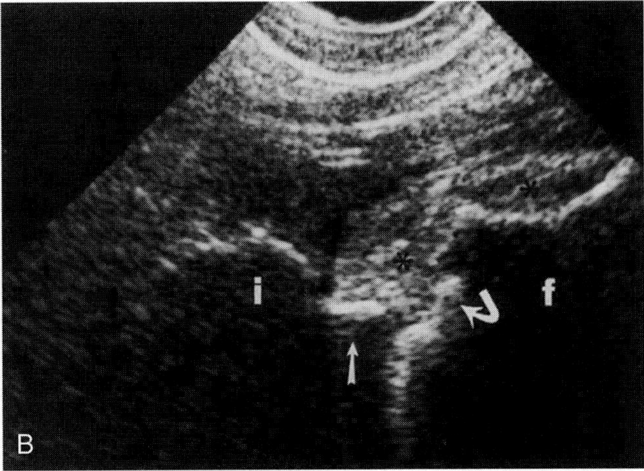

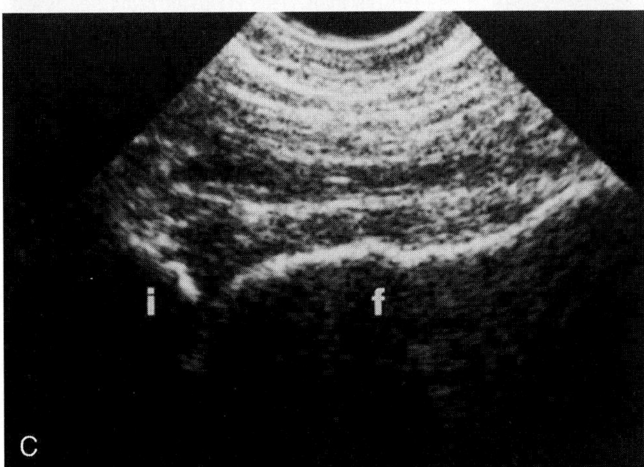

Figure 10–21 ■ **A,** Femoral neck fracture: anteroposterior radiograph. This 68-year-old female nursing home patient fell while getting out of bed. A grossly displaced fracture of the femoral neck is evident. **B,** Femoral neck fracture: longitudinal sonogram. Same patient as in **A.** The fracture (*curved arrow*) with associated capsular hematoma (*asterisks*) shows marked anterior displacement of the distal femoral neck (*f*) relative to the femoral head (*arrow*). Abbreviation: ilium (*i*). **C,** Femoral neck fracture: longitudinal sonogram of the asymptomatic femur. Same patient as in **A** and **B.** A normal smooth contour of the junction of the femoral head and neck is observed on the asymptomatic left side. The iliofemoral ligament is straight and not displaced. Abbreviations: proximal femur (*f*), ilium (*i*).

formation is becoming well established. The examiner must be aware of this syndrome, and the surface of the greater tuberosity must be closely scrutinized when there is a history of trauma. Ultrasound depicts the surface of the tuberosity with tomographic images, demonstrating a step-off deformity or angulation if a fracture is present (Patten et al., 1992). This abnormality should not be mistaken for the osseous changes seen in the greater tuberosity associated with rotator cuff disease (Chapter 7) (Wohlwend et al., 1996). High-frequency transducers are extremely important in the diagnosis of occult fracture. The technique of "sonographic palpation" is valuable in localizing the

Figure 10–22 ■ Spontaneous sternoclavicular dislocation: transverse sonogram. A 54-year-old female presented with sudden onset of sternoclavicular regional swelling. This split-screen side-by-side comparison of the sternoclavicular joints reveals asymmetric alignment of the joints, with the right clavicular head subluxed anteriorly. Abbreviations: left (*L*), right (*R*).

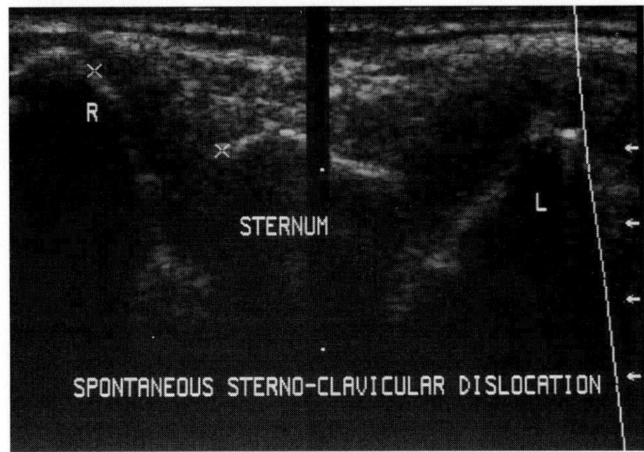

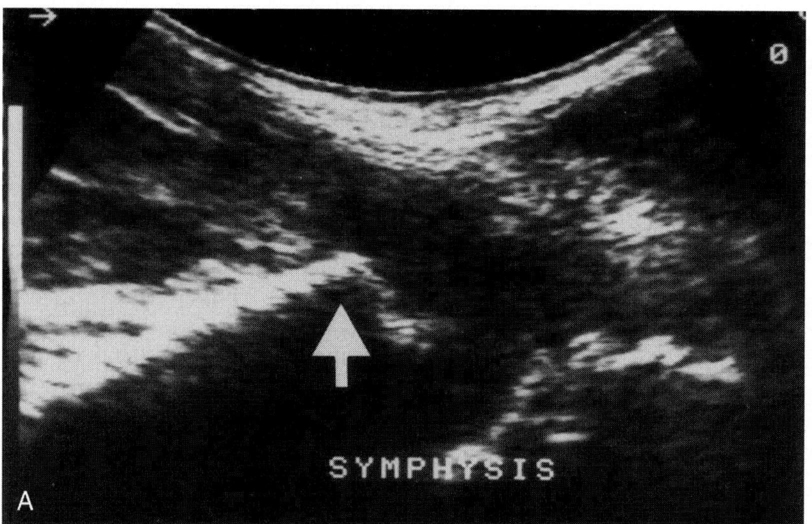

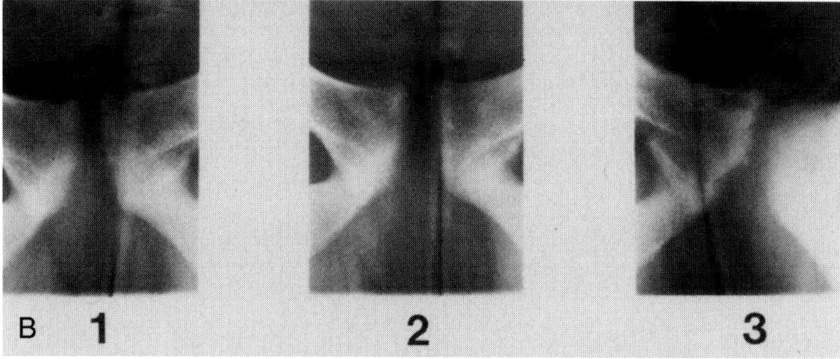

Figure 10–23 ■ **A,** Instability of the pubic symphysis: transverse sonogram. This 23-year-old professional soccer player was referred with the clinical diagnosis of adductor tendinitis. The transducer is positioned transversely over the symphysis pubis. Anterior displacement (*arrow*) of the right pubic bone is observed relative to the left. This is a common injury in soccer players due to forceful kicking. **B,** Instability of the pubic symphysis: upright differential weight-bearing views. Same patient as in **A.** This series of radiographs was obtained with weight bearing on the left leg (*1*), both legs (*2*), and right leg (*3*). Subchondral sclerosis and erosion of the inferior aspect of the symphysis are present. This technique is relatively time-consuming compared with the real-time ultrasound examination. In addition, ultrasound demonstrates the degree of anteroposterior motion, which is not evident on these radiographs.

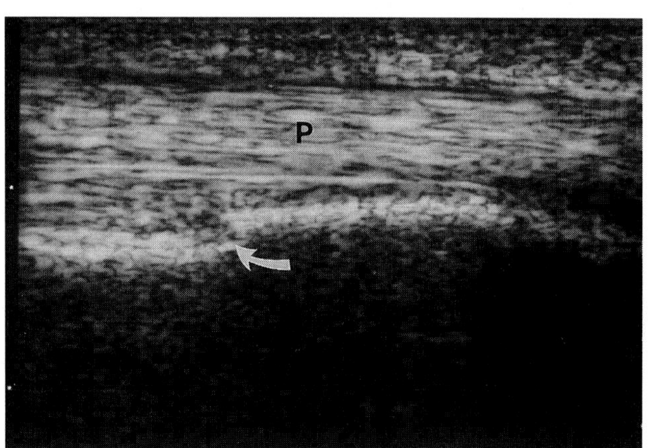

Figure 10–24 ■ Radiographically occult fracture: longitudinal sonogram. Conventional radiographs of the ankle of this 24-year-old professional hockey player, obtained after being hit with a puck, were unremarkable. A cortical step-off (*curved arrow*) indicative of fracture of the fibula is seen deep to the peroneal tendons (*P*).

Figure 10–25 ■ **A,** Freiberg infraction of the metatarsal head: longitudinal sonogram. This 19-year-old soccer player complained of left forefoot pain for 5 months. A bone scan over the lateral aspect of the foot was vaguely positive. Point tenderness was identified while scanning over the plantar aspect of the fifth metatarsophalangeal joint (*mtp*). Focal cortical irregularity (*arrow*) is identified in the fifth metatarsal head. **B,** Freiberg infraction of the metatarsal head: transverse sonogram. Same patient as in **A.** Side-by-side comparison of the fifth metatarsal heads reveals fragmentation (*open arrow*) of the subchondral bone on the left, consistent with a transchondral injury. Abbreviation: hyaline cartilage (*c*).

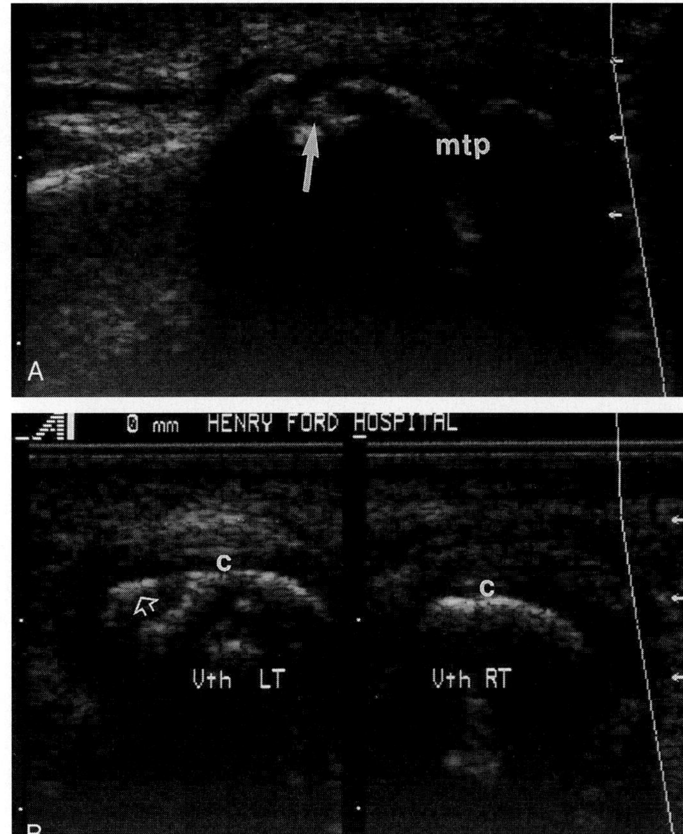

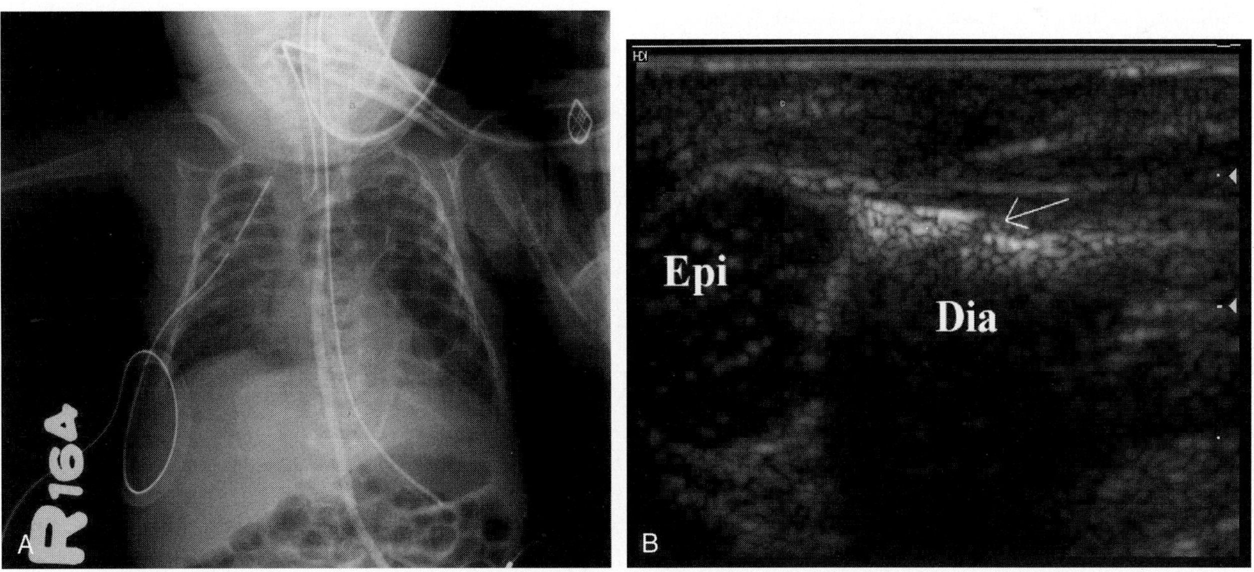

Figure 10–26 ■ **A,** Neonatal fracture: chest radiograph. Contracture of the left arm of this premature infant limited radiographic evaluation of the shoulder. There was high clinical suspicion of a shoulder dislocation. **B,** Neonatal fracture: coronal sonogram. Same patient as in **A.** A minimally displaced fracture (*arrow*) is identified in the proximal humerus. Examination of the glenohumeral joint was normal. Abbreviations: epiphysis (*Epi*), diaphysis (*Dia*).

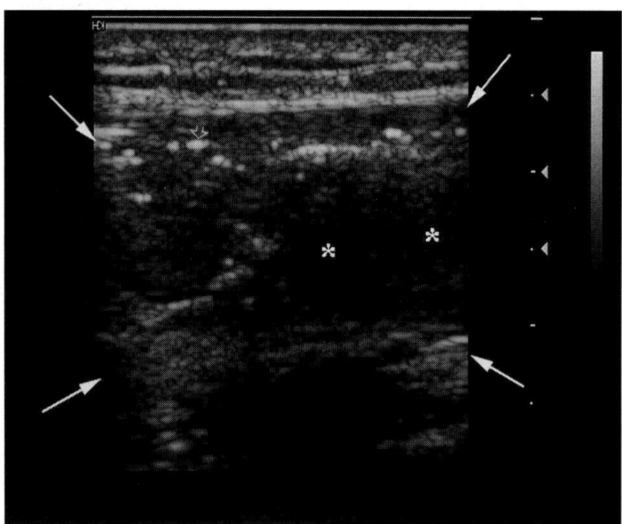

Figure 10–27 ■ Normal healing of tibial fracture: longitudinal sonogram. This 45-year-old male sustained a closed transverse fracture of the tibial diaphysis. Numerous echogenic foci (*open arrow*) are present within the callus (*arrows*) at the fracture site. Attenuation of the sound beam by these echogenic foci results in poor visualization of the deeper structures. This is compensated for in part by adjustment of the time-gain compensation (*TGC*). The intramedullary rod is not clearly visualized due to this incomplete shadowing (*).

region of interest in injuries of long bones. Often a cortical discontinuity can be identified. Observation of adjacent subperiosteal hemorrhage will confirm the diagnosis. In our institution, the sensitivity and specificity of real-time gray scale diagnosis of occult fractures of the scaphoid bone in the wrist have been approximately 80%.

Several nonimaging ultrasound techniques have also been used for the evaluation of occult fracture. Transmission ultrasound with a power output of 3 W/cm^2 has been used successfully to detect occult fractures of the scaphoid (Shenouda and England, 1987). Bone mineralization and architecture can also be evaluated using transmission ultrasound (Heaney et al., 1989). Transmission ultrasound can also be used to produce cross-sectional images in a technique called *orthographic transmission ultrasound* (Carson et al., 1977; Hentz et al., 1984, 1987). In this technique, the attenuation of the sound beam is measured, rather than the reflection, as in pulse-echo imaging. The disadvantage of this technique is that it currently requires a water path, thus limiting its use to the extremities. The differences in attenuation of sound in various soft tissues are greater than the differences in attenuation of x-rays. Therefore, greater soft tissue contrast resolution is afforded by transmission ultrasound. In vitro studies of cadaver hands have demonstrated image quality similar to that obtained with MRI. Clinical transmission ultrasound equipment is not generally available at present, but it is hoped that it will become widely available in the near future.

Gray scale and color Doppler ultrasound have both been used in assessment and follow-up of bone healing (Calliadi et al., 1993; Moed et al., 1995). Studies have focused on the healing of tibial fractures because of the tibia's limited blood supply and frequent complications of its healing process. Blood vessels are observed sonographically in the granulation tissue as early as 2 weeks after injury. Fibrous callus appears as hyperechoic tissue relative to the tibialis anterior muscle. Cartilaginous callus demonstrates small, hyperechoic speckles in the reparative tissue and signs of acoustic shadowing. Osseous callus is characterized by total reflection of the ultrasound beam. These findings have been validated in a dog study with ultrasound– pathological correlation obtained by callus biopsy (Moed et al., 1998b). Sonographic evidence of cartilaginous callus formation appears approximately 5 weeks postinjury in open tibial fractures (range, 17–65 days). Ultrasound predicted fracture healing before it was radiographically evident in all patients studied (Moed et al., 1998a). On average, ultrasound evidence of healing precedes radiographic findings by 3 months. The first examination for evaluation of tibial fracture healing is recommended 5 weeks after injury. If callus overshadows the medullary canal, the prognosis is good (Figs. 10–27 through 10–29). Bad prognostic signs include lack of acoustic shadowing, hypoechoic tissue in the fracture gap, absence of visible periosseous and periosteal vessels, lack of periosteal covering, and fluid around the tibial shaft. Patients who have been treated with an intramedullary nail will demonstrate callus overlying the nail when examined over the anterior, medial, and lateral aspects of the tibia if healing is progressing favorably. Delayed healing will not demonstrate these findings around the nail at 5 weeks. Metallic ring-down artifact will show at the fracture site (Figs. 10–30 and 10–31). Italian investigators have indicated that if only one or two vessels are visualized within the callus at 1 month and they demonstrate high resistive indices (0.8 or higher), then

Text continued on page 348

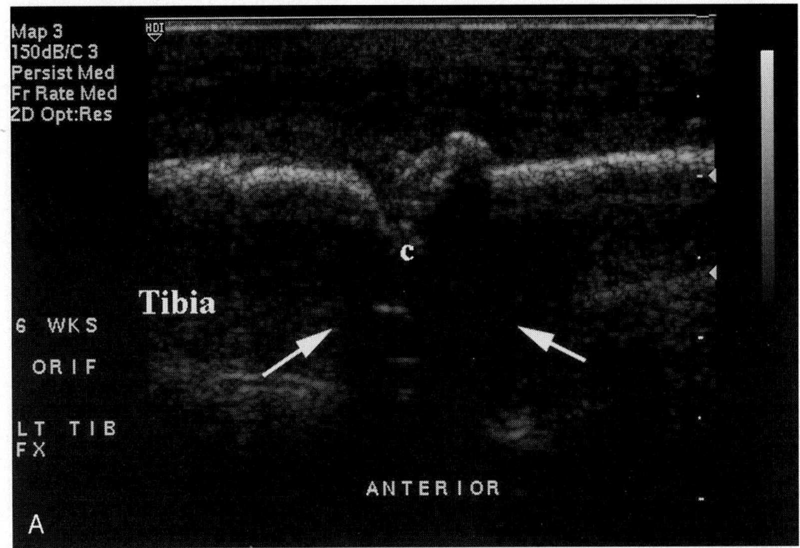

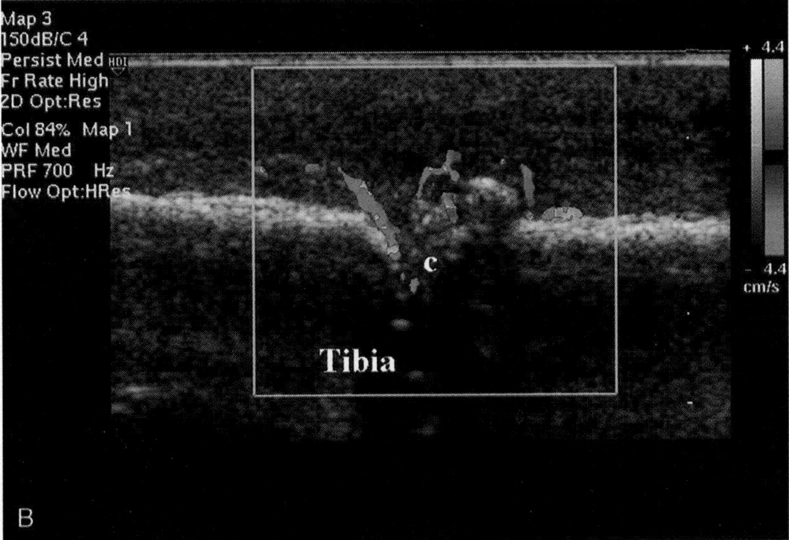

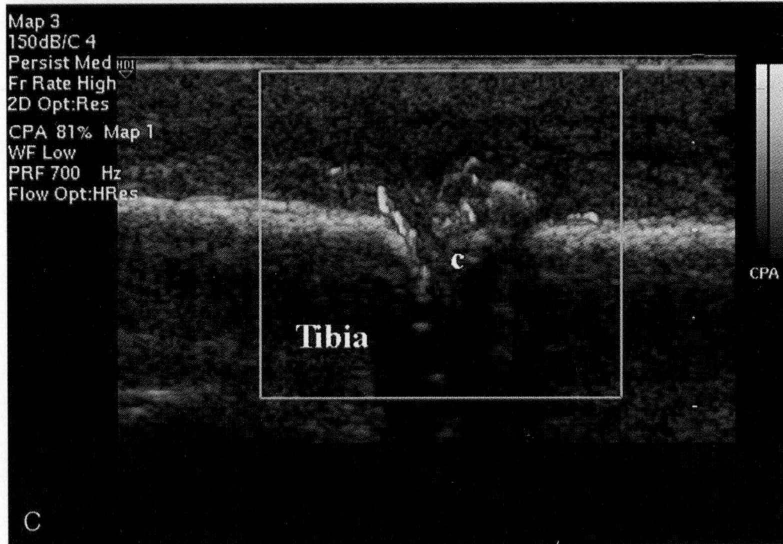

Figure 10–28 ■ **A,** Characteristics of callus vascularity: longitudinal sonogram. This 41-year-old male sustained a closed tibial fracture with compartment syndrome after being thrown from a second-floor balcony. He was treated with nonreamed intramedullary rod and fasciotomy. Six weeks after treatment, dense echogenic callus (*c*) formation with acoustic shadowing (*arrows*) is seen at the anterior aspect of the fracture site. **B,** Characteristics of callus vascularity: longitudinal sonogram with color Doppler. Same patient as in **A.** Periosteal and muscular vessels are observed supplying the callus (*c*). **C,** Characteristics of callus vascularity: longitudinal sonogram with power Doppler. Same patient as in **A.** Power Doppler provides a more accurate representation of the vessel size. Increased vascularity correlates with the ossific phase of callus formation and is a very good predictor of fracture healing.

Figure continued on following page

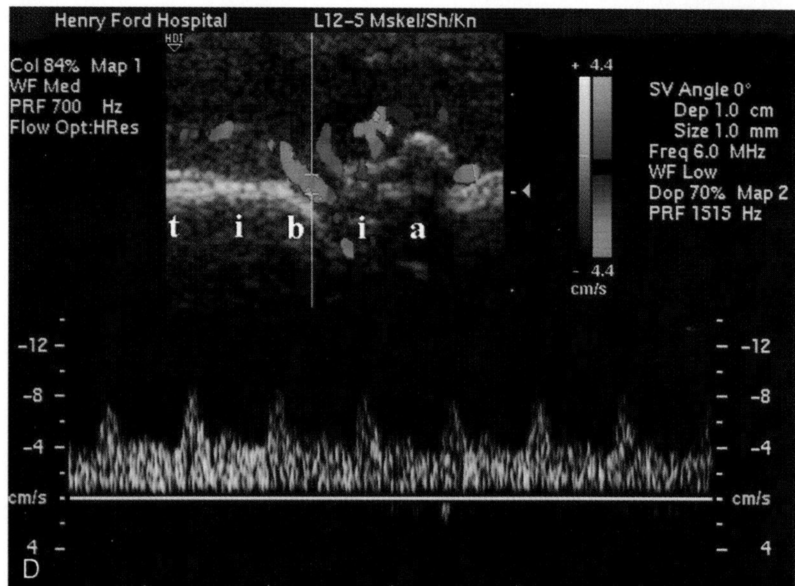

Figure 10–28 *Continued* ■ **D,** Characteristics of callus vascularity: longitudinal sonogram duplex Doppler. Same patient as in **A.** Duplex Doppler waveforms of arteries entering the callus demonstrate a low-resistance pattern. Again, this is indicative of normal healing. High-resistance vessels are reflective of poor healing.

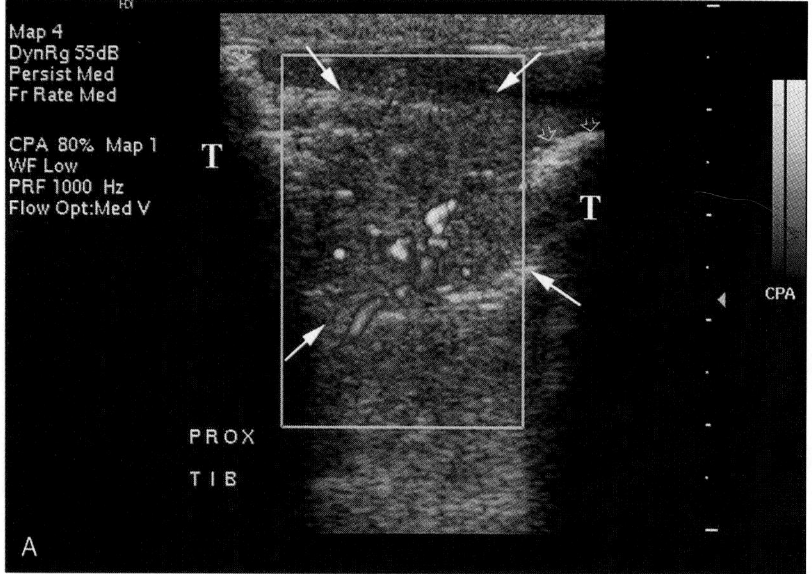

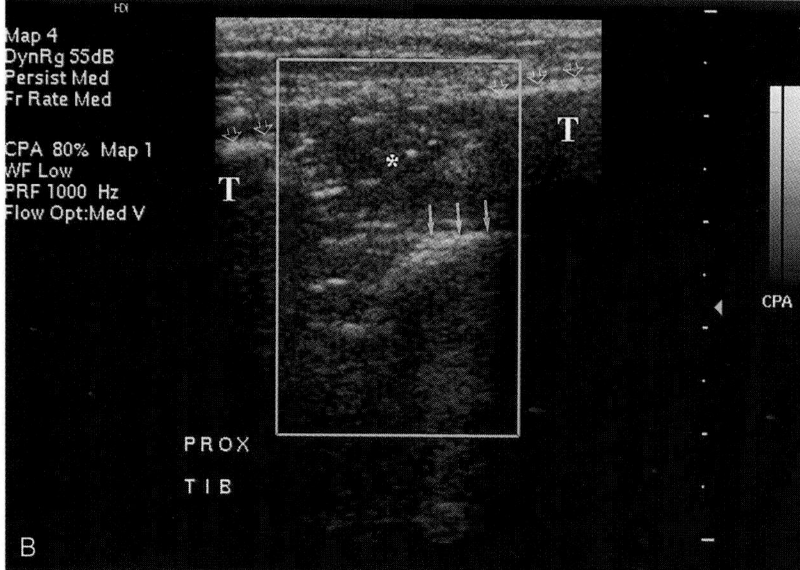

Figure 10–29 ■ **A,** Vascularity of normal fracture healing: longitudinal sonogram with power Doppler. Numerous vessels are demonstrated within the anterior aspect of the callus (*large arrows*) 6 weeks following treatment of an open tibial fracture with an intramedullary rod in this 40-year-old male. The surface of the rod is not identifiable. Abbreviations: tibial margins (*T*), tibial cortex (*open arrows*). **B,** Vascularity of normal fracture healing: longitudinal sonogram with power Doppler. Same patient as in **A.** At the medial aspect of the fracture site are numerous echogenic foci within the callus (*asterick*), but few vessels are seen. A small segment of the intramedullary rod is visualized (*arrows*). Again, note that healing at the medial aspect of tibial fractures is delayed relative to the other sides. Abbreviations: tibial margins (*T*), tibial cortex (*open arrows*).

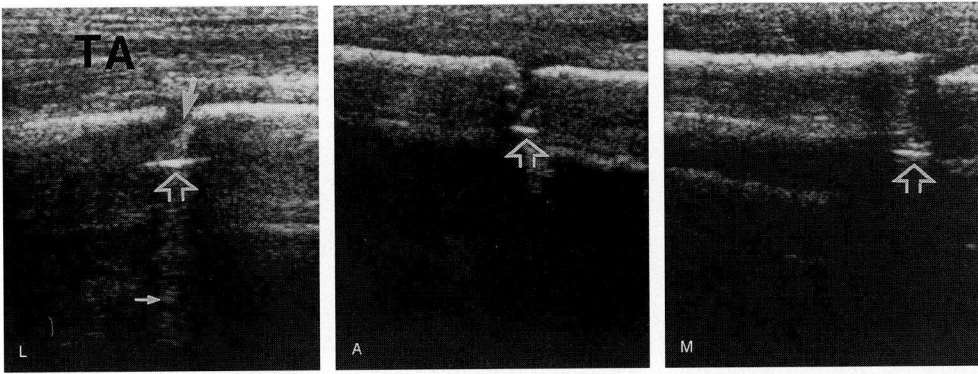

Figure 10–30 ▪ Follow-up of fracture healing: longitudinal sonograms. Six weeks after this grade I open fracture of the tibia was treated by a nonreamed intramedullary rod, radiographs showed no evidence of healing in this 37-year-old male. Longitudinal sonographic images of the lateral (*L*), anterior (*A*), and medial (*M*) aspects (*from left to right*) of the fracture site were obtained. The metallic intramedullary rod (*open arrow*) was clearly visualized on all images, identified by a clear ring-down artifact (*small arrow*). This is indicative of delayed healing at 6 weeks. Echogenicity of the callus formation within the fracture gap (*arrow*) is compared to the tibialis anterior muscle (*TA*). Normal callus formation should be at least as echogenic as the muscle.

Figure 10–31 ▪ **A,** Delayed fracture healing: longitudinal sonogram with power Doppler. Two months after an open tibial fracture was treated with a nonreamed intramedullary rod, the callus remains markedly hypoechoic in this 46-year-old female. The rod (*small arrows*) is clearly visible, with ring-down artifact (*) seen deep to the surface of the rod in this image obtained over the anterior aspect of the tibia. A single vessel (*large arrow*) is identified within the callus using power Doppler. **B,** Delayed fracture healing: longitudinal sonogram with power Doppler. Same patient as in **A.** No vessels are seen within the hypoechoic callus at the medial aspect of the fracture site. Again, ring-down artifact (*small arrows*) is seen deep to the surface of the rod (*large arrows*). Typically, the medial aspect of fractures of the tibial diaphysis is the slowest to heal.

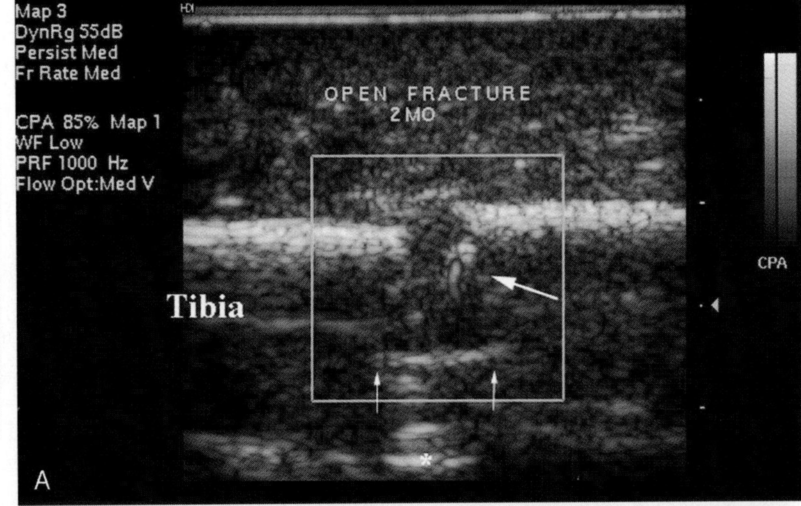

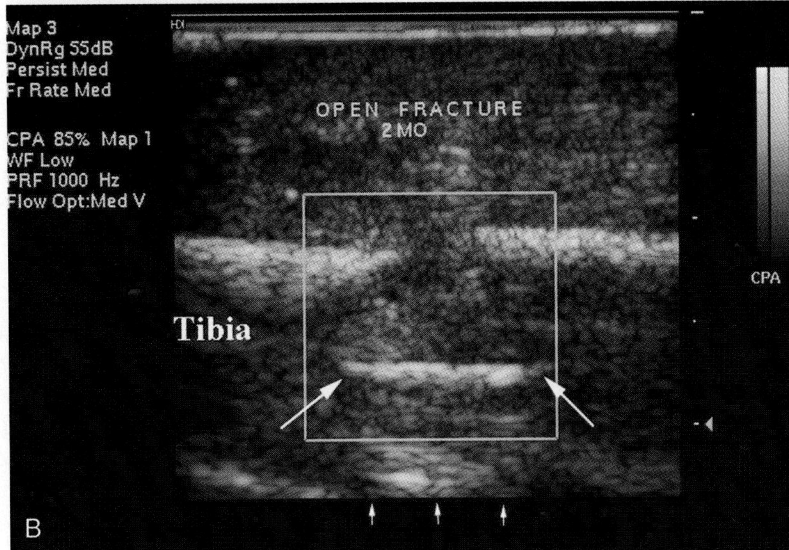

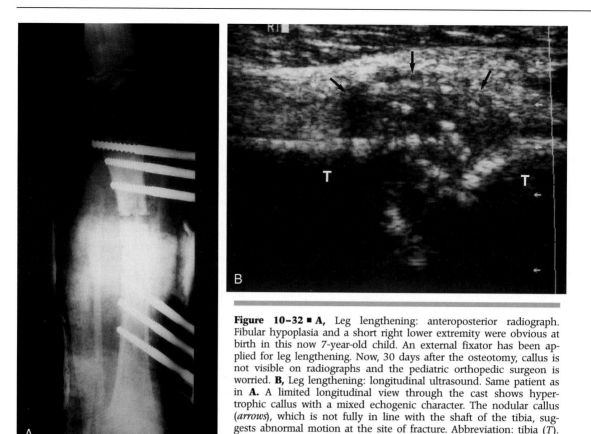

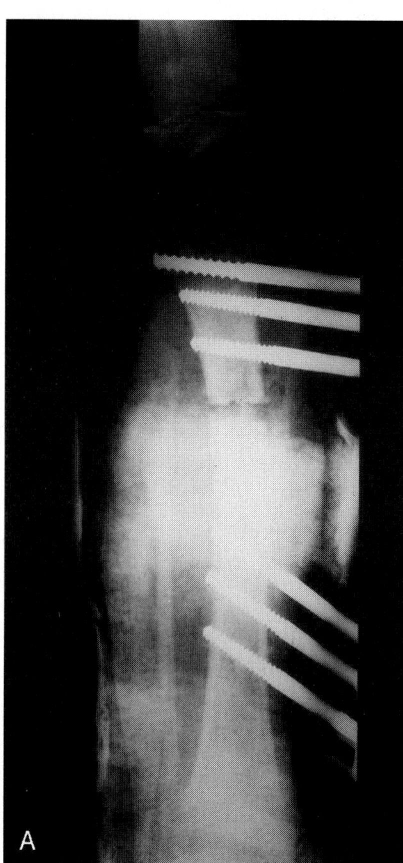

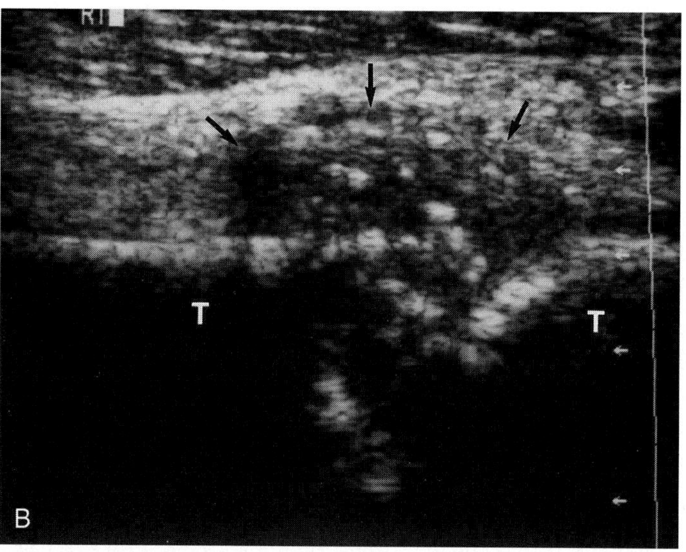

Figure 10–32 ■ **A,** Leg lengthening: anteroposterior radiograph. Fibular hypoplasia and a short right lower extremity were obvious at birth in this now 7-year-old child. An external fixator has been applied for leg lengthening. Now, 30 days after the osteotomy, callus is not visible on radiographs and the pediatric orthopedic surgeon is worried. **B,** Leg lengthening: longitudinal ultrasound. Same patient as in **A.** A limited longitudinal view through the cast shows hypertrophic callus with a mixed echogenic character. The nodular callus (*arrows*), which is not fully in line with the shaft of the tibia, suggests abnormal motion at the site of fracture. Abbreviation: tibia (*T*).

healing is in jeopardy. Fractures demonstrating poor healing are reevaluated at 7 weeks postinjury. Fractures that still lack acoustic shadowing over the medullary canal at 7 weeks postinjury have a high incidence of tibial nonunion. More aggressive treatment has been recommended in these patients. The treatment may include dynamization of an interlocking nail, placement of an exchange nail, treatment with a reamed nail, or bone grafting. The choice of treatment depends on the initial treatment and the severity of disease. Infection must always be excluded prior to any surgical intervention.

Ultrasound can also be applied in the follow-up of distraction callus formation. Distraction callus is seen only in Ilizarov external fixation applied for leg lengthening or other bone transplant procedures (Fig. 10–32). The bone formation in these cases is membranous new bone. The regenerative site in Ilizarov distraction demonstrates linear, hyperechoic structures (Fig. 10–33), as opposed to punctate foci of hyperechogenicity seen in normal cartilaginous new bone formation (Jiang et al., 1997). Because of idiosyncrasies in the rate of membranous new formation and in the tolerance of distraction, the pace of distraction must be adjusted on an individual basis. Some patients do not tolerate a 1-mm distraction rate per day. Problems are typically more accentuated in the anterior and medial aspects of the tibia, not unlike those of regular fracture healing, which is also more difficult in areas with poor vascularization. Cysts may form within the callus (Fig. 10–34). Cysts, big or small, can be aspirated under ultrasound guidance, which will facilitate healing. The cysts are typically blood-filled. Only one cyst in our series required bone grafting after repeated aspirations. This was the only cyst which yielded clear serous fluid upon aspiration. Sonography of Ilizarov leg lengthening has also been advocated to measure the distraction gap. Ultrasound has a significant advantage over radiography because it is not susceptible to image distortion through magnification (Zynamon et al., 1992).

Sonographic evaluation of bone in children is often more valuable than conventional radiography because cartilage is visualized on ultrasound images. Ossification of the growth cartilage can be detected sonographically well before it is evident on conventional radiographs (Harcke et al., 1986; Graf

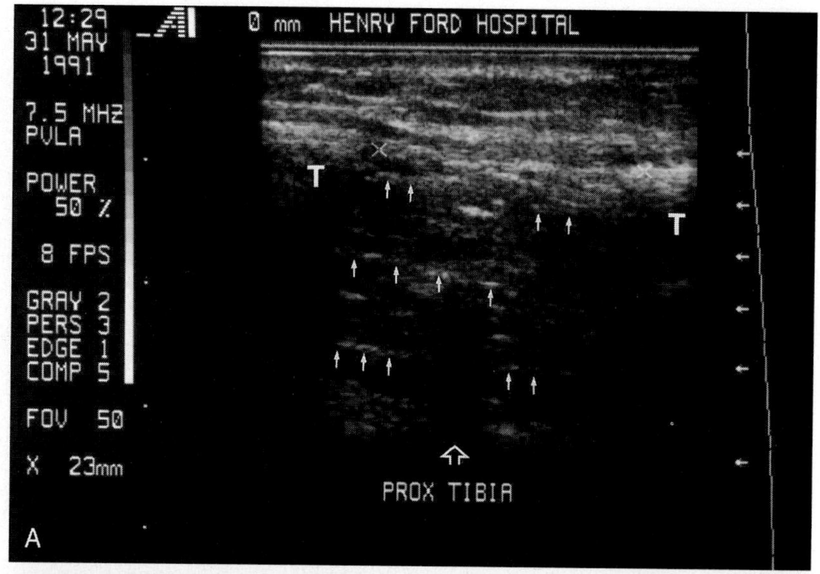

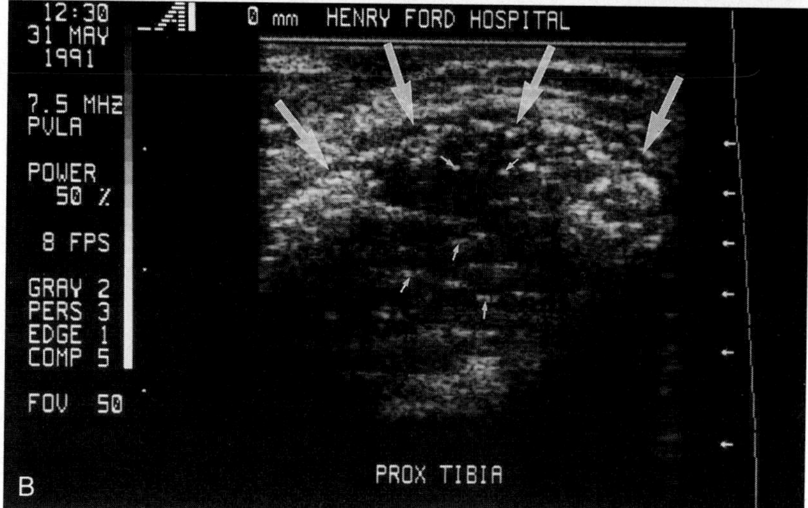

Figure 10–33 ■ A, Ilizarov distraction healing: longitudinal sonogram. In 1989, this 47-year-old male had a grade III open tibial fracture. Two years later, the fractures remained unhealed. A bone transport procedure with Ilizarov compression-distraction was required to close a large gap. This longitudinal sonogram through the proximal corticotomy shows a distraction gap of 23 mm between the tibial cortical margins (x–x). Echogenic linear striations are seen in normal healing of the Ilizarov distraction site (*arrows*). This reflects the intramembranous bone formation seen with Ilizarov distraction. Acoustic shadowing is associated with some of these echogenic striations. Abbreviation: anterior tibial cortex (*T*). **B,** Ilizarov distraction healing: transverse sonogram. Same patient as in **A.** The echogenic foci (*small arrows*) are again seen in this transverse image at the distraction site. Abbreviation: tibial periosteum (*large arrows*).

and Schuler, 1988). As discussed in Chapter 9, ultrasound is ideal for the evaluation of developmental hip dysplasia. It provides both morphological and functional information about the developing acetabulum and femoral head (Graf and Schuler, 1988; Harcke et al., 1988). Furthermore, repeat ultrasound examinations performed to follow the growth and maturation of the hip do not carry the risks associated with ionizing radiation.

Changes in the cartilaginous hip and ossification center are also seen in Legg-Calvé-Perthes disease. Until recently, arthrography (Fig. 10–35) had been the principal means of evaluating deformity of the developing femoral epiphysis. These examinations require deep sedation or general anesthesia, in addition to the risks normally associated with this invasive procedure (Suzuki et al., 1987). Ultrasound provides the same, if not more, information. Normal epiphyseal cartilage has a homogeneous, hypoechoic appearance. The smooth, spherical appearance of the developing femoral head is easily demonstrated. Ossification is identified as a stippled, echogenic region centrally within the cartilage. As growth continues, the ratio of the volume of the ossification center to the volume of unossified cartilage increases. Small intra-articular cartilage fragments are often present within the joint recesses of patients with Legg-Calvé-Perthes disease.

In addition to detection of the deformity responsible for hinge abduction, ultrasound can demonstrate deformity secondary to necrosis by measurement of the echo index (Suzuki et al., 1987). Coronal images are obtained through the midportion of the acetabulum, with the hip in 35

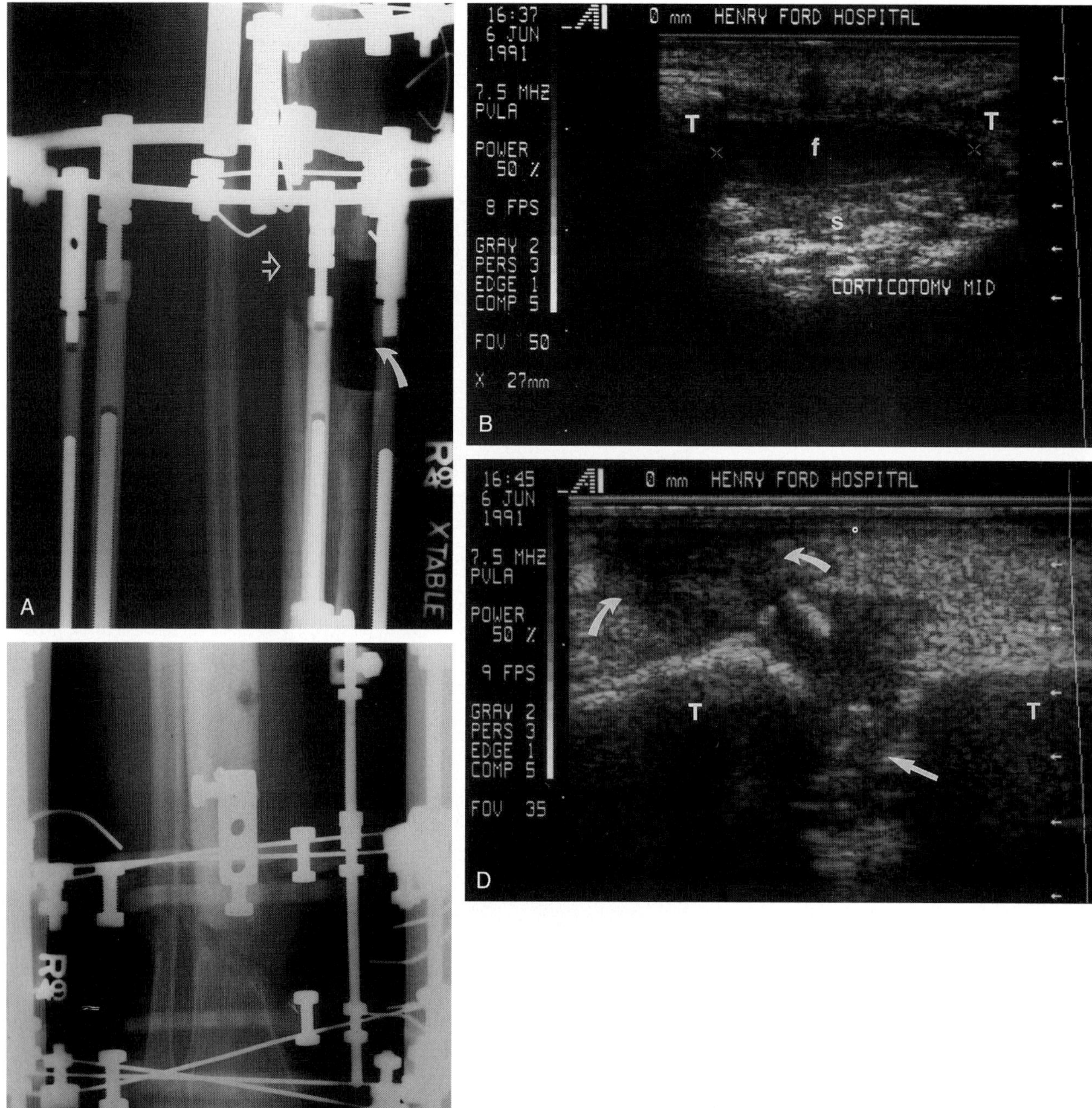

Figure 10–34 ▪ A, Abnormal Ilizarov distraction healing: conventional lateral radiograph. Ilizarov compression-distraction was utilized in the treatment of this 17-year-old male motor vehicle accident victim with a comminuted distal tibial fracture and nonunion. The proximal distraction site is shown in this lateral radiograph of the right tibia. Distraction was performed at a rate of 1.5 mm per day. Normal bone formation (*open arrow*) is seen at the posterior aspect of the distraction site but is absent anteriorly (*curved arrow*). **B,** Abnormal Ilizarov distraction healing: longitudinal sonogram. Same patient as in **A.** This longitudinal sonogram through the anterior distraction site shows an anechoic fluid collection (*f*) with normal echogenic striations (*s*) posteriorly. The fluid collection was aspirated under ultrasound guidance. When distraction is performed too rapidly, hemorrhagic fluid collections may occur. Rapid healing is observed following aspiration of these collections. Abbreviation: tibial margins (*T*). **C,** Abnormal Ilizarov distraction healing: conventional frontal radiograph. Same patient as in **A.** The compression or "docking" site of the Ilizarov device is demonstrated in the distal tibia. This is the site of nonunion. **D,** Abnormal Ilizarov distraction healing: longitudinal sonogram. Same patient as in **A.** Soft tissue abnormality superficial to the tibia (*curved arrows*) is secondary to a fistula from the infected fracture site. Mixed echogenicity callus is seen at the fracture site, which was not visible on the conventional radiographs. This fracture healed completely after resolution of the infection. Abbreviation: anterior tibia (*T*).

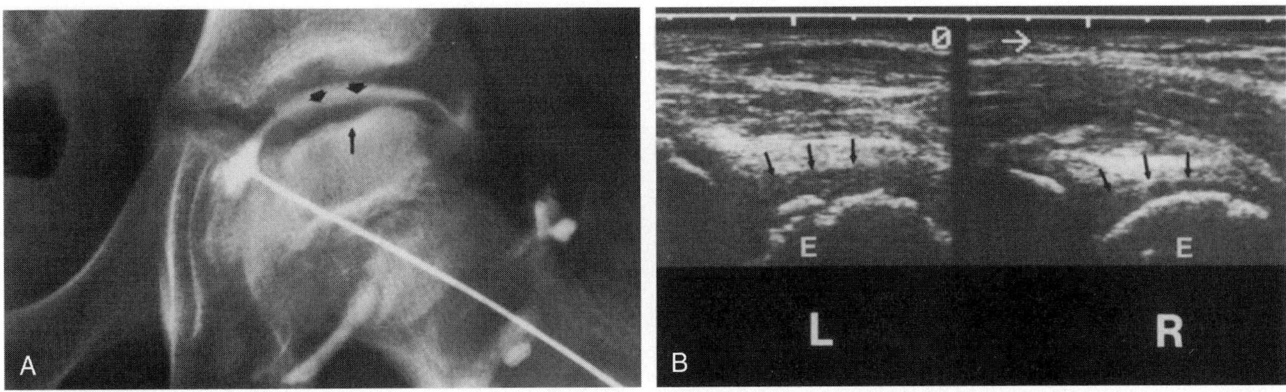

Figure 10–35 ■ **A,** Legg-Calve-Perthes disease: arthrogram. An 8-year-old boy with known Legg-Calve-Perthes disease and painful hip motion. Clinical examination demonstrated possible hinge abduction. The arthrogram shows flattening (*arrow*) of the lateral femoral head covered by intact cartilage (*thick arrows*). The density of the epiphysis is increased. **B,** Legg-Calve-Perthes disease: coronal sonogram. Same patient as in **A.** The transducer is positioned over the lateral aspect of the femoral head, with the hip in 10 degrees of adduction. The involved left hip is irregularly flattened, and the overlying cartilage (*arrows*) is thickened. No contour deformities of cartilage are observed, thus excluding hinge abduction. The information provided by the sonographic examination is identical to that provided by arthrography. The advantages of ultrasound are the noninvasive nature of the study and the ability to compare with the asymptomatic side. Abbreviations: epiphysis (*E*), left (*L*), right (*R*).

degrees of adduction. The midportion of the acetabulum can be recognized by the straight linear appearance of the iliac wing. The greatest height of the femoral epiphysis is measured from the proximal extent of the growth plate (Fig. 10–36, line A). A second measurement of the radius of the femoral head is obtained along the growth plate (Fig. 10–36, line B). The echo index is obtained by dividing the height (A) by the radius (B). A normal femoral head should be spherical; in other words,

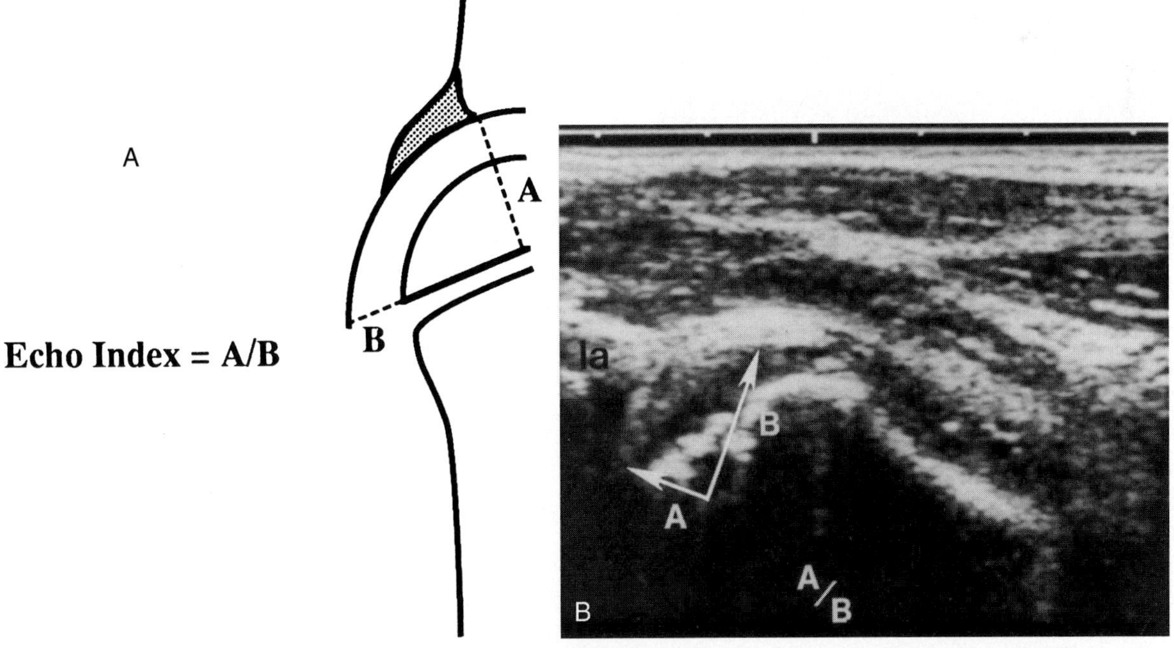

Figure 10–36 ■ **A,** Schematic diagram of the echo index measurement. **B,** Echo index of the femoral epiphysis: coronal sonogram. This 9-year-old boy was diagnosed 3 years ago with Legg-Calve-Perthes disease. This coronal image obtained with the hip in adduction demonstrates a flattened irregular femoral epiphysis. A poor prognosis is associated with flattening of the femoral head. The echo index is a valuable indicator of the degree of deformity of the femoral epiphysis, which can be used in follow-up. Abbreviation: labrum (*la*).

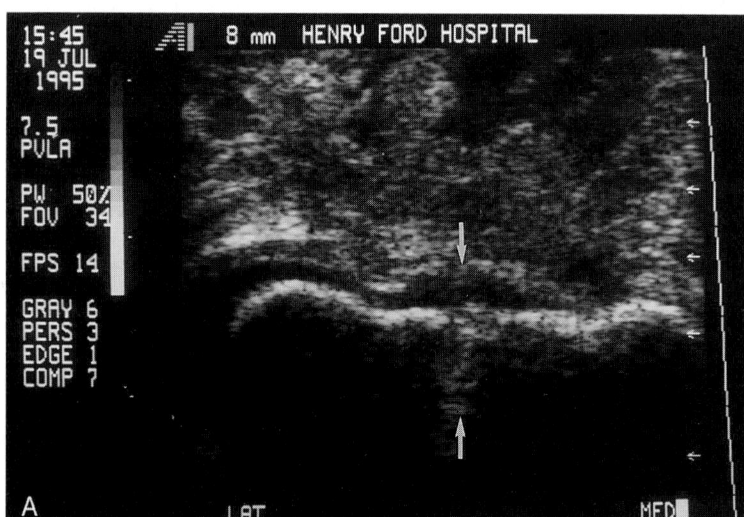

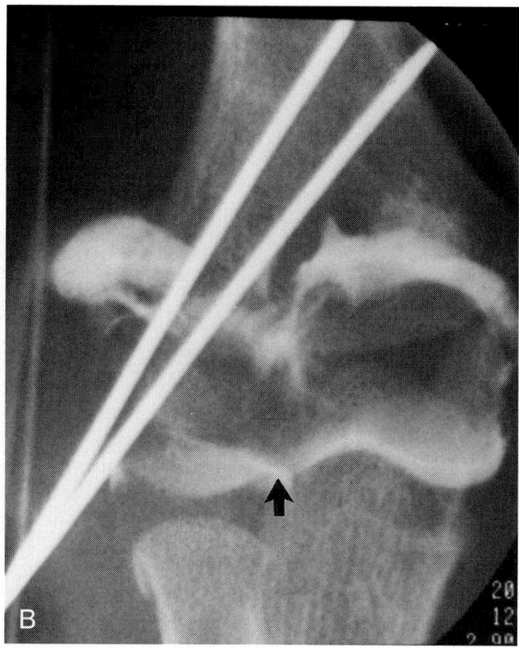

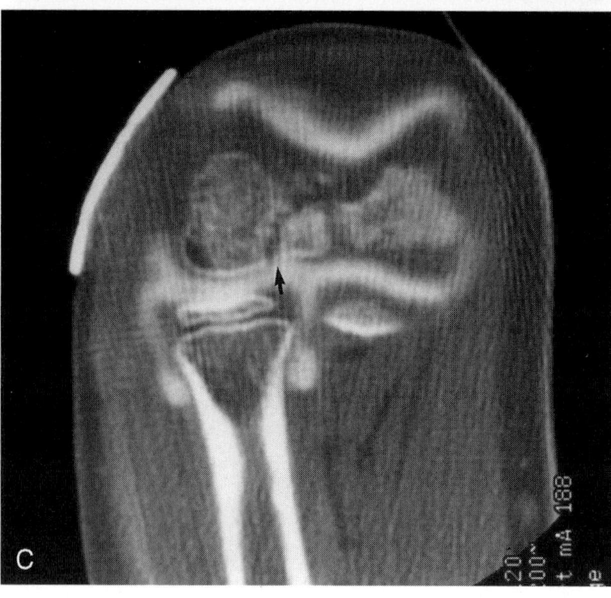

Figure 10–37 ▪ **A,** Lateral epicondyle fracture: transverse sonogram. Often in cases of lateral epicondylar fracture in children, there is a question of whether the fracture extends into the articular cartilage. In this 10-year-old boy who fell from his bike, the fracture is seen extending through bone and articular cartilage (*arrows*). **B,** Lateral epicondyle fracture: intraoperative arthrogram. Same patient as in **A.** A step-off deformity is identified (*arrow*) extending to the articular surface, requiring an open surgical procedure for fixation. **C,** Lateral epicondyle fracture: CT arthrogram. In the past, CT arthrography was the method of choice for evaluation of these fractures. Ultrasound has proven to be as effective in making the diagnosis and is less traumatic to the patient. No sedation is usually required for the ultrasound examination. In this CT arthrographic image, the cartilage defect overlying the fracture is indicated by an *arrow*.

the echo index equals 1.0. This value can be compared with the opposite side using the echo quotient, which is the echo index of the right hip divided by the echo index of the left hip. These data are valuable indicators of the degree of deformity of the femoral head and can be used in the follow-up of Legg-Calvé-Perthes disease. Orthopedic surgeons base their treatment on the degree of deformity of the cartilage and the presence of hinge abduction. The ultimate goal of therapy is maintenance of the normal spherical shape of the femoral head. Echo indexes and echo quotients are good indicators of the success of treatment over time.

The hyaline cartilage which covers the intra-articular portion of long bones can be evaluated sonographically if not shadowed by ossified structures (Chapter 8). Children have more hyaline cartilage because of the additive effect of joint cartilage and growth cartilage. Therefore, the acoustic window into their joints is larger than it is in adults. Ultrasound can be used to examine intra-articular abnormalities in children. This is particularly helpful because younger children cannot be examined by MRI without general anesthesia or deep sedation. The tomographic and dynamic capabilities of ultrasound add important information in the evaluation

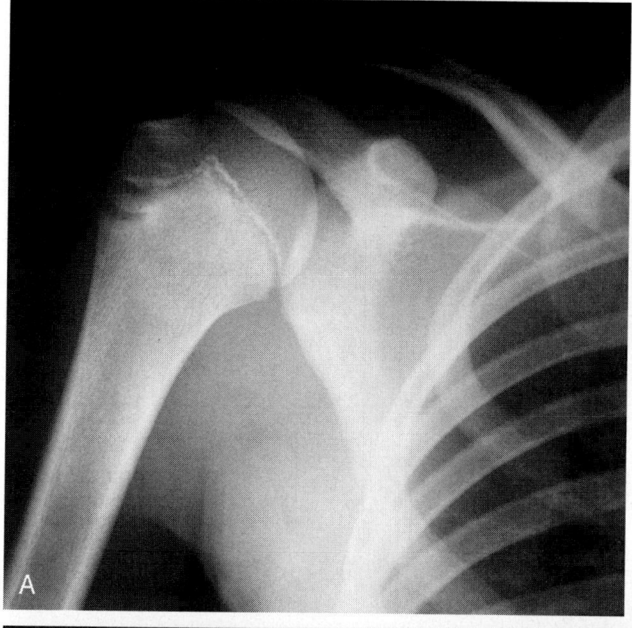

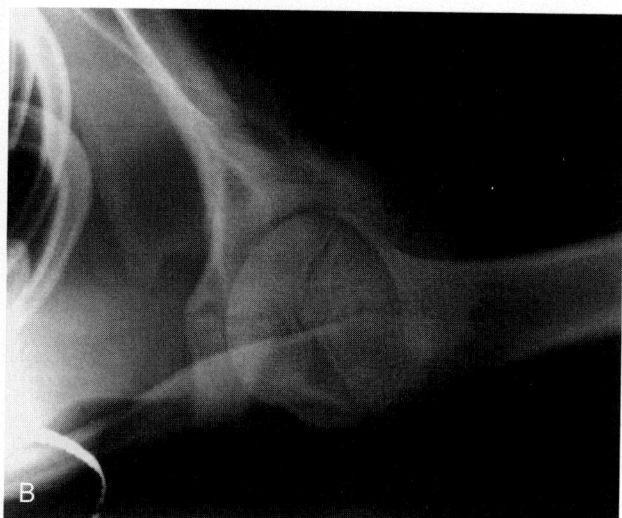

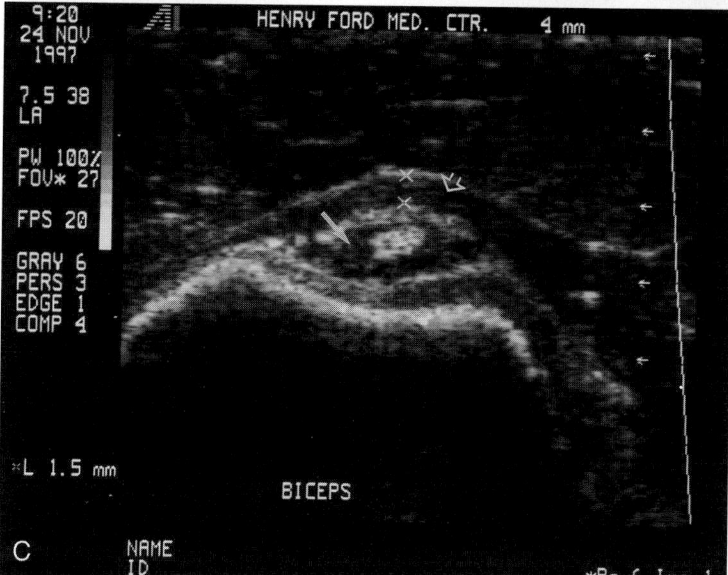

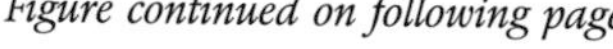

Figure 10–38 ■ A, Epiphyseal fracture: anteroposterior radiograph. This 13-year-old football player sustained a shoulder injury with pain and limitation of motion. Radiographs of the shoulder were normal. **B,** Epiphyseal fracture: axillary radiograph. Same patient as in **A.** No fracture of the humeral head is demonstrated. **C,** Epiphyseal fracture: transverse sonogram. Same patient as in **A.** An ultrasound examination was performed because of continued pain 3 weeks after the injury. The patient also complained of a clicking sensation within the joint. This transverse image obtained over the bicipital groove demonstrates increased fluid within the subacromial-subdeltoid bursa (*open arrow*) and within the biceps tendon sheath (*arrow*). **D,** Epiphyseal fracture: transverse sonogram. Same patient as in **A.** The tendons of the rotator cuff are intact. Deep to the subscapularis tendon, a fragment of cartilage and cortical bone is identified (*arrows*). Abbreviations: deltoid (*D*), subscapularis (*S*), coracoid (*C*).

Figure continued on following page

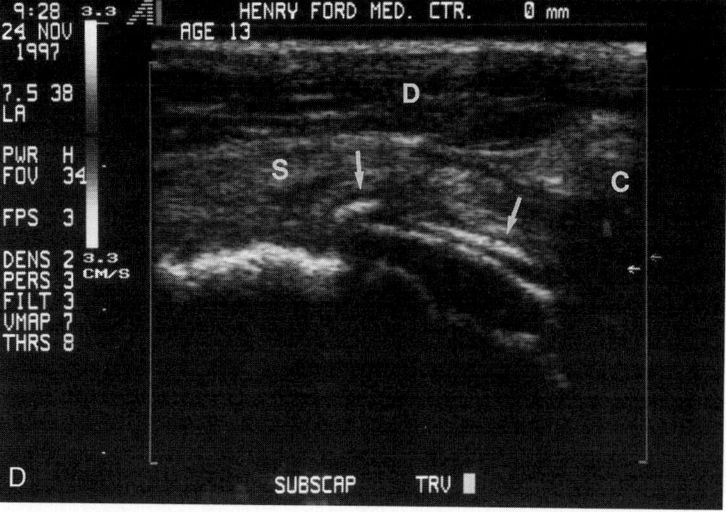

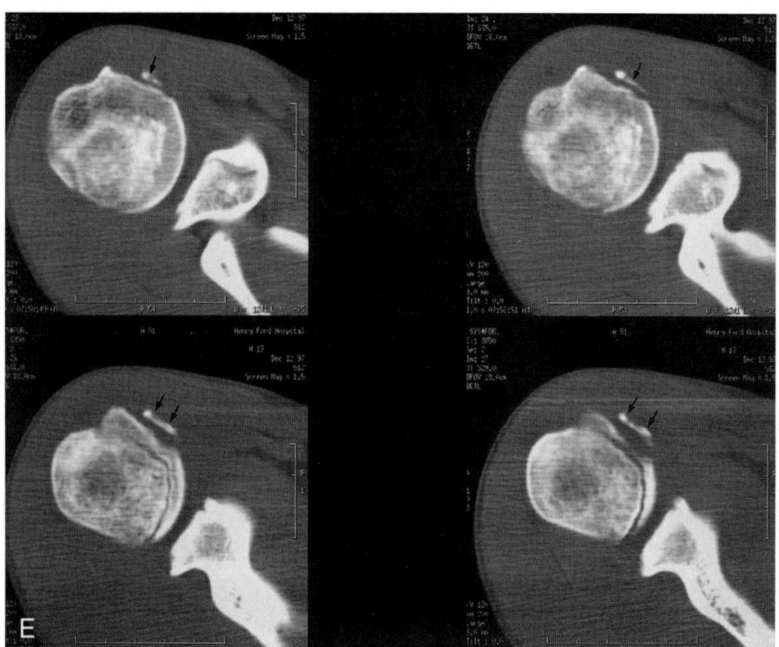

Figure 10–38 *Continued* ■ **E,** Epiphyseal fracture: CT. Same patient as in **A.** Given the ultrasound findings, a CT examination was performed. It revealed a large avulsion fracture of the anterior epiphysis (*small arrows*). Surgical exploration of the joint confirmed the presence of a large fragment of bone and cartilage attached to the subscapularis tendon.

of epiphyseal injuries. These injuries are not always visible on radiographs without introduction of contrast material (Figs. 10–37 and 10–38).

Joints may fail to develop. The diagnosis can easily be made using sonography at birth. The epiphyseal cartilage in such pseudojoints will be seen as one combined cartilage that represents the two epiphyses of those segments. Hyaline cartilage that does not form a synovial joint can be evaluated entirely without the interference of subchondral bone surfaces. This explains why ultrasound is so helpful in assisting in the diagnosis of abnormalities of the rib cage (Fig. 10–39). Tumors of the ribs are often malignant, which is the reason that imaging is critical in patients presenting with a new chest wall swelling. A significant number of benign changes are related to rib cartilage abnormalities in the adolescent because the growth spurt often accentuates congenital anomalies of rib cartilage. Ultrasound will show cartilage duplication or deformity resulting in swelling. The cartilage deformity may result in either an excavatum or a carinatum deformity. Trauma can also result in a step-off deformity of rib cartilage. These changes often worry the parents more than the adolescent. Ultrasound is a simple test to reassure parents and the referring physician (Fig. 10–40).

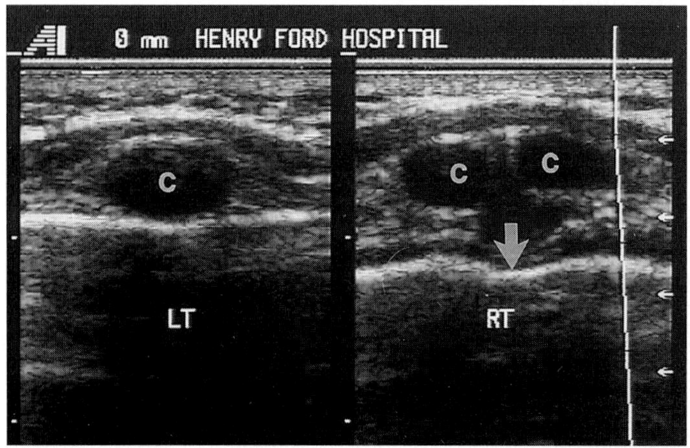

Figure 10–39 ■ Bifid costal cartilage: sagittal sonogram. A palpable chest wall mass was identified by the mother of this 4-year-old female. Her pediatrician was concerned about the possibility of a soft tissue sarcoma. This split-screen image providing side-to-side comparison reveals a bulbous bifid costal cartilage (*c*) on the right. This bulky cartilage indents the pleura (*arrow*). The contralateral normal fourth rib cartilage (*c*) is shown on the left.

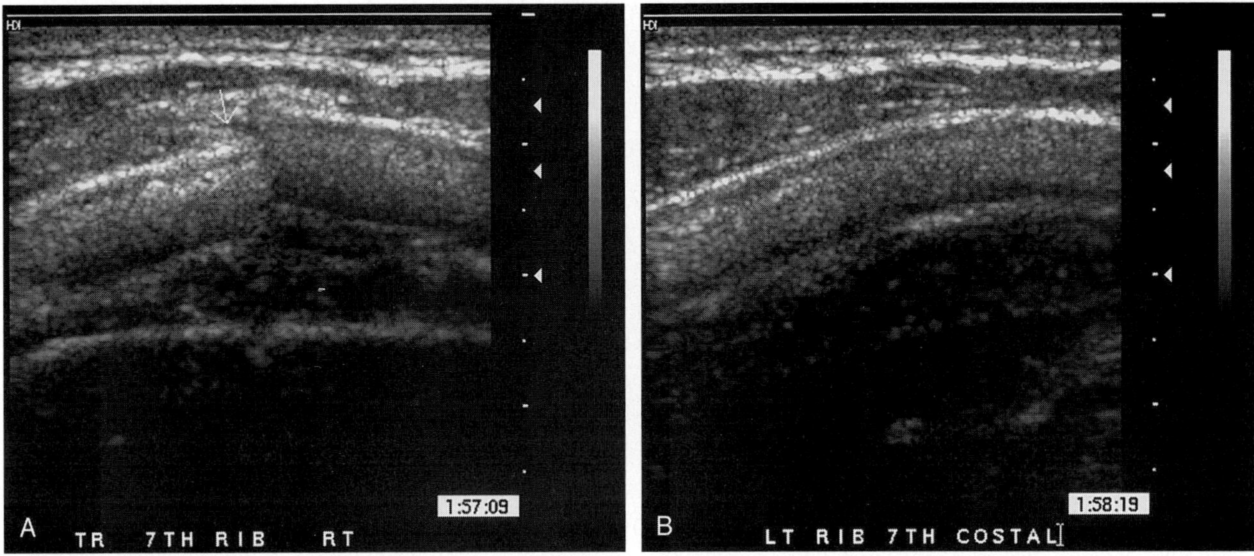

Figure 10–40 ■ **A,** Rib cartilage fracture: transverse ultrasound. A sportsman has difficulty breathing and has focal tenderness over the seventh rib after being hit in the chest. A step-off deformity is noted (*arrow*) in the cartilaginous portion of the rib. This portion of the rib is radiolucent and was therefore not detectable on x-rays. **B,** Rib cartilage fracture: transverse ultrasound. Same patient as in **A.** The contralateral normal rib cartilage has a smooth contour. (Courtesy of Jag Dhanju, RDMS, Ontario Medical Imaging, Canada.)

Measurement to Detect Abnormal Development of the Extremities

During the last half-century, many investigators have tried to develop reproducible methods for measurement of the axis of skeletal elements. Among these are retroversion of the humeral head, anteversion of the femur, and tibial torsion. Ultrasound has been proposed as a quick method to provide a rough measure of these parameters. No studies have carefully addressed the question of the relative accuracy of these methods, but estimation of the error in sonographic measurement may be as high as 20%. Therefore, we believe that the role of ultrasound is simply that of a rough screening tool. Its value in surgical planning and follow-up is very limited. CT provides the most accurate means of calculating these parameters (Hernandez et al., 1981; Berman, 1986; Aamodt et al., 1995).

Humeral Retroversion

The axis through the bicipital groove of the humeral head and the axis of the humeral epicondyles form an angle of approximately 30 degrees in normal individuals. This angle is referred to as the *angle of humeral retroversion.* Decreased retroversion of the humeral head predisposes the patient

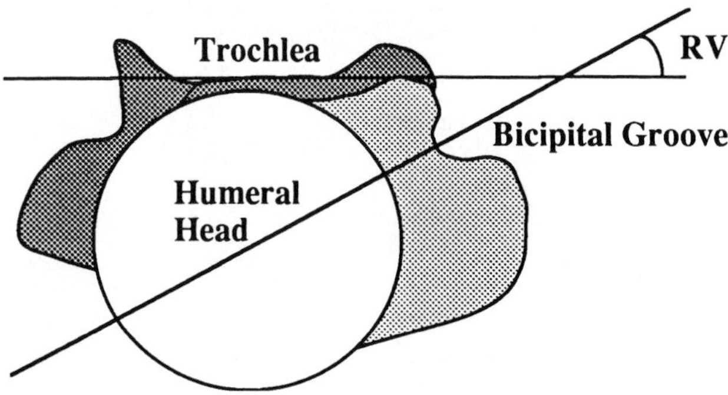

Figure 10–41 ■ Measurement of humeral retroversion: schematic representation. Abbreviation: retroversion (*RV*).

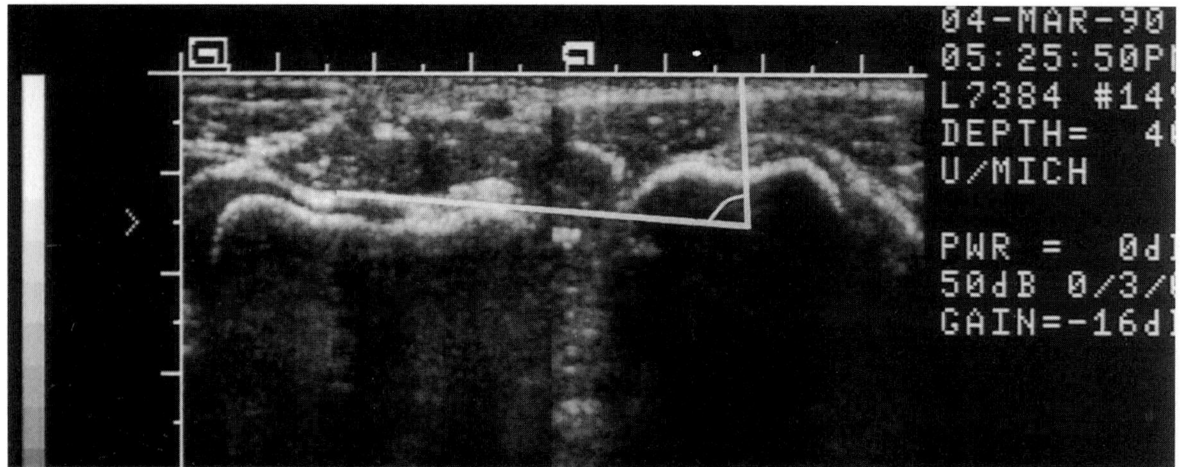

Figure 10–42 ■ Sonographic measurement of humeral retroversion. These images were obtained in a normal 7-year-old boy. A line is drawn from the center of the humeral head bisecting the bicipital groove. Another line is drawn parallel to the trochlea. The intersection of these lines yields the angle of humeral retroversion, as indicated. Sonographic measurement of humeral retroversion tends to overestimate the true angle. This method of measurement provides only a rough estimation of humeral retroversion.

to anterior dislocation of the shoulder (Graf and Schuler, 1988). Pathological retroversion can be corrected by a rotational osteotomy, which increases the degree of retroversion.

Ultrasound measurement (Figs. 10–41 and 10–42) of humeral retroversion is performed with the patient supine and the arm in the anatomical position. The greatest depth of the bicipital groove is identified on transverse images, with the transducer face parallel with the surface of the examination table. A small carpenter's level attached to the back of the transducer is very helpful in making reproducible images and accurate measurements. The second transverse image obtained is that of the distal humerus at the level of the trochlea and capitellum. Once again, the transducer face is kept parallel to the examination table. On the first image, a line is drawn from the center of the humeral head through the center of the bicipital groove. This line should be perpendicular to the transverse ligament. A line parallel to the plane of the anterior surface of the trochlea is then drawn on the second image. When these images are aligned along their border rules, the intersection of these lines yields the angle of humeral retroversion.

Femoral Anteversion

The measurement of femoral anteversion is a problem similar to that of humeral retroversion.

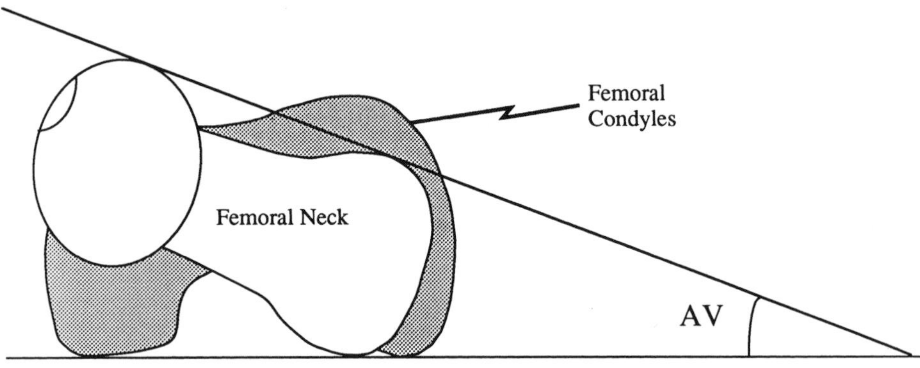

Figure 10–43 ■ Measurement of femoral anteversion: schematic representation. Abbreviation: anteversion (*AV*).

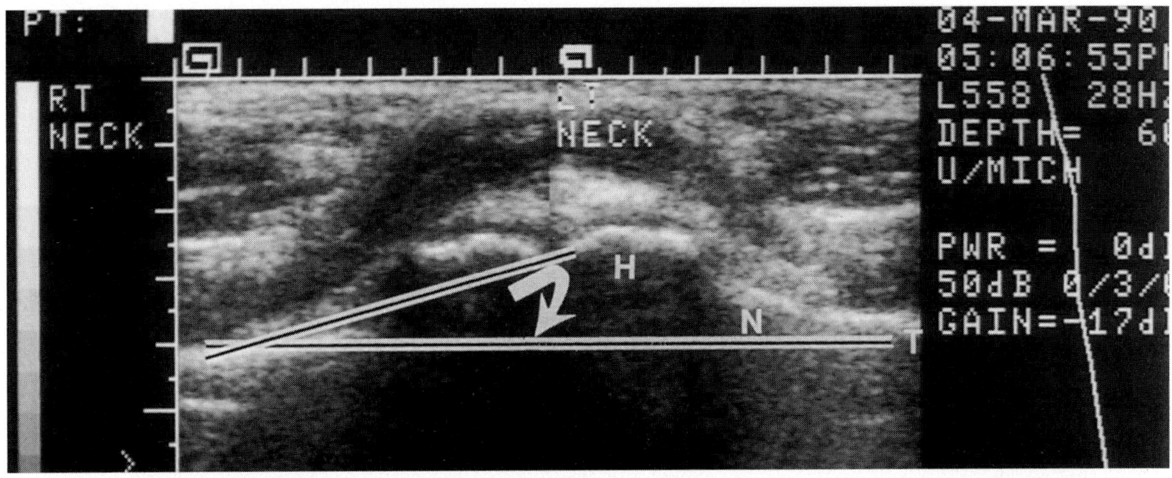

Figure 10–44 ■ Sonographic measurement of femoral anteversion. Same normal 7-year-old boy as in Figure 10-42. This split-screen image demonstrates both femoral necks, with the patient's right at the observer's left. Measurement of the angle of femoral anteversion is demonstrated on the right femur. A line is drawn parallel to the femoral neck. Its intersection with a line parallel with the border rule at the top of the image and parallel to the femoral condyles in the popliteal space defines the angle of femoral anteversion (*curved arrow*). Femoral anteversion in this case measured 13 degrees, within the normal range of 10 to 15 degrees for a well-developed child. The angle of femoral anteversion in an infant is approximately 35 degrees. This angle rapidly decreases as the child develops. Abbreviations: femoral head (*H*), femoral neck (*N*), greater trochanter (*T*).

Excessive femoral anteversion results in a toe-in deformity. Two radiographic methods are available. In a technique developed by Rippstein (1955), two radiographs are taken in special projections defined by a standard leg-positioning device. A modified device was designed by Elsasser and Walker (Dihlmann, 1985). This method yields only an estimate of femoral neck-shaft angles. CT is without question the most accurate means of evaluating femoral anteversion (Hernandez et al., 1981). Several transverse images are obtained through the femoral neck and distal femur. Lines are drawn along the plane of the femoral neck and femoral condyles, yielding the angle of femoral anteversion. The leg must be stabilized to prevent movement during the examination. The range of normal femoral anteversion is 15 to 20 degrees.

Anteversion of the femoral neck is measured sonographically in a manner similar to that of humeral retroversion (Figs. 10–43 and 10–44). The patient is supine, with the lower leg flexed 90 degrees, hanging dependently over the end of the examination table. This allows stable, reproducible positioning of the femur. A transverse image showing both the femoral head and the greater trochanter is obtained, with the transducer face parallel to the examination table. The axis of the femoral condyles is assumed to be parallel to the examination table when the patient is positioned as described earlier. The angle of femoral anteversion is obtained by drawing a line tangential to both the anterior surfaces of the femoral head and the greater trochanter. Its intersection with the border rule defining the face of the transducer yields the angle of femoral anteversion. This technique provides an estimate of femoral anteversion that will demonstrate gross pathology, but CT is the method of choice for surgical planning and follow-up (Hernandez et al., 1981; Berman, 1986).

Tibial Torsion

Lateral torsion of the tibia is responsible for the normal alignment of the foot. Normal tibial torsion is approximately 20 degrees. Tibial torsion may be increased, decreased, absent, or reversed. Abnormal tibial torsion is the most common cause of toe-in deformity in children. In the majority of cases, abnormal tibial torsion is corrected spontaneously during growth. However, in those cases in which deformity persists, measurements of tibial torsion and femoral anteversion are required to establish the site of abnormality. Corrective osteotomy can then be performed. Excessive tibial torsion is seen in patients with cerebral palsy and spina bifida (Joseph et al., 1987). Surgical correction in these cases depends on the general condition of the patient and the severity of the deformity.

Sonographic measurement (Figs. 10–45 and 10–46) is performed with the child lying prone on the examination table, with the feet extending just

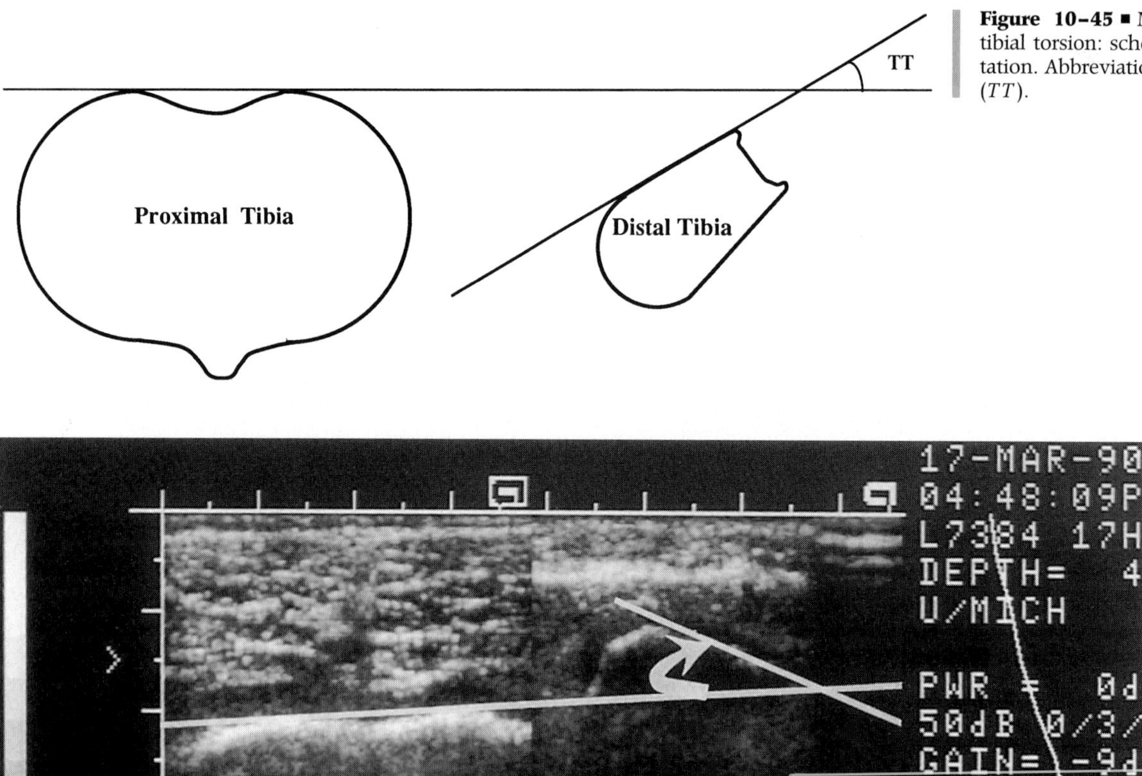

Figure 10-45 ■ Measurement of tibial torsion: schematic representation. Abbreviation: tibial torsion (*TT*).

Figure 10-46 ■ Sonographic measurement of tibial torsion. Same normal 7-year-old boy as in Figure 10-42, prone, with the feet extending freely over the end of the examination table. The proximal transverse image is obtained at the level of the tibial condyles and the distal image at the level of the tibiofibular joint. Lines are drawn parallel to the posterior surfaces of the bone. Their intersection defines the angle of tibial torsion.

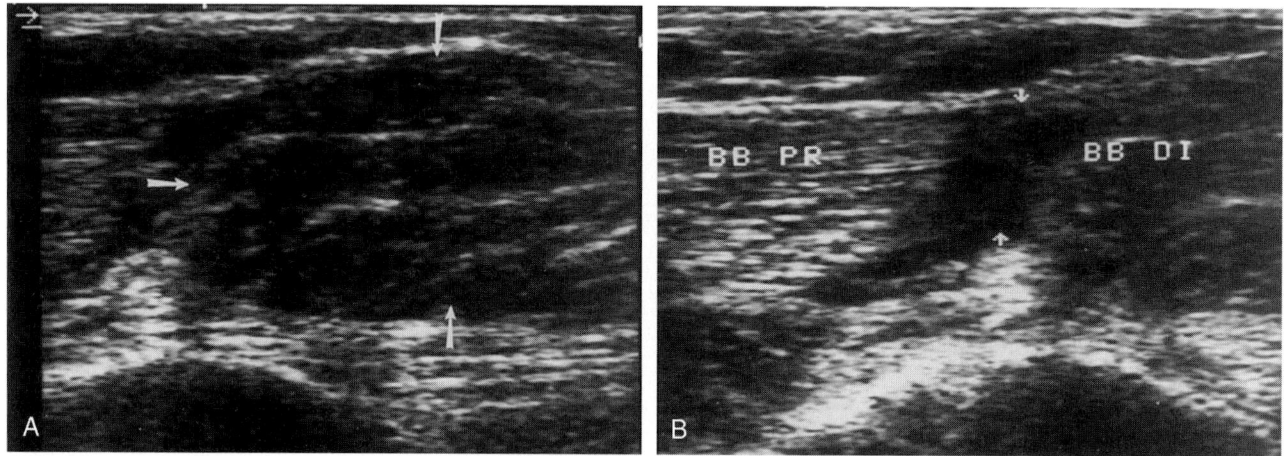

Figure 10-47 ■ **A,** Upper arm pseudotumor: longitudinal sonogram. This 60-year-old woman with a mass in the anterior upper left arm was sent for sonographic examination to evaluate the extent of presumed soft tissue sarcoma. The mass (*arrows*) has an appearance similar to that of muscle, with visualization of fibroadipose septa. **B,** The transducer was moved proximal to the mass, and a rupture of the proximal biceps muscle is demonstrated (*arrows*). The proximal (*BB PR*) and distal (*BB DI*) ends of the ruptured biceps are retracted. The distal end was more mass-like and clinically palpable, thus called a neoplasm by clinicians.

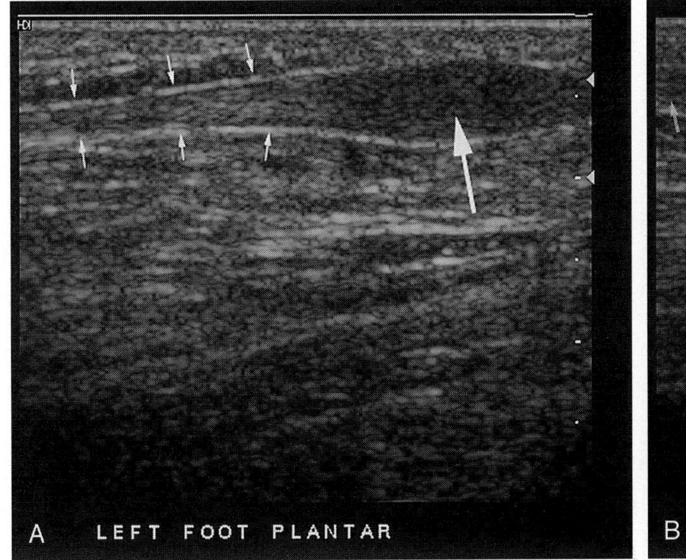

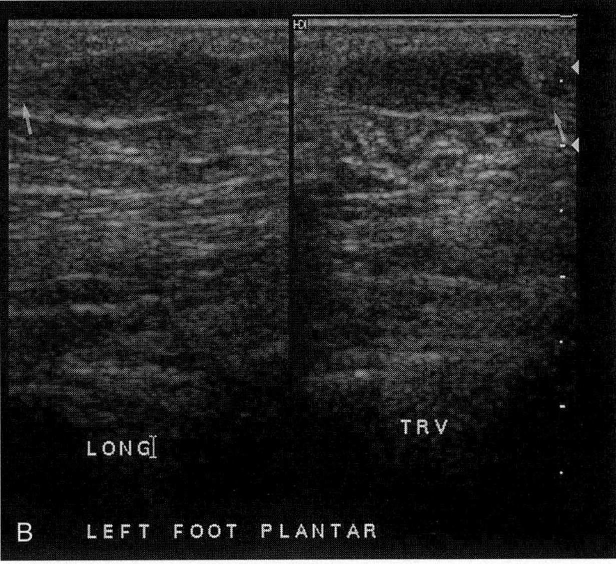

Figure 10–48 ■ **A,** Plantar fibromatosis: longitudinal sonogram. Ultrasound examination of the plantar surface of the left foot of this 34-year-old male revealed fusiform thickening (*large arrow*) of the plantar fascia (*small arrows*) with decreased echogenicity. This abnormality was rock hard on palpation, leading the patient and the clinician to suspect malignancy. However, the abnormality was limited to the plantar fascia, and the patient reported a family history of Dupuytren's contracture, leading to the correct diagnosis of Lederhose plantar fibrosis. **B,** Plantar fibromatosis: longitudinal and transverse sonograms. Same patient as in **A.** In both longitudinal and transverse planes the abnormality has a fusiform appearance, blending with the normal fascia (*arrow*). (Courtesy of Jag Dhanju, RDMS, Ontario Medical Imaging, Canada.)

beyond the end of the table. The knee and ankle can be stabilized with sandbags. Transverse images of the proximal and distal tibia are obtained, with the transducer face parallel to the examination table. The proximal image is obtained at the level of the tibial condyles, just below the joint space. Imaging of the distal tibia is done at the level of the tibiofibular joint. Figure 10–45 demonstrates the calculation of tibial torsion. The accuracy of these sonographic measurements is comparable with those obtained using CT (Joseph et al., 1987). The advantage of ultrasound in these cases is the lack of ionizing radiation. Therefore, ultrasound is preferred for long-term follow-up.

Tumors

Ultrasound has been used to examine both soft tissue (Fig. 10–47) and bone tumors, but clearly, MRI and CT provide more information about the extent of tumor involvement. MRI and CT demonstrate the full extent of local invasion, in addition to evaluating metastatic disease. Examination of neoplasia with ultrasound is limited to the soft tissue component of the mass and cortical contours of the involved bone. It can clearly demonstrate the relationship of a mass to adjacent nerves, vessels, and bone (Vincent, 1988). When the relationship of the mass to normal structures can be defined using ultrasound, the definitive diagnosis can often be established (Figs. 10–48 through 10–51). Medullary involvement of bone is not evaluated. Assessment of metastatic disease is also limited, principally to parenchymal organs. However, sonography may play a role in targeting CT or MRI examinations.

Sonography is particularly well suited for evaluating peripheral nerve lesions (Chinn, 1982; Reuter et al., 1982). It provides the ability to examine a peripheral nerve along its entire length in a few minutes, allowing targeted CT or MRI examination of the region of interest. This technique saves considerable time on the CT or MRI scanner, eliminating a screening examination. When electromyographic studies indicate the presence of a peripheral nerve lesion, ultrasound can often serve as the initial screening examination. Normal nerves are recognized as hyperechoic cords with a fascicular structure adjacent to vessels (Fornage, 1988b). These nerves are easily distinguished from tendons by their lack of motion during movement of the extremity. Flexion and extension maneuvers will

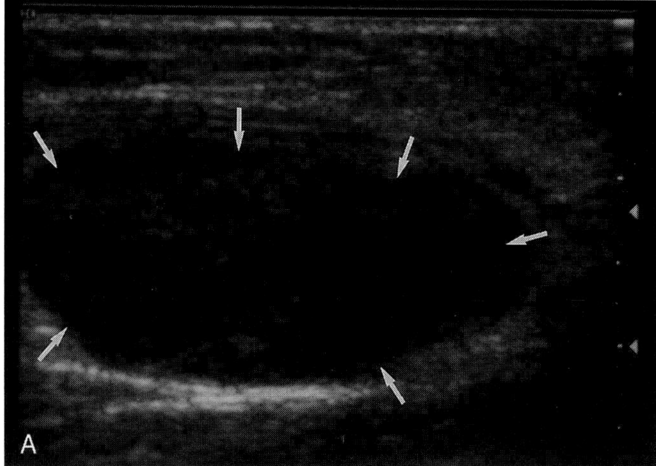

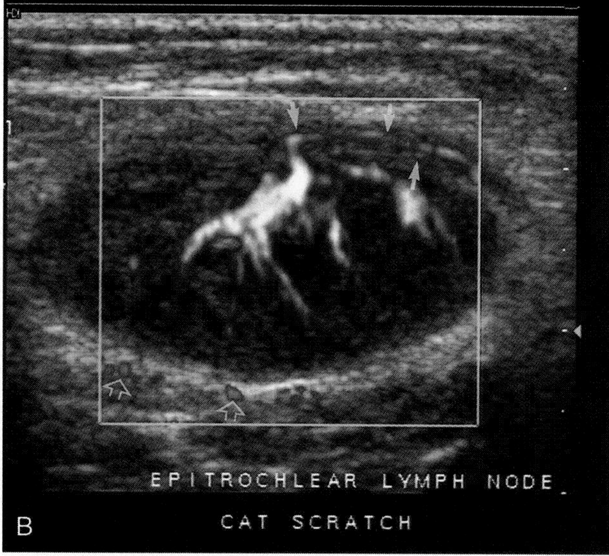

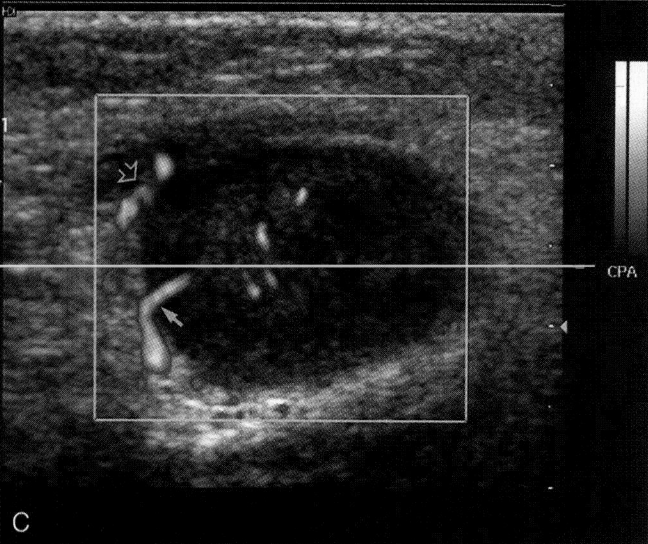

Figure 10–49 ■ A, Epitrochlear lymph node: longitudinal sonogram. This 10-year-old girl presented for evaluation of a soft tissue mass associated with the medial epicondyle of the right elbow. Sarcoma was suspected clinically. A hypoechoic, well-defined soft tissue mass (*arrows*) is identified adjacent to the medial epicondyle. **B,** Epitrochlear lymph node: longitudinal sonogram with power Doppler. Same patient as in **A.** The characteristic vascular pattern of a lymph node with an artery and a vein side by side (*arrows*), entering the hilum, is observed on this color Doppler image. Tiny capsular vessels (*open arrows*) are noted along the periphery. This highly organized vascular tree is not usually seen in neoplasms. **C,** Epitrochlear lymph node: transverse sonogram with power Doppler. Same patient as in **A.** A clearly dominant vascular pedicle (*arrow*) is identified entering the hilum. Smaller capsular vessels (*open arrow*) are again noted.

readily distinguish nerves from tendons during real-time examination. Most tumors of peripheral nerves are fusiform in shape and decreased in echogenicity relative to normal nerve tissue (Fig. 10–51). A distinction between neurofibromas and schwannomas cannot be made sonographically; both appear hypoechoic and demonstrate increased through-transmission. Schwannomas may contain cysts and grow more eccentrically along the course of the nerve. In neurofibromatosis, multiple neurofibromas are often observed in peripheral nerves, and it is not unusual to identify them in muscular branches (Fig. 10–52)

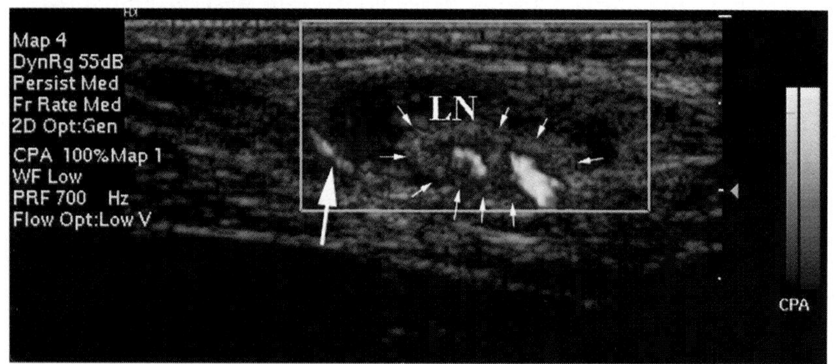

Figure 10–50 ■ Epitrochlear lymph node: transverse sonogram. A small mass was palpable at the medial aspect of the elbow in this 55-year-old female. The characteristic appearance of a reactive lymph node (*LN*) is seen in this transverse image obtained over the palpable abnormality. The vascular supply of the node, depicted with power Doppler, is seen entering through the echogenic hilum (*small arrows*). A vascular structure is noted along the periphery of the lymph node corresponding to a capsular vein (*large arrow*).

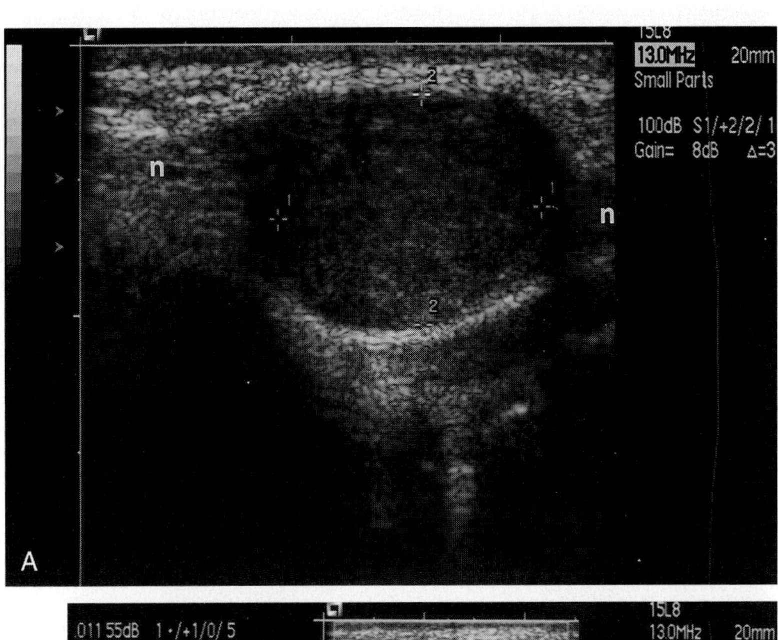

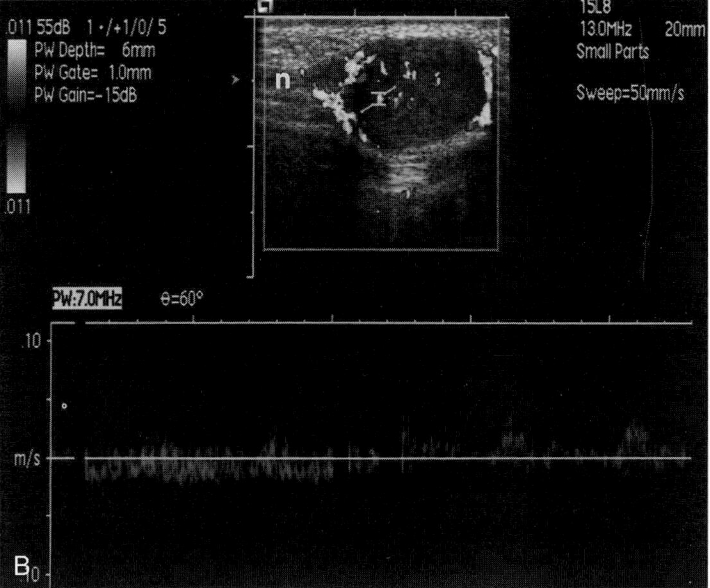

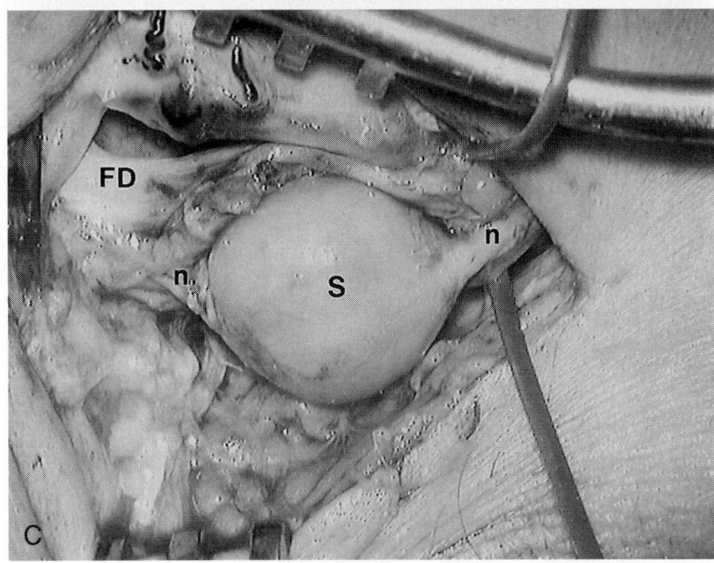

Figure 10–51 ■ **A,** Tibial nerve schwannoma: longitudinal sonogram. Focal soft tissue swelling and pain above the medial maleolus prompted this 40-year-old male to seek treatment. An ovoid, hypoechoic mass is identified in continuity with the tibial nerve (*n*). **B,** Tibial nerve schwannoma: longitudinal sonogram with power Doppler. Same patient as in **A.** Hypervascularity is noted within the mass and along the perineurium. Doppler waveforms revealed an arterial pattern with low peripheral resistance. Abbreviation: nerve (*n*). (Courtesy of B. van Holsbeeck, MD, M. Baeckelandt, MD, and L. Fidlers, MD, Stedelijk Ziekenhuis, Roeselare, Belgium.) **C,** Tibial nerve schwannoma: operative photograph. Same patient as in **A.** A well-defined schwannoma (*S*) was easily dissected free of the tibial nerve. Abbreviations: flexor digitorum (*FD*), nerve (*n*).

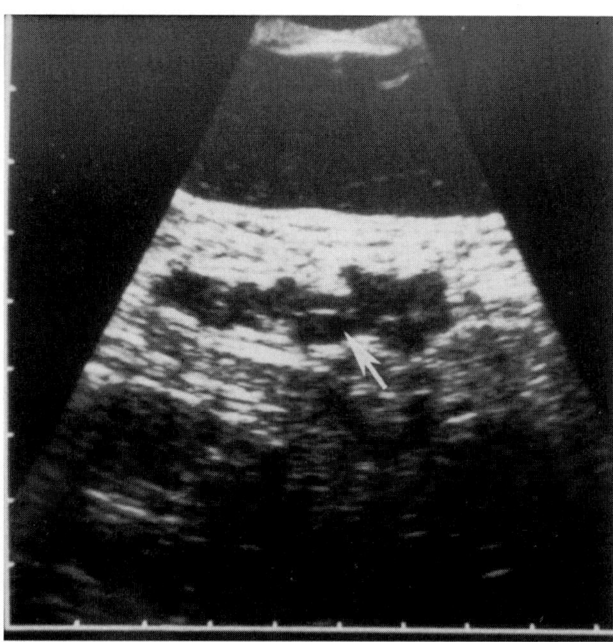

Figure 10–52 ■ Cluster of small neurofibromas: longitudinal sonogram. A mass was palpated in the right gluteal region of this 30-year-old woman with neurofibromatosis. The transducer is positioned along the length of the gluteus maximus muscle. A cluster of neurofibromas (*arrow*) is seen as a lobular mass overlying the gluteus. The finding is consistent with a plexiform neurofibroma.

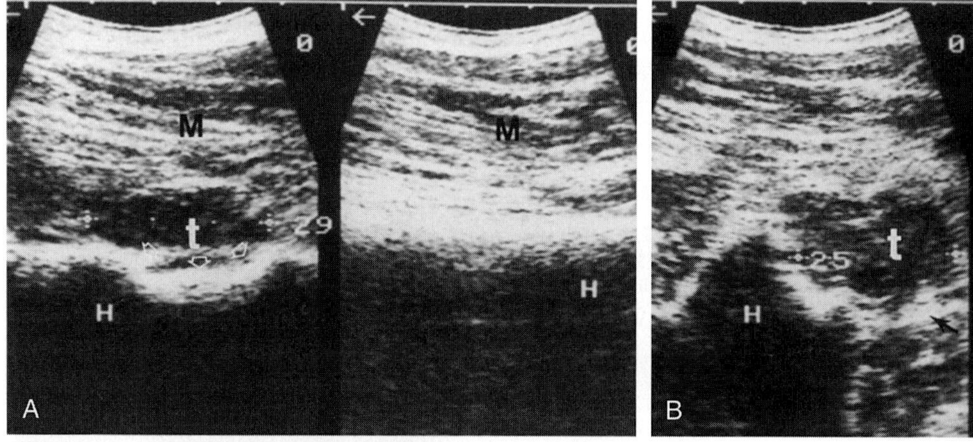

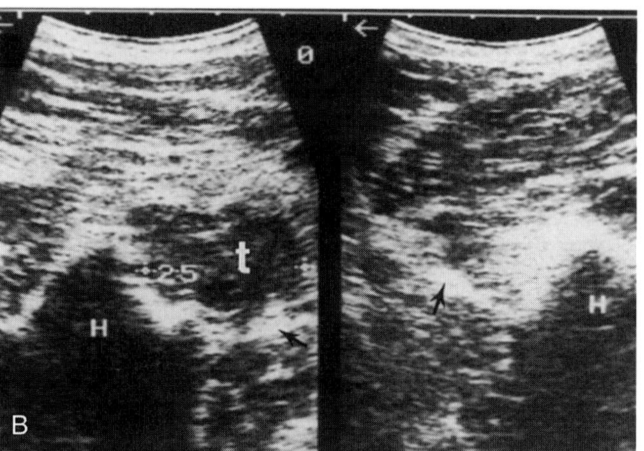

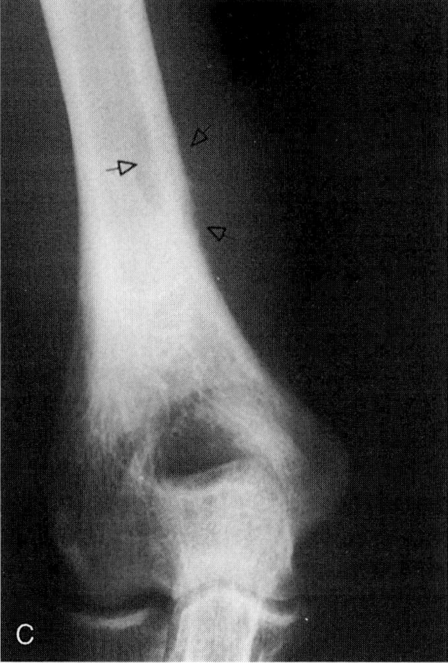

Figure 10–53 ■ **A,** Fibrosarcoma above the elbow: longitudinal sonogram. A 55-year-old man who presented with a firm mass at the medial aspect of the right distal upper arm. An ovoid hypoechoic mass (*t*) 2.9 cm in diameter is noted deep to the brachial muscle (*M*) on the left. A comparable view of the normal left arm is seen on the right. Erosion of the underlying humerus (*open arrows*) is also observed, consistent with a malignant tumor. Note that the superficial margin of the tumor is quite distinct, indicative of pseudocapsule formation. **B,** Fibrosarcoma above the elbow: transverse sonogram. Same patient as in **A.** The transducer is rotated 90 degrees; the right arm is once again on the left side of the split-screen images. The medial aspects of each arm are at the center of the figure. Immediately anterior to the ulnar nerve (*arrow*) is the previously noted fibrosarcoma (*t*) of the right upper arm. Again, invasion of the medial aspect of the humerus is noted. A normal, nondisplaced, hyperechoic ulnar nerve (*arrow*) is seen in the left arm. Abbreviation: humerus (*H*). **C,** Fibrosarcoma above the elbow: anteroposterior radiograph. Same patient as in **A** and **B**. Osseous destruction (*open arrows*) at the medial aspect of the distal humerus is associated with irregular periosteal reaction. The soft tissues are swollen, but the extent of the mass cannot be appreciated on this film.

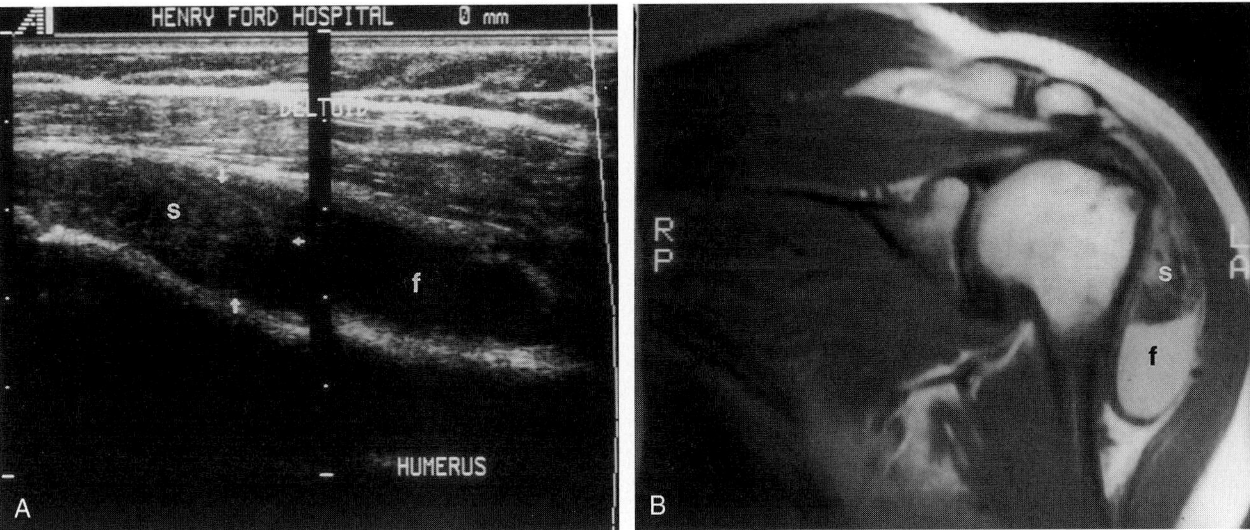

Figure 10-54 ■ **A,** Pigmented villonodular synovitis of the shoulder: longitudinal sonogram. Ultrasound examination of the shoulder of this 36-year-old female was performed for clinical suspicion of a rotator cuff tear. A large effusion (*f*) is present within the subacromial-subdeltoid bursa. A prominent nodular synovial proliferation (*s*) is also present. **B,** Pigmented villonodular synovitis of the shoulder: coronal proton density MRI. Same patient as in **A.** Nodular synovial proliferation and fluid within the bursa are identical to those demonstrated on the ultrasound examination. Synovectomy was then performed, and the histological finding of PVNS confirmed the sonographic diagnosis.

or in the subcutaneous tissues. A similar appearance has been reported in leprosy (Fornage and Nerot, 1987). Sarcomatous degeneration of neurofibromas may occur, resulting in rapid growth of the tumor, with ill-defined borders and irregular margins (Lattes, 1982; Lange et al., 1987; Reading et al., 1988). However, poor margination of a lesion is not a reliable sign of malignancy because malignant lesions may have a pseudocapsule (Fig. 10-53). Power Doppler sonography is sensitive in detecting feeding vessels. Fast-growing malignancies often have multiple feeding vessels. However, lesions with no identifiable feeding vessels are not necessarily benign.

Another good application of sonography in tumor diagnosis is in the evaluation of articular masses. Most masses in and around joints are benign. However, MRI cannot accurately distinguish those masses that are cysts from masses that are malignant and have a lot of extracellular fluid. Both processes can appear homogeneous, with high signal intensity on MRI. Synovial sarcoma and myxoid liposarcoma appear cyst-like and are often mistaken

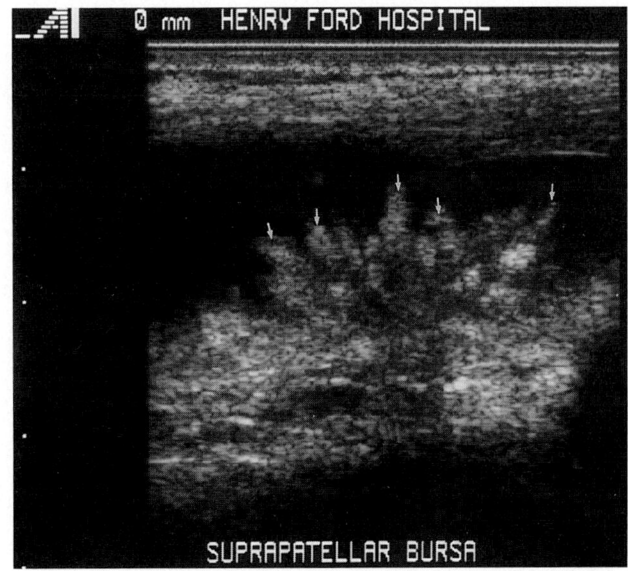

Figure 10-55 ■ Lipoma arborescens: longitudinal sonogram. Chronic massive distention of the suprapatellar bursa was observed in this 57-year-old male. This longitudinal sonographic image reveals a hyperechoic villous mass (*arrows*) within the suprapatellar bursa. A large amount of anechoic fluid surrounds this mass. At surgery this mass was identified as an intra-articular lipoma.

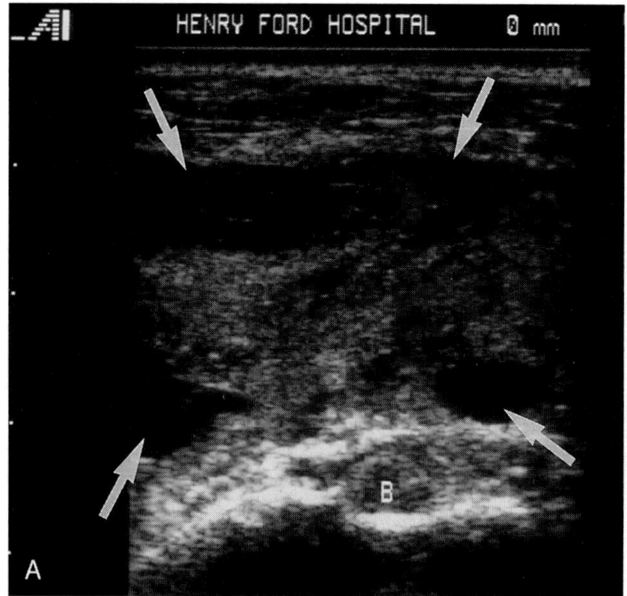

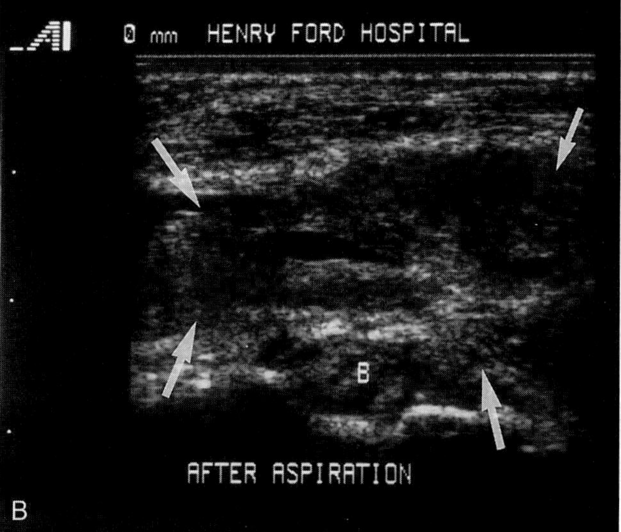

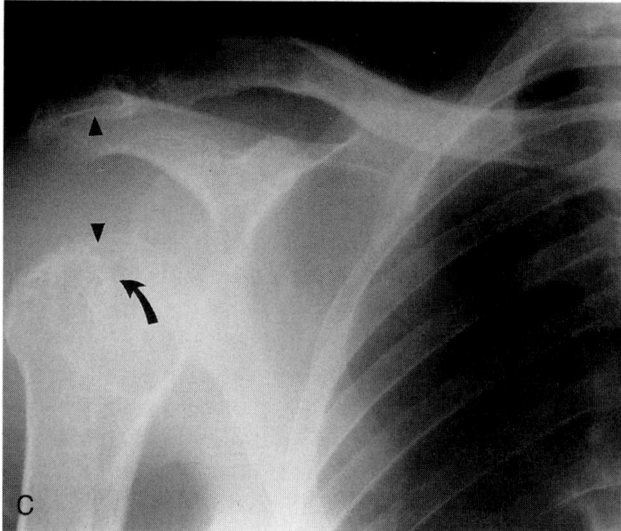

Figure 10–56 ■ **A,** Amyloidosis of the shoulder: transverse sonogram. This 66-year-old female has been on dialysis for over 10 years. She now presents with shoulder swelling and pain. Marked thickening of the subacromial-subdeltoid bursa (*arrows*) is seen with soft tissue of mixed echogenicity. Abbreviation: biceps tendon (*B*). **B,** Amyloidosis of the shoulder: transverse sonogram. Same patient as in **A.** Ultrasound-guided aspiration of the bursa yielded 50 cc of pink fluid. Following aspiration the bursa is much less distended, but regions of synovial thickening remain. Cell block analysis of the fluid revealed amyloid. **C,** Amyloidosis of the shoulder: conventional radiograph. Same patient as in **A.** Cystic changes (*curved arrow*) within the humeral head and widening of the acromiohumeral distance (*arrowheads*) are commonly seen in amyloidosis.

for benign processes, especially when they are still small. Ultrasound will demonstrate that these masses are hypoechoic, not anechoic. Atypical "cyst" location, absence of fluctuation with pressure, and calcification are absolute indications for biopsy. Tumor-like conditions of joints that can be diagnosed using a combination of ultrasound and biopsy include pigmented villonodular synovitis (PVNS), lipoma arborescens, synovial chondromatosis, osteochondromatosis, and amyloidosis. The synovium in PVNS is typically hypoechoic and often very vascular. The disease cannot be distinguished sonographically from chronic forms of inflammatory arthritis like rheumatoid arthritis and tuberculosis (Fig. 10–54) (Kaufman et al., 1982). Ultrasound-guided synovial biopsy is diagnostic. Lipoma arborescens consists of smooth nodular masses within the deep layers of the synovium or villous proliferation of synovium covering a fat pad (Fig. 10–55). As with most lipomas, their echogenicity is variable. The masses are often located within the dorsal synovial wall of the suprapatellar synovium. Osteoarticular amyloidosis presents with masses in synovium, tendon, and bone and generally demonstrates heterogeneous echogenicity (Fig. 10–56). Ultrasound examinations of the shoulder demonstrating a maximal rotator cuff thickness greater than 8 mm or the presence of hypoechoic layers between the muscle fibers of the rotator cuff have 72–79% sensitivity and 97–100% specificity for amyloidosis in the setting of long-term hemodialysis. The rotator cuff may have a feathery appearance with streaks of hyperechogenicity, and multiple rotator cuff tears are common in these patients. Deep

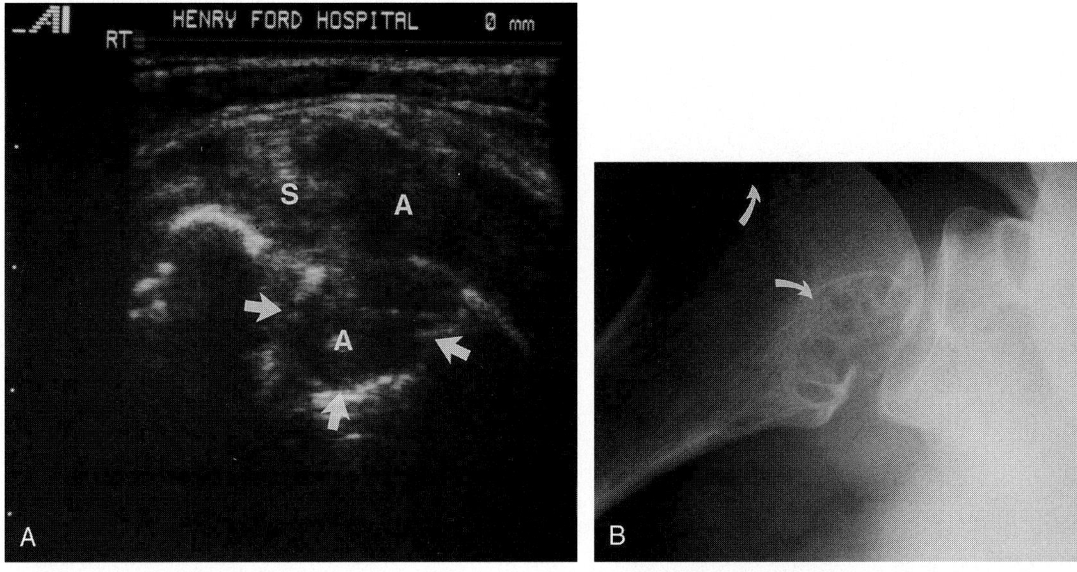

Figure 10–57 ■ **A,** Osteoarticular amyloidosis: coronal sonogram. A 62-year-old female with chronic renal failure, on hemodialysis for more than 20 years, presented with an 8-year history of right shoulder pain. This coronal image through the rotator cuff demonstrates a large lytic lesion (*arrows*) in the humeral head filled with hypoechoic material (*A*). Similar material (*A*) is present within the supraspinatus tendon. Fine needle aspiration biopsy was performed under ultrasound guidance, demonstrating amyloid. Abbreviation: supraspinatus (*S*). **B,** Osteoarticular amyloidosis: anteroposterior radiograph. Well-defined lytic lesions are present within the humeral head of this patient with proven amyloidosis secondary to long-term hemodialysis. Although this is a different patient than the one shown in **A,** the lesions are histologically identical. (Courtesy of B. Maldague, MD, Cliniques Universitaires Saint-Luc, Belgium.)

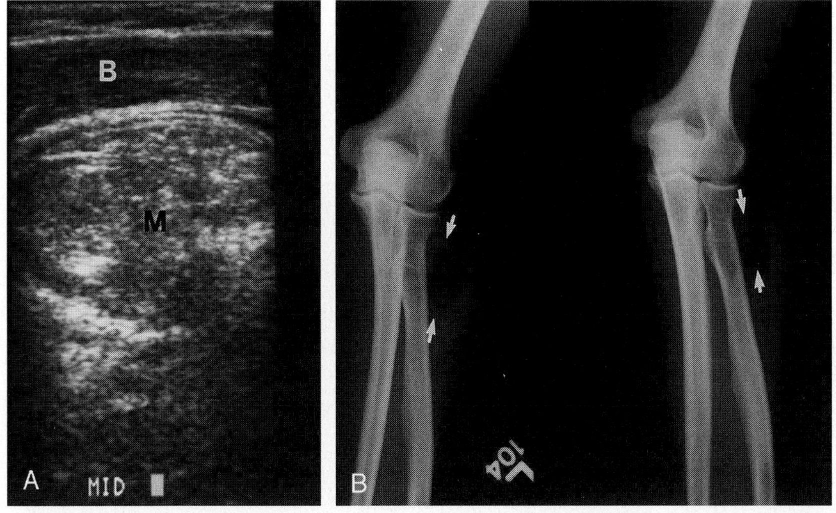

Figure 10–58 ■ **A,** Intramuscular lipoma: transverse sonogram. Pain in the left radial nerve distribution and forearm swelling were noted by this 40-year-old female. An echogenic mass (*M*) is demonstrated within the supinator muscle deep to the brachioradialis muscle (*B*). **B,** Intramuscular lipoma: conventional radiograph. Same patient as in **A.** Radiographs obtained using soft tissue technique confirm the presence of a lipoma (*arrows*) in the forearm.

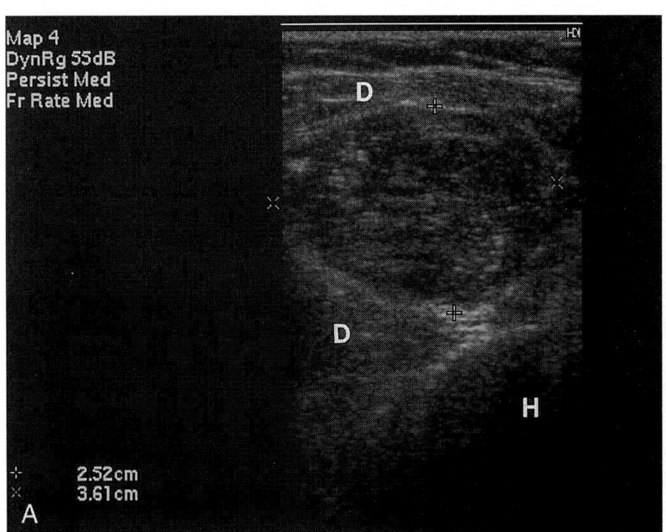

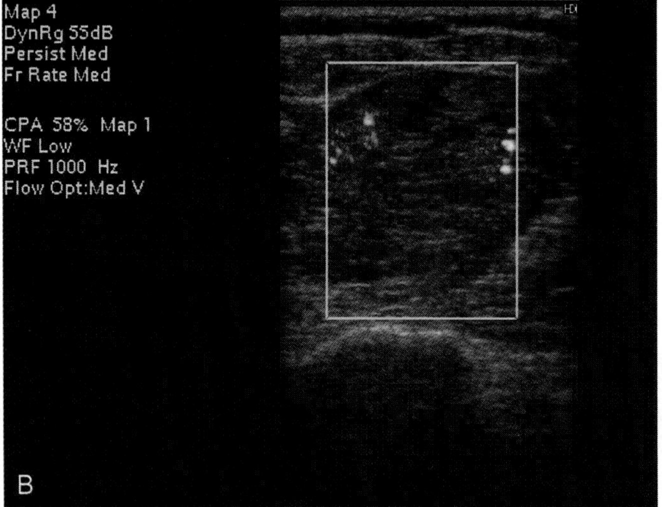

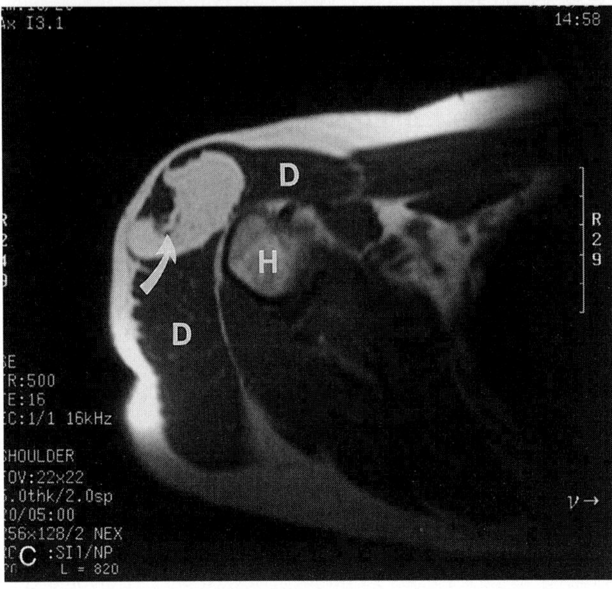

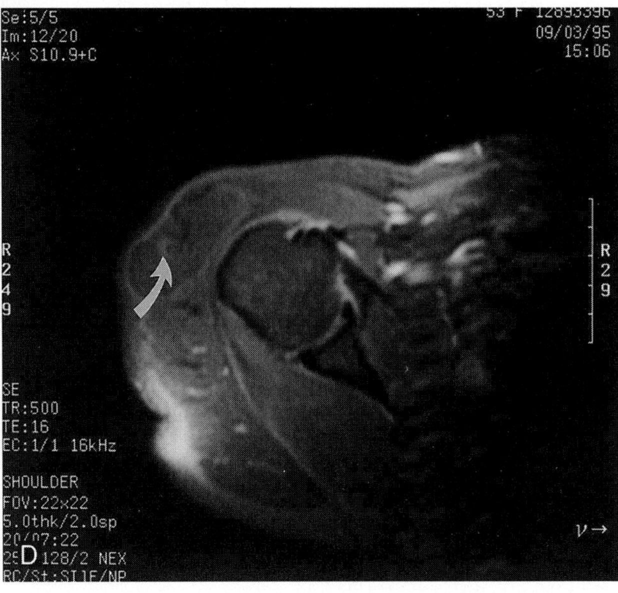

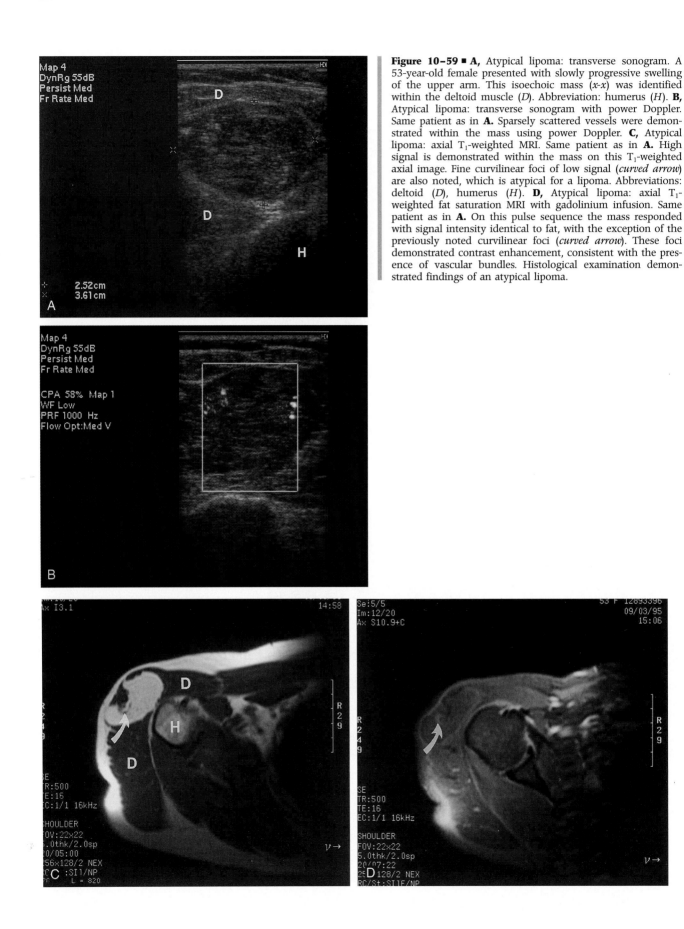

Figure 10–59 ■ **A,** Atypical lipoma: transverse sonogram. A 53-year-old female presented with slowly progressive swelling of the upper arm. This isoechoic mass (*x-x*) was identified within the deltoid muscle (*D*). Abbreviation: humerus (*H*). **B,** Atypical lipoma: transverse sonogram with power Doppler. Same patient as in **A.** Sparsely scattered vessels were demonstrated within the mass using power Doppler. **C,** Atypical lipoma: axial T_1-weighted MRI. Same patient as in **A.** High signal is demonstrated within the mass on this T_1-weighted axial image. Fine curvilinear foci of low signal (*curved arrow*) are also noted, which is atypical for a lipoma. Abbreviations: deltoid (*D*), humerus (*H*). **D,** Atypical lipoma: axial T_1-weighted fat saturation MRI with gadolinium infusion. Same patient as in **A.** On this pulse sequence the mass responded with signal intensity identical to fat, with the exception of the previously noted curvilinear foci (*curved arrow*). These foci demonstrated contrast enhancement, consistent with the presence of vascular bundles. Histological examination demonstrated findings of an atypical lipoma.

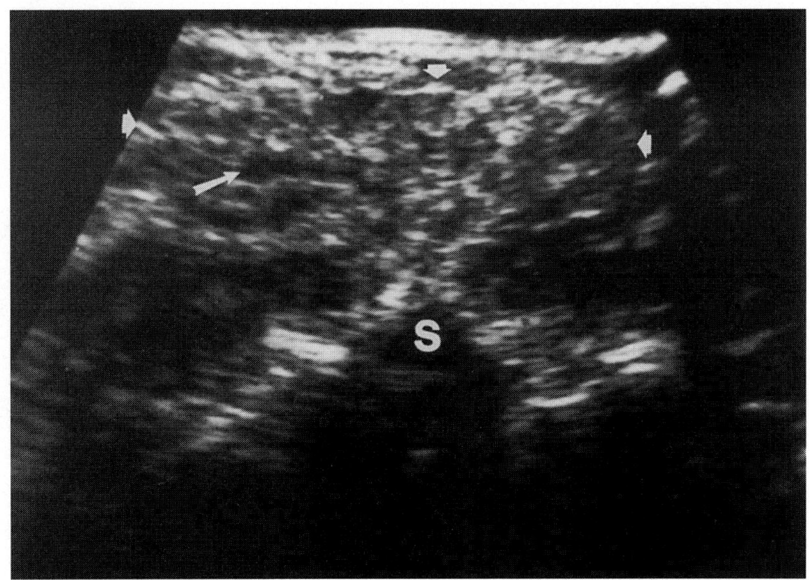

Figure 10-60 ■ Capillary hemangioma of the posterior neck: transverse sonogram. The patient is a 2-year-old boy with swelling of the posterior neck centrally. This transverse image directly over the spinous processes (*S*) demonstrates a large mass (*small arrows*) of mixed echogenicity. It is predominantly hyperechoic relative to the surrounding muscle. Surgical excision demonstrated this to be a capillary hemangioma. Hypoechoic spaces (*large arrow*) within the mass represent venous lakes. Intramuscular hemangiomas and cavernous hemangiomas would be hypoechoic relative to the surrounding muscle, unlike this capillary hemangioma.

cyst-like lesions in the articular ends of the bone are typically present (Fig. 10-57) (McMahon et al., 1991; Kay et al., 1992; Cardinal et al., 1996). Chondromatosis of the synovium is nodular and, because of calcification, frequently hyperechoic (Pai and van Holsbeeck, 1995).

Lipomas of the subcutaneous tissues may appear hyperechoic (29%) (Fig. 10-58), hypoechoic (29%), isoechoic (22%) (Fig. 10-59), or of mixed echogenicity (20%) and are always soft, pliable masses. They typically have an elongated shape and an orientation parallel to the skin (Ceulemans and van Holsbeeck, 1997). Sixty-six percent of superficial lipomas are well marginated; the remainder are poorly defined (Fornage and Tassin, 1991). Other benign tumors, such as hemangiomas (Figs. 10-60 and 10-61), can also be evaluated with ultrasound. Color Doppler studies may be valuable in identifying feeding and draining vessels, but flow within the lesion may be too slow to detect with Doppler. Power Doppler sonography has improved diagnostic accuracy. Compression imaging will demonstrate these lesions to be fluid-filled vessels. Occasionally, phleboliths may be identified within these lesions. In general, masses containing calcifications require further imaging investigation with radiographs, CT, or MRI. Intramuscular calcifications or calcifications adjacent to bone without an associated soft tissue mass, as described in Chapter 3, can safely be called myositis ossificans (Fig. 10-62) based solely on their sonographic appearance.

Bone tumors and parosteal processes can extend with mass effect upon the surrounding soft tissues. These masses are most often malignant. Hypoechoic and cyst-like soft tissue masses with calcification can be synovial sarcomas. These tumors are preferentially located in the soft tissues around the knee. When a mass has an indeterminate nature but is not vascular, ultrasound-guided biopsy can easily be performed (Reading et al., 1988). The technique employed is essentially the same as that used for the aspiration of fluid collections. Sonographic biopsy is safe, effective, and cost effective. It usually accelerates the process of diagnosis by avoiding the scheduling problems associated with CT-guided biopsy (Fig. 10-63).

Percutaneous interventions include ganglion aspiration, fine-needle aspiration, and Tru-Cut biopsy of soft tissue masses, in particular those occurring around joints, muscle biopsy in neuromuscular disorders, and fluid sampling for cultures. In the detection of local recurrences of soft tissue sarcoma, ultrasound can help differentiate scar from recurrence by guiding the biopsy needle into any growing mass (see Fig. 10-63). It is important to have a baseline postoperative study if one wants to use ultrasound in the follow-up of masses. This methodology is of particular interest in sarcoma surgery associated with metallic implants and in locally aggressive tumors that recur, such as malignant fibrous histiocytoma, liposarcoma, and desmoid tumors. Ultrasound is also useful to assist in localization of nonpalpable solid soft tissue masses (see Fig. 10-4) and vascular masses prior to surgery. Needle wire localization techniques can be used. This procedure avoids extensive soft tissue damage during surgery and positive tumor margins because of unexpected findings during the resection (Ceulemans and van Holsbeeck, 1997).

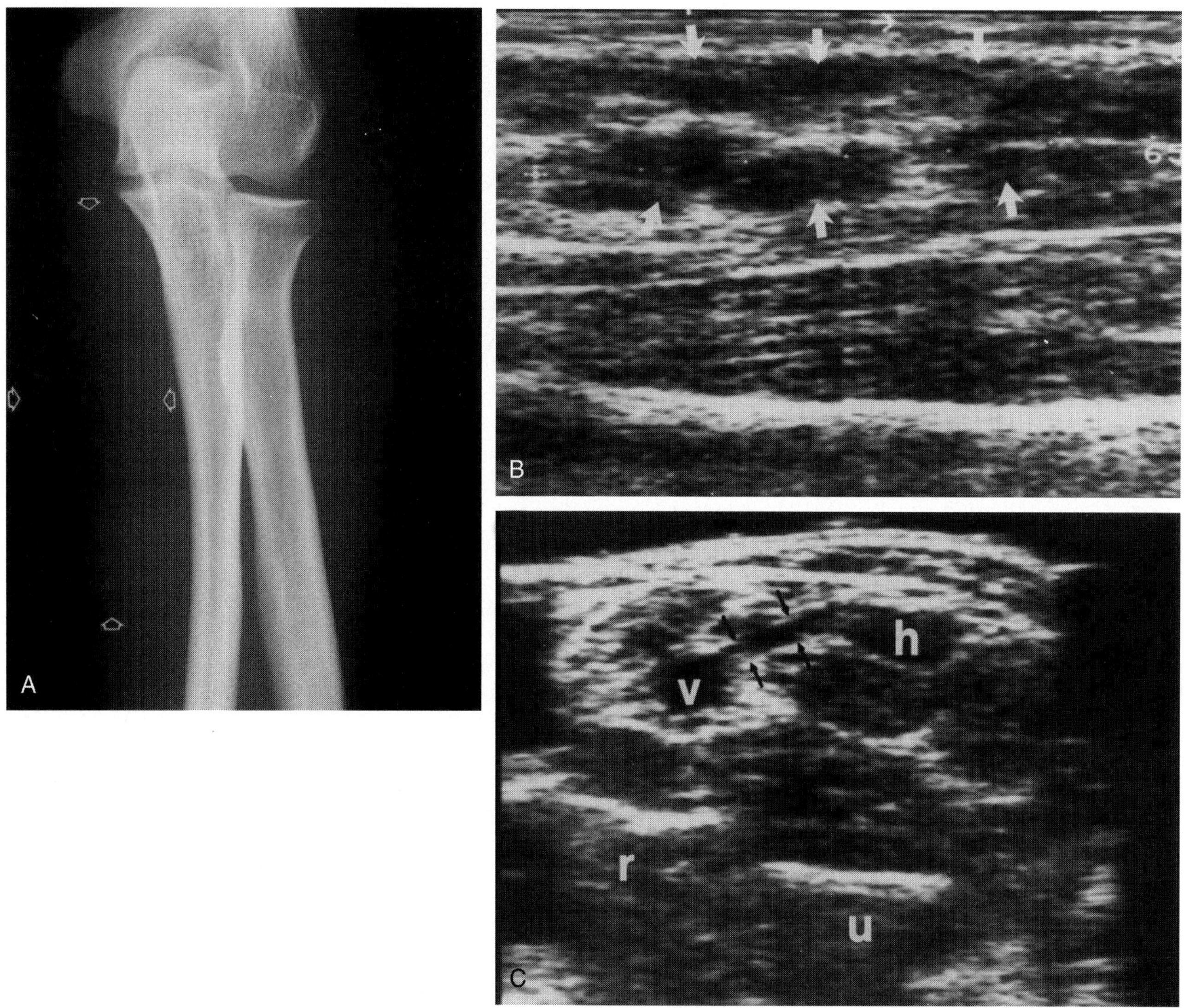

Figure 10–61 ■ **A,** Intramuscular angiomatosis: anteroposterior radiograph of the forearm. A large mass is present in the medial aspect of the left forearm of this 10-year-old boy. Multiple phleboliths (*open arrows*) are present in the soft tissues of the medial aspect of the forearm. Phleboliths may be seen in angiomatosis, hemangiomas, and lymphangiomas. **B,** Intramuscular angiomatosis: longitudinal sonogram. Same patient as in **A.** Serpiginous vessels (*arrows*) are observed extending deep into the substance of the flexor muscles. At the time of surgery, this lesion had an infiltrative appearance. However, it is a hamartoma. **C,** Intramuscular angiomatosis: transverse sonogram. Same patient as in **A** and **B.** The transducer was rotated to image transversely. A large draining vein (*arrows*) extends from the lesion (*h*) to a normal vein (*v*). Color Doppler demonstrated sluggish flow within the lesion and a normal venous signal in the vein. This image demonstrates the lesion to be limited to the superficial flexor compartment of the forearm. Abbreviations: radius (*r*), ulna (*u*).

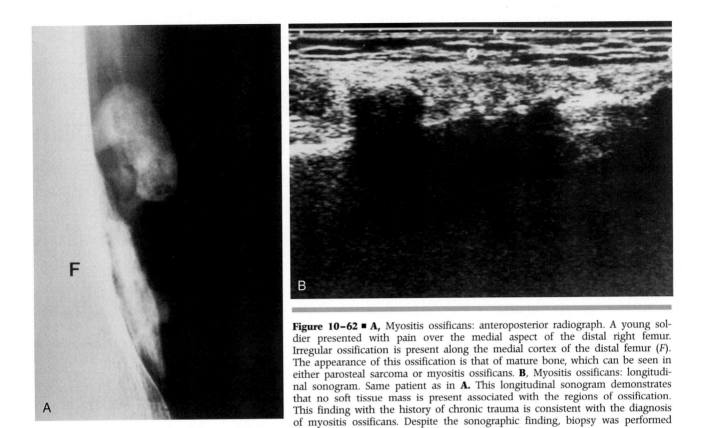

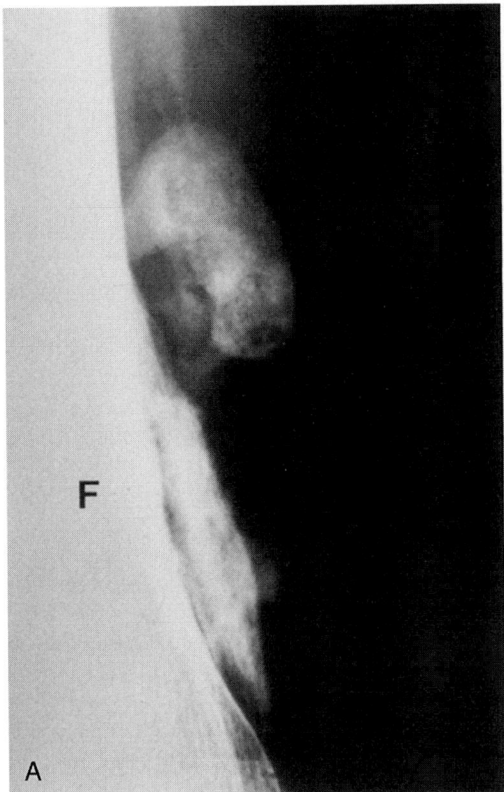

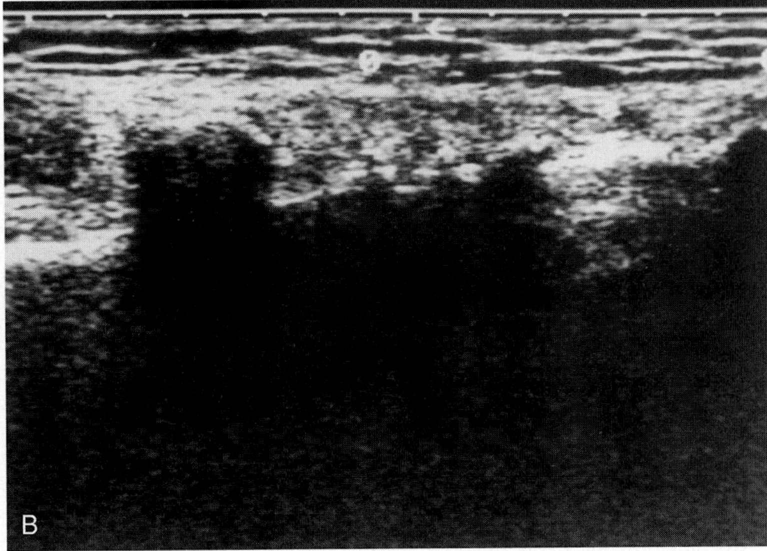

Figure 10–62 ■ **A,** Myositis ossificans: anteroposterior radiograph. A young soldier presented with pain over the medial aspect of the distal right femur. Irregular ossification is present along the medial cortex of the distal femur (*F*). The appearance of this ossification is that of mature bone, which can be seen in either parosteal sarcoma or myositis ossificans. **B,** Myositis ossificans: longitudinal sonogram. Same patient as in **A.** This longitudinal sonogram demonstrates that no soft tissue mass is present associated with the regions of ossification. This finding with the history of chronic trauma is consistent with the diagnosis of myositis ossificans. Despite the sonographic finding, biopsy was performed and the results were interpreted as myositis ossificans.

Figure 10–63 ■ Recurrence of malignant fibrous histiocytoma: transverse sonogram. Six months ago, this 85-year-old male underwent complete resection of a malignant fibrous histiocytoma from his anterior right thigh. He now presents with recurrent swelling at the surgical site. An irregular hypoechoic mass (*x-x*) is identified adjacent to the femur. A core biopsy obtained under ultrasound guidance demonstrated tumor recurrence.

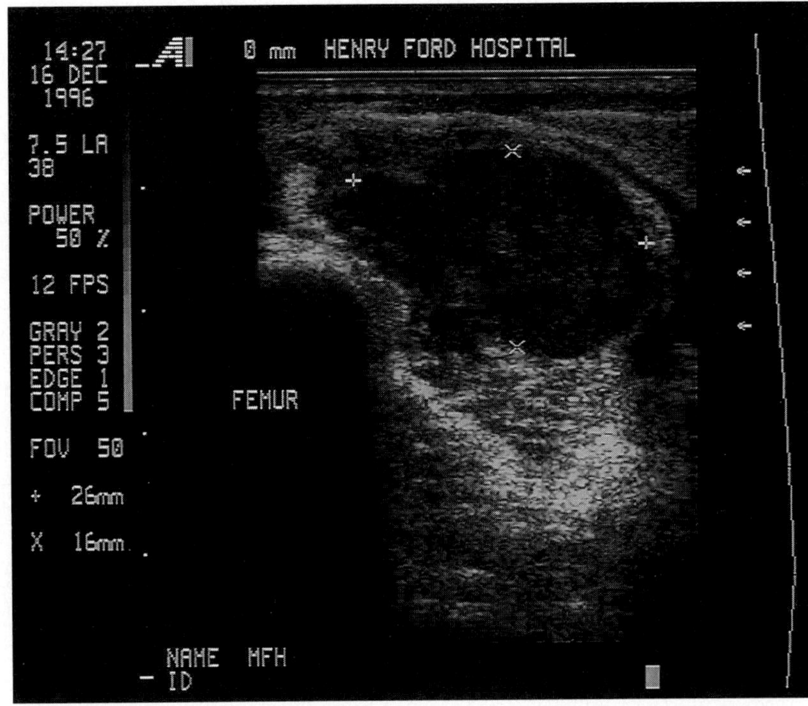

References

Aamodt A, et al: Femoral anteversion measured by ultrasound and CT: comparative study. *Skeletal Radiol* 24:105, 1995.

Abiri MM, Kirpekar M, Ablow RC: Osteomyelitis: Detection with ultrasound (work in progress). *Radiology* 169: 795–797, 1988.

Berman M: Ultrasound of the hip: A review of the applications of a new technique. *Br J Radiol* 59:13–17, 1986.

Bloom W, Fawcett DW: *A Textbook of Histology*, ed 11. Philadelphia, WB Saunders Co, 1980.

Calliadi F, et al: Color Doppler differential diagnosis between normal and delayed healing bone fractures. *Radiology* 189:209, 1993.

Cardinal E, et al: Amyloidosis of the shoulder in patients on chronic hemodialysis: Sonographic findings. *AJR* 166:153–156, 1996.

Carson PL, et al: Imaging soft tissue through bone with ultrasound transmission tomography by reconstruction. *Med Phys* 4:302–309, 1977.

Ceulemans R, van Holsbeeck M: Ultrasonography. In De Schepper AM (ed): *Imaging of Soft Tissue Tumors*. Heidelberg, Springer-Verlag, 1997.

Chiba T, et al: Ultrasonography as a method of nutritional assessment. *J Parenter Enteral Nutr* 13:529–534, 1989.

Chinn DH: Unusual ultrasonographic appearance of a solid schwannoma. *J Clin Ultrasound* 10:243–245, 1982.

Craig JG, et al: Osteomyelitis of the diabetic foot: MR imaging—pathologic correlation. *Radiology* 203:849, 1997.

Dihlmann W: *Joints and Vertebral Connections*. New York, Thieme, 1985.

Fornage BD: Glomus tumors in the fingers: Diagnosis with ultrasound. *Radiology* 167:183–185, 1988a.

Fornage BD: Peripheral nerves of the extremities: Imaging with ultrasound. *Radiology* 167:179–182, 1988b.

Fornage BD, et al: Imaging of the skin with 20-MHz US. *Radiology* 189:69, 1993.

Fornage BD, Lorigan JG: Sonographic detection and fine-needle aspiration biopsy of nonpalpable recurrent or metastatic melanoma in subcutaneous tissues. *J Ultrasound Med* 8:421, 1989.

Fornage BD, Nerot C: Sonographic diagnosis of tuberculoid leprosy. *J Ultrasound Med* 6:105–107, 1987.

Fornage BD, Rifkin MD: Ultrasound examination of the hand and foot. *Radiol Clin North Am* 26(1):109–129, 1988.

Fornage BD, Tassin GB: Sonographic appearance of superficial soft tissue lipomas. *J Clin Ultrasound* 19:215–220, 1991.

Fried AM, Coughlin K, Griffen WO: The sonographic fat/muscle ratio. *Invest Radiol* 21:71–75, 1986.

Gitschlag KF, et al: Disease in the femoral triangle: Sonographic appearance. *AJR* 139:515–519, 1982.

Graf R, Schuler P: *Sonographie am Stutz und Bewegungsapparat bei Erwachsenen und Kindern*. Weinheim, Edition Medizin VCH, 1988.

Harcke HT, et al: Ossification center of the infant hip: Sonographic and radiographic correlation. *AJR* 147: 317–321, 1986.

Harcke HT, Grissom LE, Finkelstein MS: Evaluation of the musculoskeletal system with sonography. *AJR* 150: 1253–1261, 1988.

Heaney RP, et al: Osteoporotic bone fragility. Detection by ultrasound transmission velocity. *JAMA* 261: 2986–2990, 1989.

Hentz VR, Green PS, Arditi M: Imaging studies of the cadaver hand using transmission ultrasound. *Skeletal Radiol* 16:474–480, 1987.

Hentz VR, Marich KW, Dev P: Preliminary study of the upper limb with the use of ultrasound transmission imaging. *J Hand Surg (Am)* 9:188, 1984.

Hernandez RJ, et al: CT determination of femoral torsion. *AJR* 137:97–101, 1981.

Jiang Y, Zhao J, van Holsbeeck MT, et al: Monitoring of osteogenesis in Ilizarov's leg lengthening procedures using ultrasound and radiographic examinations: Imaging and pathologic correlations. *Radiology* 205(P): 421, 1997.

Joseph B, et al: Measurement of tibial torsion by ultrasound. *J Pediatr Orthop* 7:317–323, 1987.

Kaufman RA, et al: Arthrosonography in the diagnosis of pigmented villonodular synovitis. *AJR* 139: 396–398, 1982.

Kay J, et al: Utility of high-resolution ultrasound for the diagnosis of dialysis-related amyloidosis. *Arthritis Rheum* 35:926–931, 1992.

Lange TA, et al: Ultrasound imaging as a screening study for malignant soft-tissue tumors, *J Bone Joint Surg Am* 69:100–105, 1987.

Lassau N, et al: Value of high frequency US for preoperative assessment of skin tumors. *Radiographics* 17:1559, 1997.

Lattes R: *Tumors of the Soft Tissues*. Washington, DC, Armed Forces Institute of Pathology, 1982.

Maldague B, Malghem J: Dynamic radiologic patterns of Paget's disease of bone. *Clin Orthop* 217:127–151, 1987.

McMahon LP, Radford J, Dawborn JK: Shoulder ultrasound in dialysis related amyloidosis. *Clin Nephrol* 35: 227–232, 1991.

Moed BR, et al: Ultrasound for the early diagnosis of fracture healing after interlocking nailing of the tibia without reaming. *Clin Orthop* 310:137–144, 1995.

Moed BR, et al: Ultrasound for the early diagnosis of tibial fracture healing after static interlocked hailing without reaming: Clinical results. *J Orthop Trauma* 12:206–213, 1998a.

Moed BR, et al: Ultrasound for the early diagnosis of tibial fracture healing after static interlocked nailing without reaming: Histologic correlation using a canine model. *J Orthop Trauma* 12:200–205, 1998b.

Nazarian LN, et al: Malignant melanoma: Impact of superficial US on management. *Radiology* 199:273, 1996.

Pai VR, van Holsbeeck M: Synovial osteochondromatosis of the hip: Role of sonography. *J Clin Ultrasound* 23: 199–203, 1995.

Patten RM, et al: Nondisplaced fractures of the greater tuberosity of the humerus: Sonographic detection. *Radiology* 182:201–204, 1992.

Reading CC, et al: Sonographically guided percutaneous biopsy of small (3 cm or less) masses. *AJR* 151:189–192, 1988.

Resnick D, Niwayama G: *Diagnosis of Bone and Joint Disorders*. Philadelphia, WB Saunders Co, 1988.

Reuter KL, et al: Ultrasonography of a plexiform neurofibroma of the popliteal fossa. *J Ultrasound Med* 1:209–211, 1982.

Rippstein J: Zur Bestimmung der Antetorsion des Schenkelhalses mittels zweier Rogntgenaufnahmen. *Z Orthop Ihre Grenzgeb* 86:345, 1955.

Sandler MA, Alpern MB, Madrazo BL, et al: Inflammatory lesions of the groin: Ultrasonic evaluation. *Radiology* 151:747–750, 1984.

Shenouda NA, England JPS: Ultrasound in the diagnosis of scaphoid fractures. *J Hand Surg (Am)* 220:130–136, 1987.

Suzuki S, et al: Examination by ultrasound of Legg-Calve-Perthes disease. *Clin Orthop* 220:130–136, 1987.

Tregnaghi A, et al: Ultrasonographic evaluation of the superficial lymph node metastases in melanoma. *Eur J Radiol* 24:216, 1997.

van Holsbeeck M, et al: Staging and follow-up of rheumatoid arthritis of the knee. Comparison of sonography, thermography, and clinical assessment. *J Ultrasound Med* 7:561–566, 1988.

van Sonnenberg E, et al: Sonography of thigh abscess: Detection, diagnosis and drainage. *AJR* 149:769–772, 1987.

Vincent LM: Ultrasound of soft tissue abnormalities of the extremities. *Radiol Clin North Am* 26:131–144, 1988.

Wohlwend J, et al: Sonographic evaluation of bone changes in rotator cuff disease. Scientific paper abstract presented at the American Roentgen Ray Society's annual meeting, May 5–10, San Diego, CA, 1996.

Yeh HC, Rabinowitz JG: Ultrasonography of the extremities and pelvic girdle and correlation with computed tomography. *Radiology* 143:519–525, 1982.

Zynamon A, et al: Usefulness of an acoustic edge artifact in assessment of the Ilizarov corticotomy interval. *Skeletal Radiol* 21:293, 1992.

Chapter 11
Sonography of Rheumatoid Disease

Rethy K. Chhem, M.D., Ph.D., FRCPC, and Marnix T. van Holsbeeck, M.D.

Early diagnosis, assessment of inflammation, and detection of complications of rheumatoid disease are problems that can be addressed using ultrasound. The use of noninvasive techniques is especially important in patients with rheumatoid disease. Joint aspiration and arthrography are extremely painful when performed on an inflamed joint. In addition, these procedures are associated with a significant risk of infection in this population due to immune suppression and chronic steroid therapy. Arthrography, arthroscopy, and joint aspiration must be kept to an absolute minimum in these patients (Figs. 11–1 and 11–2) (Moore et al., 1975).

Over the past 20 years, many noninvasive techniques have been proposed to assess articular involvement of rheumatoid disease. Among them are radioisotope scanning and thermography. These techniques have been of limited benefit. Most recently, MRI and sonography have come to the forefront in the noninvasive evaluation of rheumatoid disease. Given ideal conditions, both of these modalities are equally well suited for the diagnosis and follow-up of rheumatoid disease. However, as we are all aware, ideal conditions rarely exist. Sonography has a tremendous advantage over MRI in that the examination can be performed quite rapidly, within approximately 15 minutes. Rheumatoid patients cannot tolerate lying motionless on a hard table for the time required for an MRI examination. In addition, during sonographic examination, the patient may move other extremities relatively freely, and the procedure does not require sedation. Cost and availability factors also strongly favor ultrasound.

Diagnosis

The synovial membrane is an important connective tissue lining the inner surface of the joint capsule, tendon sheath, and bursa. Therefore, it is essential to understand the pathogenesis and the pathological changes seen in rheumatoid synovium in order to perform a complete scan of synovial joints.

The earliest histological finding of rheumatoid arthritis is a nonsuppurative inflammation of the synovium consisting of (Bullough and Vigorita, 1984)

- hypertrophy and hyperplasia of the synovial cells;
- infiltration of the synovial membrane by plasma cells and lymphocytes;
- lymphoid follicles;
- fibrinous exudation at the surface of the synovium and within the synovial tissue.

In rheumatoid arthritis, as in any other inflammatory arthritis, the synovium undergoes significant changes leading to the formation of a mass of synovial tissue. This is the result of edema, multiple redundant folds, and villae (Fig. 11–3A,B). All these changes vary according to the severity and chronicity of the disease (Firestein, 1994). A synovial mass in direct contact with the interface of the articular cartilage and the bare area of the bone is called pannus (Firestein, 1994). This leads to the formation of marginal erosions, which represent an essential radiological feature of inflammatory arthritis. Synovial inflammation can also be detected in bursa and tendon sheath (see Fig. 4–12).

The initial diagnosis of rheumatoid disease usually requires the correlation of the clinical history, physical examination, laboratory tests, and radiographic findings (Beecker, 1959; Ropes et al., 1959). A definitive diagnosis of rheumatoid arthritis can be made when marginal erosions are identified in the characteristic distribution on conventional radiographs. Ultrasound has been used in assessment of rheumatoid joints (Fornage, 1989, Iagnocco et al., 1992; Chhem et al., 1993; Alaasarela and Alaasarela, 1994; Coakley et al., 1994; Andronopoulos et al.,

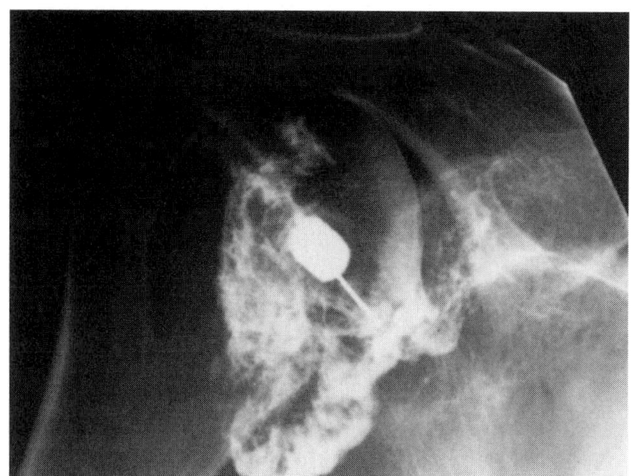

Figure 11–1 ■ Early rheumatoid arthritis: shoulder arthrogram. This single-contrast arthrogram was performed on a 56-year-old woman with a 4-month history of polyarticular arthritis predominantly in the right shoulder. Numerous filling defects indicative of synovial proliferation are noted. The rotator cuff is intact. Arthrography performed in patients with synovial inflammation is an extremely painful and usually prolonged procedure. In addition, this invasive procedure is associated with an increased risk of joint infection. Invasive procedures must be kept to a minimum in these immune-compromised patients.

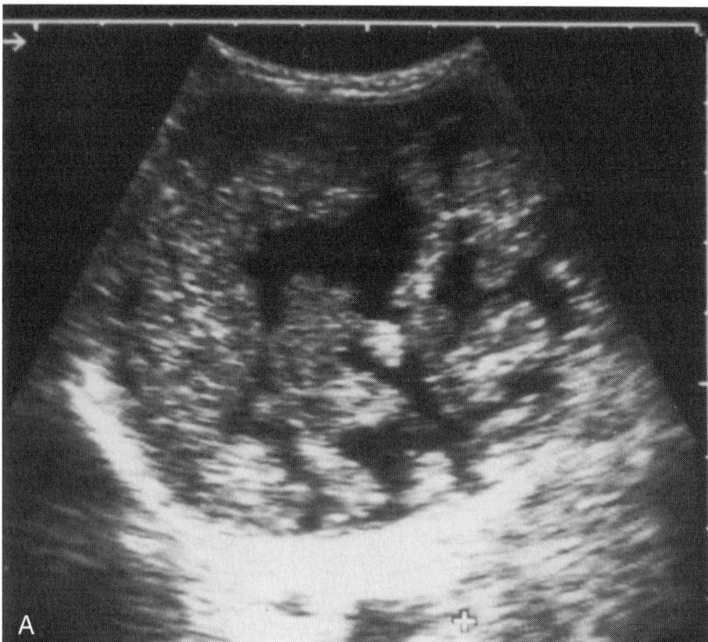

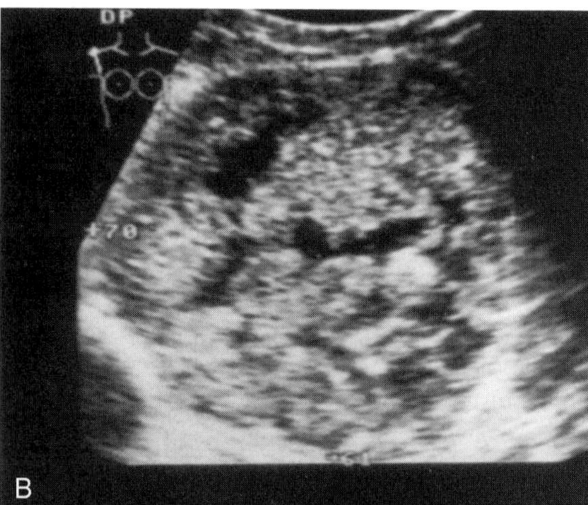

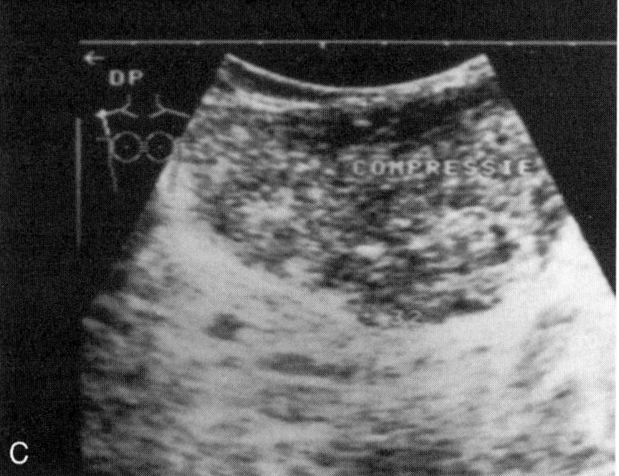

Figure 11–2 ■ **A**, Rheumatoid arthritis of the shoulder: transverse sonogram of the axillary recess of the shoulder. Same patient as in Figure 11–1. An enlarged axillary recess filled with pannus is seen on this transverse image. Villous synovial proliferation is evident within the fluid-filled joint. Sonography provides excellent noninvasive evaluation of the joint. In addition to evaluation of the synovium, the rotator cuff and biceps tendon are well evaluated during the same session. **B** and **C**, Chronic inflammation of the axillary recess of the shoulder: transverse sonograms. Same patient as in **A**. Another advantage of sonography over arthrography is the ability to quantitate synovial proliferation accurately. These two images demonstrate the necessity of compression with the transducer to measure total synovial thickness accurately. Note the marked change in the anteroposterior dimension of the axillary recess when fluid is expressed by compression.

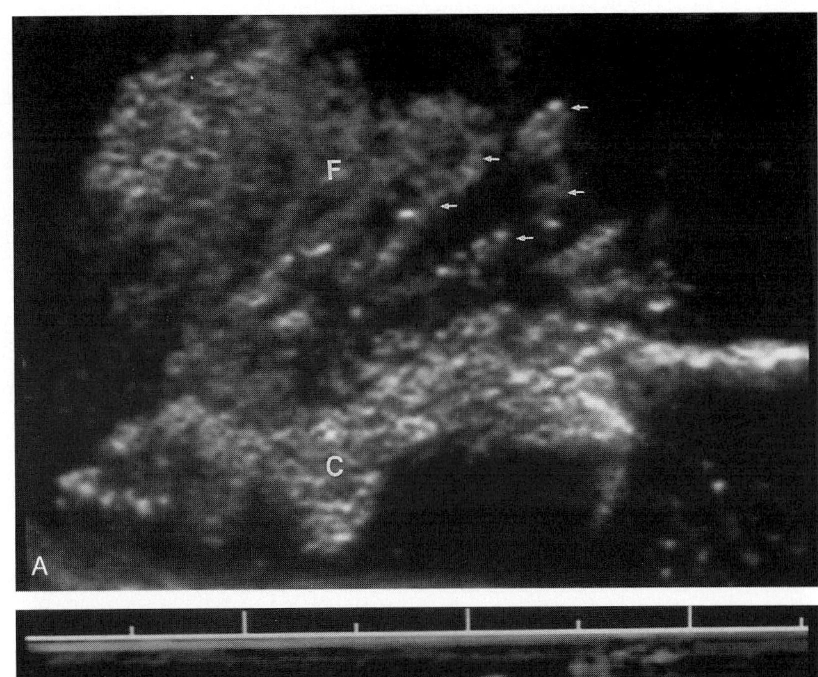

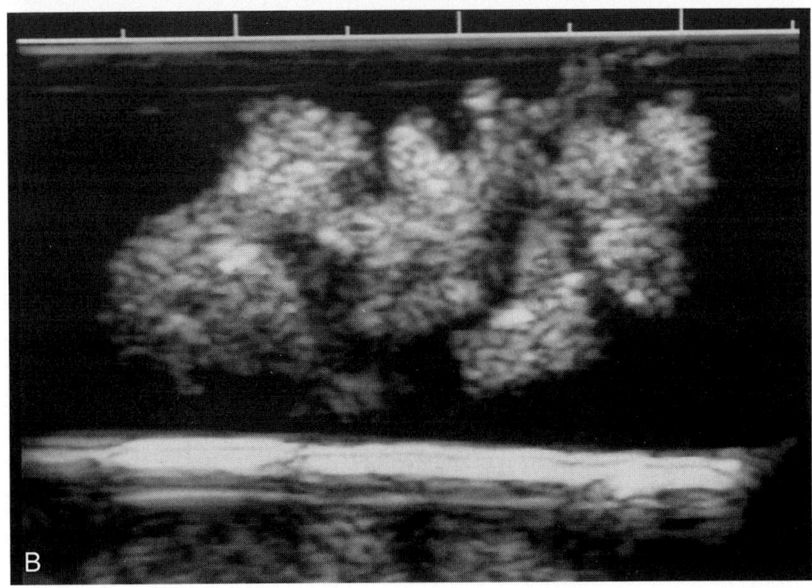

Figure 11–3 ■ **A**, Synovial hypertrophy: in vitro sonography. Synovial specimen harvested from the hip during a total joint replacement procedure for osteoarthritis. The specimen was placed in saline solution and scanned with a 10-MHz transducer. The synovium is mildly hypertrophied and appears as small, echoic villous structures (*arrows*). Because the articular cartilage is the primary site of degenerative changes, the synovium is minimally inflamed. Abbreviation: fat (*F*), capsule (*C*). **B**, Synovial pannus: In vitro sonography. Same procedure as in **A**. Marked synovial proliferation in a patient with acute rheumatoid arthritis. Synovial pannus appears as mildly echogenic nodules, which are mass-like in comparison with the noninflammatory synovium in **A**.

1995; Chhem and Beauregard, 1995; Grassi et al., 1995; Lund et al., 1995; Lehtinen et al., 1996; Ruhoy et al., 1996; Fedrizzi et al., 1997) and juvenile rheumatoid arthritis (Sureda et al., 1994). The most commonly affected joints are the metacarpophalangeal joints, the interphalangeal joints, the wrist, and the shoulders (Kelley et al., 1997) (Table 11–1). Marginal erosions are the result of chronic synovial inflammation. In the early stages of disease, a magnifying lens is helpful in identifying tiny erosions on conventional radiographs. However, detection of small erosions may be significantly delayed because they are obscured on the radiograph due to technical factors, most often patient positioning. As a result, diagnosis may be delayed for several months, and joint destruction continues untreated.

Ultrasound has proved to be extremely valuable in the early diagnosis of rheumatoid disease. It is exquisitely sensitive in detecting increased intra-articular fluid and is capable of detecting synovial proliferation before marginal erosions develop (Fig. 11–4) (Marchal et al., 1987; van Holsbeeck et al., 1988; Gielen et al., 1990). It is important to note that a normal synovial membrane cannot be demonstrated by sonography, as it blends imperceptibly with the joint capsule and the periarticular ligaments. In the early stages of active rheumatoid

Table 11-1
Epidemiology: Joint Involvement in Rheumatoid Arthritis (%)

Hands	91
Wrist	78
Shoulder	65
Knees	64
Ankle	50
Feet	43
Elbow	38
Hips	17
TMJ	8
Spine	4
Sternoclavicular	2

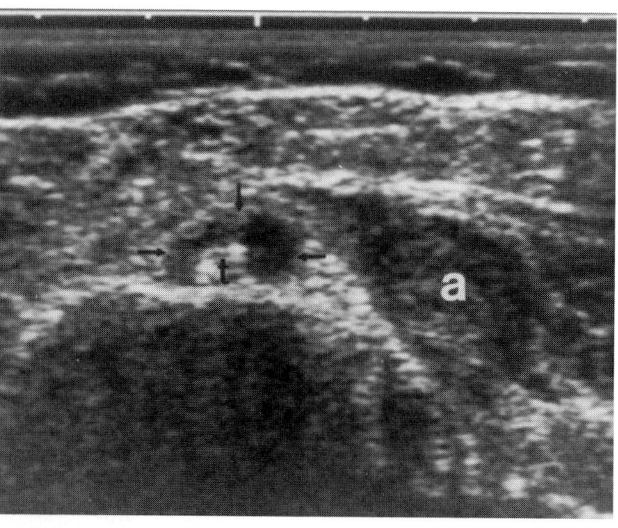

Figure 11-4 ■ Rheumatoid arthritis of the shoulder: transverse sonogram of the bicipital groove. Hypoechoic fluid and synovial proliferation (*arrows*) surround the long biceps tendon (*t*) and distend an enlarged subdeltoid bursa in this 53-year-old woman with a 2-year history of rheumatoid arthritis. An enlarged bursal recess (*a*) is pathognomonic for chronic joint disease. Often the diagnosis of rheumatoid disease can be made sonographically by the observation of an enlarged bursa with synovial proliferation several months prior to the development of marginal erosions.

disease, cartilage edema is present, which can be detected sonographically as cartilage thickening. Erosions in association with synovial proliferation are more easily detected using ultrasound (Figs. 11-5 through 11-10). A comparison of sonography with conventional radiography in the detection of erosions in the shoulder demonstrated that we could detect 27% more erosions using ultrasound.

Increased intra-articular fluid is a nonspecific finding indicative of joint pathology. Although it is nonspecific, joint effusion is a valuable indicator of active joint disease. Ultrasound has been shown to be unquestionably the best method for detection of increased intra-articular fluid and synovial proliferation (Chhem and Beauregard, 1995a). Graded compression is useful in distinguishing isolated effusion from synovial proliferation. Effusions as small as 1 mL can be detected with ultrasound (Marchal et al., 1987). Careful comparison with the contralateral joint is often helpful, but symmetrical disease may be misleading. The film of synovial fluid separating the leaves of the synovia in the joint recesses should not exceed 3 mm (Fig. 11-11).

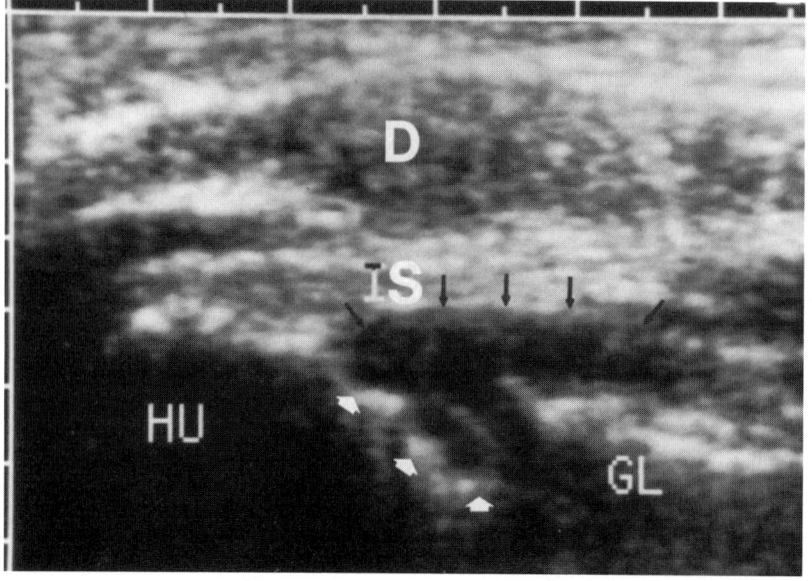

Figure 11-5 ■ Effusion in the shoulder joint: transverse sonogram of the posterior glenohumeral joint. The patient is a 39-year-old woman who developed symmetrical joint pain during pregnancy. Conventional radiographs taken after delivery were normal. Sonographic examination of the shoulder demonstrated a joint effusion with marginal erosions (*white arrows*) adjacent to the insertion of the infraspinatus tendon (*IS*). The best location to detect small effusions within the shoulder is the posterior synovial recess (*black arrows*) between the glenohumeral joint and the infraspinatus tendon. A fluid film more than 2 mm thick at this location is indicative of joint effusion. When effusion is detected in an adult without other findings, the first considerations are joint infection and rheumatoid arthritis. Aspiration is then indicated to make the definitive diagnosis. The observation of erosions in this case made the diagnosis of rheumatoid arthritis. Abbreviations: deltoid (*D*), glenoid (*GL*), humerus (*HU*).

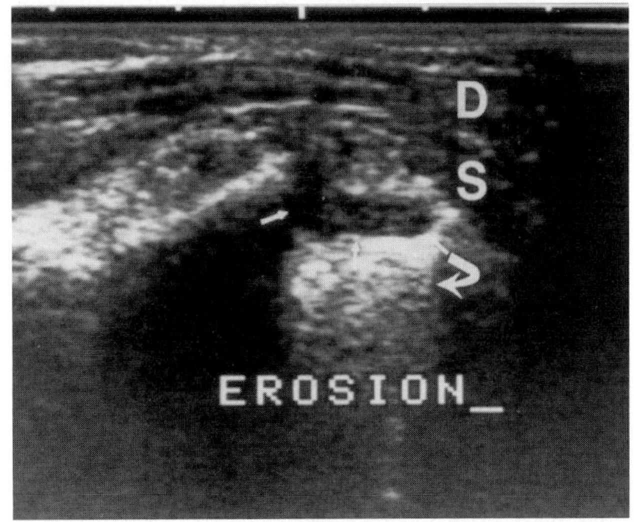

Figure 11-6 ■ Humeral head erosion: transverse sonogram. This woman has a long history of rheumatoid disease. The transducer is positioned transversely over the lateral aspect of the shoulder just inferior to the acromion. A large erosion (*small arrows*) is observed deforming the humeral head. The appearance of increase through-transmission (*curved arrow*) is frequently seen deep to large erosions. Rheumatoid erosions contain hypoechoic pannus. Along with an absence of cortical bone in the depth of the lesion, a small amount of trabecular bone may be seen. Ultrasound has been demonstrated to be more sensitive than conventional radiography in detecting marginal erosions and Hill-Sachs lesions. Abbreviations: deltoid (*D*), pannus or inflamed synovium (*S*).

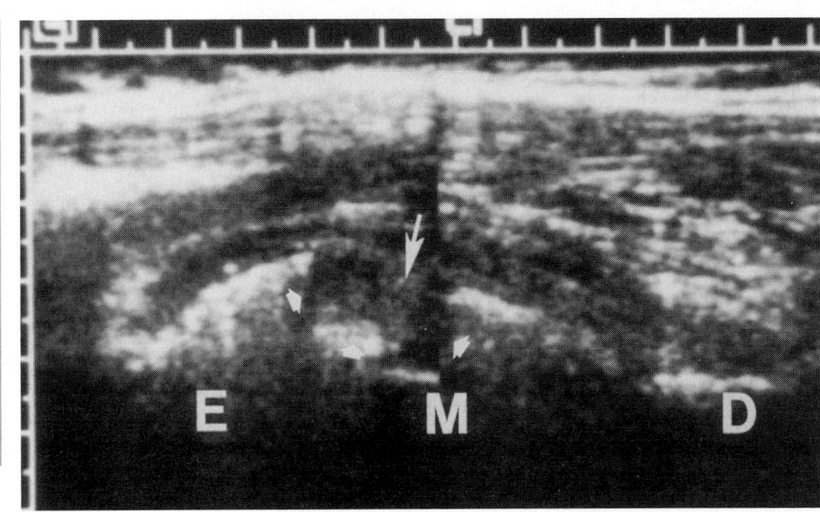

Figure 11-7 ■ Rheumatoid arthritis of the hip: longitudinal sonogram. Over the past 7 months, this 61-year-old woman experienced pain and stiffness in the right hip, which were worse in the morning. Conventional radiographs demonstrated a normal joint space and lucency in the femoral neck of unknown significance. Blind aspiration of the hip yielded a "dry tap." The transducer is positioned lateral to the femoral artery in the axis of the femoral neck. A large marginal erosion (*small arrows*) is seen in the proximal femoral neck. Hypoechoic pannus (*large arrow*) fills the erosion. This examination made the initial diagnosis of rheumatoid involvement of the hip. During the following 6 months, the patient developed a symmetrical polyarthritis. Abbreviations: diaphysis (*D*), epiphysis (*E*), metaphysis (*M*).

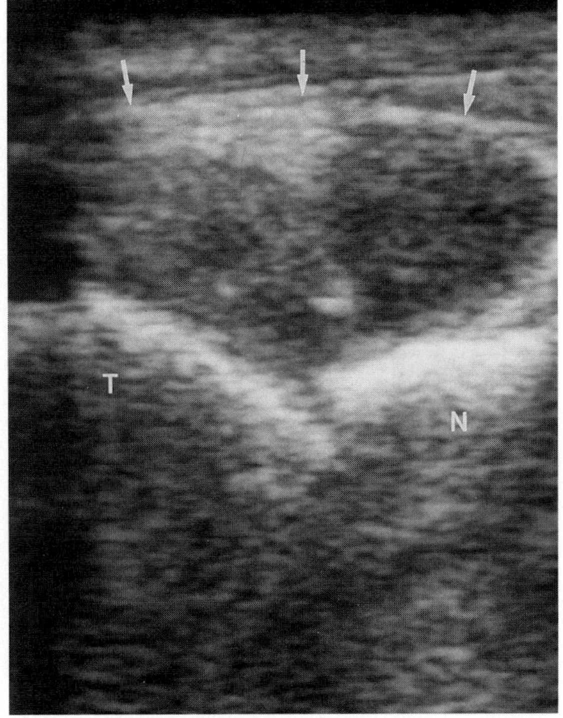

Figure 11-8 ■ Rheumatoid arthritis of the hindfoot: longitudinal sonogram. A 49-year-old female with a 2-year history of rheumatoid arthritis involving the hands and wrists, with a recent onset of pain and swelling at the dorsal aspect of the left hindfoot. Longitudinal scan of the dorsal aspect of the hindfoot shows a large effusion distending the capsule (*arrows*) of the talonavicular joint, which contained lobular echogenic material representing synovial hypertrophy. A needle biopsy of the synovial membrane was done using ultrasound guidance. The tip of the needle is demonstrated. Abbreviations: talus (*T*), navicular (*N*).

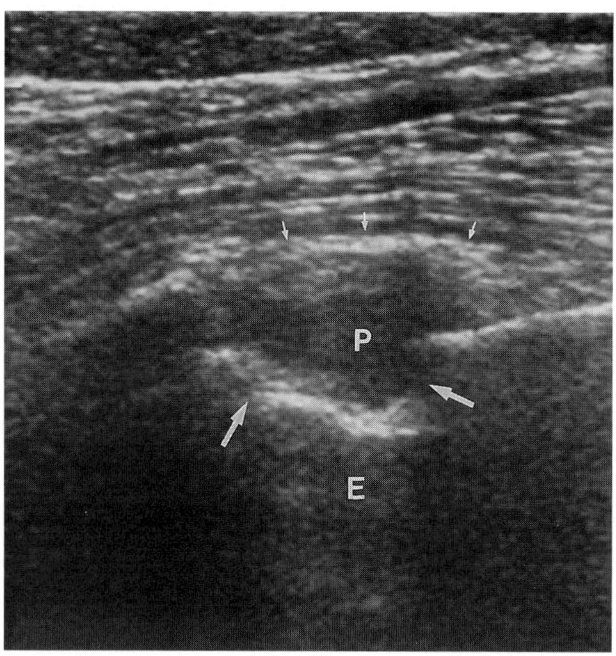

Figure 11–9 ■ Advanced rheumatoid arthritis of the elbow: coronal sonogram. A 56-year-old female with swelling and severe deformity of the elbow. She has a 14-year history of rheumatoid arthritis. Longitudinal scan of the medial aspect of the joint shows a large bone erosion (*arrows*) of the medial epicondyle containing synovial pannus and moderate distention of the joint capsule (*small arrows*). Abbreviations: pannus (*p*), medial epicondyle (*E*).

Excessive fluid resulting from an inflammatory process accumulates in articular recesses. The most important articular recesses of synovial joints affected by rheumatoid disease are summarized in Table 11–2.

Synovitis seen in rheumatoid arthritis appears as a thickening of the synovial membrane (van Holsbeeck et al., 1988; Chhem and Beauregard, 1995). Fat surrounding the inflamed synovia is increased in echogenicity. Therefore, the thickened synovial membrane has a hypoechoic appearance. Synovial thickness must be measured with firm compression applied with the transducer. This procedure expresses synovial fluid from the joint recess, allowing a reproducible measure of synovial thickness. In addition to a very irregular contour of

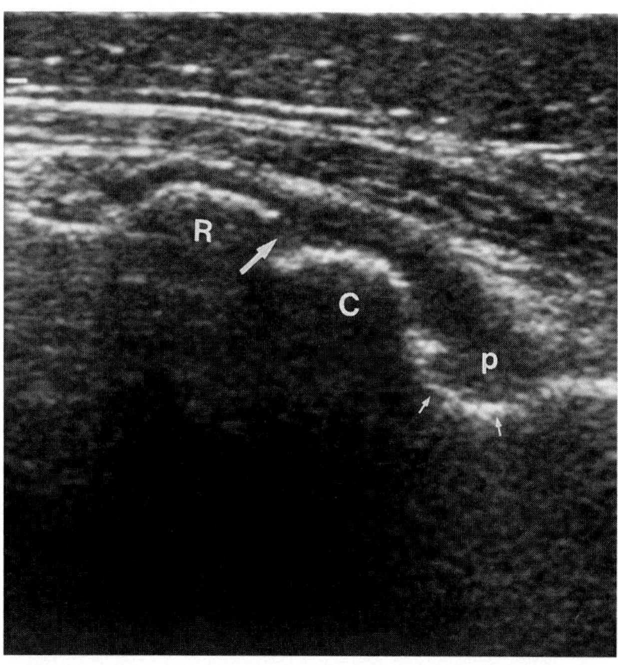

Figure 11–10 ■ Early rheumatoid arthritis of the elbow: coronal sonogram. A 46-year-old female with a recent history of rheumatoid arthritis. Longitudinal scan of the lateral aspect of the elbow. The radiocapitellar joint is well seen (*arrow*). There is a small erosion (*small arrows*) at the lateral epicondyle containing rheumatoid pannus (*p*). A moderate joint effusion is seen at the radiocapitellar and radial recess. Abbreviations: radius (*R*), capitellum (*C*).

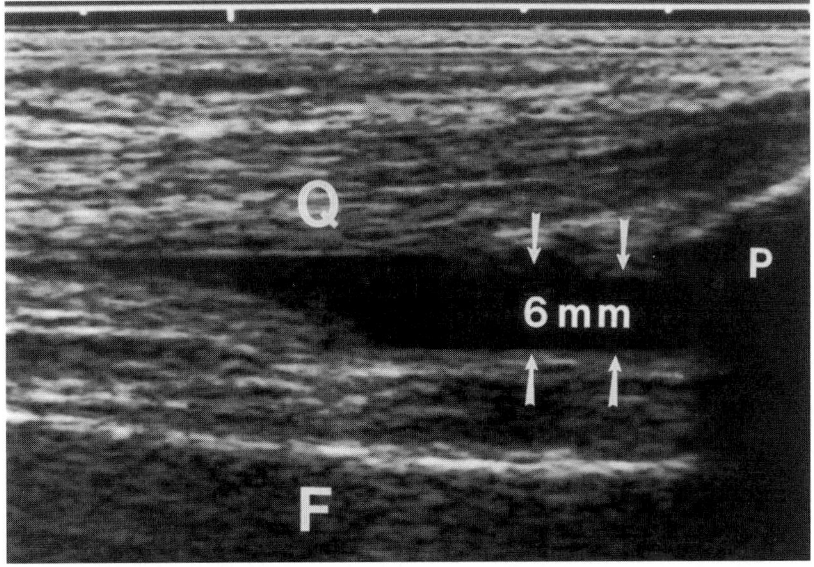

Figure 11-11 ■ Knee effusion in chondromalacia: longitudinal sonogram. A 17-year-old girl with bilateral patellar subluxation and recurrent swelling of the knees presented for sonographic evaluation. In this standard longitudinal view of the suprapatellar bursa, an anechoic fluid collection is identified within the bursa (*arrows*). The normal fluid film within the suprapatellar bursa should not exceed 3 mm. Sonography is very sensitive in detection of joint effusion. Increases in joint fluid as small as 1 mm can be detected. Effusion is a nonspecific finding seen in a wide variety of pathology, in this case chondromalacia patellae. Abbreviations: femur (*F*), patella (*P*), quadriceps (*Q*).

the synovial membrane, synechia (Fig. 11–12) between the walls of the articular recesses can be observed in late rheumatoid disease (van Holsbeeck et al., 1988). Pannus found in affected joints has the appearance of hypoechoic soft tissue masses, a pseudotumoral appearance (Fig. 11–13) (Cooperberg et al., 1978). Often it has a villous configuration and is continuous with the joint capsule. These masses can be differentiated from aggregations of proteinaceous material within the joint by their broad-based attachment to the joint capsule (Worth et al., 1986; van Holsbeeck et al., 1988).

Bursitis is also a common disease entity in rheumatoid arthritis. Subacromial-subdeltoid bursitis is the most common sonographic finding in the painful rheumatoid shoulder (Alaasarela and Alaasarela, 1994).

Cartilage edema in the early stages of rheumatoid arthritis can be detected sonographically as thickening of the articular cartilage. Electronic calipers make these measurements quite easy (Aisen et al., 1984). Normal weight-bearing cartilage ranges from 1.2 to 1.9 mm in thickness (Aisen et al., 1984; Richardson et al., 1988). Measurements of cartilage thickness greater than 2.5 mm are generally considered pathological. Chronic inflammation of the cartilage results in permanent damage to the articular surface. This is observed sonographically as blurring of the articular surface. Continued destruction of

Table 11-2
Articular Recesses

Joint	Site of Effusion Detection
Shoulder	Posterior recess
Elbow	Anterior/posterior recesses
Wrist	Prestyloid recess
Hip	Anterior recess
Knee	Suprapatellar recess
Ankle	Anterior recess

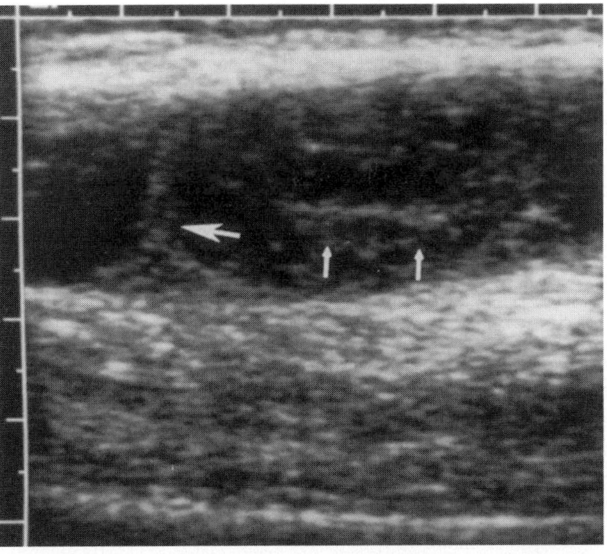

Figure 11-12 ■ Rheumatoid arthritis of the knee: longitudinal sonogram of the popliteal fossa. A large Baker's cyst is noted in the popliteal fossa. The presence of synechiae (*arrow*), synovial proliferation, and debris (*small arrows*) are characteristic findings in chronic synovitis.

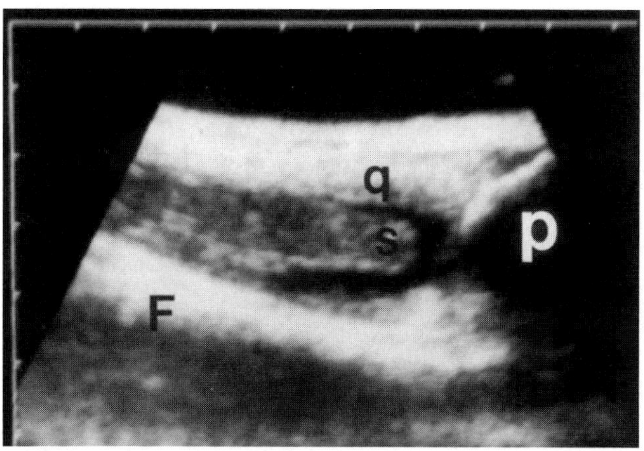

Figure 11-13 ■ Diagnosis of rheumatoid knee synovitis: suprapatellar approach. The suprapatellar bursa provides a sonographic window through which we can evaluate for joint effusion, synovial thickening, and intra-articular loose bodies. This bursa is not obscured by bone, making it ideal for ultrasound examination. In this patient with rheumatoid arthritis, a large synovial polyp (*s*) surrounded by fluid is seen extending down from the superior extent of the bursa. Abbreviations: femur (*F*), patellar base (*p*), quadriceps tendon (*q*).

the cartilage due to rheumatoid disease is seen as pitting of the articular surface and measurable thinning of the cartilage.

Marginal erosions are identified as crater-like defects in the bony contours along the edges of the articular cartilage affecting the so-called bare areas of the bone. On the ultrasound scan, the smooth, continuous echogenic line of bone is interrupted (Sarazin et al., 1996). Pannus is recognized as a hypoechoic soft tissue mass filling these erosions. As stated earlier, sonography is more sensitive than conventional radiography in the detection of these erosions. In more advanced disease, subchondral cysts can be demonstrated in the epiphysis. They may contain hypoechoic pannus.

Differential Diagnosis

Uncomplicated joint effusion, characterized by anechoic intra-articular fluid, can be seen in a wide variety of joint pathology (see Fig. 11-11). Traumatic disorders such as osteochondritis dissecans, chondromalacia patellae, patellar subluxation, medial plica syndrome, and meniscal tears are among the numerous possible etiologies. Calcium pyrophosphate dihydrate deposition disease (CPPD) is also associated with uncomplicated effusion. All of these entities are easily distinguished sonographically from rheumatoid arthritis by the absence of irregular synovial thickening.

Synovial proliferation (see Fig. 11-13) is associated with inflammatory or crystal-induced arthropathy, septic arthritis, amyloid arthropathy, pigmented villonodular synovitis (PVNS), osteochondromatosis, and hemophilic arthropathy (Table 11-3). In clinical practice, the differential diagnosis of rheumatoid arthritis most frequently includes psoriatic arthritis and Reiter's disease. Psoriatic arthritis and Reiter's disease are rarely manifested by villous synovial proliferation. However, the absence of villi attached to the irregularly thickened synovium is not a reliable means of differentiating these entities from rheumatoid arthritis. The definitive diagnosis in these cases depends on radiographic findings, laboratory data, and the clinical presentation. PVNS is another proliferative disorder involving the synovial membrane that cannot be differentiated solely by sonographic criteria. The definitive diagnosis can sometimes be made with conventional radiography, but surgical biopsy is often required to exclude synovial sarcoma. A few cases of amyloid deposition in the synovium have been detected sonographically in hemodialysis patients. It produces a slightly nodular appearance in the synovium, but no villi are present (see Fig. 14-30).

Chronic infection is a rare cause of joint effusion in combination with synovial proliferation. Tuberculosis, brucellosis, syphilis, and fungal infection all may produce sonographic findings similar to those of the inflammatory arthritides (see Table 11-3). Radiographic findings are also quite similar to those of rheumatoid arthritis. The clinical history

Table 11-3
Proliferative Synovitis: Differential Diagnosis

Rheumatoid arthritis
Septic arthritis
  Acute: Bacterial
  Subacute: Tuberculosis, fungi, brucella
Crystal induced arthropathies
Amyloid arthropathy
PVNS
Synovial osteochondromatosis
Hemophilic arthropathy

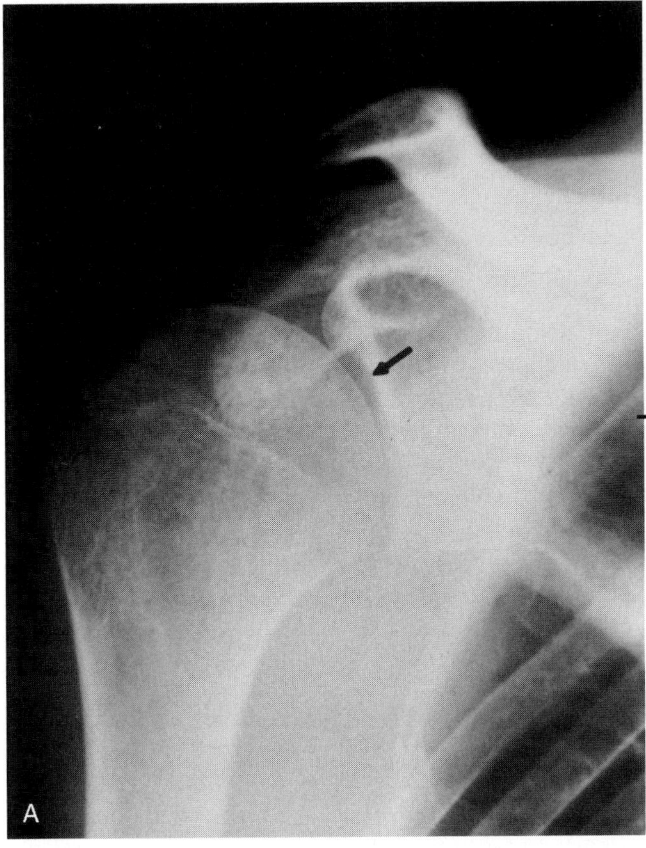

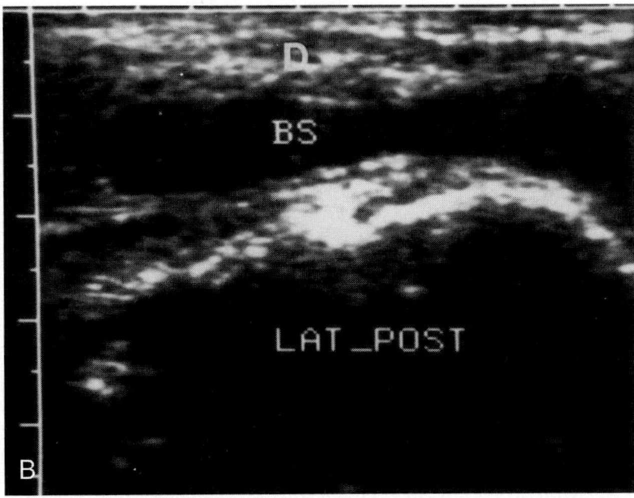

Figure 11–14 ■ **A**, Septic arthritis of the shoulder: Grashey view of the shoulder. The patient is a 31-year-old man with a renal transplant receiving cyclosporine and steroid therapy. He was afebrile, with leukocytosis and blood cultures positive for *Staphylococcus aureus.* At the time of examination, he reported right shoulder pain, but no swelling was evident. This Grashey view of the right shoulder demonstrates a vacuum phenomenon (*arrow*), generally accepted as indicating the absence of joint effusion. The remainder of the shoulder series was normal. **B**, Septic arthritis of the shoulder: coronal sonogram of the shoulder. Same patient as in **A**. Sonographic examination demonstrated a rotator cuff tear and fluid, with definite internal echos filling the subacromial-subdeltoid bursa (*BS*). Blind aspiration of the joint yielded a dry tap. Based on the ultrasound examination, the patient was taken to the operating room, and 30 mL of grossly purulent material was evacuated. Cultures grew *Staphylococcus aureus.* Abbreviation: deltoid (*D*).

and laboratory findings are suggestive of infection, but definitive diagnosis depends on aspiration of the joint and isolation of the causative organism. The presence of anechoic fluid within the joint generally reduces the suspicion of infection. However, the lack of echos within the fluid does not absolutely exclude infection. Cases of joint sepsis in which the fluid was clearly anechoic have been reported (Marchal et al., 1987). Whenever infection is suspected, joint aspiration is mandatory.

Ultrasound guidance has several advantages over fluoroscopy in joint aspiration. The major advantage is that ultrasound has the ability to localize fluid collections. If aspiration is performed using fluoroscopy, a "dry tap" does not exclude infection (Fig. 11–14). Debris within the joint may block flow through the needle, or loculations may inhibit aspiration. Sonographic guidance can direct the needle to the largest fluid-filled joint recess, avoiding vital structures. The duration of the procedure is usually not significantly longer than that of a routine ultrasound examination (McGahan, 1987).

Several small changes in aspiration technique will facilitate sonographic guidance. A linear array transducer placed within a sterile surgical glove is essential. If sterile ultrasound gel is not available, povidone-iodine or chlorhexidine gluconate skin prep solution can be substituted. Radial arrays and sector scanners make the procedure more difficult because of the varying angle of incidence of the sound beam with the needle. The needle is best visualized when the incident sound beam is perpendicular to the shaft of the needle. A 20-gauge spinal needle is routinely used for these procedures. Needles with textured surfaces are available for sonographic procedures and allow better visualization. Another trick in identifying the location of the needle tip is removal and replacement of the stylet. This pumps a tiny amount of air through the needle, producing a small bubble at the tip. The echogenic gas with shadowing is easily detected. However, this trick cannot be used more than three or four times during the same procedure. Visualization of landmarks will be obscured by shadows produced by the bubbles if it is used excessively. Aspiration technique is otherwise identical to that of a fluoroscopic approach.

Follow-up of Rheumatoid Arthritis

Previously, there were no noninvasive techniques to evaluate the activity of rheumatoid arthritis accurately in large synovial joints. Fortunately, clinical examination of small superficial joints, such as the interphalangeal joints, is a reliable means of evaluating disease activity in rheumatoid patients. Resolution of swelling in the interphalangeal joints is a reliable indicator of healing. However, it is not possible to evaluate inflammation in deep-seated joints by clinical examination. Previously, arthrotomy and biopsy were the only accurate means of evaluating deep-seated joints, but these procedures are associated with significant morbidity in this patient population. Laboratory data and conventional radiography are of little help (Desilva et al., 1986). MRI has been proposed as a noninvasive means of assessing joint inflammation (Hammer et al., 1986). Hammer et al. noted a significant change in the T_2 characteristics of the synovium after therapy, but no prospective follow-up studies over time are presently available. Also, the time required to perform the examination is usually intolerable to these patients. Thermography has shown some promise; however, it is also a difficult examination to perform. Radioisotope scanning has proved to be of questionable value. Ultrasound has demonstrated accuracy and reliability in the evaluation of joint inflammation associated with rheumatoid arthritis (Cooperberg et al., 1978; van Holsbeeck et al., 1988). This examination can be performed quickly and without discomfort. Recently, ultrasound has also been used to assess the response to therapy, whether it is systemic or local, such as intra-articular injection of somatostatin 14 into the rheumatoid knee (Coari et al., 1995). This substance inhibits the release of substance P, which significantly increases in the synovial fluid of the rheumatoid patient. Ultrasound has proven to be accurate in detecting changes in synovial proliferation by directly measuring the thickness of the synovium (Coari et al., 1995).

Adoption of a standardized technique for sonographic examination is essential. When evaluating the knee, we obtain sagittal images of the suprapatellar bursa with the patient supine and the knee flexed 30 degrees. The transducer is positioned along the length of the rectus femoris tendon, with its inferior extent touching the superior border of the patella. Two sets of images are obtained. The first set is obtained with firm pressure applied with the transducer (Fig. 11–15C), compressing the bursa between the transducer and the femur. This image allows reproducible measurement of total synovial thickness, a sum of the thicknesses of the anterior and posterior walls of the bursa. The second set of images requires two examiners. One examiner positions the transducer and the other compresses the lateral joint recesses. Compression of the lateral recesses forces fluid into the suprapatellar bursa. These images are obtained with minimal transducer pressure and provide a reliable estimation of the quantity of joint fluid (Fig. 11–15A, B).

Acute exacerbations of rheumatoid disease are accompanied by accumulation of increased intra-articular fluid and synovial thickening. Instituting appropriate therapy results in marked reduction of joint fluid within 24 hours, and approximately one-half of patients show complete resolution of joint effusion within 10 days (van Holsbeeck et al., 1988). Reduction in synovial thickness occurs almost as rapidly. A 36% decrease in mean synovial thickness was observed 10 days after initiation of steroid therapy. The rate of response has been shown to be dose related (Fig. 11–15D).

The knee is used as an example because it is a large synovial joint frequently involved by rheumatoid disease. These techniques can easily be applied to any large synovial joint. Rheumatoid disease in the shoulder is best evaluated by imaging the posterior synovial recess due to its accessibility. The transducer is oriented transversely, perpendicular to the plane of the glenoid (see Fig. 11–5). Measurements at the elbow, hip, and ankle are obtained using an anterior approach. At the elbow, images are obtained with the transducer positioned in the long axis of the radius over the radial head and the arm in extension. The hip is examined the same way an examination for transient synovitis is performed (see Fig. 11–7). The transducer is placed along the length of the femoral neck. Longitudinal images of the ankle are obtained over the anterior aspect of the tibiotalar joint.

Complications of Rheumatoid Disease

Infection

Most patients afflicted with rheumatoid arthritis are chronically immune suppressed due to steroid therapy. They are predisposed to develop joint infection,

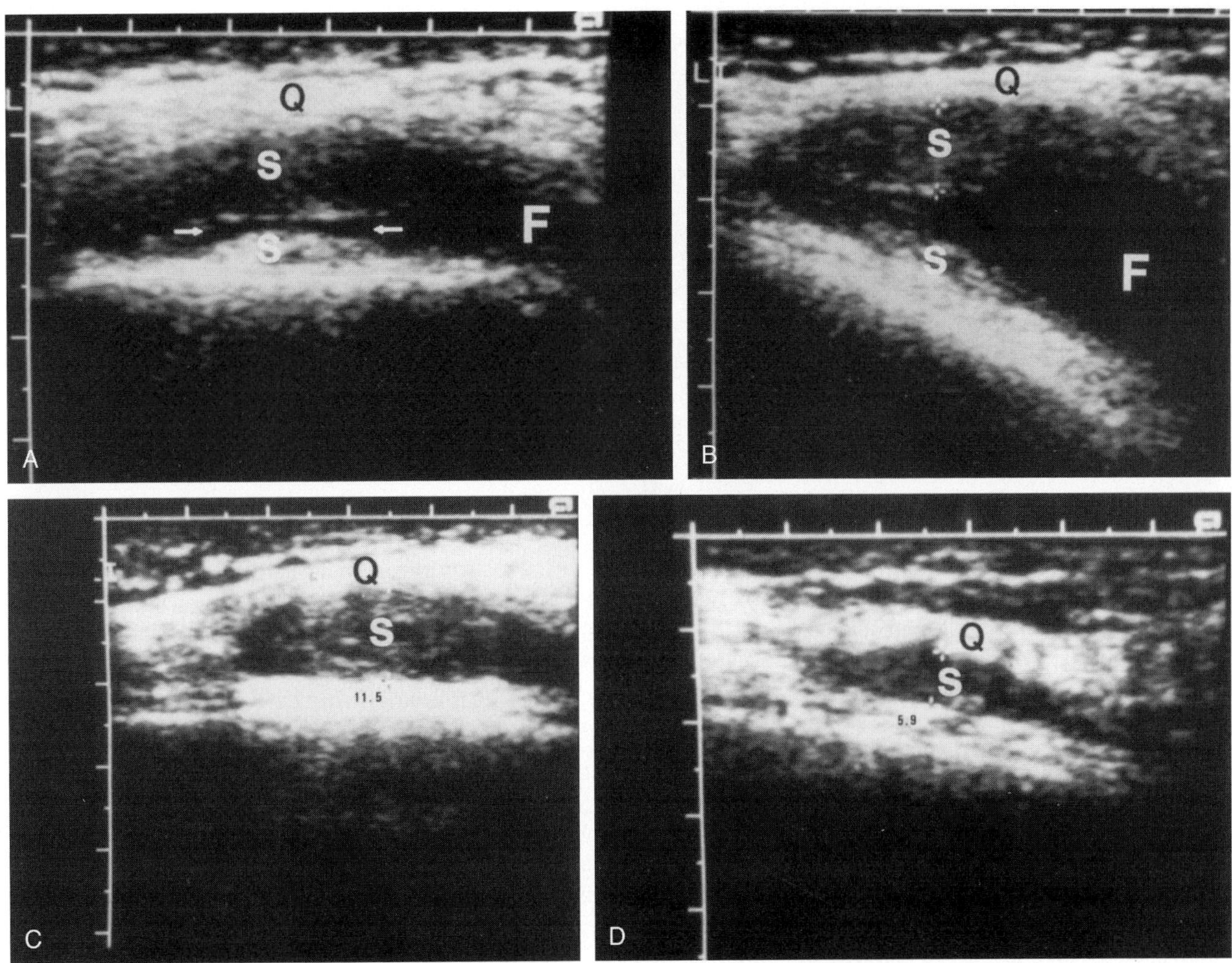

Figure 11-15 ■ **A**, Follow-up of rheumatoid synovitis: suprapatellar scan. New onset of left knee pain was reported by this patient with a history of rheumatoid arthritis for more than 10 years. This longitudinal image of the suprapatellar bursa demonstrates a small amount of fluid (*arrows*) within the bursa and marked synovial thickening (*S*). The fluid collection (*F*) increases in dimension immediately above the patella. Abbreviation: quadriceps tendon (*Q*). **B**, Accurate, reproducible estimation of the magnitude of joint effusion requires two examiners. One examiner applies pressure to the lateral joint recesses, forcing fluid (*F*) into the suprapatellar bursa. The other examiner positions the transducer. This has proved to be the best method for following the magnitude of joint effusion. Abbreviations: synovial thickening (*s*), quadriceps tendon (*Q*). **C**, The transducer has not been moved, but pressure has been applied with the transducer. All fluid has been expressed from the bursa. Pannus remains hypoechoic relative to the quadriceps tendon (*Q*) and surrounding fat despite firm compression. Total synovial thickness measured on compression images is an accurate measure of synovial proliferation and can be used to follow disease activity over time. In this case, total synovial thickness prior to therapy measures 11.5 mm. Abbreviation: synovium (*S*). **D**, Ten days after intra-articular injection of a long-acting corticosteroid preparation. Firm pressure is again applied to make an accurate measurement of the total synovial thickness (TST). A favorable response to therapy is indicated in this case by a decrease in TST to 5.9 mm. Abbreviations: quadriceps (*Q*), synovium (*S*). (From van Holsbeeck M, van Holsbeeck K, Gevers G, et al: *J Ultrasound Med* 7:561–566, 1988. Used by permission.)

which can rapidly lead to systemic sepsis if unrecognized. Ultrasound can be very valuable in the early diagnosis of joint and bursal infection in patients with rheumatoid arthritis. Prompt initiation of therapy with intravenous (IV) antibiotics and, if indicated, surgical drainage is of the utmost importance. In our experience, more than 70% of infected joints in rheumatoid patients are shoulders. This may be due to the frequent use of intra-articular steroid injections to treat shoulder pain in these patients. One series shows that in 20% of cases, more than one joint is involved (Goldenberg, 1989).

Joint and bursa infections are characterized by rapid accumulation of fluid (Figs. 11–16, 11–17)

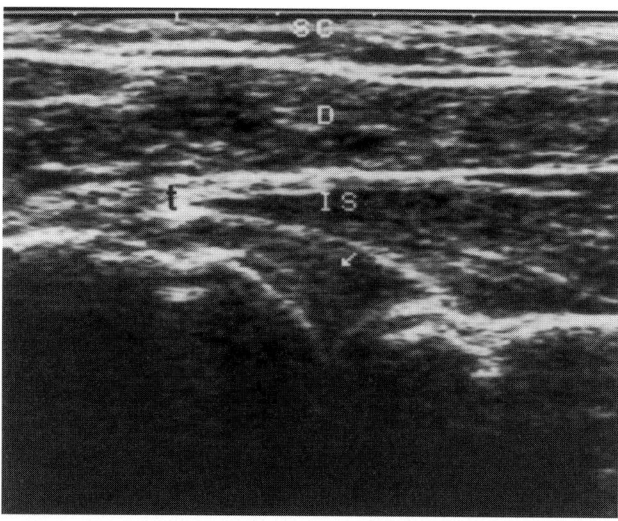

Figure 11-16 ■ Infected shoulder: transverse sonogram. A 50-year-old woman with known rheumatoid arthritis presented with increased pain and swelling of the right shoulder after an intra-articular steroid injection. The distended posterior synovial recess (*arrow*) is difficult to identify due to the isoechoic nature of the fluid within the joint. The infraspinatus muscle (*IS*) is elevated by this fluid collection. Normally, this muscle is in direct contact with the posterior glenoid and humerus. Evaluation of joint effusion in the shoulder from an anterior approach is difficult due to humeral retroversion and surrounding bony structures. A posterior approach is much more sensitive in detecting joint effusion in the shoulder. Abbreviations: deltoid (*D*), infraspinatus tendon (*t*), subcutaneous fat (*SC*).

within the infected joint or bursa. When acute swelling of an isolated joint is detected in a rheumatoid patient, infection must be suspected.

Sonography has been used to detect musculoskeletal infection (Chhem et al., 1995). The technique plays an important role in the detection of superimposed infection in patients with rheumatoid arthritis for a number of reasons:

- Evaluation of changes in the amount of effusion and degree of synovial proliferation on serial sonographic examinations;
- Detection of extension of the infection to the adjacent bursa, tendon sheath, or soft tissue; and
- Guidance of joint aspiration, which is the key examination for the confirmation of sepsis (Cardinal et al., 1997).

A sonographic sign of infection in a rheumatoid joint is marked increase in intra-articular fluid with no significant increase in synovial membrane thickness. The major differential diagnosis of septic arthritis is exacerbation of rheumatoid arthritis; the clinical

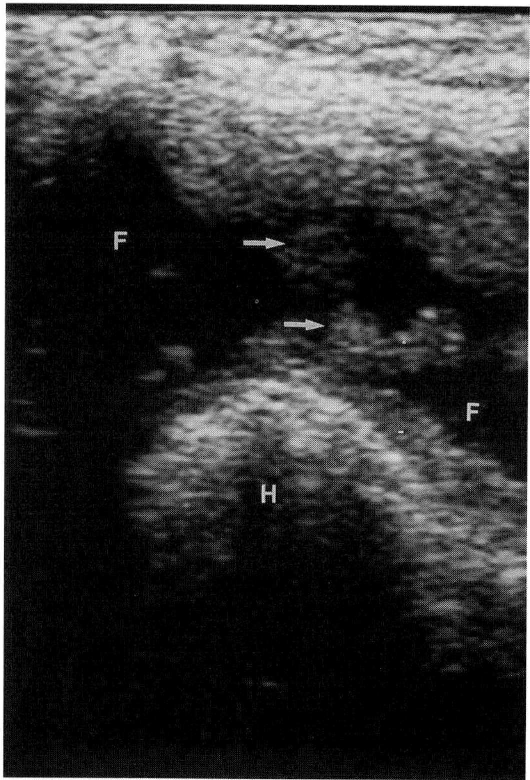

Figure 11-17 ■ Septic arthritis complicating a rheumatoid shoulder: longitudinal sonogram. A 62-year-old female patient complaining of worsening of the symptoms in her right shoulder. Longitudinal scan of the shoulder shows marked distortion of the normal anatomical landmarks of the joint due to bone destruction and malalignment. There is a large cavity filled with fluid (*F*) and synovial villi (*arrows*). The supraspinatus tendon is no longer seen because of an extensive tear. The subacromial-subdeltoid bursa communicates freely with the glenohumeral joint space. Infection was confirmed by ultrasound-guided fine needle aspiration. Abbreviation: humerus (*H*).

Table 11–4
Synovial Cyst in Rheumatoid Arthritis: Sites and Differential Diagnosis

Hand and wrist
Dorsal aspect of proximal interphalangeal joints
Metacarpal joints
Wrist joint
Flexor or extensor tendon sheath
Within carpal tunnel
Feet and ankle
Interphalangeal joints
Metatarsophalangeal joint
Distal flexor tendon sheath
Shoulder, elbow, hip, knee
Clinical differential diagnosis: bursitis, tenosynovitis, rheumatoid nodule

examination is almost always inconclusive (Goldenberg, 1989). In an exacerbation of rheumatoid disease, the joint effusion will be in proportion to the increase in synovial membrane thickness. In addition, infected fluid will have definitive internal echos in the majority of cases. However, sonographic features are not specific; therefore, prompt ultrasound-guided aspiration of the joint is mandatory. The most commonly isolated organism is *Staphylococcus aureus* (Resnick and Niwayama, 1988). When gas-producing organisms are present, gas bubbles, identified as echogenic foci with shadowing, may be observed. Despite these signs, the decision to aspirate the joint remains based on clinical criteria. The consequences of untreated joint infection in these patients are rapidly devastating. In addition to aiding the early diagnosis of infection, ultrasound can provide assistance in aspiration of the involved joint or bursa, as described earlier.

Periarticular Complications of Rheumatoid Disease

Synovial cysts are common complications of rheumatoid arthritis and may occur in any synovial joint (Table 11–4). Baker's cysts (Figs. 11–18 and 11–19) (Andronopoulos et al., 1995; Chhem and Beauregard, 1995) occur in the knee as a result of increased intra-articular fluid. Clinically, a Baker's cyst may mimic a deep vein thrombosis. Alternatively, it may may lead to venous obstruction in the calf (Palmer, 1969). Because the clinical examination is not always conclusive, sonography is very valuable in the evaluation of popliteal cysts and their complications. The most useful anatomical landmarks for the diagnosis of Baker's cyst are the medial gastrocnemius and the semimembranosus tendons. The neck of the popliteal cyst extends between these two tendons. The most dependent part of the cyst should be assessed carefully, with a search for a subtle extraluminal leak of fluid.

Other types of synovial cysts have been described in rheumatoid patients. They may arise from

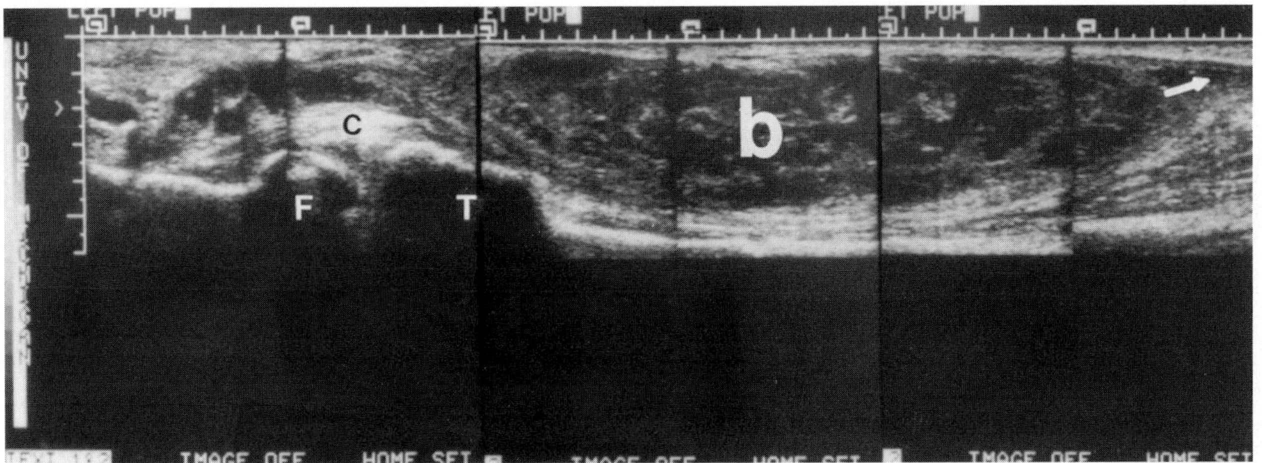

Figure 11–18 ▪ Ruptured Baker's cyst in rheumatoid arthritis: longitudinal sonogram. This 50-year-old man had a 4-month history of symmetrical polyarticular rheumatoid disease. He presented to the emergency room with acute swelling of the left calf. The results of contrast venography were negative. Ultrasound was then performed, revealing a huge rheumatoid Baker's cyst (*b*) measuring approximately 35 cm long. This huge mass is filled with hypoechoic pannus. Surrounding soft tissues are abnormally increased in echogenicity. Note that the inferior extent of the cyst appears pointed (*arrow*), a typical finding in ruptured Baker's cysts. Abbreviations: femoral condyle (*F*), posterior joint capsule (*C*), tibial condyle (*T*).

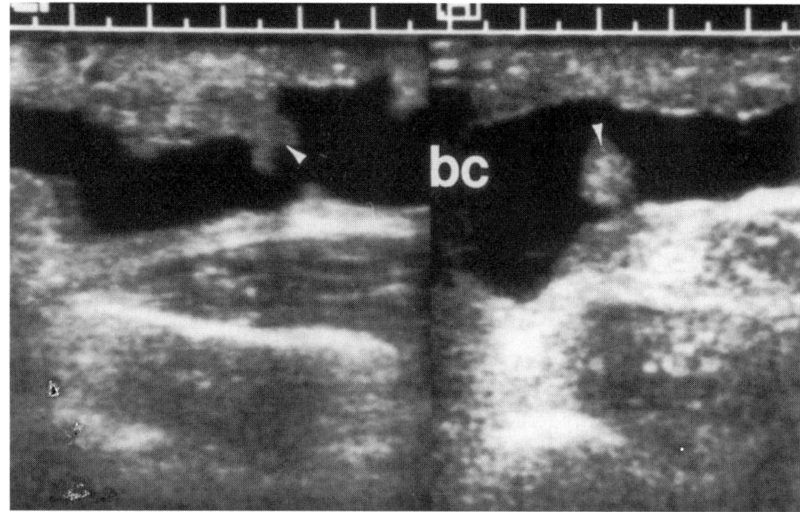

Figure 11–19 ■ Baker's cyst in amyloid arthropathy: longitudinal sonogram. This patient has been receiving chronic hemodialysis for more than 10 years. The transducer is positioned over the medial aspect of the popliteal fossa in the long axis of the leg. A Baker's cyst (*bc*) filled with anechoic fluid is noted, with irregular thickening of the synovial walls. This nodular appearance (*arrowheads*) is commonly seen in patients with amyloidosis secondary to hemodialysis.

the joints other than the knee or from the tendon sheath (Palmer, 1969; Coakley et al., 1994; Grassi et al., 1995) (see Table 11–4). Those cysts are considered abnormal extensions of an existing synovial membrane.

Bursitis can occur in inflammatory arthropathies. Bursae may be a primary site of involvement of rheumatoid disease rather than an extension of the inflammatory process to adjacent structures of the joint. Rheumatoid arthritis may affect different bursae of the extremities, namely, the medial gastrocnemius-semimembranosus, olecranon, subacromial-subdeltoid, and retrocalcaneal bursae, as well as the small bursae of the hands and feet (Resnick and Niwayama, 1988). Bursitis is a primary disease of the synovium of a bursa; it should be differentiated from the synovial herniation and the abnormal passage of joint fluid that occur in synovial cysts and from the leak of fluid in ganglia (Chhem and Beauregard, 1995a; Chhem et al., 1995b). The thickened synovial membrane in inflammatory bursitis is found in characteristic anatomical locations.

Tendon ruptures and tenosynovitis are common in rheumatoid and lupus patients. The synovial sheaths surrounding tendons are affected by rheumatoid disease in the same manner as the synovia of joints and bursae. Sonography demonstrates the characteristic irregular synovial thickening seen in joints and bursae (Figs. 11–20 through 11–23). Tendon ruptures probably result from chronic synovial inflammation with associated release of proteolytic enzymes. Inflammation within the tendon itself

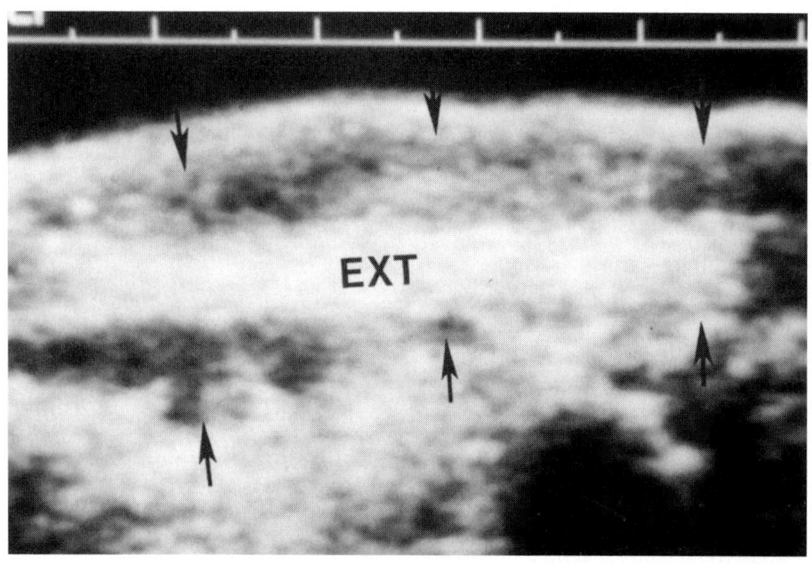

Figure 11–20 ■ Rheumatoid inflammation of the synovial sheath of the extensor pollicis longus tendon: longitudinal sonogram. Swelling over the dorsum of the right hand was noted in this 65-year-old man with rheumatoid arthritis predominating in the hands and feet. The transducer is positioned along the length of the extensor pollicis longus tendon (*EXT*). The synovial sheath (*arrows*) surrounding the tendon is markedly thickened, with an irregular appearance. Compare this appearance with that of the normal tendon sheath in Figure 11–21.

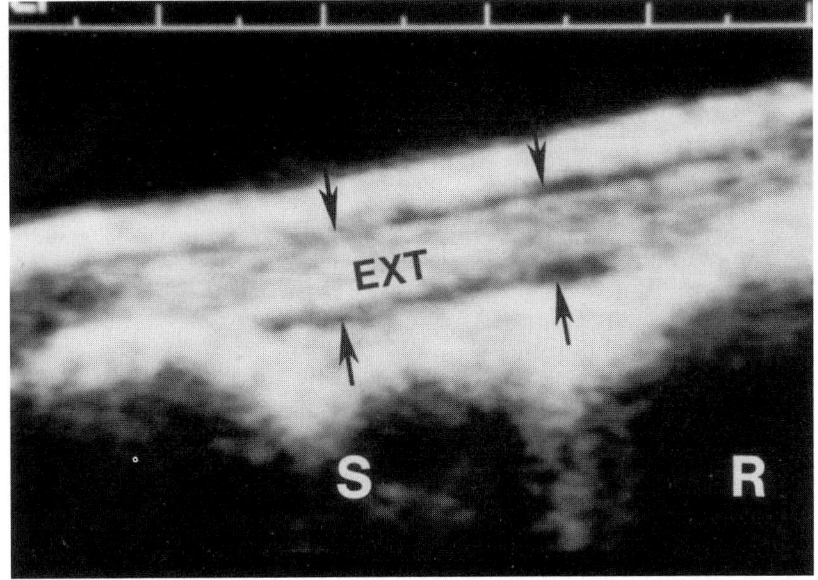

Figure 11-21 ■ Normal tendon sheath of the extensor pollicis longus tendon: longitudinal sonogram. A tendon sheath (*arrows*) of a normal 25-year-old man is shown in this longitudinal sonogram. Normal tendon sheaths are no more than 2 to 3 mm thick. Abbreviations: extensor pollicis longus (*EXT*), scaphoid (*S*), distal radius (*R*).

also causes significant weakening of the tendon. The catabolic effect of corticosteroids on mesenchymal tissues may also contribute to rupture. Supporting structures of the tendons, the vincula tendinum, may be similarly involved. This allows tendon dislocation, tendon entrapment, and further deterioration in function.

Clinical manifestations of tendon rupture and destruction of their supporting structures are most familiar in the hands. Mallet fingers, Boutonnière deformity, swan neck deformity, ulnar drift, and extensor tendon subluxations are all too familiar manifestations of rheumatoid arthritis in the hands (Smith and Kaplan, 1967; Swanson and Swanson, 1973). Ultrasound is extremely valuable in identifying sites of rupture, allowing the surgeon to plan reconstructive procedures more effectively. Longitudinal volar and dorsal scanning is most useful in detecting a tendon tear in the hand (Grassi et al., 1993). Discontinuity of the tendon is the best sign of tendon rupture (Grassi et al., 1995). Retraction of the tendon with widening of the gap between the two extremities can be best evaluated with dynamic scanning during flexion and extension (Fornage, 1989). Although tendon ruptures are most often located in the hands, they are not limited to these

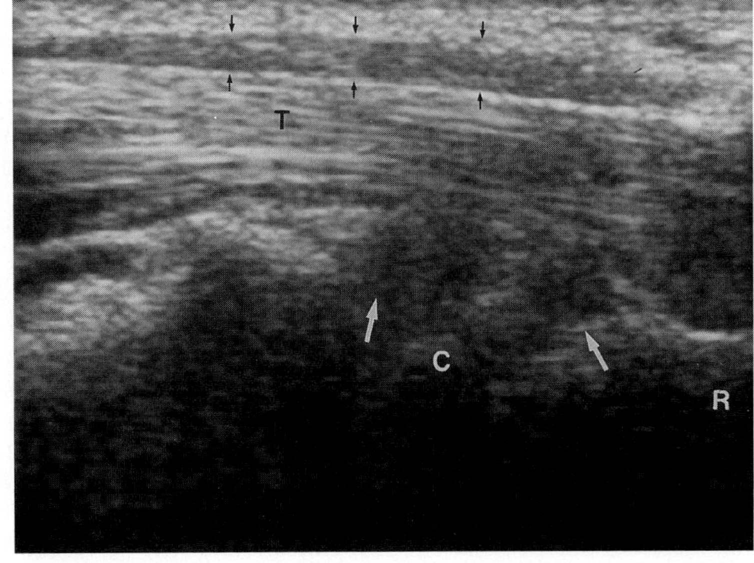

Figure 11-22 ■ Synovitis of the flexor surface of the wrist: longitudinal sonogram. A 52-year-old female with rheumatoid arthritis complains of a recent carpal tunnel syndrome. Longitudinal scan of the wrist showing the carpal tunnel structures longitudinally. The flexor tendons are normal in size and echostructure, and they have regular borders. Bone erosions (*large arrows*) are present at the radiocarpal joint. A combination of hypertrophic joint and tendon synovium at the bottom of the carpal tunnel displaces the median nerve (*arrows*) volarly. Abbreviations: carpal bones (*C*), radius (*R*), flexor tendons (*T*).

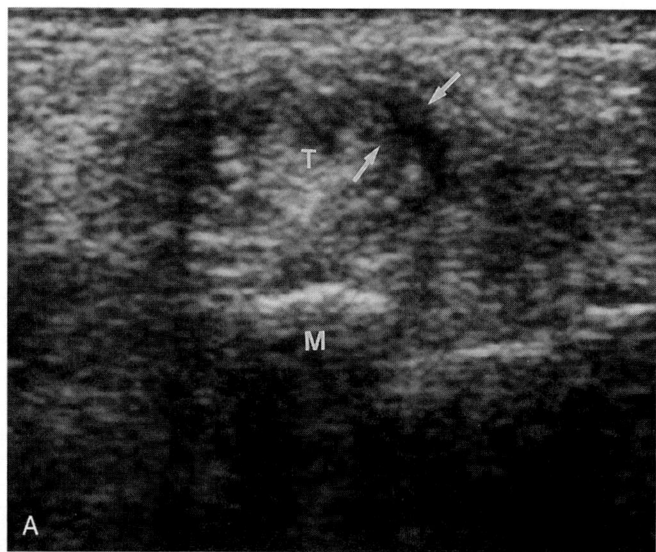

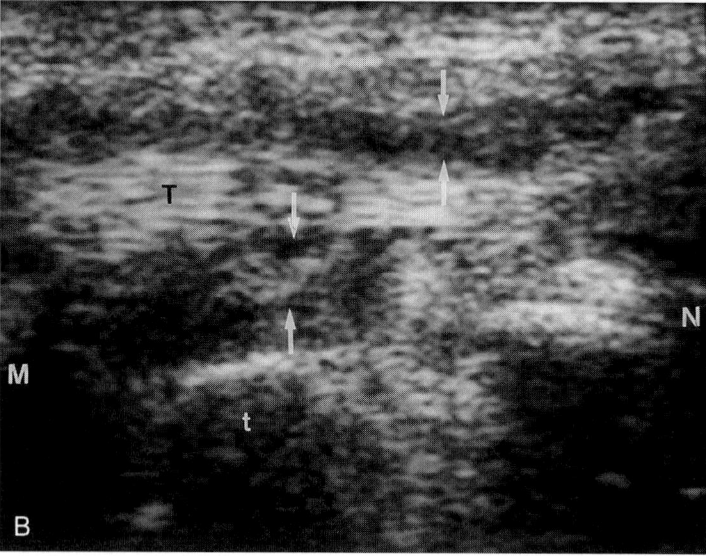

Figure 11–23 ■ **A**, Rheumatoid tenosynovitis of posterior tibialis tendon: ankle sonography. A 45-year-old female patient complains of a painful and swollen ankle, predominantly at the medial aspect of the joint. Transverse scan of the tibialis posterior tendon (*T*) at the level of the medial malleolus (*M*) demonstrates thickening of the tendon sheath (*arrows*), which is distended by synovial pannus. **B**, Rheumatoid tenosynovitis of posterior tibialis tendon: ankle sonography. Same patient as in **A**. Longitudinal scan of the posterior tibialis tendon shows a normal-sized tendon with an irregular border. The echogenicity of the tendon is preserved. The synovial sheath is thickened. Abbreviations: medial malleolus (*M*), talus (*t*), navicular (*N*).

joints. The supraspinatus, patellar, tibialis posterior (Coakley et al., 1994), and Achilles tendons are also frequent sites of rupture (Resnick and Niwayama, 1988; Alaasarela and Alaasarela, 1994). In patients with active rheumatoid disease for more than 5 years, 32% will have rotator cuff tears. These lesions are often bilateral (Fig. 11–24). According to some authors, thinning of the posterior tibialis tendon, rather than a frank rupture, contributes to the flat foot deformity (Coakley et al., 1994).

Rheumatoid nodules (Fig. 11–25) are the most common soft tissue lesion in rheumatoid arthritis. They are detected in 20–25% of patients with rheumatoid disease (Bullough and Vigorita, 1984; Resnick and Niwayama, 1988). They are located around the olecranon, the proximal ulnar, the lateral aspects of the fingers, the gluteal, and the Achilles tendon areas (Resnick and Niwayama, 1988). Rheumatoid nodules may also occur in the synovial membrane, lung, heart, and gastrointestinal tract (Bullough and Vigorita, 1984). Histologically, the nodule consists of a central area of necrotic fibrinoid material surrounded by histiocytes and chronic inflammatory cells (Bullough and Vigorita, 1984).

On ultrasound, rheumatoid nodules appear as a homogeneous hypoechoic mass (see Fig. 8–21). When they develop near a tendon, they are easily distinguished from tenosynovitis, especially when the ultrasound scan is performed in the transverse plane. Tenosynovitis appears as a target pattern, the center being the tendon itself, while a rheumatoid nodule is homogeneous and has no hyperechoic center (Chhem et al., 1993, 1995).

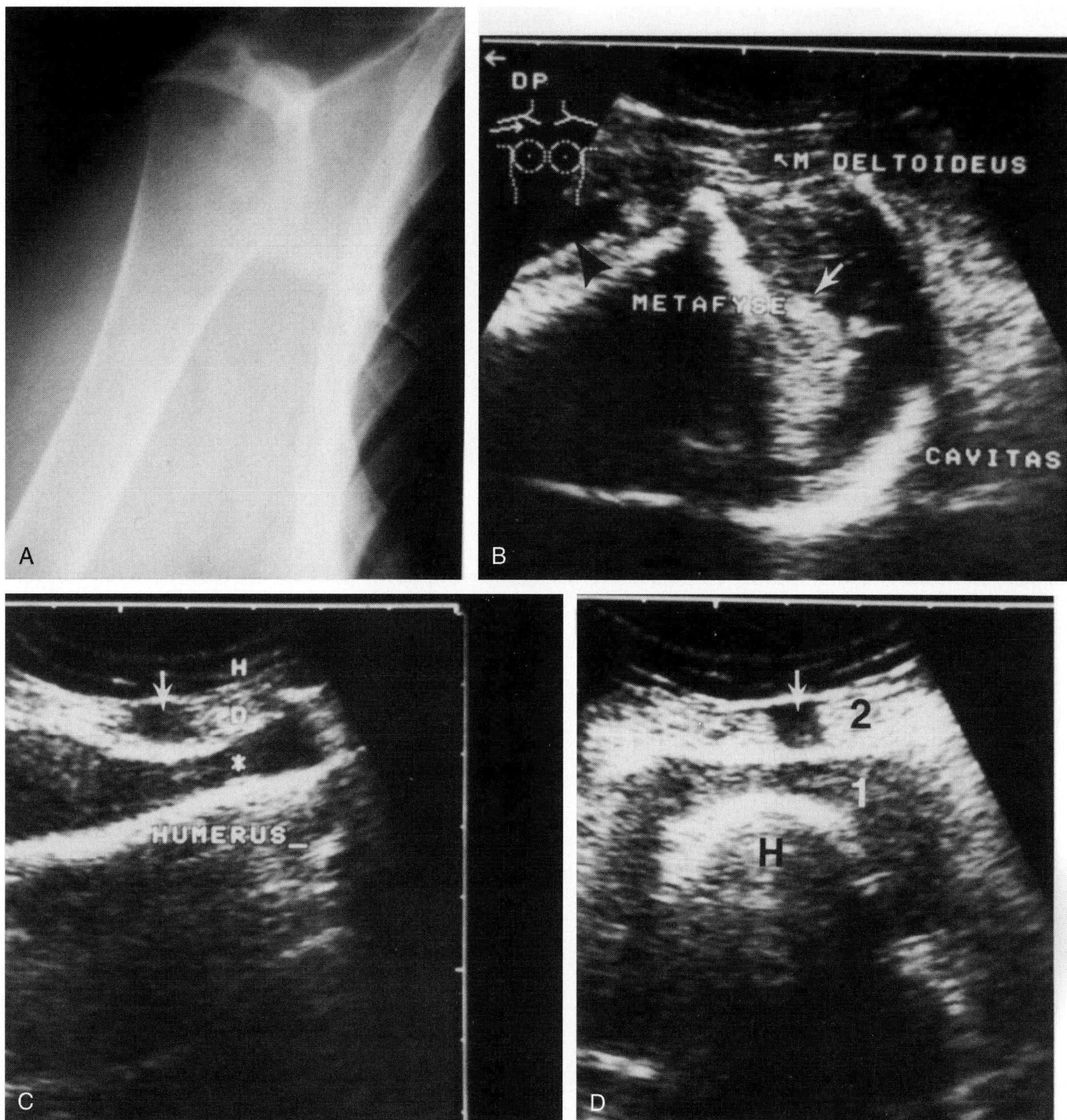

Figure 11–24 ■ **A**, Rheumatoid shoulder: radiograph of the shoulder. The patient is a 50-year-old woman with a 14-year history of rheumatoid arthritis. She presented to the emergency room with acute loss of shoulder function. A radiograph of the shoulder demonstrates a markedly deformed joint. The humeral head projects over the glenoid on both anteroposterior and Grashey views, raising the possibility of dislocation. **B**, Rheumatoid shoulder: sonogram of the shoulder. Same patient as in **A**. The transducer is positioned coronally over the lateral aspect of the shoulder. The humeral head is grossly deformed and almost completely eroded. The glenoid is also eroded, producing a pseudarthrosis within the body of the scapula. The proximal humerus and neoglenoid are in gross anatomical alignment. Deltoid muscle covers the lateral aspect of the joint. The supraspinatus is absent. Pannus (*arrow*) and fluid are identified within the joint. Fluid is also noted in the subdeltoid bursa (*arrowhead*). **C**, Rheumatoid shoulder: coronal sonogram of the shoulder. Same patient as in **A** and **B**. The transducer is moved inferior to that in **B**. A bulbous, fluid-filled subacromial-subdeltoid bursa (*asterisk*) is noted lateral to the humerus. Pressure is applied with the transducer to demonstrate that the bursa is fluid-filled. Rupture of the distal deltoid (*arrow*) is observed as a hypoechoic gap within the muscle. This accounts for the sudden loss of shoulder function. Muscle and tendon ruptures are more commonly seen in patients with rheumatoid arthritis, particularly those treated with corticosteroids. Abbreviations: deltoid (*D*), hypodermis (*H*). **D**, Rheumatoid shoulder: transverse sonogram of the shoulder. Same patient as in **A–C**. The transducer is rotated to demonstrate the cross section of the deltoid rupture (*arrow*). Two layers are identified. The superficial layer is not compressible and corresponds to the substance of the deltoid muscle (*2*). The deeper layer (*1*) was noted to be deformable, corresponding to the fluid-filled bursa. Abbreviation: humerus (*H*).

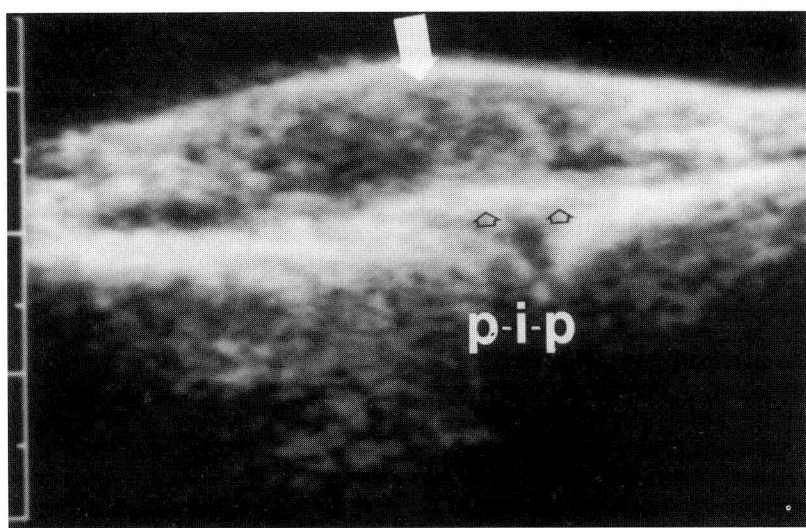

Figure 11–25 ■ Rheumatoid nodule at the finger: coronal sonogram. A 45-year-old woman with rheumatoid arthritis presents with a painful swelling over the proximal interphalangeal joint (*p-i-p*) of the left index finger. The clinical diagnosis of synovial cyst was made. This longitudinal image was obtained over the point of swelling. The joint capsule (*open arrows*) is demonstrated to be intact and nondisplaced. The nodule (*large arrow*) was composed of soft tissue without communication with the joint or tendon sheath. Surgical excision and histological analysis demonstrated this to be a rheumatoid nodule.

Secondary amyloid is a well-known complication in patients with rheumatoid arthritis (Corman et al., 1990). It occurs in 5–25% of patients with chronic rheumatoid arthritis (Resnick and Niwayama, 1988). This form of amyloidosis often affects the kidneys; in contrast, osteoarticular amyloidosis occurs more often in multiple myeloma, in chronic renal failure, and in patients on long-term hemodialysis. Deposition of amyloid substance in the synovium, joint capsule, peritendinous areas, and subcutaneous tissues is responsible for the articular manifestations of amyloidosis. Unfortunately, the clinical symptoms and findings resemble those of rheumatoid arthritis, making the distinction between these two entities very difficult. Ultrasound has been proven to be useful in the diagnosis of amyloid arthritis. Sonographic features of amyloid of the shoulder have been described in patients on chronic renal dialysis. Sonographic features associated with amyloid arthropathy of the shoulder include thickening of the rotator cuff, the synovial sheath of the biceps tendon, and the subacromial-subdeltoid bursa, as well as synovial masses, hyperechoic soft tissue nodules, a striated appearance of the cuff tendons, and intermuscular echogenic pads (Fig. 11–26; see Fig. 14–30) (Kay et al., 1992; Cardinal et al., 1996).

Ultrasound has been used in the evaluation of carpal tunnel syndrome (CTS), the most common symptom of dialysis-related amyloidosis. Sonographic findings were well correlated with the severity of CTS (Ikegaya et al., 1995). The two main sonographic criteria used in that study were the carpal tunnel width and the thickness of the palmar radiocarpal ligament.

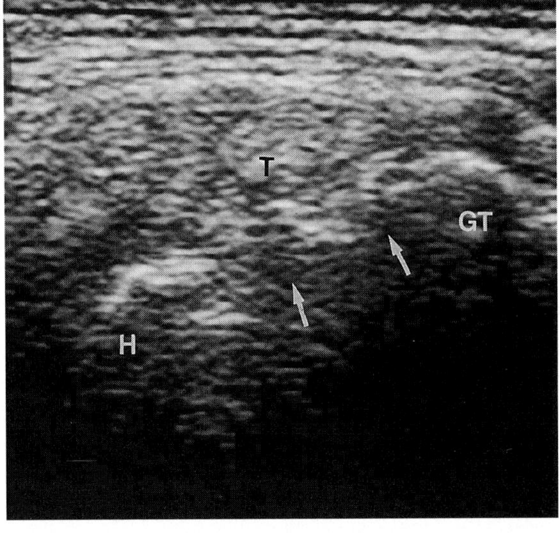

Figure 11–26 ■ Amyloid arthropathy of the shoulder: rotator cuff sonography. Longitudinal scan of the supraspinatus tendon shows marked thickening of the tendon, which became more echogenic and inhomogeneous in appearance. There are several small erosions at the bare area of the humeral head (*arrows*). Abbreviations: tendon (*T*), greater tuberosity (*GT*), humeral head (*H*).

Complications of Intra-articular Steroid Therapy

In addition to increasing the incidence of joint infection, intra-articular steroid injections can lead to destructive changes resembling joint neuropathy. The pathogenesis of this Charcot-like joint destruction is unknown but is probably multifactorial. Osteonecrosis, steroid-induced osteoporosis, intra-articular crystal deposition, steroid-induced insensitivity to pain, and a direct steroid effect on cartilage have all been implicated as causative factors (Chandler et al., 1959; Miller and Restifo, 1966; Gray and Gottlieb, 1983). In these cases, sonography demonstrates large joint effusions containing small fragments of cartilage and bone. These loose bodies are mixed with calcium hydroxyapatite crystals, which are commonly found in steroid-treated joints. Sonographic images will also demonstrate associated ligamentous and tendinous lesions.

Septic arthritis secondary to intra-articular injection of medication is a rare complication. As mentioned earlier, prompt aspiration of the joint is mandatory to exclude sepsis.

References

Adam R, et al: Arthrosonography of the irritable hip in childhood. A review of 1 year's experience. *Br J Radiol* 59:205–208, 1986.

Aisen AM, et al: Sonographic evaluation of the cartilage of the knee. *Radiology* 153:781–784, 1984.

Alaasarela EM, Alaasarela EL: Ultrasound evaluation of the rheumatoid shoulders. *J Rheumatol* 21(9):1642–1648, 1994.

Andronopoulos AP, et al: Baker's cyst in rheumatoid arthritis: An ultrasonographic study with a high resolution technique. *Clin Exp Rheumatol* 13:633–636, 1995.

Beecker HK: *Measurement of Subjective Responses.* New York, Oxford University Press, 1959.

Bullough PG, Vigorita VJ: *Atlas of Orthopaedic Pathology with Clinical and Radiologic Correlations.* Philadelphia, JB Lippincott, 1984, pp 6.14–6.22.

Cardinal E, Beauregard G, Chhem RK: Interventional musculoskeletal ultrasound. *Seminars in Musculoskeletal Radiology* 1(2):311–318, 1997.

Cardinal E, et al: Amyloidosis of the shoulder in patients on chronic hemodialysis: Sonographic features. *AJR* 166:153–156, 1996.

Chandler GN, et al: Charcot's arthropathy following intra-articular hydrocortisone. *Br Med J Clin Res* 1: 952–953, 1959.

Chhem RK, Beauregard G: Synovial diseases. In Fornage B (ed): *Musculoskeletal Ultrasound.* New York, Churchill Livingstone, 1995, pp 43–57.

Chhem RK, et al: Ultrasonography of the ankle and the hindfoot. *JCAR* 44(5):337–341, 1993.

Chhem RK, et al: Detection of musculoskeletal infection using ultrasound. *Appl Radiol* 24(10):29–33, 1995.

Coakley FV, Samanta AK, Finlay DB: Ultrasonography of the tibialis posterior tendon in rheumatoid arthritis. *Br J Rheumatol* 33:273–277, 1994.

Coari G, et al: Intra-articular somatostatin 14 reduces synovial thickness in rheumatoid arthritis: An ultrasonographic study. *Int J Clin Pharm Res* 15(1):27–32, 1995.

Cooperberg PL, et al: Gray scale ultrasound in the evaluation of rheumatoid arthritis of the knee. *Radiology* 126:759–763, 1978.

Corman LC, et al: *Rheumatology for the House Officer.* Baltimore, Williams & Wilkins, 1990, p 180.

DeSilva M, et al: Assessment of inflammation in the rheumatoid knee joint: Correlation between clinical, radioisotopic, and thermographic methods. *Ann Rheum Dis* 45:227, 1986.

Fedrizzi MS, et al: Ultrasonography in the early diagnosis of hip joint involvement in juvenile rheumatoid arthritis. *J Rheumatol* 24:1820–1825, 1997.

Firestein G: Rheumatoid synovitis and pannus. In Klippel JH, Dieppe PA (eds): *Rheumatology.* St Louis, Mosby, 1994, pp 12.1–12.4.

Fornage DB: Soft tissue changes in the hand in rheumatoid arthritis: Evaluation with ultrasound. *Radiology* 173:735–737, 1989.

Gielen JL, et al: Growing bone cysts in long-term hemodialysis. *Skeletal Radiol* 19:43–49, 1990.

Goldenberg DL: Infectious arthritis complicating rheumatoid arthritis and other chronic rheumatic disorders. *Arthritis Rheum* 32(4):496–502, 1989.

Grassi W, et al: Ultrasound examination of metacarpophalangeal joints in rheumatoid arthritis. *Scand J Rheumatol* 22:243–247, 1993.

Grassi W, et al: Finger tendon involvement in rheumatoid arthritis. *Arthritis Rheum* 38(6):786–794, 1995.

Gray RG, Gottlieb NL: Intra-articular corticosteroids. An updated assessment. *Clin Orthop* 177:235, 1983.

Hammer M, Mielke H, Wagener P: Sonography and NMR imaging in rheumatoid gonarthritis. *Scand J Rheumatol* 15:157, 1986.

Iagnocco A, Coari G, Zoppini A: Sonographic evaluation of femoral condylar cartilage in osteoarthritis and rheumatoid arthritis. *Scand J Rheumatol* 21:201–203, 1992.

Ikegaya NH, et al: Ultrasonographic evaluation of the carpal tunnel syndrome in hemodialysis patients. *Clin Nephrol* 44(4):231–237, 1995.

Kay J, et al: Utility of high resolution ultrasound in the diagnosis of dialyzed amyloidosis. *Arthritis Rheum* 35: 926–932, 1992.

Kelley W, et al: *Textbook of Rheumatology*, ed 5, vol 1. Philadelphia, WB Saunders Co, 1997, pp 893–933.

Lehtinen A, et al: Painful ankle region in rheumatoid arthritis: Analysis of soft-tissue change with ultrasonography and MR imaging. *Acta Radiol* 37: 572–577, 1996.

Lund PJ, et al: Ultrasonographic imaging of the hand and wrist in rheumatoid arthritis. *Skeletal Radiol* 24: 591–596, 1995.

Marchal GJ, et al: Ultrasonography in transient synovitis of the hip in children. *Radiology* 162:825–828, 1987.

McGahan JP: *Controversies in Ultrasound.* New York, Churchill-Livingstone, 1987.

Miller WT, Restifo RA: Steroid arthropathy. *Radiology* 86: 652, 1966.

Moore CP, Sarti DA, Lovie SS: Ultrasonographic demonstration of popliteal cysts in rheumatoid arthritis: A noninvasive technique. *Arthritis Rheum* 18:557–580, 1975.

Palmer DG: Synovial cysts in rheumatoid disease. *Ann Intern Med* 70(1):61–68, 1969.

Peck J: Ultrasound of the painful hip in children. *Br J Radiol* 50:293–294, 1986.

Resnick D, Niwayama G: *Diagnosis of Bone and Joint Disorders.* Philadelphia, WB Saunders Co, 1988.

Richardson ML, et al: Ultrasonography of the knee. *Radiol Clin North Am* 26:63–75, 1988.

Ropes MW, et al: Revision of the diagnostic criteria of rheumatoid arthritis. *Ann Rheum Dis* 18:49, 1959.

Ruhoy MK, Tucker L, McCauley RGK: Hypertrophic bursopathy of the subacromial-subdeltoid bursa in juvenile rheumatoid arthritis: Sonographic appearance. *Pediatr Radiol* 26:353–355, 1996.

Sarazin L, et al: Correlative imaging and pattern approach in ultrasonography of bone lesion: A pictorial essay. *Can Assoc Radiol J* 47:423–430, 1996.

Smith RJ, Kaplan EB: Rheumatoid deformities at the metacarpophalangeal joints of the fingers. *J Bone Joint Surg (Am)* 49:31, 1967.

Sureda D, et al: Juvenile rheumatoid arthritis of the knee: Evaluation with US. *Radiology* 190;403–406, 1994.

Swanson AB, Swanson GG: Pathogenesis and pathomechanics of rheumatoid deformities in the hand and wrist. *Orthop Clin North Am* 4:1039, 1973.

van Holsbeeck M, et al: Staging and follow-up of rheumatoid arthritis of the knee. Comparison of sonography, thermography, and clinical assessment. *J Ultrasound Med* 7:561–566, 1988.

van Holsbeeck M, Strouse P: Sonography of the shoulder: Evaluation of the subacromial-subdeltoid bursa. *AJR* 160:561–564, 1993.

Worth WD, et al: Stellenwert der Arthrosonographie in die Beurteilung der Exsudativen und Proliferativen Synovialitis. *Z Rheumatol* 45:263, 1986.

Chapter 12
Evaluation of Foreign Bodies

One of the most frequent requests made of musculoskeletal radiologists in the emergency setting is the identification and localization of foreign bodies. In an alert, cooperative adult, this task is made easier. The patient can indicate the likelihood of the presence of a foreign body, the material involved, and the general location. However, many of these patients are not alert, cooperative adults. Barefoot children possess a magnetic attraction to foreign bodies. All inquiries by the physician or parent about the accident are answered with screaming and tears. Equally challenging is the search for foreign bodies in patients involved in motor vehicle accidents. Often they are under the influence of alcohol, received intravenous (IV) analgesics, lost consciousness during the accident, or simply "hurt all over." Frequently, foreign bodies in these patients go unrecognized, even after reassessment following emergency therapy. Unrecognized foreign bodies will result in chronic draining wounds, abscesses, and persistent pain. Surrounding infection can lead to devitalization of large amounts of tissue, joint destruction, and even limb loss (Gooding et al., 1987). Other complications seen less frequently are migration of foreign bodies, metallic synovitis, and erosion into vessels with concomitant embolization.

In the evaluation for foreign bodies, radiographs alone are not adequate (Anderson et al., 1982; Gooding et al., 1987). A retrospective study of foreign bodies showed that the average time between injury and detection was 7 months. Thirty-eight percent of retained foreign bodies were overlooked on initial examination (Anderson et al., 1982). In fact, an overlooked foreign body is the second most common reason that malpractice lawsuits are filed against emergency room physicians (Schlager et al., 1991). Radiolucent foreign bodies like wood and plant thorns remain undetected most frequently (Russell et al., 1991; Flom and Ellis, 1992).

Nonradiopaque foreign bodies and patients with orthopedic implants pose the greatest challenge. These are the cases in which ultrasound is the most beneficial modality. In our experience, sonography has increased the rate of success in identifying and localizing foreign bodies by approximately 20%. Several investigators have confirmed the efficacy of ultrasound in detecting foreign bodies and their associated complications. An overall sensitivity of 95% has been cited for detection of foreign bodies using ultrasound (Crawford and Matheson, 1989). A study we conducted showed that wooden fragments embedded in cadaver feet measuring 2.5 × 1.0 mm were detected with a sensitivity of 86.7% and a specificity of 96.7%, and 5.0 × 1.0 mm fragments were detected with a sensitivity of 93.3% and a specificity of 96.7%. Three independent observers participated in this study. All examiners were unaware that they had to detect 20 foreign bodies and that 10 sham incisions had been made. The interobserver agreement was 0.77 using the *k*-statistic (Jacobson et al., 1998).

Examination Technique

A 5- or 7.5-MHz linear array transducer is recommended for these examinations due to their utility in imaging both superficial and deep foreign bodies. Examination of the superficial subcutaneous tissues requires a standoff pad. If a gel pad is unavailable or cannot be used because of a sterile field, a bag of IV fluid with the air removed will be adequate. This will eliminate near-field artifacts and help to bring the object into the optimal focal zone of the transducer. The final piece of equipment needed for the exam is an indelible marking pen (Fig. 12–1). It is extremely embarrassing when the mark indicating the location of the elusive foreign body is washed

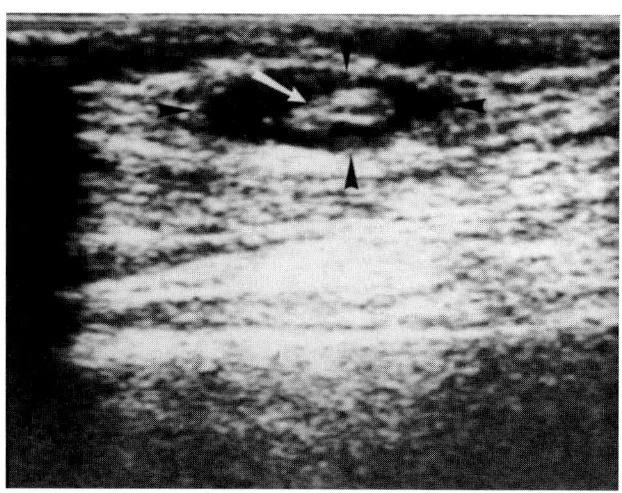

Figure 12–1 ■ Instrument breakage during arthroscopy: longitudinal sonogram of the knee. During therapeutic arthroscopy, the end of a curette was broken off in the subcutaneous tissues. Three radiographic examinations failed to demonstrate the fragment. This longitudinal image was obtained immediately superior to the suprapatellar bursa over the point of maximal tenderness. A hyperechoic foreign body (*white arrow*) is seen within the subcutaneous tissues surrounded by fluid (*black arrowheads*). The surrounding subcutaneous fat is increased in echogenicity in addition to the increased through-transmission deep to the fluid collection. No increase in intra-articular fluid was observed, thus ruling out joint infection. The skin was marked, and an instrument fragment less than 5 mm in the greatest dimension was surgically removed.

away by the surgeon while preparing the skin with an antiseptic solution. In fact, some surgeons prefer a tattoo on the skin (Graf and Schuler, 1988).

Once the foreign body is identified, its relationship to adjacent structures must be carefully documented. Defining its position relative to neighboring anatomical landmarks will make the surgeon's job much easier. In addition, the location of nearby vessels, nerves, and synovial membrane must be established, allowing the surgeon to select the most desirable approach (Fig. 12–2). These structures have a characteristic sonographic appearance (Weill,

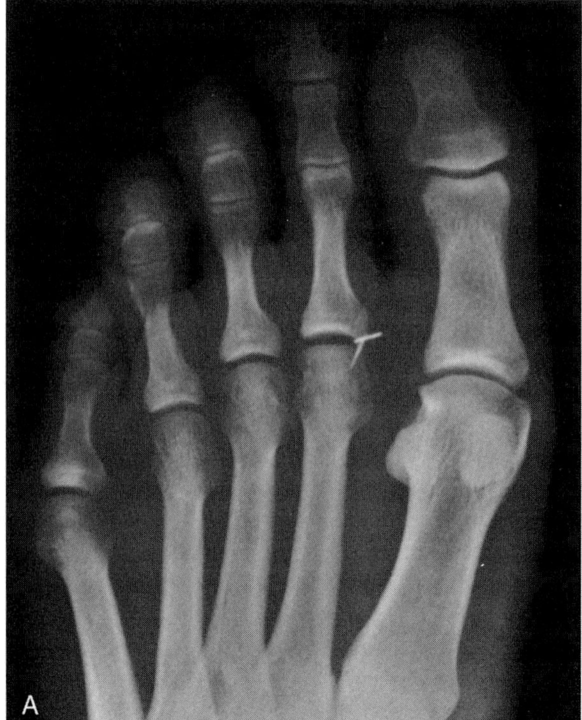

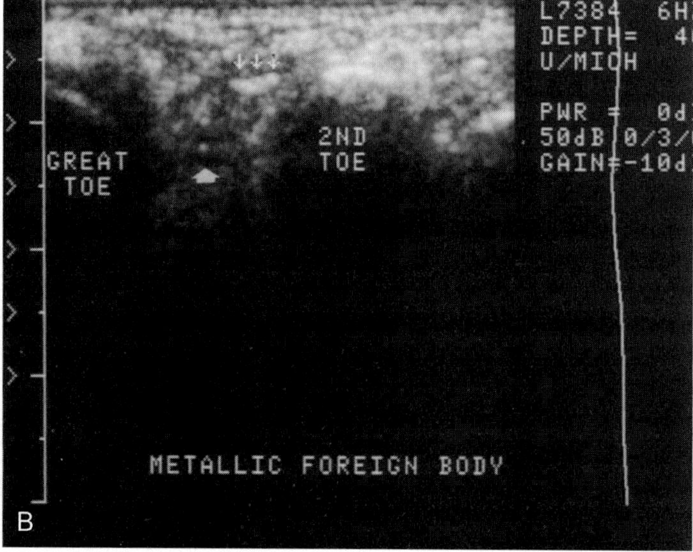

Figure 12–2 ■ **A**, Localization of a needle fragment in the foot: anteroposterior radiograph. This 28-year-old man stepped on a sewing needle lost in the carpet. The tip of the needle broke off during removal. The needle fragment is projected over the second metatarsophalangeal joint. Its relationship to the joint, vessels, and nerves is not well demonstrated on conventional radiographs. **B**, Localization of the needle fragment in the foot: transverse sonogram. A needle fragment slightly less than 1 cm long (*arrows*) is visualized as a hyperechoic line with minimal reverberation artifact. It was clearly demonstrated not to penetrate the joint capsule. The digital nerve and artery (*arrow*) are seen approximately 2 cm deep and slightly medial to the fragment. Again, the skin was marked, and surgical removal was successful.

1978; Fornage, 1988; van Holsbeeck et al., 1988). The distance separating the foreign body and these vital structures can be easily measured using the postprocessing features available on state-of-the-art ultrasound equipment. Occasionally, foreign bodies can penetrate tendons, fascia, or muscle. In these cases, real-time sonography can provide a dynamic study, which better defines the structures involved and the location of the foreign body through a range of motion (Fornage and Schernberg, 1986).

Ultrasound Versus Radiography

The standard imaging procedure used in the search for foreign bodies over the past 50 years has been conventional radiographs obtained in two projections. In the majority of cases, using this method, the diagnosis of the presence or absence of a foreign body was correct. In one large series of surgically removed foreign bodies, radiographs correctly identified metallic fragments in 100% of cases and glass in 96% of cases, but wood was correctly identified in only 15% of cases. These data would be considered quite good except for the fact that the most common foreign bodies in order of frequency are wood, glass, and metal fragments (Anderson et al., 1982). Nonradiopaque foreign bodies, such as wood, plastic, and certain types of glass, are better detected with xeroradiography or mammographic technique than with conventional radiographs (Gooding et al., 1987; Resnick and Niwayama, 1988). However, the availability of xeroradiography is rapidly decreasing, and mammographic technique can be used on only thin extremities. Conventional radiography remains the mainstay of foreign body imaging, primarily because of its wide availability, low cost, and ease of examination (Anderson et al., 1982; Fornage and Schernberg, 1986; Little et al., 1986; Gooding et al., 1987).

MRI can depict foreign bodies; the technique has been found helpful in detecting complications like abscess formation and intra-articular penetration (Donaldson, 1991; Russell et al., 1991). It may be difficult to distinguish low-signal-intensity foreign bodies from tendons, scar tissue, and calcifications (Donaldson, 1991). In a comparison study, the resolution of this technique was inferior to that of ultrasound (Mizel et al., 1994). Lack of availability and high cost further limit the usefulness of this modality. CT has sensitivity 5 to 15 times greater than that of plain radiography, but it is also less sensitive than ultrasound (Mizel et al., 1994). Additionally, the expense, use of radiation, and limited availability make CT less than optimal in the clinical detection of foreign bodies.

Ophthalmologists were the first to apply ultrasound to the detection of foreign bodies. It was found to be extremely valuable in identification and localization of minute fragments in the eye (Hassani and Bard, 1978). The absence of ionizing radiation increased the attractiveness of this modality. Gynecologists started to use ultrasound to confirm the presence and location of intrauterine devices (Cochrane, 1985). This demonstrated that depth within the body did not hamper detection of foreign bodies with ultrasound.

Ultrasound offers far more than radiography in the detection and localization of foreign bodies. Since the ability to detect an object on sonographic images is primarily a function of the difference between the acoustic impedance of the object and the surrounding tissue, objects that are radiolucent or radiopaque can be imaged quite easily. An in vivo study by Little et al. (1986) demonstrated wood fragments (Fig. 12–3) to be visualized best, followed in order by glass, plastic, and metal. Glass and metal, though intrinsically more reflective than other materials, produce considerable reverberation artifact. Most foreign bodies are associated with an acoustic shadow or a comet tail artifact (Fig. 12–4). The only exception is plant thorns, possibly because of differences in acoustic impedance relative to the surrounding soft tissues (Fig. 12–5) (Gilbert et al., 1990; Howden, 1994; Failla et al., 1995). Comet tail artifact can help to identify the foreign body, but it makes size measurement extremely difficult. This artifact can be both an aid to diagnosis and a hindrance to precise localization. Figures 12–6 through 12–11 demonstrate the sonographic appearance of various materials. Note that the diameters of the metal needles in Figure 12–9 appear to be the same, regardless of their actual size. Compare this with the sonographic appearance of the plastic IV catheters (Fig. 12–11). In vivo studies have shown sonography to be accurate in the identification and localization of foreign bodies with diameters as small as 0.5 mm (Failla et al., 1995). The smallest-diameter needle shown in Figure 12–9 is 0.3 mm, and it is clearly visualized.

Secondary signs associated with foreign bodies can aid in making the diagnosis. Surrounding hematoma or, in chronic cases, purulent material can help to outline a foreign body by providing a hypoechoic halo (see Fig. 12–3). Also, in the acute setting, air may be trapped along the path of insertion of the foreign body. This provides a trail of echogenic foci with shadowing that can be followed to the foreign body.

Text continued on page 399

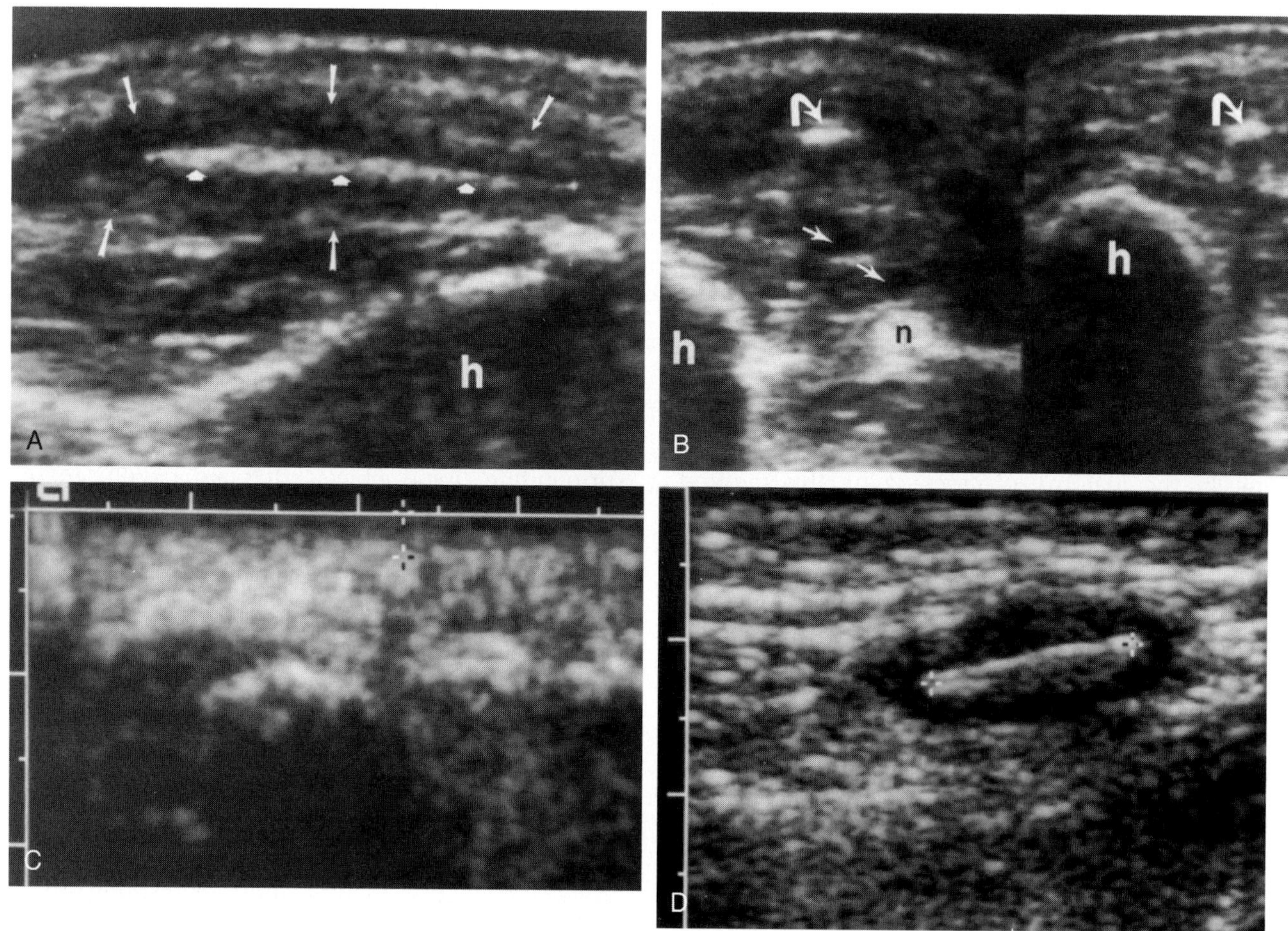

Figure 12-3 ■ **A**, Wood splinter in the elbow: longitudinal sonogram. This 35-year-old wood worker punctured the skin with a wood splinter 10 days ago. He presents with swelling and erythema over the anteromedial aspect of the elbow. The splinter (*small arrows*) is identified as a hyperechoic line surrounded by a hypoechoic fluid collection (*large arrows*). Inflammatory collections are frequently seen around wooden foreign bodies. Initially, the wood fragment is hyperechoic. As the inflammatory reaction evolves, the wood becomes progressively less echogenic. Eventually, the fragment will decompose completely in the inflammatory collection. Abbreviation: distal humerus (*h*). **B**, Wood splinter in the elbow: transverse sonogram. Same patient as in **A**. A transverse image through the middle portion of the wood splinter (*curved arrow*) is shown on the left; the distal portion is on the right. Much more purulent material is seen surrounding the middle segment of the splinter. Its relationship to the brachial vessels (*arrows*) and median nerve (*n*) is clearly demonstrated. Abbreviation: humerus (*h*). **C**, Toothpick within the heel pad of the foot: transverse sonogram. This 5-year-old boy receiving chemotherapy for leukemia stepped on a toothpick while playing yesterday. Two prior attempts at surgical localization and removal were unsuccessful. Radiographs were not helpful. Ultrasound demonstrated the toothpick fragment 0.5 cm below the skin (*t*). A mark was placed on the skin to indicate the location and orientation of the fragment. Subsequent surgical removal was simple. **D**, Wood splinter at the knee: longitudinal sonogram. The patient is a 30-year-old female who presented with a history of chronic pain over the medial aspect of the right knee, which has been present for years. The intensity of the discomfort has varied over the years but has increased over the past several months. This linear echogenic structure (+) surrounded by hypoechoic soft tissue was identified within the subcutaneous tissues of the medial right knee. Minimal shadowing is observed deep to the foreign body. Upon further questioning, the patient recalled an accident 15 years earlier in which a piece of wood was embedded beneath the skin but had been removed by her father. At surgery, a wooden foreign body surrounded by granulation tissue was removed. These wooden fragments usually decompose in an intense inflammatory reaction over a period of days or weeks. This is the most unusual presentation of a wooden foreign body we have encountered.

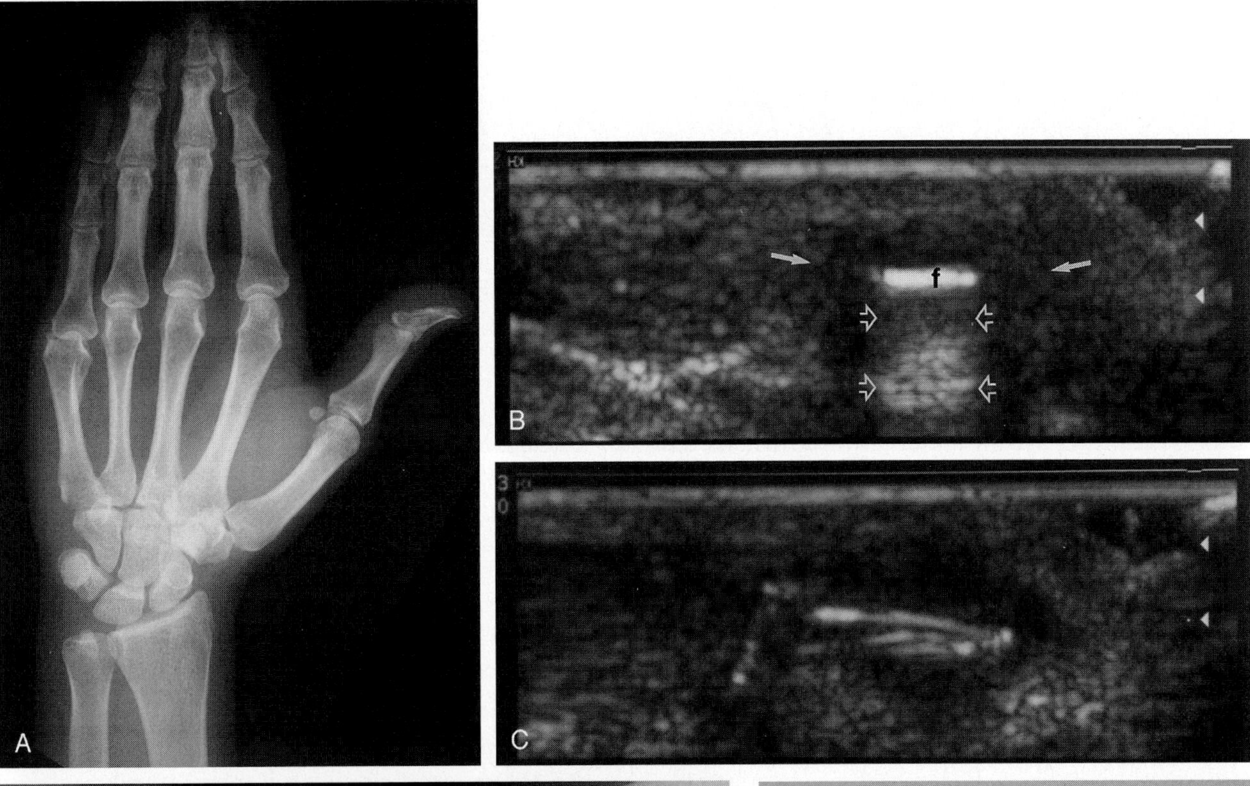

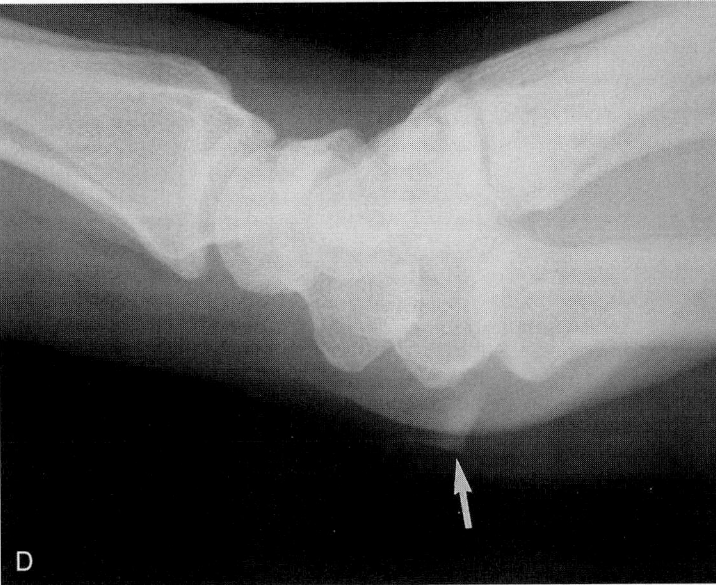

Figure 12–4 ■ **A**, Glass fragment in the thumb: anteroposterior radiograph of the hand. A 44-year-old woman, was involved in an accident 1 year ago. She does not remember the details of the accident, but she has experienced pain in her thumb since that time. Several radiographs of the hand were interpreted as negative, including the current radiograph obtained prior to the ultrasound examination. **B**, Glass fragment in the thumb: transverse ultrasound over the proximal thenar. Same patient as in **A**. A hyperechoic foreign body (*f*) stands out against a hypo-echoic background of granulation tissue (*arrows*). The deep aspect of the lesion is obscured by comet tail artifact, which is characteristic of glass foreign bodies (*open arrows*). **C**, Glass fragment in the thumb: longitudinal ultrasound over the proximal thenar. Same patient as in **A**. With the transducer aligned along the foreign body, one notices the triangular shape of the glass fragment. Comet tail artifact interferes slightly with the assessment of the contour of the fragment, but it is less bothersome in this orientation. **D**, Glass fragment in the thumb: oblique radiograph of the thenar. Same patient as in **A**. It was hard to believe that a foreign body the size of the one found on ultrasound examination could elude detection on a radiographic study. Coned-down views of the region of interest were obtained in an attempt to project the known foreign body away from the adjacent carpal bones. A large, opaque foreign body (*arrow*) is demonstrated at the volar aspect of the trapezoid on this oblique radiographic projection.

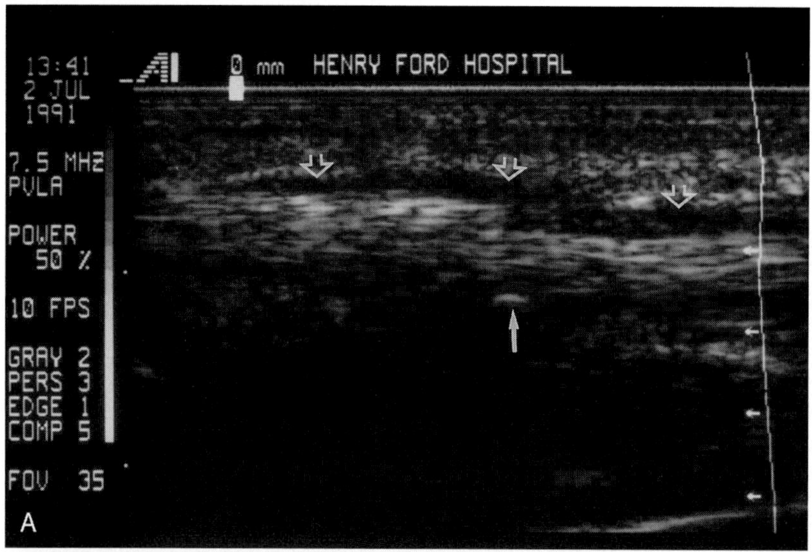

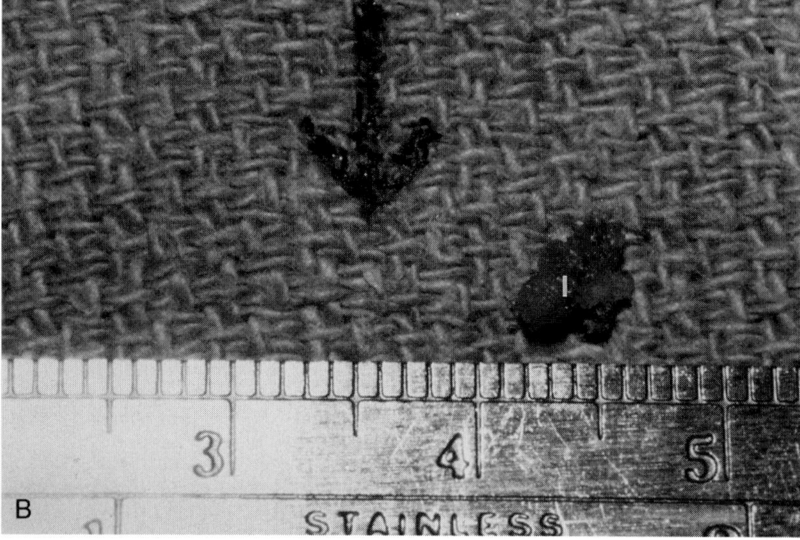

Figure 12–5 ■ **A**, Thorn-induced inflammation: longitudinal ultrasound. The middle finger of this patient has been swollen for 3 months. A puncture of the finger by a plant thorn was suspected to have been the cause of the inflammation. This ultrasound study demonstrates a tiny fragment (*arrow*) within the flexor tendon sheath at the dorsal aspect of the tendons. The location makes both clinical palpation and surgical exploration difficult. Synovial inflammation of the tendon sheath (*open arrows*) is seen as a hypoechoic layer around the tendon. **B**, Thorn-induced inflammation: specimen photograph. This thorn (*below the arrow*), which was localized with ultrasound, required a magnifying glass for removal. The inflammatory tissue (*I*) removed at surgery is much larger than the minute foreign body. Surgical removal had been previously attempted three times.

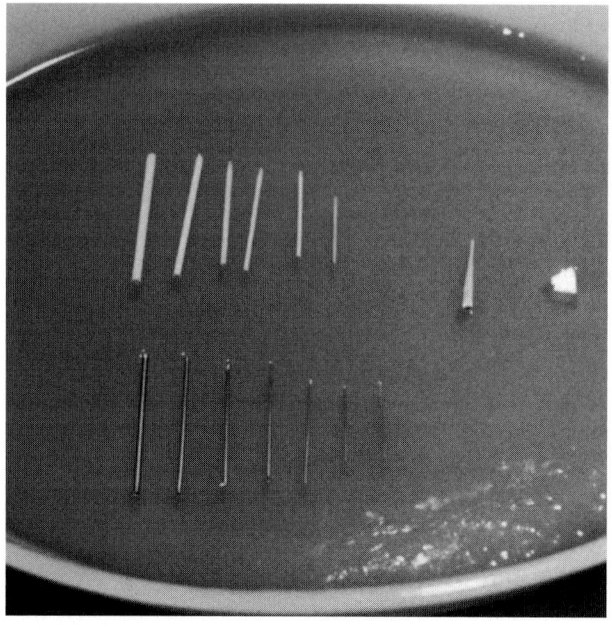

Figure 12–6 ■ Foreign body phantom. Metal needles and plastic catheters ranging in size from 14 to 30 gauge were embedded within gelatin in a glass dish. A fragment of toothpick and a small glass fragment were also included in the phantom. The ultrasound studies of the foreign bodies in this phantom are displayed in Figures 17–7 through 17–11.

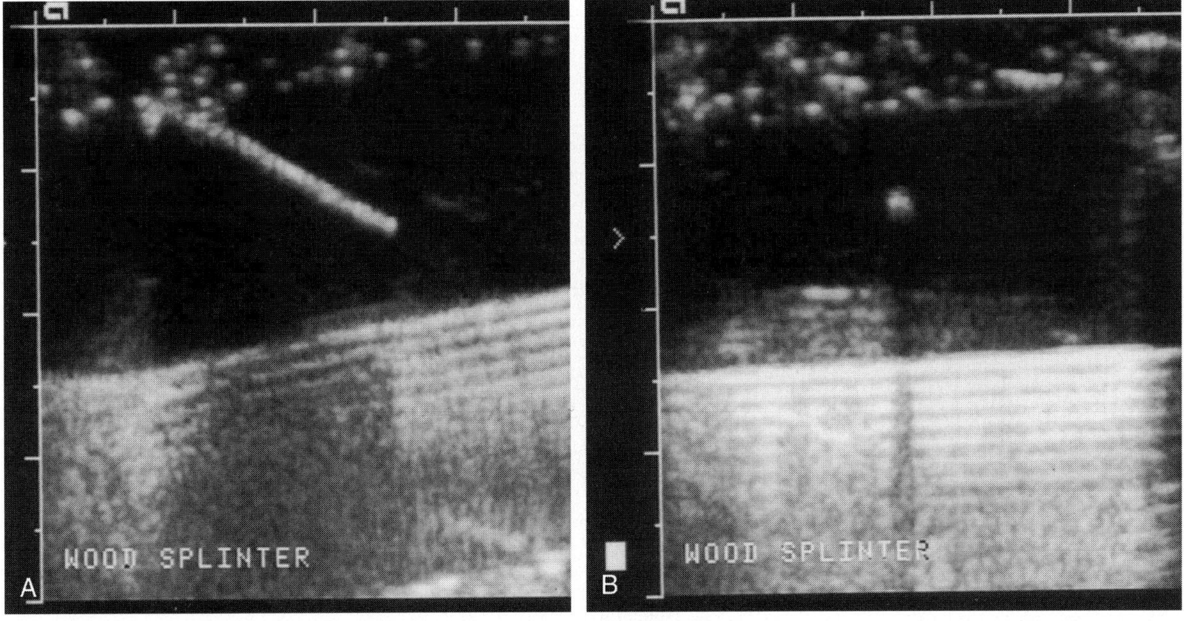

Figure 12–7 ■ Wooden splinter: longitudinal (**A**) and transverse (**B**) sonograms. The appearance of this wooden fragment is similar to that of the in vivo fragments in Figure 12–3. It appears hyperechoic without reverberation artifact. Incomplete acoustic shadowing is noted deep to this in vitro specimen. As a wooden fragment decomposes within an inflammatory collection, acoustic shadowing will no longer be observed.

Wooden fragments are hyperechoic, with acoustic shadowing deep to the object in an acute setting. This makes identification and localization quite simple. However, unlike many other types of foreign bodies, wood fragments tend to decompose quite rapidly due to the surrounding inflammatory reaction. Over the course of several days, the wooden fragment will become progressively less echogenic and finally disappear within the inflammatory collection (Graf and Schuler, 1988). These disappearing foreign bodies have misled clinicians into searching for sources of septic emboli when an

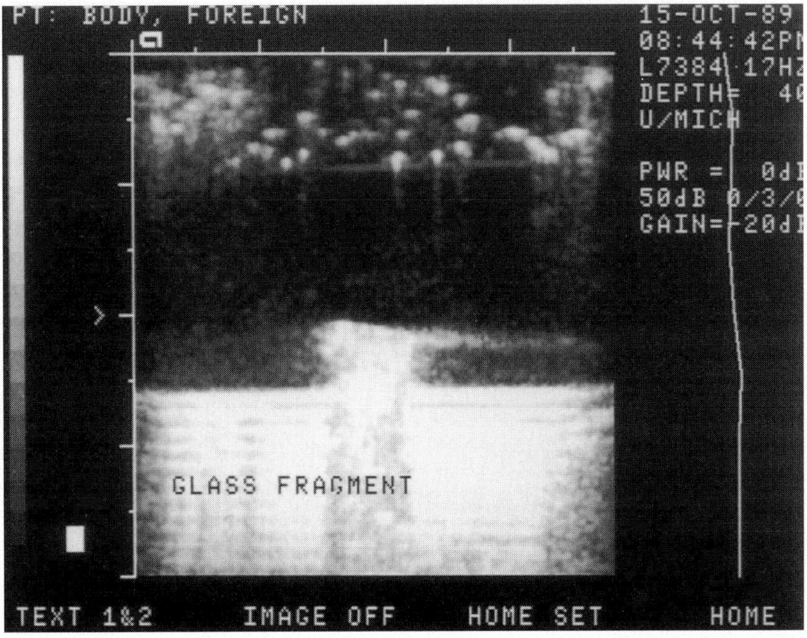

Figure 12–8 ■ Glass fragment. A striking comet tail artifact is seen deep to this glass fragment. This is often helpful in identifying glass fragments within the soft tissues. In this example, tiny echogenic foci within a layer immediately beneath the transducer face are gas bubbles in the coupling gel.

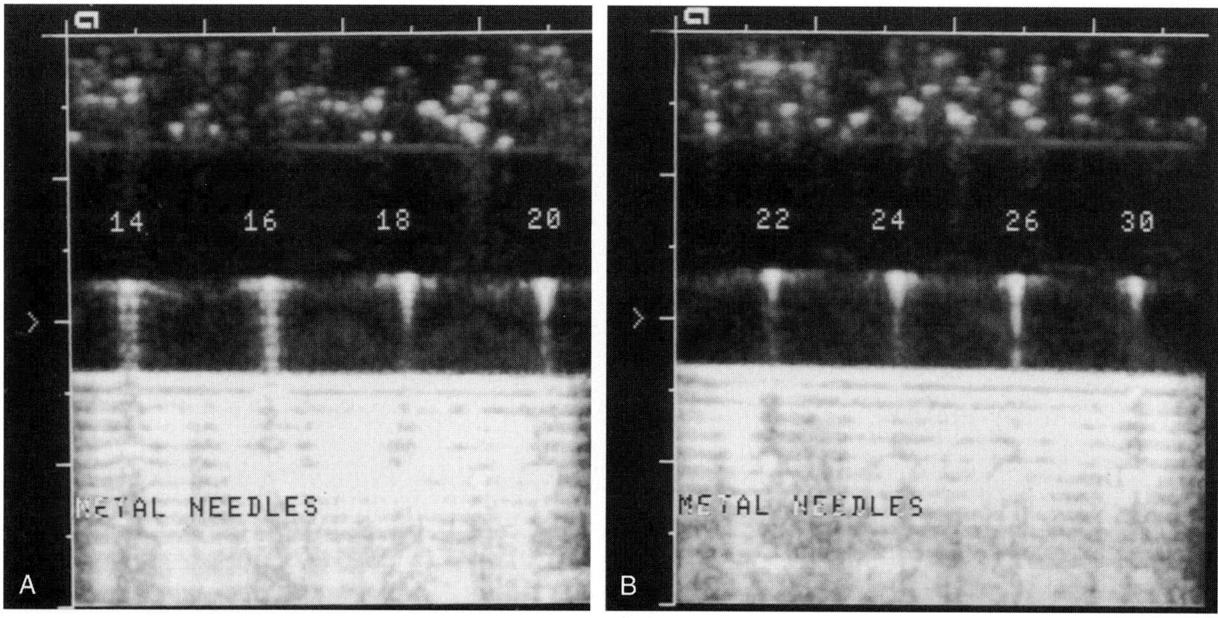

Figure 12–9 ■ **A** and **B**, Series of metal needles: transverse sonogram. These transverse images demonstrate the appearance of metallic foreign bodies of varying diameters. The 14-gauge needle has an outer diameter of 2.1 mm, and the 30-gauge needle is 0.3 mm in diameter. Note that reverberation artifact makes the 30-gauge needle appear to have the same diameter as the 14-gauge needle. This aids in the detection of small metallic foreign bodies, but realistic measurement of the dimensions of the foreign body is impossible. Metallic foreign bodies produce a comet tail artifact similar to that of glass but less striking.

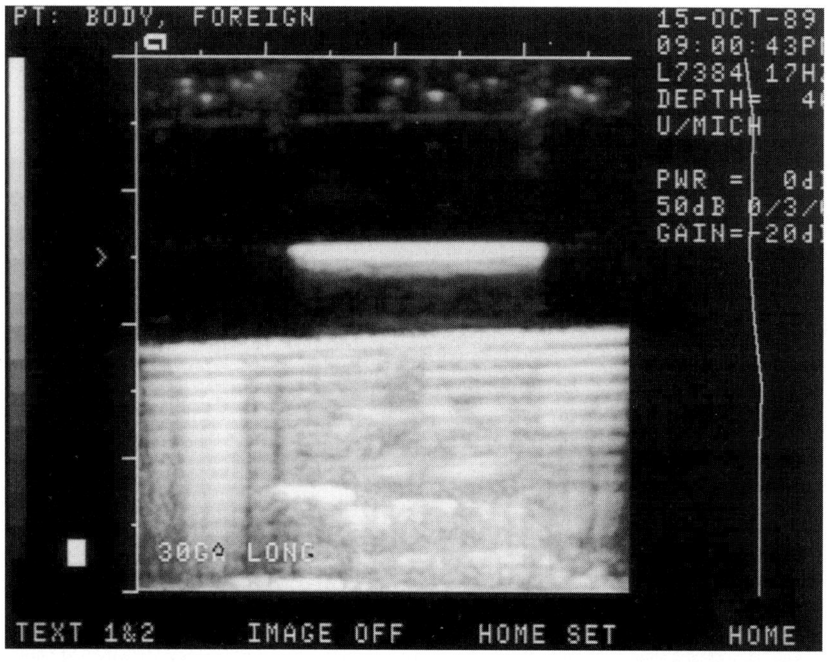

Figure 12–10 ■ A 30-gauge metal needle: longitudinal sonogram. The comet tail artifact is not as noticeable on longitudinal images due to the beam width. This appearance is also noted in vivo, as demonstrated in Figures 12–1 and 12–2B.

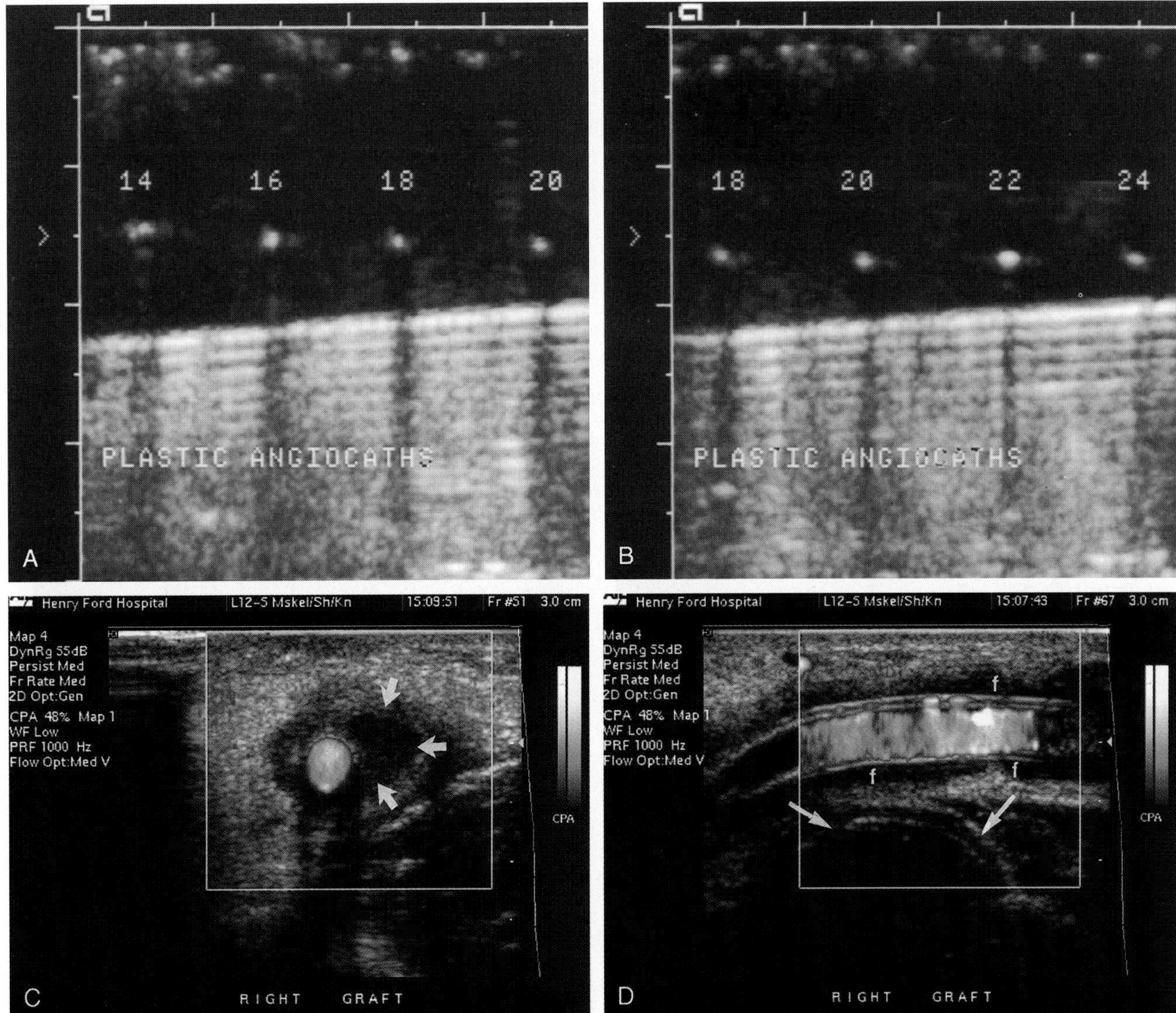

Figure 12–11 ■ **A** and **B**, Series of plastic catheters: transverse sonograms. This series of plastic catheters ranges in size from 14 to 24 gauge. Less reverberation artifact is seen with plastic catheters, allowing relative comparison of size. Acoustic shadowing is present deep to the plastic catheters, but no comet tail is seen. Compare this with the appearance of the metal needles shown in Figure 12–9. **C**, Infected vascular graft: transverse ultrasound. A dialysis patient develops acute elbow and forearm swelling. Because of fever, an ultrasound study is requested. The clinician wants to distinguish articular from periarticular inflammation. The transverse ultrasound scan of the elbow performed with a 12-MHz transducer shows a synthetic vascular graft surrounded by a hypoechoic collection (*arrows*). The power Doppler signal of normal blood flow fills the graft. The color does not spill over, as it does with regular color Doppler sonography. Refractile shadowing is noted deep to the blood vessel prosthesis. **D**, Infected vascular graft: longitudinal ultrasound. Same patient as in **C**. The transducer's orientation was changed in the long axis of the upper arm and along the vessel. Fluid (*f*) surrounds the synthetic vessel wall. The elbow joint is not infected; the normal cartilage and joint capsule (*arrows*) appear deep to the graft. Ultrasound depicts the polyester of the graft with great accuracy. Visualization of polyester and plastic is not plagued by the same artifacts as the visualization of metal and glass. In this case, the arterial wall is shown well enough to allow aspiration of the fluid under ultrasound guidance. *Staphylococcus epidermidis* grew from the abscess that surrounded the graft.

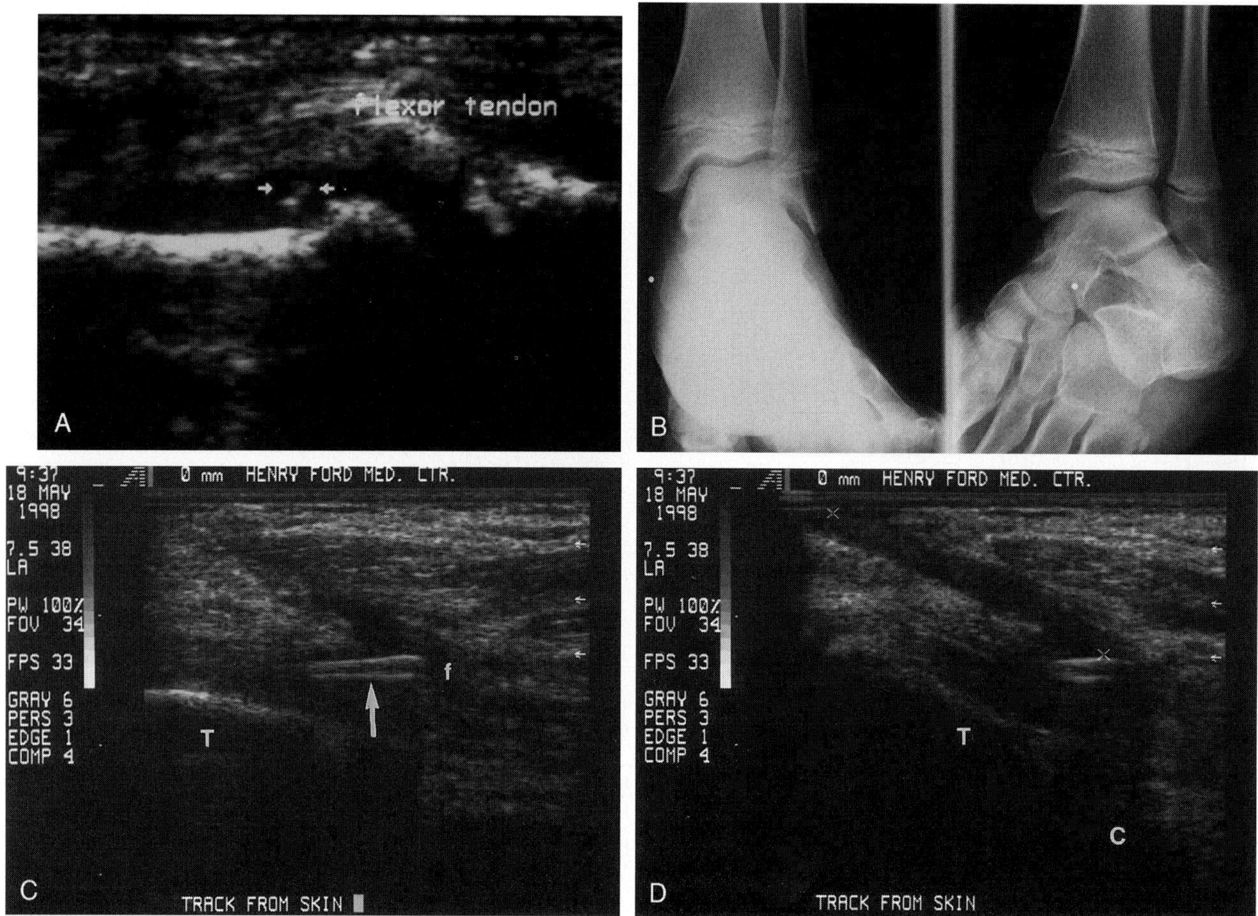

Figure 12–12 ■ **A**, Thorn-induced arthritis: longitudinal ultrasound through the flexor tendons. A child develops swelling of the proximal interphalangeal joint (*p.i.p.*) in the hand weeks after a thorn penetrated the finger. The mother removed a thorn from the dorsal surface of the finger right after the injury. The patient's X-rays are normal. A careful ultrasound exam of the extensor surface of the finger at the site of entry does not reveal a foreign body. Fluid is seen within the p.i.p. joint, however. The volar recess of the joint contains a small intra-articular body (*arrows*). Surgical removal proves that the tip of a thorn had broken off in the joint and has migrated from the dorsal to the volar aspect of the finger. **B**, Recurrent swelling of the ankle joint was observed by the mother of this child. The symptoms started after a penetrating injury in the woods and lasted for several years. Two explorative surgeries failed to discover the cause of the focal inflammation. Recently, pus had been draining from a fistulous tract at the medial aspect of the ankle. A metallic marker, shown on the radiographs, marks the skin surface erosion. **C**, The sonographer found a foreign body (*arrow*) that paralleled the talus (*T*). Fluid (*f*) makes the fragment stand out clearly. **D**, The fistula (between calipers) can be followed from the skin down to the level of the foreign body over a distance of 25 mm. The deep location of the foreign body and the oblique course of the fistula might explain why two prior surgeries had not found the piece. The fragment was thought to be located in the talo-calcaneal articulation. The third and final surgery removed a 7-mm-long thorn from the subtalar joint. Abbreviations: talus (*T*); calcaneus (*C*).

accurate clinical history is not available. Organic materials like splinters, plated wood, and thorns are very significant allergens. These foreign materials tend to induce granulomas and local infections. Synovial inflammation will often follow intra-articular penetration or penetration of the foreign body into a tendon sheath or a bursa lumen (Figs. 12–12 through 12–14). Plastic objects are slightly less echogenic than intact wood but also demonstrate acoustic shadowing. These relatively inert materials do not decompose in the surrounding inflammatory reaction. Metallic foreign bodies are hyperechoic and are associated with a significant comet tail artifact. The stiffness of the metal may cause migration of some of those materials through the soft tissues (Fig. 12–15). Pressure on the skin, muscular contractions, and respiratory motions have been known to cause migration (Harle and Beard, 1967).

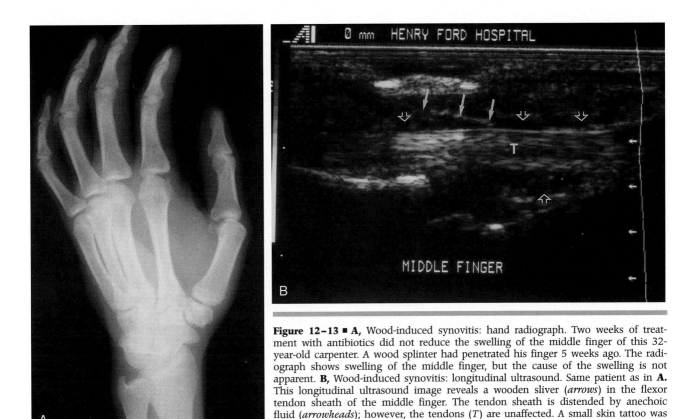

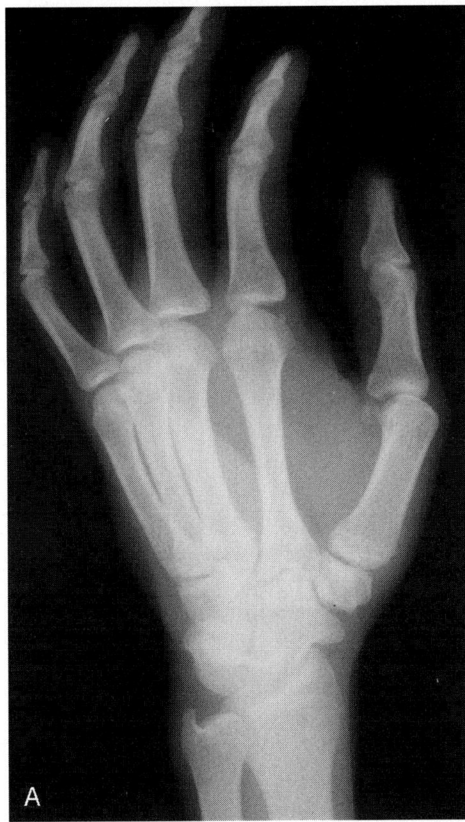

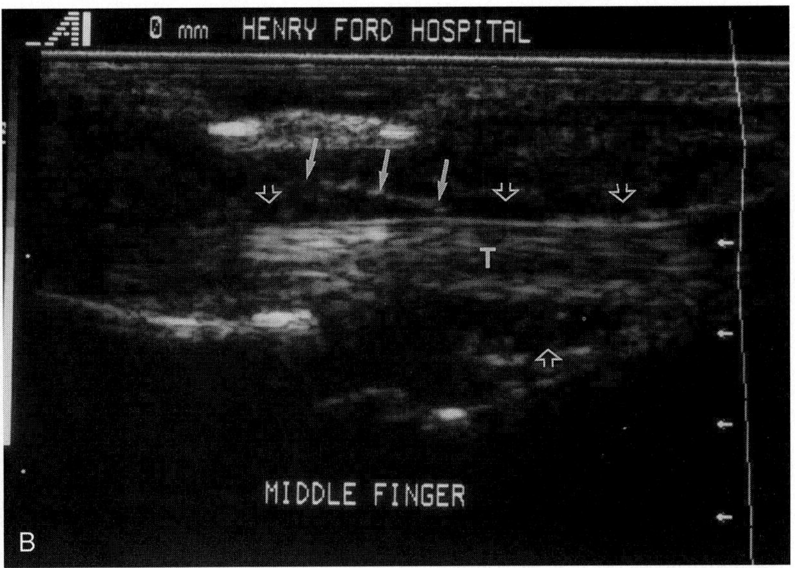

Figure 12–13 ■ **A,** Wood-induced synovitis: hand radiograph. Two weeks of treatment with antibiotics did not reduce the swelling of the middle finger of this 32-year-old carpenter. A wood splinter had penetrated his finger 5 weeks ago. The radiograph shows swelling of the middle finger, but the cause of the swelling is not apparent. **B,** Wood-induced synovitis: longitudinal ultrasound. Same patient as in **A.** This longitudinal ultrasound image reveals a wooden sliver (*arrows*) in the flexor tendon sheath of the middle finger. The tendon sheath is distended by anechoic fluid (*arrowheads*); however, the tendons (*T*) are unaffected. A small skin tattoo was placed over the foreign body, and the small fragment was then retrieved surgically. The swelling subsided almost immediately. All cultures of the tendon sheath were negative.

Figure 12–14 ■ Thorn-induced synovitis: longitudinal ultrasound. This boy fell into some shrubs, and his parents noticed gradual swelling and redness of his elbow in the region of the olecranon bursa. This longitudinal ultrasound image demonstrates a needle-like foreign body (*between the calipers*) and synovitis of the olecranon bursa (*BU*). Culture of debrided tissues after removal of the foreign body was positive for *Staphylococcus epidermidis.*

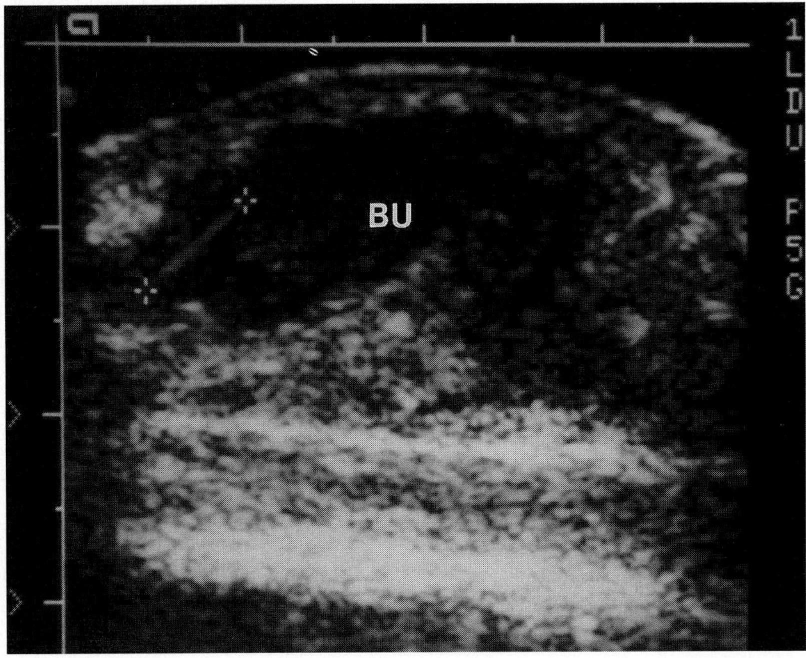

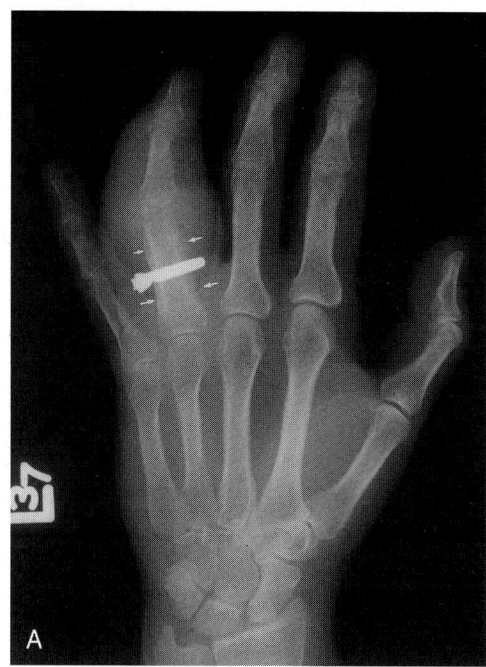

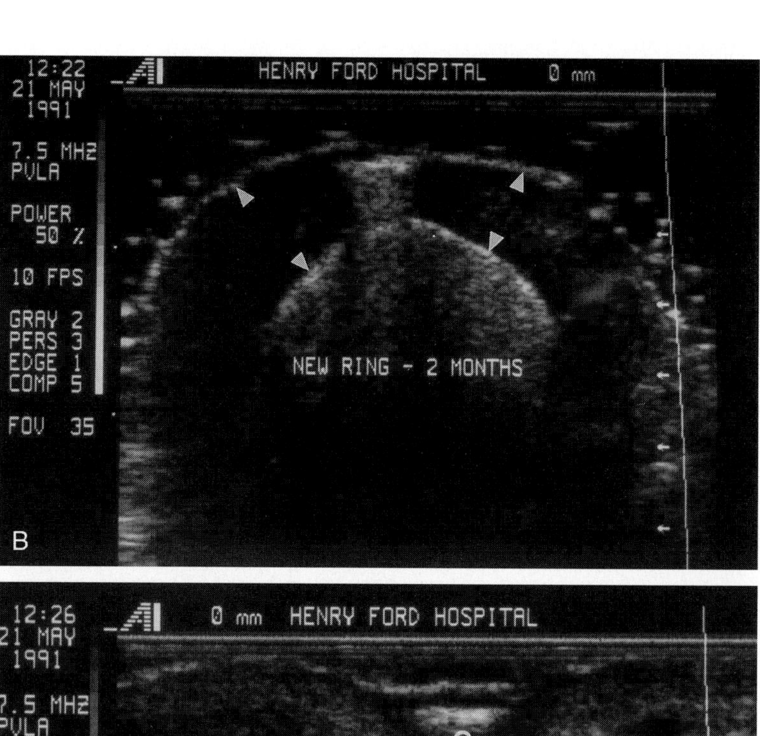

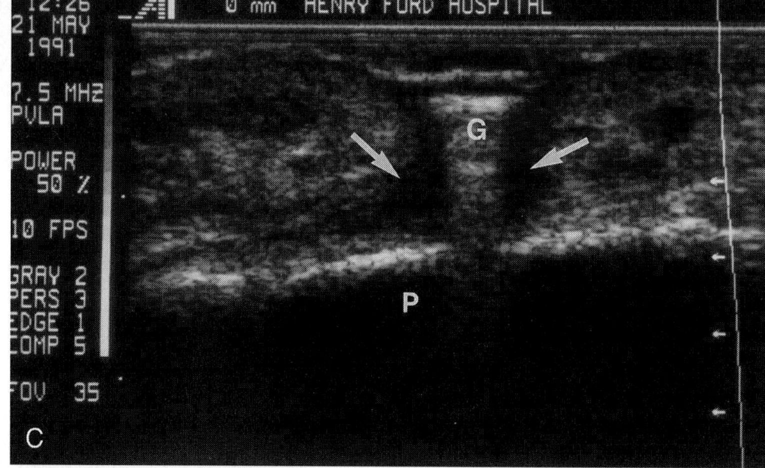

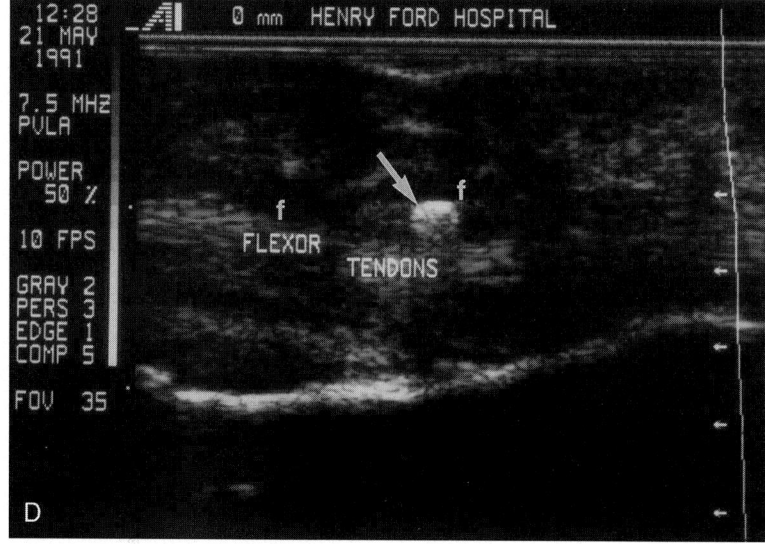

Figure 12–15 ■ **A**, Migration of a ring: hand radiograph. A homeless woman presented to the emergency department with an extremely tender and markedly swollen ring finger. Radiographs of the hand and the clinical exam did not match. The ring seen on the radiograph is not visible clinically. The woman insists that she got the new ring 2 months ago, and she blames the ring for the swelling of her finger. The emergency room physician doubts the story because he does not believe that the skin can close over a ring that quickly. Indeed, the overlying skin looks absolutely pristine. Reactive periostitis (*arrows*) is visible around the fourth middle phalanx. **B**, Migration of a ring: transverse ultrasound. The shape of the ring can be distinguished when the finger is scanned transversely over its dorsum. Reverberations make it impossible to see the tissues deeper to the dorsal surface. The ring is located 0.5 cm deep to the skin surface (*space between the arrowheads*). **C**, Migration of a ring: longitudinal ultrasound over the extensor side. Same patient as in **A**. The ring's gem (*G*) is located just below the skin surface. Fluid (*arrows*) is noted between the ring and the bone surface of the middle phalanx (*P*). **D**, Migration of a ring: longitudinal ultrasound over the flexor side. Same patient as in **C**. Longitudinal images through the flexor tendons show the segment of the ring (*arrow*) deep in the soft tissues of the volar aspect of the finger. Penetration of the flexor tendon sheath and the effusion (*f*) surrounding the tendon were treated as an emergency due to the clinical diagnosis of septic tenosynovitis. The ring was removed surgically. Pus drained from the tendon sheath, which cultured positive for *Staphylo-coccus aureus.*

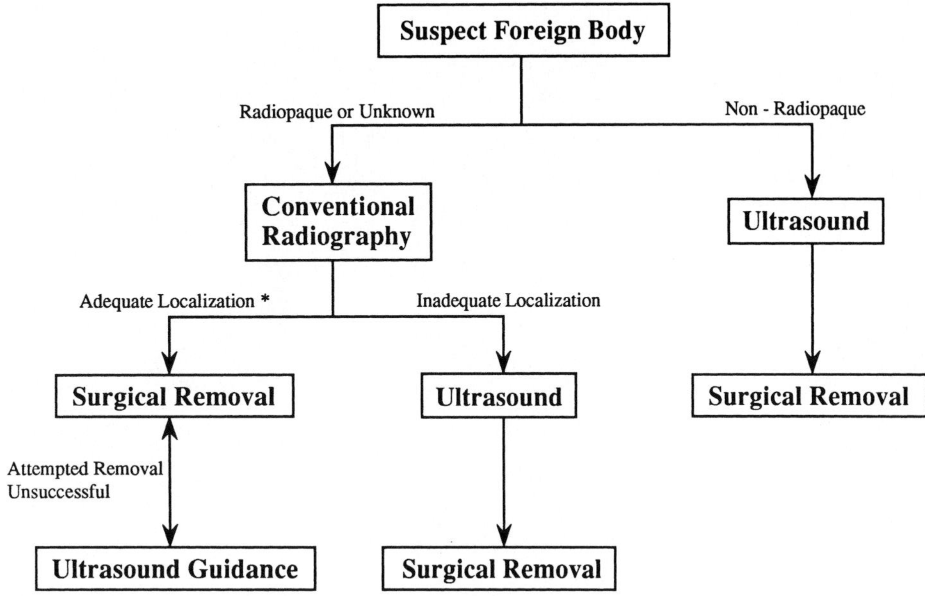

Figure 12-16 ■ Algorithm for evaluation of foreign bodies. If conventional radiographs indicate that the foreign body is in the vicinity of vital structures, ultrasound is indicated for further evaluation.

Occasionally, metal can induce synovitis. Chromium, nickel, and lead have been known to induce a sterile synovitis, which can be toxic to cartilage when a joint is involved. Around prostheses, corrosion of metals can induce sarcomas, and several case reports have been published in the literature.

Diagnostic Approach to Foreign Bodies

Sonography has been demonstrated to be clearly superior to radiography in the evaluation of foreign bodies. However, it is not practical to use ultrasound in all cases. The algorithm outlined in Figure 12-16 provides a rational, cost-effective approach to the diagnosis and localization of foreign bodies. When the clinical history indicates that the foreign body is radiolucent, ultrasound is the study of choice. Otherwise, low-kilovoltage radiography should be the first step. If radiographs do not provide adequate information, ultrasound is indicated for further evaluation. When surgical removal following conventional radiography is unsuccessful, real-time ultrasound guidance can be most helpful. Some foreign bodies are much more easily removed percutaneously, with ultrasound guidance, than surgically with classic incision and debridement (Shiels et al., 1990).

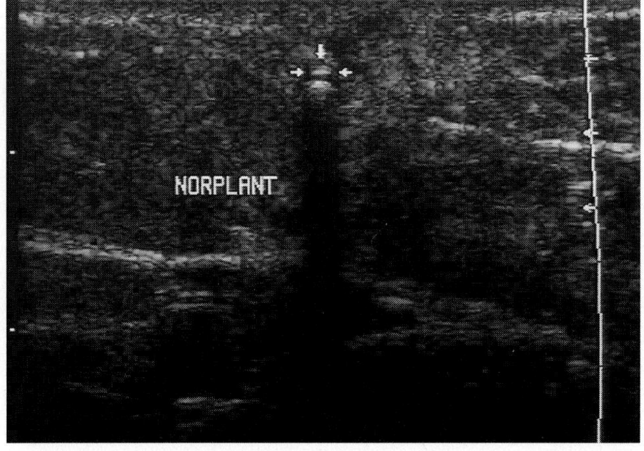

Figure 12-17 ■ Norplant: transverse ultrasound over the upper arm. A surgeon referred this 29-year-old woman for localization of a lost capsule of a Norplant contraceptive device, which had been inserted $2^1/_2$ years ago. Four capsules had been removed a month earlier, and a fifth was found in a separate surgical procedure 3 weeks later. One remaining capsule remained hidden even after a third surgical procedure. At this time, the surgeon decided to request ultrasound guidance. The small cylinder (*arrows*) is located in the thick subcutaneous fat. A narrow acoustic shadow is noted deep to the implant. The silastic Norplant capsules are accurately depicted with ultrasound. In general, the contour, structure, and size of plastic foreign bodies are imaged with few artifacts. The skin overlying this foreign body was marked over its entire length using a surgical marker and was easily removed with ultrasound guidance.

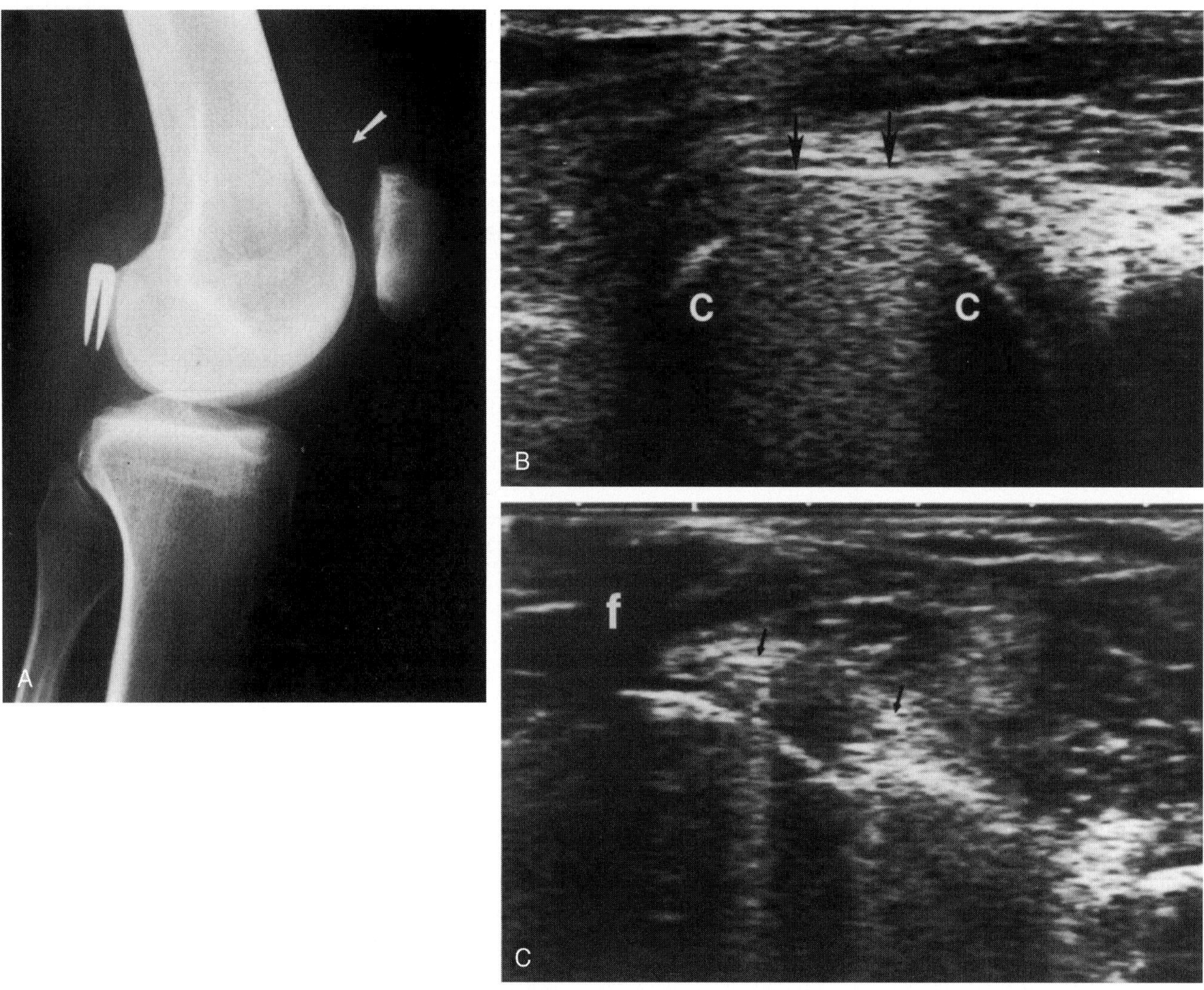

Figure 12–18 ■ **A**, Intra-articular migration of a surgical staple: lateral knee radiograph. This 22-year-old man had had ligament and posterior capsule repair $2^1/_2$ years ago. Four days ago, he reinjured the knee, and marked swelling developed immediately. Joint aspiration at the time of initial presentation yielded frank blood. The patient was referred for imaging evaluation with a complaint of decreased range of motion and increased pain. This radiograph demonstrates a joint effusion in the suprapatellar bursa (*arrow*) and a metallic staple posterior to the femoral condyles. The staple is no longer fixed in bone. The position of the staple relative to the joint space is not clear from this study; therefore, an ultrasound study was performed. **B**, Intra-articular migration of a surgical staple: longitudinal sonogram. Same patient as in **A**. The transducer is positioned over the lateral femoral condyle (*C*). A wide comet tail artifact is seen originating from the linear leg of the metal staple (*arrows*). **C**, Intra-articular migration of a surgical staple: transverse sonogram. Same patient as in **A** and **B**. The transducer is rotated 90 degrees, demonstrating both legs of the staple with comet tail artifact (*arrows*). Fluid (*f*) clearly within the joint capsule surrounds the staple, indicating its intra-articular position. The ultrasound study showed the neurovascular bundle at a safe distance. The staple was surgically removed, and the patient regained full range of motion.

Ultrasound-guided removal of Norplant contraceptive devices has been proposed (Fig. 12–17). The six silastic capsules which make up the Norplant contraceptive device can be found subdermally on the medial aspect of the upper arm about 8 to 10 cm proximal to the elbow crease. It is helpful to know that these devices are introduced through a 2-mm incision above the elbow and are placed in a radial pattern proximally, with 10- to 15-degree angle between implants. Ultrasound-guided removal can be performed through a 4-mm incision (Stein, 1996). After ultrasound localization, one can push

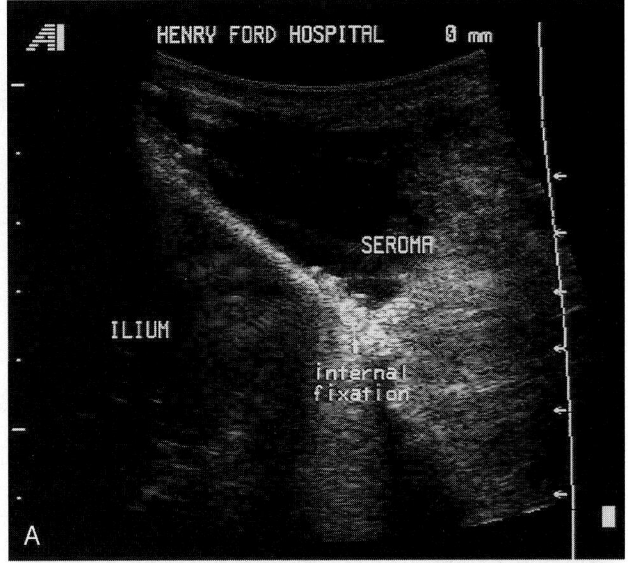

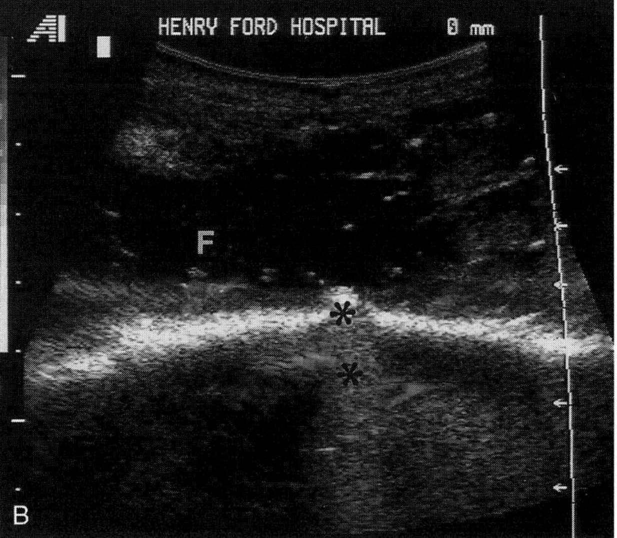

Figure 12-19 ■ **A**, Deep postoperative fluid collection: transverse ultrasound over the left ilium. Swelling and drainage at the hip persist 1 week after reconstruction of the posterior wall of the left acetabulum in this 44-year-old woman. This scan was performed with the patient laying on the nonaffected right side. A mixed-echogenicity fluid collection is located directly over the bone surface. The internal fixation material causes ring down artifact. **B**, Deep postoperative fluid collection: longitudinal ultrasound along the left ilium. Same patient as in **A**. The transducer has been rotated 90 degrees from the position in **A**. The irregular fluid collection (*F*) covers the bone and the metal (*asterisks*) on this view as well. It took only about 5 minutes to remove 500 cc of clear fluid under ultrasound guidance.

the capsules toward the incision. The tip must be grasped with a sterile mosquito forceps. It is necessary to cut the tissue sheath that has formed around the capsules (Stein, 1996).

Orthopedic Implants

Orthopedic implants are a special category of foreign bodies. Ultrasound can be very valuable in the evaluation of hardware used in internal fixation of fractures, and particularly in the evaluation of orthopedic prostheses. Problems associated with orthopedic implants can be categorized as either acute or chronic; the acute problems occur in the immediate postoperative period.

Acute Complications

Postoperative hematoma is a serious complication because it predisposes to wound sepsis. This has been well established for hip prostheses, and it can reasonably be applied to other implants as well (Wilson et al., 1973). Pelvic and spinal surgery is often complicated by significant hemorrhage due to the extent of surgery and the proximity to large vessels. Clinical examination is of little value in the detection of these hematomas, unless they are massive or very superficially located (Magnussen et al., 1988). This is due in part to the massive edema that accompanies this extensive surgery. Ultrasound is a fast, accurate, noninvasive examination for the diagnosis of postoperative hematomas (Fig. 12-18).

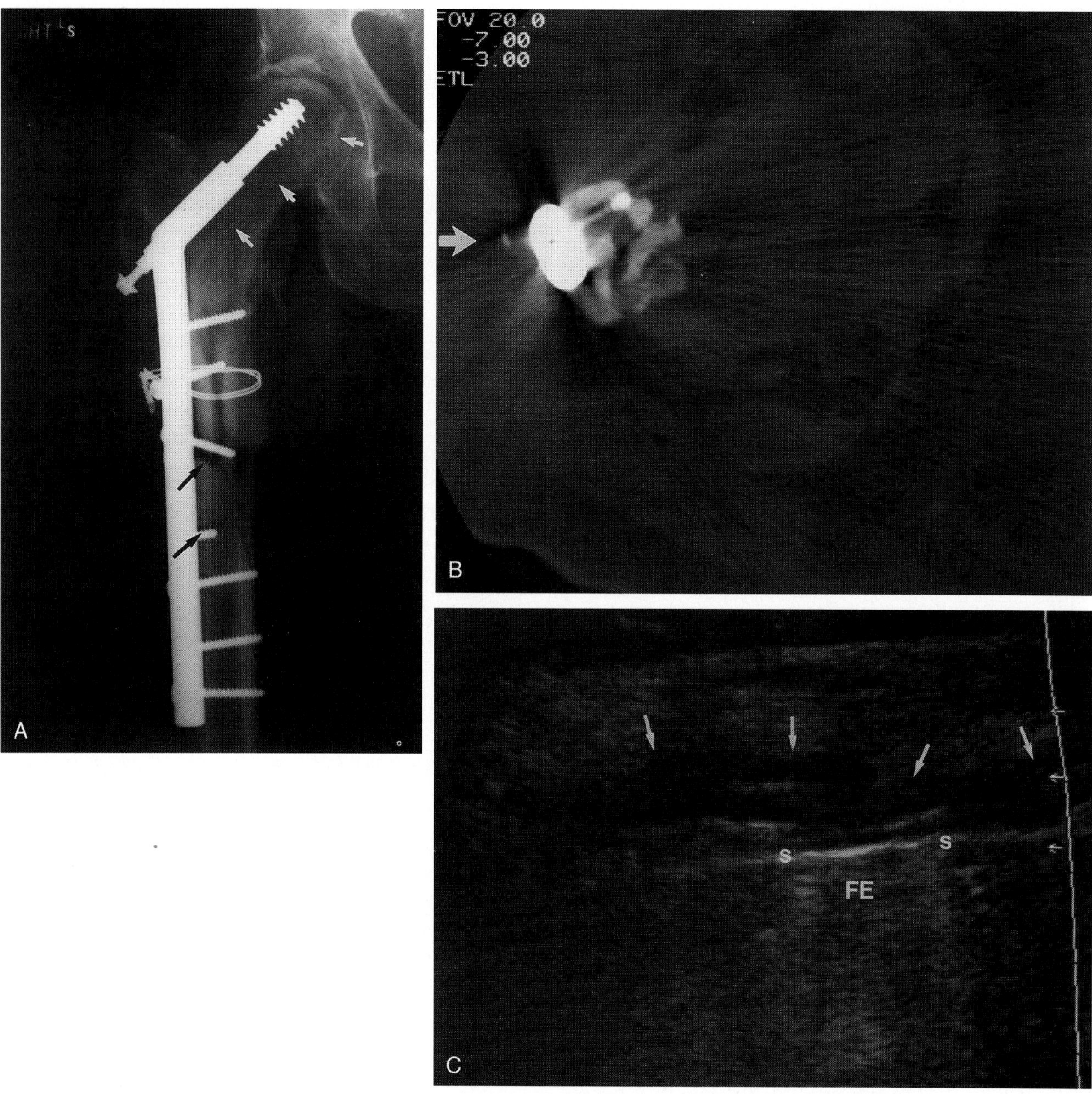

Figure 12–20 ■ **A**, Postoperative fluid: hip radiograph. A fall resulting in fracture of the right hip interrupted this 64-year-old man's travel abroad. He returned from Greece following the open reduction and internal fixation shown in this radiograph. Ten months later, he continued to experience persistent severe pain. The radiograph suggests complications. A radiolucent band is noted surrounding the prosthesis in the femoral neck and screws in the shaft of the femur (*arrows*). A dense, loose bone fragment in the subtrochanteric region may represent a sequestrum. **B**, Postoperative fluid: CT of proximal femur. Same patient as in **A**. This CT image at the level of the cerclage wires and second lag screw clarifies the location of the loose bone fragments. The metal of the hardware results in artifact (*arrow*) and obscures the soft tissue planes of the lateral thigh. **C**, Postoperative fluid: lateral thigh ultrasound. Same patient as in **A**. The transducer has been placed longitudinally over the area indicated by an *arrow* on **B**. This image along the femoral shaft (*FE*) demonstrates fluid tracking along the cortical surface of the lateral femur (*arrows*). Loose screws (*s*) are seen crossing the bone surface obliquely. Notice how the screws protrude into the soft tissues. Ultrasound accurately depicts the fluid collection, thus providing the examiner with a road map for his aspiration. Six milliliters of serosanguineous fluid was obtained and sent for culture. *Staphylococcus epidermidis* grew from the culture specimens. A repeat aspiration and culture to exclude skin contamination redemonstrated *S. epidermidis*. The CT examination was not able to demonstrate the infected fluid due to artifact. MRI would also have been limited by magnetic susceptibility artifact and would not have been able to reveal the fluid collection. The patient's hardware was removed after the second aspiration. The surgeon felt that the ultrasound study had saved the patient at least one surgical procedure. Infection of orthopedic hardware can be indolent, with few, if any, systemic signs of infection. Often the fluid aspirated does not have the appearance of pus, as in this case. Lack of fever should never stop a thorough investigation, and aspiration should be done in all equivocal cases.

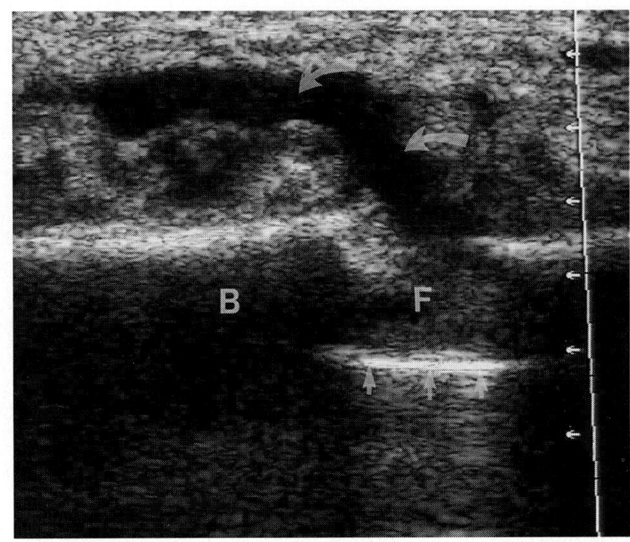

Figure 12–21 ■ Postoperative fluid: longitudinal ultrasound over the tibial diaphysis. Ultrasound study of an open tibial fracture performed 8 weeks after injury. The fracture defect (*F*) is still visible in the bone surface of the tibial diaphysis (*B*). An anechoic collection (*curved arrows*) communicates with the fracture site and with an intramedullary nail (*small arrows*) which had been placed 3 days after the injury. Aspiration of the anechoic fluid yielded pus, and routine culture was positive for *Staphylococcus epidermidis* infection. In contrast, in normal healing, callus should have been visible 8 weeks after fracture, and there should have been no fluid at the site of fracture.

Localization and aspiration can be performed rapidly (Fig. 12–19).

The distinction between superficial and deep hematomas is easily made using ultrasound (Fig. 12–19). Hematomas appear hypoechoic or anechoic, depending on their stage of evolution or resolution. Deep hematomas are located immediately over the bone surface. If the collection is separated from the prosthesis and bony structures by muscle or fascia, it is considered superficial. This distinction is important because most surgeons take both superficial and deep cultures during the surgical procedure. If the hematoma is deep and the cultures are positive, surgical or percutaneous evacuation of the collection is imperative (Magnussen et al., 1988). Management of superficial hematomas varies considerably among clinicians, depending on the condition of the patient and other clinical factors.

Persistent fluid around orthopedic implants is considered suspicious, especially when new fluid is found after the immediate postoperative period. Most fluid resorbs 2 weeks after surgery, and fluid persisting after that period is highly suspicious for infection (Figs. 12–20 and 12–21). Fever is not always present in infection complicating surgery, in part because some of the organisms involved are less virulent than the classic staphylococous aureus infection. The presence of the implant is the major predisposing factor to infection, not the virulence of the causative organism.

Chronic Complications

Infection

Even following a successful, uncomplicated postoperative period, orthopedic implants can become infected at any time (Figs. 12–22 through 12–24). Since hip prostheses are by far the most widely employed, they are most commonly infected. Whenever a patient with a prosthesis presents with fever of unknown origin or associated with pain in that area, infection is suspected. Surgeons usually perform blind or fluoroscopically guided aspiration of the joint (Resnick and Niwayama, 1988). When this yields joint fluid, the problem is solved, but a dry tap is not infrequent. Commonly, fluid surrounding a prosthesis will be irregularly distributed and loculated. The ability of ultrasound to locate periprosthetic fluid collections and guide aspiration makes it the perfect solution to the problem (Figs. 12–24 and 12–25). The sonographer must scan the entire segment of bone in which the prosthesis has been implanted. It is not unusual to see abscesses penetrating the cortex at the tip of an infected femoral stem. It is helpful to review the patient's radiographs prior to the ultrasound examination. This will assist the examiner, who will then be able to assess the position of the acetabular and femoral components and judge the length of the femoral stem. The single most reliable criterion of infection is finding an extra-articular fluid collection in continuity with the joint (van Holsbeeck et al., 1994). It is remarkable that aspiration of these collections can be positive despite a negative fluoroscopically guided joint aspiration. It seems reasonable to use ultrasound as a routine adjunct in aspiration of possibly infected hip replacements. We have never observed an infected prosthesis which was "dry" on ultrasound examination. Therefore, we feel it is not necessary to attempt aspiration in patients with a normal (less than 3.2 mm) capsule-to-bone distance if the prosthesis was placed more than 1 year prior to the

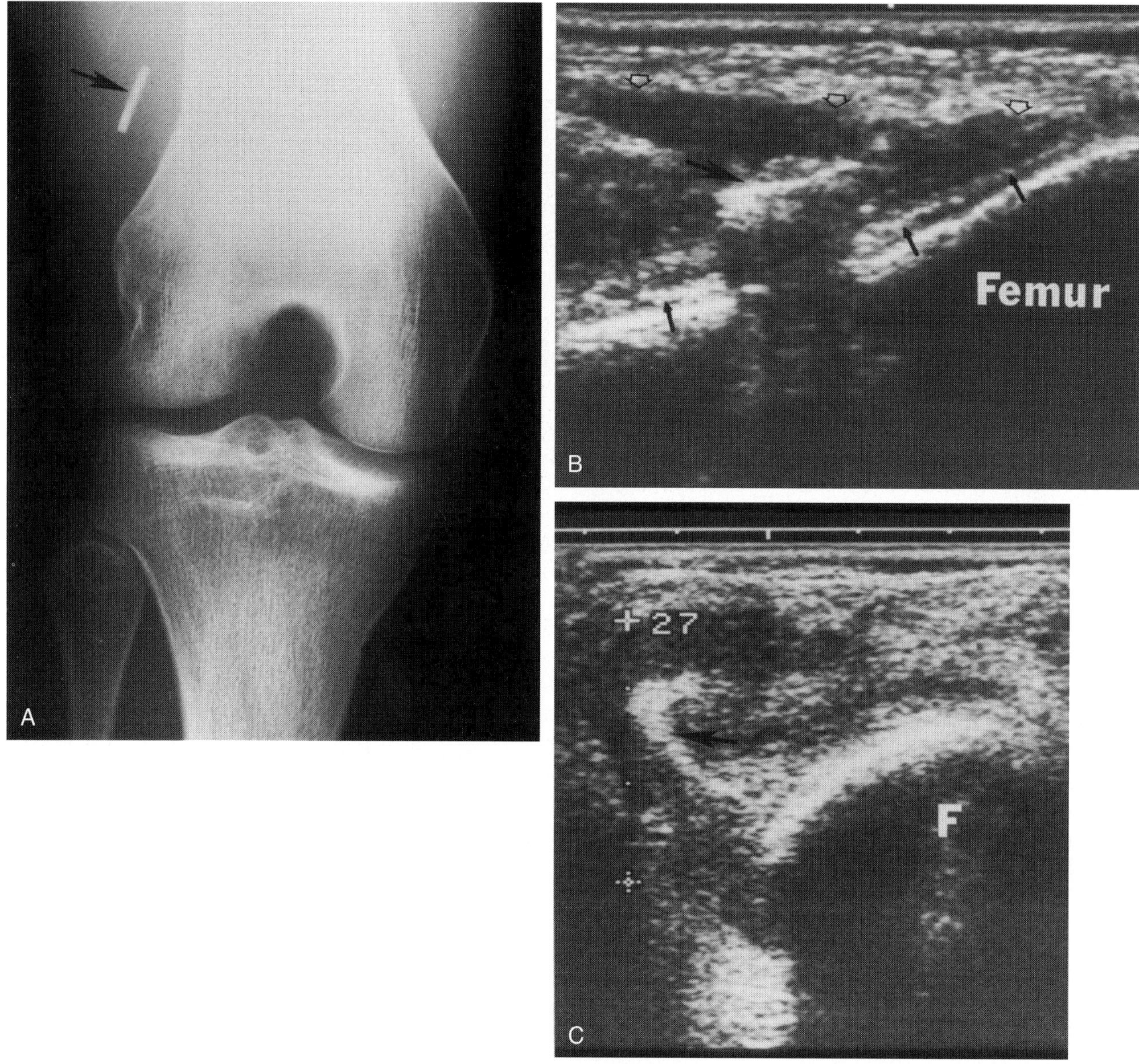

Figure 12–22 ■ **A**, Painful knee following cruciate ligament reconstruction: anteroposterior radiograph. Four months after reconstructive surgery to repair torn cruciate ligaments, this 20-year-old football player presents with pain of 2 weeks' duration on the lateral side of the right knee. A metallic foreign body (*arrow*) is identified lateral to the distal femoral metaphysis. **B**, Painful knee following cruciate ligament reconstruction: coronal sonogram. Same patient as in **A**. The transducer is placed over the lateral aspect of the distal femoral metaphysis. A linear hyperechoic foreign body (*arrow*) with associated comet tail artifact is observed. Hypoechoic fluid (*open arrows*) surrounds the foreign body. Note the periosteal thickening (*solid black arrows*) adjacent to the foreign body. This periosteal reaction was not observable on the conventional radiograph (**A**). **C**, Painful knee following cruciate ligament reconstruction: transverse sonogram. Same patient as in **A** and **B**. The metallic foreign body is seen as a curvilinear hyperechoic line with subtle comet tail artifact (*arrow*) surrounded by a hypoechoic fluid collection 27 mm in diameter. Given the duration of the pain, finding fluid with definite internal echos is highly suspicious for purulent material. No fluid was identified within the knee joint, excluding joint sepsis. At surgery, purulent material was found surrounding the foreign body. Abbreviation: femur (*F*).

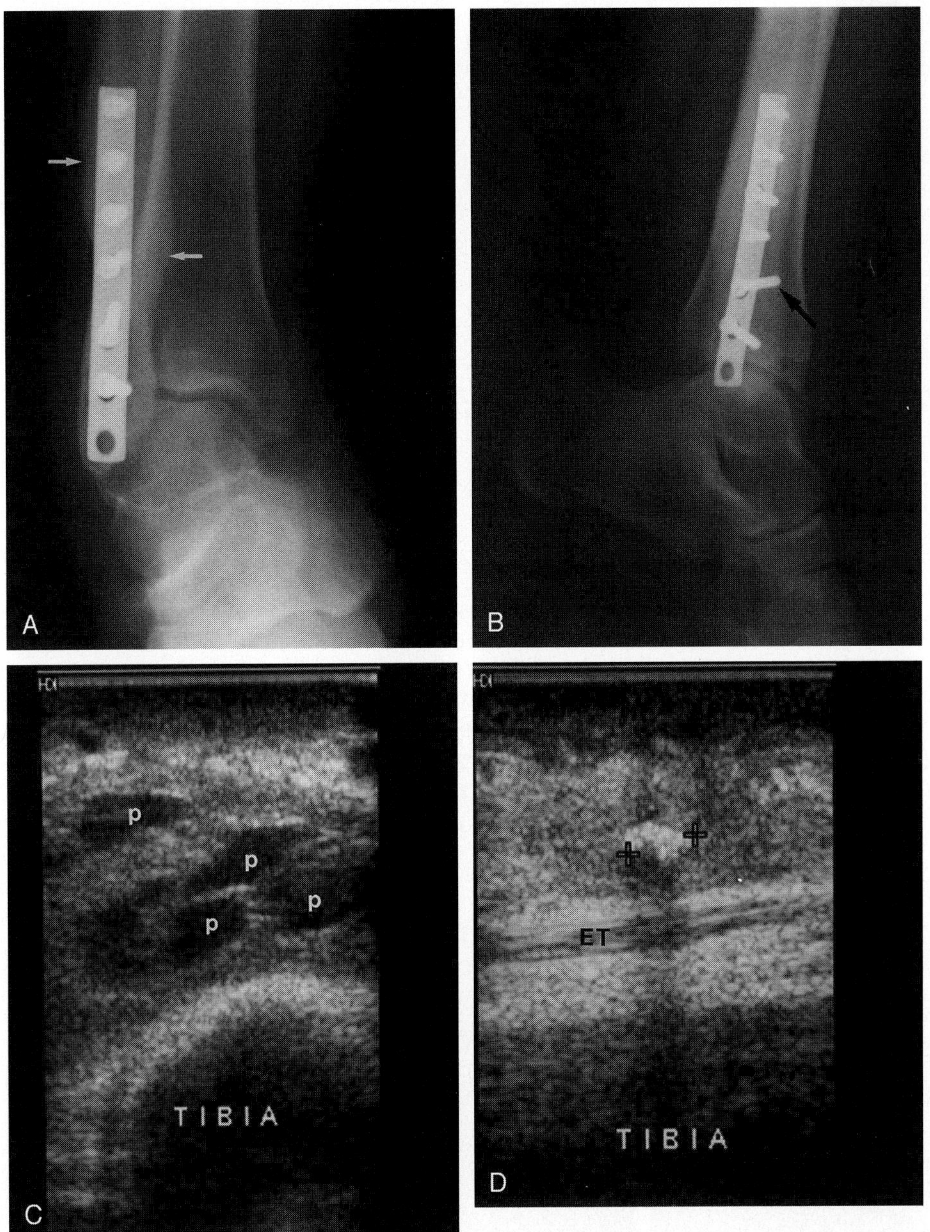

Figure 12–23 ■ **A**, Hardware-related abscess: ankle radiograph. Four days of pain and ankle swelling brought this 34-year-old woman to the orthopedic clinic. She had been treated for a Weber B-type distal fibular fracture 2 years ago. The radiographs demonstrated healing of the fibular fracture but exuberant periosteal bone apposition (*arrows*) around the distal fibula adjacent to the hardware. There were no signs of hardware loosening. **B**, Hardware-related abscess: lateral ankle radiograph. Same patient as in **A**. The lateral radiograph shows healing of the fracture. The lag screw (*arrow*) is surrounded by solid callus. Plate and screws are demonstrated, with no evidence of loosening. **C**, Hardware-related abscess: transverse ultrasound. Same patient as in **A**. A soft tissue mass is noted around the anterior and lateral aspect of the ankle. The mass appears multiloculated and contains pockets (*p*) of hypoechoic material. These loculated collections proved to be pus on ultrasound-guided aspiration. Debridement was necessary because the fluid could not be completely evacuated percutaneously. The cultures were positive for *Enterobacter cloacae*. These bacteria were resistant to penicillin and cephalosporins but sensitive to Bactrim. Ultrasound plays a significant role in confirming or excluding the diagnosis of infection. In addition, ultrasound-guided aspiration helps by identifying the causative organism and aids selection of the best antibiotic regimen through culture and sensitivity testing. This approach allows faster treatment and allows optimal antibiotic coverage during surgery. **D**, Hardware-related abscess: longitudinal ultrasound. Same patient as in **A**. A sequestrum (between the calipers) is located anterior to the extensor digitorum tendon (*ET*).

Figure continued on following page

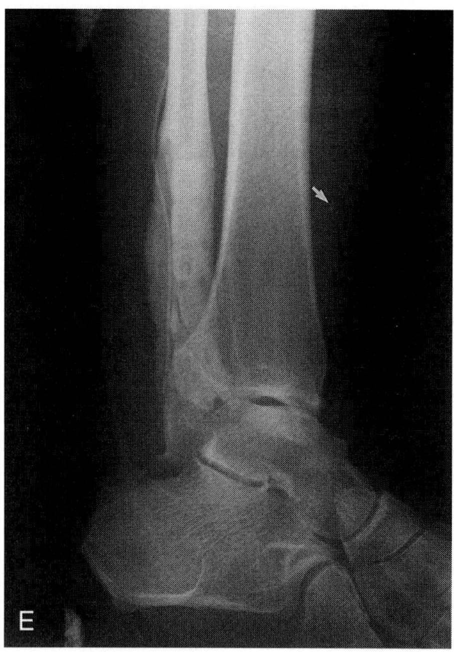

Figure 12–23 *Continued* ■ **E**, Hardware-related abscess: postoperative lateral radiograph. Same patient as in **A**. The abscess was drained, and the hardware was removed surgically. A drain is noted at the surgical site. The radiograph demonstrates bone healing, with bridging and new bone formation around the distal fibula. These findings suggest a secondary infection of the hardware, probably due to a blood-borne infection. A postoperative infection would not have allowed the fracture to heal primarily. The sequestrum (*arrow*) discovered on ultrasound has not been removed. The abscess recurred 3 days later, and resection of the sequestrum required a second surgical exploration.

ultrasound examination (van Holsbeeck et al., 1994). Infected collections tend to be more echogenic than simple joint fluid (see Fig. 12–21). Frequently, debris floating within the infected fluid can be identified.

Loosening of the Prosthesis

Modern orthopedic implants are composed of inert materials. Foreign body granulomas around these implants are rare. If present, they are usually found at the bone–cement interface (Harris et al., 1976).

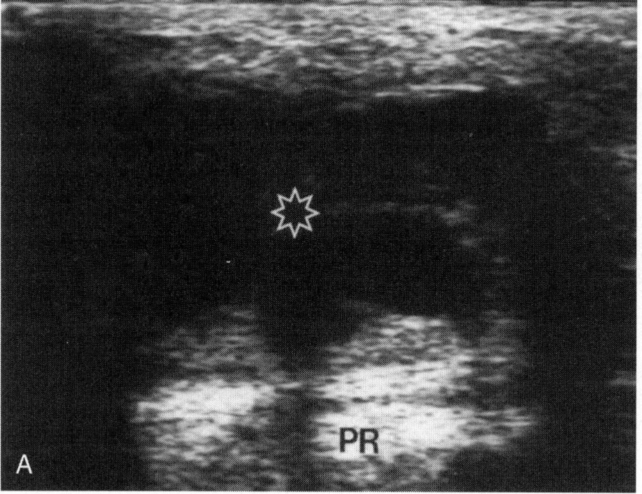

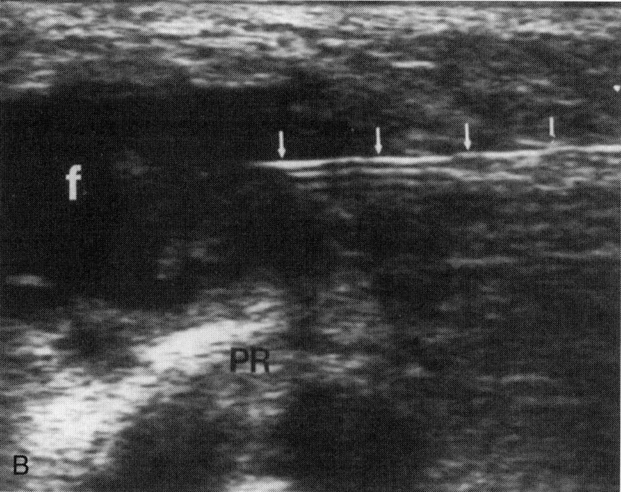

Figure 12–24 ■ **A**, Infected hip prosthesis: longitudinal sonogram. The patient is a 90-year-old woman who received a left total hip arthroplasty 2 years ago. She was observed to have deterioration in mental status accompanied by a slight fever of 2 days' duration. Chest radiographs were normal, and urine cultures were negative. Ultrasound study of the hip was requested to evaluate the prosthesis for infection. A large fluid collection (*) containing echogenic debris is identified adjacent to the femoral prosthesis (*PR*). This is clearly indicative of infection. **B**, Infected hip prosthesis: transverse sonogram. Same patient as in **A**. The fluid collection (*f*) surrounds the anterior and medial borders of the prosthesis (*PR*). Debris is again noted within the collection. A needle (*arrows*) was placed into this collection to confirm the diagnosis. A total of 80 mL of pus was removed following percutaneous placement of a drainage catheter. *Staphylococcus aureus* was the offending organism.

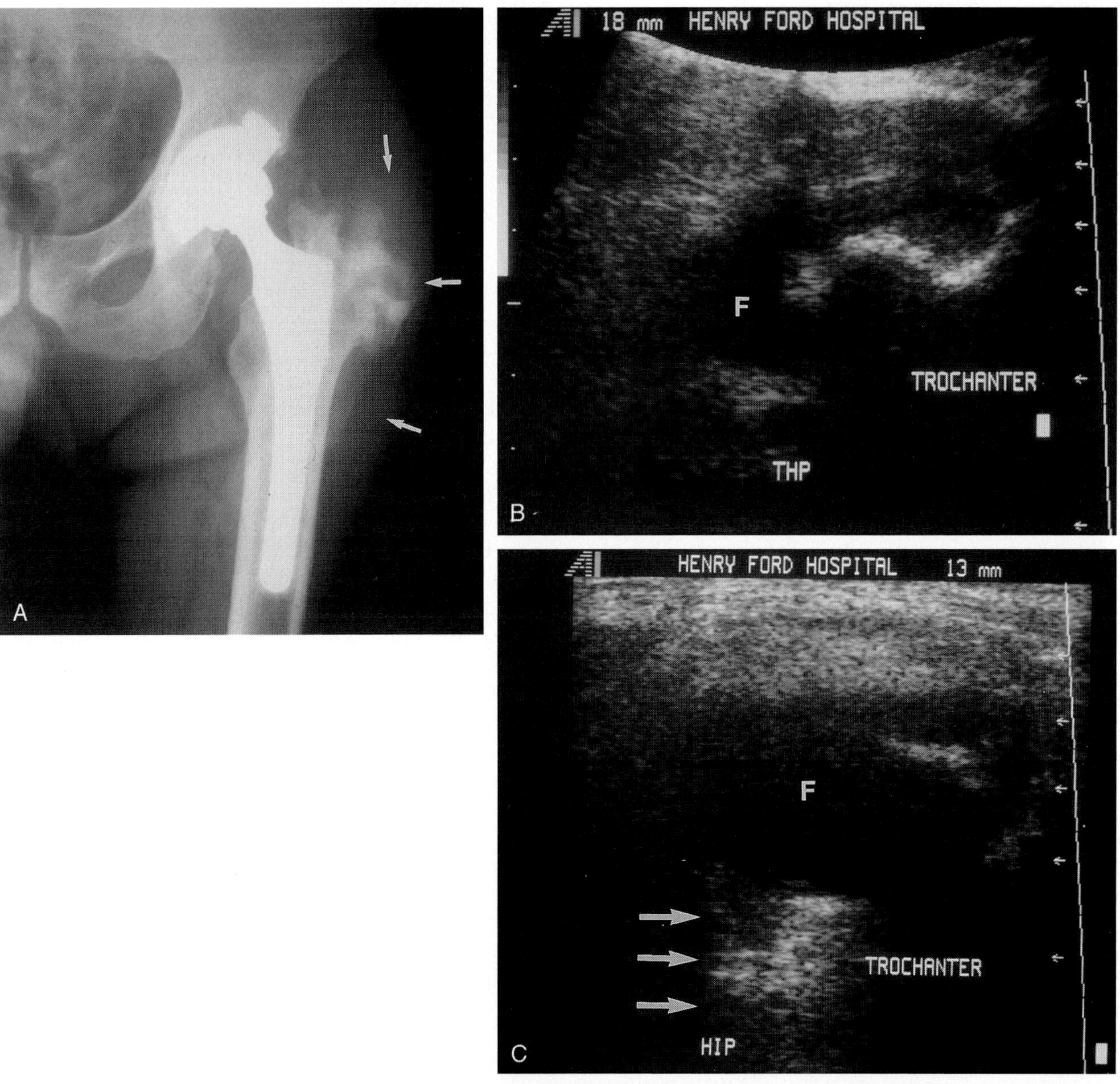

Figure 12–25 ■ **A**, Indolent hip infection: hip radiograph. An orthopedic surgeon consulted us for evaluation of a slowly growing mass over the left greater trochanter of this 40-year-old man with a total hip replacement. Noteworthy in the patient's medical history was chronic renal failure with a kidney transplant. The surgeon was concerned about the possibility of malignancy. He stated that patients with depressed immune systems are more susceptible to the development of neoplasm. The anteroposterior radiograph of the hip demonstrates hypertrophy and sclerosis of the left greater trochanter. A soft tissue mass is noted over the lateral aspect of the hip (*arrows*). **B**, Indolent hip infection: coronal hip ultrasound. Same patient as in **A**. Ultrasound examination of the lateral hip with a curved 7.5-MHz transducer reveals a soft tissue mass overlying the trochanter and neck of the total hip prosthesis (*THP*). The lesion appears hypoechoic and was not compressible over the trochanter. This tissue is suggestive of thickened synovium. The more proximal portion of the mass seems anechoic and is probably a fluid collection (*F*). **C**, Indolent hip infection: detail of a coronal sonogram over the femoral neck. Same patient as in **A**. The fluid (*F*) component of the proximal aspect of the mass is seen in more detail with the linear 7.5-MHz over the femoral neck. Increased through-transmission (*arrows*) is noted deep to the fluid. Eight milliliters of serosanguineous fluid was obtained under ultrasound guidance. The specimen was positive for *Achromobacter xylos oxidans*, and the prosthesis was subsequently removed.

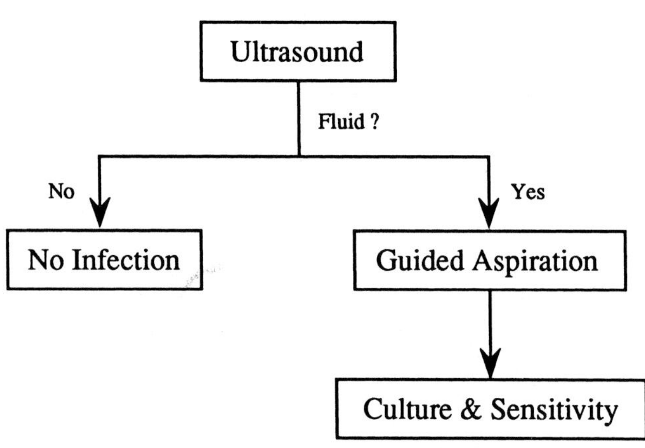

Figure 12–26 ▪ Algorithm used to evaluate joints for infection. The clinical question of joint infection most commonly arises in evaluation of hips following arthroplasty. Ultrasound's high sensitivity in detecting joint effusion makes it the best method to evaluate joints for infection. Effusions as small as 1 mL can be detected. If increased intra-articular fluid is detected, aspiration can be performed during the same session.

Granulomatous reaction in the surrounding soft tissues has not been reported. The significant complication resulting from foreign body granulomas at the bone–cement interface is loosening of the prosthesis. Motion of the prosthesis may result in pain and fracturing of the adjacent bone. These fractures may be occult on conventional radiographs due to the radiopacity of the prosthesis. Real-time sonographic examination may demonstrate mobility of the prosthesis. Fractures can also be detected as cortical discontinuity, with adjacent subperiosteal hemorrhage or periosteal new bone formation. In addition, the relationship of the acetabular and femoral components can be observed through a range of motion in real time. All fluid collections surrounding prostheses after the immediate postoperative period (2 weeks) should be considered suspicious for infection (Fig. 12–26). Prosthetic infection is rare, but the typical clinical signs of infection may be lacking. We should always be on guard for septic complications. Aseptic joint effusions do occur after arthroplasty. These effusions may be due to fracture of the polyethylene component, secondary to intra-articular wear debris or hemarthrosis. The intra-articular breakdown of cement, polyethylene, and metal, causing synovitis, becomes more likely as the prosthesis ages. The exact cause of the deterioration of the prosthetic components is still unknown. We are not always able to distinguish patients with aseptic effusions from those with septic complications. Fever and leukocytosis, present in some patients, or hyperemia detected by sonography may be indicators of infection (Fig. 12–27). The value of the clinical examination and laboratory findings is limited however, as many patients with prostheses are immune suppressed. Definitive diagnosis can only be made with fluid aspiration. This is why all symptomatic prosthetic joints with sonographic evidence of increased joint fluid are aspirated in our clinic.

Soft Tissue Erosion

Loose orthopedic hardware and penetrating screws can erode surrounding soft tissues. Metal foreign bodies can erode or occlude vessels (Leonard and Gifford, 1965; Rajamani and Fisher, 1998). Vessel thrombosis and hemopericardium have been described as the most dramatic effects of migrating hardware (Leonard and Gifford, 1965). Migrating sharp metallic foreign bodies can travel long distances and may eventually injure vital structures like the lung, esophagus, and spinal cord (Harle and Beard, 1967; Milgram, 1990). More common is erosion of tendons by screws that extend beyond the cortex (Fig. 12–28). Fraying of the posterior tibial tendon over a screw transfixing the medial malleolus and erosion of the rotator cuff by a screw transfixing a greater tuberosity fracture are relatively common complications of surgery. These complications are easy to diagnose sonographically. Irritation of a small nerve branch by a screw head or tail is also common. The treatment of those complications can be as simple as removal of the screw or replacement with a shorter screw. In some patients, the body may build its own protective barrier. Bursae can form over the sharp edges of hardware, reducing the degree of irritation (Milgram, 1990). Suture granulomas or synovitis (Fig. 12–29) secondary to foreign body irritation are relatively common complications of surgery. Simple suture removal may stop the irritation.

Summary

Ultrasound is more accurate than radiography in the detection and localization of all types of foreign

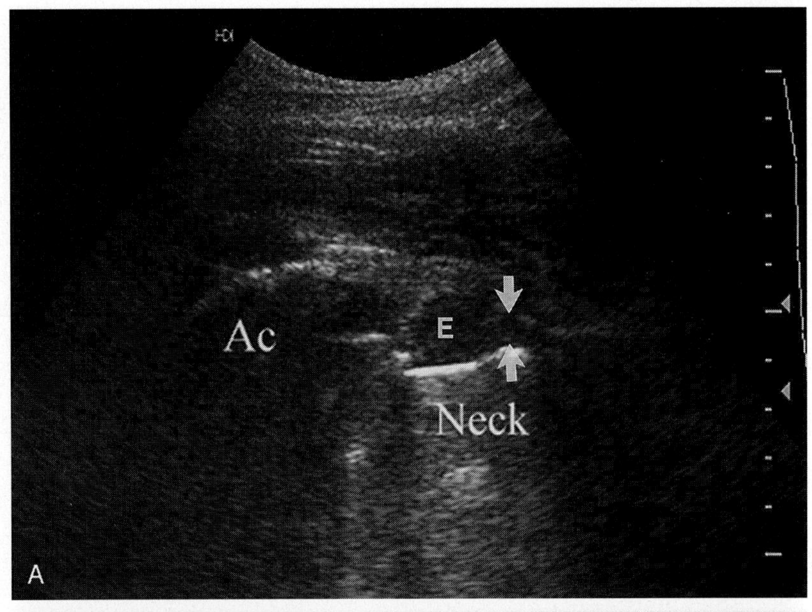

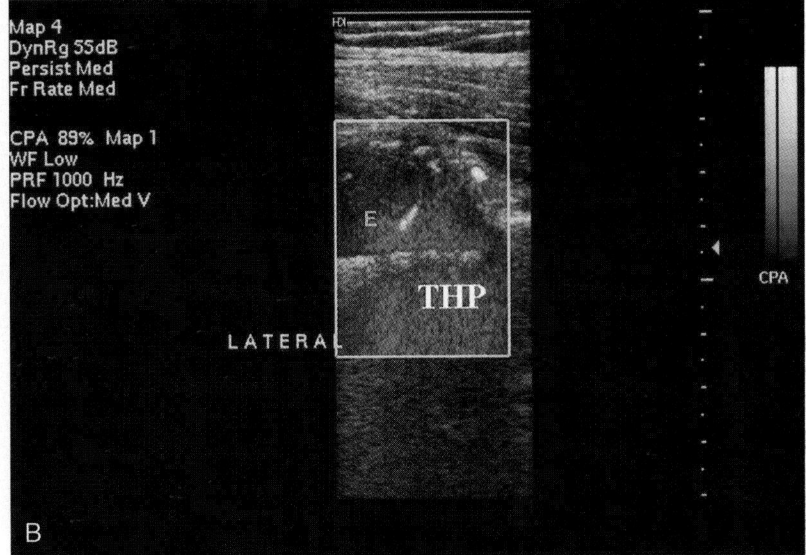

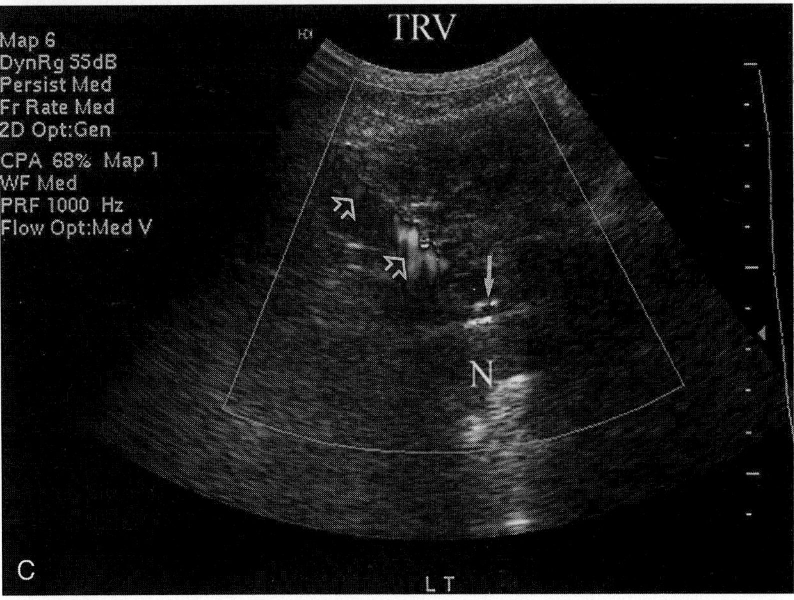

Figure 12-27 ■ **A**, Hyperemia in prosthetic hip replacement: longitudinal ultrasound. Five years after total joint replacement, this 48-year-old patient experiences acute pain of new onset in the hip after root canal surgery. The longitudinal ultrasound scan over the anterior aspect of the hip replacement shows a small effusion (*E*) over the metal femoral neck. There is separation of more than 3.5 mm (*arrows*) of the capsule from the native cortex (capsule-bone distance). Such small effusions are relatively common, and they are often aseptic due to wear debris synovitis. Abbreviation: acetabular component (*AC*). **B**, Hyperemia in prosthetic hip replacement: longitudinal ultrasound with power Doppler sonography. Same patient as in **A**. Hyperemia in the pseudocapsule of a replaced hip (*THP*) may be a sign of active infection. This scan is obtained along the metal of the femoral neck and is slightly oblique along the prosthesis. The image is focused over the junction between the metal stem and the native femoral cortex, providing easy access for ultrasound guided aspiration. The effusion (*E*) in this hip is surrounded by pulsatile flow artifacts. **C**, Hyperemia in prosthetic hip replacement: transverse ultrasound with power Doppler sonography. Same patient as in **A**. Power Doppler sonography was continued during joint aspiration. This technique facilitates the procedure, helps to avoid larger vessels, and improves visualization of the needle path by imaging tissue motion (*open arrows*). The needle type is shown over the metal of the femoral neck of the prosthesis (*N*). The fluid obtained with ultrasound guidance grew *Staphylococcus aureus*. Abbreviation: transverse orientation (*TRV*).

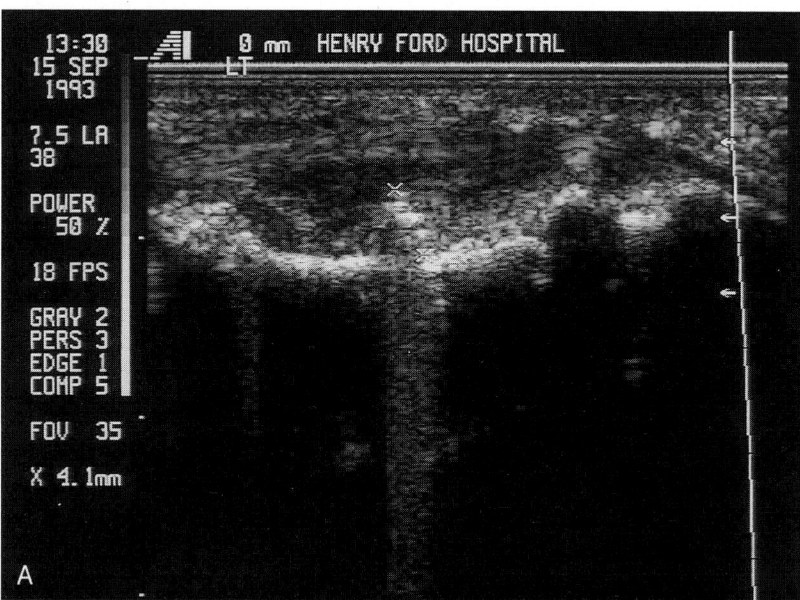

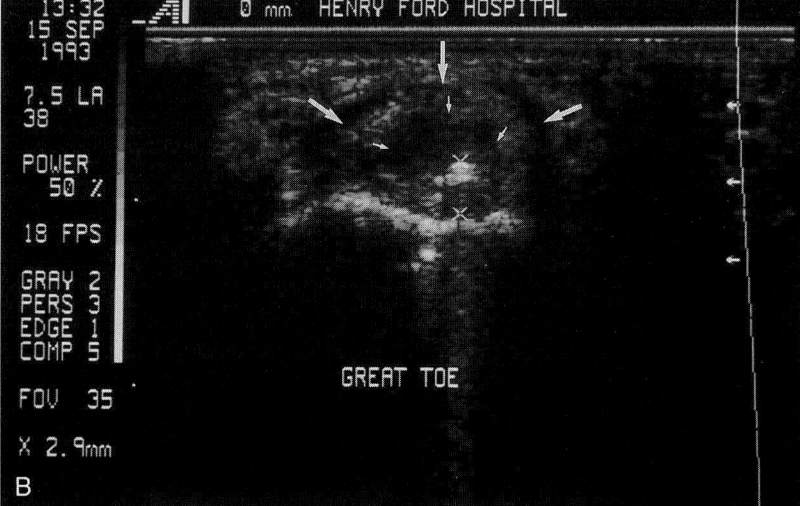

Figure 12–28 ▪ **A**, Tendon erosion by screw: longitudinal ultrasound. This middle-aged woman, who had undergone arthrodesis of the great toe with plate and screw fixation, experienced unbearable postoperative pain. The pain was greatest along the plantar aspect of the great toe. This longitudinal scan along the plantar aspect of the great toe reveals irregularity of the flexor digitorum tendon (*t*). This tendon appears to be frayed (*curved arrow*) by a protruding screw (between calipers). Four threads of the screw can be identified beyond the cortex. The total length of the protruding screw segment is 4.1 mm. The metatarsophalangeal joint is on the left side of the image, and the more distal interphalangeal joint lies at the right. **B**, Tendon erosion by screw: transverse ultrasound. Same patient as in **A**. A focal defect (*small arrows*) measuring three-fifths of the tendon's girth is identified in the central aspect of the tendon (*arrows*). The screw tip (between calipers) penetrates deep into this erosion. Removal of the screw resulted in immediate relief of the pain.

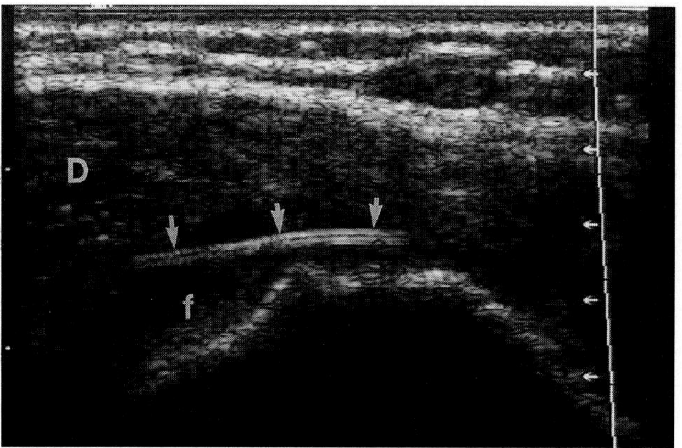

Figure 12–29 ▪ Loose suture in the shoulder: transverse ultrasound. One year after surgery, this 74-year-old man complained of constant pain in his shoulder. Ultrasound study of the rotator cuff showed retear of the supraspinatus, shoulder synovitis (*f*), and loose sutures (*small arrows*). Surgical debridement and reconstruction of the rotator cuff with placement of graft followed. Abbreviation: deltoid muscle (*D*).

bodies. In difficult cases, real-time sonographic examination can facilitate surgical removal of the foreign body. Sonography can also be very useful in the evaluation of orthopedic implants, both postoperatively and in long-term follow-up.

References

Anderson MA, Newmeyer WL, Kilgore ES: Diagnosis and treatment of retained foreign bodies in the hand. *Am J Surg* 144:63, 1982.

Cochrane WJ: Ultrasound and the intrauterine device. In Sanders RC, James AE (eds): *Principles and Practice of Ultrasonography in Obstetrics and Gynecology*. Norwalk, CT, Appleton-Century-Crofts, 1985, pp 597–602.

Crawford R, Matheson AB: Clinical value of ultrasonography in the detection and removal of radiolucent foreign bodies. *Injury* 20:341–343, 1989.

Donaldson J: Radiographic imaging of foreign bodies in the hands. *Hand Clin* 7:125–134, 1991.

Failla JM, van Holsbeeck MT, Vanderschueren G: Detection of a 0.5-mm-thick thorn using ultrasound: A case report. *J Hand Surg [Am]* 20:456–457, 1995.

Flomm LL, Ellis GL: Radiologic evaluation of foreign bodies. *Emerg Med Clin North Am* 10:163–176, 1992.

Fornage BD: Peripheral nerves of the extremities: Imaging with ultrasound. *Radiology* 167:179–182, 1988.

Fornage BD, Schernberg FL: Sonographic diagnosis of foreign bodies of the distal extremities. *AJR* 147: 567–569, 1986.

Gilbert FJ, Campbell RSD, Bayliss AP: The role of ultrasound in the detection of nonradiopaque foreign bodies. *Clin Radiol* 41:109–112, 1990.

Gooding GAW, et al: Sonography of the hand and foot in foreign body detection. *J Ultrasound Med* 6:441–447, 1987.

Graf R, Schuler P: *Sonographie am Stutz und Bewegungsapparat bei Erwachsenen und Kindern*. Weinheim, Edition Medizin VCH, 1988.

Harle TS, Beard EF: Migration of Steinman pins. *AJR* 100(3):542–545, 1967.

Harris WH, et al: Extensive localized bone resorption in the femur following total hip replacement. *J Bone Joint Surg [Am]* 58:612–618, 1976.

Hassani SN, Bard RL: Real-time ophthalmic ultrasonography. *Radiology* 127:213, 1978.

Howden, MD: Foreign bodies within finge-tendon sheaths demonstrated by ultrasound: Two cases. *Clin Radiol* 49:419–420, 1994.

Jacobson JA, et al: Wooden foreign bodies in soft tissue: Detection at ultrasound. *Radiology* 206:45–48, 1998.

Leonard JW, Gifford RW: Migration of Kirschner wire from clavicle into pulmonary artery. *Am J Cardiol* 16:598–600, 1965.

Little CM, et al: The ultrasonic detection of soft tissue foreign bodies. *Invest Radiol* 21:275–277, 1986.

Magnussen PA, Crozier AE, Gregg PJ: Detecting haematomas by ultrasound: Brief report. *J Bone Joint Surg [Br]* 70:150, 1988.

Milgram JW: *Radiologic and Histologic Pathology of Nontumorous Diseases of Bones and Joints*, vol 2. Northbrook, IL, Northbrook Publishing Co, 1990.

Mizel MS, Steinmetz ND, Trepman E: Detection of wooden foreign bodies in muscle tissue: Experimental comparison of computed tomography, magnetic resonance imaging, and ultrasonography. *Foot Ankle Int* 15:437–443, 1994.

Rajamani K, Fisher M: Bullet embolism. *N Engl J Med* 339(12):812, 1998.

Resnick D, Niwayama G: *Diagnosis of Bone and Joint Disorders*. Philadelphia, WB Saunders Co, 1988.

Russell RC, et al: Detection of foreign bodies in the hand. *J Hand Surg [Am]* 16:2–11, 1991.

Schlager D, et al: Ultrasound for the detection of foreign bodies. *Ann Emerg Med* 20:189–191, 1991.

Shiels WE, et al: Localization and guided removal of soft-tissue foreign bodies with sonography. *AJR* 155: 1277–1281, 1990.

Stein JH: *Internal Medicine*, ed 4. St Louis, Mosby–Year Book, 1996.

van Holsbeeck M, et al: Staging and follow-up of rheumatoid arthritis of the knee. Comparison of sonography, thermography, and clinical assessment. *J Ultrasound Med* 7:561–566, 1988.

van Holsbeeck MT, et al: Detection of infection in loosened hip prostheses: Efficacy of sonography. *AJR* 163: 381–384, 1994.

Weill FW: *Ultrasonography of Digestive Diseases*. St Louis, CV Mosby Co, 1978.

Wilson PD, et al: The problem of infection in endoprosthetic surgery of the hip joint. *Clin Orthop* 96: 213–221, 1973.

Chapter 13
Sonography of Pain Syndromes Following Arthroscopy

Arthroscopy has proved its value as a diagnostic and therapeutic tool with regard to knee pathology. Refinements in technique over the last 15 years have expanded its role in therapy and enabled its use in examining other joints. Its application remains primarily in the knee, but it is now being used increasingly in the shoulder, ankle, elbow, wrist, and hip (Table 13–1). All surgical procedures have an inherent risk of complications. As arthroscopy has become more sophisticated, the risk associated with these procedures has increased. Early studies by the Arthroscopy Association of North America reported an overall complication rate of 0.6%, but this reflected only first-generation procedures. A subsequent study that included second-generation procedures reported an overall complication rate of 1.8%, with the highest incidence of complications reported for lateral retinacular release (8.0%) (Fig. 13–1). Other reports have stated complication rates as high as 20% for subcutaneous lateral release (Metcalf, 1982). The range of complications includes hemarthrosis, loose bodies, infection, thromboembolic disease, instrument failure, neuromuscular deficit, and vascular injury. Many of these complications are well evaluated with ultrasound.

Pain Syndromes Following Therapeutic Arthroscopy

The vast majority of patients experience considerable improvement or complete resolution of their symptoms following arthroscopic surgery. However, a small group continue to experience pain following an arthroscopic procedure that was considered a surgical success. In some of these patients, the character of the discomfort differs from that experienced prior to surgery. Often ultrasound is helpful in evaluating these patients. Therapeutic arthroscopy is more invasive than diagnostic arthroscopy, requiring at least two access portals and frequently three (Fig. 13–2). One portal is used for viewing, and the others are used for grasping and cutting. Some orthopedic surgeons prefer a transtendinous approach for one of the portals, the Swedish technique. In this approach, access to the joint is obtained through the patellar tendon approximately 1 cm below the patellar apex. This provides access equidistant from the anterolateral and anteromedial portals. Rigidity of the tendon helps to avoid crowding of the portals. Damage to the tendon is minimized by using a sharp obturator to penetrate into the joint. Some patients develop pain and tenderness over the anterior aspect of the knee centered over the transtendinous portal.

Patellar tendinitis (Fig. 13–3) is the most frequent sonographic finding in these patients. Thickening and decreased echogenicity of the tendon may be observed for a period of up to 2 years following arthroscopy (van Holsbeeck and Introcaso, 1989). Sometimes a cleft will be observed in the tendon. These clefts are associated with significant weakening of the tendon and should be regarded as incomplete tears (Figs. 13–4 and 13–5). In all cases, Hoffa's fat pad becomes hyperechoic relative to the tendon. Often a hypoechoic tract will be noted traversing the subcutaneous fat, the tendon, and Hoffa's fat pad. This tract corresponds to the arthroscopic portal. The fat pad is under compression in both full extension and flexion. Occasionally, fat will be identified herniating through the defect in the patellar tendon. When present, the incarcerated fat prevents normal healing of the tendon.

Hoffa's fat pad is a highly vascular fibroadipose structure that extends medially and laterally to cover the anterior horns of the menisci. All of the commonly used anterior access portals pass through Hoffa's fat pad. After surgical trauma, the patient may experience chronic pain originating from the point of penetration through the fat pad. Several

Table 13–1
Approximate Distribution of Arthroscopic Procedures by Site (%)

Knee	84.7
Shoulder	12.3
Ankle	1.3
Elbow	0.9
Wrist	0.7

reports of surgical exploration of the fat pad in these patients have demonstrated foci of granulomatous reaction (Lindenbaum, 1981; Dandy, 1987). Following resection of these granulomatous lesions, symptoms resolved. Fibrosis of the fat pad at the site of surgical trauma may also occur, resulting in chronic pain. The combination of fibrosis and hyperplasia producing a sclerotic region within the fat pad and anterior retinaculum may also produce pain. In severe cases, limitation of motion will

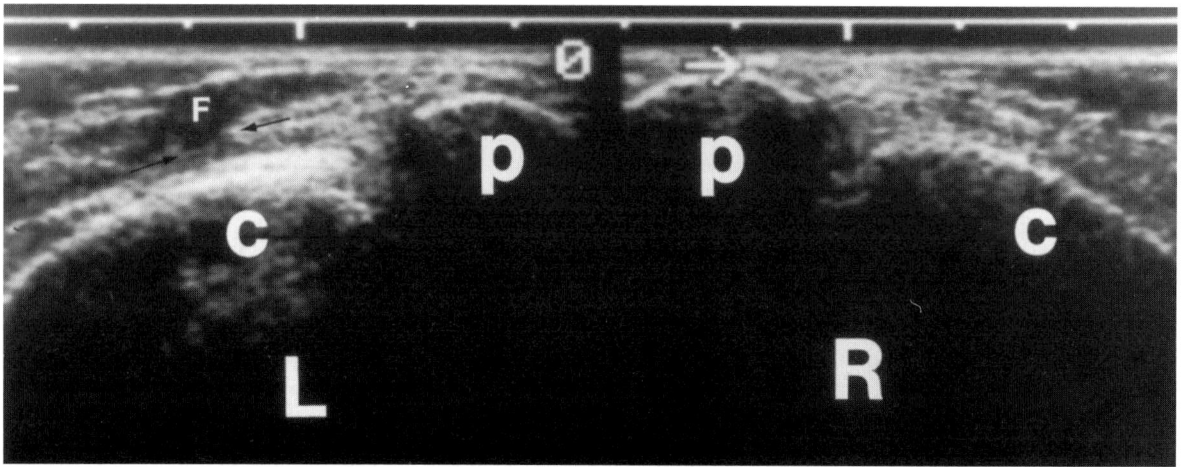

Figure 13–1 ■ Painful ganglion: transverse sonogram. The patient is a 19-year-old woman who underwent an arthroscopic lateral retinacular release 7 months ago. She presented with pain and swelling lateral to the left patella. Side-to-side comparison is provided in this split-screen image. On the left is a transverse image of the symptomatic lateral aspect of the left patellofemoral joint. The asymptomatic side is on the right. A fluid-filled cavity (*F*) is identified lateral to the patella (*p*) in direct communication with the joint through an interruption in the lateral retinaculum (*arrows*). Extravasation of synovial fluid is a common complication following arthroscopic procedures. Rarely, these collections may form fistulas to the skin. Abbreviations: lateral femoral condyle (*C*), left (*L*), right (*R*).

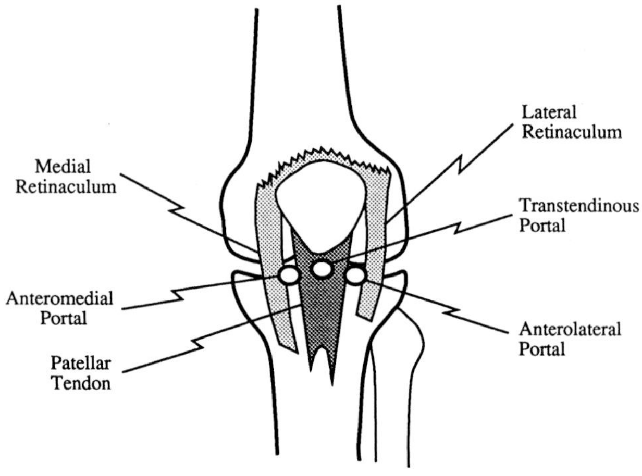

Figure 13–2 ■ Portals for therapeutic arthroscopy.

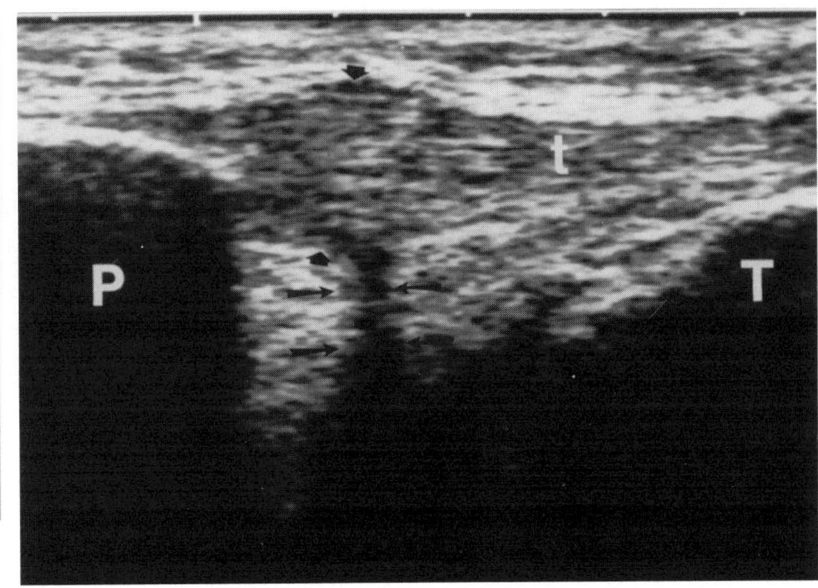

Figure 13–3 ■ Patellar tendinitis after arthroscopy: longitudinal sonogram. One and one-half years after arthroscopy, this 32-year-old male tennis player continued to have pain. This pain differed from the pain for which arthroscopy was performed and forced him to stop all athletic activity. Clinical examination revealed pain, swelling, and tenderness just below the apex of the patella. A segment of the patellar tendon (*t*) is markedly thickened (*small arrows*) and hypoechoic, indicative of patellar tendinitis. Immediately deep to the involved tendon segment is a hypoechoic tract traversing Hoffa's fat pad (*large arrows*). This is the characteristic appearance of an arthroscopic portal through the fat pad. The focal nature of the tendon abnormality associated with the transtendinous portal clearly indicates that this is a complication of the arthroscopic procedure. Abbreviations: patella (*P*), tibia (*T*).

develop (Paulos et al., 1987). Herniation of a portion of the fat pad through the extensor fascia has also been observed (Lindenbaum, 1981). Again, surgical repair is required.

Sonography will also demonstrate neuromas resulting from surgical trauma at the access portal. Cutaneous sensation over the anterior aspect of the knee is provided by the infrapatellar division of the saphenous nerve. Saphenous nerve damage is most frequently a complication of meniscal repair procedures (Fig. 13–6), but small anterior branches may be damaged in any surgical procedure. Conservative therapy that includes injection of local anesthetic and steroids is often successful. Surgical excision is rarely indicated. Cyst formation at the arthroscopic portal is not uncommon. Usually these cysts are lined by synovium and therefore are referred to as *synovial cysts*. If the wall of the cyst is predominantly fibrotic, it is called a *ganglion* (Figs. 13–7 and 13–8). These cysts typically have a pedunculated appearance with a narrow base originating at the access portal (van Holsbeeck and Introcaso,

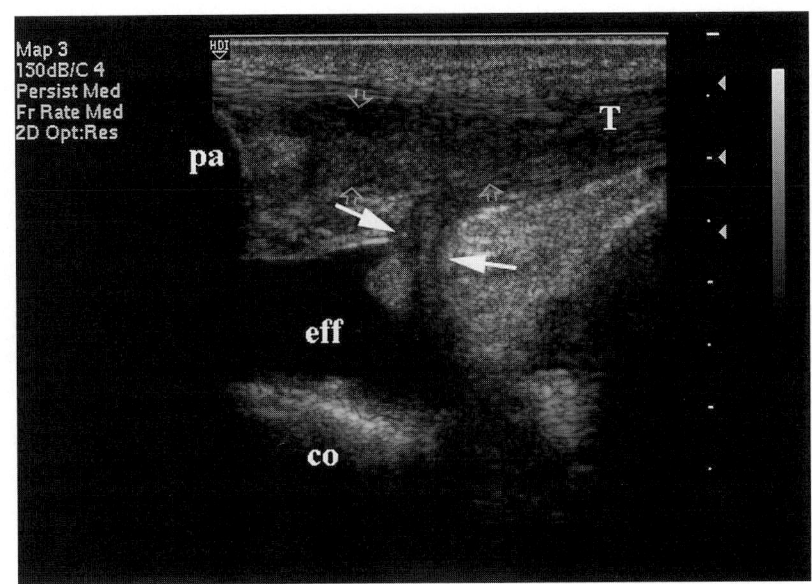

Figure 13–4 ■ Postarthroscopy knee swelling: longitudinal ultrasound. Bothered by continued knee swelling, this 35-year-old man visits the outpatient clinic six months after medial meniscectomy. Knee swelling and discomfort interfere with daily activities, and he is unhappy with the postsurgical outcome. The longitudinal view through the midline of the knee along the patellar tendon shows disruption of the fibrillar pattern of the tendon (*open arrows*), with focal edema suggestive of patellar tendinitis. The arthroscopic portal is noted through Hoffa's fat pad (*arrows*). A knee effusion (*eff*) covers the femoral condyles (*co*). The patellar tendon abnormality is worse around the apex (*pa*) of the patella.

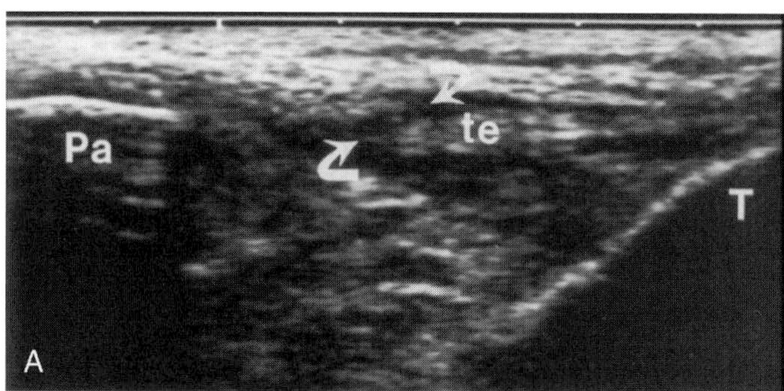

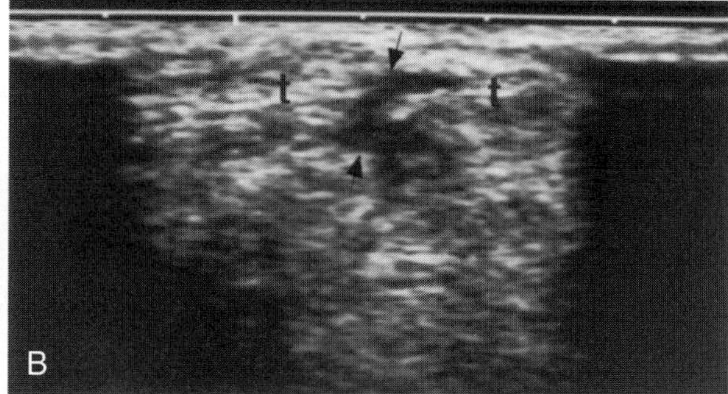

Figure 13–5 ■ **A,** Incomplete patellar tendon rupture: longitudinal sonogram. This 41-year-old man experienced pain and focal tenderness beneath the left patellar apex 8 months following therapeutic arthroscopy. He also exhibited weakened extension of the lower leg. The longitudinal image of the left patellar tendon (*te*) demonstrates a gap (*curved arrows*) in the patellar tendon at the site of the transtendinous portal. Abbreviations: patellar apex (*Pa*), tibia (*T*). **B,** Incomplete patellar tendon rupture: transverse sonogram. Same patient as in **A**. The transducer is positioned transversely over the point of maximal tenderness. A hypoechoic gap (*arrows*) is again noted in the tendon (*t*). Normal-appearing tendon is present on both the medial and lateral sides of this partial rupture.

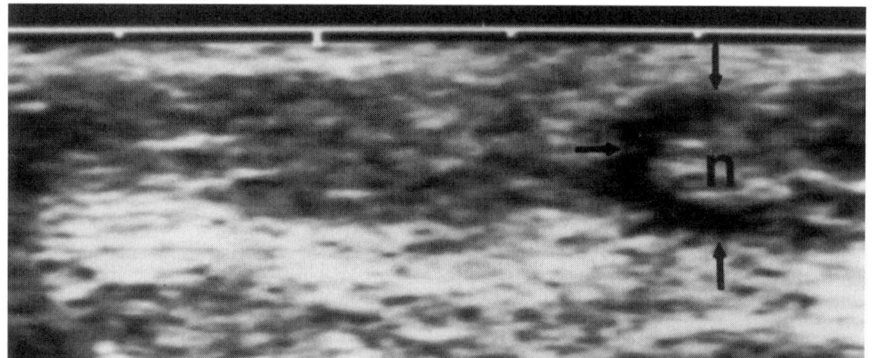

Figure 13–6 ■ Traumatic subcutaneous neuroma: transverse sonogram. This 45-year-old woman presented with pain and extreme tenderness at the medial aspect of the right knee 1½ years after arthroscopic repair of a meniscal tear. The transducer is positioned over the scar of the painful anterior medial portal. A crescentic anechoic fluid collection (*arrows*) borders a hyperechoic mass (*n*) continuous with the infrapatellar nerve. Surgical exploration revealed a neuroma of the infrapatellar nerve.

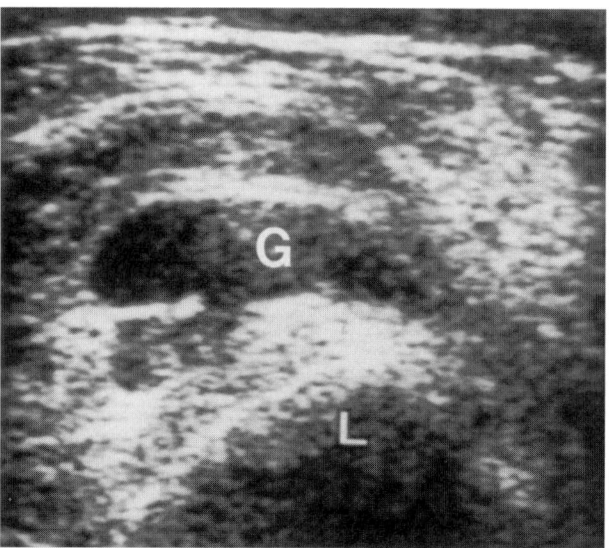

Figure 13–7 ■ Periarticular ganglion after arthroscopy: transverse sonogram. This large ganglion (*G*) was demonstrated at the anterior lateral arthroscopic portal in this 50-year-old woman. Arthroscopy was performed 2 years ago. Several months ago, the patient noted a painful swelling over the lateral femoral condyle (*L*). Surgery demonstrated a ganglion continuous with the joint at the site of the anterior lateral portal.

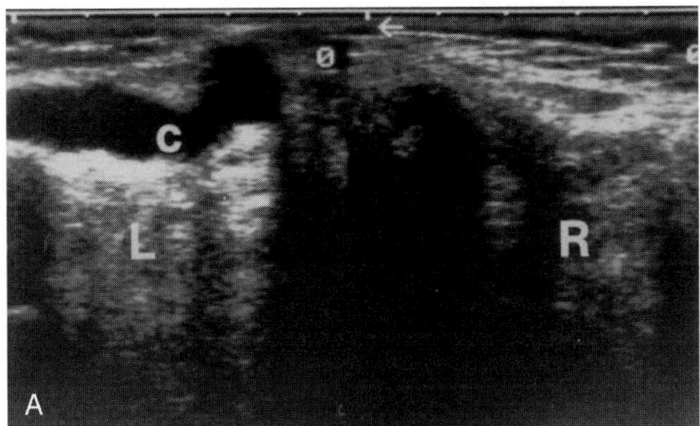

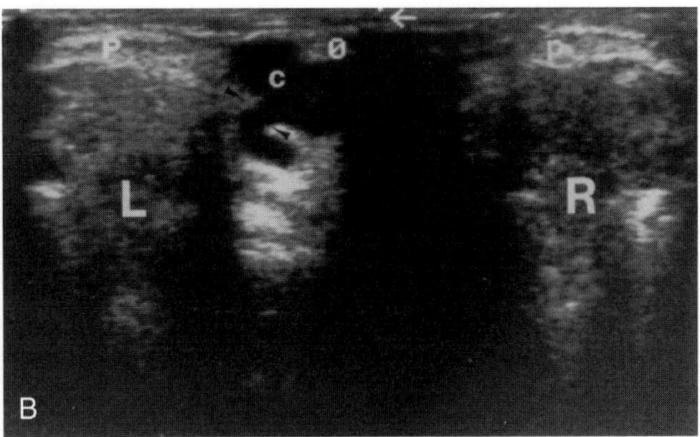

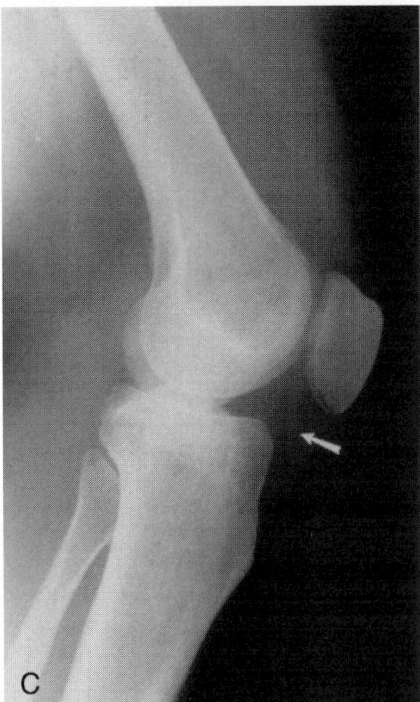

Figure 13–8 ▪ **A,** Portal ganglion: oblique sonogram. A 26-year-old woman presented with pain and swelling over the medial portal adjacent to the patellar tendon. The image on the left is an oblique image of the symptomatic left knee over the point of tenderness. A comparable image of the asymptomatic right knee is on the right. An anechoic fluid collection (*c*) continuous with the arthroscopic portal is seen. It extends laterally and superiorly through Hoffa's fat pad. Abbreviations: left (*L*), right (*R*). **B,** Portal ganglion: transverse sonogram. Same patient as in **A**. The transducer is now positioned transversely over the point of greatest swelling. Again, a split-screen comparison is provided. A point of communication with the joint through the retinaculum (*arrowheads*) is better demonstrated in this image. Abbreviations: patellar tendon (*P*), ganglion cyst (*c*). **C,** Portal ganglion: lateral radiograph. Same patient as in **A** and **B**. This lateral radiograph is essentially normal. Minimal streaky density is seen in Hoffa's fat pad (*arrow*).

1989). Fluid within these cysts is markedly hypoechoic or anechoic. Rarely, meniscal fragments or other tissue fragments may become trapped in these cysts. This is most commonly seen when a fragment slips from the grasp of a surgical instrument while being removed from the joint. An arteriovenous fistula can also develop in Hoffa's fat pad. The stab from the arthroscope may result in a communication between medium-sized vessels and may cause rapid shunting of blood (Ptasznik, 1999).

Fluid escaping from the joint at the access portals is another complication; it is easily diagnosed with sonography. During the procedure, irrigation fluid may extravasate from the joint. This is rarely significant, but when it is extensive, it has been known to result in compartment syndrome requiring fasciotomy (Peek and Haynes, 1984; Fruensgaard and Holm, 1988). Sonography is extremely valuable in the diagnosis of compartment syndrome. The diagnosis of compartment syndrome is discussed in detail in Chapter 3. Synovial fluid leaking into the subcutaneous tissues can cause significant inflammation and discomfort, sometimes mimicking venous thrombosis. Ultrasound is extremely valuable in making the definitive diagnosis in these cases. When gas is used for arthroscopy, subcutaneous emphysema, pneumoscrotum, pneumoperitoneum, and pneumopericardium may occur (Dick et al., 1978; Henderson and Hopson, 1982; Lotman, 1987). Partial airway obstruction has also been reported (Shupak et al., 1984). Cases of gas extravasation are best evaluated with conventional radiographs.

Vascular complications following arthroscopy are predominantly cases of deep venous thrombosis (Cohen et al., 1973; Walker and Dillingham, 1983). The incidence of deep venous thrombosis is greatest in patients more than 50 years of age and when

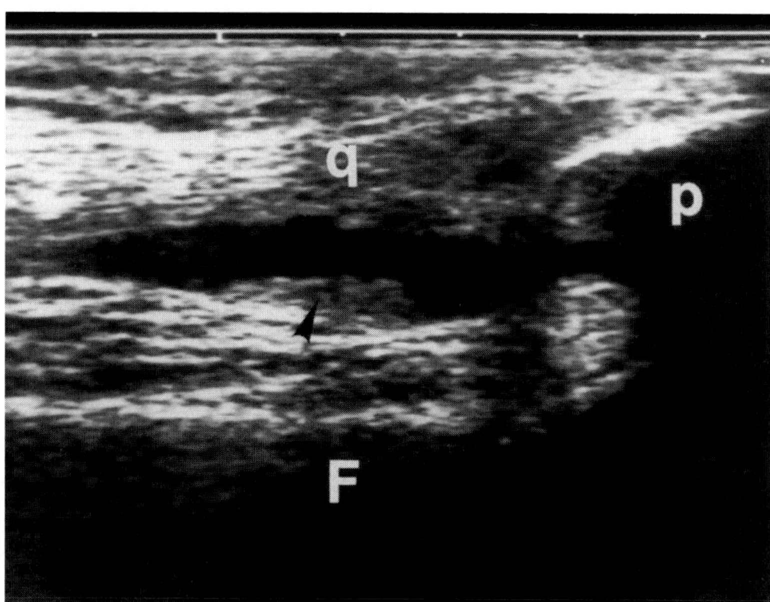

Figure 13-9 ▪ Hemarthrosis following arthroscopy: longitudinal sonogram. This 30-year-old soccer player had arthroscopic medial meniscectomy 5 days ago. He was admitted for increased swelling of the knee and slight fever. A large effusion is noted in the suprapatellar bursa. Several blood clots (*arrowhead*) were noted moving freely within the joint. Joint aspiration was performed and yielded frank blood. Cultures were negative. Abbreviations: femur (*F*), patella (*p*), quadriceps (*q*).

tourniquet time exceeds 1 hour (Sherman et al., 1986). This has become an increasing problem as arthroscopic procedures have become more sophisticated and as the duration of these procedures has increased. Doppler techniques and compression ultrasound examination for deep venous thrombosis have demonstrated their value (Lensing et al., 1989). The absence of a Doppler signal alone may not be adequate to make the diagnosis of deep venous thrombosis. In cases of very slow flow, a Doppler signal may not be detected due to filter threshold. Compression examination should be used to confirm the absence of a Doppler signal. If a vein is not compressible when pressure is applied with the transducer, thrombus must be present.

Arterial pseudoaneurysm is a very rare complication of arthroscopy (Kvist and Ksaergaard, 1979; Sherman et al., 1986). It occurs secondary to perforation of the posterior joint capsule by sharp instruments, adjacent to the popliteal vessels. Some of these accidents have resulted in death or amputation (Sherman et al., 1986). If a diagnostic test is required, the correct diagnosis is quickly established with sonography. Ultrasound images will demonstrate a popliteal mass continuous with the artery. A Doppler signal may be absent within the aneurysm due to thrombosis. Mural thrombus will be seen as hypoechoic material layering peripherally or completely filling the pseudoaneurysm. Emergent excision and graft placement are indicated because the natural history of these vascular lesions is inevitable rupture.

Instrument breakage (see Fig. 12-1) is a complication that has decreased in incidence recently, perhaps due in part to refinement of instrument design (Sprague, 1989). It is most often associated with partial lateral meniscectomy procedures. When fragments are located in the peripheral recesses of the joint or subcutaneous tissues, ultrasound can be of significant benefit. The approach to these situations is identical to that used for any foreign body, as outlined in Figure 12-16. However, if instrument fragments are located deep within the joint, conventional radiography is the examination of choice. Instrument fragments tend to have sharp edges, causing them to remain fixed in location when deep within the joint. In contract, tissue fragments may become lost within the joint during arthroscopy. Meniscal fragments or pieces of osteophyte lost within the joint will migrate to the peripheral synovial recesses. Once sequestered within the synovial recesses, they are easily detected with sonography (see Fig. 8-46).

Hemarthrosis is the most common complication following both therapeutic and diagnostic arthroscopy. To be considered a complication, bleeding into the joint must be of sufficient magnitude to require intervention (Fig. 13-9). Significant hemarthrosis requires evacuation for two reasons: formation of adhesions and infection. Often untreated hemarthrosis will result in the formation of adhesions within the joint during the process of resolution. Adhesions may limit the range of motion of the joint and may cause chronic pain. A second

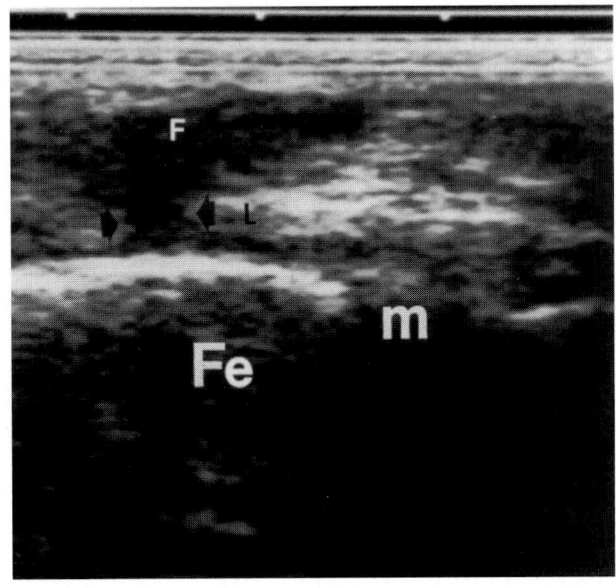

Figure 13–10 ■ Medial collateral ligament rupture secondary to arthroscopy: coronal sonogram. Four days after an arthroscopic medial meniscectomy, this 35-year-old man presented with a complaint of progressively increasing swelling over the medial aspect of the knee. The proximal aspect is at the observer's left. A disruption (*arrows*) is noted in the medial collateral ligament (*L*). Fluid (*F*) extends through the gap and pools beneath the skin in the subcutaneous tissue. Acute ruptures of the medial collateral ligament may be due to excessive valgus stress applied during the procedure or an overaggressive incision. Abbreviations: femur (*Fe*), meniscus (*m*).

surgical procedure is required to lyse these adhesions. Capsular rupture is one cause of hemarthrosis. Often these lesions go unrecognized. Involvement of the medial collateral ligament is a severe form of capsular rupture that greatly reduces joint stability. Rupture of the medial collateral ligament during an arthroscopic procedure is rare but may result from excessive valgus stress applied in an attempt to visualize the medial compartment more clearly (Fig. 13–10). Peripheral extension of the meniscectomy incision into the medial collateral ligament can also result in rupture. Infection is the second most common complication of arthroscopic procedures. The risk of infection is considerably increased when hemarthrosis is present. Therefore, evacuation of significant intra-articular hemorrhage is recommended. In these cases, sonography is used to detect and characterize abnormal intra-articular fluid collections. Ultrasound is exquisitely sensitive in detecting increased intra-articular fluid, far more sensitive than aspiration (van Holsbeeck et al., 1988). If needed, ultrasound guidance can be provided for aspiration to obtain fluid for culture.

Pain Following Diagnostic Arthroscopy

The spectrum of complications related to diagnostic arthroscopy is identical to that of therapeutic arthroscopy. They differ only in incidence. Fewer complications are seen following diagnostic procedures because they tend to be less invasive and tourniquet times are considerably shorter. As stated earlier, the two most frequent complications are hemarthrosis and infection.

Pain that persists following a normal diagnostic arthroscopic procedure is usually not attributable to a complication of the procedure. It is more likely that the cause of the pain lies outside of the diagnostic range of the arthroscope. Arthroscopy is excellent for the evaluation of intra-articular pathology, but it cannot evaluate the periarticular structures. Examination of the posterior horns and the peripheral areas of the menisci is limited and requires extensive manipulation through multiple ports (Weisman and Sledge, 1986). This increases the risk of complications.

Ultrasound and MRI have great utility in the evaluation of the periarticular tissues. Low cost, wide availability, and capability for dynamic examination make ultrasound the favored examination for periarticular structures. Sonography can evaluate posterior and peripheral meniscal lesions far better than arthroscopy. Meniscal cysts associated with small degenerative meniscal tears are particularly well evaluated by ultrasound (Coral et al., 1989). These lesions are completely overlooked by arthroscopy. Sonography has demonstrated that these lesions occur far more frequently than was previously thought. Peripheral meniscal lesions are commonly associated with collateral ligament and capsular injuries. These lesions are easily evaluated in the same ultrasound examination. In acute injury, small hematomas within the substance of the collateral ligaments can be demonstrated. Chronic intrasubstance injury of the medial collateral ligament (type

I and II lesions) is also well demonstrated. These lesions are discussed in detail in Chapter 6. Overall, sonography is excellent for the evaluation of lesions that lie outside of the diagnostic range of arthroscopy. The role of MRI often complements that of ultrasound. In knee imaging, MRI will assist in evaluating subacute or chronic anterior cruciate ligament tears and uncomplicated meniscal tears. In the shoulder, MRI arthrography may still be better than ultrasound in evaluating labral pathology; however, this type of arthrography is invasive and labor intensive and comes at a cost that society may not be willing to pay routinely. The choice between MRI, ultrasound, and diagnostic arthroscopy is a complicated one often made by the referring physician. Imagers should assist in making a choice between different diagnostic techniques. The choice should be driven by cost efficiency, and the chosen procedure should be minimally invasive.

References

Cohen SH, et al: Thrombophlebitis following knee surgery. *J Bone Joint Surg* [*Am*] 55A:106–112, 1973.

Coral A, van Holsbeeck M, Adler R: Imaging of meniscal cysts of the knee in three cases. *Skeletal Radiol* 18: 451–455, 1989.

Dandy DJ: *Arthroscopic Management of the Knee*, ed 2. New York, Churchill-Livingstone, 1987.

Dick W, et al: Complications of arthroscopy. A review of 3714 cases. *Arch Orthop Trauma Surg* 92:69–73, 1978.

Fruensgaard S, Holm A: Compartment syndrome complicating arthroscopic surgery: Brief report. *J Bone Joint Surg* [*Br*] 70:146–147, 1988.

Henderson CE, Hopson CN: Pneumoscrotum as a complication of arthroscopy. *J Bone Joint Surg* 8:1238–1240, 1982.

Kvist E, Ksaergaard E: Vascular injury complicating meniscectomy. Report of a case. *Acta Chir Scand* 145: 191–193, 1979.

Lensing AWA, et al: Detection of deep-vein thrombosis by real-time B-mode ultrasonography. *N Engl J Med* 320:342–345, 1989.

Lindenbaum BL: Complications of knee joint arthroscopy. *Clin Orthop* 160:158, 1981.

Lotman DB: Pneumoperitoneum and acidosis during arthroscopy with CO_2. *Arthroscopy* 3:185–186, 1987.

Metcalf RW: An arthroscopic method for lateral release of subluxating or dislocating patella. *Clin Orthop* 167:9, 1982.

Paulos LE, et al: Infrapatellar contracture syndrome, an unrecognized cause of knee stiffness with patellar entrapment and patella infera. *Am J Sports Med* 15: 331–341, 1987.

Peek RD, Haynes DW: Compartment syndrome as a complication of arthroscopy: A case report and a study of interstitial pressure. *Am J Sports Med* 12:464–468, 1984.

Ptasnik R: Ultrasound in acute and chronic knee injury. *Radiol Clin North Am* 37(4):797–830, 1999.

Sherman OH, et al: Arthroscopy—"no problem surgery." *J Bone Joint Surg* [*Am*] 68:256–265, 1986.

Shupak RC, Shuster H, Funch R: Airway emergency in a patient during CO_2 arthroscopy: Report of a case. *Anesthesiology* 60:161–172, 1984.

Sprague NF: *Complications in Arthroscopy*. New York, Raven Press, 1989.

van Holsbeeck M, et al: Staging and follow-up of rheumatoid arthritis of the knee. *J Ultrasound Med* 7:561–566, 1988.

van Holsbeeck M, Introcaso J: Ultrasound follow-up of knee arthroscopy. *Orthop Today* 9:10, 1989.

Walker RH, Dillingham M: Thrombophlebitis following arthroscopic surgery of the knee. *Contemp Orthop* 6: 29–33, 1983.

Weissman BNW, Sledge CB: *Orthopedic Radiology*. Philadelphia, WB Saunders Co, 1986.

Chapter 14 Interventional Musculoskeletal Ultrasound

Ultrasound detects abscesses (Loyer et al., 1996) and diagnoses septic complications of surgery (van Holsbeeck and Introcaso, 1992; van Holsbeeck et al., 1994). Within joints, sonography can distinguish simple effusion from synovial inflammation, and in patients with soft tissue tumor, ultrasound can separate solid cellular masses from vascular tissue and tumor necrosis (Rubens et al., 1997). Because of these unique features, we choose ultrasound to guide our procedures in most soft tissue processes. Recent technological developments have made it possible to sample tissues with minimal invasiveness. Noteworthy in that respect are thin coaxial bone and soft tissue biopsy needles specifically designed to allow maximum visibility in the ultrasound field of view and color Doppler sonography and vibration technology to detect needle placement. There is no limit to the size of the lesion that can be sampled. Practically, this means that if a lesion can be seen with ultrasound, it can be targeted for biopsy using ultrasound (Rubens et al., 1997). Often our choice between aspiration needles and biopsy devices is based entirely on the findings of the ultrasound exam.

Examination Technique

The equipment used for an interventional musculoskeletal ultrasound study is a combination of equipment used for a routine musculoskeletal ultrasound study and equipment needed for arthrography. High-frequency transducers with a center frequency of 5 MHz and above are needed. Those transducers may be equipped with a biopsy guide for convenience. In our practice, we use 7.5-, 10-, and 13-MHz transducers with a linear footprint and a 5-MHz curved linear array transducer. The last transducer may be necessary for optimal beam penetration in larger patients and for deep-seated structures. This is important for imaging the popliteal space, the hip, and the posterior shoulder (Gaucher et al., 1997). High elevational frequency is critical in the choice of transducers. These transducers provide sharper definition of the margins of the lesion. Transducers focused at different depths are best suited for this type of examination. If these transducers are not available, the examiner should know the depth at which transducers are focused. Standoff pads are not recommended because of the difficulty of working under sterile conditions.

A full ultrasonographic examination should be completed first (Rubens et al., 1997). This study must show the mass or the area in which the procedure is planned. This will allow us to mark the field that must be prepared for the procedure. Mass characterization with ultrasound is highly dependent upon technical factors. The transducer selected should be appropriate for the size and depth of the abnormality. The focal zone should be centered at the depth of the lesion, and the gain settings should be adjusted to allow differentiation of simple cysts and solid masses. Settings should not be so high that too many echoes are placed within simple cysts. This is important in musculoskeletal imaging because higher-frequency transducers will often show internal echos within cysts due to significant frequency dependent backscatter. By the same token, power and time gain compensation settings should not be too low to prevent recognition of internal echos that are truly present in a mass. A rate of over 12 frames per second is necessary to avoid missing lesions between successive frames during scan sweeps.

Using coordinates, one can indicate the preferred access route. There is no single correct method for performing interventional procedures with ultrasound imaging guidance. We can use either freehand scanning with or without a needle guide. The equipment on hand and the experience of the physician performing the procedure will often determine selection of the technique.

In patients with small lesions, it may be advisable to follow the route of the needle entry. A transducer with small footprint, a transducer cover, and sterile gel will then be needed for the procedure. If the needle entry is aligned with the transducer, one may be able to follow the entire shaft of the needle. Once the needle is in the lesion, it is necessary to check the location of the needle tip in the transverse plane to avoid inappropriate placement secondary to partial volume averaging. Transverse images will show the needle as a single dot. Prior to biopsy or aspiration, this dot should be located in the center of the mass. We puncture the skin away from the transducer in order to work as sterilely as possible. Others may choose to enter the skin next to the footprint of the transducer, with the needle shaft and transducer shaft in parallel.

Local anesthetic is necessary to decrease pain during the procedure. Isotonic solutions avoid the stinging that normally accompanies injection of Lidocaine. The local anesthetic is applied generously along the course that will be traversed by the biopsy needle. Take care not to inject air bubbles because they may obscure the region of interest. Ultrasonic guidance can be used to aid infiltration of anesthetic around the mass. This is important when the lesion is expected to have several neural elements in or around the lesion. Also, in performing bone biopsies under ultrasound guidance, it is important to infiltrate the periosteum excessively at the biopsy site because of the hypersensitivity of the periosteal envelope. Application of a local anesthetic (Emla cream), which is resorbed transdermally under cover of a patch, may be very helpful in young children. This patch is applied approximately 45 minutes prior to the procedure. The perception of a needle will stop all cooperation in most children under 6 years of age. Therefore, we perform the procedure rapidly in these children without further local anesthesia once the patch starts to work.

A small incision is often required before introduction of a 16-gauge or larger biopsy needle. A coaxial needle system does not always require a skin incision. A surgical blade (No. 10, for example) and suture material should be available in case the opening created causes esthetic problems afterward. Aspirations are performed with 1- or 2-inch needles or with spinal needles for deeper-seated structures. It may be necessary to resort to longer needles, such as Ciba or Wescott needles, in patients with morbid obesity. A variety of systems are available for soft tissue and synovial biopsy. The Tru-Cut needle is easily visible sonographically; it has centimeter marks to follow the depth of penetration. The needle can be pushed up to the edge of the targeted lesion; the biopsy guillotine must be pushed into the lesion and the system then fired. Become familiar with the throw-length of your biopsy system. This will allow you to sample the tissues of interest and avoid vital structures. Bone biopsy needles end in a cylindrical "corkscrew" (Fig. 14–1) at the tip. The teeth cut into the bone when a rotary motion is applied to the ends of the needles. For large specimens we use the Craig needle; for precision biopsies and smaller samples we use Geremia needles. A variety of single-use histology needles are now available from a large number of suppliers. All of these needles are designed so that the core sampled from the bone is held in the shaft during withdrawal. It can then be pushed out with a stylet, which is part of the sterile package.

Specimens should be sent to the pathology department for cytological or histological examination, depending on the size of the specimen. At least one sample should be sent to the microbiology laboratory. We do this routinely for both fluid and solid samples unless we are dealing with tumor recurrence or if imaging studies have shown precisely what type of histology to expect.

Applications

Aspiration of Soft Tissue

In both trauma and infection, one may find fluid in the soft tissues. This fluid can accumulate in different anatomical regions. Aspiration may be indicated for a variety of reasons (Loyer et al., 1996). In some cases, aspiration is done to relieve pain; in other cases, it is done because of infection or the risk of infection. In cases with equivocal diagnostic findings (Fig. 14–2), aspiration is required to obtain a sample for cytological examination.

Hematoma

Pain is often the leading symptom in soft tissue hematomas. The hematoma can be subcutaneous, intramuscular, subperiosteal, or within a synovial space. The mass often appears as a mixed echogenicity lesion (Fig. 14–3) because of the mixture of liquid, fibrous material, and coagulum. The blood in soft tissue hematomas often coagulates; in joints, however, blood clot is rarely found. Intrasynovial hemorrhage will often demonstrate fluid-fluid layering because of sedimentation. Such sedimentation can be shown sonographically by demonstrating the presence of fluid with different echogenicity; the

Figure 14–1 ■ **A,** Bone biopsy needle: needle tip with stylet in place. The needle and stylet are pushed as one unit through skin, hypodermis, and muscle. The stylet is removed after it has been anchored in the periosteum. Note the characteristic "corkscrew tip" (*curved arrows*) of the bone biopsy needle. **B,** Bone biopsy needle: needle tip that enters the bone. Once the stylet has been removed, the bone biopsy needle cuts a path through the bone under the pressure of the examiner's hand. The pressure is applied while rotating the needle clockwise. After the biopsy, the needle is removed by a gentle pull and counterclockwise movement.

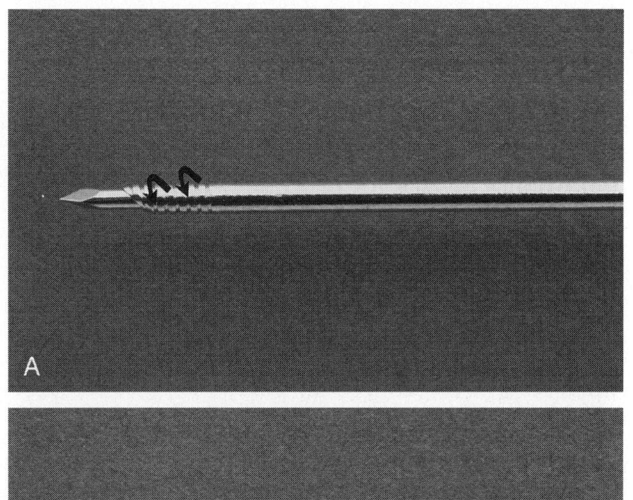

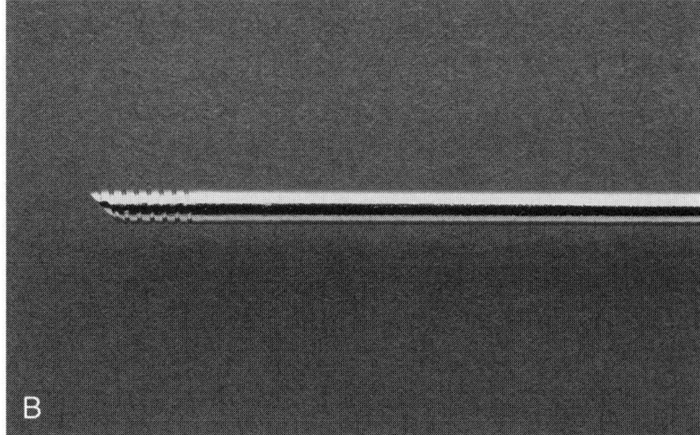

Figure 14–2 ■ **A,** Organized venous thrombus containing calcification: longitudinal sonogram. A 42-year-old man presented with chronic pain and swelling of the calf. Ultrasound images demonstrate a tubular structure (*arrows*) of mixed echogenicity with multiple foci of acoustic shadowing (*open arrows*). **B,** Organized venous thrombus containing calcification: longitudinal sonogram. Under ultrasound guidance, a needle aspiration was performed, which yielded organized thrombus with foci of calcification. Needle (*arrows*).

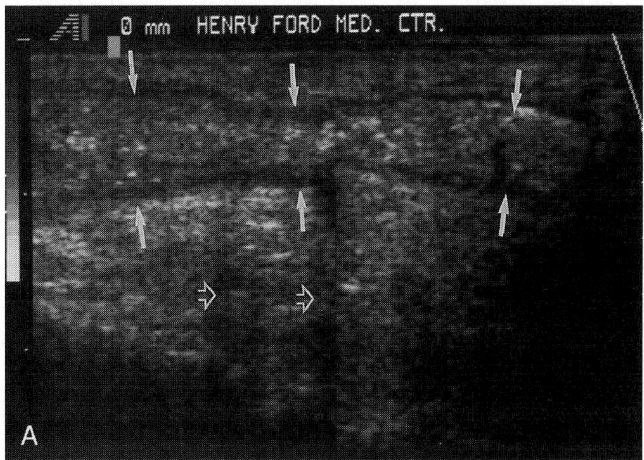

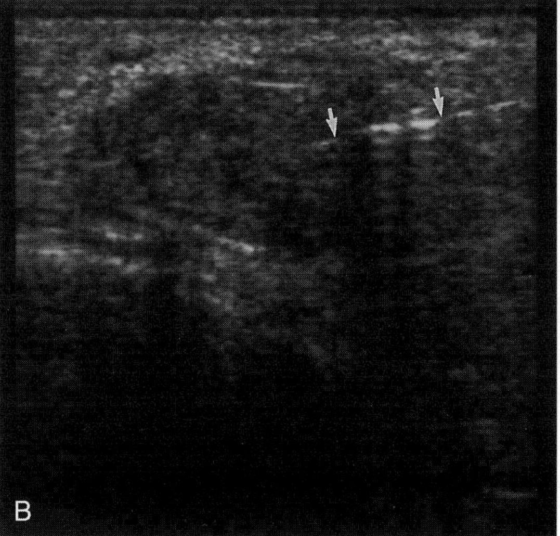

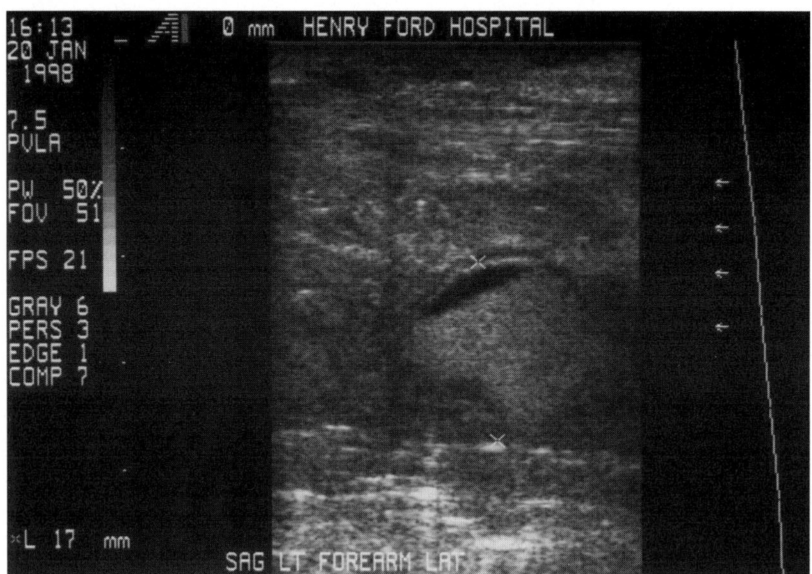

Figure 14–3 ■ Forearm hematoma: longitudinal sonogram. The patient is a 33-year-old male after a motor vehicle accident who suffered fractures of the radius and ulna. He was treated with open reduction, internal fixation, and an iliac free flap graft. Over the course of 2 weeks following the operation, the circumference of the forearm markedly increased, and he developed an acute compartment syndrome. The ultrasound examination demonstrates several fluid collections containing fluid-fluid levels (*x*). These fluid pockets were aspirated under ultrasound guidance, relieving the compartment syndrome.

sedimented red blood cells are shown by a bottom layer of higher echogenicity. Fat can appear as a third layer in cases of lipohemarthrosis. Fat-fluid separation is not unique to joints (Fig. 14–4). For example, it can be seen in any intrasynovial hemorrhage, as well as in bursal trauma and sometimes in subcutaneous bleeding.

Indications for aspiration include bleeding that causes compartment syndrome, postoperative bleeding of an open wound, and hematomas with pain or associated with fever. Contraindications are hematomas that may accompany primary tumors of bone and soft tissue and hematomas that have a good chance of being infected secondary to aspiration. Technically, aspiration is easy to perform. Because of their variable depth, hematomas are often aspirated using freehand technique. Ideally, the needle is 16-gauge or larger because of the thickness of the fluid. Drainage catheters placed for prolonged use are contraindicated; the risk of secondary infection is too high. Repeated needle aspiration is preferable to catheter evacuation. We mark the hematoma with a surgical marker over the skin (Fig. 14–5). Put the transducer over the swelling with the longitudinal axis along the greatest length of the mass, and make two marks on either side of the probe. Now

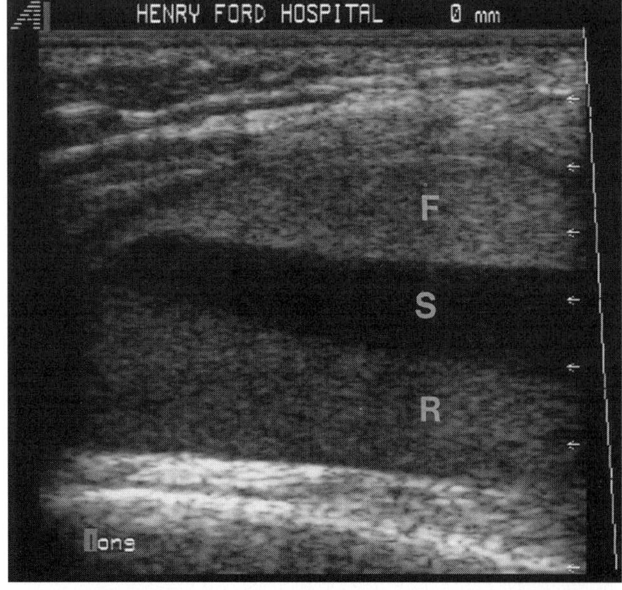

Figure 14–4 ■ Lipohemarthrosis with a hematocrit level: longitudinal sonogram. This 17-year-old girl suffered a patellar dislocation while playing soccer. A longitudinal sonographic image obtained over the suprapatellar bursa demonstrates a hyperechoic layer of fat (*F*) floating on top of a hematoma (serum, *S*; RBCs, *R*) with a hematocrit level.

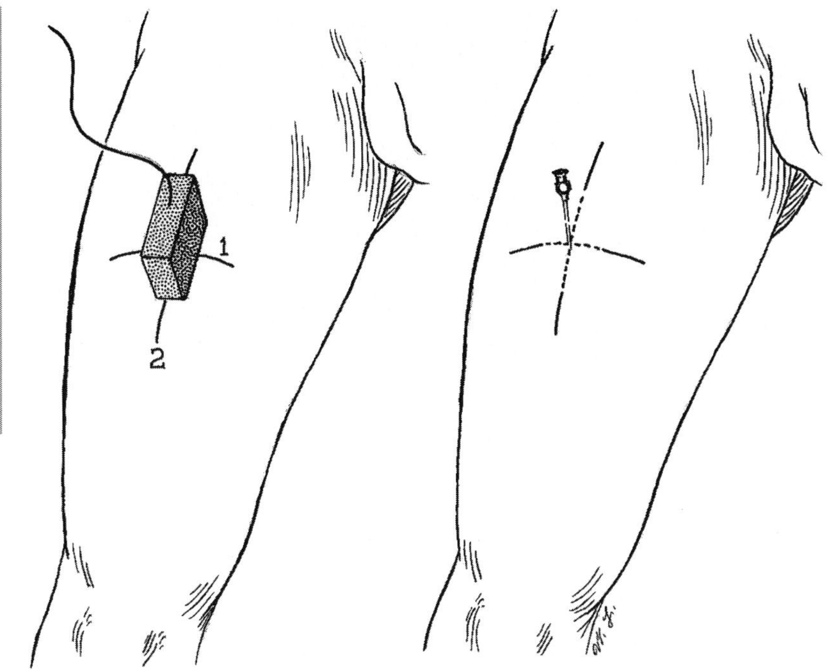

Figure 14–5 ■ Diagram of safe aspiration technique. Put the transducer over the mass or hematoma and measure the distance from the skin to the center of the lesion. In this illustration, we first placed the transducer over the swelling in the transverse axis of the lower extremity. Marks were made on both sides of the transducer at the site of the greatest transverse diameter of the mass (*1*). Now put the transducer crosswise, find the maximum length of the lesion, and repeat the skin marking (*2*). Take the transducer away, and connect the lines. Aim the needle at the intersection of your coordinates. Enter the tissues at a right angle to the original scanning planes and push the needle as deep as you measured the center of the mass to be at the start of the study.

put the transducer crosswise, find the maximum width, and repeat the skin marking. Remove the transducer and connect the lines. Aim the needle at the center of the coordinates. Enter the tissues at right angles to the original scanning planes. Send the samples for culture in all cases, particularly with postoperative hematomas and posttraumatic hematomas with skin lesions. The macroscopic appearance of the fluid may be deceptive.

Seroma

Posttraumatic or postsurgical fluid collections in obese patients deserve special attention. In a large number of these patients, hematomas will develop between the fascia and hypoderma. Vessels perforate the fascia at right angles. Because of differences in tissue elasticity, shear forces will rupture vessels at the interface between fascia and subcutaneous fat. Lesions can develop after a fall, after a motor vehicle accident, or after surgery. These fluid collections often persist; sometimes they are detected because of pain or residual deformity years after the injury. Sonography shows hypoechoic, and most often anechoic, fluid collections that have no discernible wall (Fig. 14–6). The location over the fascia is characteristic. In some fluid collections, one may be able to detect fat lobules that have broken loose from the surrounding subcutaneous layer. Ultrasound is very helpful in detecting the extensions of the collection prior to compression. When aspirated, the fluid appears straw-colored, with low viscosity. Large quantities of fluid, sometimes more than 1 L, can be present in the thigh. The mixture of fragmented fat and blood may interfere with normal blood coagulation. This would explain the frequency of seromas in the subcutaneous layer around the hips of obese women. The aspiration technique used for hematomas can be applied to seromas as well. The choice of needle is less critical. A 19-gauge spinal needle can be used because of the low viscosity of the fluid. Lateral compression of the thigh is often necessary to empty the collection in its entirety. Try to evacuate all the fluid detected on the ultrasound scan. More than one puncture may be necessary.

Abscess and Phlegmon

Aspiration of a soft tissue abscess is often done for diagnostic reasons. If the symptoms are suggestive and the diagnosis of infection is strongly suspected, it may be helpful to aspirate some pus to prove the presence of infection and obtain a specimen for culture and sensitivity analysis. The fluid will be of mixed echogenicity. In contrast to hematomas and seromas, the wall of an abscess will be thick, sonographically detectable, and often more echogenic than the content of the abscess. Abscesses may mimic solid tissue, and color Doppler ultrasound is often required to distinguish the pus from the surrounding granulation (Rubens et al., 1997). Color Doppler and power color Doppler show numerous capillaries in the wall of the abscess and in the surrounding soft tissues but not in the pus collections.

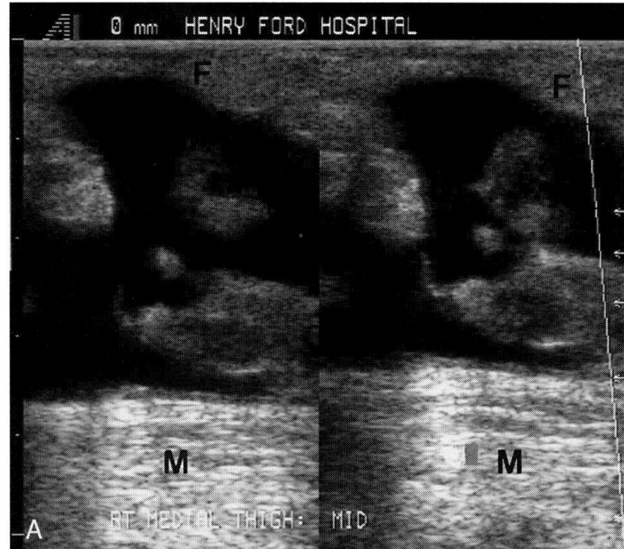

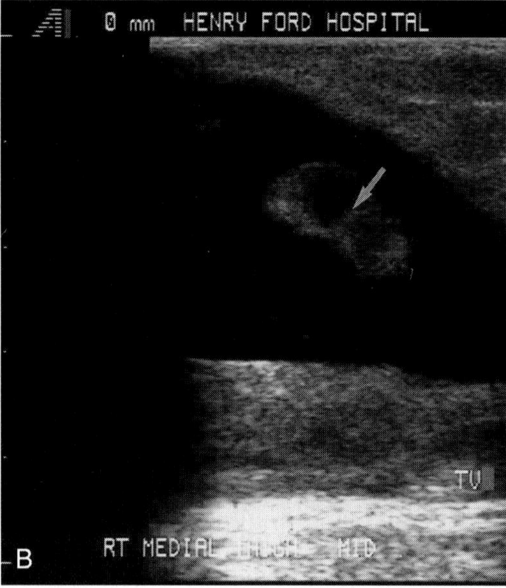

Figure 14–6 ■ **A,** Seroma with clumps of fibrinous debris: longitudinal sonogram. This split-screen image from an ultrasound examination of the thigh of a 50-year-old morbidly obese woman was obtained 7 months after a motor vehicle accident. Compression was applied while obtaining the image on the right. Note the movement of fibrinous debris within this seroma. Typically, these collections occur along the surface of the fascia where it contacts the subcutaneous fat. The persistence and appearance of this seroma are not unusual in morbidly obese patients. Abbreviations: muscle (*M*), fat (*F*). **B,** Seroma with clumps of fibrinous debris: transverse sonogram. Same patient as in **A**. Fibrinous debris (*arrow*).

The fluid pockets may be small and contain debris, lacking the usual through-transmission characteristics of larger collections (Rubens et al., 1997). Color Doppler ultrasound will provide a road map for the procedure. One should avoid hyperemic areas and aspirate collections that do not show vascular flow. The tissue around abscesses is hypersensitive. Ample local anesthesia should precede the aspiration. A large-caliber needle is necessary. Pus can be difficult to evacuate. A percutaneous drain may be introduced under ultrasound guidance. It can be left in place if the fluid is not located in a synovial space. Manual pressure around the transducer may be helpful to evacuate as much pus as possible. The aspiration of phlegmons is similar to that of abscesses. The sonographic image shows little surrounding fibrous tissue in these lesions.

Calcium

Calcific deposits can be present in the soft tissues for years, causing few symptoms. Often, however, an acute inflammatory reaction may occur (Resnick and Kang 1988). The pain caused by calcium hydroxyapatite crystals can be excruciating. In these patients, tendons and surrounding soft tissue, and often synovial tissue as well, may be inflamed. Calcific bursitis of the subacromial-subdeltoid bursa in the shoulder has been known to cause acute disease in the shoulder in middle-aged sedentary women. The calcifications can be removed with needle aspiration (Farin, 1996). Ultrasound is particularly helpful when the calcific material is toothpaste-like or liquid (Fig. 14–7). Injecting small amounts of corticosteroids at the location of the calcification can prolong pain relief.

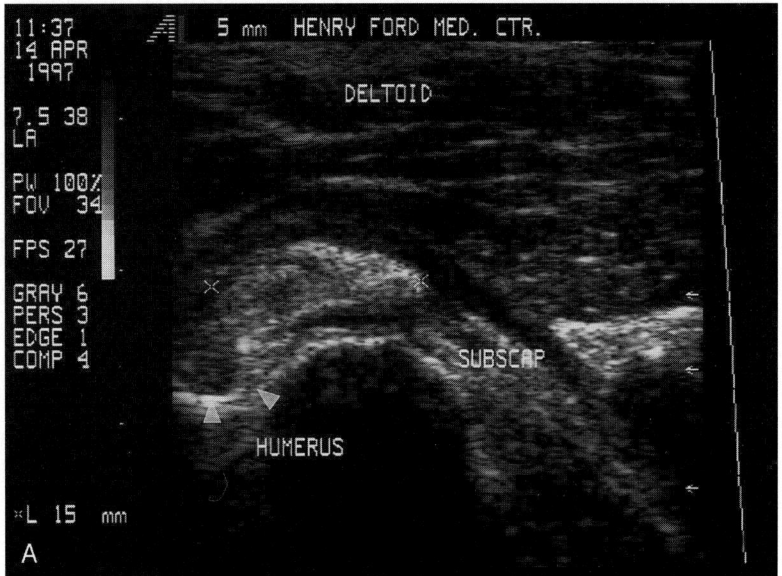

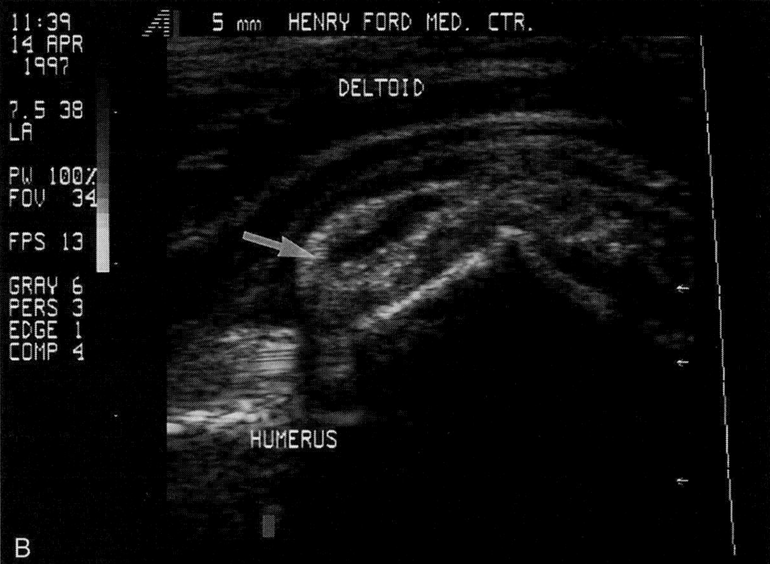

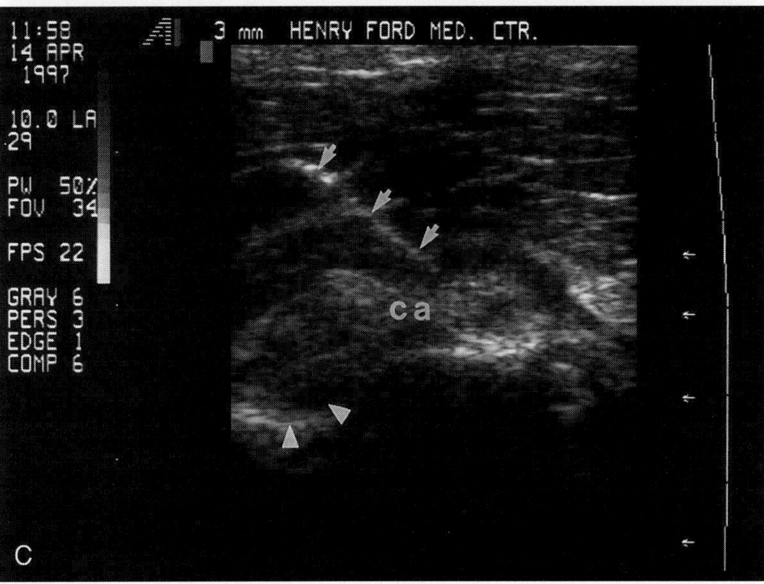

Figure 14–7 ■ **A,** Calcific tendinitis and bursitis: transverse sonogram. Upon awakening in the morning, this 36-year-old postal worker could not move his right arm due to pain in the shoulder. He was treated with an intra-articular steroid injection, which temporarily relieved the symptoms. Two weeks later, he again presented with severe limitation of motion. Ultrasound examination demonstrates an oval, hyperechoic structure (*X*) within the lateral subscapularis tendon. Bicipital groove (*arrowheads*). **B,** Calcific tendinitis and bursitis: longitudinal sonogram. Same patient as in **A**. Hyperechoic material (*white arrow*) consistent with calcification is present within the subdeltoid bursa. **C,** Calcific tendinitis and bursitis: transverse sonogram. Same patient as in **A**. A 20-gauge spinal needle (*small arrows*) is guided into the calcific material (*ca*) within the bursa. The needle indents the calcium deposit. Bicipital groove (*arrowheads*).

Figure continued on following page

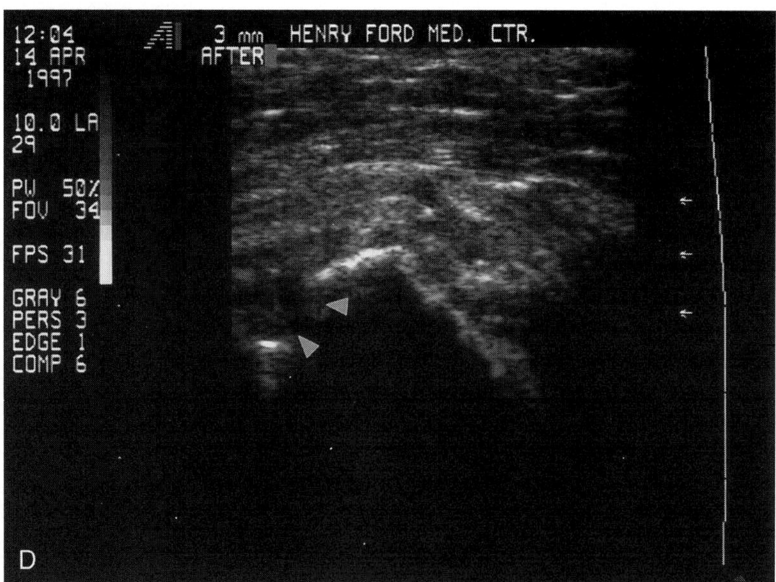

Figure 14–7 *Continued* ■ **D,** Calcific tendinitis and bursitis: transverse sonogram. Same patient as in Figure **A.** After aspiration of approximately 4 cc of calcific debris, the mass is no longer visualized. The patient returned to limited work the following day. One week later, he was asymptomatic and resumed a normal work schedule. Bicipital groove (*arrowheads*).

Cellulitis

Diffuse changes may be present in the subcutaneous fat layer in patients with signs of infection (Loyer et al., 1996) (Fig. 14–8). Instead of fluid collections, one may find extravasation of fluid along septal lines and between fat lobules. This fluid often seems easy to aspirate, but dry taps are the rule under these circumstances. The recommended procedure is injection and reaspiration. This technique has also been used to remove hard concrements of calcium from tendon tissue (Farin, 1996) and in ruling out infection after joint replacement surgery.

The sonographer places two needles in the inflammatory mass (Fig. 14–9A, B). It is best to attempt aspiration at the lesion edge. Do not rupture bullae or vesicles. One needle can be used to inject nonbacteriostatic saline in the hypoderma, and a second 16-gauge needle can be used to reaspirate what has been injected. In cases of infectious cellulitis, flushing saline through the subcutis will wash up bacteria for culture in about 20% of cases (Stevens, 1995).

Aspiration of Joint

Joint aspiration has long been used by rheumatologists, orthopedic surgeons, and other physicians who developed the technical skills necessary to aspirate joints blindly. The technique has been used to diagnose inflammation of joints with greater accuracy. Blind aspirations in inflamed and infected joints are often successful. One can become familiar with bony landmarks and develop skill in performing these aspirations. The technique is difficult if it is used by an inexperienced examiner or in patients with bony landmarks hidden by adipose tissue. In addition, in some cases, the aspiration will fail because the indication for the procedure was not strict enough and the clinical exam was poorly performed. Blind aspiration, then, may pose a dilemma: Did the examiner miss the joint and did the needle deflect during the procedure, or was there simply no abnormal fluid production? Large synovial joints contain no more then 0.1 cc of viscous fluid, and this fluid is difficult to aspirate even with the needle placed intra-articularly during aspiration of a joint with or without fluid. The needle can become stuck in cartilage, synovium, or joint capsule, and there is no way to determine this during a blind aspiration. A large intra-articular fluid collection is rarely a problem, but adhesions will form if the collection is due to infection and if the infection is subacute or chronic (van Holsbeeck et al., 1994). Encapsulated fluid collections are, of course, more difficult to aspirate. The fibrinous material in septic joints may clog the needle, resulting in a falsely negative joint aspiration.

Difficulties with blind aspiration have been significant enough to encourage the development of more sensitive aspiration techniques. Up to about 10 years ago, fluoroscopically guided aspiration was popular. The bony landmarks were shown in detail, and the joint aspirations were more accurate with this technique. The procedure is still hampered by one important limitation: The examiner may see the bony boundaries of the joint, but he or she does not see the joint capsule and consequentially cannot detect the fluid to be aspirated.

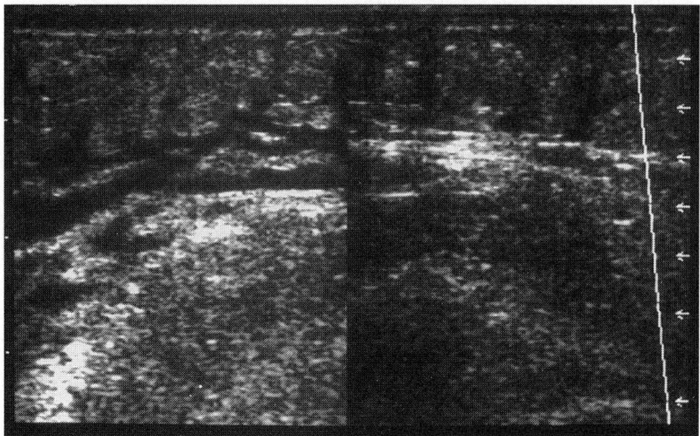

Figure 14–8 ■ Cellulitis: transverse sonogram. A 44-year-old female presented with swelling and redness of the right buttock following hip surgery. The right side of this split-screen image shows a corresponding area of the asymptomatic left buttock. Shown on the left is increased echogenicity and thickening of the subcutaneous fat in the inflamed region. A double-needle technique was utilized with ultrasound guidance. Sterile saline was injected through one needle and simultaneously aspirated through the second needle. *Streptococcus* grew in culture.

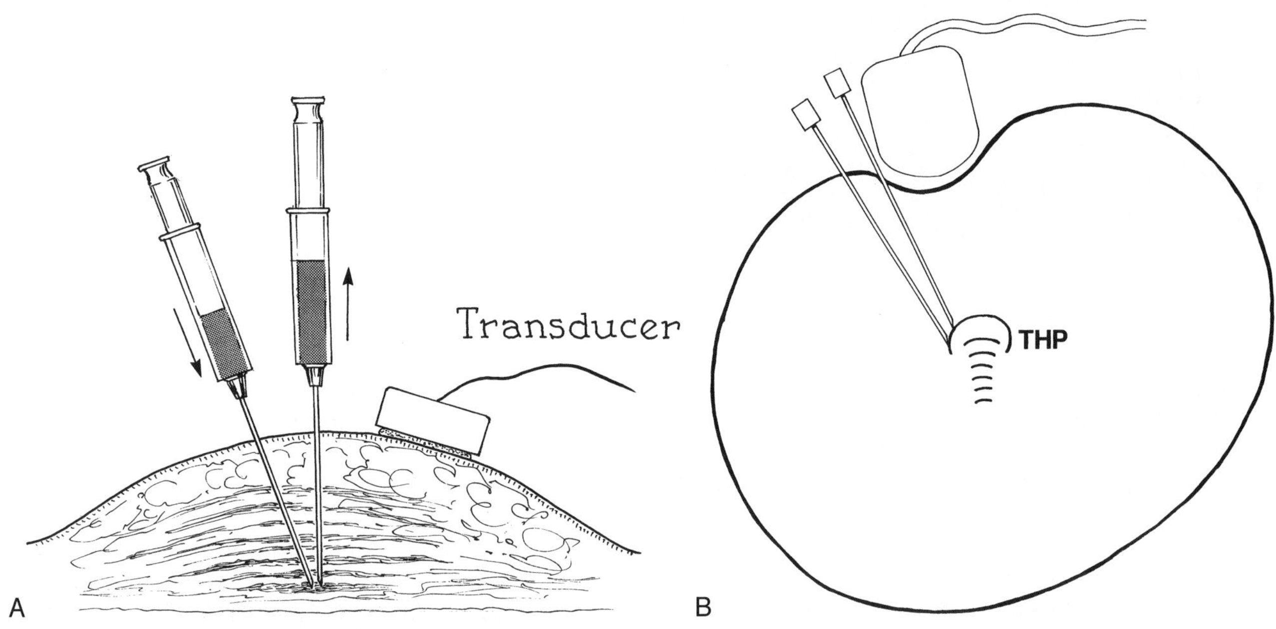

Figure 14–9 ■ **A,** Diagram of double-needle aspiration in the diagnosis of cellulitis. The technique consists of the placement of two needles in the edematous soft tissues. Sonography can assist in placing the needle tips close together. In the diagram, the needles have been positioned within one of the hypoechoic layers of the subcutis. Syringes are then used to inject nonbacteriostatic saline and to reaspirate the fluid that has passed through the soft tissues. In cases of infectious cellulitis, the flushing of saline through the subcutis will wash up bacteria for culture in about 20% of cases. **B,** Diagram of double-needle aspiration of a total hip replacement. Patients with loosening of a joint replacement need preoperative aspiration to exclude infection prior to revision surgery. In some patients with a "dry" initial joint tap, the clinician may insist on reaspiration because of a high clinical suspicion of sepsis. The diagram shows how two needles can be placed for injection and reaspiration of nonbacteriostatic saline. The bevels of both spinal needles face the metal of the femoral stem of the hip prosthesis (*THP*). The ring down artifact of the stem makes it easy to localize this landmark prior to aspiration.

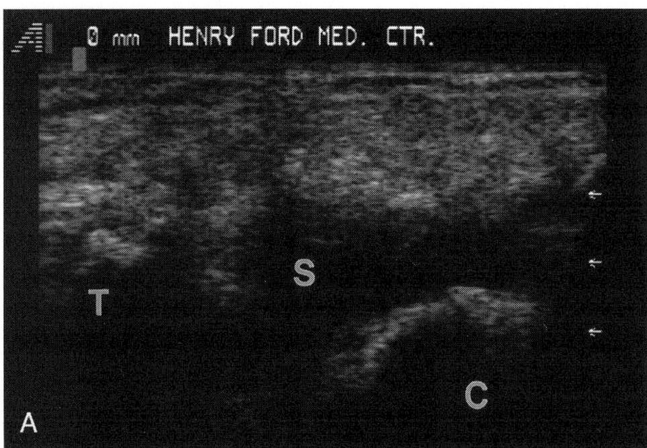

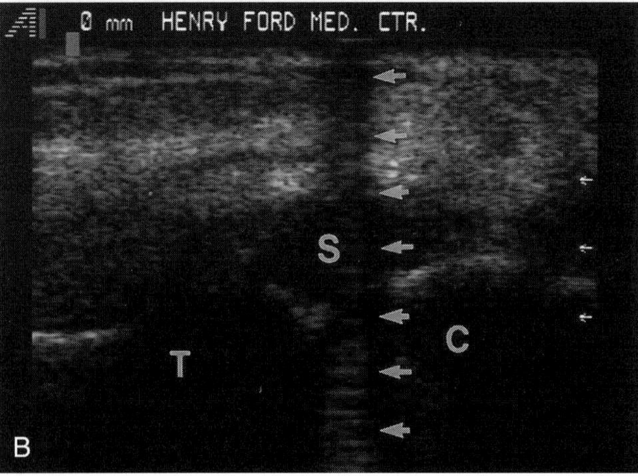

Figure 14–10 ■ **A,** Lyme arthritis of the subtalar joint: coronal sonogram. Hypoechoic swelling of the synovium (*S*) of the subtalar joint is demonstrated. Abbreviations: talus (*T*), calcaneus (*C*). **B,** Lyme arthritis of the subtalar joint: coronal sonogram. Same patient as in **A**. A ring-down artifact (*small arrows*) is projected along the planned path of needle aspiration. This artifact was created by placing a paper clip on the skin beneath the transducer. Abbreviations: synovium (*S*), talus (*T*), calcaneus (*C*).

In our practice, we developed an approach involving routine aspiration of all joints using ultrasound. The equipment and technical skills used in this procedure are no different from those used to aspirate fluid collections in the abdomen and breast. The needle placement has to be absolutely sterile because of the devastating course that infections can take in joints (Rubens et al., 1997).

The joint is scanned prior to the procedure. The sonographer screens the capsule and maps the presence of fluid within the recesses. The largest pocket or the most easily accessible fluid is then marked for aspiration. Because of the importance of a sterile procedure, we often choose the method with coordinates. Once the coordinates are drawn, we often check the accuracy of joint delineation by putting a metal marker on the intersection. A forceps or an open paper clip can be used. The transducer over the metal creates an artifact characterized by ring down; it shows us the path that the needle is supposed to follow (Figs. 14–10 and 14–11).

Arthrogram trays that are used for fluoroscopically guided procedures can be used for these ultrasound procedures. Without a prepared tray, the examiner can aspirate if the skin is adequately sterilized and after the application of local anesthesia. After disinfection of skin with Betadine or isopropyl alcohol, there is a recommended waiting time of approximately 2 minutes. The local anesthetic can be applied after the use of an occlusive local anesthetic patch or an isotonic solution of Lidocaine to relieve the burning caused by the injection of Lidocaine.

An 18-gauge spinal needle 7.5 cm in length is appropriate for most deep-seated joints. The wrist, ankle, and elbow joints can be aspirated using 3-cm-long 21-gauge needles. If the system of coordinates is used, it is mandatory to follow the same path as the ultrasound beam at the time of marking. This will be perpendicular to the surface of the bone because that is the way joints are scanned. Most aspirations are quick and efficient because we only aspirate those joints which show abnormal effusion. Rarely, when the first aspiration attempt fails, a repeat puncture may require direct needle visualization (Fig. 14–12). Some centers use sterile transducer covers and sterile gel. We often bathe the

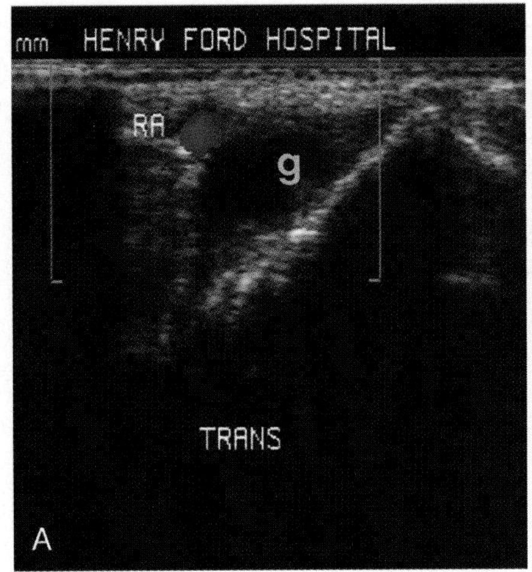

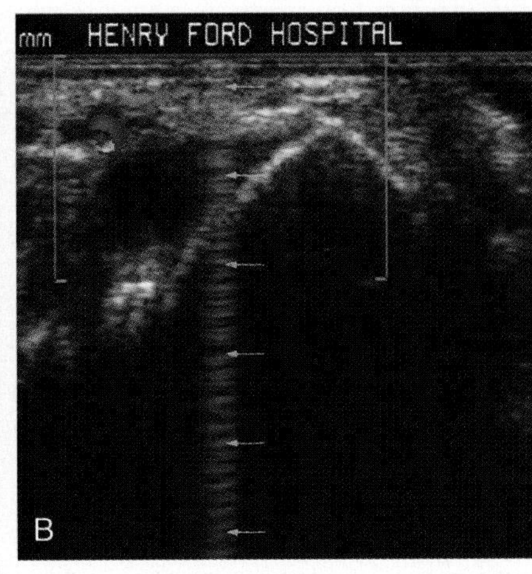

Figure 14-11 ■ **A,** Snuff box ganglion aspiration: transverse sonogram. A 5-mm-diameter ganglion (*g*) is noted, interposed between the radial styloid and the radial artery (*RA*). **B,** Snuff box ganglion aspiration: transverse sonogram. The path (*arrows*) for needle aspiration was carefully planned using a paper clip as a guide.

transducer in a concentrated alcohol solution for several minutes; then we sterilize the handle. The wet footprint of the transducer acts as a coupling medium, and puncture under ultrasound guidance can then be done, bypassing the need for sterile gel. Small transducers designed for intraoperative use are ideal for this purpose. Our experience with over 100 joint infections has taught us that infection appears with hypoechoic or anechoic fluid in a distended capsule. However, we have seen three examples of joint infection with initially negative ultrasound images. We postulate that in those patients, the pain may have been caused by inflammation of the joint capsule and was possibly related to thrombosis of vessels in the synovium. There are two strategies that can be used. All the infections we observed had fluid on the scan 1 or 2 days after the onset of pain. The easiest approach in cases of a negative study but strong clinical suspicion is to recommend a repeat scan after 2 days, if pain persists. The other option is to use a saline washout of the joint. Double-needle technique will then be necessary (Fig. 14-13). Sonography can confirm the intra-articular position of the needle. We have had few cases that were positive with double-needle technique and negative on initial joint aspiration.

Joint fluid is always sent for aerobic, anaerobic, fungal, and mycobacterial cultures. Gram stain and

Figure 14-12 ■ Baker cyst aspiration: transverse sonogram. A 26-year-old woman had several episodes of phlebitis-like symptoms in her leg. Sonography showed that repetitive rupture of a Baker cyst (*cy*) had occurred. The orthopedic surgeon requested aspiration of the cyst to exclude an inflammatory etiology. The cell count from this fluid showed normal synovial fluid, however. Abbreviations: needle (*arrows*), medial gastrocnemius muscle (*ga*).

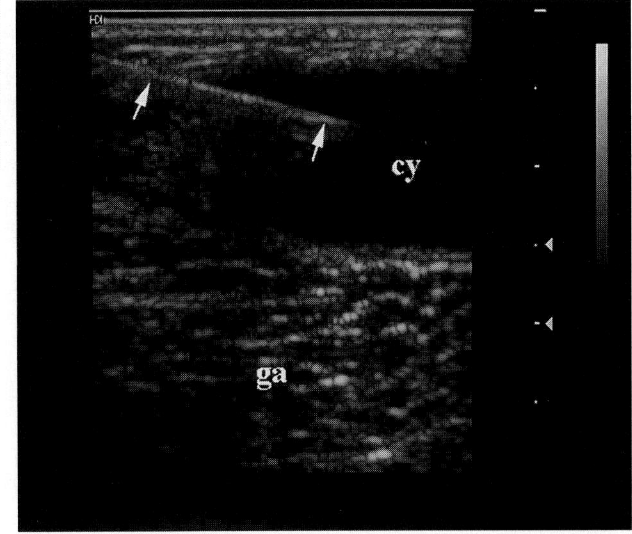

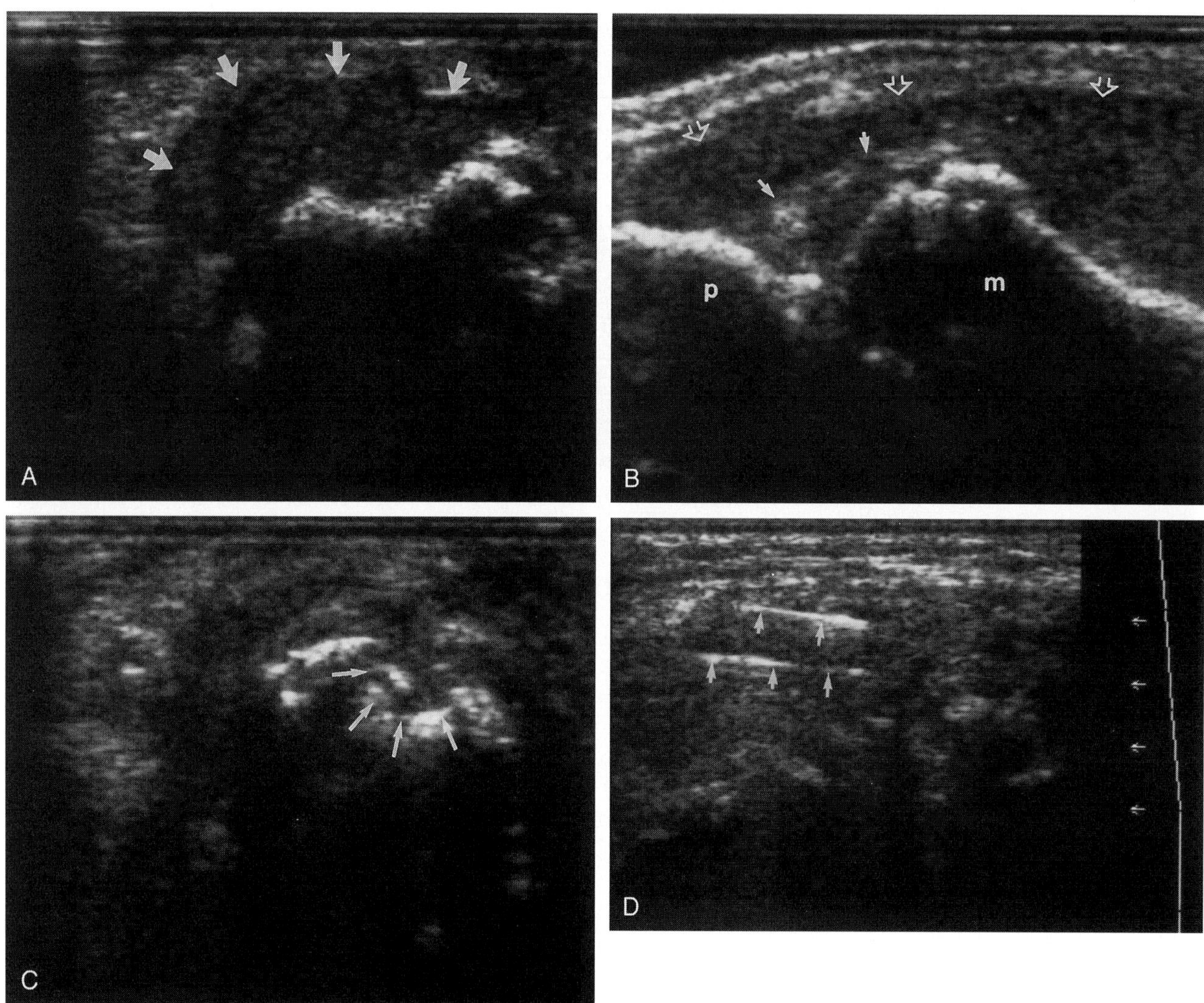

Figure 14–13 ■ **A,** Gout: transverse sonogram. A 62-year-old woman with diabetes mellitus presented with diffuse swelling of the forefoot, and was unable to flex her big toe. Blind aspiration of the metatarsophalangeal joint did not yield fluid. This transverse sonogram over the proximal phalanx shows hypoechoic swelling (*arrows*) superficial to bone. **B,** Gout: longitudinal sonogram. Same patient as in **A**. Hypoechoic swelling (*open arrows*) tracks along the length of the metatarsal, extending over the metatarsophalangeal joint. Slightly more echogenic material is present within the joint capsule (*arrows*). Abbreviations: metatarsal (*m*), phalanx (*p*). **C,** Gout: transverse sonogram. Same patient as in **A**. This transverse image over the metatarsal head shows erosive changes (*arrows*). **D,** Gout: transverse sonogram. Same patient as in **A**. Ultrasound-guided aspiration was performed at the location shown in **C** using the double-needle (*arrows*) technique. Numerous urate crystals were present within the aspirate.

a cell count should be done if sufficient fluid is available. The two last tests are very important if the fluid looks inflamed or infected. The quick reading provided by these tests allows the start of treatment, often on the day of admission. Macroscopic screening of the fluid may also provide valuable information. Normal joint fluid clots when in contact with the glass recipient. Inflammatory fluid is less viscous and does not clot in most cases. Hold the fluid up to your laboratory coat. If you cannot read your name on the coat, that suggests inflammation and the presence of too many white cells. In true infection, the pus will obscure the whiteness of your coat. Inflamed synovium is hypervascular; therefore, it is not uncommon for the synovium to bleed when you pass through it. Infection will then be recognized because of the gold tint of the hemorrhage. Be ready to be surprised by unexpected culture results. It is a good idea to discuss unusual or unexpected culture results with the microbiologist. One of the germs with special requirements for culture is *Neisseria gonorrhoeae*. If you suspect this common monoarticular disease, a chocolate agar or a modified Thayer-Martin

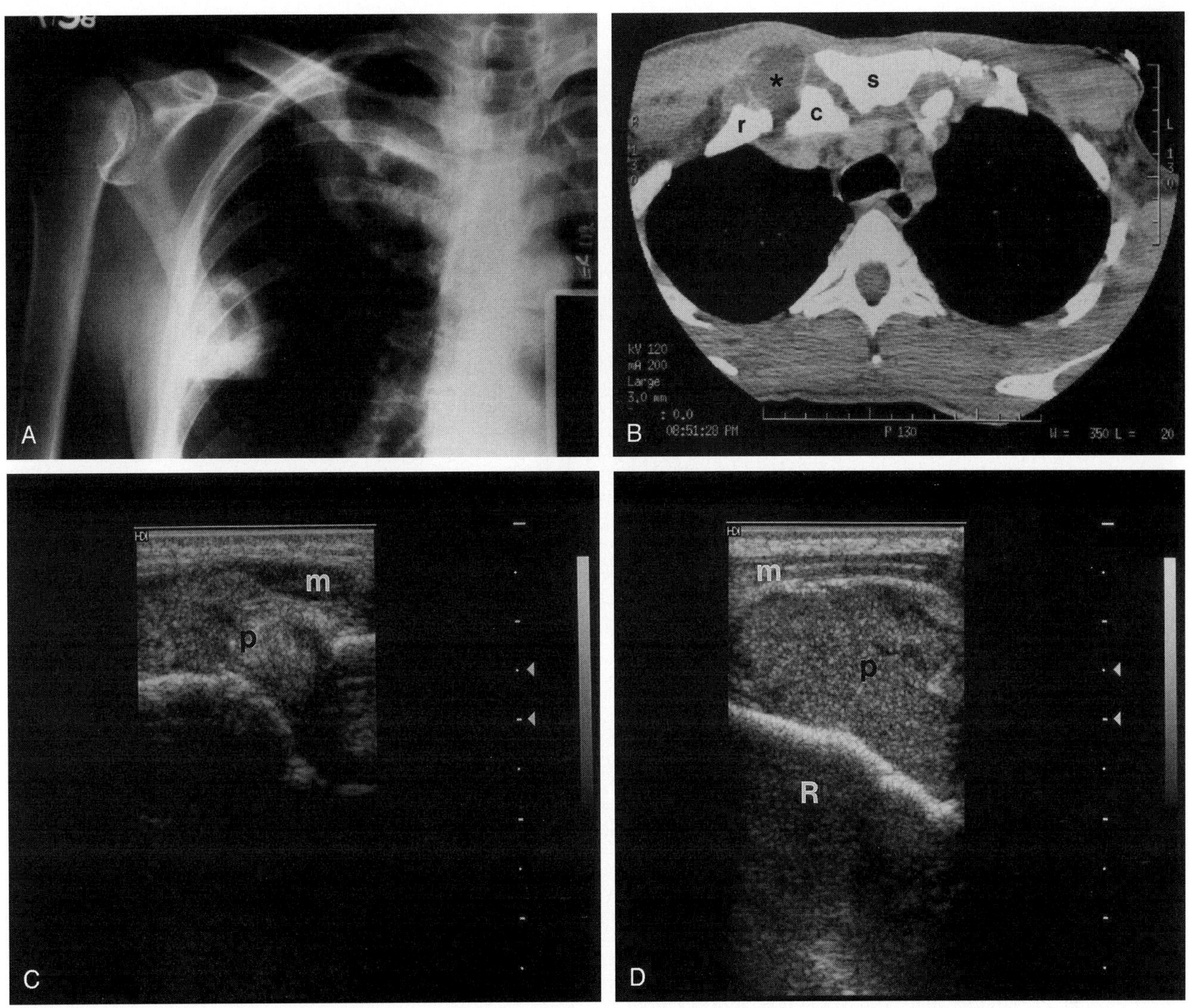

Figure 14–14 ■ **A,** Infected sternoclavicular joint: conventional radiograph. This 30-year-old intravenous drug abuser presented with painful swelling over the right anterior chest wall. A peripheral cavitary pulmonary mass is noted in the right upper lobe. In addition, there is erosion of the head of the clavicle and hyperostosis of the sternocostoclavicular joint. **B,** Infected sternoclavicular joint: CT. Same patient as in **A**. A fluid attenuation mass (*) is demonstrated arising from the right sternoclavicular joint anteriorly. Abbreviations first rib (*r*), clavicle (*c*), sternum (*s*). **C,** Infected sternoclavicular joint: transverse sonogram. Same patient as in **A**. This image was obtained at the level of the sternoclavicular joint. Purulent material (*p*) appears hyperechoic relative to the adjacent pectoralis muscle (*m*). **D,** Infected sternoclavicular joint; transverse sonogram. Same patient as in **A** approximately 1.5 cm inferior to the image in **C**. The synovial space of the sternocostoclavicular joint is grossly distended, covering the anterior medial aspect of the first rib (*R*). Abbreviation: pectoralis muscle (*m*).

plate should be available for direct inoculation of the aspirate. Direct plating is necessary because the gonococcus is extremely susceptible to drying. Remember to avoid using wood sticks and swabs with cotton fibers. These swabs contain fatty acids, which are inhibitory to the gonococcus. Calcium alginate or Dacron swabs are preferable for specimen collection. Roll the swab in a Z pattern across the agar surface. One plate per culture is recommended. Transport to the microbiology lab should be fast. If this cannot be done immediately, a CO_2 tablet should be placed in a plastic bag with the plate. This bag will then have to be incubated at 37°C until the time of transport.

Cultures for *Mycobacterium* may turn positive 1 month after aspiration. Several cultures of orthopedic hardware have grown *M. Xenopi.* Cultures of water in certain hospitals have been positive for this atypical species of *Mycobacterium* as well. Awareness of this newly recognized hospital infection and identification of cases within our own hospital have caused us to add these cultures to our protocol

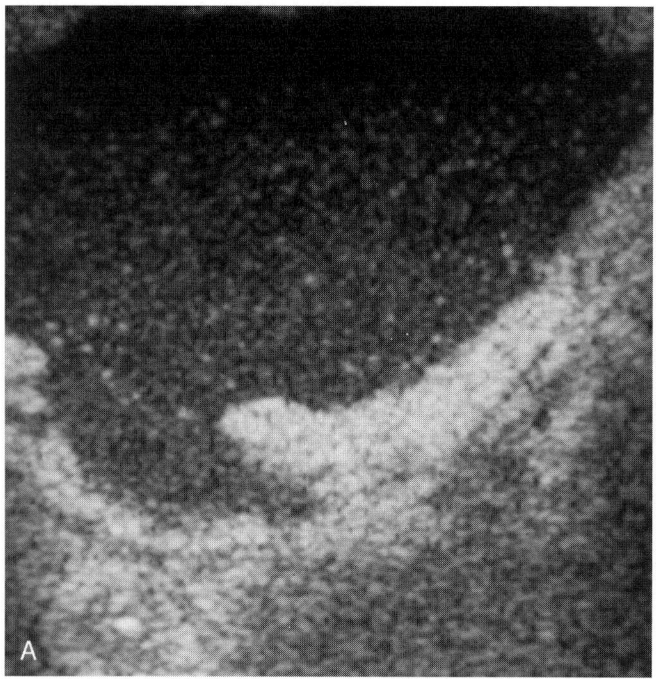

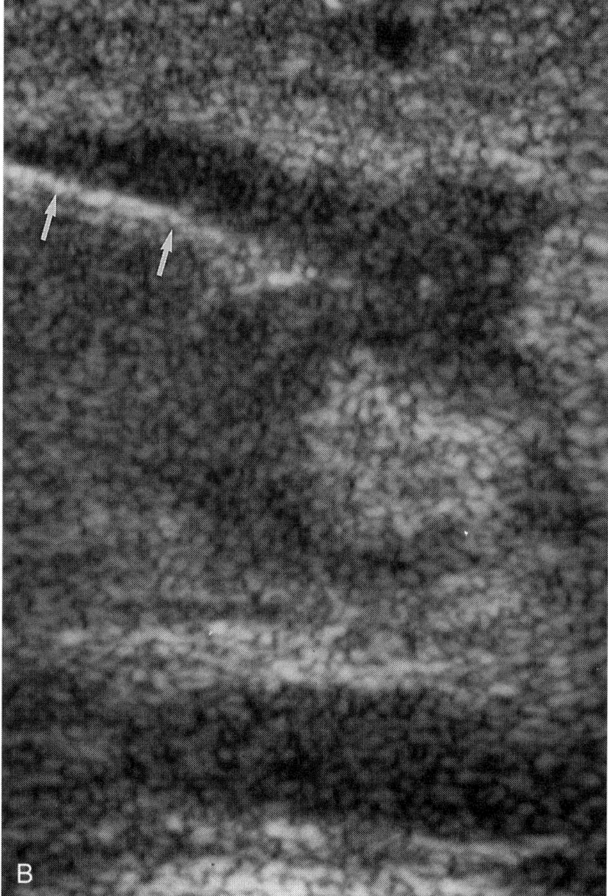

Figure 14–15 ■ **A,** Septic prepatellar bursa: transverse sonogram. This 75-year-old male with severe peripheral vascular disease, CHF, and leg ulcers complained of acute diffuse swelling of the right leg and fever. He had received prophylactic antibiotic therapy. A large, heterogeneous fluid collection is demonstrated in the prepatellar bursa with a debris-fluid level. This bursa was not clinically palpable. It was aspirated under ultrasound guidance four times. Each sample was culture negative but demonstrated numerous gram-positive diplococci. Antibiotic treatment was ultimately changed to vancomycin, with resolution of the infection. **B,** Septic prepatellar bursa: transverse sonogram. Same patient as in **A**. This sonogram shows the needle (*arrows*) in place during the procedure. Aspiration of the supernatant fluid was easy to perform under ultrasound guidance. The synovial lumen has now collapsed, and at this time it is no longer possible to withdraw fluid. The hypoechoic structure deep to the needle is synovial wall edema. This edema can be the cause of the negative blind taps of inflamed joints.

except in cases of obvious acute and purulent infection. Another joint infection on the rise is Lyme disease. The culture and detection of this *Borrelia burgdorferi* infection requires special attention as well. Research studies show that the diagnosis of Lyme disease has improved with the introduction of polymerase chain reaction (PCR). This process, which allows the unlimited reproduction of DNA fragments of microorganisms, is helpful in the detection of *Borrelia* infection (Shutzer, 1992; Desjardin, 1998). Other infections, which are difficult to diagnose by culture, such as tuberculosis, chlamydia, herpes, and gonococcal infections, may also benefit from this new development in genetic engineering.

Most infections show hypoechoic fluid containing particles suspended in the effusion. A very characteristic infection will have strongly echogenic dots suspended in the fluid. We think that these dots are aggregates of fibrin and white blood cells. Be aware, however, that several authors, including us, have observed anechoic septic effusions (Marchal et al., 1987; Gaucher et al., 1997; van Holsbeeck et al., 1994). Absence of echos in the effusion does not exclude infection. More rare are infections characterized by a homogeneous hyperechoic effusion. We have observed this only during aspiration when the effusion was complicated by hemorrhage or in very superficial collections (Figs. 14–14 and 14–15). When in doubt, one can use color Doppler ultrasound to determine whether a mass contains fluid. Color Doppler ultrasound identifies the fluid component in a mass by a color flash artifact generated by swirling complex debris (Rubens et al., 1997).

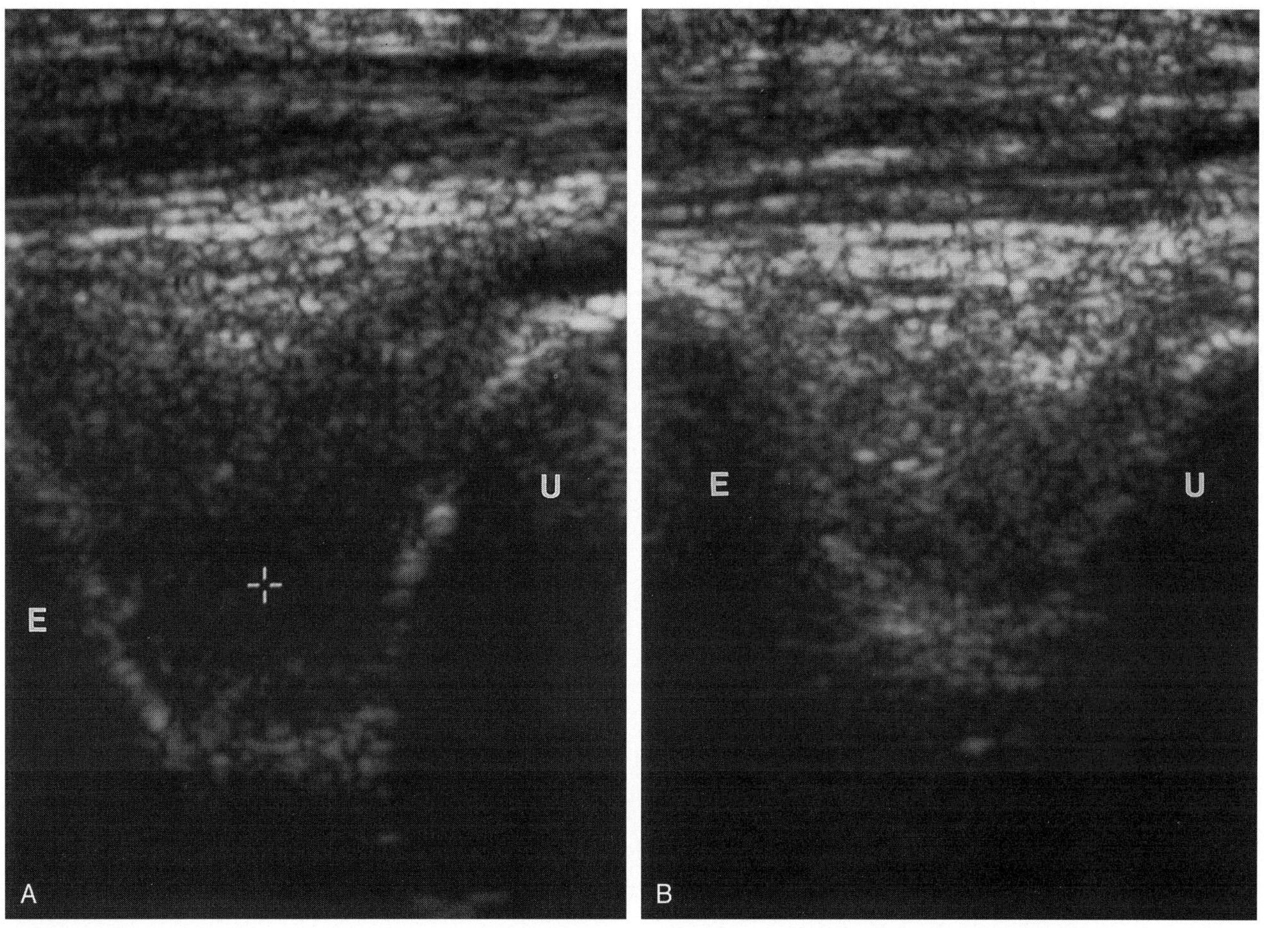

Figure 14–16 ■ **A,** Reactive inflammatory arthropathy of the elbow: coronal sonogram. The patient is a 24-year-old male who presented with a 3-day history of pain and swelling involving the right elbow. He reported no recent trauma. Laboratory studies revealed an elevated white blood cell count and sedimentation rate. This coronal image obtained over the lateral epicondyle and joint space reveals hypoechoic swelling of the joint space (+) with displacement of the joint capsule. Abbreviations: medial epicondyle (*E*), ulna (*U*). **B,** Inflammatory arthropathy of the elbow: coronal sonogram. Same patient as in **A**. This image was obtained at the same position, following the aspiration of 4 cc of turbid fluid from the joint under ultrasound guidance. The hypoechoic fluid layer is no longer visualized, but echogenic thickening of the joint capsule persists. Gram stain and cultures were negative. Numerous WBCs (26,500/mm^3) were present in the fluid. Review of the patient's medical records revealed a history of prior gonococcal infection. Urinary tract cultures revealed chlamydia. Abbreviations: medial epicondyle (*E*), ulna (*U*).

Sonographic aspiration of joints is an elegant, fast, and reliable technique. The test can be ordered in equivocal clinical cases (Figs. 14–15 through 14–17) and can be performed on prosthetic joints and after other foreign body implants (van Holsbeeck et al., 1994) (Figs. 14–18 and 14–19). Because ultrasound is so accurate (Figs. 14–20 through 14–23) in localizing the fluid, it seems to be the correct choice in the workup of pediatric joint infections. Children do not allow hesitation during aspiration (Fig. 14–24). Ultrasound also avoids contamination of deep-seated compartments. Contamination can occur in infection of bursae or tendon synovium; by localizing the septic synovium superficial to the joint, one avoids seeding the infection into bone or joint (Figure 14–21). Moreover, ultrasound limits fluoroscopy and radiation exposure, and it can be used to evaluate complications of pregnancy (Fig. 14–25). Above all, we have noted that the number of unnecessary punctures and unwanted explorative surgeries has decreased dramatically since the introduction of this technique. The diagnosis is far more accurate and can now be made in hours rather than days or weeks; the average time from admission to the start of treatment is significantly shorter compared to the presonography era. Ultrasound-guided aspiration has a palliative effect, which can be helpful in addition to its diagnostic usefulness (Kesteris, 1996). Arthrocentesis of hip effusions in children with transient synovitis has

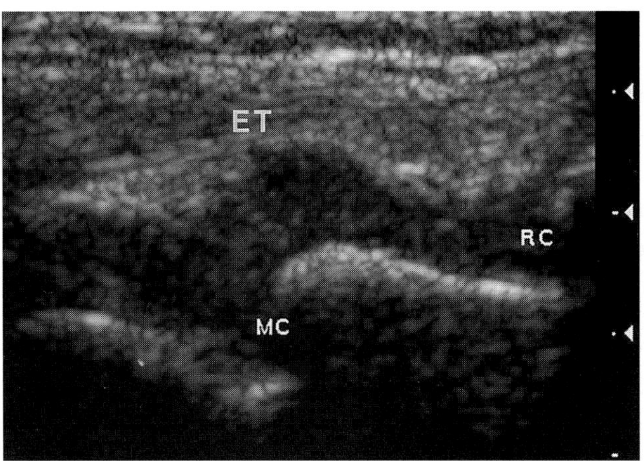

Figure 14–17 ■ Gonococcal arthritis: longitudinal sonogram. Acute painful swelling of the right wrist awakened this 17-year-old female. She has no active wrist flexion or extension. The distal aspect of the midcarpal joint (*MC*) is displayed at the left on this image obtained over the dorsum of the wrist. A homogeneous, hypoechoic layer is present superficial to the carpal bones and joints. A needle was guided into the midcarpal joint, and aspiration was attempted. It yielded no fluid. Therefore, a small amount of fluid was injected into the joint and reaspirated. Cultures of this fluid were positive for *Neisseria gonorrhoeae.* The homogeneous hypoechoic layer probably represents the edematous capsulosynovial membrane. Abbreviations: radiocarpal joint *(RC)*, extensor tendon (*ET*).

been shown to reduce the size of the effusion for as long as 4 days after the aspiration, resulting in significant reduction of symptoms. Thus far, aspiration has not been shown to be effective in reducing the incidence of childhood Legg-Calvé-Perthes disease; however, studies are ongoing (Kesteris, 1996).

Injection of Joints and Soft Tissue

An inflamed joint, tendon, or bursa can be injected under ultrasound guidance using a technique similar to the aspiration just described. The preparation, puncture, and needle guidance are identical. Because of the even greater risk of infection, we are extremely careful not to contaminate the sterile field. The structure to be infiltrated is localized first, and the skin is then marked. The technique using coordinates is the safest, and it is therefore the technique we choose first. If deemed necessary, ultrasound guidance can be used, with a sterile cover over the transducer. Gel is then squeezed into the plastic cover bag, and sterile gel is applied over

Sonographic Appearance of the Prosthetic Hip

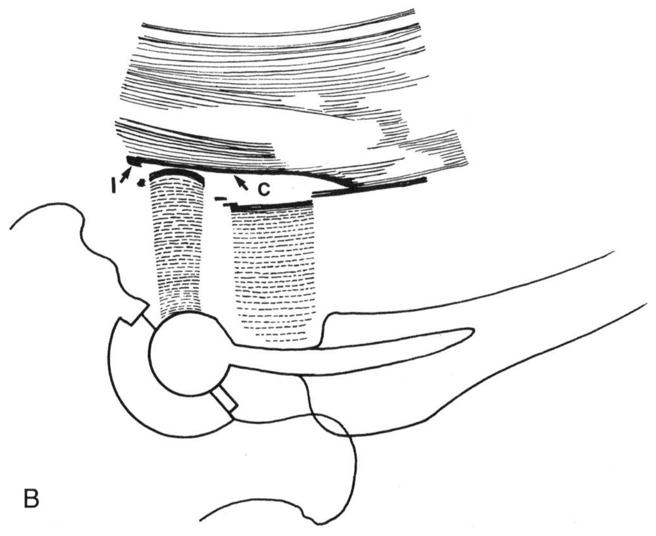

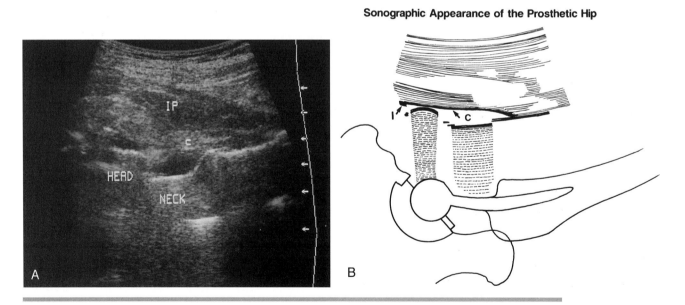

Figure 14–18 ■ **A,** Normal total hip arthroplasty: longitudinal sonogram. The transducer is aligned along the femoral neck of this normal hip arthroplasty prosthesis, which was placed 1 year ago. The hyperechoic pseudocapsule (*c*) lies on the same plane as the native femoral cortex. The metal prosthetic head and neck are separated from the pseudocapsule by a hypoechoic layer. This is the normal appearance of a hip prosthesis after healing. Abbreviation: iliopsoas (*IP*). **B,** Total hip arthroplasty prosthesis. In this diagram, the upper portion represents the sonographic image of the prosthesis obtained by scanning anteriorly. The anatomical representation of the prosthesis is depicted immediately below, in the lateral projection. Abbreviations: anterior lip of the acetabulum (*l*), joint pseudocapsule (*C*). (Reprinted with permission from van Holsbeeck MT: Detection of infection in loosened hip prostheses: Efficacy of sonography. *AJR* 163:381–384, 1994.)

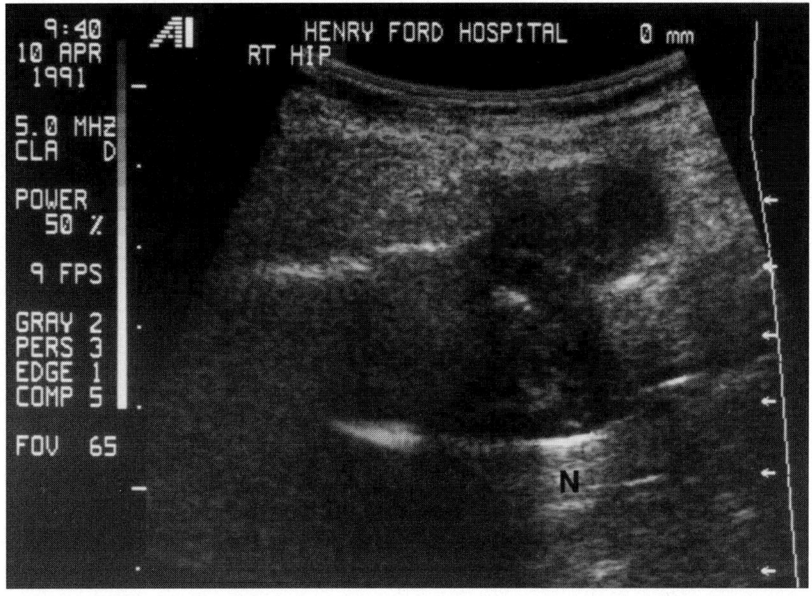

Figure 14–19 ■ Chronic infection of a hip prosthesis: longitudinal sonogram. Seven years after a total hip arthroplasty, this 70-year-old man presented with increasing pain in the right hip. This longitudinal sonogram demonstrates increased intra-articular fluid extending through a defect in the joint pseudocapsule. The joint was aspirated twice under ultrasound guidance. Atypical mycobacteria were cultured from the aspirates. Abbreviation: prosthetic femoral neck (*N*). (Reprinted with permission from van Holsbeeck MT: Detection of infection in loosened hip prostheses: Efficacy of Sonography. *AJR* 163:381–384, 1994.)

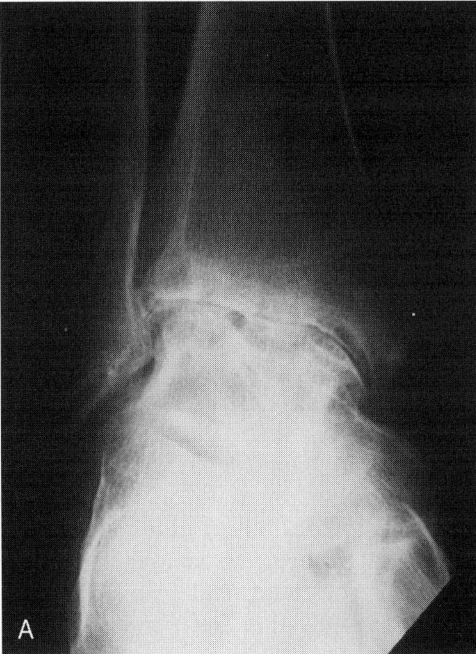

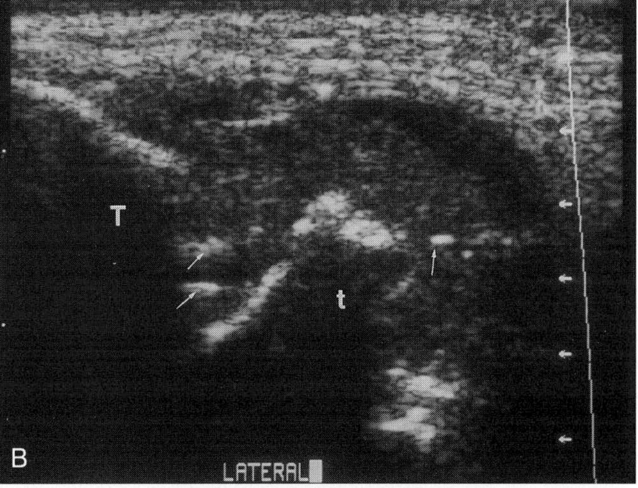

Figure 14–20 ■ **A,** Septic arthritis of the ankle: anteroposterior radiograph. Characteristic changes of chronic arthropathy of the ankle are demonstrated on this radiograph of a 28-year-old male with hemophilia and AIDS. He complains of a recent change in the character of his ankle pain and has developed a fever. **B,** Septic arthritis of the ankle: longitudinal sonogram. Over the lateral aspect of the tibiotalar joint, a hypoechoic swelling of the joint cavity is demonstrated. Several hyperechoic foci (*arrows*) are noted, suggesting infection. Aspiration was performed, and 5.5 cc of purulent material was obtained. Gram stain and cultures were positive for *Staphylococcus aureus.* This aspiration would have been very difficult with a blind tap or with fluoroscopic guidance. It might not have been possible to get the fluid at all. Abbreviations: tibia (*T*), talus (*t*).

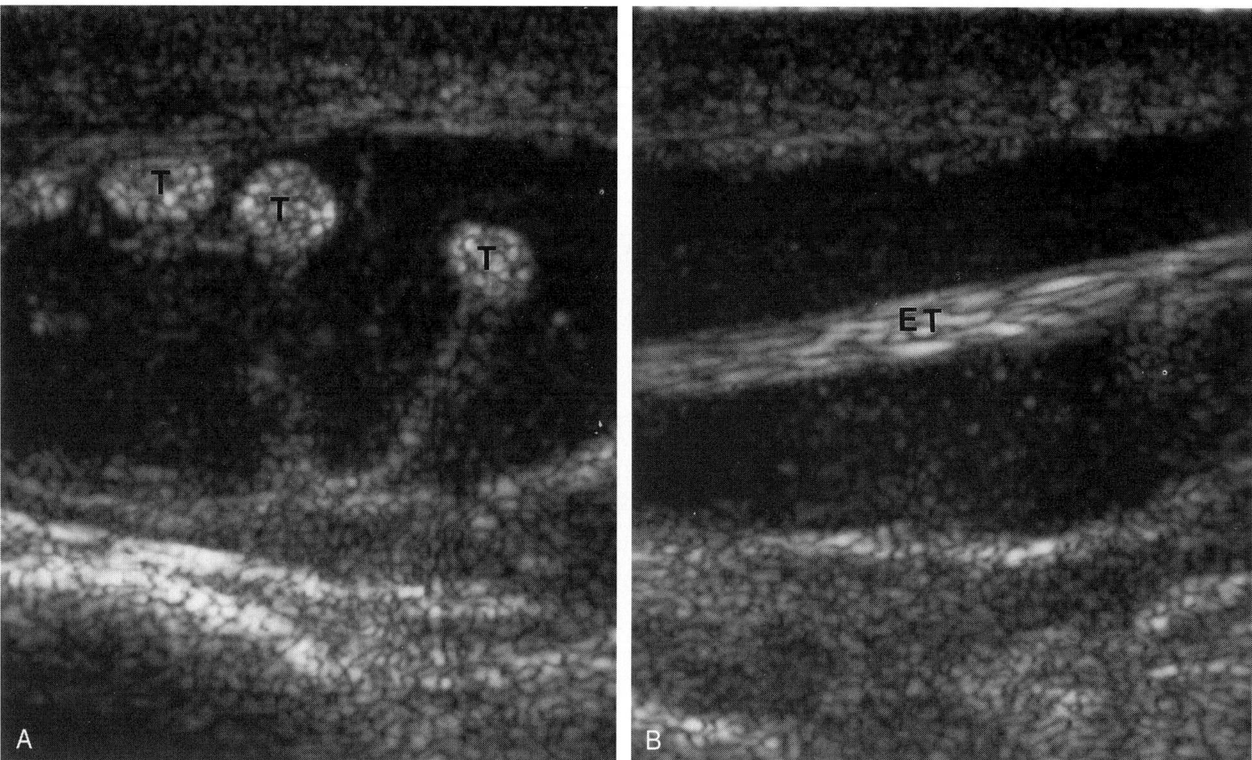

Figure 14–21 ■ **A,** Septic tenosynovitis: transverse sonogram. An 82-year-old diabetic female presented with increasing swelling and pain over the dorsum of the foot during the past week. An ovoid hypoechoic mass with septations surrounds the extensor digitorum tendons (*T*). **B,** Septic tenosynovitis: longitudinal sonogram. A normal-appearing tendon is surrounded by a hypoechoic fluid collection, which contains numerous punctate echogenic foci. Aspiration was performed under ultrasound guidance. Cultures yielded *Nocardia asteroides.* Abbreviation: extensor tendon (*ET*).

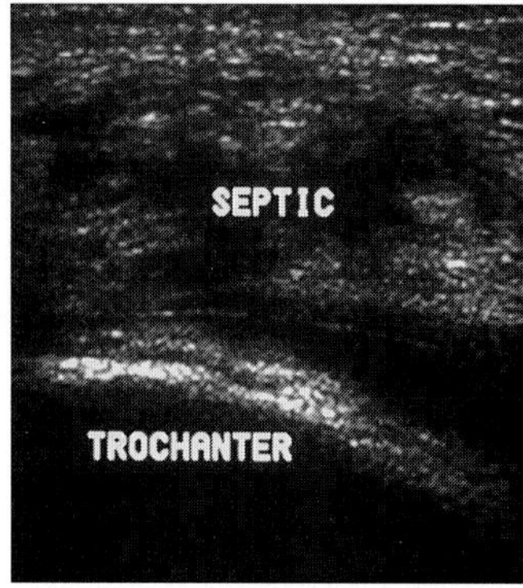

Figure 14–22 ■ Associated septic arthritis and bursitis: coronal sonogram. This 51-year-old diabetic had a total hip arthroplasty 1 year ago. He now presents with a red, swollen left thigh. Increased intra-articular and bursal fluid is nearly anechoic but demonstrates irregular margins. This is not uncommon in septic arthritis. Ultrasound guidance was utilized for aspiration of the bursal fluid, yielding purulent material with 100,000 WBC/mm^3. Gram stain and cultures were positive for *Staphylococcus aureus.* The hip prosthesis was removed 2 days later, but the patient died 2 weeks later from disseminated intravascular coagulation.

the skin. Several indications exist for this method. One application involves the precise injection of a mixture of Lidocaine and Marcaine into a synovial space or around an anatomical trigger point. This method allows the clinician to confirm or exclude a diagnosis. Suppose that a physiatrist attributes shoulder pain in one of his patients to bursal inflammation. Ultrasound-guided injection of the bursa can confirm the synovial inflammation of the bursa. If the pain was caused by the bursa, it should subside after local anesthesia. Pain that persists must be due to other causes. Another application is the injection of intra-articular, intrabursal, or peritendinous corticosteroid solutions for symptomatic treatment of pain. The injection with ultrasound guidance increases the chances of success. It has been shown that ultrasound can guide needles into spaces with millimeter accuracy (Marchal et al., 1987). With the needle in place, one can use color flow during the injection. The location of the color

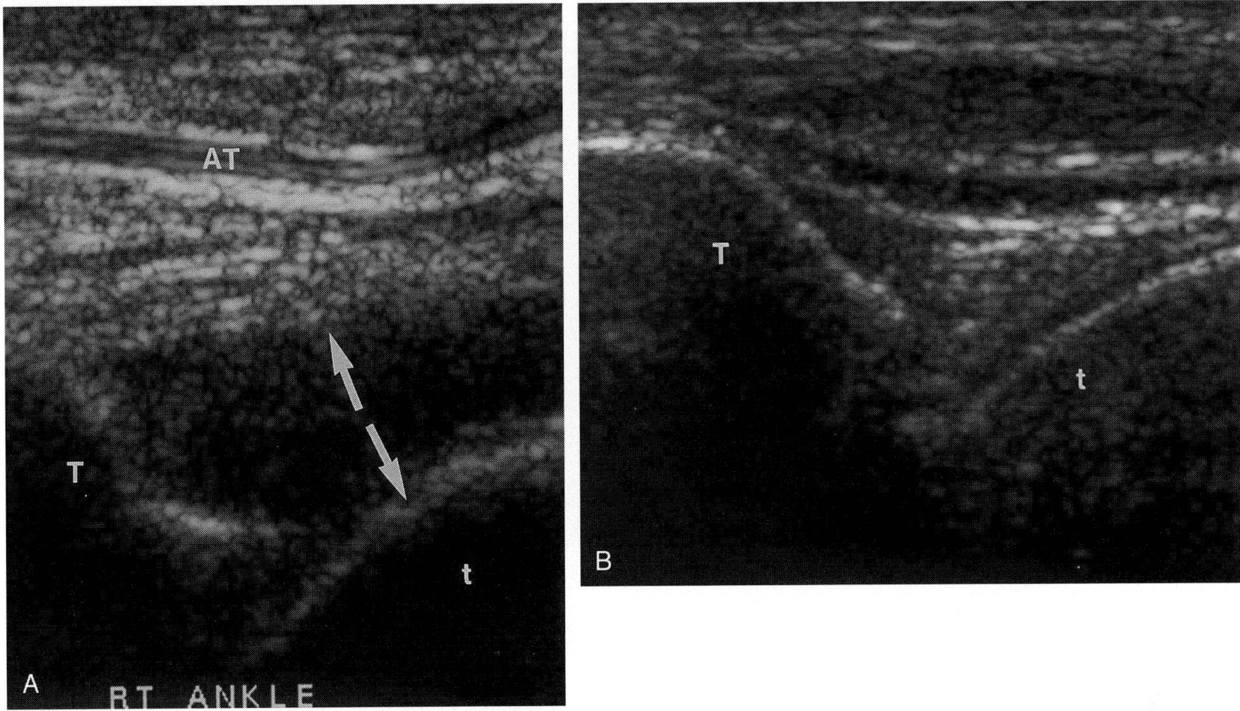

Figure 14–23 ■ **A,** Ankle effusion: longitudinal sonogram. The patient is a 55-year-old male after a liver transplant with chronic renal failure who presents with a 2-day history of redness, swelling, and pain in the right foot and ankle. He also reports fevers and chills. A hypoechoic distention of the anterior tibiotalar joint capsule (*between the arrows*) is noted on this longitudinal sonogram. Aspiration was performed under ultrasound guidance, which yielded numerous urate crystals. Abbrevia-tions: anterior tibia (*T*), talus (*t*), anterior tibial tendon (*AT*). **B,** Ankle effusion: longitudinal sonogram. For comparison, a normal configuration of the anterior tibiotalar joint is demonstrated in this volunteer. Abbreviations: anterior tibia (*T*), talus (*t*).

Figure 14–24 ■ Hip joint effusion: longitudinal sonogram. A 15-year-old female presented with a 2-day history of pain in the right hip. Side-to-side comparison on these images demonstrates anterior displacement of the joint capsule (*c*) by a hypoechoic fluid layer. Joint aspiration under ultrasound guidance yielded 4.5 cc of clear yellow fluid and resulted in immediate of symptoms relief. The Gram stain and cultures were negative. On fluid analysis, 8900 WBC/mm^3 were demonstrated. These findings are consistent with reactive synovitis. The patient was observed clinically, without further treatment or recurrence of symptoms.

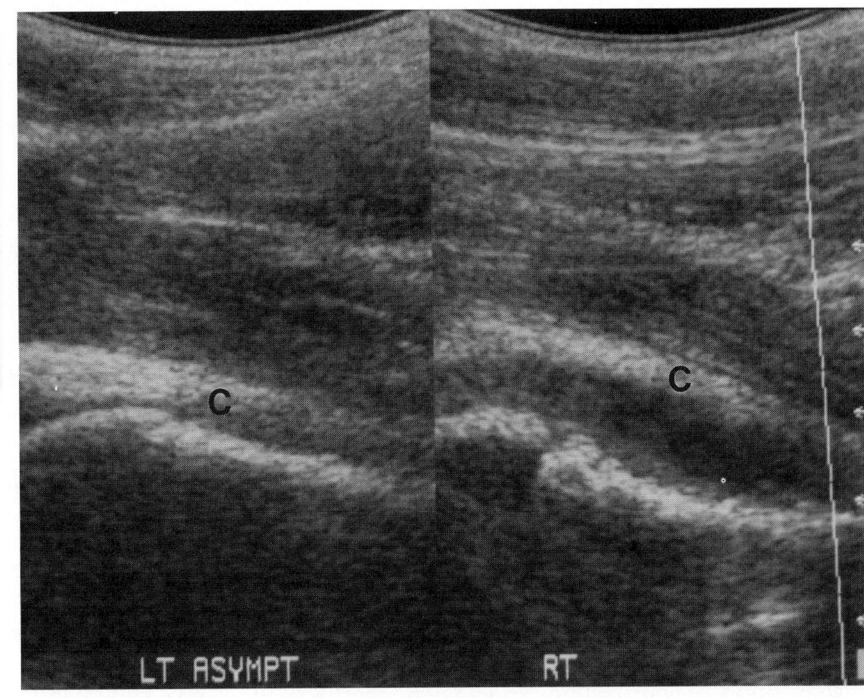

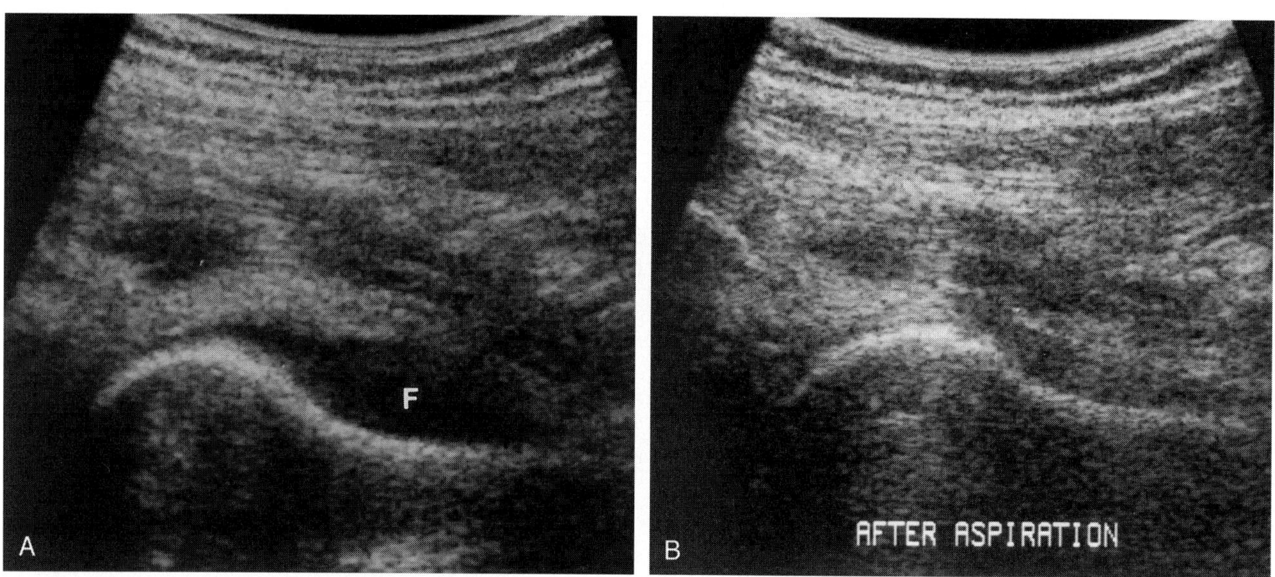

Figure 14–25 ■ **A,** Juvenile rheumatoid arthritis: longitudinal sonogram. A pregnant 15-year-old female presented with new-onset right hip pain. Her past medical history was unremarkable. Hypoechoic fluid (*F*) distends the anterior joint capsule. It was aspirated under ultrasound guidance, and clear, nonviscous fluid was obtained. Although the Gram stain and cultures were negative, the fluid contained 12,700 WBC/mm^3. The right hip pain recurred several months later, accompanied by recurrent hip joint effusion. In addition, joint effusions were present in the left hip and knee. All three joints were aspirated; fluid demonstrated inflammatory cells, without evidence of infection. Postpartum, a left hip synovectomy was performed. Histological changes within the synovium were suggestive of rheumatoid synovitis. Radiographic findings remained negative. **B,** Juvenile rheumatoid arthritis: longitudinal sonogram. Same patient as in **A**. Following joint aspiration, a normal relationship of the joint capsule relative to the femoral neck was observed.

jet will confirm that the placement of the needle is correct.

The *brisement procedure* (Andrén and Lundberg, 1965), which has benefits in adhesive capsulitis and frozen shoulder disease, can be performed with fluoroscopic or sonographic guidance. The procedure consists of joint distention requiring slow, intermittent injection of larger and larger volumes of saline solution mixed with Lidocaine. The physician who performs the procedure should allow some of the fluid to return into the syringe after injection of each bolus (Resnick and Kang, 1988). With the needle slightly withdrawn, the patient is instructed to move the arm. Some authors have forced up to 100 mL into the joint capsule. Typically, the capsule will be disrupted and the procedure is then halted. The most common locations for disruption are the subscapularis recess and the bicipital tendon sheath. Physiatrists have recommended postprocedural physical therapy. A slightly modified brisement procedure can be performed under ultrasound guidance. First, we localize the joint capsule and then inject 1 cc of Lidocaine under sonographic visualization of joint filling. The easiest approach to the shoulder joint capsule is from the dorsal aspect. The needle enters the infraspinatus recess in the axial plane, with the transducer placed transversely over the posterior glenohumeral joint and the needle traversing the deltoid lateral to the transducer. The first injection is followed by a mixture of 20 cc of Marcaine 0.75%, 1 cc of epinephrine, and 1 cc or 40 mg Triamcinolone. The injection can be followed in real time with ultrasound. This technique guarantees proper intra-articular placement of the fluid. In a number of patients, pain relief will be immediate and may be prolonged, probably because of the effect of the long-acting steroid. A remarkable improvement in joint mobility is often noted as a very favorable result of the brisement procedure.

Synovial Biopsy

Arthritis can be a manifestation of several systemic and local diseases. In many instances the diagnosis can be made by biopsy of the synovium. This technique formerly required arthrotomy or arthroscopic surgery for accurate needle placement. A few rheumatologists have been practicing synovial

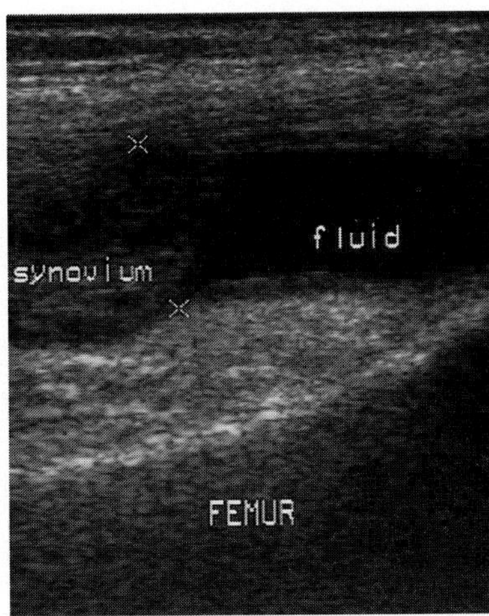

Figure 14–26 ▪ Reactive arthritis: longitudinal sonogram. This 39-year-old male reported a 6-month history of pain and swelling of the knee. His past medical history was remarkable for prior chlamydial urinary tract infection. A moderate anechoic effusion is present in the suprapatellar bursa, with hypoechoic synovial thickening noted in the superior bursal recess. Ultrasound, unlike MRI, is able to distinguish edematous or swollen synovium from fluid.

biopsy by blind puncture (Schumacher and Kulka, 1972).

The practice of synovial biopsy in combination with ultrasound has opened a whole new realm in articular examination. Joints that are swollen but have little intra-articular fluid can now be examined in far more detail. Sonography reveals those areas with swollen and diseased synovium and joint capsule noninvasively (Van Vugt, Van Dalen, and Bijlsma, 1997) (Figs. 14–26 and 14–27). We feel that synovial biopsy is indicated in cases with hypoechoic joint swelling but with negative joint aspiration or with edema which is difficult to sample with sonographically guided aspiration of the joint. Power Doppler sonography has shown increased capillary flow within the hypoechoic synovial lining (Breidahl et al., 1998). Breidahl and coworkers proved that a significant proportion of the hypoechoic mass represents vascularized synovium rather than complex fluid. The needle can be directed into these hyperemic, swollen soft tissues, and a selective sample can be obtained (Rubens et al., 1997; Van Vugt, Van Dalen, and Bijlsma, 1997) (Figs. 14–28 through 14–30). Infections like tuberculosis cause tissue necrosis; ultrasound allows us to sample perfused, viable synovium and permits accurate diagnosis of chronic granulomatous diseases.

Figure 14–27 ▪ Candida parapsilosis synovitis: transverse sonogram. Five years after a total hip replacement, this 63-year-old man developed pain and swelling of the left hip and proximal thigh. He was afebrile and had a normal WBC count. Markedly irregular synovial proliferation (*S*) is demonstrated on this transverse image obtained over the neck of the prosthesis. A moderate amount of hypoechoci fluid (*F*) is present around the prosthesis. The aspirated fluid cultured positive for *Candida parapsilosis.* Synovial biopsy was also positive. (Reprinted with permission from van Holsbeeck MT: Detection of infection in loosened hip prostheses: Efficacy of sonography. *AJR* 163:381–384, 1994.)

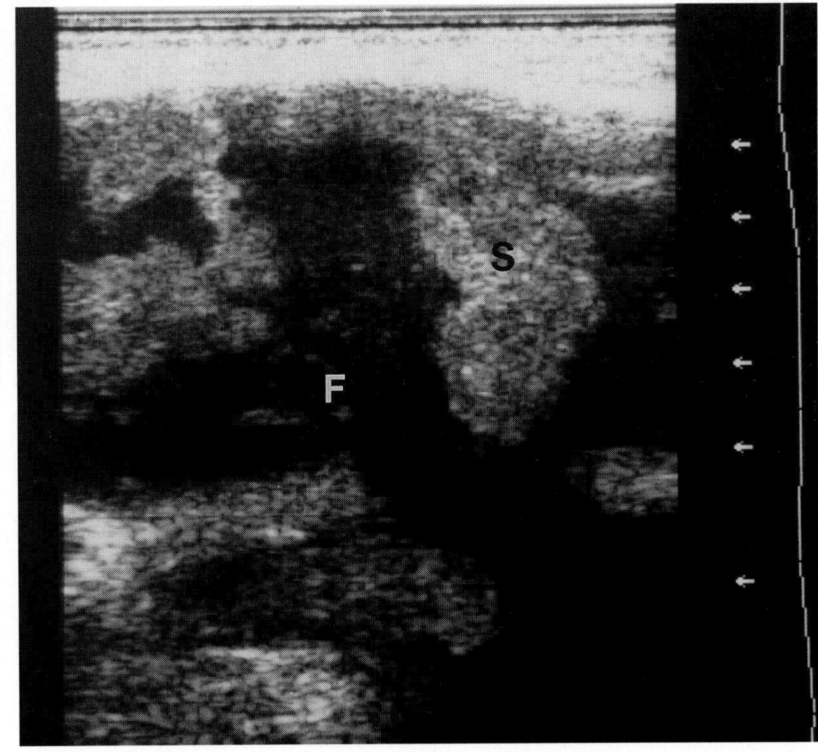

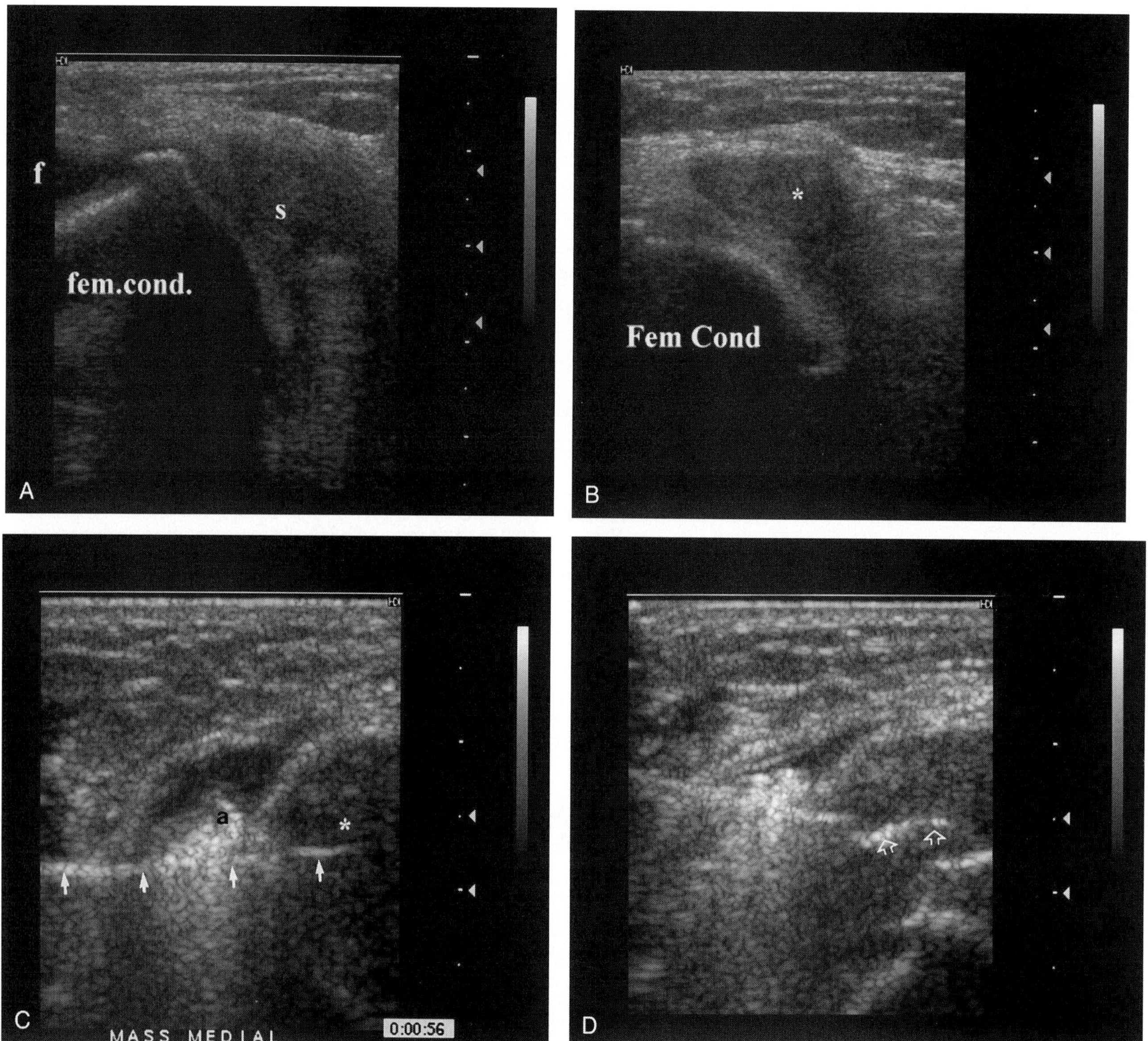

Figure 14–28 ■ **A,** Reparative granuloma of the joint synovium: transverse sonogram. A nodular soft tissue structure is demonstrated adjacent to the medial femoral condyle (*fem. cond*) of the left knee of this 54-year-old female with systemic lupus. This nodule was noted to be mobile under real-time imaging. Abbreviations: soft tissue mass (*S*), intra-articular fluid (*f*). **B,** Reparative granuloma of the joint synovium: transverse sonogram. Same patient and imaging position as in **A**. This image demonstrates movement of the soft tissue mass, which was mobilized by palpation. Palpation helped to localize this mass lying within the joint capsule. Abbreviations: synovial mass (*), medial femoral condyle (*Fem Cond*). **C,** Reparative granuloma of the joint synovium: transverse sonogram. Same patient and imaging position as in **B**. A core biopsy needle (*arrows*) is shown entering the synovial mass (*). A small amount of echogenic air (*a*) was introduced into the joint when lidocaine was injected to anesthetize the synovium. **D,** Reparative granuloma of the joint synovium: transverse sonogram. Same patient and imaging position as in **C**. As the core biopsy needle is withdrawn, an echogenic tract (*arrows*) is noted within the synovial nodule.

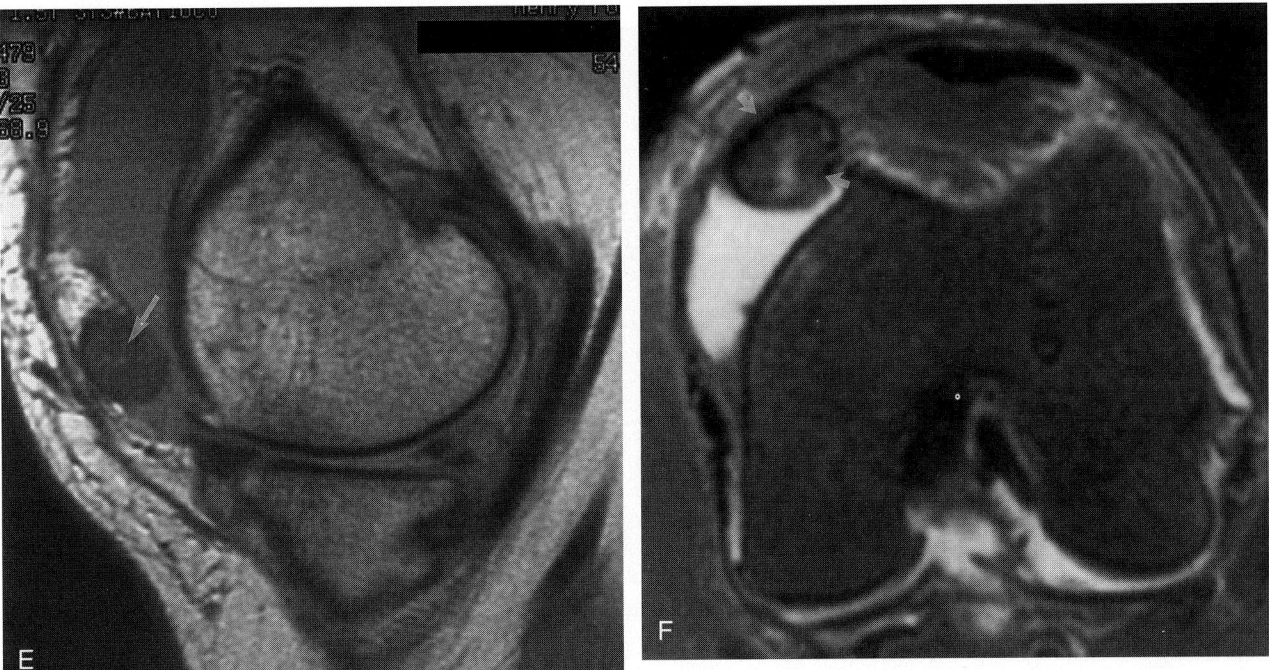

Figure 14–28 *Continued* ■ **E,** Reparative granuloma of the joint synovium: sagittal MRI image. Proton-density-weighted MRI image obtained sagittally through the knee of the same patient. An ovoid mass (*arrow*) with mixed-signal characteristics is noted in the medial joint recess. Note the degenerative disease in the medial knee compartment and the posterior medial meniscal tear. **F,** Reparative granuloma of the joint synovium: axial MRI image. Same knee examined with an axial T_2-weighted image with fat suppression. The signal intensity of the mass (*arrows*) is mixed. The lesion appears well circumscribed relative to the intra-articular fluid. The lesion was diagnosed as a reparative granuloma in the synovium after histological analysis of the tissue specimen obtained with ultrasound guidance.

The small caliber of the needle and the reduction of resulting trauma have increased the situations in which needle biopsy can be used in the diagnosis of articular disease. The technique has been successfully applied in examination of the wrist, ankle, elbow, hip, knee, and shoulder. Procedures can be done for both inpatients and outpatients, and repeat biopsies are readily performed when indicated. This may be necessary in the absence of characteristic lesions in the initial specimen, in suspected focal conditions such as gout or granulomatous infection, or in the occasional case of an inadequate initial result (Schumacher and Kulka, 1972).

The patient is brought to the examining room with an intravenous line in place. The procedure can be performed by one examiner (Van Vugt, Van Dalen, and Bijlsma, 1997). Ideally, though, two examiners should work together. One examiner can prepare and handle the transducer; the other one can set up the sterile biopsy kit, disinfect the skin, inject the local anesthesia, make an incision, and engage the needle. One percent Lidocaine is used for local anesthesia. Patients who are apprehensive are premedicated with 5 to 10 mg Valium intramuscularly or intravenously and Oxymorphone (0.5 mg) or with an initial dose of 25 mg Demerol intravenously. The local anesthetic is applied widely both subcutaneously and intramuscularly. The injection of Lidocaine is done with progressively longer needles. When the joint capsule is entered, one should first try to aspirate joint fluid and send it for cultures. At the end, the joint capsule is infiltrated and 1–2 mL of anesthetic is placed within the joint cavity as well. Wait a couple of minutes before proceeding. The next step requires a small skin incision. We use a No. 10 surgical blade and make an opening approximately 3 mm wide. This incision leaves enough maneuverability for our 16-gauge biopsy needle. A variety of needles can be used. One should become familiar with at least one biopsy set. The Tru-Cut (Cook) is an easy-to-use, disposable system. There is no cannula, and repeated sampling requires additional punctures. The Monopty (Bard) biopsy system is also disposable. It provides an equally good sample of synovium and capsule but is somewhat more difficult to use. It has the advantage of working through a cannula, several samples can be obtained, and only one initial

Text continued on page 453

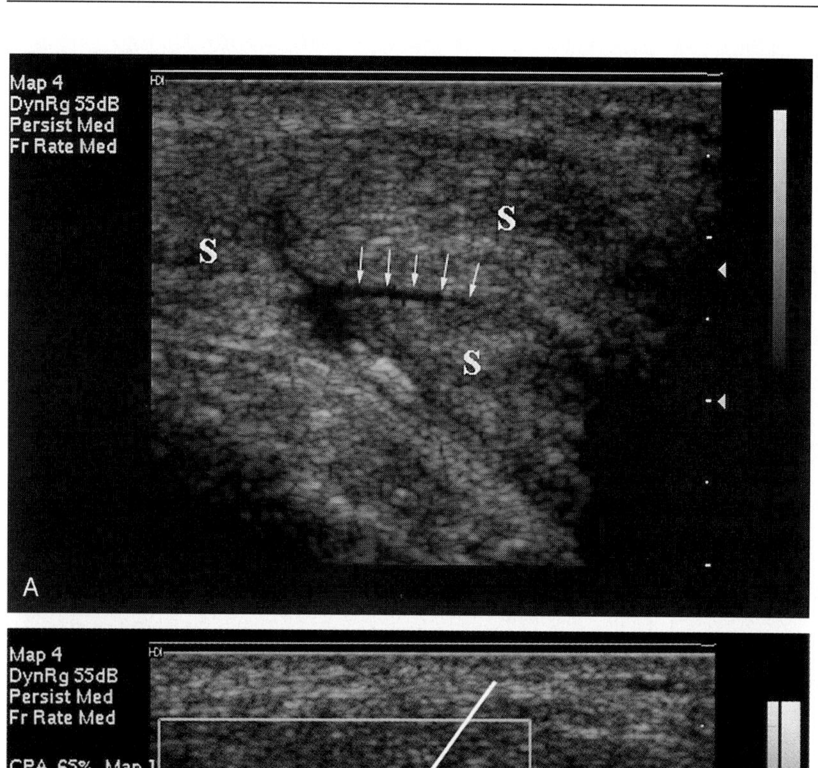

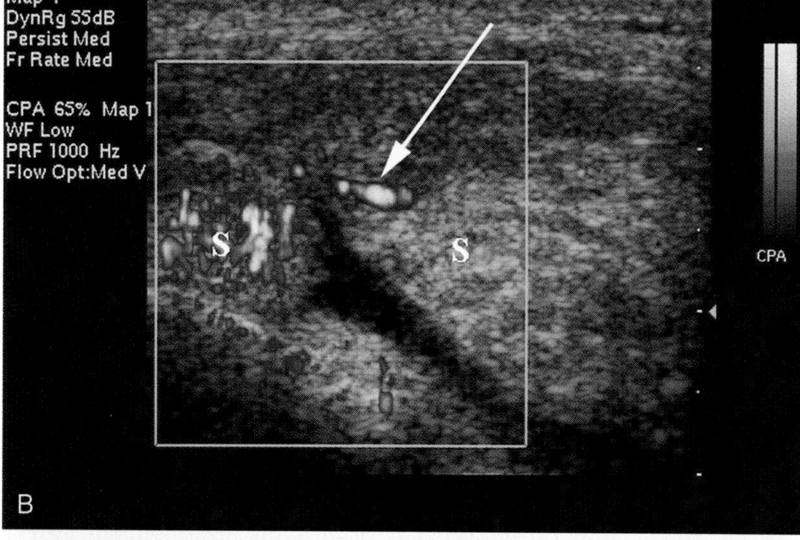

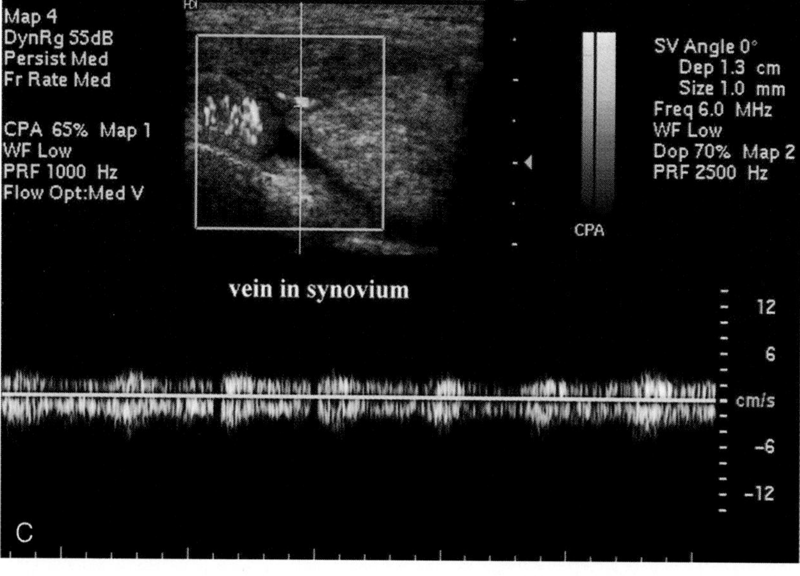

Figure 14–29 ■ **A,** Synovial lipomatosis: transverse sonogram. Isoechoic synovial masses are noted within the suprapatellar bursa of this 32-year-old male presenting with chronic swelling of the right knee. A linear anechoic structure (*arrows*) is present within the synovial mass. Abbreviation: synovium (*S*). **B,** Synovial lipomatosis: transverse sonogram. Same patient and imaging location as in **A**. Power Doppler imaging of this region demonstrates the synovial masses (*S*) to be quite vascular. The linear anechoic structure shown on the initial image demonstrates flow (*arrow*). **C,** Synovial lipomatosis: transverse sonogram. Same patient and imaging location as in **A**. The duplex Doppler waveforms obtained by sampling the vessel are characteristic of a vein.

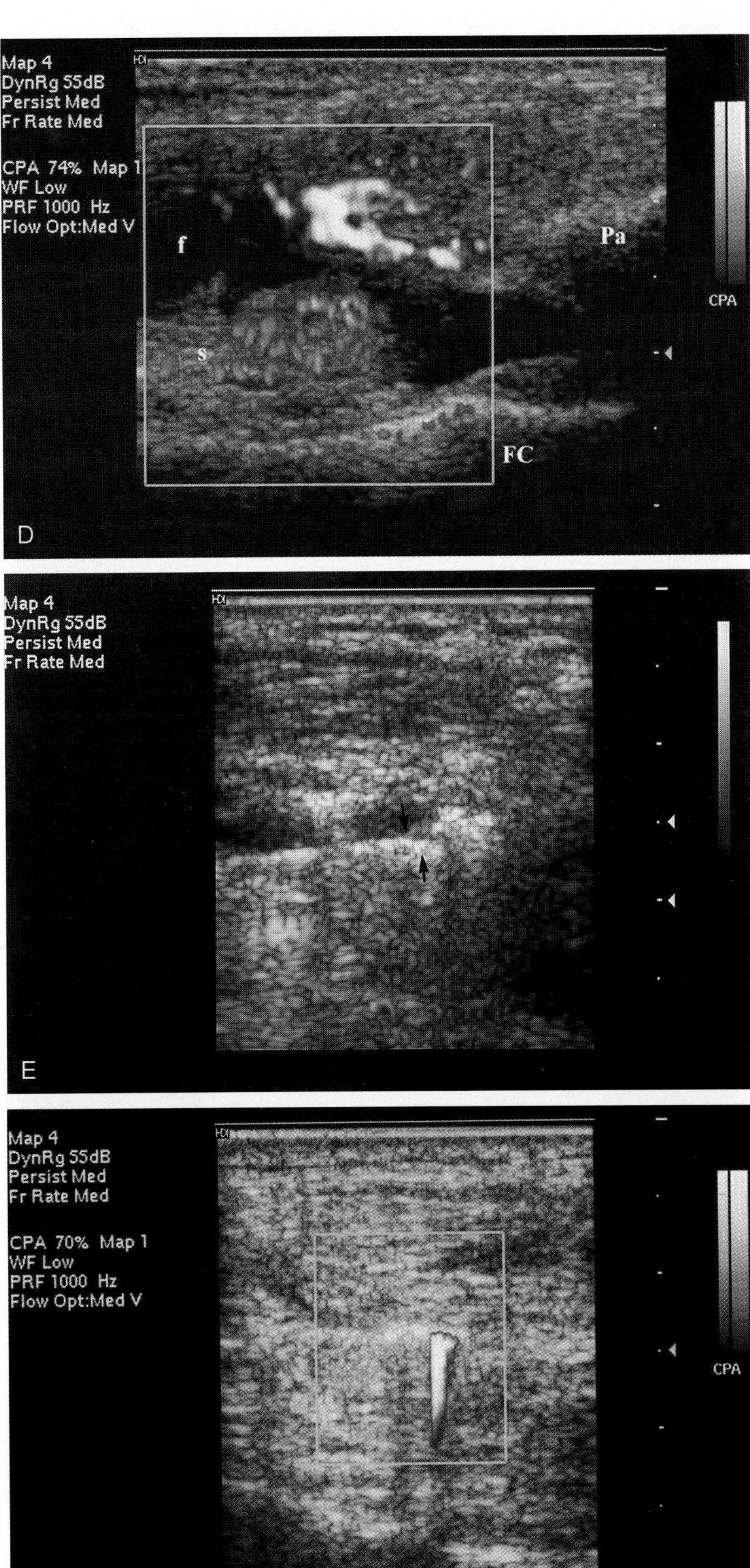

Figure 14–29 *Continued* ■ **D,** Synovial lipomatosis: longitudinal sonogram. Same patient and imaging location as in **A**. Power Doppler helps to define the extent of synovial proliferation and differentiate it from intra-articular fluid. Abbreviations: base of patella (*Pa*), distal femoral condyle (*FC*), fluid (*f*), synovium (*s*). **E,** Synovial lipomatosis: transverse sonogram. Same patient and imaging location as in **A**. A core biopsy needle is introduced into one of the synovial masses. Visualization of the needle tip (*arrows*) is difficult. **F,** Synovial lipomatosis: transverse sonogram. Same patient and imaging location as in **A**. Subtle movement of the needle tip while using power Doppler indicates the tip of the needle by a bright-colored comet tail. Histological examination showed fatty tumoral infiltration of the joint synovium.

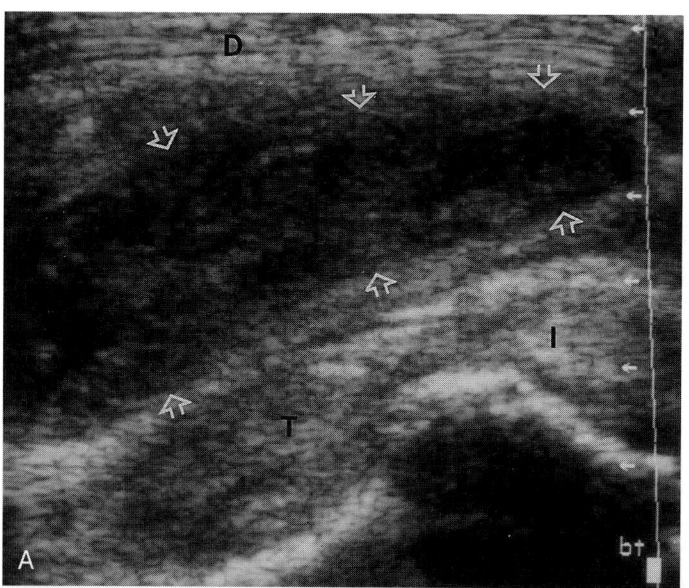

Figure 14–30 ■ A, Synovial amyloidosis: coronal sonogram. A large hypoechoic synovial mass (*open arrows*) is demonstrated deep to the deltoid muscle (*D*) and superficial to the infraspinatus (*I*) and teres minor (*T*) tendon. **B,** Synovial amyloidosis: coronal sonogram. Same patient and imaging location as in Figure **A**. In the top series of three images, a bone biopsy needle is advanced toward an erosion in the humeral head. The specimen was composed of nondiagnostic fibrous tissue. The bottom row of three images show sampling of the hypoechoic synovial mass using a core biopsy. An angle for the needle was chosen to optimize exposure of the cutting surface to the synovial mass. **C,** Synovial amyloidosis: histologic section, Congo red stain. Histological examination of the synovial specimen demonstrated homogeneous acellular material with intense staining by Congo Red, characteristic of amyloid.

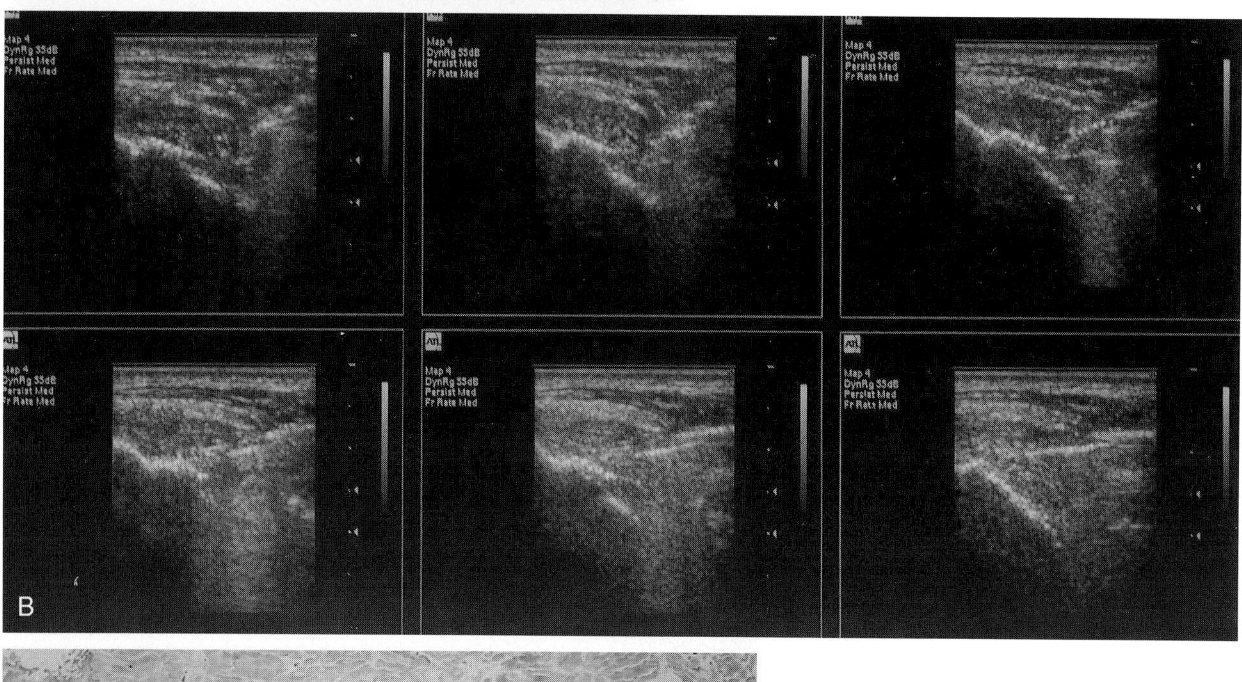

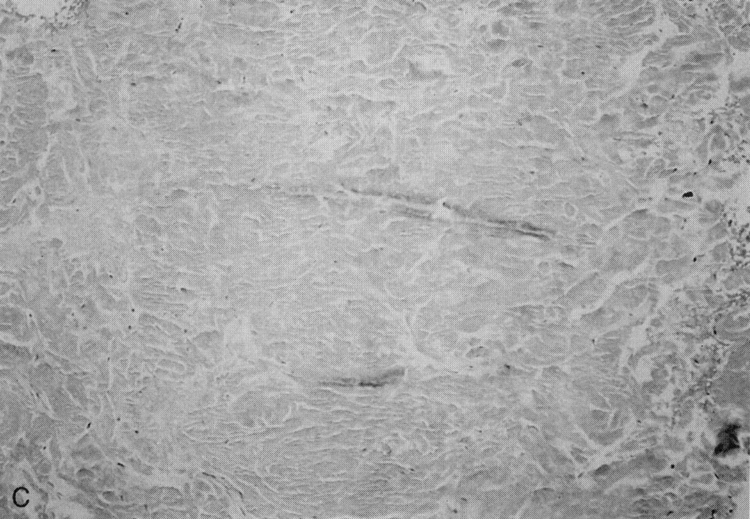

skin and muscle puncture is needed. The Parker-Pearson needle is a reusable system which has proven to be efficacious and minimally invasive (Schumacher and Kulka, 1972). This needle uses a 14-gauge cannula, which allows repeat biopsies without repeat tissue injury. The use of ultrasound guidance helps to reduce the invasiveness of the procedure. The shortest path to the joint can be chosen, and vessels and nerves can be avoided. The samples can be taken from the most suspicious-looking segments of the capsular structures of the joint. Thickness, edema, and microvascularity are the parameters used to judge the abnormality of the soft tissues of the joint.

The needles that we use have a throw length of approximately 1 cm. It is important to know the exact length of the notch in the distal needle. This will allow you to avoid vital structures and adjust the position of the needle. Ultrasound measurement is accurate, and it allows us to position the needle across the joint capsule. Halt the needle tip a few millimeters outside the capsule; then fire the biopsy gun. The specimen should be obtained across the capsular structures. Open the notched segment in the biopsy needle upon withdrawal and examine the specimen. A good synovial specimen will be pink; a failed biopsy may show a yellow-white fibrinous exudate, fat, or necrotic material. In order to reduce sampling error, one should take three to eight specimens from various parts of the inflamed synovium. Biopsy samples are placed in a plastic container half filled with neutral buffered formalin. Absolute alcohol is used only when gout is suspected. An additional sterile container is used for transport of at least one specimen for tissue culture. Saline may be used to suspend the tissue in this container. Do not allow the tissues to dry, and transport them to the laboratory quickly. In addition to light microscopic examination, the specimens can be subjected to electron microscopy, bacterial and viral tissue cultures, and immunofluorescence studies.

At the end of the procedure, the patient is advised to rest the biopsied joint until the following day. We examine the joint a few hours later and prior to discharge. The percentage of patients with complications is estimated at less than 1%. Intra-articular hemorrhage is the only complication that we have observed. Prolonged immobilization of the limb until resolution of symptoms is then recommended (Schumacher and Kulka, 1972).

Histological examination has proven to be valuable in making the diagnosis of pigmented villonodular synovitis, synovial osteochondromatosis, pseudogout, gout, hemochromatosis, ochronosis, pyogenic arthritides, gonococcal arthritis, tuberculosis, and coccidioidomycosis. These specimens may be pathognomonic. The combination of histological and microbiological examinations is often diagnostic in unusual infectious arthritides. In other patients, the diagnosis can be established when microscopic and clinical findings are combined. Conditions in this group include rheumatoid arthritis, sarcoidosis, systemic lupus erythematosus, Reiter's syndrome, and osteoarthrosis. In a minority of patients, the biopsy findings are nonspecific and do not lead to establishment of a diagnosis (Schumacher and Kulka, 1972).

Synovianalysis is increasing in popularity. It often allows a final diagnosis, confirmation of the suspected diagnosis, or reclassification of disease. The technique offers major diagnostic assistance in 40% of biopsies (Schumacher and Kulka, 1972).

Ultrasound Guided Core Biopsy

Soft Tissue Mass

Core biopsy of soft tissue masses has long been practiced in the diagnosis of malignancies of the extremities. Clinicians often biopsy these lesions blindly when they have sufficient data to suggest that the tumor arises from the soft tissues, does not transilluminate, and is suspected to be malignant. Sometimes the biopsy will be planned because the tumor shows equivocal characteristics on imaging studies. One example is the atypical lipoma. The drawbacks of blind biopsy are obvious: difficulty in targeting the lesion, the risk of neurovascular injury, and the risk of compartment contamination. Core biopsy in combination with ultrasound can avoid these problems. The technique has been called "tissue sparing" (Rubens et al., 1997). The diagnostic yield of the biopsy is higher because we can biopsy the solid components of the tumor and avoid tumor necrosis and hemorrhage. Color Doppler sonography is a valuable aid during the procedure. The technique helps us avoid taking a biopsy specimen from an aneurysm, arteriovenous fistula, or a nerve tumor. At the same time, the technique helps us select tissue which is well perfused and viable (Rubens et al., 1997).

Indications for this type of biopsy include all soft tissue tumors with potentially malignant characteristics. These include large tumors, tumors that are hard and solid during palpation, tumors with an inhomogeneous MRI signal, and tumors with hypervascularity, multiple feeding vessels and necrosis on CT, MRI, or ultrasound studies.

The preparations prior to biopsy have been described above. A variety of core biopsy needles can be used. We use the same systems as for synovial biopsy. It is important to collect the tissue aseptically. Try to include material from both the center

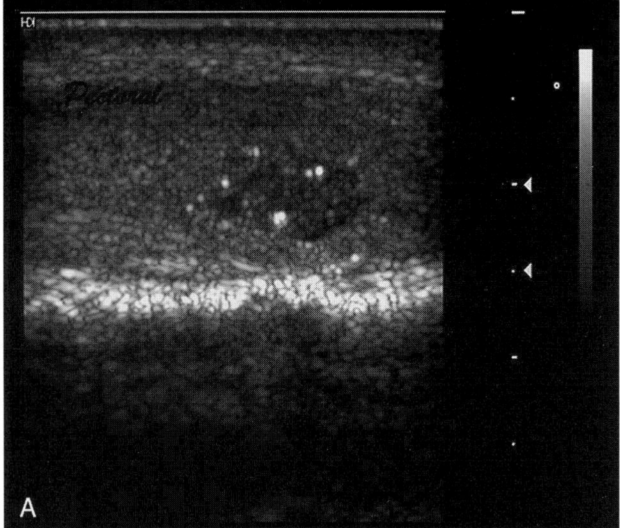

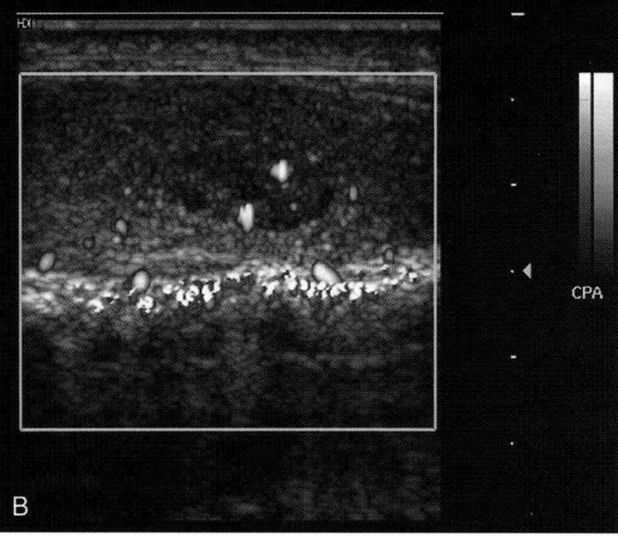

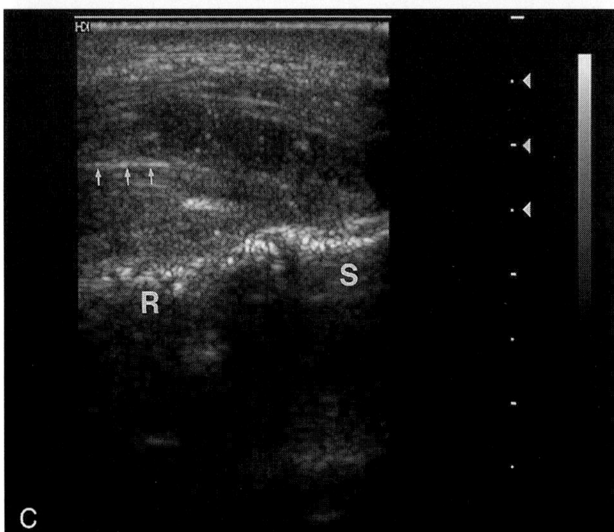

Figure 14–31 ■ **A,** Pyomyositis of the pectoralis muscle: transverse sonogram. One week following transureteral prostatectomy, this 80-year-old male presented with acute swelling of the right pectoralis muscle. This transverse image demonstrates loss of the normal pennate muscle architecture with marked swelling of the muscle. A nodular mixed echogenic structure is noted centrally. **B,** Pyomyositis of the pectoralis muscle: transverse sonogram. Same patient and imaging location as in **A**. Power Doppler imaging demonstrated hyperemia of the periosteum of the first rib. **C,** Pyomyositis of the pectoralis muscle: transverse sonogram. Same patient and imaging location as in Figure **A**. Direct aspiration of the mass was unsuccessful. Therefore, nonbacteriostatic saline was injected and aspirated, and a tissue specimen was obtained. Cultures were positive for *Klebsiella,* and a histological examination showed acute inflammation of muscle compatible with pyomyositis. Abbreviations: needle (*arrows*), first rib (*R*), sternum (*S*).

and the edge of the lesion, and avoid areas of liquefaction. One specimen should be sent in a container on sterile gauze moistened with sterile, nonbacteriostatic saline, and at least one specimen should be sent in a container with formalin. Aspiration-reaspiration should be used in combination with biopsy if infection is suspected (Fig. 14–31).

Bone Lesion

Recently, we discovered the usefulness of ultrasound in the biopsy of certain bone lesions. This may appear contradictory since the internal structure of bone is invisible under pulsed Doppler ultrasound. However, lesions may be visible if they are subperiosteal or cortical in location and if they destroy the bone cortex. Lesions associated with subperiosteal breakthrough can also be considered for ultrasound biopsy. Ultrasound will be used if possible because of the ease of ultrasound localization of tumors (Fig. 14–32) and because of the comfort for both patient and examiner during ultrasound-guided procedures (Fig. 14–33). In lesions with an intact cortical shell, the procedure is more involved than that in soft tissue biopsy because of the sensitivity of the periosteum. The patient should be kept NPO the night of the procedure and blood coagulation tested the next morning. Sedation is often necessary because of the depth of the biopsy and the sensitivity of the bone envelope. An intramuscular injection of Valium is given approximately half an hour before the procedure. An intravenous line is placed and a pulse oximeter applied to one finger prior to the start of the procedure. In sensitive patients, 0.25 mg Oxymorphone is injected intravenously at the start of the procedure. Dose increments of up to 0.5 mg can be given during the

Text continued on page 458

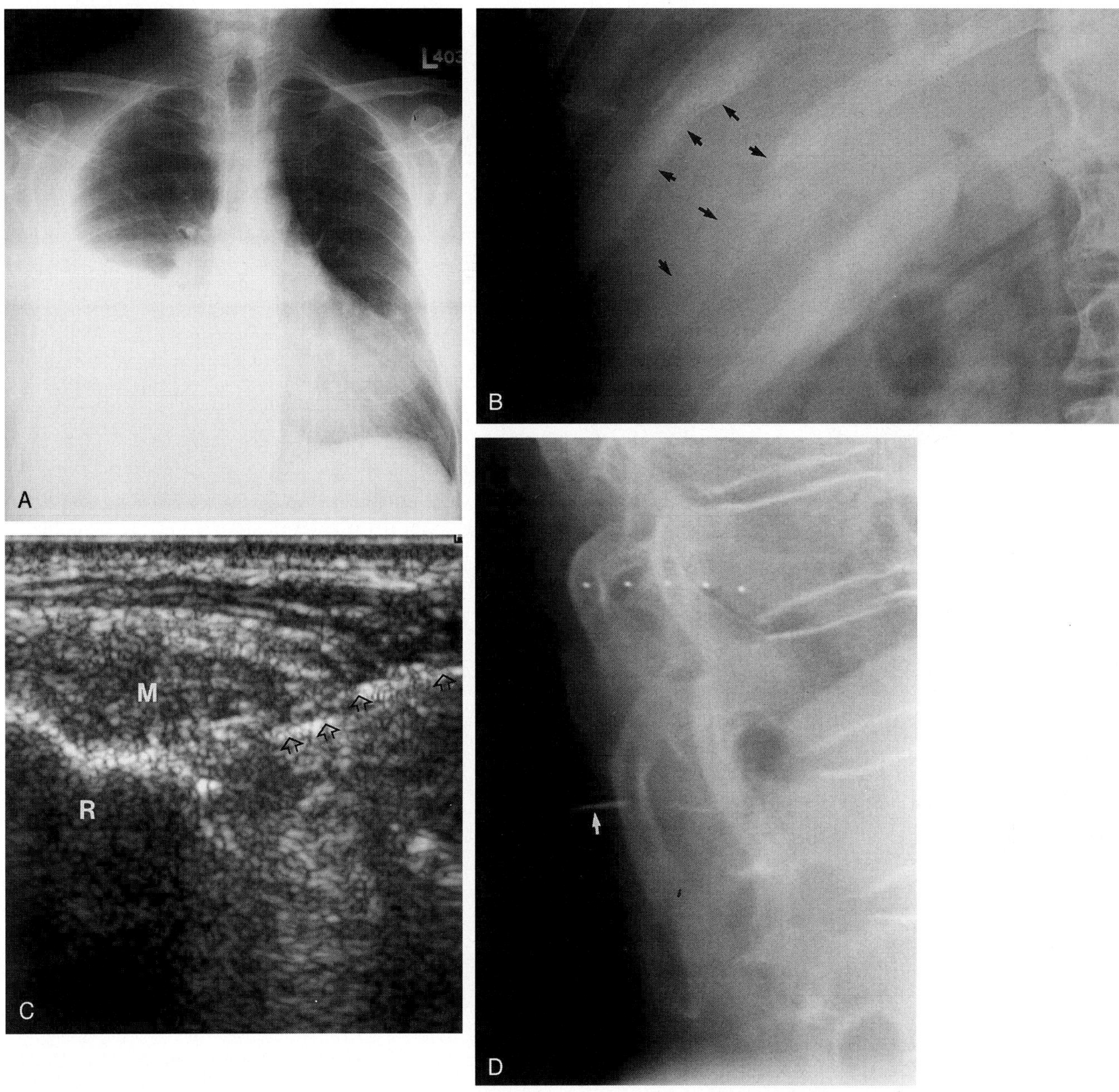

Figure 14–32 ■ **A,** Mesothelioma: chest radiograph. The patient is a 75-year-old pipe fitter who presented with right upper quadrant pain. A large right pleural effusion is present. **B,** Mesothelioma: rib detail radiograph. Same patient as in Figure **A**. Erosion of the posterolateral aspects of the right ninth and tenth ribs is demonstrated (*arrows*). **C,** Mesothelioma: longitudinal sonogram. Same patient as in **A**. This image, obtained with the transducer aligned along the length of the eroded tenth rib, demonstrates a soft tissue mass (*M*) associated with the rib (*R*). A core biopsy needle (*open arrows*) is seen entering the soft tissue mass from the right. The needle "guillotine" is in the open position. Cortical bone lesions are easily biopsied under ultrasound guidance. **D,** Mesothelioma: lateral spot fluoroscopic image. Same patient as in **A**. Often, fluoroscopic guidance is not very valuable for biopsy of superficial cortical lesions. A needle (*arrow*) is anchored in a soft tissue mass. The lesion itself was not identifiable on the tangential radiograph. The serial dots in the image represent a measurement scale for digital fluoroscopy. Histological exam of the specimen was diagnostic for mesothelioma.

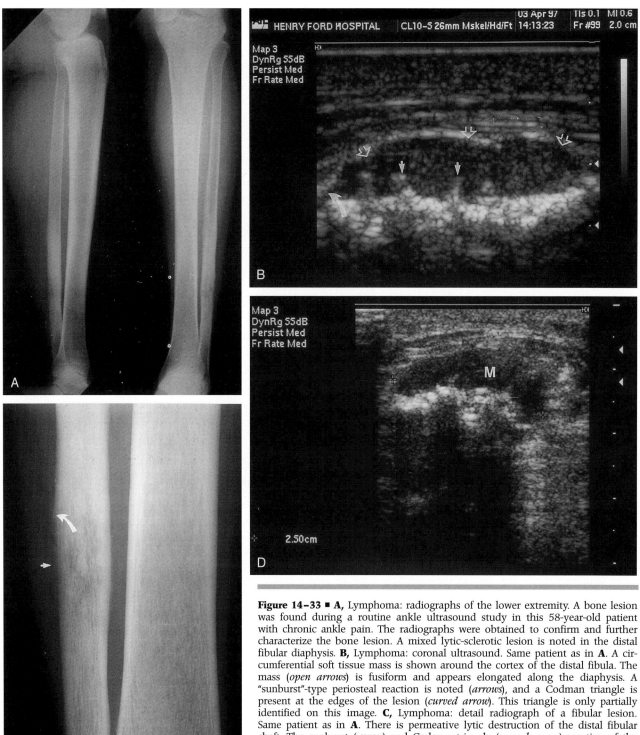

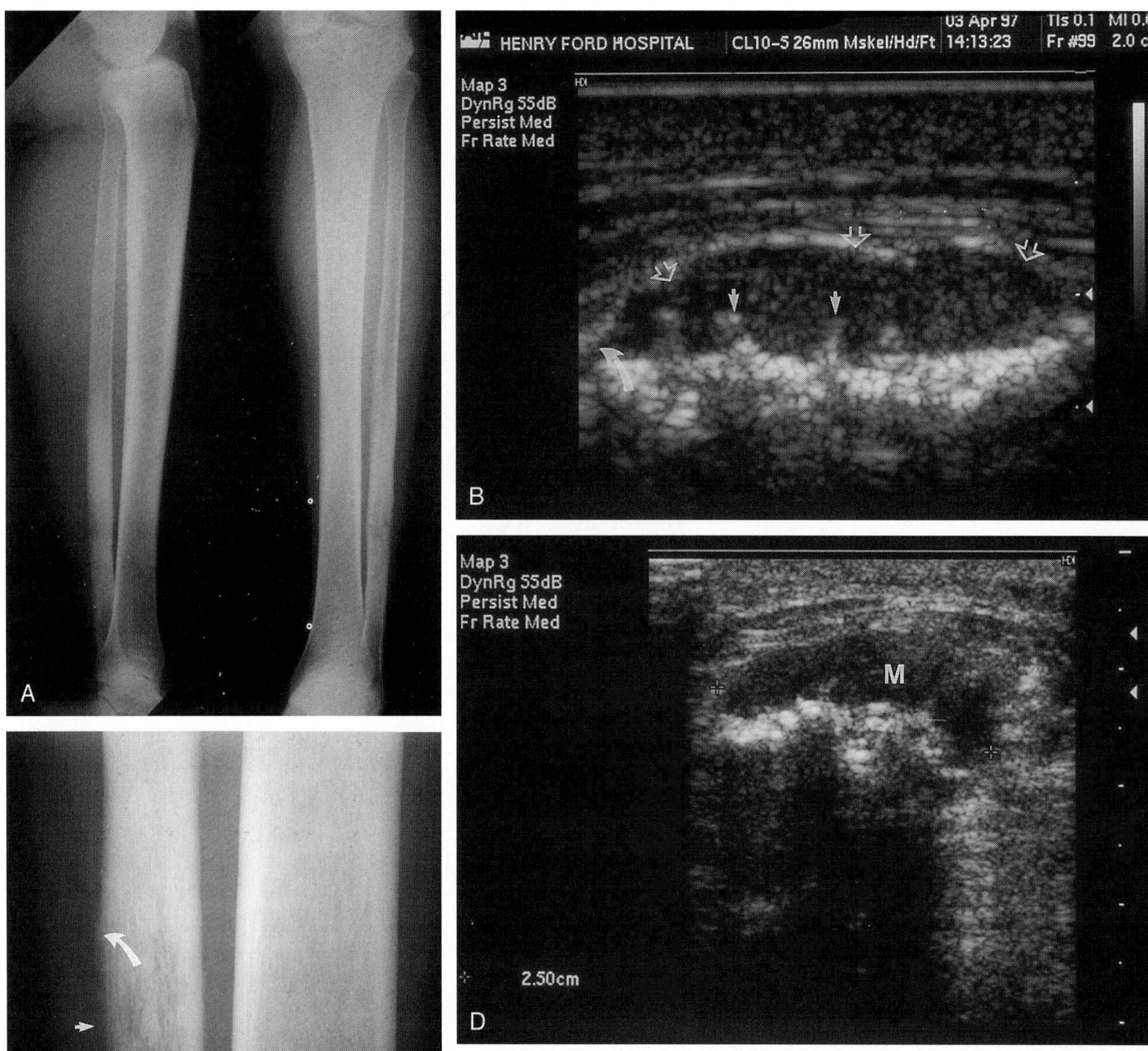

Figure 14–33 ■ **A,** Lymphoma: radiographs of the lower extremity. A bone lesion was found during a routine ankle ultrasound study in this 58-year-old patient with chronic ankle pain. The radiographs were obtained to confirm and further characterize the bone lesion. A mixed lytic-sclerotic lesion is noted in the distal fibular diaphysis. **B,** Lymphoma: coronal ultrasound. Same patient as in **A**. A circumferential soft tissue mass is shown around the cortex of the distal fibula. The mass (*open arrows*) is fusiform and appears elongated along the diaphysis. A "sunburst"-type periosteal reaction is noted (*arrows*), and a Codman triangle is present at the edges of the lesion (*curved arrow*). This triangle is only partially identified on this image. **C,** Lymphoma: detail radiograph of a fibular lesion. Same patient as in **A**. There is permeative lytic destruction of the distal fibular shaft. The sunburst (*arrow*) and Codman triangle (*curved arrow*) reaction of the periosteum are clearly identified. **D,** Lymphoma: transverse ultrasound. Same patient as in **A**. A kidney-shaped hypoechoic mass (*M*) surrounds an irregular cortex and periosteum. The mass measures 2.5 cm between the calipers.

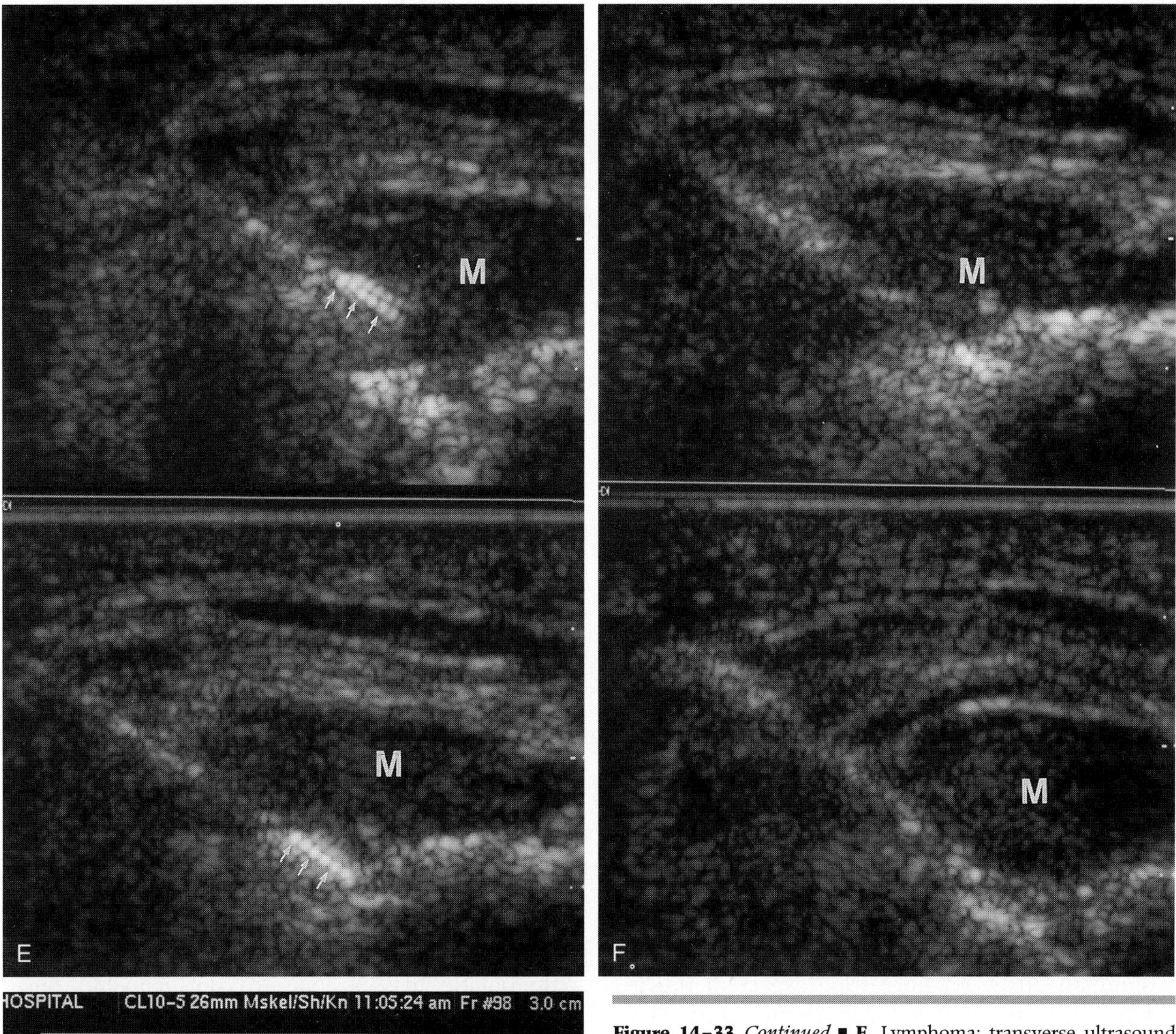

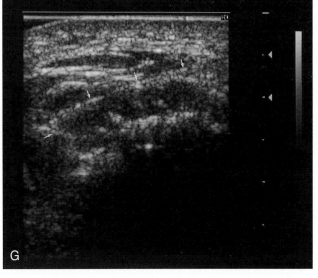

Figure 14–33 *Continued* ■ **E,** Lymphoma: transverse ultrasound during a biopsy. Same patient as in **A**. A bone biopsy needle traverses the soft tissue mass (*M*) and approaches the bone surface (*top image*). The needle then enters the periosteum (*bottom image*). Note the corkscrew threads on the distal end of the biopsy needle (*small arrows*). **F,** Lymphoma: transverse ultrasound during a biopsy. Same patient as in **A**. Force must now be applied, and the needle is turned into the bone, manually rotating a handle at the opposite end of the needle. The bone biopsy needle traverses the periosteum (*top image*) and disappears in the cortex (*bottom image*). **G,** Lymphoma: transverse ultrasound during wire localization. Same patient as in **A**. The center of the mass was marked with a harpoon-like (*small arrows*) localizing wire prior to surgical removal. Histopathological examination of the bone biopsy sample and of the surgical specimen showed large B-cell lymphoma. Staging of this non-Hodgkin lymphoma was negative for other disease locations. The patient underwent chemotherapy and radiation and was free of disease $1\frac{1}{2}$ years later.

procedure. Additional local anesthesia should be applied in and around the periosteum. Bone biopsy needles with irregular teeth at the tip can be screwed into the bone. The stylet or trocar is removed as soon as the bone surface is reached. Simultaneous pushing and rotation of the needle into the lesion advances the needle. The needle is placed about 1 cm deep into the tumor and then withdrawn. It should be pulled back gently to avoid self-inflicted injury. The sterile biopsy packet contains a metallic stylet with a blunt tip to remove the bone core from the biopsy needle.

Most biopsies can be done with the elegant, thin, and disposable OSTEOCUT needle (EZM). Very distant lesions may need a more complicated coaxial biopsy needle. The Geremia needle allows us to take sufficient samples of deep-seated bone structures in a minimally invasive fashion. The larger Craig bone biopsy set is used only if the pathologist needs large specimens and the lesion is located superficially. A discussion of the individual case with the pathologist prior to the procedure is always helpful.

Lesions that have destroyed the cortex completely are easier to sample, and conscious sedation will not be necessary for most patients (Rubens et al., 1997). In metastatic lesions and lesions with a soft tissue component smaller than 3 cm, fine-needle aspiration with 22-gauge needles will often suffice (Civardi et al., 1994; Rubens et al., 1997). For lesions with a soft tissue mass greater than 3 cm and for sarcomas, 14- to 18-gauge core biopsy needles are necessary (Logan et al., 1996).

In cases of a single lytic lesion, specimens must be sent to the microbiology and pathology laboratories simultaneously. An interesting aspect of procedures in bone and joint radiology is the need for a procedure with combined biopsy and aspiration in some lesions. All bone lesions, which could represent infection, need such intervention. This often requires the use of ultrasound and fluoroscopy during the same procedure.

First, the workup of such lesions requires a detailed examination of the bone marrow with MRI. The location of fluid can be assessed with intravenous Gadolinium using fat-suppressed T_1-weighted images. At the beginning of the procedure, ultrasound can locate fluid, if present, in the soft tissues around the bone. Aspiration of fluid and Gram stain can end the study quickly if the test is positive. In other patients, ultrasound will help find the cloaca, and the intraosseous abscess can then be found easily by pushing a needle through the cloaca in the direction of the abscess. In many cases of chronic osteomyelitis, there will be fluid in the bone that has not yet emerged. The bone biopsy will then require fluoroscopy to guide the biopsy needle in the direction of the presumed cavern in the bone. When the needle enters the cavity, a sudden drop in resistance will occur. The core-filled bone biopsy needle must then be removed and the tissue specimen submitted for histological exam. Afterward, a spinal needle must be introduced and directed in the tract of the prior bone biopsy. This tract appears as a round defect in the cortex on magnification fluoroscopy. The thin biopsy needle must enter the ring-like cortical lucency. The needle follows the biopsy path easily once it enters the defect. Ultrasound may be of assistance during the procedure if fluoroscopy does not localize the cortical defect adequately. In most instances, ultrasound finds biopsy tracts easily. The needle is then pushed through the biopsy tract into the cavern caused by infection. Pus is sent for culture and Gram stain. Biopsies are of the utmost importance in cases with equivocal imaging findings. It is not always possible to distinguish osteomyelitis with a large pus collection from a tumor with significant tissue necrosis.

Presurgical Hookwire Localization

Most soft tissue lesions are easily palpable, and the surgeon will need preoperative imaging only for diagnostic reasons and for staging of a tumor. However, there are small lesions that the surgeon cannot palpate (Fig. 14–34). Modern cross-sectional imaging techniques are so sensitive that they may help detect small nerve tumors, ganglia, or other symptomatic masses that are not palpable. Small masses can be extremely tender if they irritate major nerve branches or contain multiple nerve endings. The patient may then insist on having the lesion removed.

Prior to removal of a small lesion, we are often asked to mark the mass sonographically. The procedure consists of careful scanning in both the longitudinal and transverse planes. We then sterilize the field and rescan the extremity under sterile conditions. Most often, the transverse plane is used. The shortest and safest path through the soft tissues is chosen, and a Hookwire is placed along that path. The Hookwire is the type of wire used in mammography localization. Ultrasound ensures correct placement in masses that can be as small as 1 cm (Rubens et al., 1997). The wire is opened by removing its metallic cover when ultrasound shows it to

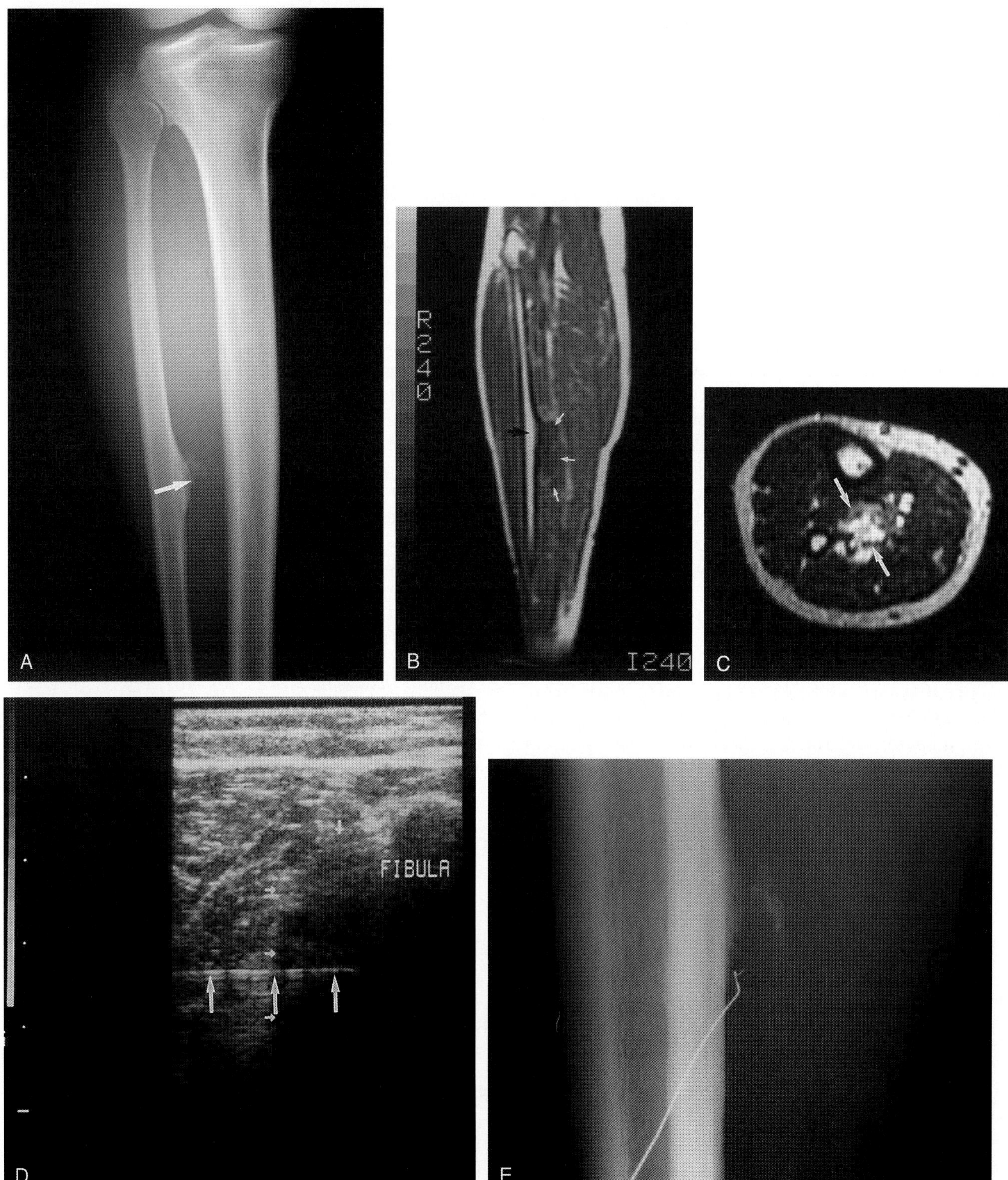

Figure 14–34 ■ **A,** Wire localization of parosteal mass: frontal radiograph. This 23-year-old male presented with pain in the right calf. Several years earlier, he had had a below-knee amputation of the left leg for treatment of a synovial sarcoma. A partially calcified parosteal mass (*arrow*) is noted, associated with the middiaphysis of the fibula. **B,** Wire localization of a parosteal mass: T_1-weighted coronal image. Normal marrow signal (*black arrow*) is demonstrated in the fibula adjacent to this cortical and parosteal lesion (*white arrows*). **C,** Wire localization of a parosteal mass: T_2-weighted axial image. The parosteal mass measures 2.7 cm in the greatest transverse dimension and is located in the deep posterior compartment. Since this mass (*arrows*) was not palpable, the surgeon requested image-guided localization in order to reduce the extent of the surgical exposure. **D,** Wire localization of a parosteal mass: transverse sonogram. Sonographic imaging was performed over the deep lateral posterior compartment. A wire localization needle (*large arrows*) was advanced into the lesion (*small arrows*). **E,** Wire localization of a parosteal mass: fluoroscopic spot radiograph. This image confirms the position of the localizing wire. The mass was cleanly excised, and histological analysis demonstrated myositis ossificans.

be in the center of the mass. The end of the wire is firmly placed over the skin and affixed with a transparent window adhesive. The patient is sent to the operating room, and the wire is prepared as part of the operating field. This technique minimizes tissue damage; it allows a small, esthetically acceptable skin incision and reduces time in surgery considerably.

Image Guided Surgery

Ultrasound's role in guiding musculoskeletal procedures is limited. Sonographers have removed certain foreign bodies using ultrasound. We have found it most useful in removing pieces of gravel or metallic foreign bodies. Removal of pieces of glass is more delicate and requires a combined approach of ultrasound and surgery. Wood can be removed, but only when the injury is fresh. Splinters and thorns that have been causing granulation for weeks cannot be removed as one piece, and they often disintegrate upon removal.

The percutaneous removal of foreign bodies requires sterile preparation of the transducer, skin cleansing with iodine and alcohol, and sterile instruments that can grab the foreign body. Make sure that you have a set of instruments available: forceps, alligator and Kocher, for example. Two pairs of hands are useful during the procedure. The sonographer handles the transducer and the grasping instrument. Another person can handle sterile solutions, gauze, transducer, and instruments.

The procedure begins with sonographic localization of the foreign body. The most superficial end of the foreign body is marked. A small dot can be marked on the skin with a sterile marker to locate this point. A skin incision is made that will allow the instrument to enter the cutis and subcutaneous tissues. The instrument is then guided toward the foreign body, using ultrasound to guide it and establish the road map. The transducer is removed if and when the piece has been firmly grasped. Make sure that the skin incision is wide enough to allow extraction without injury, and proceed with removal. Careful rescanning of the surface to make sure that all material has been removed always follows foreign body removal.

Tumor ablation has been performed percutaneously as well. An alcohol solution can be used to induce necrosis in posttraumatic neuromas and in Morton's neuromas. Ultrasound is the preferred imaging method because of its superior spatial resolution and its ability to show and follow the normal nerve into the mass. This allows us to target nerve lesions with great accuracy and without causing damage to the normal nerve feeding the lesion. Pathological lymph node removal and extraction of recurrent melanoma have been done for diagnostic purposes. These few examples demonstrate what is possible with ultrasound guidance: faster and more accurate procedures that save tissue and reduce costs. However, much more is possible and remains unexplored. Better communication between orthopedic surgeons and imagers may soon lead to new percutaneous procedures. We anticipate that the following procedures may be done percutaneously and with ultrasound guidance: tendon, ligament, and capsular release, loose body removal, and meniscal and rotator cuff repair.

References

Andrén L, Lundberg BJ: Treatment of rigid shoulders by joint distention during arthrography. *Acta Orthop Scand* 356:45, 1965.

Breidahl WH, et al: Power Doppler sonography in tenosynovitis: Significance of the peritendinous hypoechoic rim. *J Ultrasound Med* 17:103–107, 1998.

Chhem RK, Kaplan PA, Dussault RG, et al: Ultrasonography of the musculoskeletal system. *Radiol Clin North Am* 32:275, 1994.

Civardi G, et al: Lytic bone lesions suspected for metastasis: Ultrasonically guided fine needle aspiration biopsy. *J Clin Ultrasound* 22:307, 1994.

Desjardin LE, et al: Comparison of the ABI System and Competitive PCR for quantification of IS 6110 DNA in sputum during treatment of tuberculosis. *J Clin Microbiol* 36:1964–1968, 1998.

Farin PU: Consistency of rotator-cuff calcifications: Observations on plain radiography, sonography, computed tomography, and a needle treatment. *Invest Radiol* 31:300, 1996.

Gaucher H, et al: Échographie articulaire pédiatrique. Aspects de la pathologie synoviale. *J Radiol* 78: 1123–1138, 1997.

Kesteris U: The effect of arthrocentesis in transient synovitis of the hip in the child: A longitudinal sonographic study. *J Pediatr Orthop* 16(1):24–29, 1996.

Lindblad S: Recent progress in the study of synovitis by macroscopic and microscopic examination—a review. *Scand J Rheumatol* 17(76):27–32, 1988.

Logan PM, et al: Image guided percutaneous biopsy of musculoskeletal tumors: An algorithm for selection of specific biopsy techniques. *AJR* 166:137, 1996.

Loyer EM, et al: Imaging of superficial soft-tissue infections: Sonographic findings in cases of cellulitis and abscess. *AJR* 166:149, 1996.

Marchal GJ, et al: Ultrasonography in transient synovitis of the hip in children. *Radiology* 162:825–828, 1987.

Resnick D, Kang HS: *Internal Derangements of Joints.* Philadelphia, WB Saunders Co, 1988, chap 12.

Rubens DJ, et al: Effective ultrasonographically guided intervention for diagnosis of musculoskeletal lesions. *J Ultrasound Med* 16:831–842, 1997.

Schumacher HR, Kulka JP: Needle biopsy of the synovial membrane. *N Engl J Med* 286:416–419, 1972.

Shutzer SE: Diagnosing Lyme disease. *Am Fam Physician* 45(5):2151–2156, 1992.

Stevens DL (ed): Skin, soft tissue, bone and joint infections. In Mandell GL (ed chief): *Atlas of Infectious Diseases,* vol 2. Philadelphia, Churchill Livingstone, 1995, pp 1–5.

van Holsbeeck M, Introcaso JH: Musculoskeletal ultrasonography. *Radiol Clin North Am* 30:907, 1992.

van Holsbeeck MT, et al: Detection of infection in loosened hip prostheses. *AJR* 163:381–384, 1994.

Van Vugt RM, van Dalen A, Bijlsma JWJ: Ultrasound guided synovial biopsy of the wrist. *Scand J Rheumatol* 26:212–214, 1997.

Chapter 15
Sonography of the Shoulder

Ronnie Ptasznik, MBBS, FRANZCR

Introduction

The shoulder joint is probably the most accessible joint for sonography in the adult. Most shoulder joint syndromes are not related to an erosive or degenerative arthropathy but are in fact caused by pathological changes in the periarticular soft tissues of the joint. Conventional radiographs remain the mandatory first step in the investigation of patients presenting with shoulder pain, as the clinical signs and symptoms of rotator cuff syndromes are nonspecific. Neoplasms of either bone or soft tissue can mimic rotator cuff pathology, as can erosive or degenerative arthropathies of the glenohumeral joint (Crass and Craig, 1988).

Up to 7% of patients presenting with shoulder pain have rotator cuff calcifications (Faure and Daculsi, 1983). Conventional radiographs may demonstrate an os acromiale, ossification of the coracoacromial ligament, excessive downward-sloping or low-lying acromion, downward-sloping coracoid, prominent greater tuberosity (usually posttraumatic), or hypertrophic changes in the acromioclavicular joint, all factors predisposing to impingement. Superior subluxation of the glenohumeral joint resulting in an acromial humeral distance of less than 6 mm is specific for the presence of a rotator cuff tear. Conventional radiographs may show irregular, sclerotic, or cystic changes in the greater tuberosity or undersurface of the acromion, suggesting rotator cuff degeneration. However, radiography is unable to make a definitive diagnosis in the majority of cases (Fig. 15–1) (Gold et al., 1993).

Other diagnostic modalities, such as arthroscopy or MRI/CT arthrography are expensive, time-consuming, and invasive. While arthrography is accurate in the detection of full-thickness tears it is inaccurate in the assessment of tear size and cannot detect bursal surface partial-thickness tears. Arthrography also cannot distinguish between a normal tendon and one that is dysfunctional but intact (Hall, 1986). MRI has difficulty distinguishing tears from degeneration of the cuff (Stiles and Otte, 1993).

Ultrasound has the added advantage of offering a dynamic examination enabling an assessment of both the range of movement and muscular coordination about the joint. Sonography has been increasingly employed in the assessment of the shoulder and rotator cuff since the mid-1980s (Crass et al., 1984; Bretzke et al., 1985; Mack et al., 1985; Middleton et al., 1984, 1985, 1986; Patee and Snyder, 1988; Mellerowicz et al., 1990).

Clinical Aspects

Patients presenting with shoulder pain, including those complaining of a painful arc and pain worsening at night, may in fact have a variety of underlying complaints. These include syndromes involving rotator cuff attrition such as rotator cuff tendinitis, tendinopathy, partial- and full-thickness rotator cuff tears, and syndromes not involving cuff attrition such as cervical nerve root compression, acromioclavicular joint inflammation, calcific tendinitis, fractures, and adhesive capsulitis. Sixty percent of shoulder abnormalities have been attributed to rotator cuff disease (Hawkins, 1989). Arthroscopic studies suggest that 10% of painful shoulders are due to full-thickness tears, with the majority of the remainder consisting almost entirely of partial-thickness tears, bursal thickening, and tendinitis (Brenneke and Morgan, 1992) .

Most rotator cuff pathology is related to cuff fiber failure (Matsen, Arntz, and Lippitt, 1998). Epidemiological (Codman 1934) and pathological (Ozaki, 1988) studies have shown that the incidence of rotator cuff fiber failure and resulting rotator cuff tears increases with age. Rotator cuff tears are un-

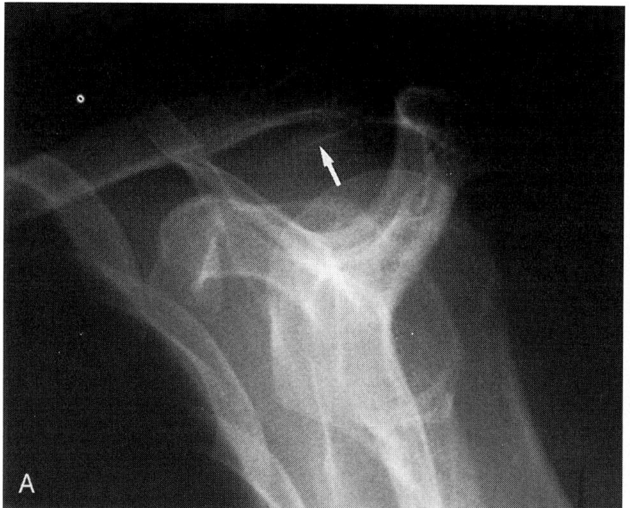

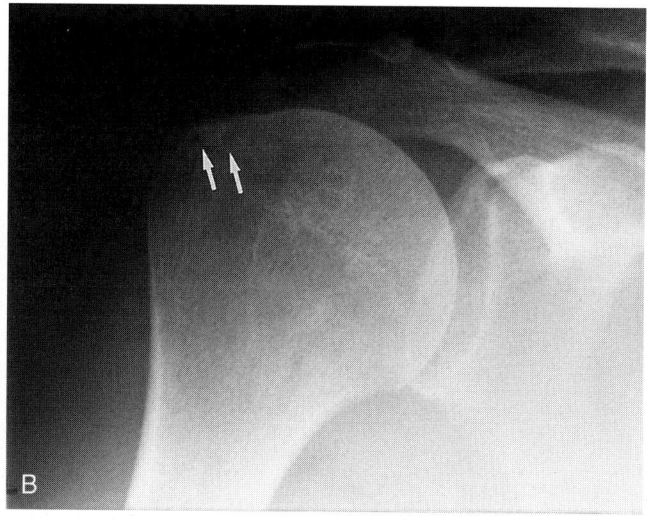

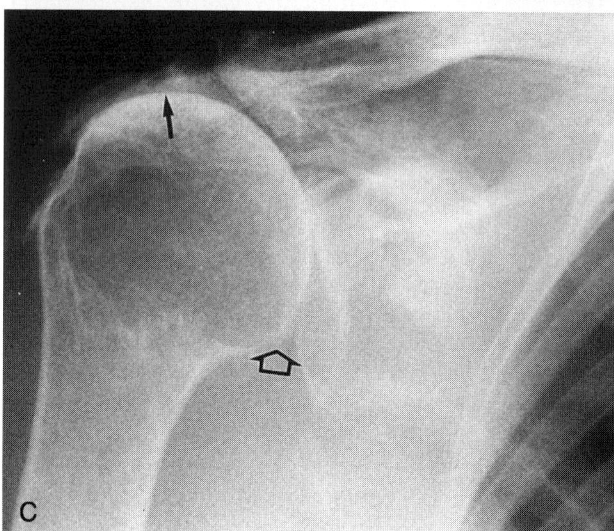

Figure 15-1 ■ **A,** Impingement syndrome: shoulder radiograph. A 56-year-old person presents with a painful arc. Lateral X-ray of the shoulder joint with 15 degrees of down tilt, the so-called outlet view. The anterior acromion slopes inferiorly (*arrow*), a finding associated with impingement syndrome. **B,** Impingement syndrome: shoulder radiograph. Severe shoulder pain awakens this 68-year-old man every night. This has been going on for at least 1 month. An anteroposterior X-ray of the shoulder demonstrates cystic and sclerotic changes at the greater tuberosity (*arrows*), a finding associated with rotator cuff degeneration. **C,** Impingement syndrome: shoulder radiograph. This 85-year-old man complains of chronically restricted and painful shoulder movement. An anteroposterior X-ray of the shoulder demonstrates obliteration of the subacromial space, eburnation, and rounding of the greater tuberosity (*arrow*) associated with superior subluxation of the glenohumeral joint (*open arrow*), findings characteristic of a massive chronic rotator cuff tear.

common below the age of 30, start increasing in frequency after the age of 40, affect about 40% of the population in the seventh decade of life, and are present in the majority of the population over 70 years of age (Katthagen, 1989). Cuff fiber failure probably commences as a degenerative process, tendinopathy, and progresses through partial-thickness tears to full-thickness tears of the rotator cuff, generally involving first the supraspinatus tendon and then multiple tendons. Cuff fibers may fail a few at a time, giving rise to a clinical presentation often misinterpreted as bursitis or tendinitis. Neer coined the term *impingement* in 1972 (Neer, 1972).

There is no comparable tendon, such as the supraspinatus of the rotator cuff, which is situated between two bones (the head of the humerus and the acromion), that can be compressed as if between pincers. Forward flexion is the most common movement of the upper body. As the humerus is raised, the supraspinatus tendon immediately abuts against the coracohumeral ligament and the anterior edge of the acromion. This compression leads to both mechanical irritation and ischemia. These combined insults, if prolonged, cause degenerative changes (tendinopathy). The tendinopathy and consequent fiber failure impair an important rotator cuff function: stabilization of the humeral head at the glenoid and humeral depression. As a result, there is an increased tendency for impingement as the humerus is elevated unopposed by deltoid contraction, leading in turn to further attrition of the rotator cuff. The tendinopathy and rotator cuff tears generally commence in the so-called critical zone of the supraspinatus tendon, an area of relative avascularity located approximately 0.5–1 cm proximal to the distal tendon insertion upon the greater tuberosity.

Isolated subscapularis tears are uncommon and have been described as a component of the pathology seen in recurrent dislocation of the shoulder (DePalma et al., 1967) and in sudden violent contractions of the subscapularis during adduction and internal rotation. These tears have been detected by ultrasound (Dragoni et al., 1994). Tears of the infraspinatus tendon are almost never seen in isolation.

Impingement has been classified into three stages by Neer. Stage 1 involves edema and hemorrhage in the bursa and the rotator cuff. Stage 2 is characterized by fibrosis, thickening of the subacromial soft tissue, and sometimes partial rupture of the rotator cuff. In Stage 3 there is complete rupture of the rotator cuff. The impingement syndrome frequently occurs before the age of 25, especially in young athletes engaged in repetitive, frequent throwing motions (e.g., volleyball, tennis, badminton, javelin, and swimming) (Neer, 1972) Treatment programs designed to decrease impingement pathophysiology in young people have not always had good long-term results. This has led to the observation that impingement pathophysiology may coexist with or be secondary to primary instability.

In patients presenting with impingement-like symptoms below the age of 35, instability should be considered the primary disorder until proven otherwise. It should be remembered that not everyone who has shoulder pain and dysfunction has impingement syndrome, and not everyone who has impingement has primary impingement syndrome (Stiles and Otte, 1993).

Instrumentation

High-resolution linear array transducers are essential. A minimum frequency of 7.5 MHz is required. Recently, the introduction of broad-bandwidth technology with improved electronic focusing has further improved spatial and contrast resolution. Ten and even 12 MHz transducers are now becoming commonplace. Sector scanners, curved linear array scanners, and all other transducers with a diverging ultrasound beam are not acceptable. They are limited by poor near-field resolution and are more prone to anisotropy, as only a small percentage of tendon fibers in the center of the image provide specular reflection.

Examination Technique

A detailed knowledge of the complex anatomy and pathology related to the rotator cuff and the glenohumeral joint is essential (Katthagen, 1989; Middleton, 1992; Mack and Matsen, 1995). The examination is recorded on film. Our protocol is to record 15 standard "slices" followed by a dynamic assessment of glenohumeral movement relative to the acromion process of the scapula. The technique is a modification of that described by Mack et al. (1995). It is essential that the radiologist issuing the report has also examined the patient. Reports based solely on a review of static sonogram photographs have been shown to be highly inaccurate (Drakeford et al., 1990).

Patient Position

The examination commences with the patient sitting facing the examiner on a rotating chair or stool. A built-in foot rest is an advantage, as it encourages the correct degree of elbow flexion. A back rest encourages an erect posture, which enhances visualization of the rotator cuff and the biceps tendon.

Slice 1: Biceps Transverse

The patient sits with the elbow flexed to 90 degrees, the forearm half pronated resting gently on the lap, and the fingers pointing toward the opposite knee. This causes slight internal rotation at the glenohumeral joint, bringing the bicipital groove into an anterior position. The examiner can hold the ipsilateral wrist of the patient to allow fine tuning of the bicipital groove's position.

The long head of the biceps brachii (LHB) originates at the supraglenoid tubercle and glenoid labrum in the superiormost portion of the glenoid. The origin of the tendon is not visible during an ultrasound examination. The intra-articular portion of the LHB is easily identified on transverse scans as an oval-shaped echogenic structure forming a sonographic anatomical landmark between the tendons of the subscapularis anteromedially and the supraspinatus posterolaterally. The tendon can be followed inferiorly as it travels obliquely to enter the bicipital groove deep to the echogenic transverse humeral ligament.

The transducer is oriented transversely and placed on the upper arm of the patient directly over the bicipital groove. The bicipital groove and its contained tendon are easily located on axial scans of the humeral head lying between the lesser and greater tuberosities (Fig. 15–2).

Slice 2: Biceps Longitudinal

The transducer is then oriented perpendicularly between the tuberosities to obtain longitudinal images of the tendon. The longitudinal view of a normal tendon reveals a fine fibrillary pattern. The fibrillary pattern should be seen with a modern 7.5-MHz

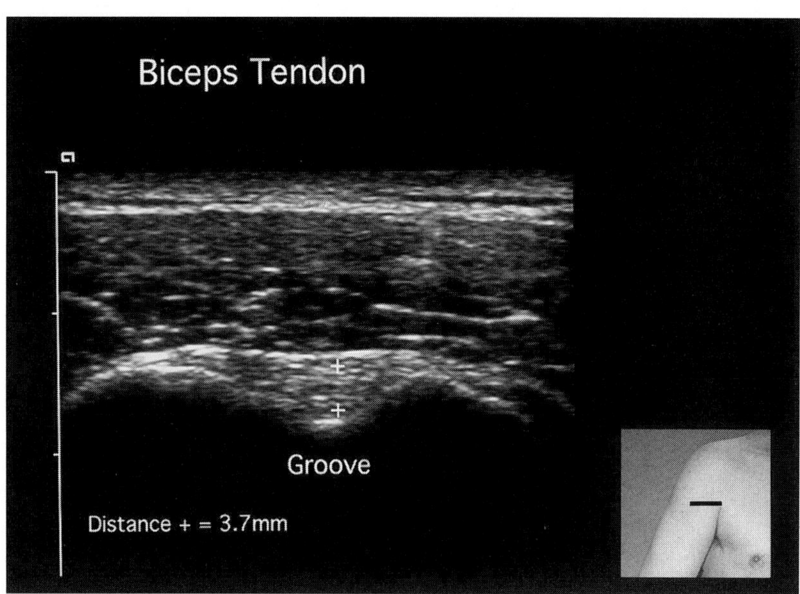

Figure 15–2 ■ Normal biceps tendon: transverse sonogram. An asymptomatic 24-year-old medical student. Transverse view of normal biceps tendon within the bicipital groove. The tendon is a rounded, echogenic structure 3.7 mm in depth (+).

transducer in even the largest patients. It is usually necessary to angle superiorly, "heel to toe," in order to visualize the tendon in an orthogonal manner (Fig. 15–3). Absence of the fibrillary pattern is always abnormal.

Slice 3: Subscapularis Transverse

The position of the transducer does not generally require alteration. The patient's elbow is placed against the ipsilateral iliac crest, and the glenohumeral joint is placed in external rotation.

The subscapularis tendon has a convex superficial margin and is outlined by an echogenic layer representing subdeltoid fat. The subscapularis tendon forms an acute angle at its insertion on the lesser tuberosity. The apex of this angle, in the neutral position prior to external rotation, points toward 11 o'clock when the right shoulder is examined and 1 o'clock when the left shoulder is examined. Following full external rotation at the glenohumeral joint, this orientation should be 7 o'clock and 5 o'clock, respectively. Failure to point below the

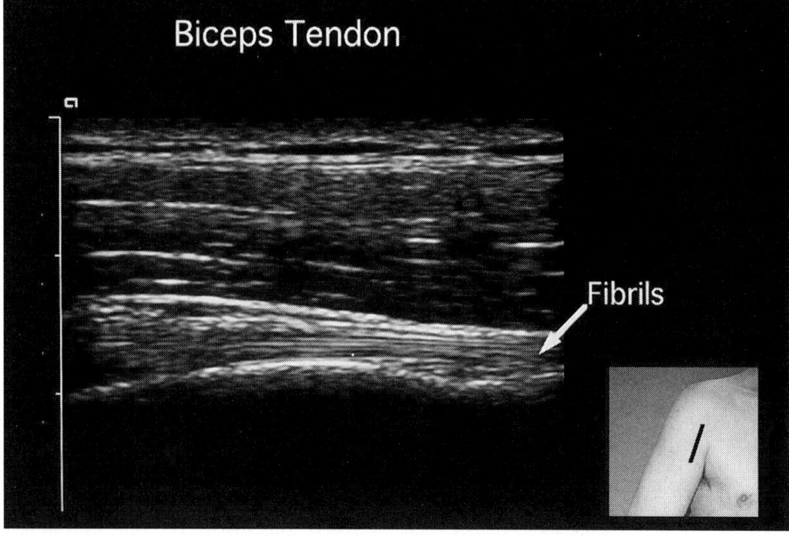

Figure 15–3 ■ Normal biceps tendon: longitudinal sonogram. Same person as in Figure 15–2. A fine fibrillar pattern is evident throughout the length of the long biceps tendon (*arrow*). The subacromial bursa is a potential space between the tendon and the overlying deltoid muscle.

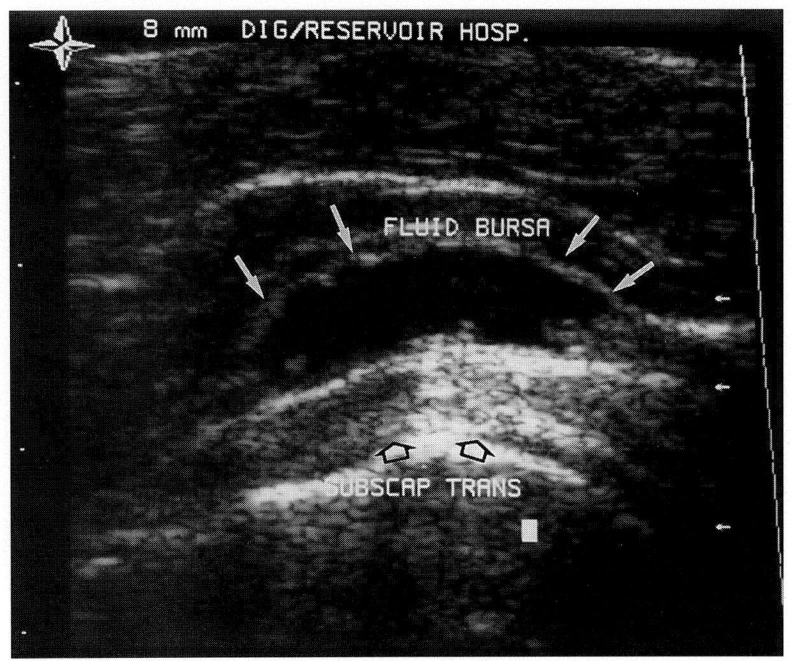

Figure 15–4 ■ Bursal fluid: transverse sonogram. This 53-year-old man presents with shoulder weakness and pain upon forward arm elevation. Symptoms started spontaneously about 6 weeks ago. Bursal fluid (*arrows*) is seen with a full-thickness tear of the rotator cuff (not shown). The fluid was only detected superficial to the subscapularis tendon (*open arrows*) during external rotation.

horizontal (i.e., 9 and 3 o'clock) on either side is abnormal and reflects a restriction in the range of movement in external rotation (this is discussed in greater detail in the later section dealing with adhesive capsulitis).

The subacromial subdeltoid bursa is located superficial to the tendon, deep to the subdeltoid fat, and should not measure more than 2 mm in thickness. In the neutral position, small amounts of fluid within the bursa tend to collect within a subcoracoid recess, outside of the field of view. Following external rotation, this recess is obliterated, and any fluid present is forced laterally, superficial to the subscapularis tendon. This may be the only maneuver that displays bursal fluid (Fig. 15–4)

The humeral cortex deep to the tendon may be slightly scalloped. This is a normal anatomical variant. In this position, the transducer is swept superiorly and then inferiorly in order to cover the entire tendon.

Slice 4: Subscapularis Longitudinal

The glenohumeral joint is kept in external rotation, and the transducer is rotated 90 degrees. The subscapularis tendon appears as a convex cuff of tissue following the convex contour of the underlying humerus. Small amounts of subacromial bursal fluid, when present, will collect inferiorly. The longitudinal view aids in the detection of this fluid. Further, tears of the subscapularis tendon tend to be along the axial plane. The longitudinal view displays the sudden transition to a thinner structure more clearly, indicating the presence of a tear that may not be readily apparent on axial scanning.

Slice 5: Acromioclavicular Joint

The arm is returned to the neutral position. The transducer is oriented along the coronal plane. Commencing at the lateral edge of the acromion, the transducer is moved slowly medially until the acromioclavicular joint is visualized. The clavicular cortical surface is usually positioned slightly superior to that of the acromion. The joint capsule is readily identified and is usually closely applied to the periarticular surface of the clavicle. The origin of the deltoid muscle on the outer clavicle and acromion can be identified adjacent to the joint. There is great variation in the ultrasound appearance of the joint with age, among patients, and even among the joints of the same patient. However, fragmentation of the periarticular cortex is always abnormal and may indicate previous trauma or osteolysis.

Careful note should be taken of any localized tenderness to sonographic palpation, particularly if the clavicular capsular insertion is stripped off the clavicle (Fig. 15–5). These findings generally indicate clinically significant inflammation within the joint. If gentle motion at the glenohumeral joint provokes bulging of the acromioclavicular joint capsule, it

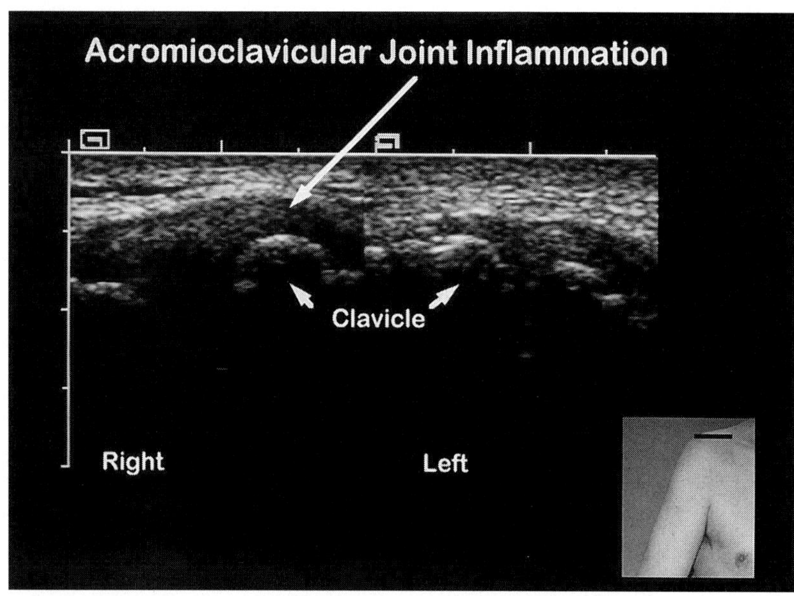

Figure 15–5 ■ Acromioclavicular joint inflammation: coronal Sonograms. A retired 33-year-old football player, has difficulty throwing a ball. Comparison of the normal left and abnormal right acromioclavicular joints in this patient, who presents with a painful arc and focal tenderness noted over the right acromioclavicular joint. The right joint capsule is distended (*long arrow*) and displaced from the clavicle (*short arrows*).

implies an abnormal communication between the two joints, indicating superior subluxation of the glenohumeral joint, erosion of the acromioclavicular joint capsule, and impending rotator cuff arthropathy. This is the ultrasound equivalent of the arthrographic "geyser sign" (see Fig. 15–29).

Slice 6: Infraspinatus Muscle/Posterior Glenoid Labrum

The patient's hand is placed on the contralateral shoulder. The patient is rotated 90 degrees, and the transducer is oriented in the axial plane until the head of the humerus is seen adjacent the posterior glenoid labrum. The deeper fibers of the infraspinatus muscle should be no more than 2 mm from the labrum; a greater distance than this indicates the presence of a joint effusion (Fig. 15–6). Fluid in the bursa, if present, may be seen superficial to the infraspinatus, but if bursal fluid is seen in this location, the total amount of fluid present within the bursa is likely to be large. A depression in the normally rounded contour of the humeral head at this

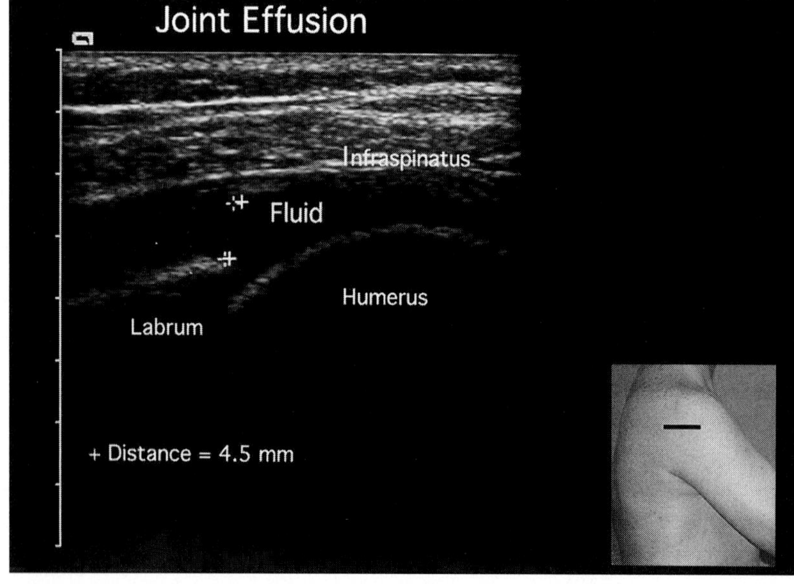

Figure 15–6 ■ Joint effusion: transverse sonogram. Same patient as in Figure 15–4. Posterior transverse view of the inferior glenoid labrum and the infraspinatus muscle. The deep fibers of the infraspinatus tendon are displaced 4.5 mm from the inferior glenoid labrum, indicating the presence of joint fluid. Note the normal rounded contour of the posterior humeral head at this level and compare it with Figure 15–7.

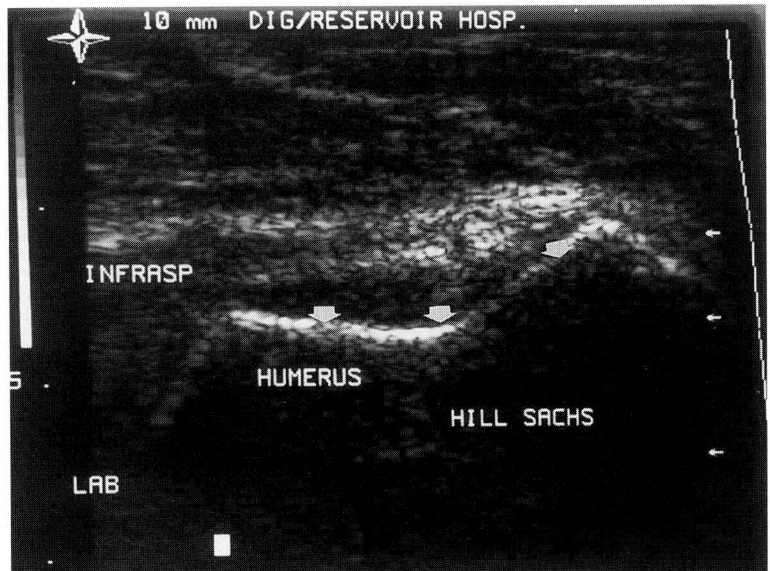

Figure 15–7 ■ Hill-Sachs defect: transverse sonogram. Painful shoulder in a 28-year-old football player. Hill-Sachs lesion in a patient with recurrent anterior dislocation of the glenohumeral joint. Same transducer position as in Figure 15–6. *Arrows* indicate the presence of a depressed fracture of the posterior humeral head.

level indicates the presence of a Hill Sachs deformity (Fig. 15–7). On occasion, ganglion cysts may be observed in the spinoscapular notch, medial the glenoid.

Slice 7: Infraspinatus Tendon

Next, the transducer is moved further laterally past the musculotendinous junction of the infraspinatus and the tendon, and its insertion comes into view. Radiographically occult calcification may be seen in this location. A notch in the bone is commonly seen deep to the musculotendinous junction. This is a normal finding, but it may be accentuated in throwing athletes. We do not routinely image teres minor, as pathology involving this tendon is exceedingly rare.

Slice 8: Supraspinatus Transverse Hyperextended, Internal Rotation

The patient's arm is put into full internal rotation and hyperextension, with the dorsum of the hand placed in the small of the back. There should be no air gap between the cubital fossa and the lateral chest wall. This position can best be explained to the patient by asking him or her to reach for the opposite back pocket. Sufficient internal rotation should be applied to place the biceps tendon in a bottom corner of the screen.

The full internal rotation/hyperextension view places the rotator cuff under stress and helps accentuate cuff defects. In this position, the supraspinatus tendon becomes an anterior structure, emerging from underneath the cover of the acromion, and is therefore generally superior to the neutral or shrug position, where most of the tendon is hidden (Crass et al., 1987). In most patients, the echogenicity of the supraspinatus tendon is greater than that of the deltoid muscle.

Correct orientation is achieved when the imaging plane shows crisp definition of the bone surface and a sharp outline of the cartilage of the humeral head. Patients who have adhesive capsulitis may not be able to tolerate this position. Any tendon seen posterolateral to the biceps tendon should be considered supraspinatus tendon. Any tendon tissue lying anteromedially is subscapularis tissue.

Scanning commences superiorly at the level of the coracoacromial ligament and continues inferiorly to the level of the greater tuberosity, where no more tendon is visible and the roughened bone of the greater tuberosity is readily distinguishable from the smooth, cartilage-covered bone deep to the supraspinatus tendon. Hard copy should be taken at a level where both the tendon and the underlying humeral cortex are optimally in focus (Fig. 15–8).

An apparent hypoechoic gap is often seen on either side of the biceps. This space is the "rotator cuff interval" formed by the coracohumeral ligament passing superficially over the biceps tendon and merging with the subscapularis tendon medially and the supraspinatus tendon laterally. This gap may be as large as 3 mm on either side of the biceps.

A 1-mm-thick obliquely oriented line, its superficial end oriented medially, is often observed ap-

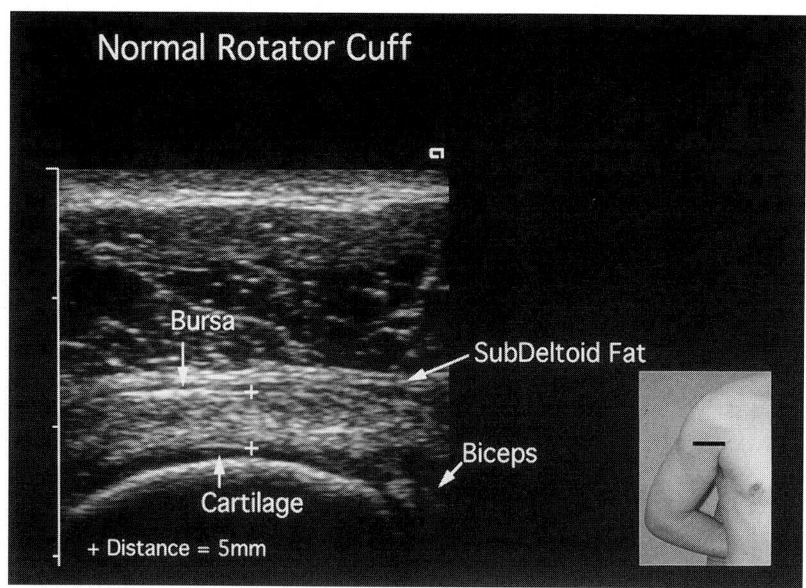

Figure 15-8 ■ Normal supraspinatus tendon: transverse sonogram. Same patient as in Figure 15-2. Transverse view taken with the patient in full internal rotation. The biceps tendon marks the anteromedial border of the supraspinatus tendon. The subacromial bursa is a hypoechoic layer deep to the echogenic subdeltoid fat, and the hyaline cartilage represents a second hypoechoic layer deep to the tendon possessing a weak interface with the overlying tendon in a normal patient.

proximately 2.5 cm posterior to the biceps. This represents the supraspinatus–infraspinatus interface (Fig. 15-9). The bone deep to the tendon should be smooth.

A thin, hypoechoic layer deep to the tendon approximately 1 mm thick represents the hyaline cartilage. Strong enhancement of the cartilage–tendon interface is abnormal and indicates the presence of an excessive amount of joint fluid.

In the young person, tendon parenchyma is composed of homogeneous medium-level echoes. With age, there is progressive fibrofatty replacement of the tendon parenchyma, which produces high-level echos and disorganization of fiber orientation. For this reason, a diagnosis of tendon disruption based solely on regions of increased echogenicity is often unreliable. The tendon displays a convex superficial margin; only minor undulations are acceptable as a normal finding.

As with the subscapularis and infraspinatus tendons, a 2-mm hypoechoic layer superficial to the tendon represents the subacromial bursa, which is

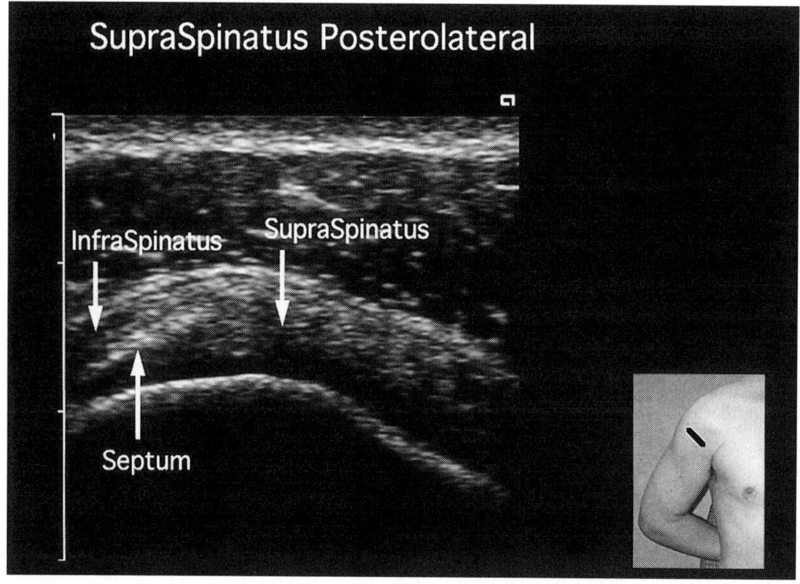

Figure 15-9 ■ Normal supraspinatus tendon: transverse sonogram. Same figure as in Figure 15-2. The scan of Figure 15-8 is extended more posteriorly. The posterolateral extent of the supraspinatus tendon is marked by an oblique echogenic septum (*middle arrow*), posterior to which is the infraspinatus tendon.

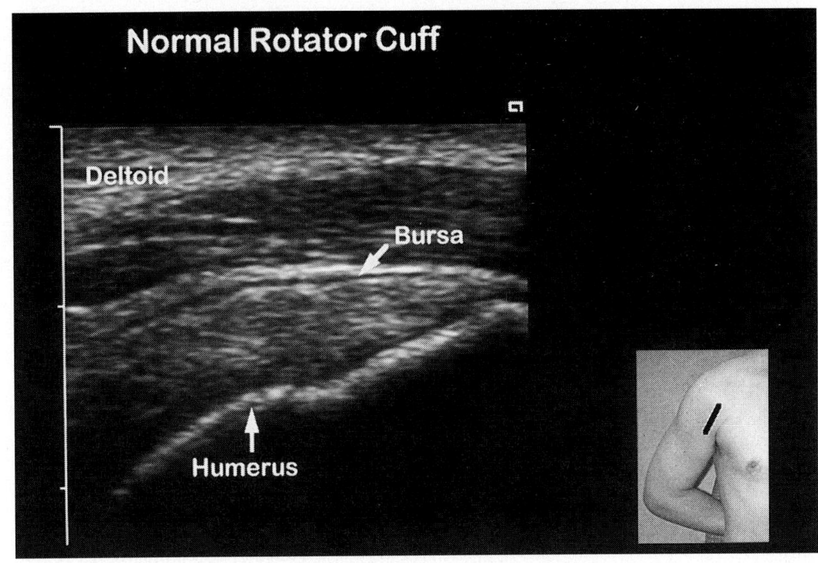

Figure 15–10 ▪ Normal supraspinatus tendon: longitudinal sonogram. Same patient as in Figure 15–2. The supraspinatus tendon is located deep to the subacromial bursa. Note the "parrot's beak" appearance of the supraspinatus tendon in this view and the smooth appearance of the humeral cortex deep to the tendon.

covered by the subdeltoid fat stripe. Occasionally, one can appreciate the supraspinatus tendon being formed from two distinct cones of tendon bundles. The more cephalad bundle arises from the anterior part of the muscle belly and converges into a cylindrical tendon which maintains an anterior position. Slightly distally, a second tendon arises from the middle of the muscle belly. The tendon is flat, tapers posteriorly, and infiltrates the undersurface of the cylindrical tendon. A hypoechoic band of muscle tissue may sometimes be seen separating the flat and cylindrical parts of the tendon; it should not be mistaken for a rotator cuff tear (Turrin and Capepello, 1997). The normal tendon measures approximately 6 mm in thickness (SD = 1.1 mm) and should be similar in thickness to the overlying deltoid muscle (5.9 mm; SD = 1.3 mm); greater thicknesses may occasionally be seen in athletes (Crass and Craig, 1988). There should be no significant difference in thickness between the dominant and nondominant extremities (Collins et al., 1987). Rotator cuff thickness in women and older patients tends to be less than that of younger active men.

Slice 8: Comparison Views, Supraspinatus Transverse Hyperextension, Internal Rotation

The screen is split, and comparison views of the supraspinatus tendon at the level described above are abtained. Any significant difference in the thickness of the tendons is noted and may provide supportive evidence of disuse atrophy or tendinitis (see Fig. 15–16).

Slice 9: Supraspinatus Longitudinal Hyperextended Internal Rotation

The transducer is rotated 90 degrees from the position described in slice 7. The position of extreme internal rotation promotes visualization of the majority of the proximal supraspinatus tendon from underneath the acromion. The supraspinatus tendon has an outline that has been likened to that of a parrot's beak. It has a convex superficial margin that tapers to a point at its distal insertion on the greater tuberosity. This position optimizes assessment of the tendon parenchyma.

The normal thickness of the supraspinatus tendon is 6 mm (SD = 1.1 mm) measured 1 cm proximal to the insertion of the distal supraspinatus (Bretzke et al., 1985). The underlying humeral cortex does not parallel the tendon outline but has a sloping surface distal to the rounded humeral head oriented superficially toward the apex of the greater tuberosity. This smooth, sloping surface is devoid of hyaline cartilage (Fig. 15–10). Once again, the potential space of the subacromial bursa and the subdeltoid fat lie superficial to the tendon.

Slice 10: Subacromial Bursa

The transducer is shifted laterally and distally, scanning parallel to the long axis of the humeral diaphysis just distal to the supraspinatus insertion and deep to the deltoid muscle distal to its origin from the lateral edge of the acromion. In this position, the subacromial subdeltoid bursa lies immediately superficial to the bone, extending distally to the deltoid insertion. Bursal thickness should be no greater

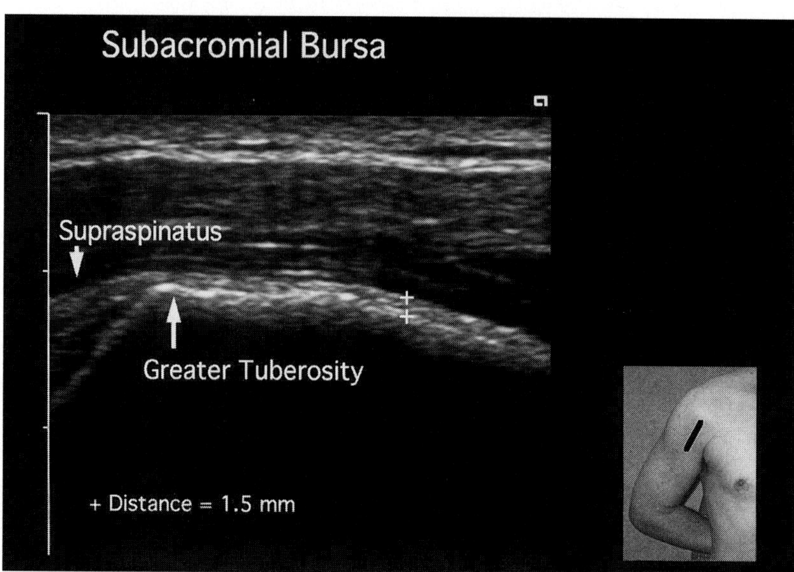

Figure 15-11 ■ Normal subacromial bursa: longitudinal sonogram. Same patient as in Figure 15-2. The normal bursa is 1.5 mm thick and lies distal to the greater tuberosity and the supraspinatus insertion. As elsewhere in the rotator cuff, the deltoid muscle lies immediately superficial to the bursa.

than 2 mm. A normal bursa does not contain fluid (Fig. 15-11).

Slice 11: Supraspinatus, Transverse Partial Internal Rotation (Shrug Position)

The patient's arm is brought alongside the body, with the glenohumeral joint kept in less severe internal rotation. The forearm is pronated, and the patient's thumb is directed posteriorly. Prior to scanning the supraspinatus, the examiner should review the subacromial bursa distal to the supraspinatus insertion, as small amounts of bursal fluid that were not previously visible may be expressed into this location during this maneuver, Any volume of fluid that was visible in this location previously also tends to increase.

While the previous position is superior for the assessment of tendon texture, the "shrug" position is superior for the assessment of tendon contour, as the tendon is less "on stretch" and any subtle tendon contour alterations may be visible only in this position (see Fig. 15-22). Extension of the glenohumeral joint while maintaining internal rotation may, on occasion, potentiate this effect.

If the patient's hand is held with the examiner's free hand, the glenohumeral joint may be slowly rotated, enabling a better evaluation of the rotator cuff interval, which may often appear hypoechoic due to the anisotropy caused by the extreme internal rotation of the previous position. Such slow, controlled rotation may also help distinguish between tendon and the less mobile bursal tissue, enabling identification of small tears.

Slice 12: Supraspinatus Tendon, Longitudinal Partial Internal Rotation (Shrug Position)

The patient is kept in the same position, but the transducer is rotated 90 degrees. Again, subtle alterations in tendon contour are best appreciated in this position.

Slice 13: Dynamic Scanning

The patient's elbow is flexed to 90 degrees, and he or she is guided into active forward flexion and abduction of the glenohumeral joint (Farin et al., 1990). The degree of humeral depression that occurs in association with these movements is evaluated. Failure of humeral depression is a predisposing factor for impingement. The supraspinatus tendon and subacromial bursa are scanned while passing beneath the acromion and coracoacromial ligament. The smooth flow of the tendon beneath the acromion in a normal patient can be likened to the flow of water over a fall. Attention should be paid to any "bunching" or cogwheel hesitation of the rotator cuff tendons (Collins et al., 1987) or gradual distention of the bursa (Farin et al., 1990). These observations are correlated with the onset of any pain reported of by the patient or any sensation of crepitus that can be appreciated by the examiner transmitted through the transducer.

The patient is not allowed to rotate the glenohumeral joint internally or externally while abducting

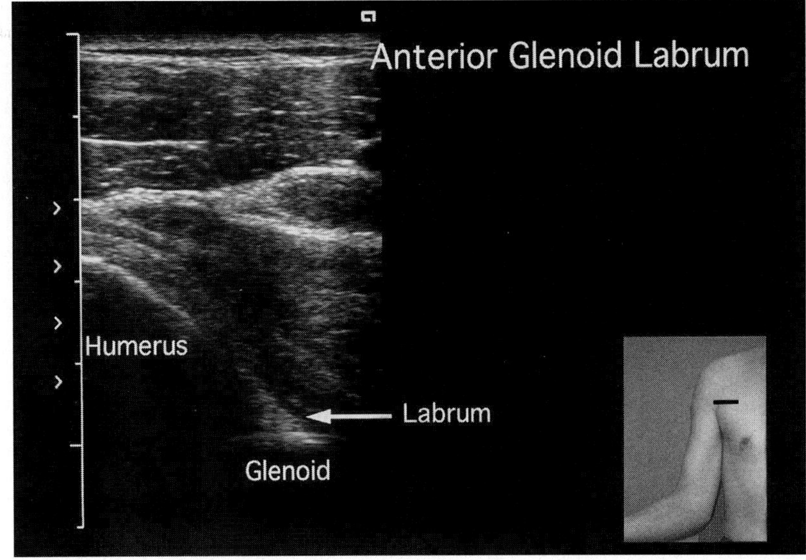

Figure 15-12 ■ Normal anterior glenoid: transverse sonogram. Same patient as Figure 15-2. The arm is held in external rotation, and the transducer is pressed firmly against the anterior joint space. The *arrow* indicates a triangular homogeneous, echogenic structure, the labrum, with its base attached to the linear echogenic glenoid fossa.

or forward flexing, as this "trick" maneuver may avoid impingement.

Slice 14: Instability Assessment

In carefully selected patients, an attempt can be made to detect instability lesions. These patients are generally under 35, are athletic, and present with shoulder pain and symptoms suggestive of instability such as "clicking" or a history of shoulder dislocation. On physical examination the "apprehension" test may be positive.

A Hill-Sachs lesion may be detected posteriorly, just lateral to the position for scanning the posterior glenoid labrum. The humeral head at this level should have a rounded contour. A Hill-Sachs lesion appears as a sudden depression in the bony contour. Small, radiographically occult lesions less than 1 cm may be detected (see Fig. 15-7).

The anterior glenoid labrum is best seen with the patient supine, the arm adducted, and the elbow flexed. The transducer is placed transversely approximately midway between the acromion and the axilla. Passive rotation of the glenohumeral joint readily identifies the immobile anterior glenoid labrum as a triangular echogenic structure smaller than the posterior glenoid labrum (Fig. 15-12). The anterior capsule may be identified as it passes over the labrum. In larger patients, a 5-MHz transducer may be required to demonstrate this relatively deep structure.

The superior glenoid labrum is difficult to visualize. The transducer is placed in the coronal plane, posterior to the obtuse angle formed by the acromion and clavicle and angled laterally and inferiorly.

Joint Fluid

The presence of joint fluid is a common but nonspecific finding. Joint fluid is readily demonstrated within the biceps tendon sheath. The biceps tendon sheath communicates with the joint, and as it is in a gravity-dependent position during the ultrasound examination, it will distend with any joint fluid that may be present. The fluid tends to collect medially (Fig. 15-13).

The most common cause of biceps sheath fluid is adhesive capsulitis. Approximately 40% of patients with this condition exhibit fluid within the sheath. The cause of this condition is not known, but it may be related to intra-articular adhesions trapping the small amount of intra-articular fluid normally present within the sheath. Other causes of joint or biceps sheath fluid include rotator cuff tears, inflammatory arthropathy, trauma, infection, and bicipital tenosynovitis.

Joint fluid may also be detected in the posterior synovial recess of the glenohumeral joint, between the posterior glenoid labrum and the deep fibers of the infraspinatus. Any separation of these structures of more than 2 mm indicates the presence of joint fluid (van Holsbeeck et al., 1990) (see Fig. 15-6).

Axillary scans of the glenohumeral joint have been advocated as a sensitive method for the detection of intra-articular fluid (Koski, 1989). The distance

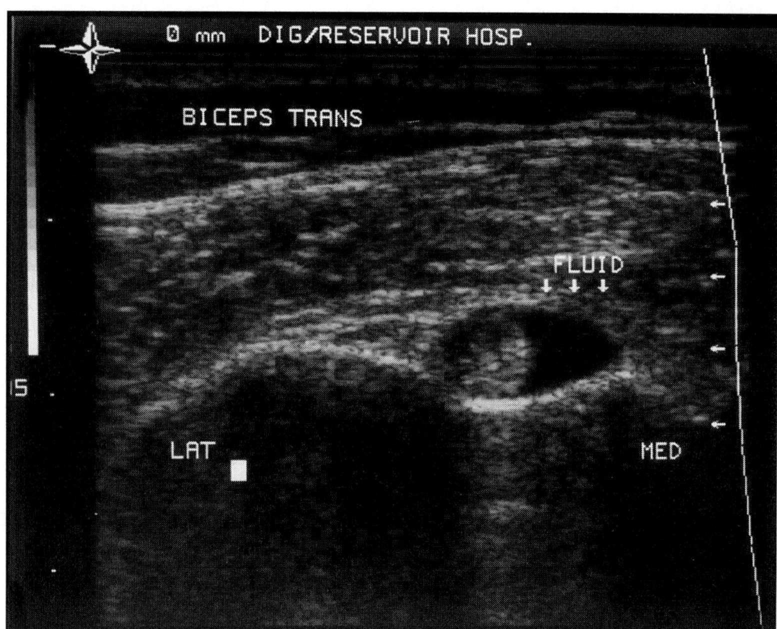

Figure 15-13 ■ Adhesive capsulitis: transverse sonogram. A 50-year-old female presents with shoulder pain of 4 months' duration that is worse at night, with an increasing restriction in her range of movement. The transducer is aligned transversely over the distal biceps groove. *Small arrows* indicate a small amount of fluid within the biceps tendon sheath; this rim of fluid almost always appears medially (*MED*). Arthrography demonstrated the characteristic picture of adhesive capsulitis.

between the humerus and the joint capsule is measured at the axilla with the arm in 90 degrees of abduction. The criterion for intra-articular effusion is an anechogenic space between the bone and joint capsule of more than 3.5 mm, or a difference of 1 mm or more between the right and the left joints (Koski, 1991). Axillary scanning is likely to be more sensitive, as the axillary recess is redundant, with the arm adducted. Any fluid present tends to collect there due to its dependent position when the patient is sitting upright.

However, as any fluid present is often readily detected, either within the biceps tendon sheath or between the posterior glenoid labrum and the infraspinatus tendon, we do not routinely use this technique. We employ it mainly when the clinical history indicates that joint fluid may be present but it has not been found in the above two locations. For example, it is used in the assessment of possible rheumatoid involvement of the shoulder joint.

Rotator Cuff Disease

There is a steady increase in the incidence of rotator cuff tears with age. The majority of patients over the age of 60 will have a rotator cuff tear, either full or partial thickness. Many of these tears are asymptomatic or may only present with shoulder pain after many years of quiescence. As mentioned previously, Neer described a pathological progression of rotator cuff degeneration commencing with tendinitis, fibrosis, partial-thickness tears, full-thickness tears, and, finally, rotator cuff arthropathy. Most of these stages can be successfully assessed with ultrasound.

Impingement

During forward flexion and abduction of the glenohumeral joint, the supraspinatus muscle, aided by the remainder of the rotator cuff and the biceps tendon, acts as a humeral depressor to stabilize the head of the humerus in the glenoid. Without this counteraction, the humeral head will be uplifted by deltoid contraction, causing impingement of the supraspinatus and the subacromial bursa against one or more components of the coracoacromial arch. The coracoacromial arch is composed of five basic structures: distal clavicle, acromioclavicular joint, anterior one-third of the acromion, coracoacromial ligament, and anterior one-third of the coracoid process.

Failure of humeral depression is the major precipitating cause of impingement (Lanzer, 1988). The subacromial-subdeltoid bursa surrounding the shoulder has both a lubricating and a shock-absorbing function. The bursa may distend with fluid and, if the process is chronic, thicken due to hypertrophy of the synovium and subsynovial fat (Gold et al., 1993). Stretching of small nerve fibers within the thickenened bursal tissues results in pain upon motion and provides less space for the rotator cuff during movement because of the thickened, inflamed tissues described above. Patients complain of pain, especially when sleeping on the affected

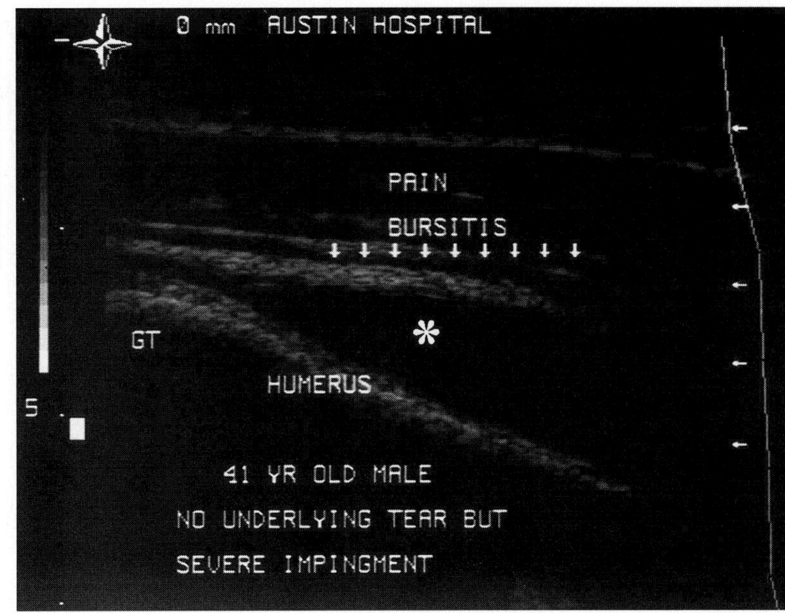

Figure 15-14 ■ Subacromial-subdeltoid bursitis: longitudinal sonogram. A 41-year-old female aerobics instructor complains of an 8-day history of pain in the shoulder aggravated by lifting the arm. The ultrasound scan demonstrates a grade 1 impingement lesion. The rotator cuff was intact. The subacromial bursa distal to the supraspinatus insertion at the greater tuberosity (*GT*) is distended with fluid (*), but there is no synovial proliferation. The distended bursa is tender to sonographic palpation (*PAIN*).

side and when initiating movement in either forward flexion or abduction (Figs. 15-14 and 15-15).

Poor humeral depression may be due to poor muscle coordination or weakness. The latter may be due to trauma, inflammation, or tears involving the rotator cuff, the most important component of which is the supraspinatus tendon. Once impingement develops, a vicious circle can become established whereby impingement causes trauma, inflammation, and tendinopathy, predisposing to further tearing of the supraspinatus tendon, which in turn worsens the severity of the impingement, causing further damage to the rotator cuff (Butters and Rockwood, 1988).

Tendons with these degenerative inflammatory changes are more susceptible to tears. Therefore, acute tears in healthy cuffs are extremely rare and are usually the result of high-velocity trauma. The average age of persons with rotator cuff tears is approximately the sixth decade of life. An area of relative avascularity 1 cm proximal to the point of insertion on the greater tuberosity has been described. This has been termed the *critical zone*. The changes of attrition leading to tearing almost always

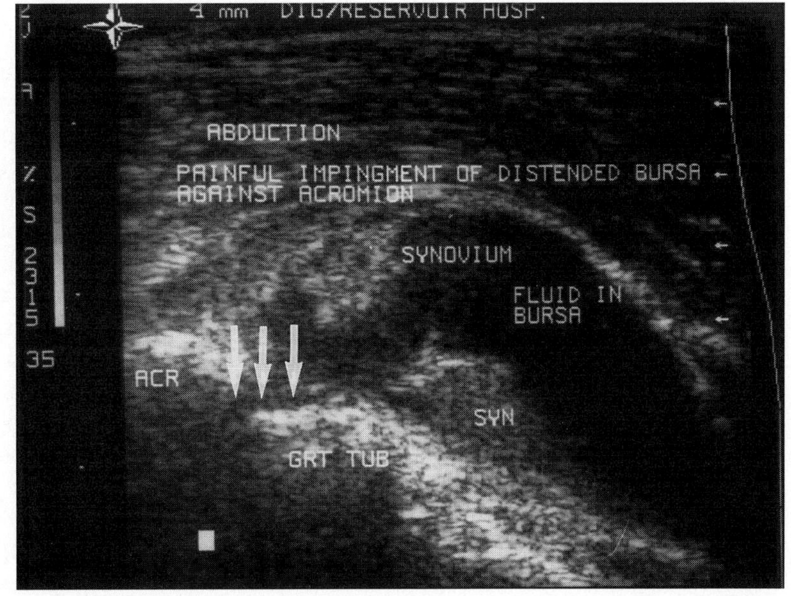

Figure 15-15 ■ Severe subacromial bursitis: longitudinal sonogram. A 52-year-old man presents with increasing shoulder pain over a 2 month period. The subacromial bursa distal to supraspinatus insertion is grossly distended by fluid; there is marked synovial proliferation (*SYNOVIUM, SYN*). The distended, thickened bursa fails to pass between the narrow gap (*arrows*) between the acromion (*ACR*) and the greater tuberosity (*GRT TUB*). The gap is narrowed by poor humeral depression in this patient with a large full-thickness rotator cuff tear.

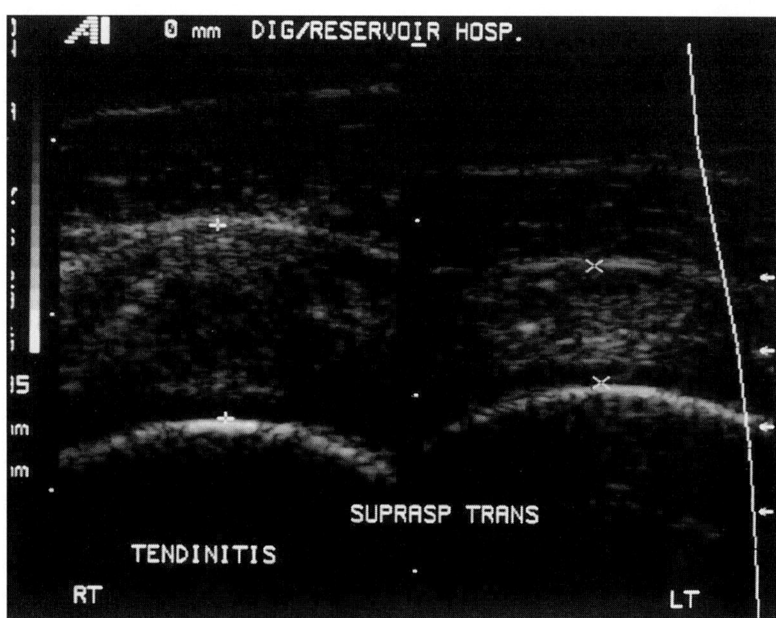

Figure 15-16 ■ Tendinitis: transverse sonogram. A 28-year-old man with a 1-week history of moderate shoulder pain on attempted forward flexion. Transverse views of both supraspinatus tendons. The tendon on the patient's right (*RT*) is more than 2 mm thicker than the tendon on the asymptomatic contralateral side. The findings are compatible with a grade I impingement lesion.

occur in this region and may be observed by ultrasound (Rathbun and Macnab, 1970). As described above, with experience, a subjective assessment of the adequacy of humeral depression may be made during the dynamic phase of the ultrasound examination.

Subacromial impingement is defined as distention of the subdeltoid bursa against the outer edge of the acromion during abduction (or forward flexion) from the adducted position (Farin et al., 1995b) or bunching (or buckling) of the supraspinatus tendon during abduction (or forward flexion) against the outer edge of the acromion (Collins et al., 1987; Drakeford et al., 1990). Impingement is rarely an isolated finding. There are usually secondary changes within the supraspinatus tendon or the subacromial bursa. The presence of a fluid collection alone in the subacromial-subdeltoid bursa has been used as a further criterion for the presence of early-stage impingement syndrome, i.e., Neer grade 1 (see Fig. 15-14). The presence of thickening within the subacromial bursal soft tissues in the presence of an intact cuff implies a grade 2 impingement lesion. Primary bursitis, which is seen in rheumatoid arthritis, tuberculosis, gout and pyogenic infections, must be excluded before a diagnosis of early-grade impingement can be made (Farin et al., 1990). Thickening of the rotator cuff (tendinitis) has been correlated with stage 1 impingement, and thinned, echogenic cuffs (fibrosis) have been correlated with stage 2 impingement lesions (Crass et al., 1988). Van Holsbeeck described other criteria for the grading of impingement based on ultrasound images (van Holsbeeck et al., unpublished):

Stage 1: bursal thickness of 1.5 to 2.0 mm
Stage 2: bursal thickness over 2 mm
Stage 3: partial- or full-thickness tear of the rotator cuff

It is important to understand that ultrasound can only assess the first 90 degrees of motion in forward flexion and abduction. In addition, proximal subacromial impingement, occurring after the supraspinatus has passed under the acromion and out of the examiner's field of view, cannot be assessed. MRI is required for this purpose.

Tendinitis

As described by Neer (1972), tendinitis is most commonly observed in patients under the age of 30. The patients are often engaged in athletic activity, which they now feel to be restricted during a particular range of movement, most commonly forward flexion or abduction. Tendinitis produces no reliable morphological changes in the supraspinatus tendon, but often the tendon is obviously thickened compared to the asymptomatic contralateral side. A difference in tendon thickness of more than 2 mm compared to the contralateral side has been suggested as a criterion for tendinitis (Fig. 15-16) (Dondelinger, 1995). Other authors have suggested an increase of more than 2.5 mm or one-third the thickness of the contralateral normal tendon (Crass et al., 1988). In our practice, a difference of 1.5 mm in the appropriate clinical context is considered highly suspicious of a grade 1 impingement lesion.

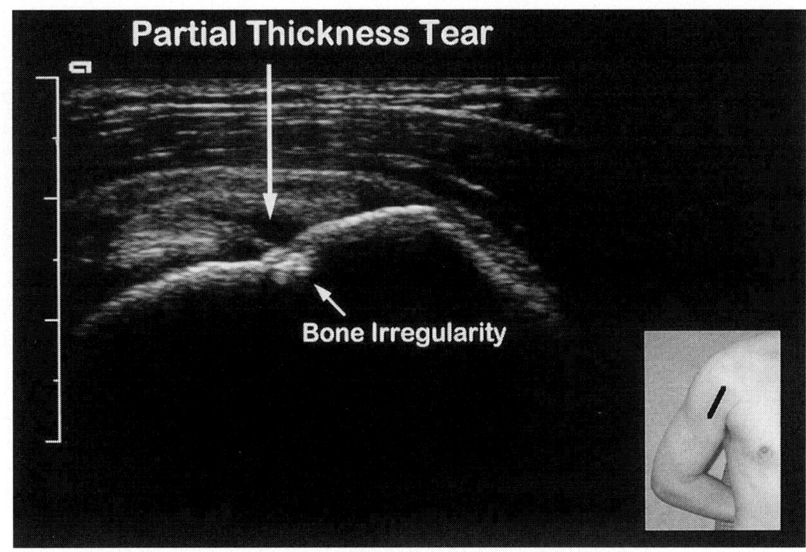

Figure 15-17 ■ Partial-thickness tear of the supraspinatus tendon: longitudinal sonogram. Physiotherapy was tried in this 33-year-old man who had had 3 months of continued shoulder pain. He reported no improvement in his symptoms after several sessions. A focal sonolucent defect at the articular surface of the supraspinatus tendon contains an oblique echogenic stripe centrally (*long arrow*); the underlying humeral cortex is focally eroded (*small arrow*).

A mild coexistent subacromial bursitis is also often present in these patients. It has been reported that power Doppler, which is angle independent and offers an extended dynamic range over that provided by conventional color Doppler imaging, is more sensitive to changes in perfusion at the microvascular level and therefore can depict the soft tissue hyperemia present in rotator cuff tendinitis. However, the technique relies on a subjective assessment of increased regional perfusion, and no quantitative parameter is applicable to the technique (Newman et al., 1994). The supraspinatus tendons are symmetrical in size in young, asymptomatic patients and, there is no relationship between tendon size and the dominant arm. Tendon thickness greater than 8 mm should be treated with suspicion, although comparison with the contralateral side is more reliable than absolute measurements. Tendinitis is a reversible condition, and a follow-up examination when the patient is asymptomatic will often show symmetrically sized tendons.

Tendinopathy

Tendinopathy was not described by Neer but represents regions of mucinous degeneration accompanied by microscopic tears within the tendon. The condition is identical to that found in the more common patellar tendinopathy, or "jumper's knee" (Katthagen, 1989). Tendinopathy and tears of the supraspinatus tendon almost always occur in this critical zone. Sonographically, the region of tendinopathy appears as a focal, hypoechoic region, seen in two planes, devoid of any normal fibrillary pattern, that is often tender to sonographic palpation. The underlying humeral cortex is normal. It is likely that tendinopathy represent a pre-tear state.

Rotator Cuff Tears

Rotator cuff tears may be classified as either full or partial thickness. Full-thickness tears allow communication between the glenohumeral joint and the subacromial bursa. Partial-thickness tears are tears of the rotator cuff that do not result in this abnormal communication.

Partial-Thickness Tears

Partial thickness tears fall into three categories:

1. Bursal surface tears
2. Intrasubstance tears
3. Articular surface tear

Tears of the rotator cuff almost always begin in the critical zone of the supraspinatus tendon. Articular surface partial-thickness tears account for up to 80% of partial-thickness tears detected during ultrasound examination, although they are said to represent no more than 40% of all partial-thickness rotator cuff tears. Two criteria have been described to depict partial thickness tears:

1. A mixed hyper- and hypoechoic focus in the critical zone of the supraspinatus tendon (Fig. 15-17).
2. A hypoechoic lesion visualized in two orthogonal imaging planes, with either articular or bursal extension (Fig. 15-18) (van Holsbeeck et al., 1992).

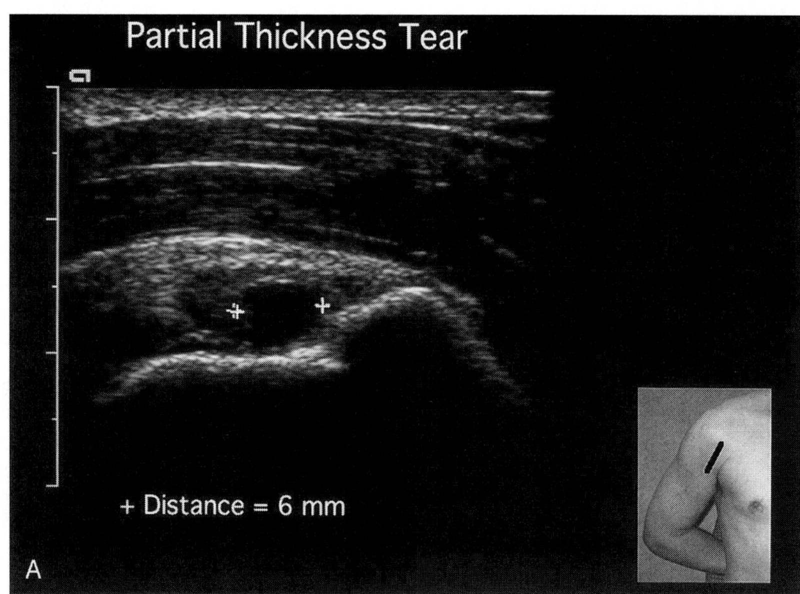

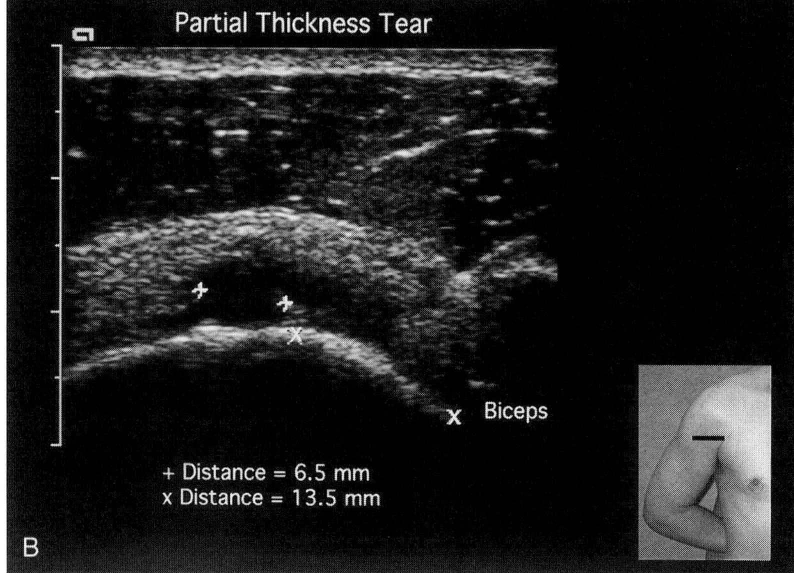

Figure 15-18 ■ **A,** Articular side partial-thickness tear: longitudinal sonogram. A 30-year-old male who presents with shoulder pain and has a painful arc at clinical examination. A 6 mm sonolucent defect at the articular surface of the supraspinatus tendon is noted on this longitudinal scan. **B,** Articular side partial-thickness tear: transverse sonogram. Same patient as in **A**. The same anechoic defect is noted on the transverse section. The partial-thickness tear is located in the most common location, within 15 mm of the biceps tendon and within 10 mm of the distal tip of the supraspinatus insertion. Visualization of the lesion in two orthogonal planes gives extra support to the diagnosis.

Using these criteria, the sensitivity of ultrasound in the depiction of partial-thickness tears is 93% and the specificity is 94%. The positive predictive value is 82%, and the negative predictive value is 98% (van Holsbeeck et al., 1995). A third criterion has also been successfully applied by some authors: the presence of a large, dominant linear echogenic focus within the substance of the cuff, with or without an associated decrease of cuff thickness (Wiener and Seitz, 1993). In 85% of patients with partial-thickness tears, associated soft tissue and bony abnormalities are found. Seventy percent of partial-thickness tears are associated with regions of irregularity within the anterior greater tuberosity. These range from small defects in the cortex to bone fragmentation and bone spurs. The cause of this humeral irregularity seen in both full- and partial-thickness tears is not understood. It has been postulated that the humeral cortex may suffer direct trauma from loss of the protective thickness of the rotator cuff. It is also possible that an inflammatory response arising as a result of the damaged tendon may directly cause bony erosion.

Sixty-six percent of patients with partial-thickness tears have small biceps tendon sheath effusions, and small bursal fluid collections have been detected in 25% of patients. False-positive results may be avoided by recognizing echoes of normal tendon within hypoechoic lesions.

The exact nature of the central hyperechoic area, which is surrounded by a hypoechoic zone, is not known. It has been postulated to result from the separation of the retracted distal segment of the tendon from the surrounding tissue; the separation results in a new interface within the tendon. Joint fluid is thought to penetrate the tendon substance and surround this torn edge of tissue, explaining the hyper-hypoechoic ultrasound features (van Holsbeeck et al., 1995), but a similar echogenic structure has been described in normal, asymptomatic tendons and has been postulated to represent an edge of the coracohumeral ligament where it interfaces with the supraspinatus tendon (Ptasznik, 1997). Flattening of the normally convex superficial contour of the rotator cuff has been described as a further criterion for a partial-thickness tear (Hodler et al., 1988). However, we have found flattening to be a difficult criterion to apply objectively. Indeed, it had a prospective sensitivity of only 42% in the study in which it was described, which increased to a retrospective sensitivity of 100% after the ultrasound examinations were reviewed with the knowledge of the surgical findings.

Partial-thickness tears may be tender to sonographic palpation. Articular surface tears may be associated with a small amount of fluid within the biceps tendon sheath, but a large amount of fluid within the subacromial-subdeltoid bursa should raise the suspicion of a sonographically occult full-thickness tear.

Bursal surface tears are the next most commonly observed partial-thickness tears seen on ultra-sound. They generally appear as hypoechoic, concave defects located at the bursal surface of the tendon. They are often extremely tender to sonographic palpation.

Intrasubstance tears are rarely seen and should not be confused with distal prolongation of supraspinatus muscle tissue beyond the outer edge of the acromion. Confusion can be avoided if the defect is viewed in two planes. Distal prolongation of muscle tissue will be shown to be continuous with proximal muscle tissue, whereas the true intrasubstance tear will be shown as a small, rounded or oval-shaped, hypoechoic defect seen both longitudinally and transversely.

Full-Thickness Tears

Full-thickness tears may be classified according to the number of tendons involved or according to their size. The size of a full-thickness tear is estimated from images recorded in both the axial and sagittal planes. The plane in which the tear is larger is used for classification purposes. As the supraspinatus tendon measures on average 2.5 cm in width, tears greater than 2.5 cm extending posteriorly from the biceps tendon must involve the infraspinatus. Van Holsbeeck and Wiener have both reported that the accuracy of ultrasound in the determination of rotator cuff size is acceptable. Therefore, this modality is useful in the preoperative planning of tendon repair. Both authors used slightly different criteria. Van Holsbeeck (1996) proposed four categories:

1. Partial-thickness tears
2. Small full-thickness tears of less than 2 cm in the anteroposterior direction over the greater tuberosity
3. Large full-thickness tears of 2–4 cm
4. Massive full-thickness tears of more than 4 cm

Wiener also proposed 4 categories (Wiener and Seitz, 1993). The plane in which the tear was largest was used for classification purposes:

1. Partial-thickness tears
2. Small tears (those under 1 cm in the maximum dimension)
3. Large tears (those 1–3 cm in the maximum dimension)
4. Massive tears (those greater than 3 cm in the maximum dimension)

Full-thickness tears exhibit a variety of appearances on ultrasound, and the sonographic signs of a full-thickness tear can be divided into primary and secondary categories. A primary finding is absolute evidence of a full-thickness tear. A secondary finding is merely supportive (Middleton, 1989; Dondelinger, 1995).

Primary Signs

Primary signs of full-thickness tears include the following:

1. Absence of rotator cuff
2. Focal nonvisualization of the cuff
3. Hypoechoic or anechoic cleft in the cuff
4. Direct joint communication through a tendon gap with a distended subacromial-subdeltoid bursa
5. Naked tuberosity (focal apposition of the deltoid muscle on the greater tuberosity)
6. Compression of tendon
7. Herniation of the deltoid muscle or of the subacromial-subdeltoid bursa in the cuff

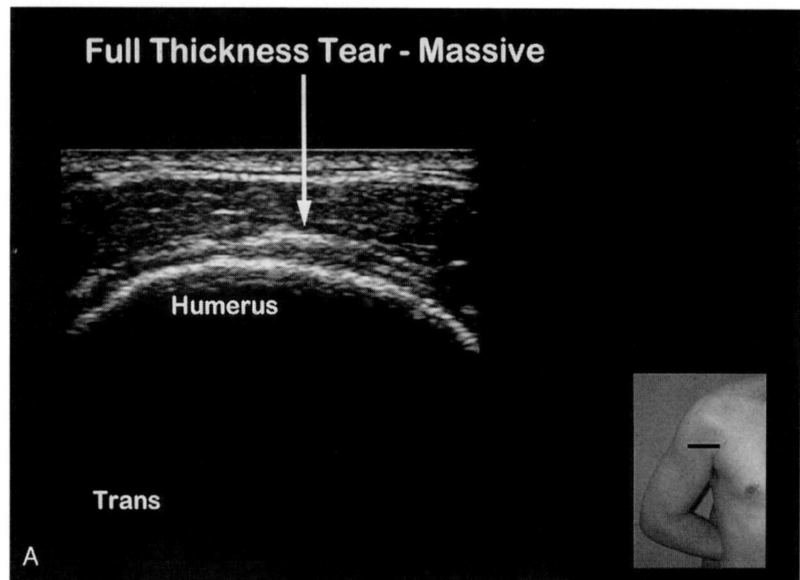

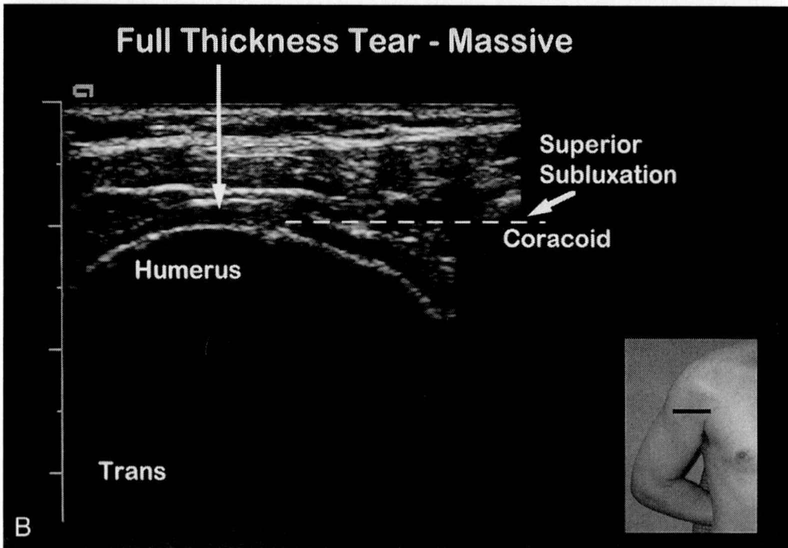

Figure 15-19 ■ **A,** Massive full-thickness tear: transverse sonogram. This 82-year-old female has shoulder pain which increases at night. No appreciable cuff tissue is visible. A thin soft tissue layer lies between the humeral head and the deltoid (*arrow*). This represents thickened bursal tissue and should not be mistaken for cuff. **B,** Massive full-thickness tear: transverse sonogram. Same patient as in **A**. A short, curved echogenic focus with posterior acoustic shadowing represents the coracoid process (*short arrow*). The humeral head is subluxed anteriorly and superiorly and now lies at the same level as the coracoid process.

Absence of Rotator Cuff

In massive rotator cuff tears, little or no tendon remnant can be seen covering the humeral head. These tears almost always involve the entire supraspinatus tendon, commencing immediately posterior to the bicipital groove and extending posteriorly to involve a majority of the infraspinatus tendon. The torn tendon retracts proximally beneath the acromion process, and the deltoid muscle becomes closely opposed to the humeral head. In this circumstance, the deep surface of the deltoid muscle maintains its convex contour because, with no intervening cuff tissue, it exactly parallels the contour of the humeral head. The subscapularis tendon is less frequently involved, and the biceps tendon, if intact, is generally severely degenerated. A thin layer of soft tissue may cover the humeral head, but it represents thickened bursal tissue, not cuff. Passive movement may help distinguish between thickened bursal tissue and cuff remnant.

The humeral head may be subluxed superiorly relative to the coracoid and acromial processes (Fig. 15-19), and the humeral contour appears rounded on the longitudinal view due to wasting of the greater tuberosity (Fig. 15-20). Joint and bursal fluid may be present. Humeral depression is weak, and crepitus under the transducer may be appreciated secondary to bone-on-bone impingement.

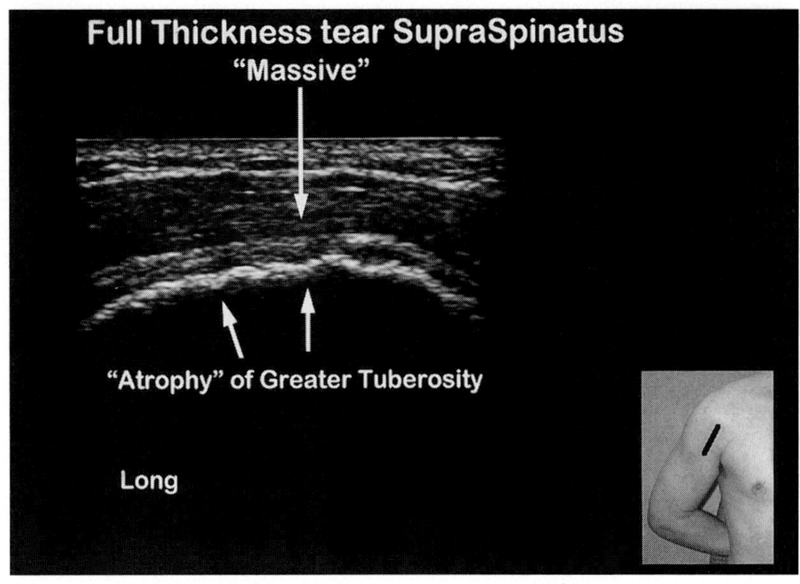

Figure 15-20 ■ Chronic massive full-thickness tear (*long arrow*): longitudinal sonogram. Pain flares up intermittently in the shoulder of this 75-year-old man. His shoulder has been bothering him for years. The greater tuberosity is atrophic and has taken on a more rounded contour. Note the irregular cortical outline (*short arrows*).

Focal Nonvisualization of the Cuff

These tears are smaller than massive rotator cuff tears, but where the cuff is absent, the bursa is in contact with the humeral head. Almost all of these tears are located distally and anteromedially in the critical zone of the supraspinatus tendon, within 1 cm proximal to the distal greater tuberosity and within 1 cm posterior to the bicipital groove. The underlying humeral cortex may be irregular deep to the tear; joint and bursal fluid is usually present. (Fig. 15-21).

Hypoechoic or Anechoic Cleft in the Cuff

These tears are smaller still, with the cuff defect filling either with fluid or with thickened bursal tissue (Fig. 15-22).

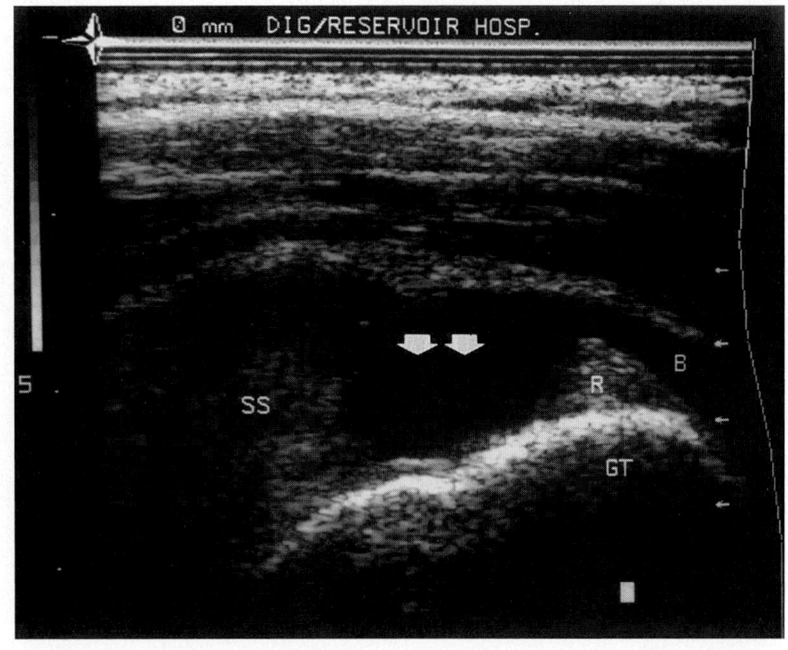

Figure 15-21 ■ Focal nonvisualization of the cuff: longitudinal sonogram. Focal pain over the deltoid insertion brings this 49-year-old woman to the doctor. The discomfort in her shoulder girdle started about 3 months ago. A sonolucent, fluid-filled cuff defect (*arrows*) is noted in the cuff over the anatomical neck of the humerus. The supraspinatus tendon has retracted proximally (*SS*), leaving a small tendon remnant (*R*) attached to the distal tip of the greater tuberosity (*GT*). The defect is in direct continuity with the distended bursa (*B*). The defect represents a small full-thickness tear in the rotator cuff.

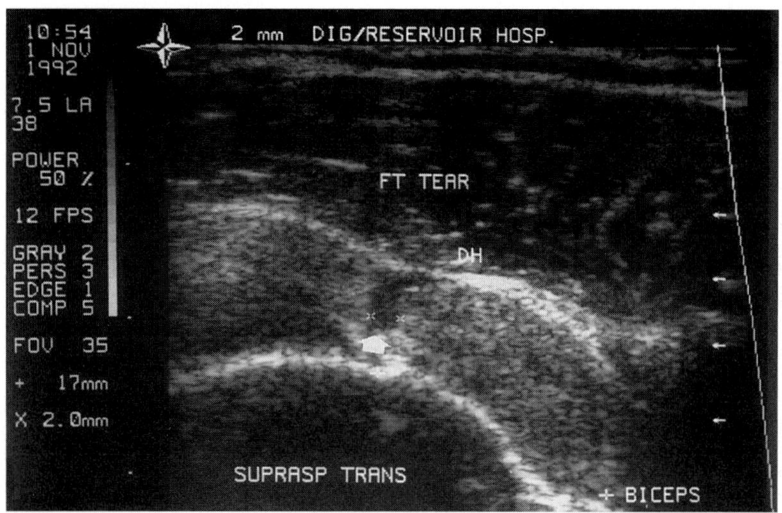

Figure 15-22 ■ Small full-thickness tear: transverse sonogram. A 49-year-old woman complains of discomfort for 2 months in her shoulder. A 2 mm hypoechoic cleft (*arrow*) interrupts the arc-shaped supraspinatus tendon approximately 17 mm posterior to the biceps tendon. The bursal surface of the tendon possesses a concave contour. Abbreviation: deltoid herniation (*DH*).

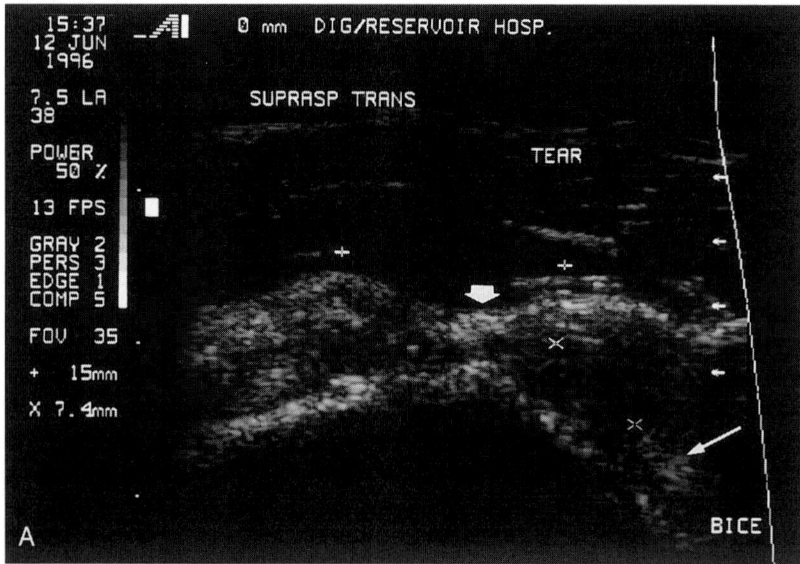

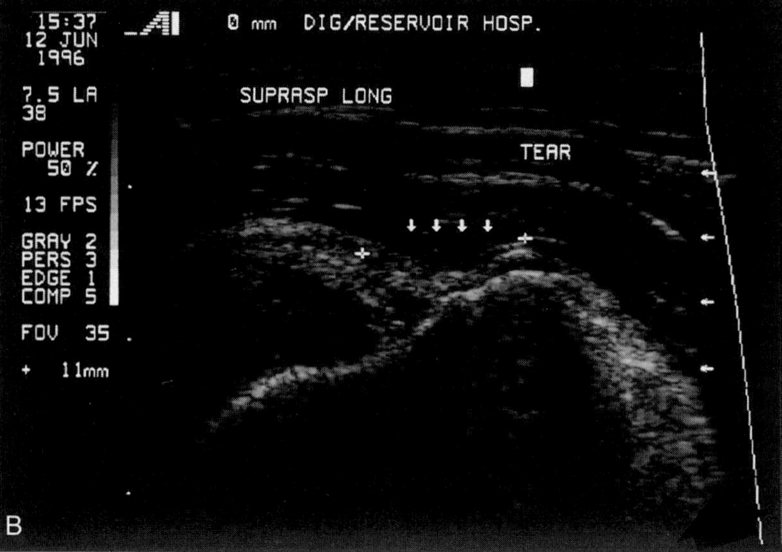

Figure 15-23 ■ **A,** Deltoid herniation: transverse sonogram. Unbearable shoulder pain at night is the cause of chronic insomnia and distress in this 53-year-old woman. The bursal surface of the supraspinatus tendon has a deep concave contour (*thick white arrow*) representing a 15 mm tear 7.4 mm posterior to the biceps tendon (*thin white arrow*). The deltoid fills the space left behind by the torn supraspinatus. **B,** Deltoid herniation: longitudinal sonogram. Same patient as in **A**. An 11 mm concave bursal contour extends to the distal tip of the greater tuberosity (*short white arrows*).

Figure 15–24 ■ **A,** Full-thickness tear of a subscapularis tendon: transverse sonogram. This 50-year-old man has pain when lifting objects, and his examination shows a painful arc for several months in a row. A 10 mm sonolucent defect is found in the subscapularis tendon (*arrow*). The image was obtained without transducer pressure. **B,** Full-thickness tear of a subscapularis tendon: transverse sonogram. Same patient as in **A**. Compression applied on the transducer collapses a segment of the tendon. A more extensive tear shows with this technique (25.1 mm, *arrows*).

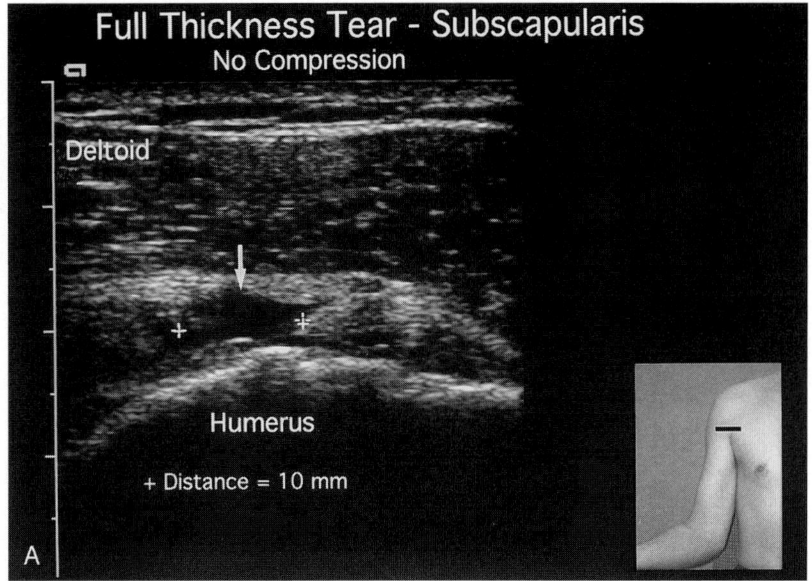

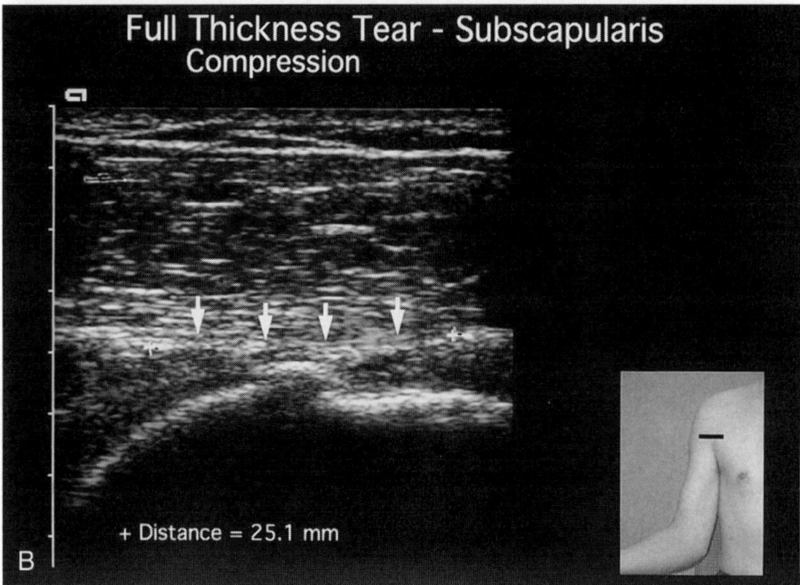

Herniation of the Deltoid Muscle or of the Subacromial-Subdeltoid Bursa in the Cuff

Both the deep surface of the deltoid and the subacromial-subdeltoid bursal contour become concave, rather than showing the usual convex appearance. The concavity should be deep, i.e., greater than 50% of the tendon thickness in order to differentiate a full-thickness tear from a partial-thickness, bursal surface disruption. The tissue deep to the deltoid herniation is granulation tissue, thickened bursa, and scar tissue. (Fig. 15–23) (Hodler et al., 1988). The echogenicity of this tissue may be iso-, hypo-, or hyperechoic with respect to the remaining cuff (Fig. 15–23).

In smaller full-thickness tears associated with minimal retraction, only minimal change in the contour of the deep Deltoid surface is seen. This may be a subtle concavity or focal flattening. In these cases, differentiation from a partial-thickness tear cannot be made with any confidence (Middleton, 1992).

Compression of the Tendon

The normal rotator cuff cannot be compressed. In many cases of full-thickness tear, the resulting gap fills with fluid and debris, and the convex superior margin of the cuff appears to be maintained. In larger patients, the difference in texture between intact cuff and debris may be difficult to appreciate, but it becomes evident as compression with the transducer is applied and the torn segment of tendon collapses against the underlying bone (Fig. 15–24). In very small tears, while the tendon may

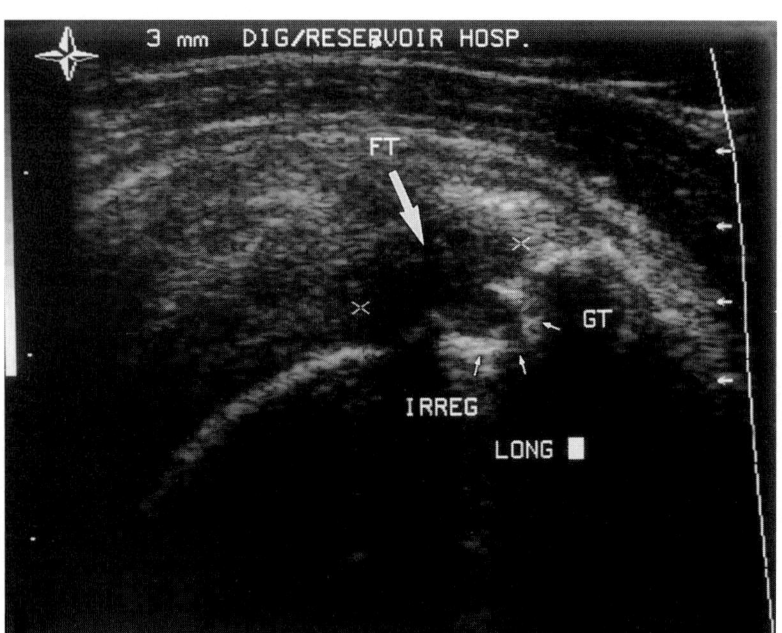

Figure 15-25 ■ Cortical irregularity in a rotator cuff tear: longitudinal sonogram (*LONG*). A 58-year-old man who has pain in his shoulder when lifting overhead and when he rolls on his shoulder at night. A 12 mm sonolucent defect representing a full-thickness tear (*FT*) extends through the supraspinatus tendon from its bursal to its articular surface (*large arrow*). Focal bony irregularity (*IRREG*) is present at the base of the tear (*small arrows*). Abbreviation: greater tuberosity (*GT*).

not compress, small echogenic foci, most likely representing debris from the tear, can be seen being squeezed through the interstices of the tendon.

Secondary Signs

Secondary signs of full-thickness tears include the following:

1. Cortical irregularity of the greater tuberosity (Fig. 15-25)
2. Subacromial-subdeltoid bursitis (see Figs. 15-4 and 15-15)
3. Cartilage sign (Fig. 15-26)
4. Effusion in the biceps tendon sheath
5. Glenohumeral joint effusion

Other Observations in Tears

In one study of 144 shoulders, greater tuberosity irregularity was found in 36 of 40 full-thickness tears, but 12 shoulders had irregularity without rotator cuff tears (Wohlwend et al., 1996).

Reports in the earlier literature suggested that focal hyperechoic foci within the rotator cuff may be reliably used as a criterion for the diagnosis of a rotator cuff tear (Crass and Craig, 1988). However, subsequent researchers have found this sign to be unreliable and nonspecific, and its use is no longer considered appropriate (Ahovuo et al., 1989b; Middleton, 1989).

Only a small percentage of tears of the rotator cuff involve predominantly (6% of all tears) or exclusively (2% of all tears) the subscapularis tendon. These tend to occur in cases of recurrent dislocation or in patients with a history of either forcible abduction and external rotation or direct anterior trauma.

Ultrasonography has been shown to have sensitivity of 82% and specificity of 100% in the detection of these tears (86% of full-thickness tears and 67% of partial-thickness tears) (Farin and Jaroma, 1996). However, detection of subscapularis tears requires the arm to be externally rotated when the study is performed. False-negative findings generally occur in patients with adhesive capsulitis or osteoarthritis in whom full external rotation may not be possible.

The sonographic findings of subscapularis tears are similar to those seen in tears of the supraspinatus tendon, although articular surface partial-thickness tears seem difficult to identify with sonography. Biceps tendon dislocations are found in 57% of patients with full-thickness tears of the subscapularis tendon. This is due to the close relationship of the coracohumeral and transverse humeral ligaments with the subscapularis tendon. These ligaments are also the major anatomical structures preventing dislocation of the biceps tendon.

Pitfalls

Errors of sonographic interpretation have been classified into four categories (Middleton et al., 1986):

1. Normal anatomy mimicking an abnormality
2. Soft tissue abnormalities confusing the echo pattern

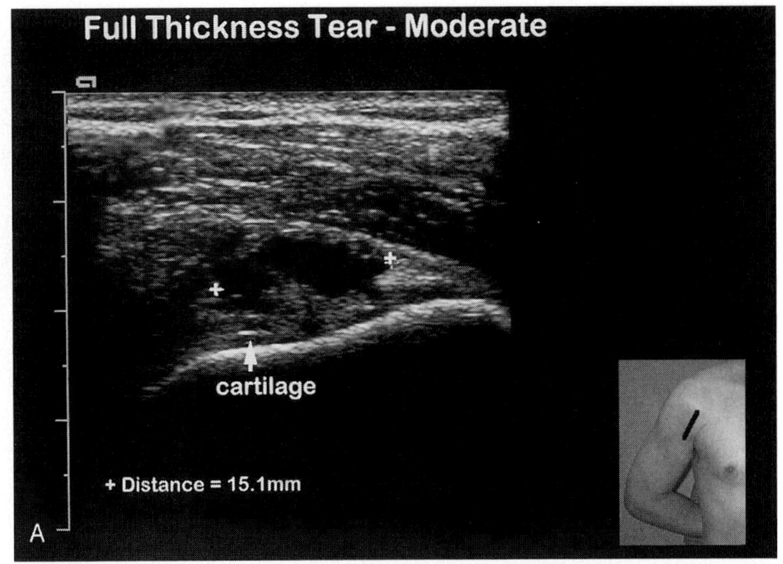

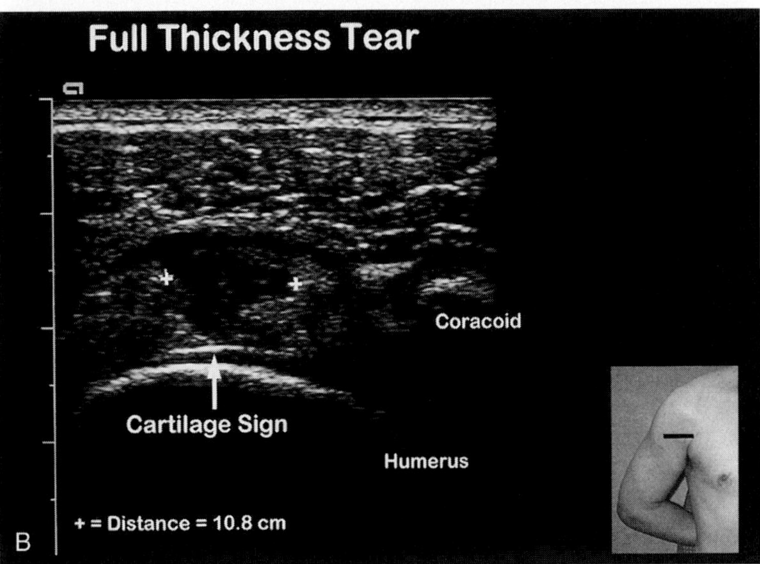

Figure 15-26 ▪ A, Cartilage sign: longitudinal sonogram. This 63-year-old woman complains of pain in her shoulder for 6 months. Now she is worried because of increasing restriction in her range of motion. The hyaline cartilage (*arrow*) displays a strong echogenic interface at the base of the sonolucent tear on this view. This is due to acoustic enhancement afforded by the overlying fluid-filled tear. The cartilage sign displays the distal extent of the hyaline cartilage covering the humeral articular surface; this sign can be displayed only if the tear extends proximally enough and uncovers joint surface. **B,** Cartilage sign: transverse sonogram. Same patient as in **A**. Note that on the transverse view, the humeral head lies well below the level of the coracoid process: a sign of a small full-thickness tear. The interface with the cartilage is focally very echogenic (*arrow*).

3. Bony abnormalities distorting the normal landmarks
4. Inherent limitations of the technique

Normal Anatomy Mimicking an Abnormality

In most patients, the echogenicity of the supraspinatus tendon is greater than that of the deltoid muscle. The relative echogenicity of the rotator cuff decrease with age, and the cuff may become isoechoic with the deltoid. On transverse views of the anterior cuff, the biceps tendon appears as an echogenic focus between the supraspinatus and subscapularis tendons. This echogenic focus should not be confused with a calcium deposit or a region of scarring.

Normally, a hypoechoic region is present on either side of the biceps tendon. This is the rotator cuff interval, and it should not be confused with a tendon disruption (Fig. 15-27) (Brandt et al., 1989). The normal anterior cuff is thickest anteriorly. The anterior cuff averages 6 mm in diameter and the posterior cuff 3.6 mm (Bretzke et al., 1985). This normal posterior thinning of the cuff should not be misinterpreted as a tear. Posterior thinning should be symmetric and gradual in both shoulders, whereas tears manifest as an abrupt transition between normal and abnormal areas. Isolated posterior cuff tears are also quite rare.

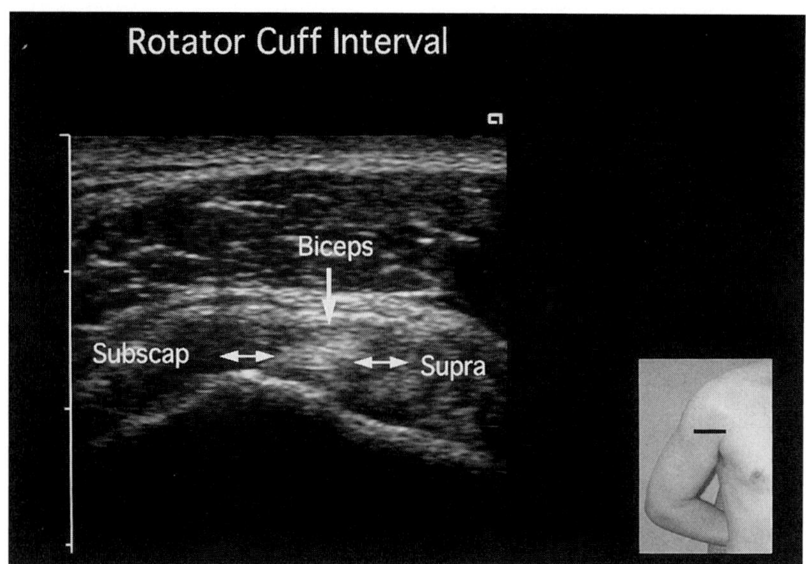

Figure 15-27 ■ Rotator cuff interval: transverse sonogram. Same patient as in Figure 15-2. The transducer is positioned over the intracapsular biceps tendon. The biceps tendon (*arrow*) appears as an echogenic focus separated from both the subscapularis tendon medially (*Subscap*) and the supraspinatus tendon laterally (*Supra*) by a short, variable sonolucent region, the rotator cuff interval.

The echogenicity of the rotator cuff in young, athletic persons is often quite homogeneous. With age and decreasing physical activity, the rotator cuff shows mild focal inhomogeneities. These lack an abrupt transition from the rest of the cuff, and the appearance is symmetrical with that of the contralateral side. This probably represents progressive fibrofatty infiltration of the tendon and is not pathological.

Soft Tissue Abnormalities Confusing the Echo Pattern

Calcific tendinitis most often produces a well-defined echogenic focus associated with posterior acoustic shadowing. This is not always the case. On occasion, confusing ill-defined, faint echogenic foci only slightly more echogenic than the surrounding tendon, obscuring tendon detail, may be detected.

Electronic transducers, employing multiple focal zones, may obscure the acoustic shadowing resulting from calcific tendinitis. In these cases, a single focal zone should be used to distinguish between calcium or linear areas of increased echogenicity within the tendon. If doubt persists, a single anteroposterior film of the shoulder in external rotation should confirm the presence of calcium within the supraspinatus tendon. Shadowing resulting from calcium deposits within the rotator cuff may mimic a tear (Drakeford et al., 1990).

Bony Abnormalities Distorting the Normal Landmarks

The superficial contour of the supraspinatus tendon may follow the contour of an underlying depressed fracture simulating a rotator cuff tear. Severe fractures may grossly distort the relationships of the rotator cuff tendon, making interpretation difficult.

Inherent Limitations of the Technique

The part of the rotator cuff lying proximal and deep to the acromion cannot be imaged by ultrasound. Hence, inferior osteophytes arising from the acromioclavicular joint and causing impingement cannot be detected. Imaging the cuff with the arm in the extended/internal rotation position or asking the patient to shrug back the shoulders and sit up straight brings more of the cuff into view, but the entire cuff can never be visualized. Fortunately, most rotator cuff pathology occurs in the terminal 1.5 cm of tendon, the critical zone, which can almost always be seen.

It should be noted that the supraspinatus tendon inserts at the distal aspect of the greater tuberosity. Small tears may cause the tendon to retract from this attachment but still maintain its convex contour. Subtle alterations in contour may be missed if the tendon is kept at "full stretch," with the arm in extreme internal rotation. For this reason, it is good practice to reexamine the supraspinatus tendon with the arm internally rotated but adducted.

Some patients may be able to rotate the arm internally to such an extent that the biceps tendon cannot be seen on the screen. A significant portion of the supraspinatus tendons' critical zone will therefore not be assessed or will be obscured by anisotropy. In such cases, the patient is asked to drop the hand to the seat of the chair or alongside the body, where the arm can be slowly rotated externally to ensure visualization of the entire supraspinatus.

In large patients, parenchymal detail may be lost due to acoustic impedance. In such cases, strong downward pressure by the transducer should be applied to detect a compressible, fluid-filled tendon defect which may be obscured by noise. A normal tendon does not compress. Occasionally, muscle bundles penetrating the cuff may simulate tears when scanned transversely, as they appear as rounded hypoechoic defects. Their true nature becomes readily apparent when the "lesion" is scanned longitudinally and the muscle bundles can be traced proximal to the acromion. Shadowing arising from fibrous septa in the subcutaneous fat or deltoid muscle may give the appearance of a lesion in the deeper rotator cuff. Anisotropy resulting from oblique scanning of tendon fibrils may simulate pathology. The transducer should be gently rocked to ensure that the suspected abnormality is constant, and all pathological foci should be recorded in two orthogonal planes.

Rarely, an acute full-thickness tear may be represented as a localized area of decreased echogenicity in a tendon with a bulging, convex outer border. This appearance has been shown to represent a hematoma in a fresh tear (Hodler et al., 1988).

In elderly patients with chronic disuse atrophy generally due to a chronic erosive arthropathy such as rheumatoid arthritis, the supraspinatus tendon may be so grossly thinned as to mimic total absence of cuff.

Sensitivity/Specificity of Ultrasound

Several studies have reported relatively poor sensitivity of ultrasound in the detection of rotator cuff tears (Burk et al., 1983; Brandt et al., 1989; Miller et al., 1989; Vick and Bell, 1990; Misamore and Woodward, 1991; Nelson et al., 1991). These studies have discouraged generalized acceptance of the technique (Hall, 1989). However, it is now generally accepted that accurate sonography of shoulder joint is both operator and equipment dependent and that the operator's learning curve is steep (Takagishi et al., 1996). Many of the above studies were performed with inexperienced sonographers using 5-MHz or sector scanners (Burk et al., 1983; Brandt et al., 1989; Miller et al., 1989; Nelson et al., 1991). Patient positioning in some cases was not optimal (Vick and Bell, 1990), and the patient's arm was not placed in hyperextension and internal rotation. In at least one study, the type of equipment used was not listed (Misamore and Woodward, 1991). Further, a large number of different criteria for rotator cuff tear have been published. The selection of inappropriate criteria such as hyperechoic foci have contributed to diagnostic error (Hodler et al., 1988; Mack et al., 1988; Patee and Snyder, 1988; Ahovuo et al., 1989b; Middleton, 1989, 1992; Kural et al., 1991).

Studies in anatomical specimens have demonstrated that focal hyper- or hypoechoic changes in otherwise homogeneous echogenic tendons do not necessarily show a full-thickness tear of the rotator cuff (Ahovuo et al., 1989a; Brandt et al., 1989). Several authors have now reported sensitivity and specificity in excess of 90% for the detection of both full- and partial-thickness tears. Ultrasound has also been shown to be accurate in evaluating the size and site of rotator cuff tears (Farin et al., 1996b).

One study using appropriate criteria for the diagnosis of full-thickness tears (contour absence or nonvisualization) reported good results for the detection of full-thickness tears (sensitivity of 95%, specificity of 93%) but poorer results in the detection of partial-thickness tears (41% and 91%, respectively). However, this study employed a 5-MHz transducer and used focal echogenicity as a criterion of partial-thickness tears. This again stresses the importance of adequate equipment and appropriate criteria to achieve good results even when the technique is clearly adequate (Brenneke and Morgan, 1992).

Conventional Radiographs

Radiographs of the shoulder are an integral part of the imaging assessment of shoulder pain. Occasionally, a destructive lesion, fracture, arthropathy, or faint calcification that would be difficult to detect on ultrasound examination may be detected.

Sclerosis and irregularity of the greater tuberosity on radiographs should be taken as strong evidence of a rotator cuff tear. If there is corresponding sclerosis and irregularity of the undersurface of the acromion, a rotator cuff tear is invariably present. Other findings include inferior acromioclavicular and biceps groove osteophytes and flattening of the anatomical neck of the humerus. An acromiohumeral distance of less than 6 mm is also characteristic of a full-thickness tear of the rotator cuff.

Rotator Cuff Arthropathy

Neer coined the term *rotator cuff arthropathy* (Neer et al., 1983). This term refers to an end-stage destructive arthropathy, said to occur in 4% of all full-thickness tears, similar in radiographic appearance to an end-stage crystal deposition arthropathy but

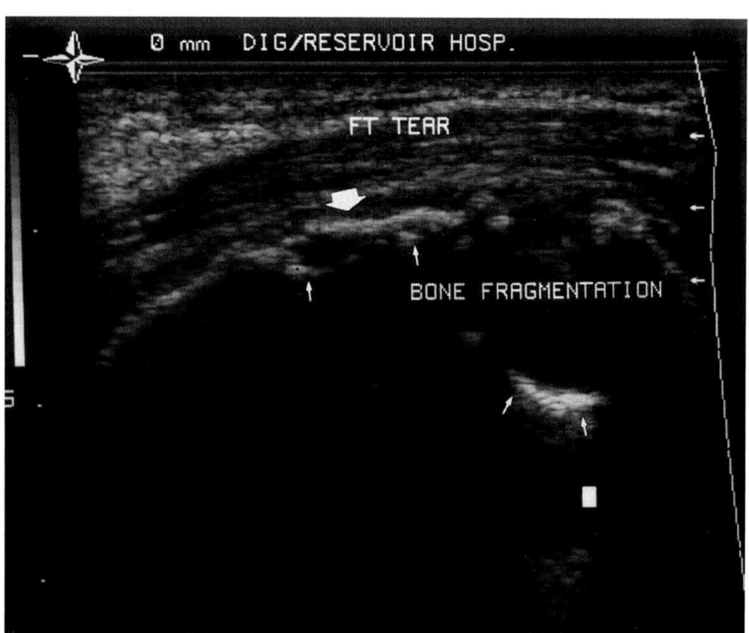

Figure 15-28 ▪ Rotator cuff arthropathy: longitudinal sonogram. After a long history of a documented rotator cuff tear, this 73-year-old man presents with 9 months of progressive restriction of shoulder movement. The rotator cuff and hyaline articular cartilage are entirely absent. Atrophied deltoid muscle (*large arrow*) lies flush to an irregular, pitted, fragmented humeral cortical surface (*small arrows*). Abbreviation: full-thickness tear (*FT TEAR*).

resulting from a chronic, massive rotator cuff disruption. The hallmark appearances are superior subluxation of the humerus in the glenohumeral joint, sclerosis, cystic change, and fragmentation of the cortical humeral surface.

Neer proposed a pathogenesis related to a neglected rotator cuff tear, secondary mechanical instability, and alteration of normal synovial nutrition. The ultrasound appearance of rotator cuff arthropathy includes superior subluxation of the humeral head, fragmentation, deep pitting or other irregular changes in the contour of the humeral head, and loss of normal hypoechoic cartilage (Fig. 15-28). Superior subluxation is best assessed by noting the position of the humeral head relative to the coracoid process (see Fig. 15-19B) (Wiener and Seitz, 1993). Superior subluxation of the humeral head may lead to erosion of the inferior acromioclavicular joint capsule. During a glenohumeral arthrogram, contrast will track superiorly into the acromioclavicular joint, producing a *geyser sign* that is pathognomonic for rotator cuff arthropathy. On ultrasound examination in these patients, the acromioclavicular joint capsule appears grossly distended, and passive movement of the glenohumeral joint leads to visible movement of debris within the acromioclavicular joint. We have termed this motion the *ultrasonic geyser sign*. Recognition of this sign is important, as the distended acromioclavicular joint may be mistaken for a ganglion. An attempt to excise this "ganglion" leads to a persistently draining sinus (Fig. 15-29).

Calcific Tendinitis

Calcific tendinitis is most commonly an idiopathic primary condition, but it may also be secondary to other disease processes including end-stage renal failure, tumoral calcinosis, vitamin D intoxicosis, and collagen-vascular diseases (Hayes and Conway, 1990). The condition is characterized by deposition of calcium, predominantly hydroxyapatite, in the rotator cuff and biceps tendon. The most frequent site is the supraspinatus tendon (Fig. 15-30) (Goldman, 1989). The pathogenesis of the condition in the supraspinatus tendon is thought to be related to the critical zone of the tendon, a relatively hypovascular area located 1 cm from its insertion. It has been postulated that fibrocartilaginous metaplasia with a propensity to calcify may occur in response to the relative hypoxia found in this location (Uthoff et al., 1976; Neer, 1990).

In our experience, the coexistence of a rotator cuff tear and calcific tendinitis is rare. The reason for this negative correlation is not understood. As most tears are located in the critical zone of the supraspinatus tendon, it is tempting to speculate that the two represent mutually exclusive responses to a hypoxic event, perhaps instigated by impingement, either metaplasia or disruption.

The clinical presentation is variable. Patients may present acutely or with a history of chronic or recurrent shoulder pain. Calcium deposition within tendons may be asymptomatic in one-third of the cases (Bosworth, 1941). The natural history of the

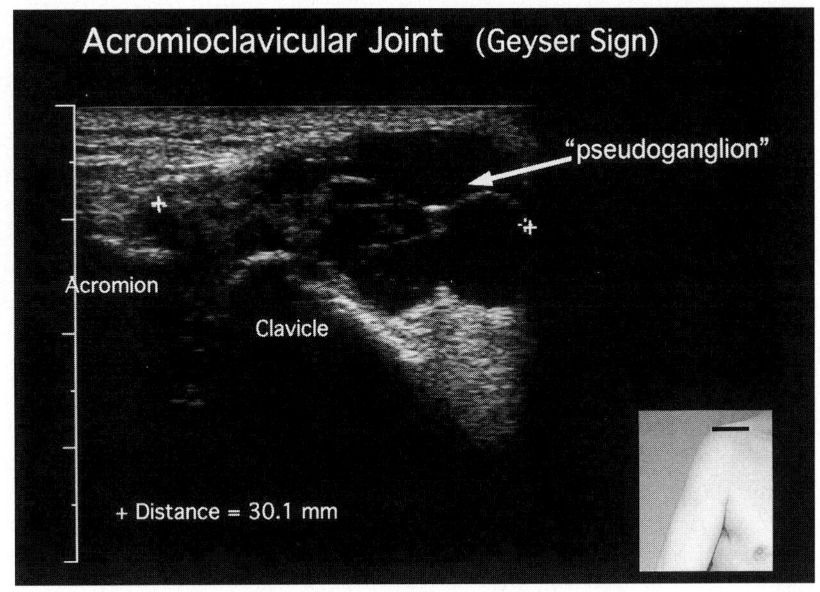

Figure 15-29 ■ Pseudoganglion of the acromioclavicular joint: coronal sonogram. A 72-year-old man presented with a fluctuant mass lying superficial to his acromioclavicular joint. A 3 cm multiloculated, fluid-filled mass (*arrow*) arises from the acromioclavicular joint. Passive movement of the glenohumeral joint provoked movement within the mass. Ultrasound examination also revealed a massive full-thickness tear of the rotator cuff associated with signs of rotator cuff arthropathy, including gross superior subluxation of the humeral head.

condition has been described as occurring in three stages (Moseley, 1969):

Stage 1: The silent phase or formative phase. The calcium deposit within the tendon is sharply defined, and symptoms are minimal.

Stage 2: The mechanical or resorptive phase. The deposit liquefies and is radiographically less well defined (Farin and Jaroma, 1995).

Stage 3: Adhesive periarthritis. The calcium deposits are associated with an adhesive bursitis. The diminished range of movement associated with this condition can be assessed by ultrasound and is similar to the deficit seen in adhesive capsulitis.

Three types of calcification can be found by ultrasonography:

1. A hyperechoic focus with a well-defined shadow (79%)
2. A hyperechoic focus with a faint shadow (14%)
3. A hyperechoic focus with no shadow (7%)

Types 2 and 3 can be classified as "slurry," which corresponds to the resorptive phase, or stage 2. Using this classification, ultrasound has been found

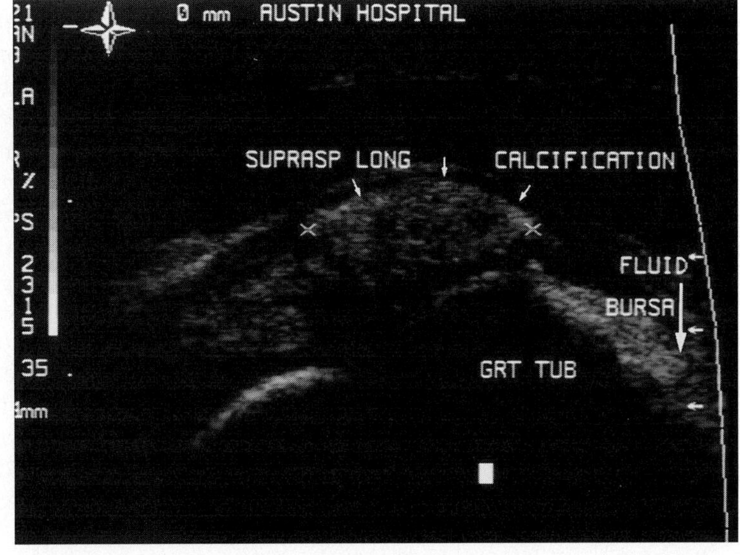

Figure 15-30 ■ Calcific tendinitis and bursitis: longitudinal sonogram. A 28-year-old woman presents with a 2 day history of incapacitating shoulder pain and with gross restriction in range of shoulder movement. A weakly shadowing 13 mm echogenic focus (*small arrows*) is present, within the distal supraspinatus tendon (*SUPRASP LONG*) just proximal to the distal tip of the greater tuberosity (*GRT TUB*). The calcium deposit protrudes into the adjacent subacromial bursa (*single long arrow*), which is thickened and contains fluid.

to be more reliable than plain films in predicting the consistency of rotator cuff calcifications. Slurry calcifications found on ultrasound have been proved to be nearly liquid in 93% of cases and can be successfully aspirated (Farin, 1996a).

Bursal calcifications are better seen on ultrasound, but small and scattered deposits are better seen on plain X-rays. Ultrasound is also reliable in localizing calcifications seen on X-ray to a particular tendon. Overall, in the assessment of calcifications in the cuff or bursal system, ultrasonography showed a sensitivity of 94% and a specificity of 99%. Acoustic shadowing is best seen using a minimum number of focal zones.

Avulsion fractures of the greater tuberosity may mimic rotator cuff calcification. Bone fragments tend to be more sharply defined, with echogenic characteristics similar to those of the bony cortex elsewhere. The calcium excites an inflammatory reaction within the rotator cuff leading to tendon edema, poor humeral depression, and impingement. Any calcium that ruptures into the subacromial bursa causes a severe exacerbation of symptoms (Neer, 1990). This group of patients may be the most debilitated of all by their pain.

The thickened, edematous tendon, poor humeral depression, impingement, and bursitis can all be assessed by ultrasound. Calcium deposits may be seen within the thickened, inflamed bursa. Aspiration of the calcium deposit during this phase, using a freehand, ultrasound-guided technique, has been shown to be effective in providing pain relief in these patients (Bradley et al., 1995; Farin et al., 1996a). Pain relief may be achieved even though the calcium deposit may be only partially aspirated. This may be due to a combination of decreased intratendinous pressure and production of localized bleeding, aiding resorption and dispersion of the remaining calcified material.

At 1 year of follow-up, ultrasound-guided aspiration was shown to decrease the size of the calcium deposit in 74% of cases, including 28% of cases in which the calcium deposit disappeared completely. The study by Farin et al. (1996a) resulted in an excellent clinical result in 74% of patients and moderate clinical result in 10%.

In stage 3 of calcific tendinitis, the calcium may exist in either a hard or a soft form, depending on the stage of resorption. The hard stage is easily recognizable. Echogenically it is similar to a gallstone, producing a strong echogenic interface with posterior acoustic shadowing. It is important to be aware of the condition so as not to confuse this shadowing with a tendon tear. The soft form is less strongly echogenic and poorly shadowing, and may appear similar to fibrofatty replacement within the tendon. Fibrous tissue in muscles and tendons may shadow. Careful correlation with plain films is therefore always mandatory.

The tendon may be grossly swollen compared to the asymptomatic contralateral side. Humeral depression is weak, and visible impingement against the outer edge of the acromion is often observed. Calcific bursitis reveals a bursa which generally appears thickened. There may be significant synovial proliferation, and the bursa is filled with echogenic debris, evidence of a powerful inflammatory response.

Ultrasound is often more sensitive than radiographs in detecting calcium deposits within the subscapularis or biceps tendon, where the calcium may be obscured by the underlying humeral shaft.

Acromioclavicular Joint

Acromioclavicular joint inflammation often presents clinically in a similar fashion to rotator cuff disorders. The patient also has a painful arc and has difficulty sleeping at night. Sonographic assessment of the acromioclavicular joint presents some difficulty, as there is a great variation in the appearance of the joint with age among patients and even among the joints of the same patient.

Degenerative changes within the joint producing osteophytic lipping are common and are generally asymptomatic. Asymmetry in joint space distances may be observed and is likely to reflect previous sprains of the acromioclavicular ligaments. Gross instability of the joint is best assessed by conventional radiographs with weight bearing.

Ultrasound is more sensitive than X-rays in the detection of grade 1 sprains of the acromioclavicular joint. The joint capsule may be distended by hematoma or fluid (Lind et al., 1989). Significant focal tenderness to sonographic palpation has proved the most reliable indicator of acromioclavicular joint inflammation. Generally, the joint capsule can be followed laterally, stripping the periosteum from the medial clavicular head (see Fig. 15–5). Occasionally, the visible portion of the clavicular head may appear eroded. The absence of these signs in the presence of tenderness on sonographic palpation should not eliminate the diagnosis of acromioclavicular joint inflammation. The majority of these patients do well with an injection of a local anesthetic/ steroid into the joint. This is most easily accomplished under fluoroscopic control.

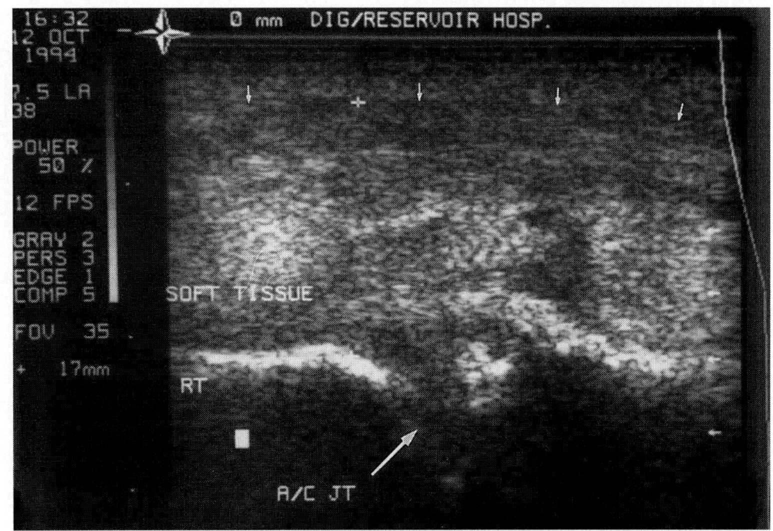

Figure 15–31 ■ Septic arthritis of the acromioclavicular joint: coronal sonogram. A 54-year-old man with 2 days of fever, increasing pain, and tenderness related to the acromioclavicular joint. The acromioclavicular joint capsule is grossly distended (*small arrows*) by soft tissue material, and early erosive change was noted at the articular surfaces of the joint (*long arrow*). Aspiration revealed pus.

Ultrasound examination can also distinguish between septic arthritis of the joint and traumatic avulsion of the deltoid insertion from its origin along the acromion and clavicle adjacent to the joint. In these cases, injection of steroids is contraindicated (Fig. 15–31).

Suprascapular Nerve Compression

Suprascapular nerve entrapment may be caused by anomalies of the suprascapular notch, fractures of the scapula, and ganglia pressing on the nerve. Ultrasound has been shown to play a role in the diagnosis of the last condition. Patients present with pain, weakness of external rotation and abduction, and wasting of the infraspinatus muscle. These patients may be difficult to differentiate clinically from those with rotator cuff lesions. Ultrasound will demonstrate a cystic structure at the base of the scapular spine at the spinoscapular notch (Takagishi et al., 1991) (see Figs. 8–29 through 8–32).

Fractures of the Greater Tuberosity

Minor fractures of the greater tuberosity can be either avulsion or depressed. Depressed fractures may result from direct trauma. Avulsion fractures usually arise in younger patients who have had an acute distraction avulsion injury at the glenohumeral joint (Fig. 15–32). In these younger patients, the bony supraspinatus attachment may give way prior to tendon rupture (Matsen and Arntz, 1990). These fractures may be less than 1 cm in diameter and are often radiologically occult. They may appear as a subtle region of increased technetium uptake on nuclear medicine bone scan.

The clinical presentation is identical to that of rotator cuff syndrome, except that there is often focal tenderness that can be localized to the microfracture by sonographic palpation. The distinction between fracture and rotator cuff tear is important, as the treatment and prognosis are significantly different (Hammond, 1991; Patten et al., 1992). The pain may be chronic. We have seen one patient who had persistent pain for 1 year following the trauma and who was found to have a focus of inflammatory synovial proliferation surrounding the avulsed bony fragment. A highly echogenic joint effusion that swirls with motion is evidence of a lipohemarthrosis, indicating the probable presence of an intra-articular fracture (Steiner and Sprigg, 1992). The fat in a lipohemarthrosis may also originate from the synovial membrane, capsuloligamentous structures, or intra-articular fat pads. The sonograms may reveal a fat-fluid level with a hyperechoic upper band of fat and a lower hypoechoic band of blood. If the joint is immobilized, three layers may be evident representing fat (superior hyperechoic), serum (intermediate anechoic) and blood cells (inferior hypoechoic) (Bianchi et al., 1995). Ultrasound has been successfully used to diagnose a Salter-Harris type 1 fracture in the unossified epiphysis of an agitated neonate suffering from mild respiratory distress following a spontaneous assisted vaginal delivery in the footling position (Fisher et al., 1995).

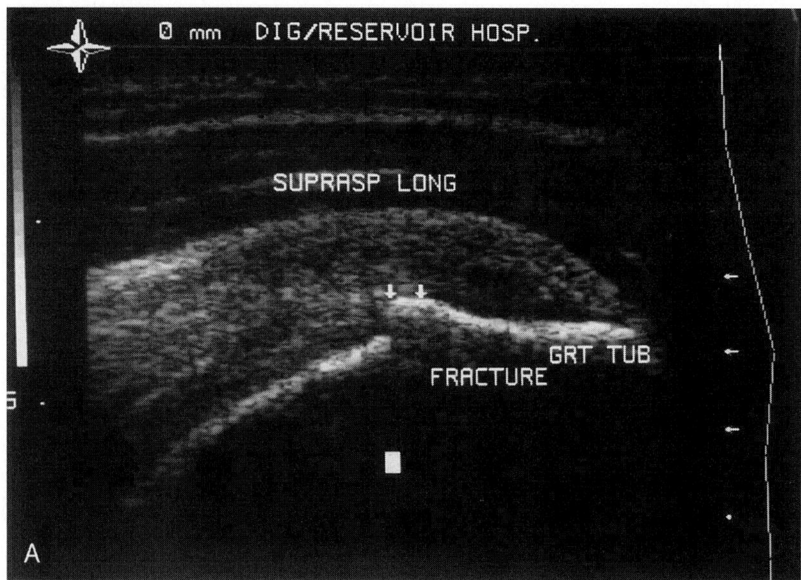

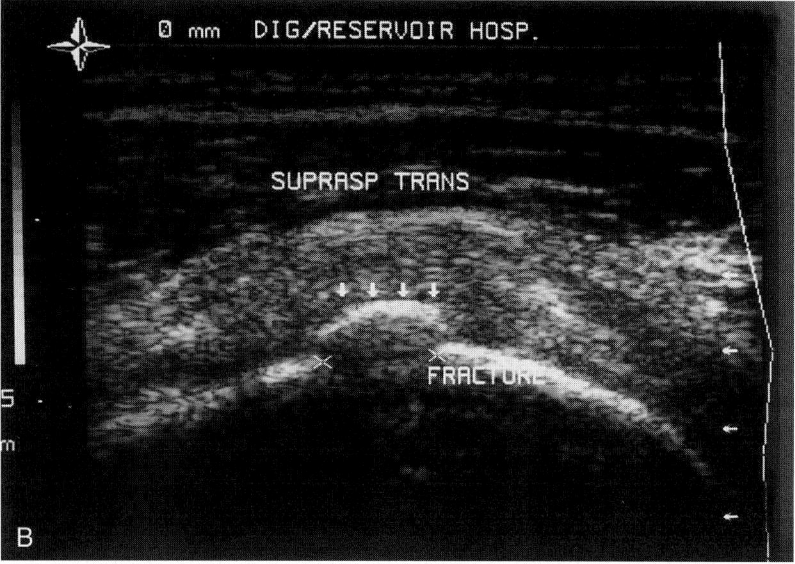

Figure 15–32 ■ **A,** Avulsion fracture: longitudinal sonogram. A 27-year-old female attempted to stop a fall while rollerblading; she braced herself with her outstretched arm and felt a sudden sharp pain in the shoulder. The greater tuberosity (*GRT TUB*) is displaced (*arrows*), and a step-off deformity is noticed at its surface. Abbreviation: supraspinatus (*SUPRASP LONG*). **B,** Avulsion fracture: transverse sonogram. Same patient as in **A**. Transverse images demonstrate a 0.5 cm avulsion fracture (*small arrows*) arising from the insertion of the supraspinatus tendon just distal to the humeral articular surface. The fracture was radiographically occult. Abbreviation: supraspinatus (*SUPRASP TRANS*).

Subacromial Bursa

The subacromial-subdeltoid bursa is the largest bursa in the body. It acts as a joint between the rotator cuff and the overlying acromion and deltoid muscle. Fluid within the bursa dissipates friction between these structures. The subdeltoid and subacromial components of the bursa are contiguous in approximately 95% of patients. Anteriorly, the bursa covers the bicipital groove and the rotator cuff interval. Fluid within the bursa in this location should not be confused with joint fluid contained within the biceps tendon sheath (Fig. 15–33). The bursa is separated from the joint by the rotator cuff. Full-thickness tears of the cuff therefore allow communication between the bursa and joint.

The normal bursa is no more than 2 mm thick, including a thin, hypoechoic layer of fluid located between the two opposing sides of the bursa (Fig. 15–11) (van Holsbeeck and Introcaso, 1989). Fluid within the bursa tends to accumulate in one of three locations:

1. Distal to the lateral edge of the greater tuberosity just distal to the supraspinatus insertion, where it appears as a tear-shaped thickening of the bursa lying against the proximal humeral diaphysis. Fluid tends to collect here transiently after the arm is returned to the patient's side

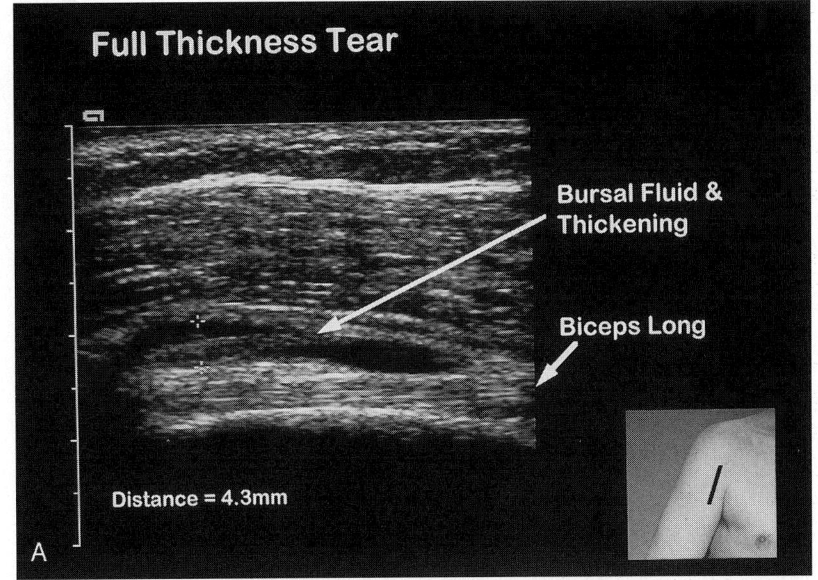

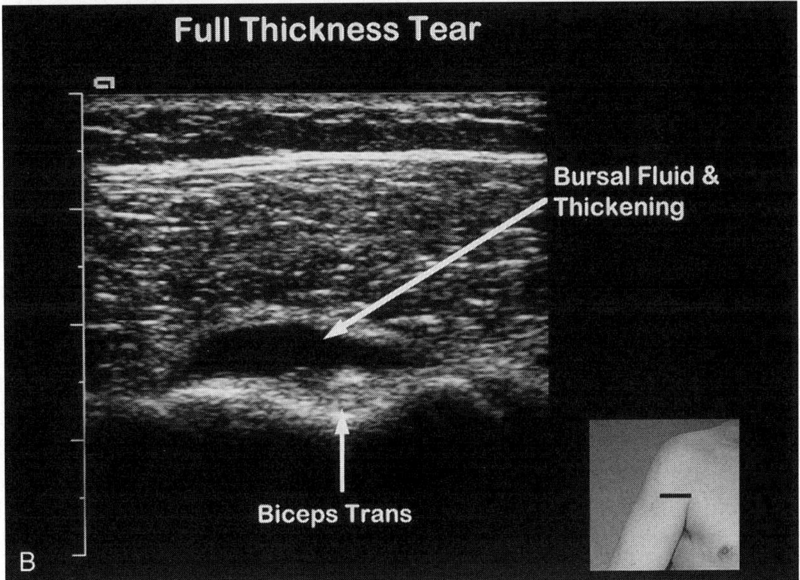

Figure 15-33 ■ **A,** Bursal fluid: longitudinal sonogram. A 64-year-old man with a full-thickness tear of the rotator cuff. Fluid covers the anterior long biceps tendon but does not surround the tendon. **B,** Bursal fluid: transverse sonogram. Same patient as in **A**. The thickened subacromial-subdeltoid bursa covers the anterior shoulder; the bursa is distended by fluid (*long arrows*). The effusion in the bursal lumen extends both medially and laterally beyond the bony margins of the biceps groove.

from the extreme internal rotation position while internal rotation is maintained (Fig. 15-34). Care must be taken to examine the bursa distally at the level of the deltoid insertion, as fluid may accumulate in this gravitationally dependent position.

2. Anterior to the subscapularis tendon during external rotation. Fluid is "pumped" into this location by obliteration of the subcoracoid recess, where fluid accumulates with the arm in internal rotation (see Fig. 15-4).
3. Anterior to the bicipital groove. As the examination commences in this position, an early indication of the likelihood of a rotator cuff tear may be noted (see Fig. 15-33).

Bursal distention has been divided into two types: communicating and noncommunicating abnormalities (van Holsbeeck and Strouse, 1993). These will now be discussed.

Communicating Abnormalities

In symptomatic patients, the presence of bursal fluid has been found to have a specificity of 96% for the diagnosis of rotator cuff tears (Hollster et al., 1995). Other authors have reported specificities of 90% (van Holsbeeck and Strouse, 1993) and 87% (Hollister et al., 1995). The detection of both joint effusion and bursal effusion improved the specificity of rotator cuff tear to 99% (Hollister et al., 1995).

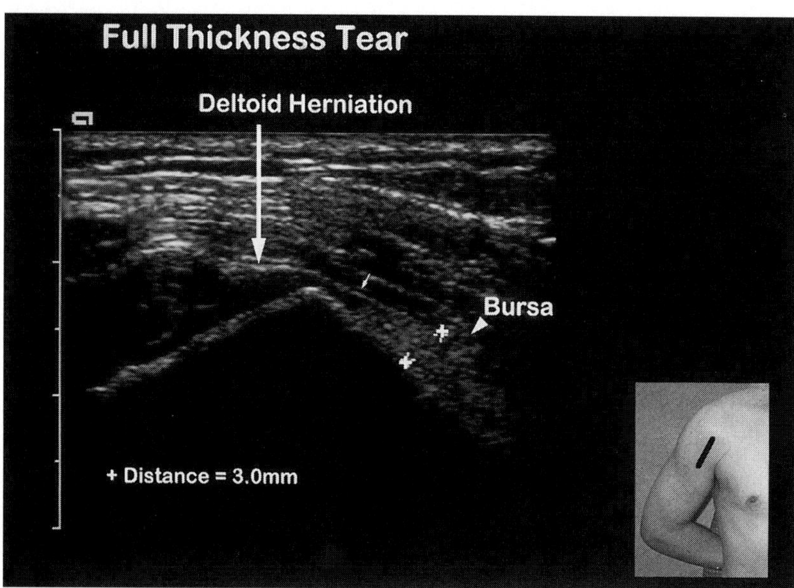

Figure 15-34 ■ Rotator cuff tear with bursal fluid: longitudinal sonogram. A 66-year-old female with a small full-thickness tear of the supraspinatus tendon. A significant alteration of the distal supraspinatus contour is present (deltoid herniation—*long arrow*). The subacromial bursa distal to the supraspinatus insertion contains some fluid (*small arrow*) and is thickened.

Awareness of the high specificity of combined bursal and joint effusions for rotator cuff tears should help reduce false-negative diagnoses by increasing the sonologist's level of suspicion in difficult or equivocal cases. In asymptomatic shoulders, the incidence of isolated joint effusions is 6.9%, that of isolated bursal fluid collections is 3.4%, and that of combined bursal and joint fluid collections is 1.7%.

Fluid within both bursa and joint in the presence of a full-thickness tear of the rotator cuff is due to direct communication between the two compartments through the defect, akin to the positive findings during a single-contrast arthrogram. Fluid in a partial-thickness tear is most likely due to direct mechanical irritation of the bursa by impingement or fenestrations within the partially torn cuff, allowing the communication. In full-thickness tears, the volume of fluid within the bursa is far greater than that seen in partial-thickness tears or impingement.

Noncommunicating Distention/Thickening of the Rotator Cuff

Hemorrhagic Bursitis

This condition results from a direct blow to the bursa. Initially the bursa is hyperechoic, but it becomes progressively more hypoechoic over several days as the blood products are broken down.

Impingement Syndrome

The bursa is progressively irritated by chronic trauma resulting from repetitive friction against the acromion or the coracoacromial ligament. The synovial lining of the bursa is thickened, and the bursa may contain fluid (see Fig. 15–14). The amount of fluid found in this condition is considerably less than that seen in full-thickness tears and corresponds to the grade 1 and 2 impingement lesions described by Neer (bursal hemorrhage and edema). These grade 1 and 2 lesions are often accompanied by an edematous supraspinatus tendon (see Fig. 15–16). Any larger collection of fluid in the absence of an inflammatory arthropathy should be taken as extremely strong evidence for the presence of a full-thickness tear of the rotator cuff (grade 3 lesion). Subacromial-subdeltoid bursitis related to impingement syndrome is not always anechoic; it can present as a thickened wall and solid contents without fluid. The focal bursal thickening may be tender to sonographic palpation. During dynamic testing, the thickened bursal tissue may be seen to "bunch up" against the outer edge of the acromion, failing to pass beneath. The commencement of this bunching coincides with the onset of the painful arc.

Arthropathies and Infiltrative Disorders

Infective, seropositive, and seronegative arthropathies lead to synovial wall proliferation and thickening of the bursa. Polymyalgia rheumatica, hydroxyapatite, and calcium deposition (Fig. 15–35) can also cause inflammation of the bursa, which is quite severe in the last case. In amyloidosis, as will be discussed, bursal thickening may be so profound that the patient's shoulders take on a contour akin to that of shoulder pads such as those worn by American football players.

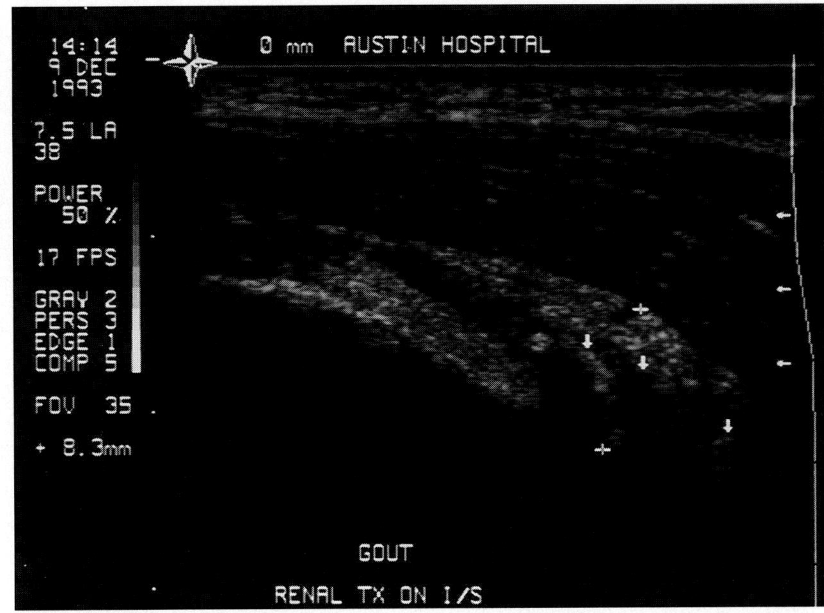

Figure 15-35 ■ Uric acid-related synovitis: longitudinal sonogram. A 30-year-old dialysis patient who has a previous history of renal transplantation and has been on immunosuppressive drugs presents with sudden onset of severe shoulder pain. A longitudinal view of the subdeltoid bursa distal to the supraspinatus insertion reveals a thickened, tender bursa containing numerous shadowing calcific foci (*small arrows*). The patient was subsequently shown to be suffering from gout.

Septic bursitis is usually not associated with septic arthritis, but it may be difficult to distinguish between these entities clinically. Arthrocentesis has traditionally been employed to exclude joint infection, but it involves the risk of introducing organisms into a sterile joint if infection was present only in the periarticular tissues. Ultrasound can obviate the need for arthrocentesis by visualizing a complex bursal fluid collection and demonstrating the absence of intra-articular fluid (Lombardi et al., 1992).

In chronic tears, especially those that are asymptomatic, bursal fluid is rarely found, although the bursa itself may be slightly thickened. In many patients who have chronic, asymptomatic full-thickness tears, the finding of bursal fluid, indicating the presence of bursal inflammation, is the most likely explanation for the onset of symptoms.

Postoperative Assessment

The symptomatic postoperative patient may be suffering from recurrent tear of the rotator cuff, adhesive capsulitis, tendinitis, or impingement. Arthrographic assessment of a possible recurrent rotator cuff tear following surgery is problematic, as postoperative adhesions may cause a false-negative result. A positive result may be meaningless, as a completely watertight closure does not appear to be essential for a good functional result, which is probably more dependent on subacromial decompression and restoration of a mechanically effective cuff (Calvert et al., 1986). While a watertight closure may not be essential, detection of a large, recurrent tear is important, as it will invariably lead to further narrowing of the subacromial space and continuing pain and put the patient at potential risk for the development of rotator cuff arthropathy (Crass et al., 1996).

Ultrasound has been used successfully to assess the postoperative shoulder (Mack et al., 1988). Patients with intact tendons have been found to have better function and range of movement than those with recurrent tears, and the degree of functional loss was related to the size of the recurrent defect (Harryman et al., 1991). Recurrent tears are common. They have been reported in up to 20% of patients who had a small preoperative defect confined to the supraspinatus tendon and in up to 50% of patients with preoperative defects involving more than one tendon (Harryman et al., 1991).

Ultrasound assessment in the postoperative patient is a challenge. In many cases, a confident diagnosis of recurrent tear can be made. However, in many instances, several technical difficulties will lead to many equivocal examinations, i.e., it can be difficult to exclude a recurrent tear. The sonographic appearance of postoperative shoulders is virtually never normal (Crass et al., 1986). There is always a loss of soft tissue planes surrounding the rotator cuff and abnormally increased echogenicity in the tendon. Altered echogenicity should therefore never be used as a criterion for recurrent tear. The increase in tendon echogenicity is thought to

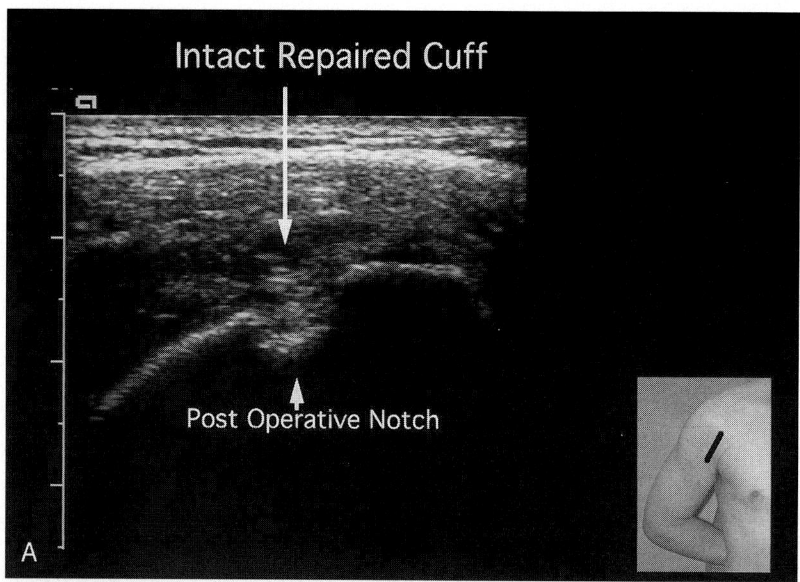

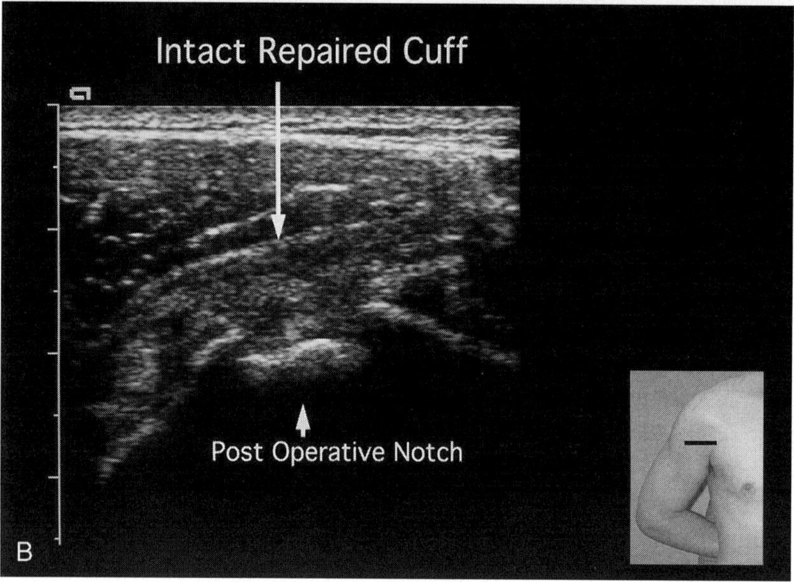

Figure 15-36 ■ **A,** Rotator cuff repair: longitudinal sonogram. Six months following a repair, this 52-year-old male has an intact rotator cuff. A shallow postoperative notch in the humeral neck is noted just proximal to the greater tuberosity. The notch is 4 mm (*small arrow*). An intact tendon is inserted into the notch (*long arrow*). Note the flattened tendon contour and the poor delineation between the supraspinatus tendon and the overlying deltoid muscle as a result of loss of the subdeltoid fat. **B,** Rotator cuff repair: transverse sonogram. Same patient as in **A**. The anteroposterior diameter of the postsurgical groove in the proximal humerus is less than 1 cm.

be due to persistent disorganization and irregularities in the collagen bundles. These changes have been documented to persist for up to 6 years following the surgical repair (Crass et al., 1986). Following rotator cuff surgery, whether open or via arthroscopy, clear definition of the soft tissue planes, particularly the curved, echogenic plane of the subdeltoid fat superficial to the subacromial bursa, may be severely impaired. The sonographic appearance of the supraspinatus tendon never returns to normal. The intact postoperative tendon is often thinned; a mild concave contour is common, and echogenicity is altered (usually increased) (Furtschegger and Resch, 1988). In addition, the operative details are often not available, making it difficult to distinguish between postoperative deformity, scarring, and pathology.

A characteristic sonographic abnormality of the acromial contour has been described following acromioplasty (Mack et al., 1988). The normally well-defined, rounded margins of the anterior inferior acromion are replaced by a less distinct, irregular surface with an amputated edge. Acromioplasty generally allows visualization of a greater proportion of the proximal supraspinatus tendon, which is usually hidden under the acromion.

Optimally, the torn tendon will be implanted in bone at the level of the greater tuberosity. However, if sufficient viable cuff is not available, the surgeon will often fashion a trough in the head of the

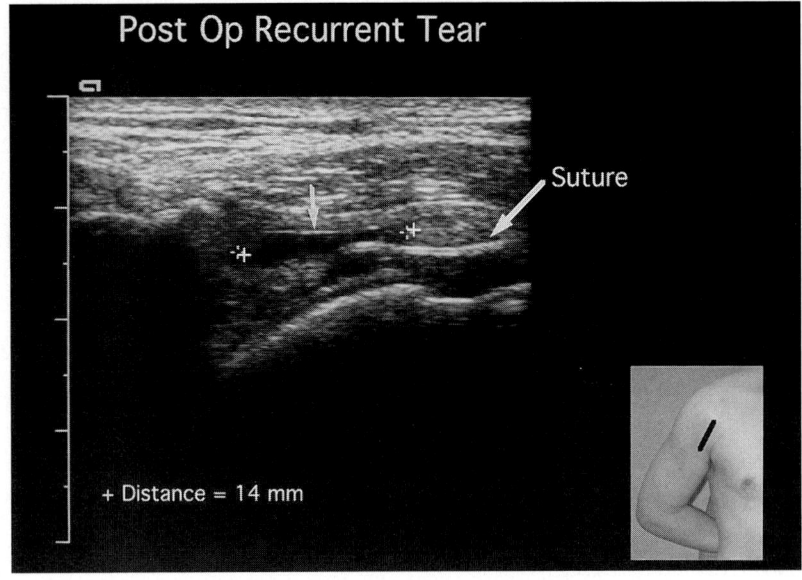

Figure 15–37 ■ Retear of supraspinatus tendon: longitudinal sonogram. Recurrent full-thickness tear of the supraspinatus tendon in a 40-year-old male. A 14 mm cuff defect is present (*small arrow*). The torn end of a suture protrudes into the cuff defect, casting a weak reverberation artifact (*large arrow*).

humerus within the sulcus adjacent to the humeral articular surface. The position is variable, depending on the difficulty of mobilizing the supraspinatus tendon, but it is usually located lateral to the biceps groove. It is into this notch that the retracted torn edge of the supraspinatus tendon is placed under maximal tension (Fig. 15–36). As a result, some bare bone in the region of the greater tuberosity may be acceptable in the postoperative patient, and it does not necessarily indicate the presence of a recurrent tear. Suture material casting a reverbation shadow may be seen. Bony fragments may be seen in the subacromial space and may account for recurrent impingement.

The contour of the supraspinatus tendon is no longer a totally reliable indicator of pathology. The tendon is often scarred and reduced in volume and may possess a slightly concave contour, but it is still intact. A postoperative baseline study for comparison is invaluable but rarely available.

Visualization of a definite cuff defect or gap is required before a recurrent tear can be diagnosed with certainty (Fig. 15–37) (Crass et al., 1986). Other reliable signs of a recurrent tear are absence of the cuff, large amounts of extra-articular fluid within the remnants of the subacromial bursa, and retraction of the supraspinatus tendon from the surgical trough (Fig. 15–38).

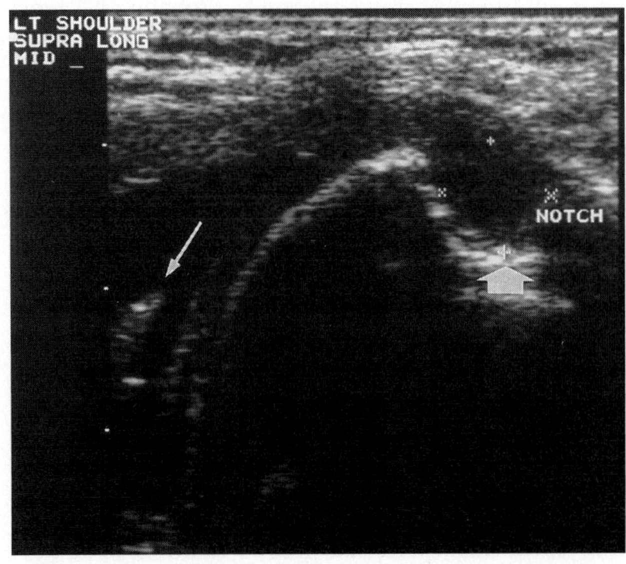

Figure 15–38 ■ Full-thickness retear: longitudinal sonogram. Recurrent full-thickness tear of the supraspinatus tendon in a 45-year-old female. The postoperative notch contains only fluid (*short thick arrow*). The retracted edge of the retorn tendon can be seen 2.5 cm proximally surrounded by fluid (*long thin arrow*).

The sensitivity of ultrasound in detecting postoperative rotator cuff tears has been reported at 100%, specificity 90%, and overall accuracy 98% (Mack et al., 1988). Dynamic scanning enables an assessment of the adequacy of any acromioplasty that may have been performed and will differentiate secondary adhesive capsulitis from a recurrent tear. It will also help detect recurrent tears in difficult cases by distinguishing between the mobile supraspinatus tissue and the relatively immobile deltoid muscle, which may have similar echogenicity in the postoperative patient.

Long Head of Biceps Tendon (LHB)

Normal Anatomy

The long head of the biceps brachii originates at the supraglenoid tubercle and glenoid labrum in the most superior portion of the glenoid. The cross-sectional dimensions of the tendon change during its course, but it measures a maximum of 4.7 mm in depth within the groove. It courses obliquely across the top of the humeral head into the bicipital groove. On average, the tendon is 9 cm in length, becoming musculotendinous near the insertion of the deltoid.

The LHB is intra-articular but extrasynovial. The synovial sheath, which communicates directly with the glenohumeral joint, ends in a blind pouch at the end of the bicipital groove.

LHB Function

The LHB is a weak flexor, abductor, and external rotator of the glenohumeral joint. Probably its most important function at the glenohumeral joint is to act as both an active and a static humeral head depressor. It is therefore important in preventing impingement.

Soft Tissue Restraint

The LHB is restrained at three principal levels along its course in the arm. The intra-articular portion runs underneath the coracohumeral ligament that lies between and strengthens the interval between the subscapularis and supraspinatus, the so-called rotator cuff interval. It is an integral part of the cuff and capsule and can be distinguished only by sharp dissection.

The chief restraint to medial dislocation of the LHB within the proximal groove is the medial portion of the coracohumeral ligament close to its insertion on the lesser tuberosity, not the transverse humeral ligament, as has been traditionally taught (Slatis and Aalto, 1979). The main structure containing the tendon within the groove, further distally, below the top of the tuberosity, is the tendinous expansion from the insertion of the sternocostal portion of the pectoralis major, the falciform ligament. It crosses the tendon, inserting predominantly onto the lateral lip of the groove.

Osseous Anatomy and Pathoanatomy

The bicipital groove is formed between the lesser and greater tuberosities. The mean value of the medial wall angle is 56 degrees. There is a wide variation in groove width but a constant ratio of 1.6 between the width of the groove at its lips and the width at a point equal to half of its depth. The average depth of the groove is 4.3 mm. Grooves less than 3 mm in depth are regarded as shallow (Farin et al., 1995a). The groove is positioned at approximately 15 degrees posterior to the midsaggital plane of the humerus when in the anatomical position.

From the quadruped to the erect biped, there has been progressive anteroposterior flattening of the thorax, resulting in an increased angle that the scapula forms with the thorax and relatively lateral displacement of the scapula. This results in a greater degree of medial rotation of the humerus for the human hand to reach the midline, which in turn causes the LHB to ride against the lesser tuberosity.

As a result, a low medial wall angle predisposes to medial dislocation. Similarly, a narrow groove with a sharp medial wall or osteophyte at the aperture traumatizes the tendon, predisposing to bicipital tenosynovitis and rupture. Spurs on the floor of the groove may erode the tendon. A posteriorly placed groove puts the tendon at greater risk for impingement against the anterior edge of the acromion on forward flexion.

Pathology

In acute progressing to chronic bicipital tenosynovitis, a spectrum of gradual pathological changes have been described. Initially there is edema of the tendon, with progressive cellular infiltration of the synovial lined sheath. In the chronic stage there is fraying of the LHB, synovial proliferation, fibrosis, and, ultimately, replacement of tendon fibers by fibrous tissue. After rupture or dislocation, granulation and fibrous tissue have been found occupying the groove.

In all LHB dislocations or subluxations, the tendon dislocates medially, either superficial or deep to

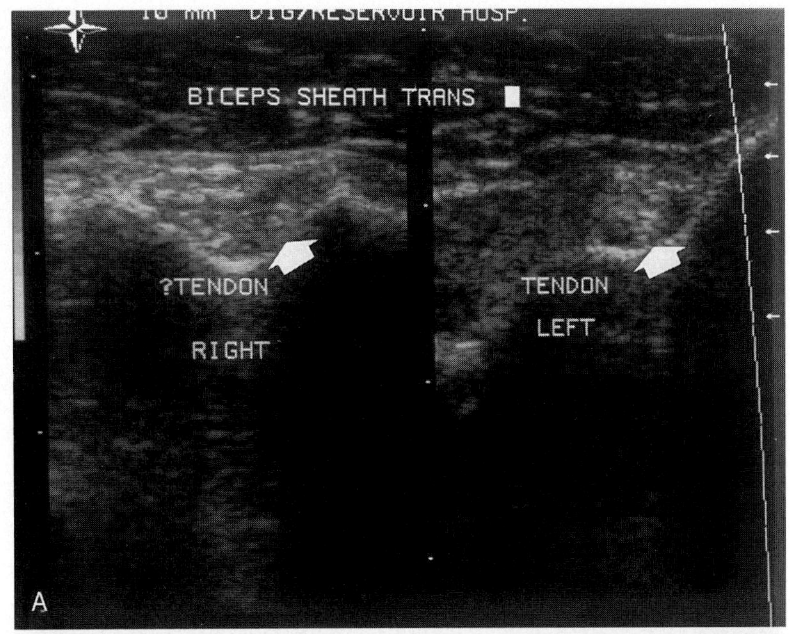

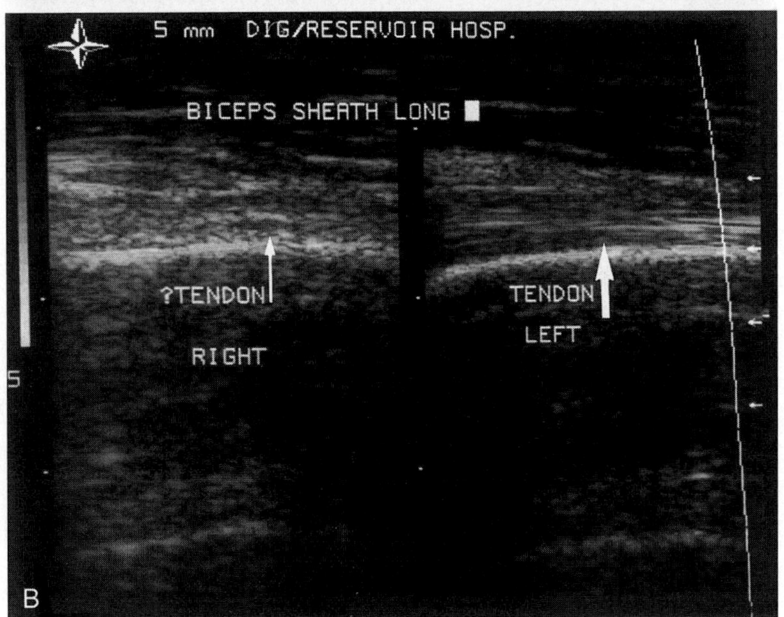

Figure 15-39 ■ A, Full-thickness tear of the long biceps tendon: transverse view. Shoulder symptoms suddenly increased in this 68-year-old man who had a known rotator cuff tear. Weakness in his shoulder did not allow him to raise his arm. A transverse section through both bicipital grooves in this patient shows rounded echogenic structures (*short thick arrows*). **B,** Full-thickness tear of the long biceps tendon: longitudinal view. Same patient as in **A**. Only the groove on the left contains a true tendon showing a normal fibrillar pattern (*long thick arrow*). The groove on the right contains disorganized fibrous tissue devoid of fibrillar pattern (*long thin arrow*). Longitudinal views are the most useful in detecting the full extent of tendon retraction.

the subscapularis tendon following degeneration of the subscapularis tendon and the coracohumeral ligament in the region of the lesser tuberosity (Farin et al., 1995a). Acute traumatic dislocations rarely occur. The LHB and its enveloping synovial sheath are often affected by any inflammatory, infectious, or traumatic process involving the glenohumeral joint.

Sonographic Findings

The intra-articular portion of the LHB is easily identified on transverse scans as an oval-shaped, echogenic structure forming a sonographic anatomical landmark between the tendons of the subscapularis anteromedially and the supraspinatus posterolaterally (see Fig. 15-27). The tendon can be followed inferiorly to enter the bicipital groove.

The longitudinal view of a normal tendon reveals a fine fibrillary pattern (see Fig. 15-3). The fibrillary pattern should be seen with a modern 7.5 MHz transducer in even the largest patients. It is usually necessary to angle superiorly in order to visualize the tendon in an orthogonal manner.

Absence of the fibrillary pattern is always abnormal. It indicates that the tendon is severely degenerated, ruptured, or dislocated and that it has been replaced by fibrous and granulation tissue (Fig. 15-39) (Farin et al., 1995a). The "empty groove" sign

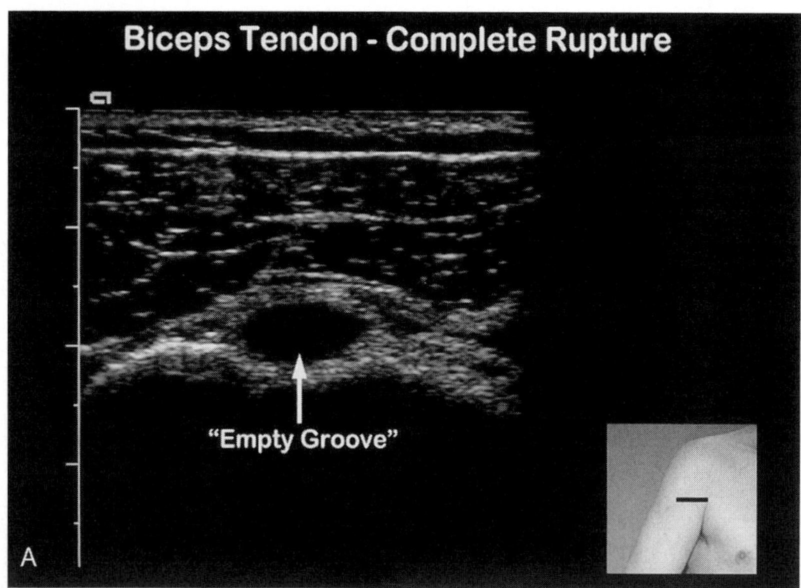

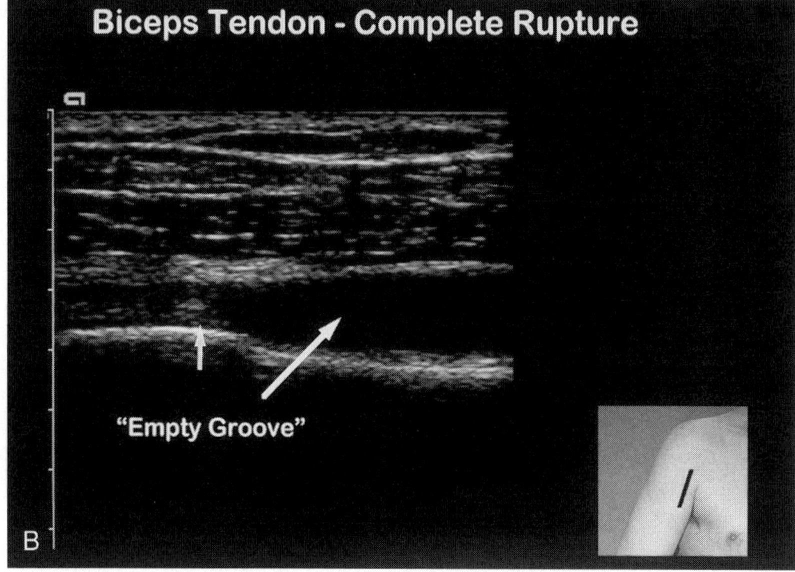

Figure 15-40 ■ **A,** Acute complete rupture of the long biceps tendon: transverse sonogram. While this 57-year-old man was lifting a heavy object, he experienced a sudden snap in the upper arm. This transverse view of the midportion of the groove demonstrates an "empty groove"; the biceps tendon sheath is distended with fluid (*arrow*). **B,** Acute complete rupture of the long biceps tendon: longitudinal sonogram. Same patient as in **A**. Imaging along the length of the tendon demonstrates the point of rupture (*short arrow*) of a degenerate tendon with a poor fibrillar pattern. The sheath distal to the rupture is distended with fluid (*long arrow*).

previously described is, in our experience, applicable only in acute LHB ruptures (Fig. 15-40). Fluid within the sheath is a pathological but nonspecific finding (Middleton, 1992; Paavolainen and Ahovuo, 1994). It may be seen in any condition that causes a joint effusion, any cause of synovitis, and adhesive capsulitis. Ninety percent of patients with fluid in their biceps tendon sheath have pathology elsewhere in the glenohumeral joint. For this reason, we do not diagnose bicipital tenosynovitis unless the tendon itself is enlarged or if the amount of fluid surrounding the tendon is out of proportion to that present within the rest of the joint (Fig. 15-41). Small volumes of fluid collect medially within the sheath, and if one scans medially to the tendon in the longitudinal plane, a tear-shaped, blind-ending synovial sac can be visualized. Echogenic debris within a large sheath collection, particularly in the setting of trauma and in the absence of findings elsewhere, has often indicated the presence of a previously undetected intra-articular fracture. The volume of sheath fluid tends to be large in full-thickness tears (Fig. 15-41) and small in adhesive capsulitis and articular surface partial-thickness tears.

Fluid within the sheath must be carefully differentiated from fluid within the subacromial-subdeltoid bursa, which lies superficially between the sheath and the deltoid muscle (see Fig. 15-33). The combination of fluid within the sheath and within

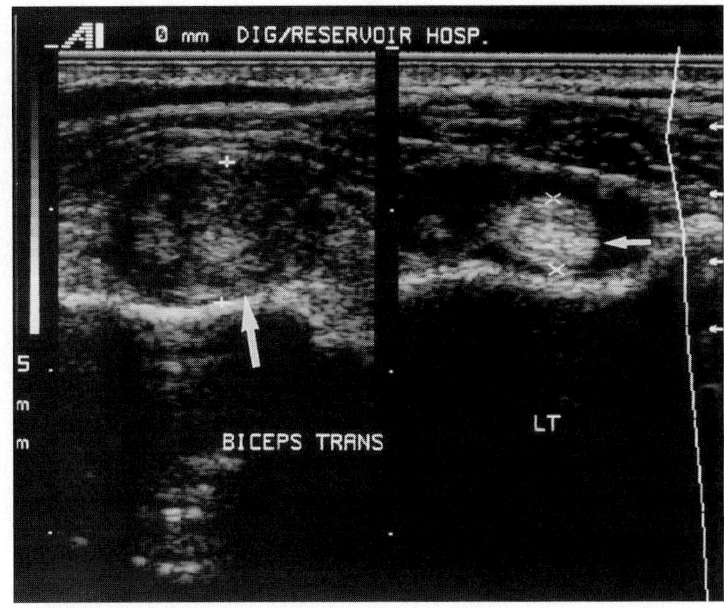

Figure 15–41 ■ Bicipital tendonitis: transverse sonogram. This 41-year-old man presents with a painful arc and focal tenderness upon palpation of the bicipital groove. Left–right comparison of the long biceps tendons in one patient. The tendon of the right shoulder is grossly edematous and surrounded by a thin rim of fluid measuring 9.5 mm in thickness (*large arrow*) compared to 4.5 mm on the left (*small arrow*). The tendon on the left is surrounded by joint fluid within its sheath, as the patient had a large rotator cuff tear on that side.

the bursa is virtually pathognomonic of a full-thickness tear of the rotator cuff.

The biceps tendon sheath may contain osteochondral loose bodies (Fig. 15–42) or may be involved with synovial chondromatosis. On occasion, the biceps tendon or its sheath may calcify. Dissecting synovitis or synovial cysts may be associated with chronic rotator cuff tears, rheumatoid arthritis, or following local steroid injections. They appear on ultrasound examination as a loculated collection of fluid causing an outbulging from the side of the biceps tendon sheath (Farin, 1996b).

Thickening of the bursa (>2 mm) superficial to the tendon generally indicates the presence of impingement, but it may also be seen in any condition that causes generalized synovial proliferation (e.g., rheumatoid disease, amyloidosis). The bursa distinguishes itself from the synovial sheath of the biceps

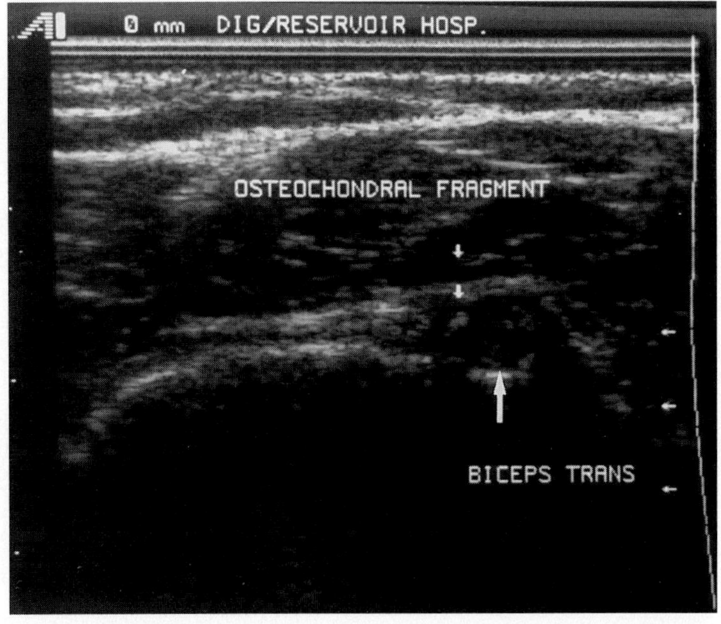

Figure 15–42 ■ Osteochondral fragment: transverse view. A 25-year-old man presents with intermittent locking of the glenohumeral joint several weeks after trauma to the shoulder girdle. The distal biceps groove contains a 3 mm weakly shadowing, echogenic focus representing an osteochondral fragment (*deep to the small arrows*) lying adjacent to the biceps tendon (*large arrow*).

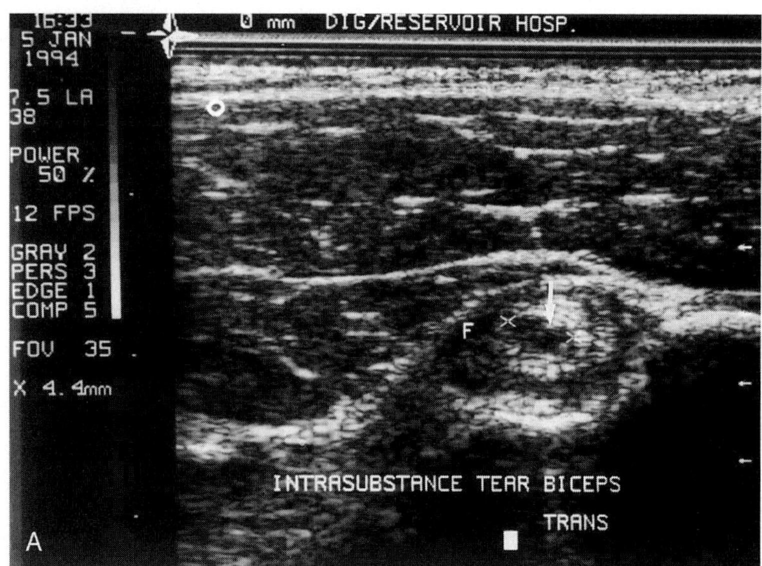

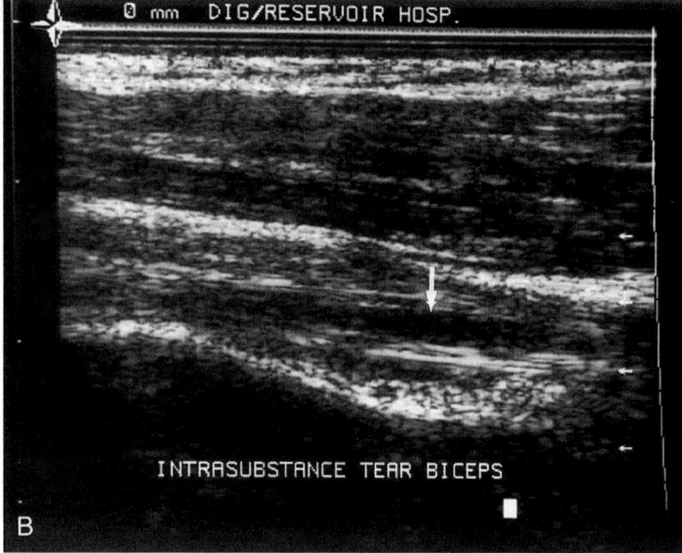

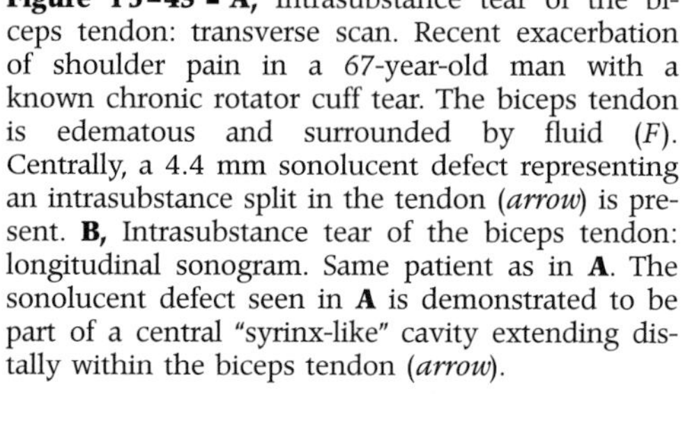
Figure 15–43 ■ **A,** Intrasubstance tear of the biceps tendon: transverse scan. Recent exacerbation of shoulder pain in a 67-year-old man with a known chronic rotator cuff tear. The biceps tendon is edematous and surrounded by fluid (*F*). Centrally, a 4.4 mm sonolucent defect representing an intrasubstance split in the tendon (*arrow*) is present. **B,** Intrasubstance tear of the biceps tendon: longitudinal sonogram. Same patient as in **A**. The sonolucent defect seen in **A** is demonstrated to be part of a central "syrinx-like" cavity extending distally within the biceps tendon (*arrow*).

by its location. The bursa extends medial and lateral to the biceps groove; the biceps tendon sheath, by contrast, does not.

Full-thickness tears of the LHB are easily identified by a sudden disruption of the fibrillary pattern, but partial-thickness tears can also be identified. Intrasubstance tears, producing a syrinx-like cavity within the tendon, are not uncommon (Fig. 15–43).

Evaluation of the osseous anatomy is straightforward. The depth and medial wall angle of the groove can be measured directly. Bony spurs may be seen arising from both the floor and the medial wall of the groove (Fig. 15–44). Almost all patients with a shallow, irregular groove possessing spurs have a coexistent rotator cuff tear, and the biceps tendon, if intact, will be grossly degenerate. Displacement of the biceps tendon is an uncommon and unrecognized cause of shoulder pain (DePalma, 1983). Dislocations, in our experience, always occur medially, deep or superficial to the subscapularis, and in most cases are associated with a full-thickness tear of the supraspinatus tendon, but they can also occur following the application of a heavy load (Fig. 15–45). We have also seen several cases of bilateral congenital subluxation seemingly secondary to shallow medial wall angles (Fig. 15–46).

The displacement may be either subluxation or dislocation. The displacement may be intermittent, and the patient may complain of a snapping sensation. Farin et al. (1995a) described a dynamic

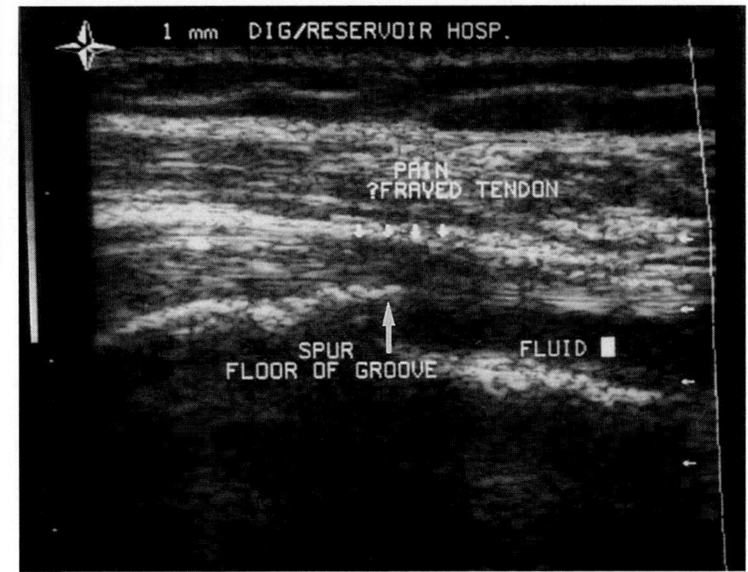

Figure 15-44 ■ Impingement by osteophyte: longitudinal sonogram. This 69-year-old man presents with a 2 month history of sharp pain localized to the bicipital groove that is worsened by forward flexion of the arm. A 5 mm bony spur arises from the floor of the bicipital groove and impinges directly on the biceps tendon (*large arrow*). There is focal loss of fibrillar pattern indicative of tendon fraying (*small arrows*) corresponding to the patient's point of maximal tenderness (*pain*); fluid (*fluid*) is noted along the floor of the bicipital groove.

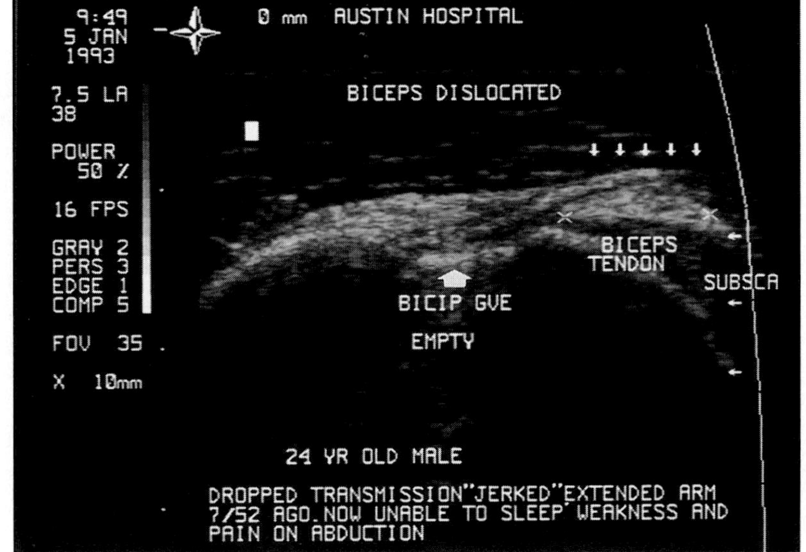

Figure 15-45 ■ Biceps dislocation: transverse sonogram. Transverse scan of the bicipital groove in a 24-year-old man presenting with anterior shoulder pain following an attempt to catch a heavy object. The bicipital groove (*BICIP GVE*) is empty (*short thick arrow*), and the biceps tendon is dislocated medially (*short arrows*) deep to the subscapularis tendon (*SUBSCA*).

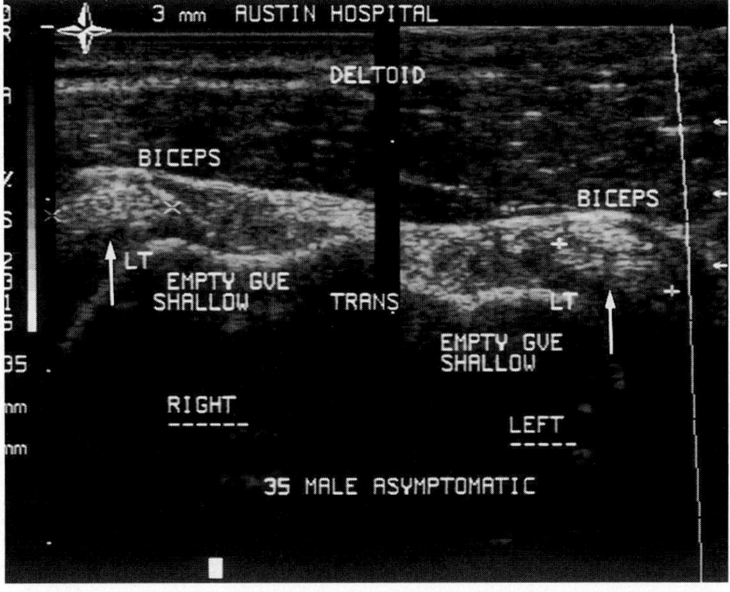

Figure 15-46 ■ Congenital dislocation of both biceps tendons: transverse sonogram. Ultrasound scan of both bicipital grooves in an asymptomatic 35-year-old man. Both grooves are symmetrically shallow and "empty" (*EMPTY GVE*). The biceps tendons are both located medially deep to the subscapularis (*arrows*).

method of detecting intermittent displacement of the biceps tendon. This was performed by placing the humerus in external rotation while observing the biceps tendon in real time in the transverse view at the level of the biceps groove. In positive cases the test can be repeated to demonstrate to-and-fro medial displacement of the tendon. *Subluxation* is defined when at least part of the biceps tendon was displaced over the lesser tuberosity at the groove level. *Dislocation* is the term used when the entire tendon lies outside the groove. If the patient has adhesive capsulitis, the dynamic test cannot be employed effectively.

Biceps tendon displacement is usually associated with a full-thickness tear of the rotator cuff. The subscapularis tendon is commonly involved, and the coracohumeral and transverse humeral ligaments are generally found to have ruptured or degenerated.

The falciform ligament of the pectoralis major can be identified. The LHB, when torn or avulsed, prolapses anteriorly out of the groove.

As the biceps tendon forms a readily recognizable landmark, most authorities have traditionally recommended that its identification mark the commencement of any ultrasound examination of the shoulder. Our experience has shown this to be a fortuitous choice, as with the aid of modern high-frequency equipment, the biceps tendon has become a window on shoulder pathology. An abnormal tendon warns of the likelihood of pathology elsewhere in the cuff. A normal tendon and overlying bursa often predict a normal examination.

Adhesive Capsulitis

Adhesive capsulits is a condition of unknown etiology that affects both sexes but shows a predilection for perimenopausal women. There may be a history of prior shoulder immobilization, but in many cases there is no obvious antecedent cause. The diagnosis is generally a clinical one based on findings made during the physical examination. However, in our experience, it is often difficult to distinguish clinically between adhesive capsulitis and an impingement syndrome in some patients. In many cases adhesive capsulitis is unquestionably present, but it masks the underlying and possibly precipitating rotator cuff tear.

The discovery of an underlying tendon tear has important prognostic implications as well as therapeutic considerations, especially if one is considering distention arthrography as a method of treatment. Adhesive capsulitis has a characteristic arthrographic appearance consisting of a generalized reduction in joint volume capacity particularly affecting the axillary and subscapular recesses. Irregularity of the capsular insertion may also be observed. Ultrasound cannot, of course, visualize the adhesions or assess the reduction in joint volume, but a diagnosis of adhesive capsulitis can be made based on a characteristic restriction in the range of movement.

Ryu et al. (1993) described the following criteria for the diagnosis of adhesive capsulitis to be applied after observing the movement of the supraspinatus tendon underneath the acromion during abduction:

1. Continuous limitation of sliding movement
2. Continuous visualization of the supraspinatus tendon during lateral elevation of the arm

An ancillary finding was a biceps tendon sheath effusion.

In our experience, external rotation seems to be the movement first and most severely affected (Fig. 15–47), followed by abduction and internal rotation, with forward flexion the least diminished movement. In rotator cuff disorders the pattern is often reversed, with forward flexion most severely affected if impingement is present, and with very little effect on the range of movement in internal and external rotation. Recent data suggest that the incidence of rotator cuff tears in patients with adhesive capsulitis is lower than the incidence of rotator cuff disease in the general population (van Holsbeeck et al., 1997).

In more severely affected cases, careful distinction needs to be made between cessation of movement in forward flexion and abduction due to impingement or cessation due to a mechanical block caused by intra-articular adhesions. In the former case the limitation is due to pain, and slight assistance to the patient by the examiner can usually complete the movement. In the case of adhesive capsulitis the range of movement at the glenohumeral joint cannot be increased by any method, and any further abduction of the arm that may be observed is usually due to scapulothoracic rotation. This "trick" movement can be detected by ultrasound, as the humerus will not move relative to the acromion on the screen.

It is our practice to offer distention arthrography to patients who we feel have adhesive capsulitis based on the above criteria (Fig. 15–48). Fluoroscopy is the method of choice for advancing a needle into the glenohumeral joint, but in adhesive capsulitis the joint capsule is contracted superiorly, anteriorly, and inferiorly. Difficulty may be encountered in injecting contrast into the joint from an anterior approach. In such cases, a technique of sonographic control of needle placement into the joint

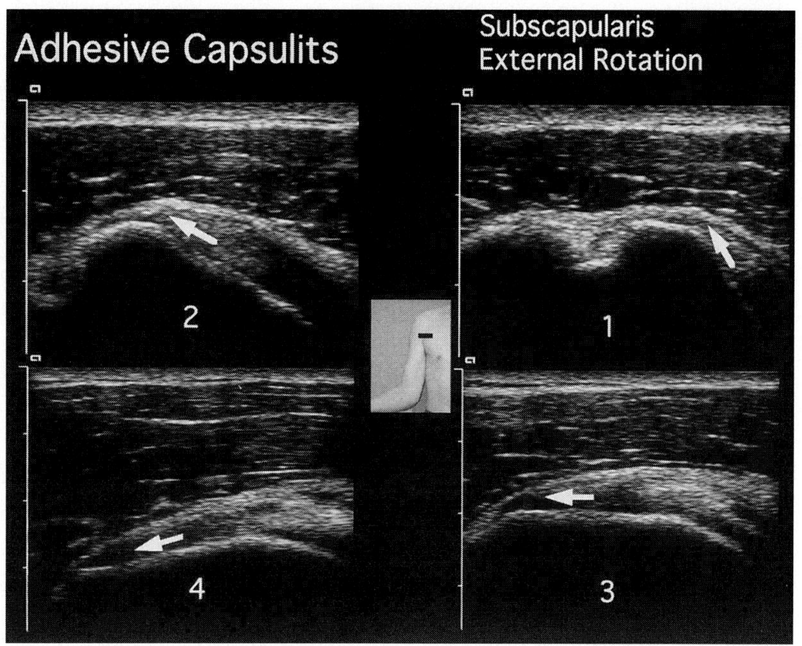

Figure 15-47 ▪ Adhesive capsulitis: dynamic ultrasound study. Assessment begins with a transverse scan of the bicipital groove in the neutral position. (*1*) In this position, the bursal surface of the subscapularis tendon forms a V with the underlying humeral cortex, the apex of the V being the tendons' insertion at the lesser tuberosity. The apex of the V on the right side points to 11 o'clock (*arrow*). In a normal patient with progressive degrees of external rotation, the apex of the V points to 10 o'clock (*2*), then 9 o'clock (*3*), and finally 7 o'clock (*4*). In patients with adhesive capsulitis, external rotation is blocked prior to attaining the 9 o'clock position; most patients with this condition fail to progress beyond 10 o'clock.

employing a posterior approach has been described (Cicak et al., 1992).

Instability

The shoulder joint, consisting of the large spherical head of the humerus articulating with the small, shallow glenoid fossa, is inherently unstable. Ligamentous and capsular restraints are considered the major passive mechanisms of joint stability. However, the role of the active dynamic stabilizers, including the supraspinatus tendon and the tendon of the LMB, is receiving increasing recognition.

The significance of the Bankart lesion in the incidence of posttraumatic shoulder instability is well

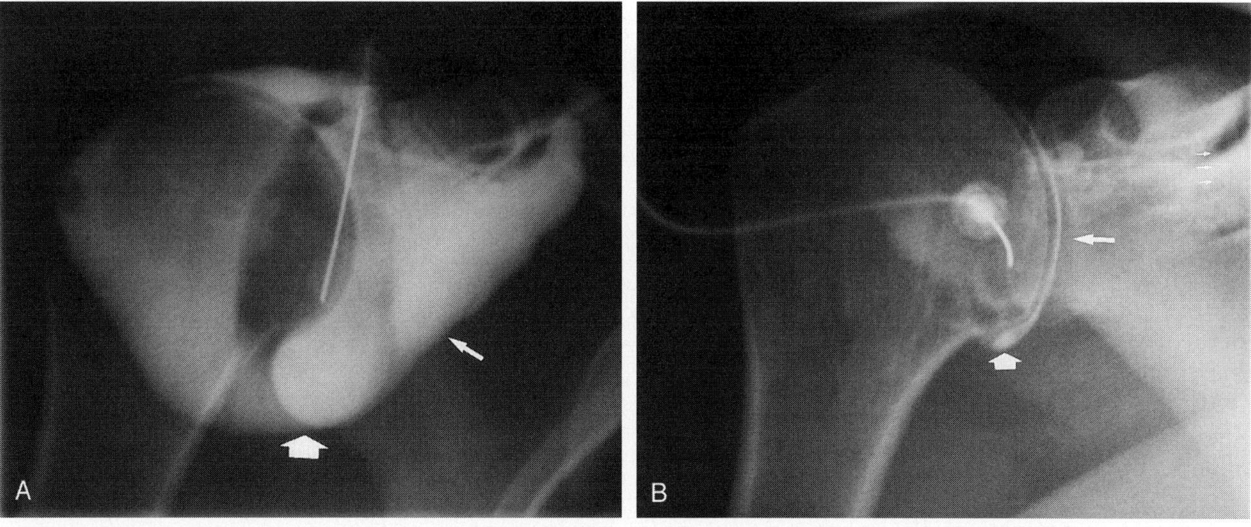

Figure 15-48 ▪ **A,** Normal shoulder: arthrography. Note the capacious axillary (*short thick arrow*) and subscapularis recesses (*short thin arrow*). **B,** Adhesive capsulitis: arthrography. A 50-year-old woman with increasing discomfort at night and with restriction in the range movement. An arthrogram was performed during hydrodilatation. Note the tightly constricted axillary recess (*short thick arrow*) and the obliterated subscapularis recess (*short thin arrow*). The capsule has ruptured following the administration of only a few milliliters of fluid (*small arrows*). The diagnosis of adhesive capsulitis had been predicted with dynamic sonography.

established, raising the possibility that disruption of the capsular mechanism also disturbs muscle coordination.

Jerosch et al. (1993) described a technique for documenting the extent of passive glenohumeral translation using ultrasound. They also demonstrated an increase in passive translation following the injection of intra-articular lidocaine, suggesting that the glenohumeral joint capsule has proprioceptive capability as part of a physiological feedback mechanism. Further work is required to establish if the normal ranges of glenohumeral translation established by this study can be used to assess the presence of glenohumeral instability in clinical patients (anteroposterior translation 6.8 ± 3.2 mm; downward translation 2.7 ± 2.1 mm). The technique is potentially less observer dependent and less clinically subjective than clinical examination (Jerosch et al., 1993).

Some instability lesions can be readily demonstrated by ultrasound examination. Small Hill-Sachs deformities, representing depressed fractures of the posterior humeral head against the anterior glenoid in an anterior dislocation, often radiographically occult, can be detected by scanning posteriorly at the level of the posterior glenoid labrum. At this level, the humeral cortical surface should be smooth and round. A Hill-Sachs deformity, as discussed previously, appears as a wedge-shaped shallow depression (Fig. 15–49). A shallower cortical erosion of the posterior humerus has been observed in posterior glenoid impingement. This impingement can lead to bone defects, partial tears of the posterior cuff, and posterior labral pathology. The disease is relatively common in baseball players.

Occasionally, fragmentation of the underlying glenoid, representing an associated Bankart lesion, may be seen by scanning anteriorly and transversely over the anterior glenoid labrum (Fig. 15–50). Tears in the anterior glenoid labrum appear as echogenic linear foci similar to those seen in disrupted knee menisci (Fig. 15–51) (Rasmussen et al., 1995). Reverse Bankart lesions causing depressed fractures of the lesser tuberosity may also be identified. Acute posterior dislocation is frequently misdiagnosed. The average interval between injury and correct diagnosis is 1 year. The subtlety of the radiographic abnormalities, which can easily be overlooked on a conventional anteroposterior view, is one of the causes of delayed diagnosis. Additional views may be difficult to obtain due to patient discomfort.

A method of evaluating posterior instability and dislocation of the shoulder using ultrasound has been described (Bianchi et al., 1994). The technique involves assessing the distance between the glenoid and the humeral head in the symptomatic shoulder and comparing it with the same parameter in the normal contralateral side. Distances greater than 20 mm indicate dislocation, whereas distances between 12 and 18 mm are more indicitative of subluxation. Either an anterior or a posterior approach may be used. The technique also involves a dynamic examination in an attempt to provoke and assess the severity of any intermittent mild subluxation. Traction on the glenohumeral joint has been used to enable an assessment of joint stability. Even though the superior glenoid labrum can be visualized from a superior approach, behind the clavicular head, we have not been able to demonstrate superior labrum anterior to posterior (SLAP) lesions.

Arthropathy

Gross irregularity of the humeral cortical surface deep to the rotator cuff indicates the presence of an arthropathy that may be degenerative or erosive. Correlation with plain films is required to complete the diagnosis. Significant thickening of the subacromial bursa associated with cortical erosions indicates the presence of either a seropositive or a seronegative arthropathy. There may be associated joint effusions or erosion at the acromioclavicular joint. Ultrasound examination can differentiate between shoulder involvement in a patient who has a known erosive arthropathy and unrelated incidental rotator cuff pathology.

Rheumatoid Arthritis

Up to 60% of rheumatoid patients have shoulder pain (Petersson, 1986). The inflamed, thickened synovium of the glenohumeral joint in rheumatoid arthritis erodes the rotator cuff, and inflammation of the acromioclavicular joint or subacromial bursa may cause impingement (Weiss et al., 1975; Watson, 1985). Conventional radiographic examination of the shoulder is generally negative in the early stages of the disease, as the erosive changes visible on X-ray examination are a relatively late finding. A rational decision on the treatment of shoulder pain in rheumatoid arthritis depends on an accurate assessment of its cause and the extent of rheumatoid involvement.

Ultrasound has been shown to reveal more precise knowledge of painful shoulder conditions than clinical examinations or radiographs and has been shown to reveal inflammatory conditions at early

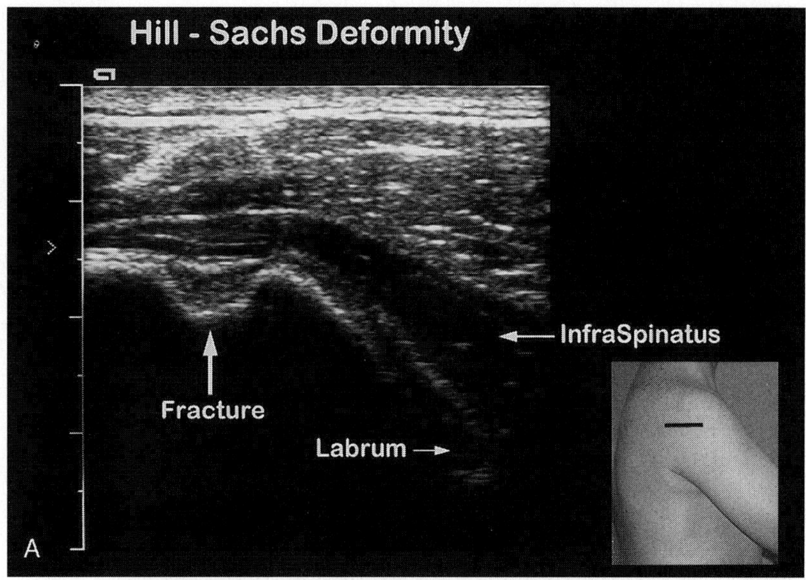

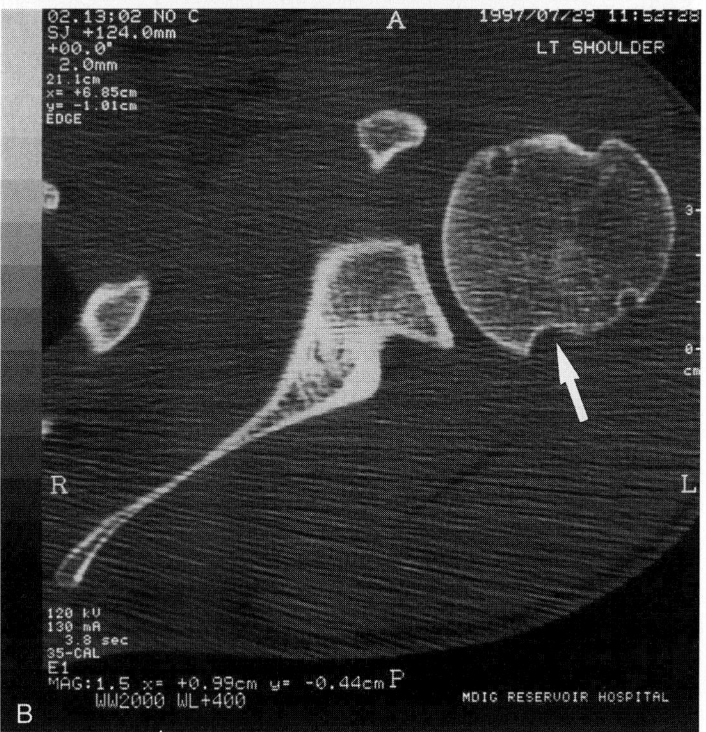

Figure 15-49 ■ **A,** Hill-Sachs deformity: transverse sonogram. This 27-year-old man has a history of recurrent anterior shoulder dislocation. View of the posterior humeral cortex at the level of the posterior glenoid labrum (*short thin arrow*). A shallow, depressed fracture is present (*long thick arrow*) deep to the infraspinatus tendon (*long thin arrow*). The posterior humeral head at this level should be perfectly round. **B,** Hill-Sachs deformity: CT scan. Same patient as in **A**. The impaction fracture of the humeral head is clearly seen (*arrow*). An associated displaced fracture of the coracoid process is present anteriorly.

stages of rheumatoid arthritis, when no radiographic changes are evident. In patients with rheumatoid arthritis and symptomatic shoulders, the most common findings are subacromial-subdeltoid bursitis (69%) and glenohumeral synovitis (57%). Other conditions that can be detected are supraspinatus tendinitis, biceps tendinitis, and, in advanced cases, hyaline cartilage thinning (Alasaarela and Alasaarela, 1994).

The accuracy of ultrasound for the detection of shoulder joint effusions has been shown to have a sensitivity of 85% when an axillary approach is used (Koski, 1991). Ultrasound is also 27% more sensitive in the detection of early erosions of the humeral head than conventional radiography (Fig. 15-52) (van Holsbeeck and Introcaso, 1990) and may be able to detect early cartilage edema.

Measurements of cartilage thickness greater than 2.5 mm are pathological. Cartilage thickness decreases in the later stages of the disease. Rheumatoid erosions may contain hypoechoic pannus. The technique also shows promise as a test to evaluate

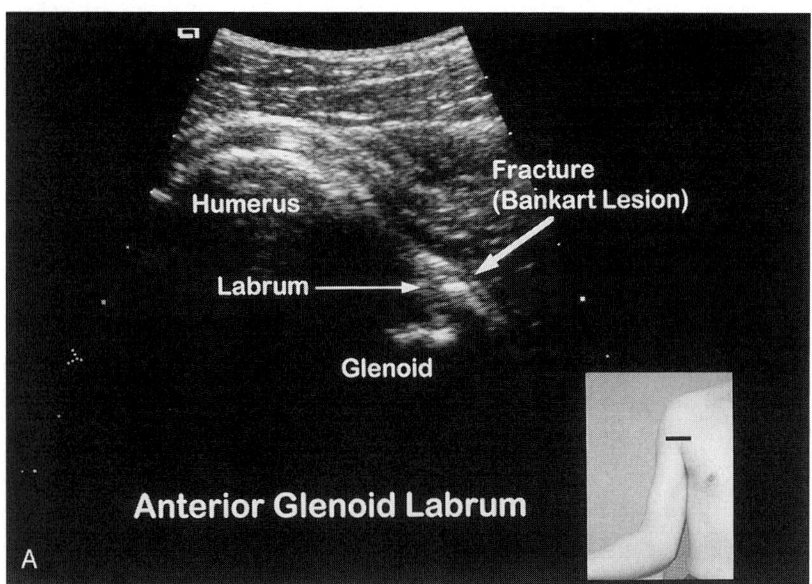

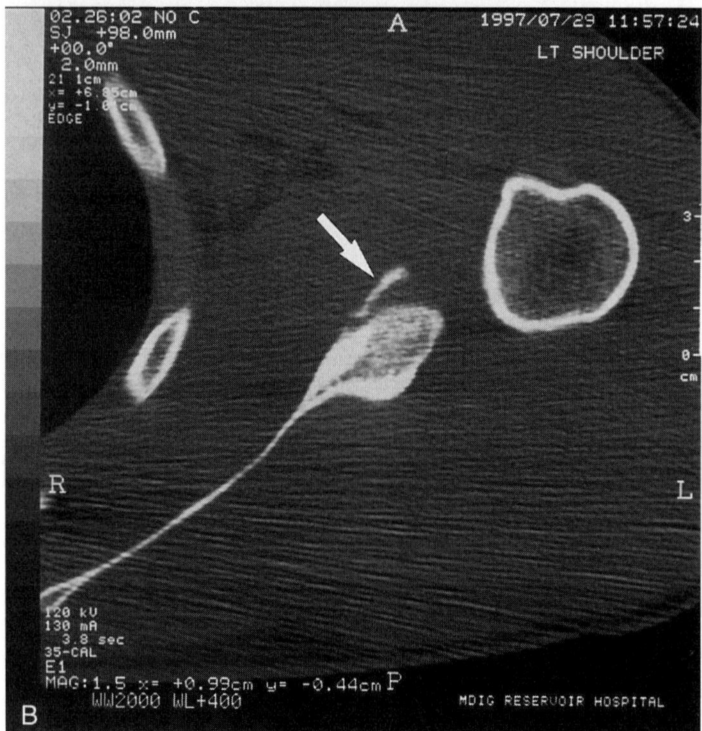

Figure 15-50 ■ **A,** Bankart lesion: transverse sonogram. Same patient as in Figure 15-49. View of the anterior glenoid labrum (*thin arrow*) obtained with the arm in external rotation. A small, detached fracture of the anterior glenoid causing weak posterior acoustic shadowing is present (*thick arrow*). **B,** Bankart lesion: CT scan. Same patient as in **A**. A CT scan confirms a detached fracture arising from the anterior glenoid (*arrow*).

the response of the active rheumatoid shoulder to therapy by demonstrating a decrease in synovial thickness. Synovial thickening is best measured by firm compression applied by the transducer (van Holsbeeck and Introcaso, 1990; Chhem, 1994).

Ultrasound is a valuable adjunct in the preoperative assessment of rotator cuff integrity in patients who have end-stage glenohumeral erosive arthropathy and require joint replacement.

Amyloid

Infiltration of the rotator cuff, subacromial bursa, capsule, and bone of the glenohumeral joint seems to be an unavoidable complication of long-term dialysis (Bardin et al., 1985; Brown et al., 1986). The amyloid protein deposited is a β_2 microglobulin, a form of amyloid specific to patients on long-term hemodialysis. After approximately 10 years of he-

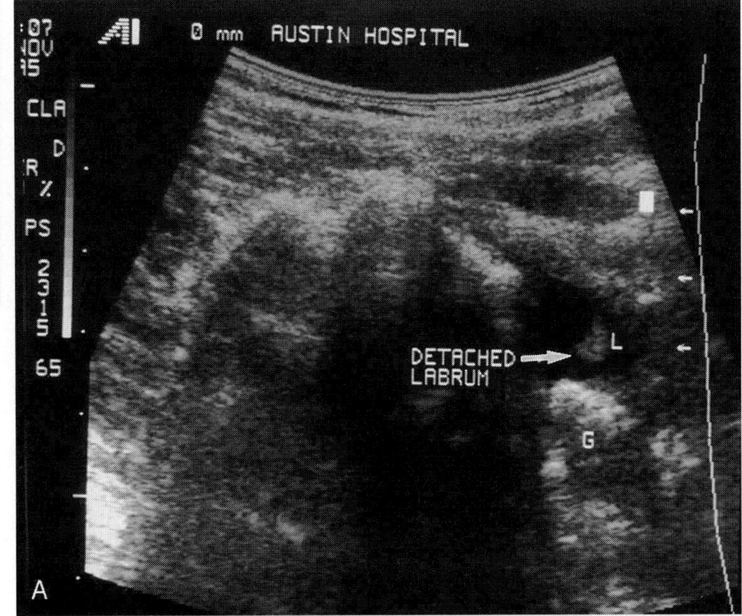

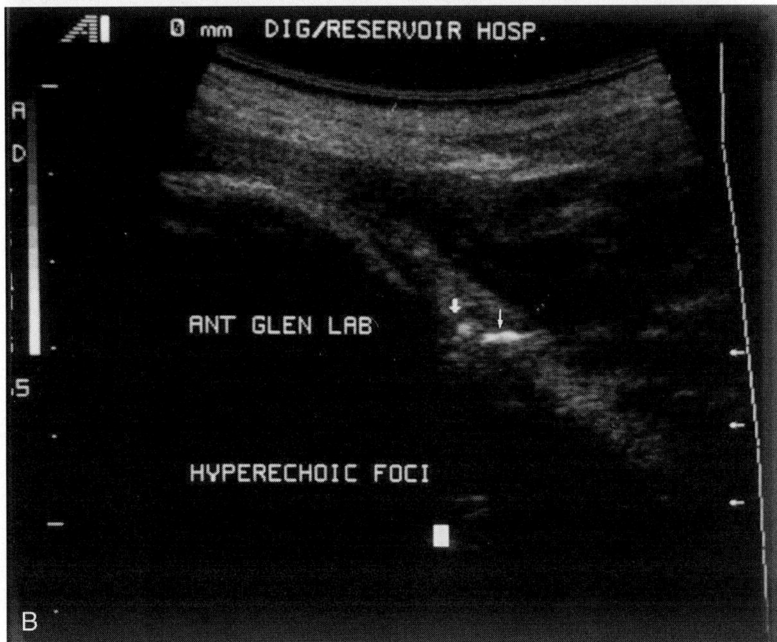

Figure 15–51 ■ **A,** Detached anterior labrum: transverse sonogram. A 23-year-old football player with a history of recurrent shoulder dislocation. The transducer is positioned over the anterior glenohumeral joint just distal to the coracoid. This view of the anterior glenoid labrum demonstrates the detached anterior glenoid labrum (*arrow, L*) surrounded by fluid and lying separate from the glenoid (*G*). **B,** Anterior glenoid labral tear: transverse sonogram. Same patient as in **A**. Small, echogenic foci are seen within the base of the triangular anterior glenoid labrum (*ANT GLEN LAB*).

modialysis, patients begin to present with a variety of complaints, most commonly shoulder pain syndrome, carpal tunnel syndrome, flexor synovitis of the hand, spondyloarthropathy, and lytic bone lesions. Shoulder pain syndrome is the most frequent complaint, occurring in up to 50% of patients on long-term dialysis (Laurent et al., 1983).

The ultrasound changes in the rotator cuff are considered highly characteristic (McMahon et al., 1991; Kay et al., 1992). The tendons of the rotator cuff, especially the LHB, the subscapularis tendon, and the supraspinatus tendon are directly infiltrated and thickened. A thickness of more than 7 mm (excluding cartilage thickness) in a dialysis patient is considered specific (Fig. 15–53) (Cardinal et al., 1996). Prior to thickening, the tendons exhibit a nonuniform parenchyma with focal areas of both increased and decreased echogenicity (Ptasznik et al., 1996).

The synovial sheath of the LHB tendon is, on average, more than 3 mm thick in affected patients. (normal thickness <1 mm). Thickening of the syn-

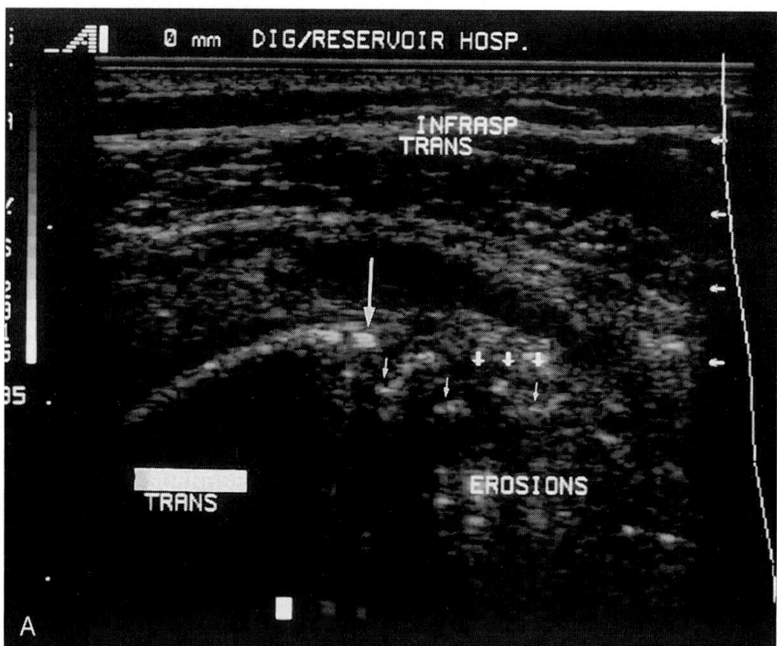

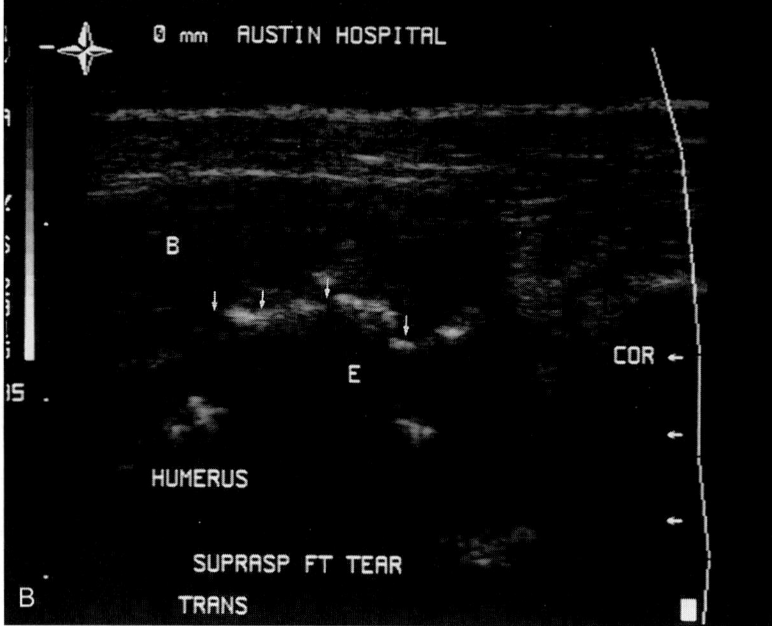

Figure 15-52 ▪ A, Inflammatory disease of the shoulder: transverse sonogram. Rheumatoid disease started about 2 years ago in this 51-year-old woman. She now begins to complain about shoulder discomfort and morning stiffness. Early rheumatoid disease involving the shoulder joint. Transverse scan of the posterior humeral head deep to the infraspinatus. There is an abrupt transition between the smooth curve of the humeral head (*large arrow*) and a shallow, irregular surface representing erosions (*small arrows*). The erosive arthropathy was not visible on the films. **B,** Inflammatory disease of the shoulder: transverse sonogram. End-stage rheumatoid disease in a 60-year-old woman with known chronic severe rheumatoid disease who has significantly reduced range of shoulder movement. The transducer over the anterior shoulder shows a massive full-thickness tear of the cuff. A grossly eroded humeral head (*small arrows*) is subluxed superiorly, lies at the level of the coracoid process, and is covered by thickened bursal tissue (*B*). Abbreviation: erosions (*E*).

ovial sheath is seen as a noncompressible, hypoechoic halo surrounding the biceps tendon (Fig. 15-54). The biceps tendon itself is not thickened in the early stages, but the fibrillary pattern appears enhanced due to the improved through-transmission of sound by the thickened sheath.

The subacromial bursa becomes grossly thickened, on average more than 8 mm, and measurements exceeding 2 cm are not uncommon (Fig. 15-55). The bursa can become distended by fluid and may contain internal septations. The thickened bursa accounts for the prominent "shoulder pads" seen in these patients clinically.

Punched-out lytic lesions of the humeral head, usually containing hypoechoic masses (amyloidomas), are common. The amyloidomas may also be intra-articular or periarticular.

Sonographic abnormalities may be detected in symptomless joints (Coari et al., 1996). As these patients present a surgical risk for even the most minor procedures, ultrasound offers an early, specific, and noninvasive method to detect the pres-

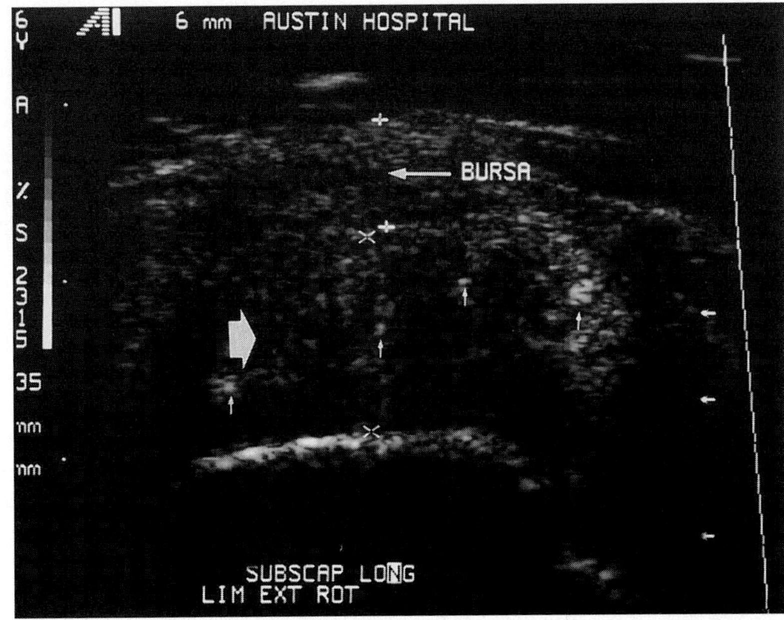

Figure 15-53 ■ Dialysis-related amyloid arthropathy: transverse sonogram. Rotator cuff from a postmortem specimen taken from a patient who had been on dialysis for 20 years and had histologically proven amyloid infiltration of the rotator cuff. The supraspinatus tendon is hypoechoic and thickened (*short thick arrow*), measuring 13 mm in thickness; the overlying bursa is also thickened (*thin arrow*) and infiltrated, measuring 5 mm in thickness. Scattered foci of increased echogenicity are present throughout the thickened tendon (*small arrows*).

ence and extent of amyloid infiltration and to monitor the efficacy of any treatment that may be employed in the future.

Anatomical Variations

Anatomical variations are occasionally encountered and may lead to false-positive findings. Apparent erosions deep to the infraspinatus tendon are not uncommon. These seem to be larger in throwing athletes. Some of these changes have been diagnosed as "bare areas" and have been considered a normal anatomical variant. Others may represent minor forms of posterior glenoid impingement. On occasion, erosions that are quite narrow and relatively deep may be seen deep to the critical zone of the supraspinatus tendon (which is intact). These erosions are usually symmetrical, with similar erosions found on the contralateral side.

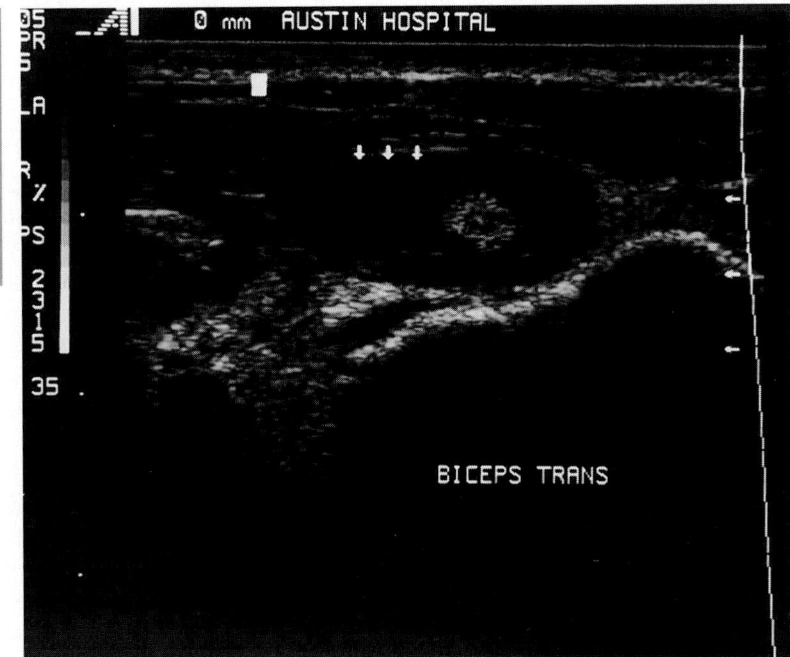

Figure 15-54 ■ Dialysis-related amyloid arthropathy: transverse scan. This hemodialysis patient reports increasing stiffness in his shoulders; he has difficulty raising his shoulders as well. The patient has been on dialysis for 12 years and is now 45 years of age. The transducer is positioned over the distal bicipital groove. Early stages of cuff infiltration. The biceps tendon is normal but is surrounded by hypoechoic, noncompressible material (*small arrows*), representing amyloid, grossly distending the biceps tendon sheath.

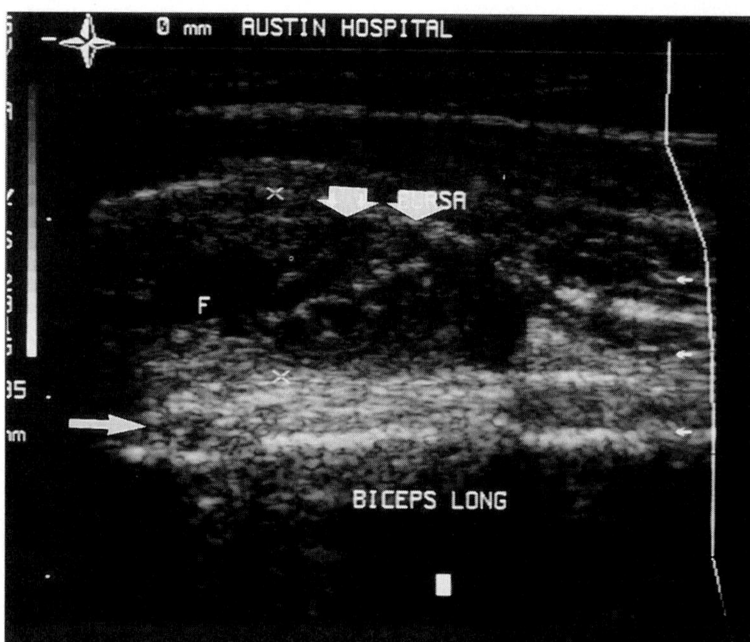

Figure 15-55 ▪ Dialysis-related amyloid arthropathy: longitudinal sonogram. A 53-year-old man with an 18-year history of hemodialysis presents with intractable shoulder pain. The transducer is aligned along the biceps tendon groove (*long arrow*). The subacromial bursa is grossly thickened (12 mm), lying superficial to the biceps tendon. Pockets of fluid (*F*) are found within the infiltrated, thickened bursa (*short thick arrows*). Abbreviation: subacromial bursa (*SA*).

Bursal thickness greater than 2 mm may often be seen in large individuals.

Reporting Method

The report should be concise, mentioning all relevant positive as well as relevant negative findings. The size of any rotator cuff tear, the number of tendons involved, the estimated age of the tear (acute or chronic), the degree of retraction, and the quality of the remaining tendon should all be described. It should be noted that there is a tendency for ultrasound to underestimate the size of large tears (Hodler et al., 1988). This may be due to the release of pressure that occurs after the surgeon incises the roof of the subacromial bursa. Associated findings such as the volume of any joint or bursal fluid, the degree of bursal thickening, the status of the biceps tendon, the humeral cortical surface, any humeral subluxation, and the type of restriction in the range of glenohumeral movement should all be described. The relevant negative findings to be mentioned depend on the presenting clinical syndromes. For example, the study may rule out instability, impingement, calcific tendinitis, and so on.

Ultrasound versus MRI

Because of its reasonable cost and good patient compliance, ultrasound should be the method of first choice in the imaging assessment of rotator cuff pathology if the study is performed by a competent sonographer (Hodler et al., 1991; Bachman et al., 1997). The sensitivity of the technique, in experienced hands using appropriate equipment, rivals that of MRI in the detection of large full-thickness tears of the rotator cuff and exceeds that of MRI in the detection of small full-thickness and partial-thickness tears. Intra-articular injection of gadolinium improves the sensitivity and specificity of MRI but adds to its cost and complexity (Zlatkin et al., 1989; Hodler et al., 1992). Ultrasound does not require intra-articular injection of contrast material and is far less expensive. Most examinations can be completed in less than 15 minutes. Ultrasound technology is freely available and readily accessible and enables comparison to the contralateral side if clinically appropriate. Patient compliance is better with ultrasound, as claustrophobia is not an issue and painful immobilization of the upper limb for long periods is not required.

The dynamic component of the examination enables assessment of the adequacy of humeral depression and detects both impingement and evidence of adhesive capsulitis. Ultrasound is more sensitive in the detection of calcium deposits within distal tendons (Hodler et al., 1991).

MRI is less operator dependent and can depict early changes in rotator cuff impingement or tendon degeneration not visible by sonography. The changes of tendinitis are nonspecific and difficult to distinguish from those of tendon degeneration, partial-thickness tears, or the magic angle phenomenon in normal patients (Gold et al., 1993). MRI should be reserved for patients in whom ultrasound is technically difficult, such as obese patients, those who are immobile, those with suspected instability lesions of the labrum or joint capsule, or those with suspected proximal subacromial impingement, i.e., deep to the acromioclavicular joint.

In practice, the exact role of each of these modalities depends on the expertise of the persons performing the examinations in any particular institution (Lawson and Middleton, 1991).

Ultrasound versus Arthrography

Ultrasound offers the following advantages over arthrography: better definition of the extent and location of a tear, detection of bursal surface and intrasubstance partial-thickness tears, no radiation, less expense, painless dynamic assessment of impingement, and examination of the contralateral side and the subacromial bursa.

Conclusion

A range of management options exist for patients with signs and symptoms referable to the rotator cuff. A spectrum of rotator cuff pathology exists, ranging from early tendon and bursal inflammation through partial-thickness tears to full-thickness tears and eventual rotator cuff arthropathy. Knowledge of the precise pathology that is present, its extent, and the quality of the remaining cuff tissue is essential for optimal management.

Ultrasound has been shown to be a rapid, low-cost, accurate technique in the detection and grading of pathology involving the tendons of the rotator cuff. A negative sonogram obtained by experienced sonologists has been correlated with a good prognosis and a short duration of symptoms.

Accurate, confident choices can be made between conservative options, arthroscopy, and limited and extensive open surgical techniques. This, in turn, enables a preoperative assessment of the patient's prognosis and, by allowing accurate presurgical planning, minimizes patient morbidity (Seitz et al., 1989; Wiener and Seitz, 1993).

Finally, despite the many uses for ultrasound in the shoulder, it should be pointed out that any complete evaluation of a shoulder complaint should include initial adequate radiographs that will often provide substantial information about bone and soft tissue pathology, on occasion making it unnecessary to pursue more advanced imaging studies (Creen and Norris, 1994).

References

Ahovuo J, Paavolainen P, Bjorkenheim JM: Ultrasonography in lesions of the rotator cuff and biceps tendon. *Acta Radiol* 30(3):253–255, 1989a.

Ahovuo J, Paavolainen P, Homstrom T: Ultrasonography of the tendons of the shoulder. *Eur J Radiol* 9:17–21, 1989b.

Alasaarela EM, Alasaarela ELI: Ultrasound evaluation of painful rheumatoid shoulders. *J Rheumatol* 21(9):1642–1648, 1994.

Bachman GF, et al: Diagnosis of rotator cuff lesions: Comparison of US and MRI on 38 joint specimens. *Eur Radiol* 7(2):192–197, 1997.

Bardin T, et al: Synovial amyloidosis in patients undergoing long term hemodialysis. *Arthritis Rheum* 28:1052–1058, 1985.

Bianchi S, et al: Sonographic evaluation of lipohemarthrosis: Clinical and in vitro study. *J Ultrasound Med* 14: 279–282, 1995.

Bianchi S, Zwass A, Abdelwahab: Sonographic evaluation of posterior instability and dislocation of the shoulder. *J Ultrasound Med* 13:389–393, 1994.

Bosworth BM: Calcium deposits in the shoulder and subacromial bursitis: A survey of 122 shoulders. *JAMA* 116:2477–2482, 1941.

Bradley M, Bhamra M, Robson MJ: Ultrasound guided aspiration of symptomatic supraspinatus calcific deposits. *Br J Radiol* 68:716–719, 1995.

Brandt TD, et al: Rotator cuff sonography: A reassessment. *Radiology* 173:323–327, 1989.

Brenneke SL, Morgan CJ: Evaluation of ultrasonography as a diagnostic technique in the assessment of rotator cuff tendon tears. *Am J Sports Med* 20(3):287–289, 1992.

Bretzke CA, et al: Ultrasonography of the rotator cuff: Normal and pathologic anatomy. *Invest Radiol* 20:311–315, 1985.

Brown EA, Arnold IR, Gower PE: Dialysis arthropathy: Complication of long term treatment with hemodialysis. *Br Med J* 292:163–166, 1986.

Burk DL, et al: Rotator cuff tears: Prospective comparison of MR imaging with arthrography, sonography and surgery. *AJR* 153:87–92, 1983.

Butters KP, Rockwood CA: Office evaluation and management of the shoulder: Impingement syndrome. *Orthop Clin North Am* 19(4):755–765, 1988.

Calvert PT, et al: Arthrography of the shoulder after operative repair at the torn rotator cuff. *J Bone Joint Surg [Br]* 68B:147–150, 1986.

Cardinal E, et al: Amyloidosis of the shoulder in patients on chronic hemodialysis: Sonographic findings. *AJR* 166:157–162, 1996.

Chhem RK: Advantages and limitations of ultrasound in the evaluation of the rheumatoid shoulder. *J Rheumatol* 21(9):1591–1592, 1994.

Cicak N, Matasovic T, Bajraktarevic T: Ultrasonic guidance of needle placement for shoulder arthrography. *J Ultrasound Med* 11(4):135–137, 1992.

Coari G, et al: Sonographic findings in haemodialysis—related chronic arthropathy. *Eur Radiol* 6(6):890–894, 1996.

Codman EA: *The Shoulder*, ed 2. Boston, Thomas Todd, 1934.

Collins RA, et al: Ultrasonography of the shoulder: Static and dynamic imaging. *Orthop Clin North Am* 18:351–360, 1987.

Crass JR, Craig EV: Noninvasive imaging of the rotator cuff. *Orthopedics* 11:57–64, 1988.

Crass JR, Craig EV, Feinberg SB: Clinical significance of sonographic findings in the abnormal but intact rotator cuff: A preliminary report. *J Clin Ultrasound* 16: 625–634, 1988.

Crass JR, Craig EV, Feinberg SB: Letter to the editor. *AJR* 147:647, 1996.

Crass JR, Craig EV, Feinberg SB: Sonography of the postoperative rotator cuff. *AJR* 146:561–564, 1986.

Crass JR, Craig EV, Feinberg SB: Ultrasonography of rotator cuff tears: A review of 500 diagnostic studies. *J Clin Ultrasound* 16:313–327, 1988.

Crass JR, Craig EV, Feinberg SM: The hyperextended internal rotation view in rotator cuff ultrasonography. *J Clin Ultrasound* 15:416–420, 1987.

Crass JR, et al: Ultrasonography of the rotator cuff: Surgical correlation. *J Clin Ultrasound* 12(8): 487–491, 1984.

DePalma AF: *Surgery of the Shoulder*, ed 2. Philadelphia, JB Lippincott Co, 1983, pp. 270–272.

DePalma AF, et al: The role of subscapularis in recurrent anterior dislocation of the shoulder. *Clin Orthop* 54:35–39, 1967.

Dondelinger RF: *Peripheral Musculoskeletal Ultrasound Atlas*, ed 2. New York, Thieme, 1995, p 65.

Dragoni S, et al: Isolated partial tear of subscapularis muscle in a competitive water skier. *J Sports Med Phys Fitness* 34(4):407–410, 1994.

Drakeford MK, et al: A comparative study of ultrasonography and arthrography in evaluation of the rotator cuff. *Clin Orthop* 253:119–122, 1990.

Farin PU: Consistency of rotator cuff calcifications. *Invest Radiol* 31(5):300–304, 1996a.

Farin PU: Sonography of the biceps tendon of the shoulder: Normal and pathologic findings. *J Clin Ultrasound* 24(6):309–316, 1996b.

Farin PU, et al: Medial displacement of the biceps brachii tendon: Evaluation with dynamic sonography during maximal external shoulder rotation. *Radiology* 195: 845–848, 1995a.

Farin PU, et al: Rotator cuff calcifications: Treatment with ultrasound guided percutaneous needle aspiration and lavage. *Skeletal Radiol* 25(6):551–554, 1996a.

Farin PU, et al: Shoulder impingement syndrome: Sonographic evaluation. *Radiology* 176:845–849, 1990.

Farin PU, et al: Shoulder impingement syndrome: Sonographic evaluation. *Radiology* 195:845–848, 1995b.

Farin PU, et al: Site and size of rotator cuff tear. Findings at ultrasound, double contrast arthrography, and computed tomography arthrography with surgical correlation. *Invest Radiol* 31(7):387–394, 1996b.

Farin PU, Jaroma H : Sonographic detection of tears of the anterior portion of the rotator cuff (subscapularis tendon tears). *J Ultrasound Med* 15(3):221–225, 1996.

Farin PU, Jaroma H: Sonographic findings of rotator cuff calcifications. *J Ultrasound Med* 14(1):7–14, 1995.

Faure G, Daculsi G: Calcified tendinitis: A review. *Ann Rheum Dis* 42(suppl):49–53, 1983.

Fisher NA, et al: Ultrasonographic evaluation of birth injury to the shoulder. *J Perinatol* 15(5):398–400, 1995.

Furtschegger A, Resch H: Value of ultrasonography in preoperative diagnosis of rotator cuff tears and postoperative follow-up. *Eur J Radiol* 8:69–75, 1988.

Gold RH, Seger LL, Yao L: Imaging shoulder impingement. *Skeletal Radiol* 22:555–561, 1993.

Goldman AB: Calcific tendinitis of the long head of the biceps brachii distal to the gleno-humeral joint: Plain film radiographic findings. *AJR* 153:1011–1016, 1989.

Green A, Norris TR: Imaging techniques for glenohumeral arthritis and glenohumeral arthroplasty. *Clin Orthop* 307:7–17, 1994.

Hall F: Ultrasonographic evaluation of the rotator cuff and biceps tendon (letter). *J Bone Joint Surg [Am]* 68(6): 950–951, 1986.

Hall FM: Sonography of the shoulder. *Radiology* 173:310, 1989.

Hammond I: Unsuspected humeral head fracture diagnosed by ultrasound (letter). *J Ultrasound Med* 10(8): 422, 1991.

Harryman DT, et al: Repairs of the rotator cuff. Correlation of functional results with integrity of the cuff. *J Bone Joint Surg [Am]* 73(7):982–989, 1991.

Hawkins R: Rotator cuff tears. Presented at the orthopaedic symposium on rotator cuff tears, Antwerp, Belgium, February 24–25, 1989.

Hayes CW, Conway WF: Calcium hydroxyapatite deposition disease. *Radiographics* 10:1031–1048, 1990.

Hodler J, et al: MRI and sonography of the shoulder. *Clin Radiol* 43:323–327, 1991.

Hodler J, et al: Rotator cuff disease: Assessment with MR arthrography versus standard MR imaging in 36 patients with arthroscopic confirmation. *Radiology* 182: 431–436, 1992.

Hodler J, et al: Rotator cuff tears: Correlation of sonographic and surgical findings. *Radiology* 169:791–794, 1988.

Hollister MS, et al: Association of sonographically detected subacromial/subdeltoid bursal effusion and intraarticular fluid with rotator cuff tear. *AJR* 165:605–608, 1995.

Jerosch J, et al: Does the glenohumeral joint have proprioceptive capability? *Knee Surgery, Sports Traumatology, Arthroscopy* 1(2):80–84, 1993.

Katthagen B-D: *Ultrasonography of the Shoulder*. New York, Thieme, 1989, pp 3–4.

Kay J, et al: Utility of high resolution ultrasound for the diagnosis of dialysis related amyloidosis. *Arthritis Rheum* 35:926–932, 1992.

Koski JM: Axilla ultrasound of the glenohumeral joint. *J Rheumatol* 16(5):664–667, 1989.

Koski JM: Validity of axillary ultrasound scanning in detecting effusion of the glenohumeral joint. *Scand J Rheumatol* 20:49–51, 1991.

Kurol M, Rahme H, Hilding S: Sonography for diagnosis of

rotator cuff tear. Comparison with observation at surgery in 58 shoulders. *Acta Orthop Scand* 62(5): 465–467, 1991.

Lanzer WL: Clinical aspects of shoulder injuries. *Radiol Clin North Am* 26(1):157–160, 1988.

Laurent G, Calemard E, Charra B: Dialysis-related amyloidosis. *Kidney Int Suppl* 33(24):32–34, 1983.

Lawson TL, Middleton WD: MRI and ultrasound evaluation of the shoulder. *Acta Orthop Belg* 57(suppl 1):62–69 1991.

Lind T, et al: Sonography in soft tissue trauma of the shoulder. *Acta Orthop Scand* 60(1):49–53, 1989.

Lombardi T, Sherman L, van Holsbeeck M: Sonographic detection of septic subdeltoid bursitis: A case report. *J Ultrasound Med* 11(4):159–160, 1992.

Mack LA, et al: Sonographic evaluation of the rotator cuff. Accuracy in patients without surgery. *Clin Orthop* 234:21–27, 1988.

Mack LA, et al: Sonography of the postoperative shoulder. *AJR* 150:1089–1093, 1988.

Mack LA, et al: US evaluation of the rotator cuff. *Radiology* 157(1):205–209, 1985.

Mack LA, Matsen FA III: Rotator cuff. *Clin Diagn Ultrasound* 30:113–135, 1995.

Matsen FA, Arntz CT, Lippitt SB: Rotator cuff. In Rockwood CA, Matsen FA III (eds): *The Shoulder*, ed. 2, vol II. Philadelphia, WB Saunders Co, 1998, pp 755–839.

McMahon LP, Radford J, Dawborn JK: Shoulder ultrasound in dialysis related amyloidosis. *Clin Nephrol* 35:227–232, 1991.

Mellerowicz H, Stelling E, Kefenbaum A: Diagnostic ultrasound in the athlete's locomotor system. *Br J Sports Med* 24(1):31–39, 1990.

Middleton WD: Status of rotator cuff sonography. *Radiology* 173:307–309, 1989.

Middleton WD: Ultrasonography of the shoulder. *Radiol Clin North Am* 30(5):927–940, 1992.

Middleton WD, et al: Ultrasonography of the rotator cuff: Technique and normal anatomy. *J Ultrasound Med* 3(12):549–551, 1984.

Middleton WD, et al: Sonographic detection of rotator cuff tears. *AJR* 144:349–353, 1985.

Middleton WD, et al: Pitfalls of rotator cuff sonography. *AJR* 146(3):555–560, 1986.

Miller CL, et al: Limited sensitivity of ultrasound for the detection of rotator cuff tears. *Skeletal Radiol* 18: 179–183, 1989.

Misamore GW, Woodward C: Evaluation of degenerative lesions of the rotator cuff. *J Bone Joint Surg [Am]* 73(5):704–706, 1991.

Moseley HF: *Shoulder Lesions*, ed 3. Baltimore, Williams & Wilkins, 1969, pp 99–118.

Nelson MC, et al: Evaluation of the painful shoulder. *J Bone Joint Surg [Am]* 73(5):707–715, 1991.

Neer CS II: Anterior acromioplasty for the chronic impingement syndrome of the shoulder. *J Bone Joint Surg [Am]* 54:41–50, 1972.

Neer CS II: *Shoulder reconstruction*. Philadelphia, WB Saunders Co, 1990, pp 427–433.

Neer CS II, Craig EV, Fukuda H: Cuff tear arthropathy. *J Bone Joint Surg [Am]* 65:1232–1244, 1983.

Newman JS, et al: Detection of soft-tissue hyperemia: Value of power Doppler sonography. *AJR* 163: 385–389, 1994.

Ozaki J, et al: Tears of the rotator cuff of the shoulder associated with pathological changes in the acromion. *J Bone Joint Surg [Am]* 70(8):1224–1230, 1988.

Paavolainen P, Ahovuo J: Ultrasonography and arthrography in the diagnosis of tears of the rotator cuff. *J Bone Joint Surg [Am]* 76A(3):335–340, 1994.

Patee GA, Snyder SJ: Sonographic evaluation of the rotator cuff: Correlation with arthroscopy. *Arthroscopy* 4(1): 15–20, 1988.

Patten RM, et al: Nondisplaced fractures of the greater tuberosity of the humerus: Sonographic detection. *Radiology* 182:201–204, 1992.

Petersson CJ: Painful shoulders in patients with rheumatoid arthritis. Prevalence, clinical and radiological features. *Scand J Rheumatol* 15:275–279, 1986.

Ptasznik R: The echogenic nidus in partial thickness tears: What is it? In Proceedings of the Royal Australian College of Radiology, annual scientific meeting, Adelaide, Australia, August 1997.

Ptasznik R, et al: Ultrasound findings in dialysis related amyloid deposition. Presented at the 96th annual meeting of the American Roentgen Ray Society, 1996. Absract in *AJR* (Suppl) 166(3):138.

Rasmussen OS, et al: Ultrasonic evaluation of the glenoid labrum: Correlation with arthroscopy. *J Ultrasound Med* 14:41, 1995.

Rathbun JB, Macnab I: The microvascular pattern of the rotator cuff. *J Bone Joint Surg [Br]* 52:540, 1970.

Ryu KN, et al: Adhesive capsulitis of the shoulder. *Medicine* 12(8):445–449, 1993.

Seitz WH, Froimson AI, Shapiro JD: Chronic impingement syndrome. The role of ultrasonography and arthroscopic anterior acromioplasty. *Orthop Rev* 18(3): 364–375, 1989.

Slatis P, Aalto K: Medial dislocation of the tendon of the long head of the biceps brachii. *Acta Orthop Scand* 50:77–80, 1979.

Steiner GM, Sprigg A: The value of ultrasound in the assessment of bone. *Br J Radiol* 65:589–593, 1992.

Stiles RG, Otte MT: Imaging of the shoulder. *Radiology* 188:603–613, 1993.

Takagishi K, et al: Ganglion causing paralysis of the suprascapular nerve. Diagnosis by MRI and ultrasonography. *Acta Orthop Scand* 62(4):391–393, 1991.

Takagishi K, et al: Ultrasonography for diagnosis of rotator cuff tear. *Skeletal Radiol* 25:221–224, 1996.

Turrin A, Capepello A: Sonographic anatomy of the supraspinatus tendon and adjacent structures. *Skeletal Radiol* 26:89–93, 1997.

Uthoff H, Sarkar K, Maynard J: Calcifying tendinitis: A new concept of its pathogenesis. *Clin Orthop* 118:164–168, 1976.

van Holsbeeck MT: Sonographic measurement of rotator cuff size. Presented at the 96th annual meeting of the American Roentgen Ray Society, 1996. Abstract in *AJR* (Suppl) 166(3):178.

van Holsbeeck MT: et al: Rotator cuff changes in cadavers

and asymptomatic adults: A vision on the future of rotator cuff imaging: Unpublished work.

van Holsbeeck MT, et al: Sonographic detection and evaluation of shoulder joint effusion. *Radiology* 177:214, 1990.

van Holsbeeck MT, et al: US depiction of partial thickness tear of the rotator cuff. *Radiology* 197:443–446, 1995.

van Holsbeeck MT, Introcaso JH: Sonography of the postoperative shoulder. *AJR* 152:202, 1989.

van Holsbeeck MT, Introcaso JH: *Musculoskeletal ultrasound.* Chicago, Mosby–Year Book, 1990, pp 231–244.

van Holsbeeck MT, Kolowich PA, Introcaso JH: Sonographic appearance of partial thickness tears of the rotator cuff (abstract). *Radiology* 185:144, 1992.

van Holsbeeck MT, Strouse PJ: Sonography of the shoulder: Evaluation of the subacromial-subdeltoid bursa. *AJR* 160:561–564, 1993.

van Holsbeeck MT, Vanderschueren G, Wohlend JR: Shoulder sonography in adhesive capulitis. Presented at the 83rd annual meeting of the Radiological Society of North America, Chicago, December 1997.

Vick CW, Bell SA: Rotator cuff tears: Diagnosis with sonography. *AJR* 154:121–123, 1990.

Watson M: Major ruptures of the rotator cuff. *J Bone Joint Surg [Br]* 67:618–624, 1985.

Weiss JJ, et al: Rotator cuff tears in rheumatoid arthritis. *Arch Intern Med* 135:521–525, 1975.

Wiener SN, Seitz WH: Sonography of the shoulder in patients with tears of the rotator cuff: Accuracy and value for selecting surgical options. *AJR* 160:103–107, 1993.

Wohlwend J, et al: Sonographic evaluation of bone changes in rotator cuff disease. Presented at the scientific session of the AJR scientific meeting, session 17, May 7, 1996. Abstract 184 in *AJR* (Suppl) 166:89.

Zlatkin MB, et al: Rotator cuff tear: Diagnostic performance of MR imaging. *Radiology* 172:223–229, 1989.

Chapter 16
Sonography of the Elbow, Wrist, and Hand

Clinical examination of the elbow, wrist, and hand is much easier than examination of the shoulder. These joints are much more accessible due to their superficial nature. The majority of injuries in these regions involve bone and are therefore usually well evaluated with conventional radiographs. However, ultrasound is valuable in the diagnosis of muscle, tendon, and ligament pathology in these regions. In selected cases, ultrasound may even be helpful in the diagnosis and staging of cartilage injury. When the radiographic examination is normal, ultrasound is indicated to evaluate persistent pain and swelling.

The Elbow

Indications for Scanning

The most common type of soft tissue pathology of the elbow is epicondylitis (Figs. 16–1 and 16–2). Tendinitis of the proximal radial extensors (tennis elbow) and proximal ulnar flexors (golfer's elbow) are often confused with joint pathology due to their close proximity. Lateral epicondylitis is encountered more frequently. Biceps and triceps tendinitis may also be mistaken for joint pathology. These entities are clearly best evaluated with ultrasound because calcifications are seen only in advanced disease (Fig. 16–3). At the same time, the examiner can evaluate for evidence of intra-articular pathology.

Joint effusion, although nonspecific, is a clear indicator of joint pathology (Figs. 16–4 through 16–8). The most frequently observed joint pathology in the absence of radiographic findings is cartilaginous loose bodies (Frankel, 1998). Often these loose bodies are found in the anterior, posterior, or annular joint recesses (Figs. 16–9 through 16–14). In young patients, they are often caused by cartilage shedding at the site of an osteochondral or chondral injury involving the capitellum humeri. The osteochondral type of these lesions has long been known as *Panner's lesion*. Valgus alignment of the elbow puts the patient at increased risk. Panner's disease is common in baseball pitchers, and it is included in the differential diagnosis of "Little League elbow." The mechanism of injury is a valgus force on the elbow causing rupture of the ulnar collateral ligament or avulsion of the medial epicondylar apophysis. Abnormal widening of the joint space at the medial aspect is accompanied by narrowing of the lateral joint spaces. In cases of acute injury, lateral impaction on the capitellum in valgus alignment results in failure of the subchondral bone of the distal humerus (Fig. 16–15). The overlying cartilage may be cracked along the edges of the subchondral fracture. If the cartilage fails, the osteochondral fragment will loosen and may float freely in the synovial fluid. Cartilage derives its nutrition from surrounding joint fluid. Therefore, the free cartilage fragment may grow into a larger loose body within the joint. This growth explains why most loose bodies do not fit their original donor site. Examination using transducer frequencies of 10 MHz and above reveals the hyaline nature of some of these loose bodies. Hyaline cartilage can be observed at the periphery of the calcified matrix (see Fig. 16–13). A hyperechoic segment is typically identified in association with the hyaline cartilage. This corresponds to the portion which has calcified or the fragment of avulsed subchondral bone. The region surrounding this linear echogenic structure appears hypoechoic, corresponding to hyaline cartilage from the articular donor site.

Text continued on page 521

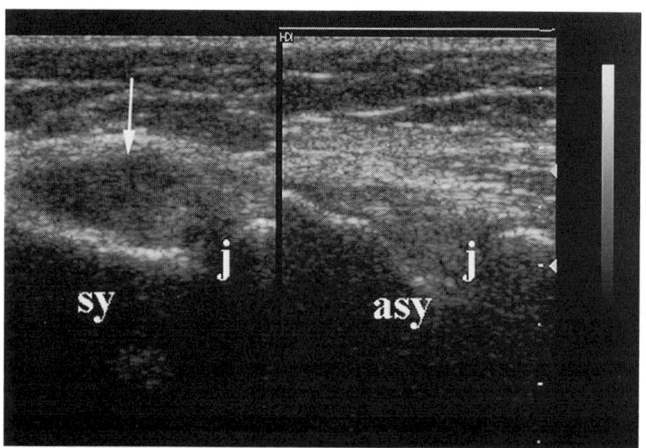

Figure 16–1 ■ Lateral epicondylitis: coronal sonogram. A 37-year-old male window washer presented with a 3-month history of right elbow pain. Point tenderness was detected with the transducer over the lateral epicondyle. This split-screen image demonstrates the symptomatic (*sy*) right lateral extensor tendons immediately proximal to the joint space (*j*). The tendon origin is thickened and hypoechoic (*arrow*) relative to the normal asymptomatic side (*asy*).

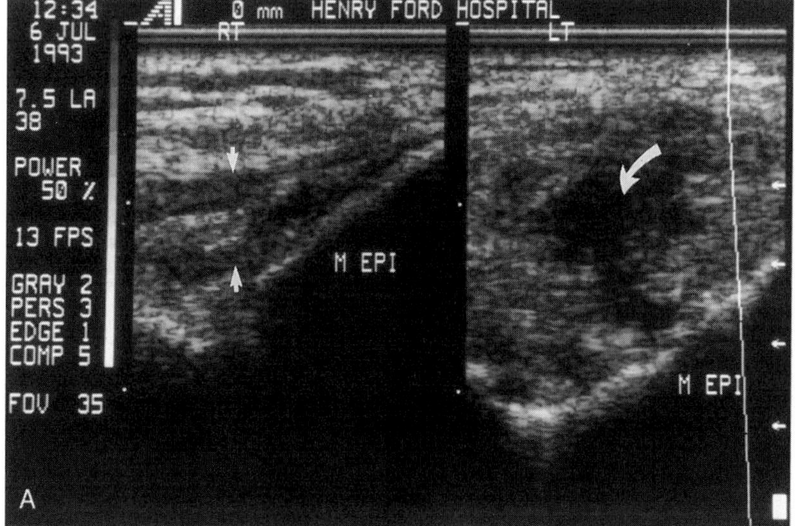

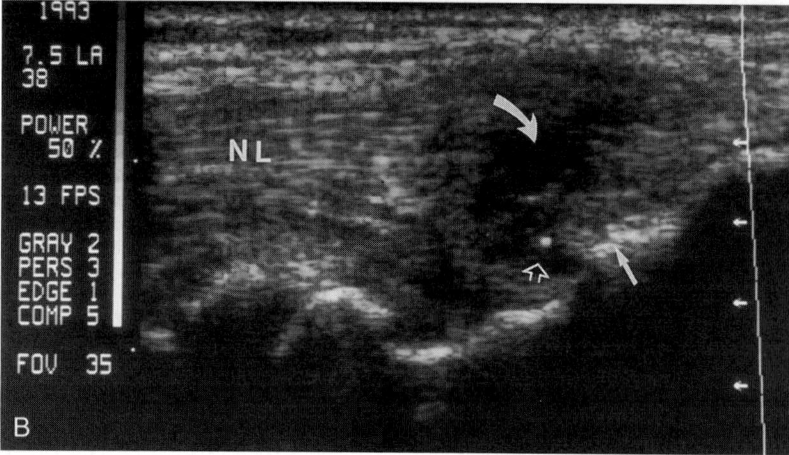

Figure 16–2 ■ **A**, Medial epicondylitis: coronal sonogram. This 28-year-old professional baseball player complained of pain in the medial left elbow for 2 weeks. The clinical diagnosis was a torn ulnar collateral ligament. However, this split-screen coronal sonogram demonstrates discontinuity and swelling (*curved arrow*) of the left flexor tendon origin displayed on the right. The normal right flexor tendon origin (*small arrows*) is shown on the left. Note that the proximal aspect of the joint is at the right of each image. **B**, Medial epicondylitis: coronal sonogram, magnified view. Same patient as in **A**. The classic appearance of epicondylitis consists of a partial-thickness tear (*curved arrow*) in the tendon origin, which in chronic cases is associated with calcification (*open arrow*) and epicondylar bone spurs (*straight arrow*). Note the contrast between the normal portion of the tendon (*NL*) on the left side of the image and the focal abnormality in the tendon origin on the right. In this case, the partial-thickness tear of the tendon is slightly more extensive than is usually seen.

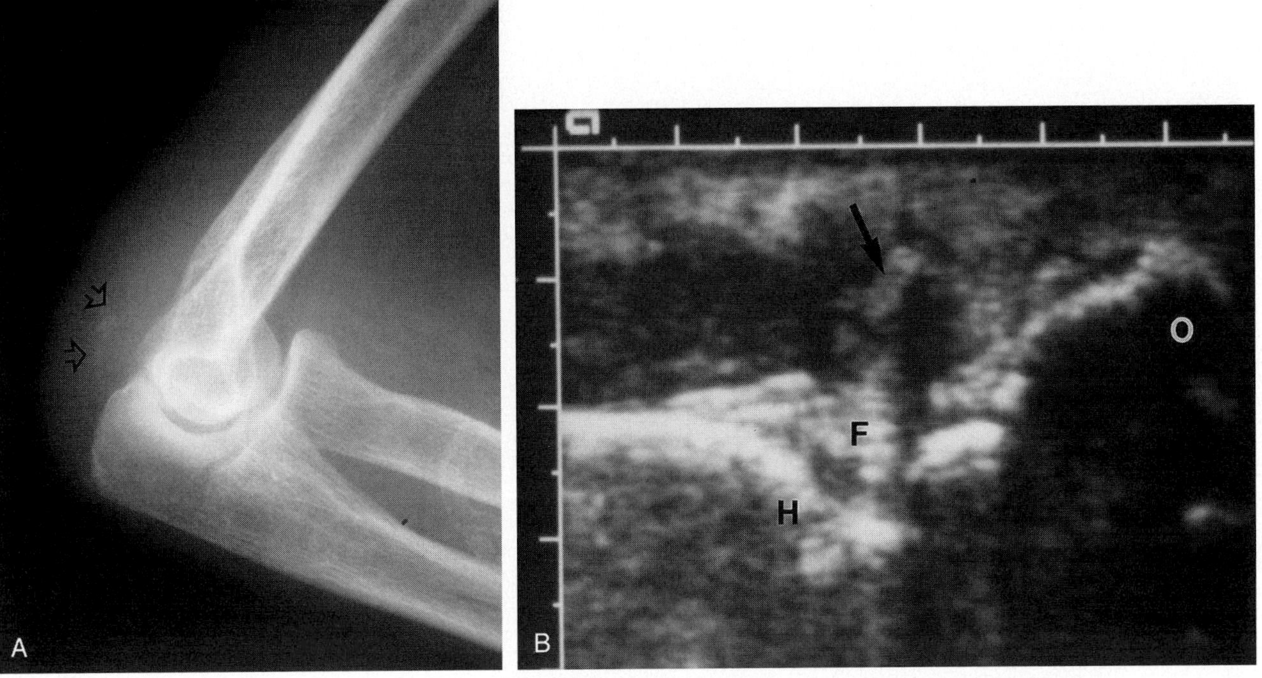

Figure 16–3 ■ **A**, Calcific tendinitis: conventional radiograph, lateral projection. Sudden onset of focal posterior elbow pain prompted this 69-year-old dialysis patient to seek treatment. Soft tissue swelling and calcification (*open arrows*) are seen in the region posterior to the elbow joint. The differential diagnosis includes avulsion of the triceps tendon, intra-articular loose bodies, and bursal or tendinous calcification. **B**, Calcific tendinitis: sagittal sonogram. Same patient as in **A**. This sagittal sonogram in the region of the triceps tendon insertion onto the olecranon (*O*) demonstrates that the calcification (*arrow*) lies within the tendon. The normal posterior fat pad (*F*) is partially obscured by the acoustic shadow of the calcification. Abbreviation: distal humerus (*H*).

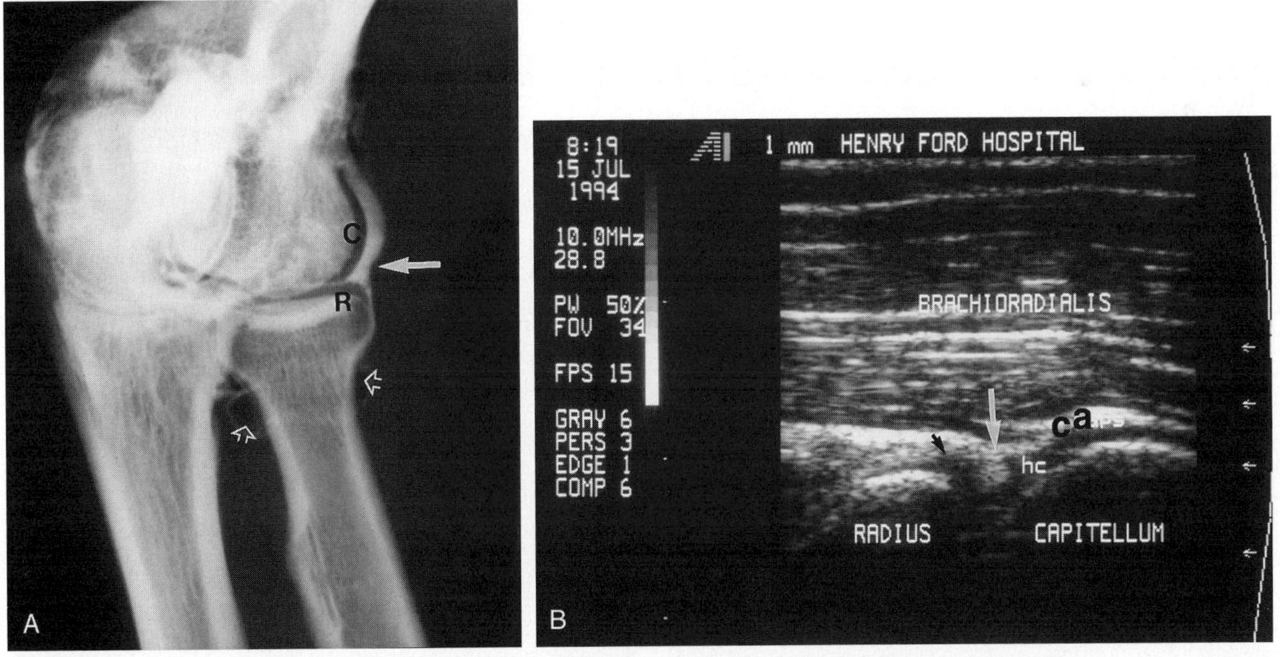

Figure 16–4 ■ **A**, Normal elbow: arthrogram. This 25-year-old male tennis player presented with diffuse elbow pain. Note the smooth contours of the radiolucent cartilage of the capitellum (*C*) and the radial head (*R*), as well as the contour of the joint capsule paralleling the cartilage surface. A capsular fold (*white arrow*) is present at the level of the joint space. Also note the annular recess of the joint (*open arrows*) surrounding the radial head. **B**, Normal elbow: sagittal sonogram. Same patient as in **A**. Well-defined contours of the hyaline cartilage covering the radial head (*small black arrow*) and capitellum (*hc*) are demonstrated. The echogenic joint capsule (*ca*) tightly approximates the cartilage surfaces, folding in at the level of the joint space (*white arrow*).

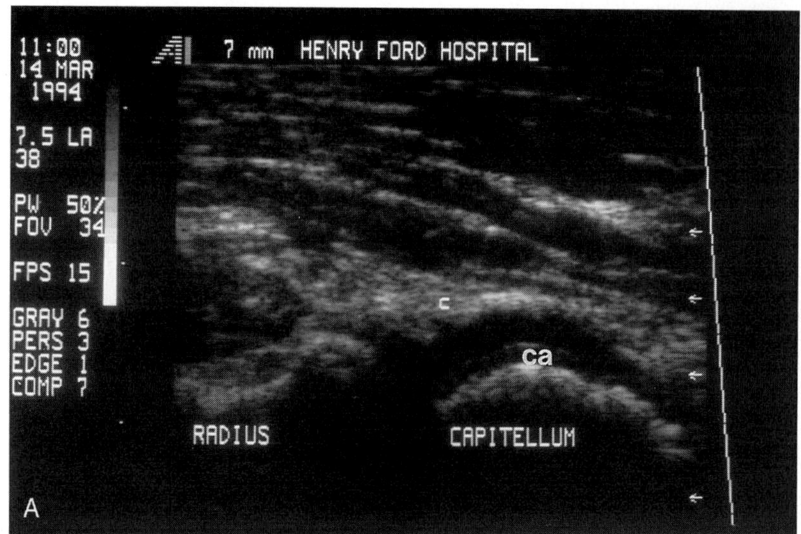

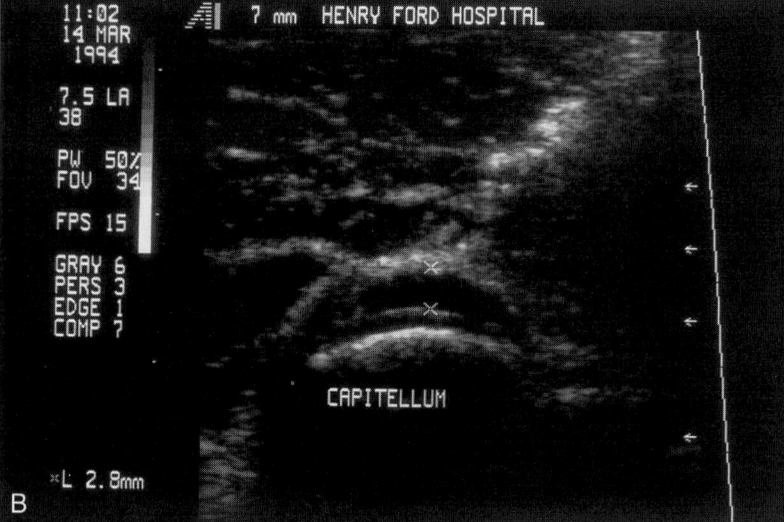

Figure 16–5 ■ **A**, Elbow effusion: longitudinal sonogram. A 42-year-old female presented with pain in her right elbow after a fall. This longitudinal image demonstrates elevation of the joint capsule (*c*) off of the articular cartilage (*ca*) by an anechoic fluid collection. Note the sharply defined interface at the surface of the cartilage. **B**, Elbow effusion: transverse sonogram. Same patient as in **A**. Again, the surface of the articular cartilage of the capitellum is clearly demonstrated by a sharp hyperechoic line much thinner than the joint capsule. Anechoic fluid separates the two structures (×–×).

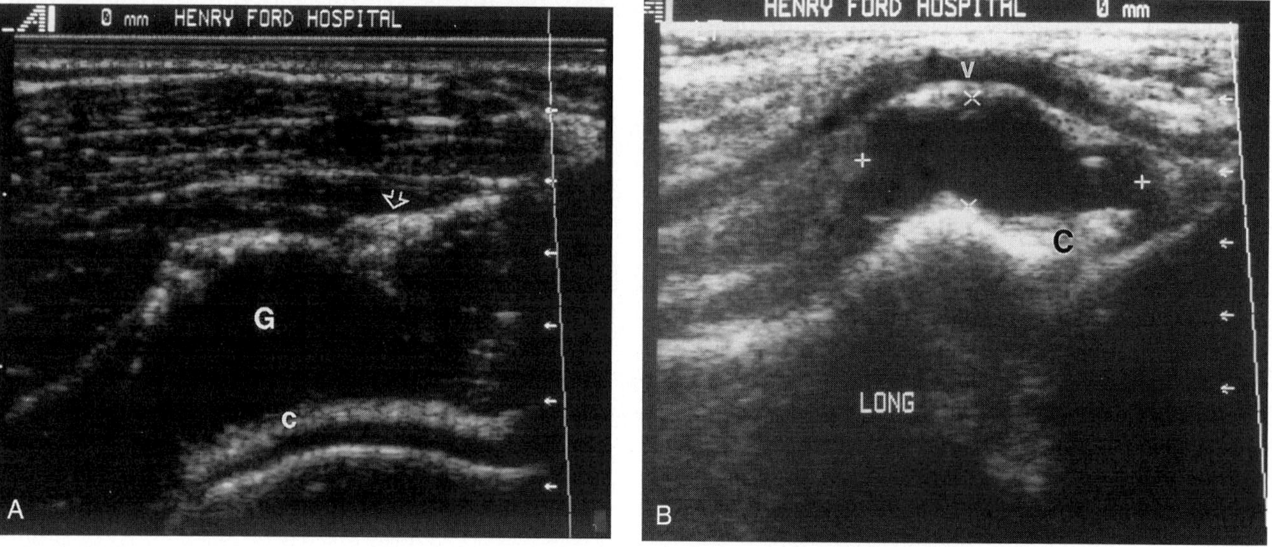

Figure 16–6 ■ **A**, Periarticular ganglion: transverse sonogram. This 30-year-old female complained of pain and tingling in the left radial nerve distribution. The echogenic joint capsule (*c*) is closely opposed to the articular cartilage of the capitellum. A fluid collection superficial to the joint capsule is identified. Aspiration of this collection yielded gelatinous fluid found in a ganglion (*G*). Radial nerve (*arrow*). **B**, Periarticular ganglion: longitudinal sonogram. Same patient as in **A**. This image confirms the extracapsular location of the fluid collection. Note the vessel (*v*) draped over the ganglion. Abbreviation: joint capsule (*C*).

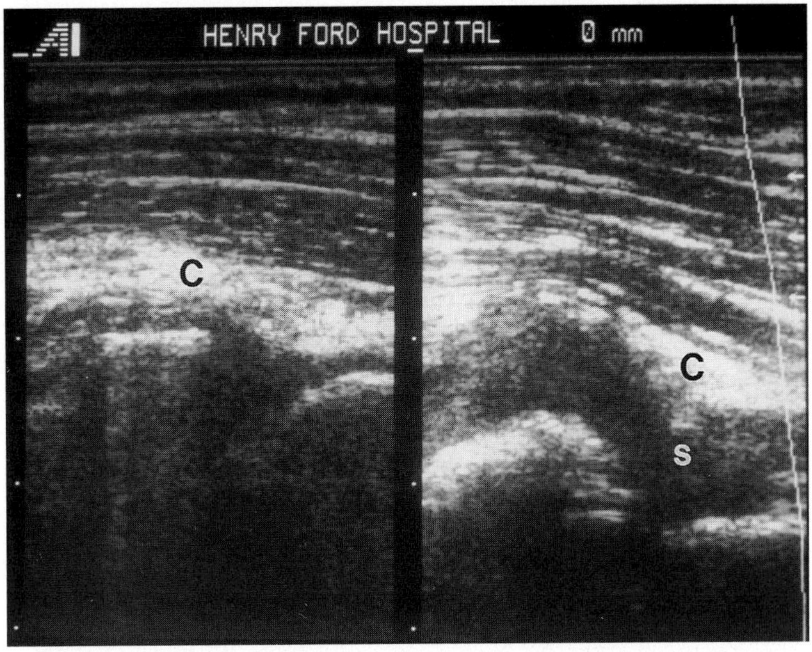

Figure 16–7 ■ Rheumatoid arthritis and synovitis of the elbow: longitudinal sonogram, split screen. A 52-year-old female presented with chronic right elbow pain. The image on the left is the asymptomatic left elbow imaged over the anterior lateral aspect. Note that the joint capsule (*C*) is closely apposed to the joint surfaces. On the symptomatic side, there is a moderate amount of hypoechoic soft tissue (*s*) separating the joint capsule from the bone surface. This tissue was not compressible when pressure was applied with the transducer. This finding suggested synovial edema or pannus rather than fluid.

It is possible to diagnose associated ulnar collateral ligament tears as well (Fig. 16–16). A normal collateral ligament connects the distal humerus to the ulna and can be found deep to the flexor origin. It is identified as a layered structure. The injuries we have found are more common at the origin, over a narrow groove in the humerus located distal, slightly posterior, and deep to the medial epicondyle.

Major nerve branches pass adjacent to the elbow joint. It is important to become familiar with the location of these nerves. This knowledge of anatomy is helpful when ultrasound is utilized to perform small interventions in the region of the elbow. Interventional procedures should be planned with a safe margin from neurovascular bundles. Ultrasound-guided invasive procedures are very safe because an instantaneous road map can be drawn to avoid nerves and arteries. Power Doppler is very useful in this regard. For examiners who are less familiar with the regional anatomy, it is easy to remember that major nerve branches are often accompanied by arteries.

Nerves have a characteristic appearance on ultrasound (Silvestri, 1995). Small, echogenic dots are noted within larger nerves on transverse images (Fig. 16–17). A fascicular pattern is noted on longitudinal views. Hypoechoic bundles contrast with hyperechoic interfaces. Anatomical detail improves significantly when transducer frequencies above 10 MHz are used. In scanning nerves, one should be aware that the echogenicity of an anatomical structure depends on the attenuation of the ultrasound beam by surrounding tissues. The echogenicity of a nerve imaged in muscle is very different from its echogenicity when imaged in the vicinity of joints (Fig. 16–18).

Trauma plays a major role in the pathology of nerves in the elbow (Fig. 16–19). The ulnar nerve seems particularly vulnerable, possibly because of its superficial location in a narrow bone tunnel. Injury to ligamentous structures in the elbow allows the ulnar nerve to sublux or even dislocate. Anterior and medial subluxation of the ulnar nerve relative to the medial epicondyle has been observed. Elbow flexion seems to accentuate the abnormality (Fig. 16–20). Surgical procedures to reroute the ulnar nerve have been tried.

Peripheral nerve tumors along the course of a nerve are easily detected. Nerve tumors may be fusiform, oval-shaped, or round and are often hypervascular. Neurofibromas and schwannomas are usually hypoechoic. Schwannomas may be cystic or may contain multiple small cystic spaces (Fig. 16–21). Ultrasound's higher spatial resolution is better than that of MRI in demonstrating this characteristic internal structure, which can be pathognomonic for schwannoma (neurilemmoma). It

Text continued on page 524

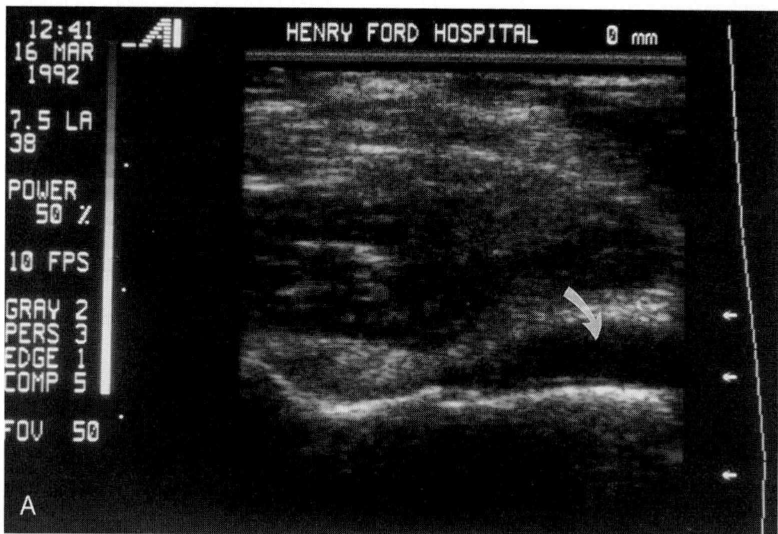

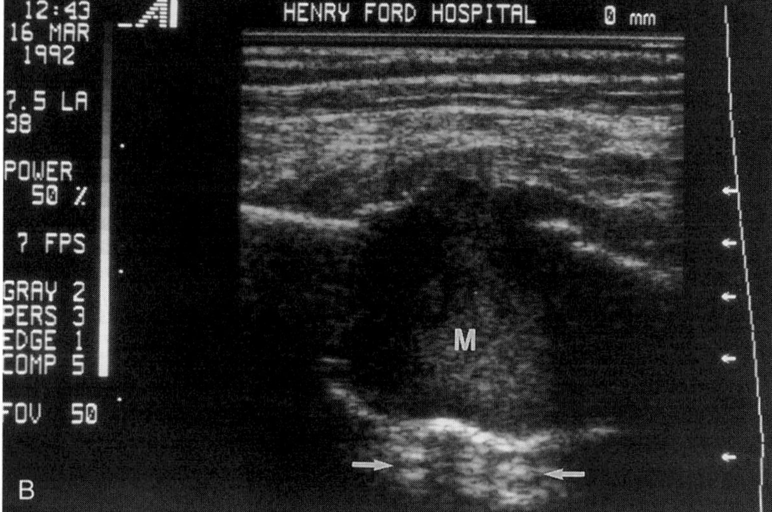

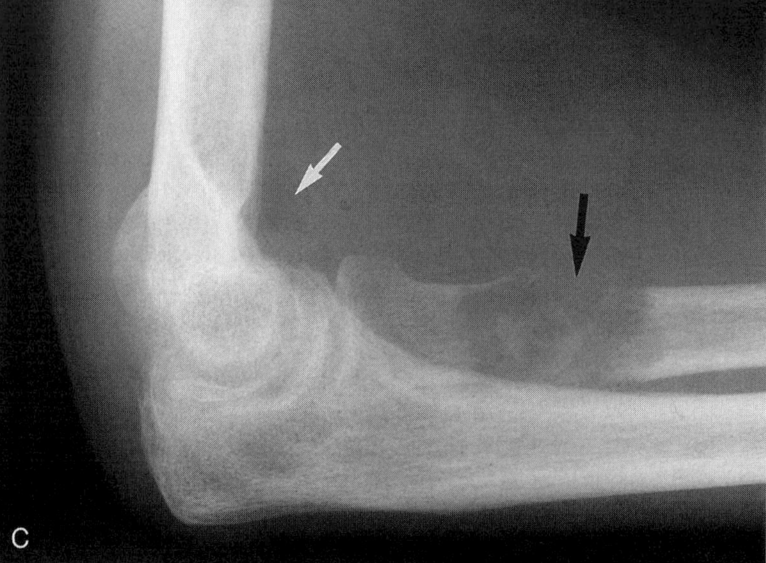

Figure 16-8 ■ **A**, Reactive elbow joint effusion: transverse sonogram. An otherwise asymptomatic 62-year-old male presented with right elbow pain of recent onset. This transverse image of the right elbow demonstrates a layer of anechoic fluid (*curved arrow*) elevating the joint capsule off of the capitellum. **B**, Reactive elbow joint effusion: longitudinal sonogram. Same patient as in **A**. The proximal portion of the radius was examined, as shown in this longitudinal image. A region of cortical destruction with a hypoechoic soft tissue mass (*M*) was identified. Increased through-transmission (*arrows*) is seen deep to the mass. **C**, Reactive elbow joint effusion: conventional radiograph. Same patient as in **A**. The destructive lesion (*black arrow*) involving the proximal radius is confirmed on this ra-diograph. A positive anterior fat pad sign (*white arrow*) is noted, consistent with the joint effusion demonstrated by the ultrasound examination. Surgical biopsy revealed plasmocytoma. Joint effusions may result from both intra-articular and periarticular pathology. A conventional radiographic examination should always precede the ultrasound examination.

Figure 16–9 ■ **A**, Intra-articular loose bodies: longitudinal sonogram, supinated forearm. A 52-year-old tennis player presented with decreased range of motion and loss of strength in the right elbow. Fluid (*f*) is identified in the anterior joint recesses and the annular recess (*curved arrow*). **B**, Intra-articular loose bodies: longitudinal sonogram, pronated forearm. Same patient as in **A**. A large loose body (*arrows*) migrated into the annular recess when the patient moved the forearm into pronation. It is common for loose bodies in the elbow to move in and out of the field of view when the patient changes from pronation to supination during the ultrasound examination.

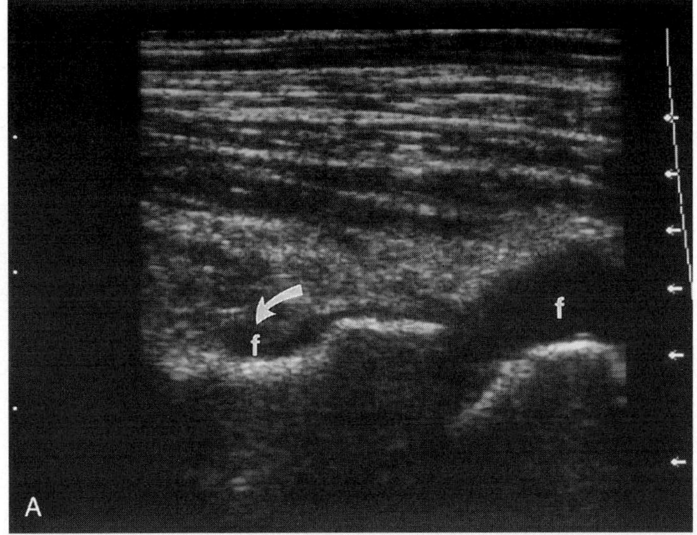

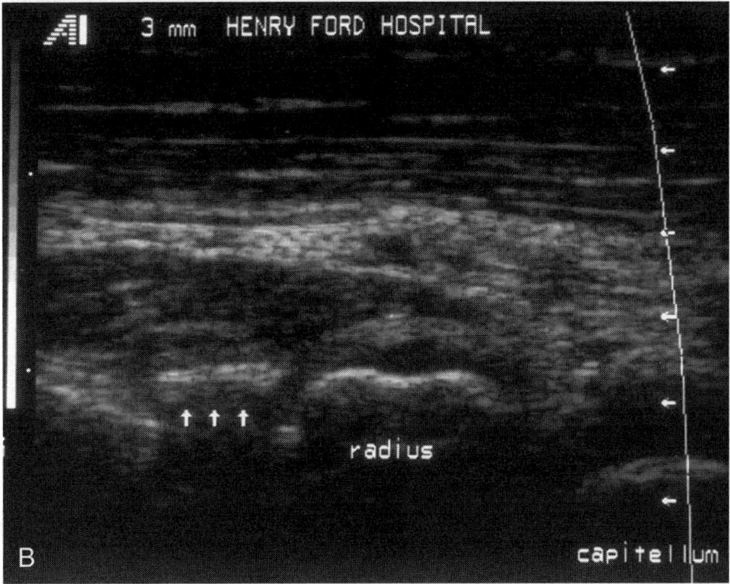

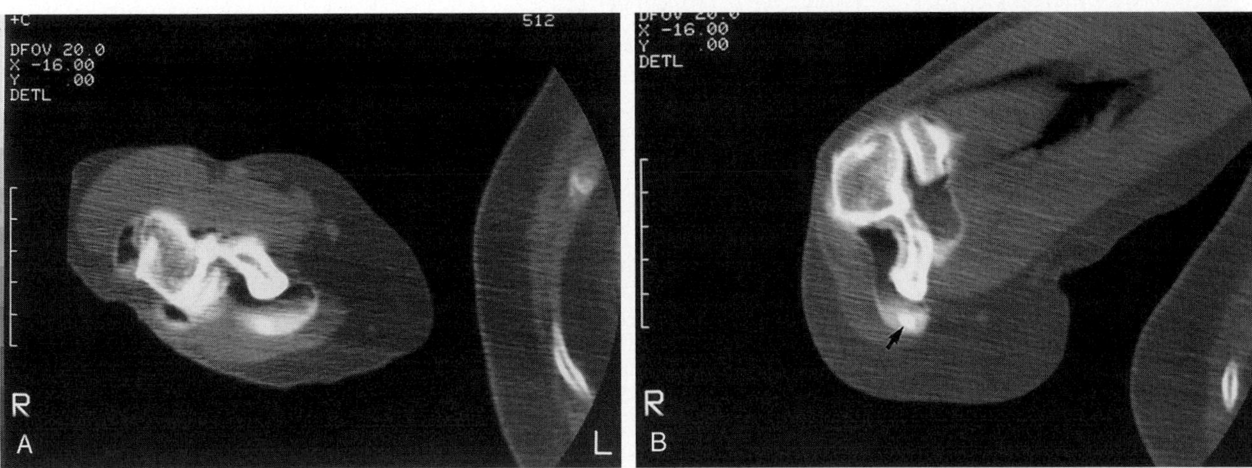

Figure 16–10 ■ **A**, Mobility of intra-articular loose bodies: CT arthrography of the forearm in supination. A double-contrast CT arthrogram performed in this patient with chronic elbow pain demonstrates a dilated medial recess but no loose body. **B**, Mobility of intra-articular loose bodies: CT arthrography of the forearm in supination. Same patient as in **A**. However, when the patient was rescanned with the forearm pronated and placed over the abdomen, a loose body (*arrow*) was identified in the medial recess. Due to greater imaging contrast, ultrasound is the preferred imaging modality for the identification of loose bodies in the elbow.

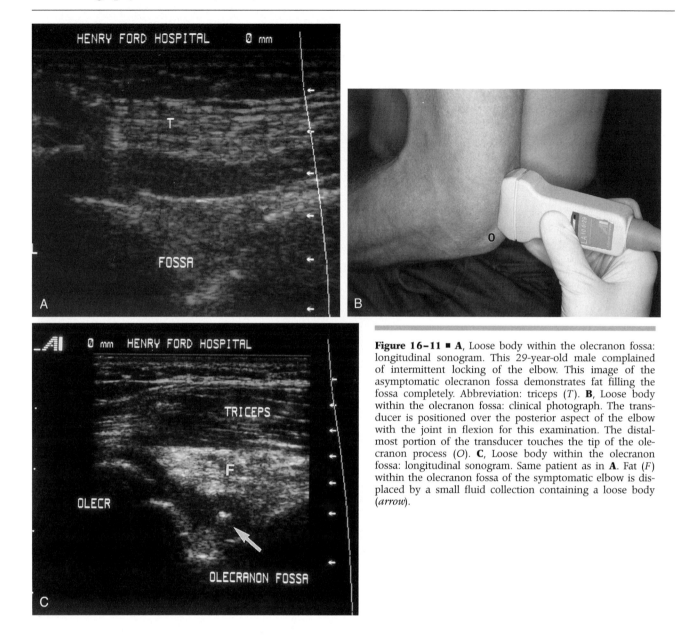

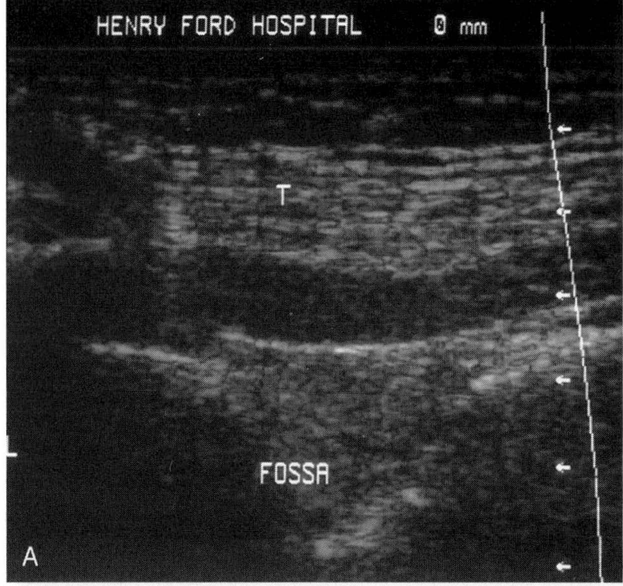

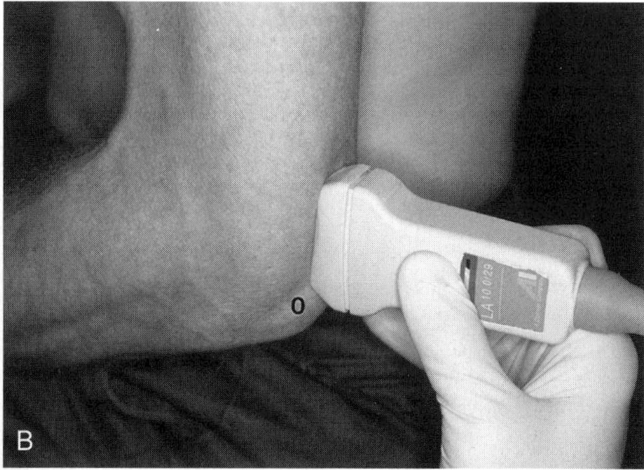

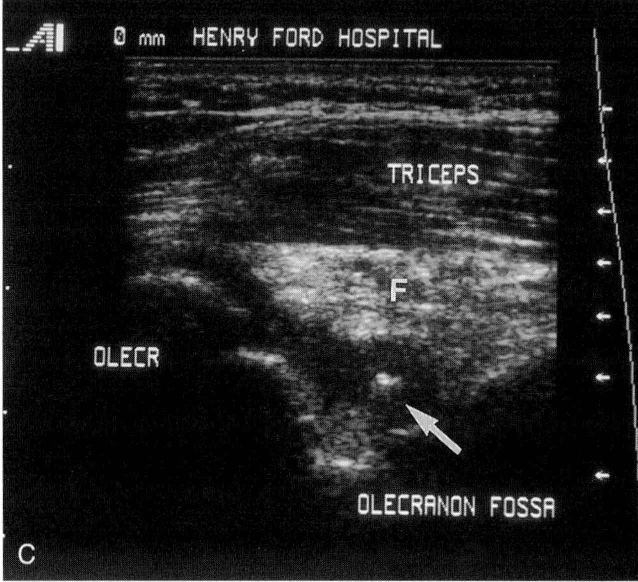

Figure 16–11 ■ **A**, Loose body within the olecranon fossa: longitudinal sonogram. This 29-year-old male complained of intermittent locking of the elbow. This image of the asymptomatic olecranon fossa demonstrates fat filling the fossa completely. Abbreviation: triceps (*T*). **B**, Loose body within the olecranon fossa: clinical photograph. The transducer is positioned over the posterior aspect of the elbow with the joint in flexion for this examination. The distal-most portion of the transducer touches the tip of the olecranon process (*O*). **C**, Loose body within the olecranon fossa: longitudinal sonogram. Same patient as in **A**. Fat (*F*) within the olecranon fossa of the symptomatic elbow is displaced by a small fluid collection containing a loose body (*arrow*).

is possible to identify a tumor as a nerve tumor by demonstrating continuity of the lesion with the nerve. We have observed the junction between the tumor and the normal nerve to appear like a "rat tail" in schwannomas, whereas neurofibromas are more fusiform. Characteristically in schwannomas, one can identify the normal nerve bundles along the tumor eccentrically (Fig. 16–22). In contrast, neurofibromas appear centrally entwined within the nerve structure (Box 16–1). These are anecdotal observations. Further prospective studies will be required to document the diagnostic reliability of ultrasound in distinguishing schwannomas from neurofibromas. This differential diagnosis seems useful, as schwannomas can be removed by simple

Box 16–1
Differential Characteristics

Schwannoma and Neurilemmoma

- Sometimes cystic or multicystic
- Normal nerve found along the lesion (rat tail)
- Surgery easy

Neurofibroma

- Intertwined with nerve
- Surgery more complicated

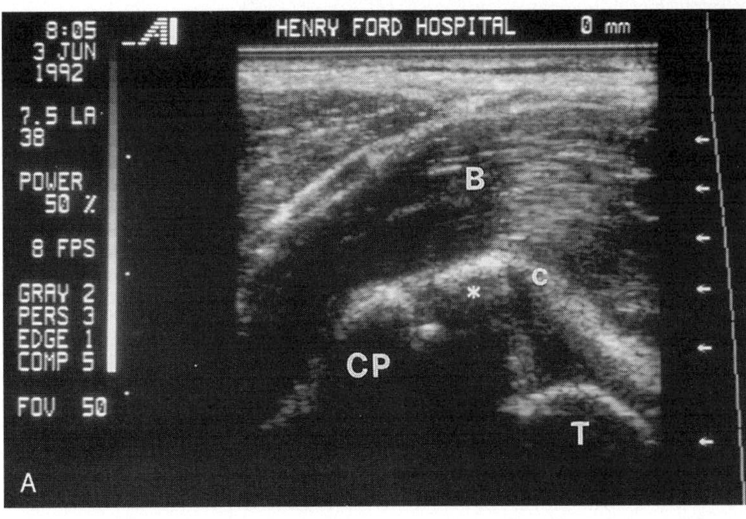

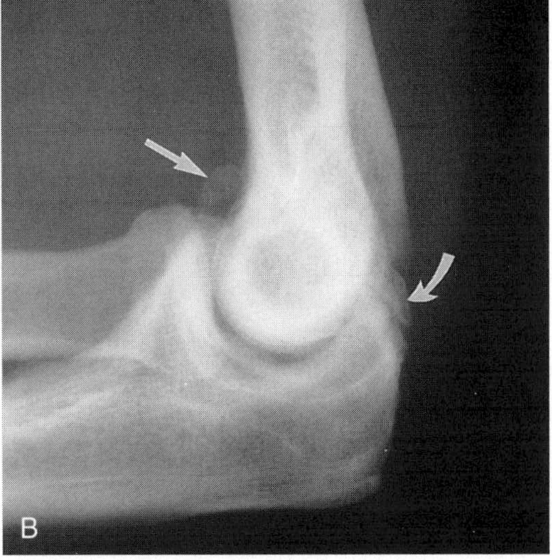

Figure 16–12 ■ **A**, Loose bodies within a dry joint: longitudinal sonogram, anterior recess. A 38-year-old retired baseball player cannot flex the elbow greater than 30 degrees. A hyperechoic loose body (*) displaces the joint capsule (*c*). In some patients, no joint effusion accompanies loose bodies. In these cases, it is very difficult to mobilize the loose body. Identification of the loose body then depends on appreciation of the deformity of the contour of the joint capsule and acoustic shadowing deep to the loose body. Abbreviations: brachialis muscle (*B*), coronoid process (*CP*), trochlea (*T*). **B**, Loose bodies within a dry joint: conventional radiograph. Same patient as in **A**. The radiograph demonstrates the calcified loose body (*arrow*) in the anterior recess adjacent to the tip of the coronoid process. Note the old fracture of the tip of the olecranon process (*curved arrow*).

enucleation, while neurofibromas need more complicated reconstructive surgery if they involve major nerve branches.

Plexiform neurofibromas in neurofibromatosis tend to follow the course of nerves but may extend into adjacent regions. Like other benign nerve tumors, they are also hypoechoic and extend like sausages along large nerve segments. The nerve appears thickened into a convoluted mass which has been likened to a "bag of worms." Neurofibrosarcomas are very rare; we have not encountered them in our large series of peripheral nerve tumors. Sarcomas tend to be large, very vascular masses. Areas of central necrosis are common.

Capsular and synovial processes can cause periarticular swelling. Therefore, they may be mistaken clinically for soft tissue tumors. In these cases, ultrasound can demonstrate the benign character of these masses. Arthritis and ganglia can cause significant soft tissue swelling around the elbow. The diagnosis with ultrasound is straightforward. Homogeneous hypoechoic or anechoic fluid indicates the benign character of these masses (see Fig. 16–6). Typical ganglia have a narrow communi-

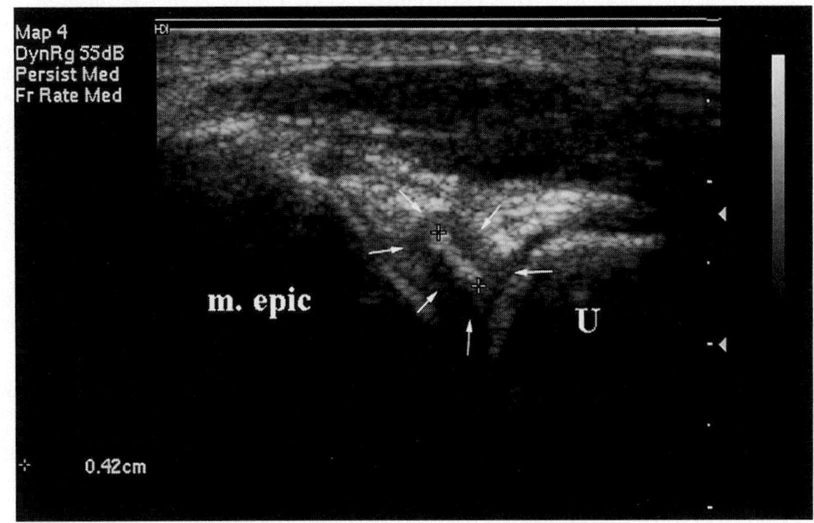

Figure 16–13 ■ Loose bodies within a dry joint: longitudinal sonogram. Elbow pain and crepitation caused this 35-year-old auto mechanic to seek treatment. New high-frequency transducers allow visualization of both the echogenic calcified portion of the loose body (+) and the hypoechoic peripheral hyaline cartilage (*arrows*). Abbreviations: medial epicondyle (*m. epic*), proximal ulna (*U*).

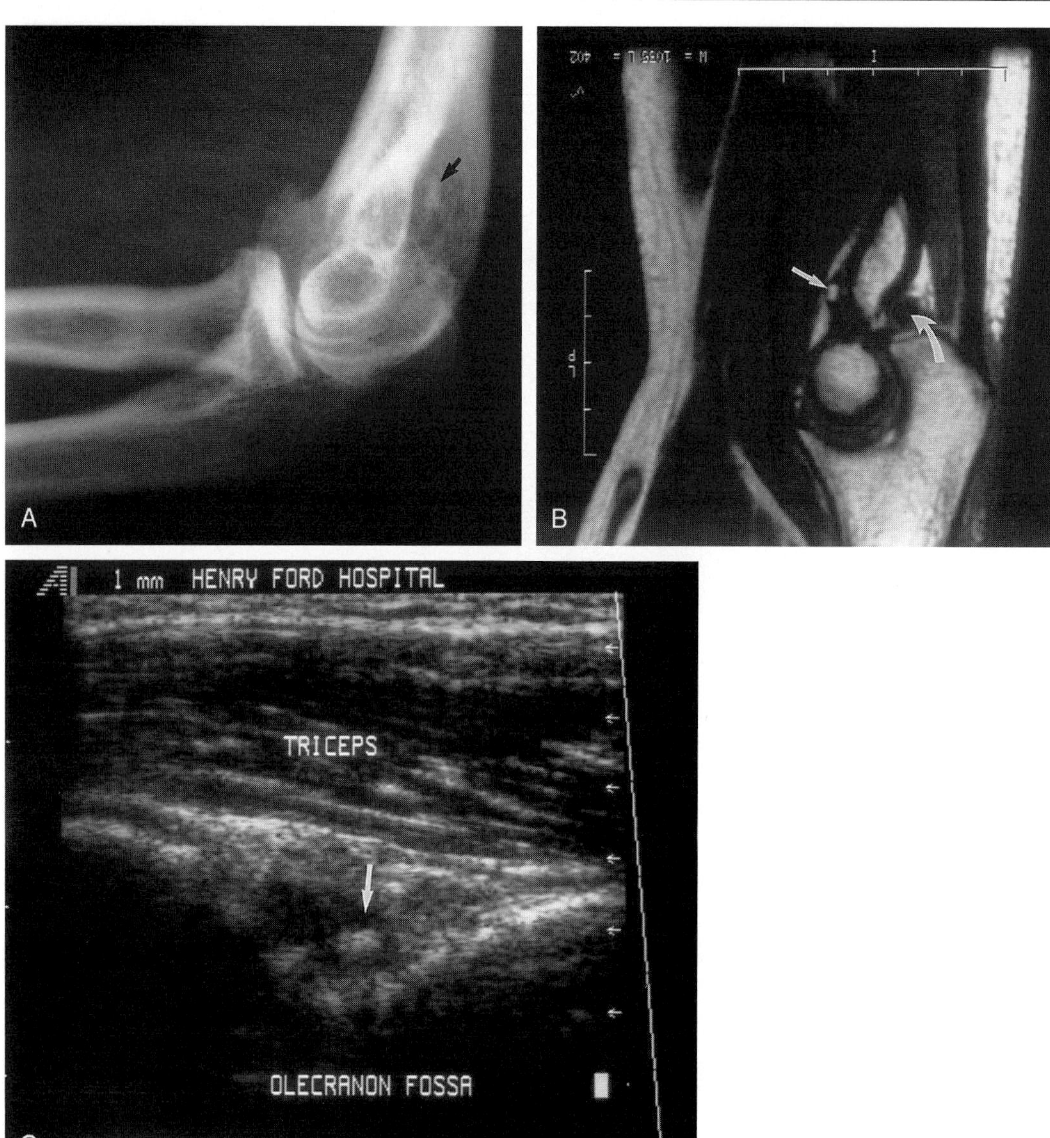

Figure 16–14 ■ **A**, Imaging of loose bodies: conventional radiograph. Conventional radiographs were obtained of this 34-year-old man with limited extension of the elbow. Often, due to radiographic projection, loose bodies in the olecranon fossa (*black arrow*) may be mistaken for bone islands. **B**, Imaging of loose bodies: T_1-weighted MRI. Same patient as in **A**. A small loose body containing marrow (*straight arrow*) is easily identified within the anterior joint recess. However, the large loose body (*curved arrow*) resulting in limitation of the range of motion is much less easily identified within the posterior recess due to the signal void resulting from its dense calcification and cartilage. **C**, Imaging of loose bodies: longitudinal sonogram. Same patient as in **A**. The central echogenic focus (*arrow*) of the calcified portion of the loose body is easily seen on this ultrasound image. The surrounding hypoechoic zone corresponds to noncalcified hyaline cartilage.

cation with the tendon sheath or joint synovium. Their content is typically homogeneous. Compartmentalization with thick, fibrous septae is common. Ganglia forming within nerve sheaths have also been observed. The fluid, if aspirated, is very thick and gelatinous. Aspiration may alleviate pain or reduce the functional impairment of the compressed nerve. If aspiration is performed for treatment, we recommend a multidirectional approach with multiple puncture holes using the largest possible needle. This will result in more damage to the thick, fibrous capsule and the internal septae, reducing the likelihood of recurrence.

A challenging clinical diagnosis to establish is the rupture or partial rupture of the distal biceps tendon (Figs. 16–23 and 16–24). In full-thickness tears of the distal biceps, the tendon retracts above the antecubital fold. The tendon typically retracts in a folded pattern, and retraction may not be demonstrable in a straight line. Partial-thickness tears are

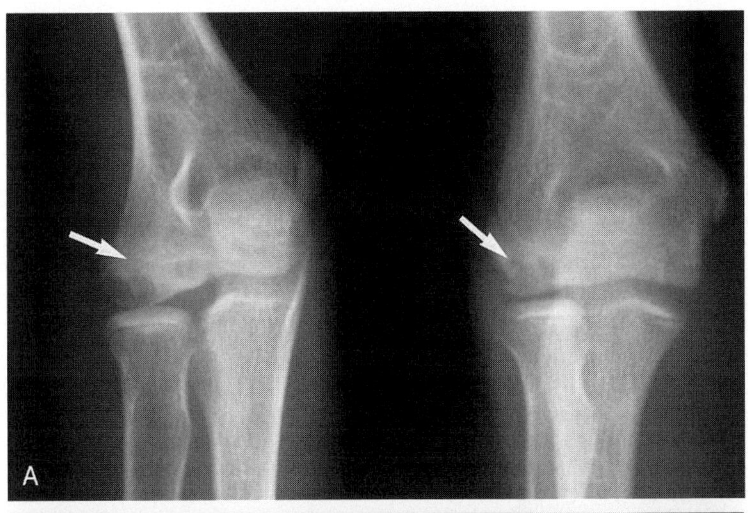

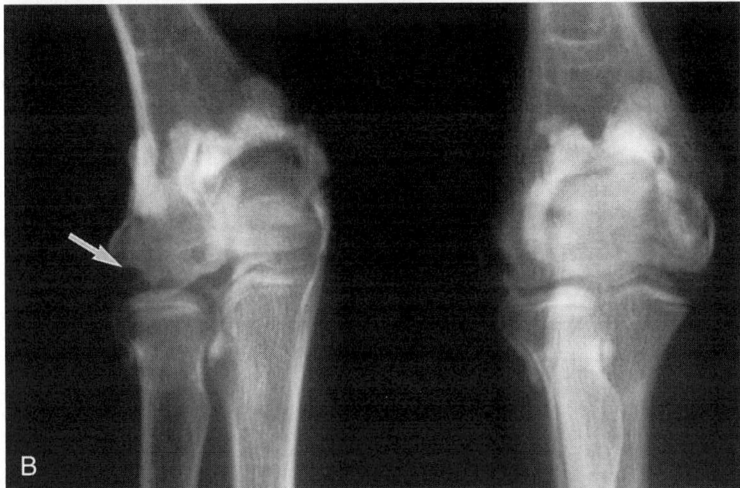

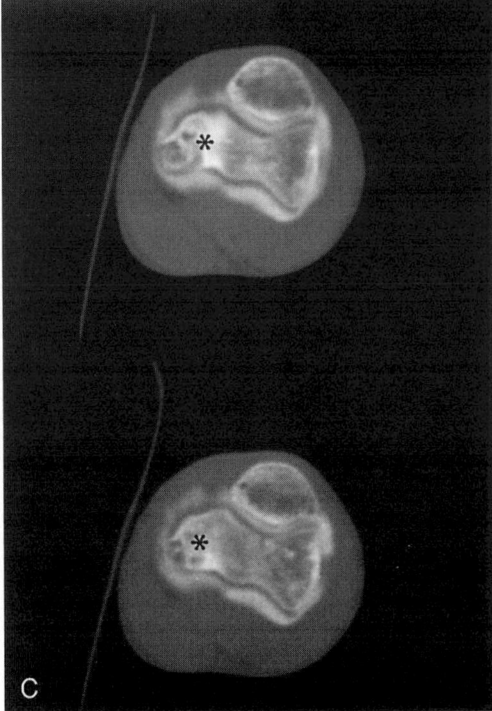

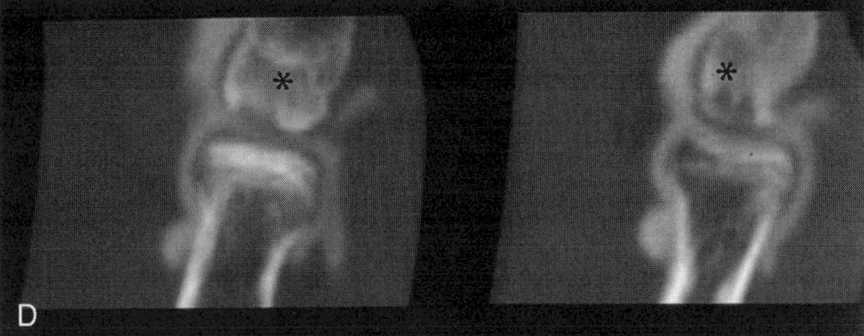

Figure 16–15 ■ **A**, Panner's disease of the capitellum: conventional radiograph. This 11-year-old Little League baseball player has pain in his elbow while pitching. These radiographs demonstrate a mixed lytic-sclerotic focus (*arrows*) in the capitellum. **B**, Panner's disease of the capitellum: single-contrast arthrogram. Same patient as in **A**. It is very difficult to evaluate this lesion (*asterisks*) further on this single-contrast arthrogram. The clinical question of the integrity of the overlying cartilage could not be answered reliably. **C**,**D**, Panner's disease of the capitellum: CT arthrogram. Same patient as in **A**. Evaluation of the curved surface of the hyaline cartilage covering this lesion (*asterisks*) is difficult on these axial images. Sagittal reconstructions do not add significantly to the evaluation of the cartilage.

Figure continued on following page

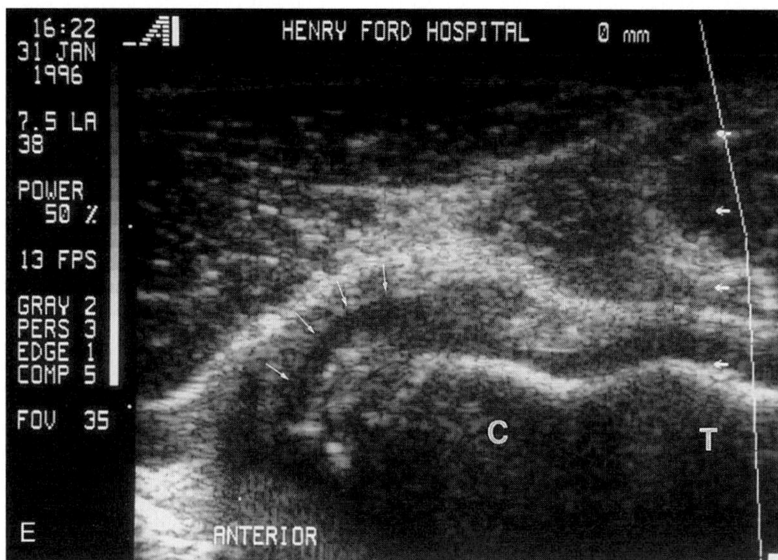

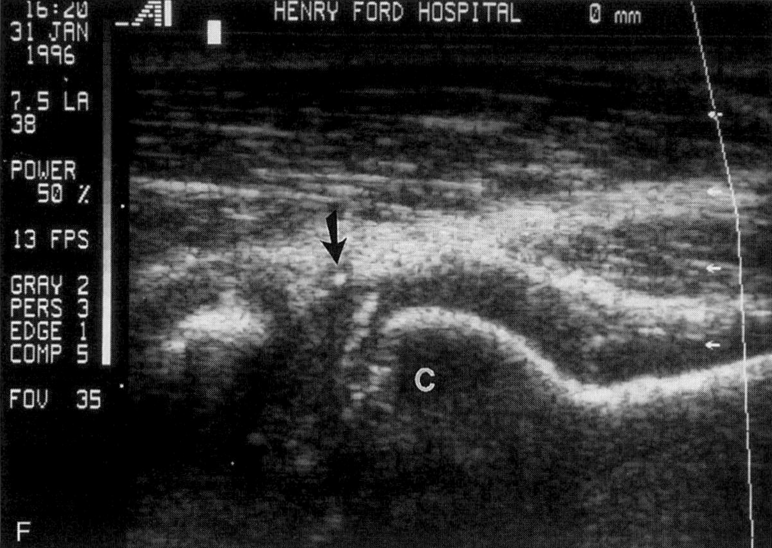

Figure 16–15 *Continued* ■ **E**, Panner's disease of the capitellum: transverse sonogram. Same patient as in **A**. The transverse ultrasound image demonstrates the cartilage (*arrows*) overlying the lesion to be intact. Abbreviations: capitellum (*C*), trochlea (*T*). **F**, Panner's disease of the capitellum: longitudinal sonogram. Same patient as in **A**. When the elbow was examined in the longitudinal plane, a thin, mobile flap of cartilage (*black arrow*) was identified in the vicinity of the capitellum (*C*). The most common cause of loose bodies in the elbow is trauma to the capitellum, which is often seen in baseball players.

far more difficult to diagnose. The tears occur close to the radial tuberosity. In its normal anatomical course, the distal biceps tendon folds in between the proximal radius and ulna, and it is not possible to follow the tendon down to the tuberosity in the supinated elbow. Incomplete tears can often be shown by pronating the elbow and scanning the radial tuberosity through the extensor compartment. Surgical exploration and reattachment on the radial tuberosity is often necessary to regain full elbow strength. Equally important is the diagnosis of a triceps tendon tear. Missing a tear of the triceps tendon can lead to permanent loss of elbow extension. Patients undergoing hemodialysis and kidney transplantation seem particularly prone to this type of injury. Ultrasound typically shows discontinuity of the tendon just proximal to the tip of the olecranon (Fig. 16–25A). Surgical reattachment is the treatment of choice.

Technical Guidelines and Scanning Technique

Examination of the elbow is initiated by evaluation of the anterior synovial recess. If no fluid is found within the anterior synovial recess, intra-articular pathology is unlikely. For the examination, the patient sits facing the examiner, with the arm lying slightly flexed on the examination table. Imaging is performed with the transducer in the long axis of the arm. Normally, a hypoechoic layer of hyaline cartilage no greater than 1 mm in thickness is identified surrounding the subchondral bone surfaces of the elbow joint (see Fig. 16–4). Examination of the medial and lateral epicondyles is performed next. Careful side-to-side comparison of the dimensions and echogenicity of the tendons is most important (see Figs. 16–1 and 16–2). The patient places the palmar surfaces of the hands together, with the arms

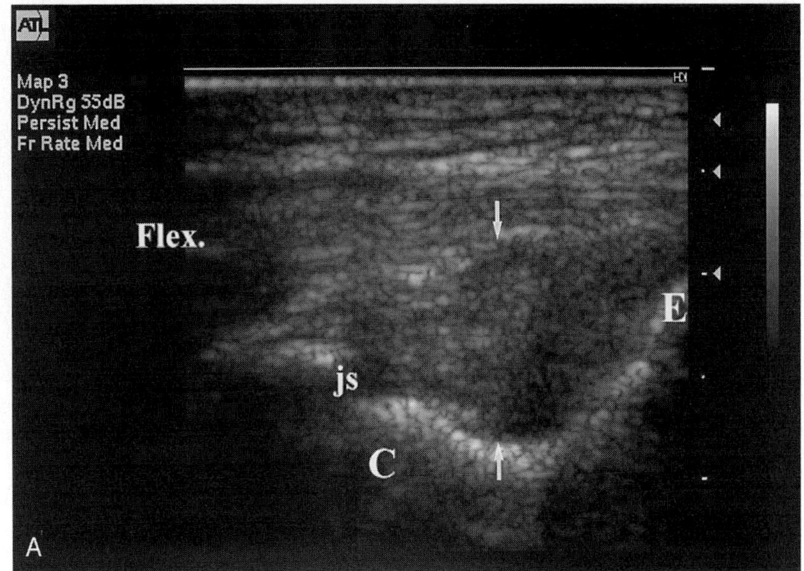

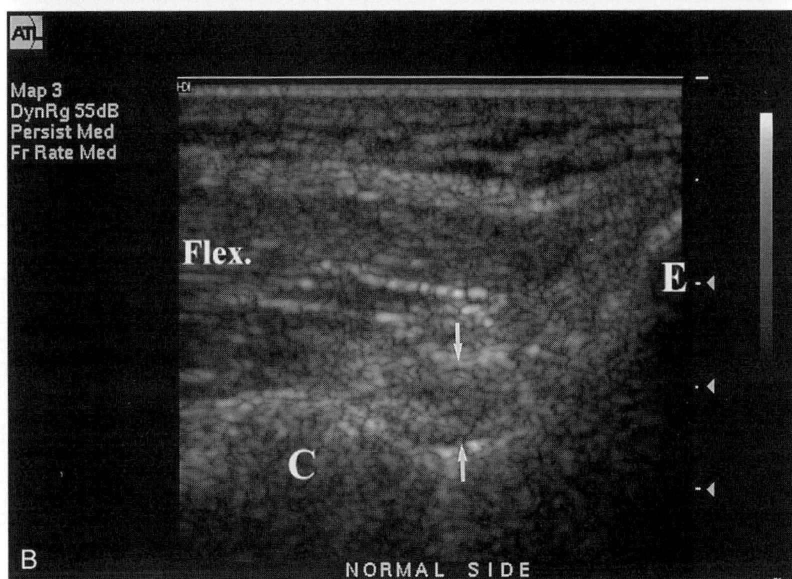

Figure 16–16 ■ **A**, Medial collateral ligament injury: longitudinal sonogram. An abnormally swollen medial collateral ligament (*arrows*) is demonstrated in this longitudinal image of the right elbow of a 22-year-old professional baseball player who complains of chronic elbow pain. Abbreviations: medial epicondyle (*E*), medial condyle (*C*), joint space (*js*), flexor muscles (*Flex.*). **B**, Medial collateral ligament injury: longitudinal sonogram. Same patient as in **A**. The patient's asymptomatic left elbow demonstrates a thinner, homogeneously echogenic anterior bundle of the ulnar collateral ligament (*arrows*). Laxity or tear of the ulnar collateral ligament results in the Panner lesion described in Figure 16–15. Abbreviations: medial epicondyle (*E*), medial condyle (*C*), flexor muscles (*Flex.*).

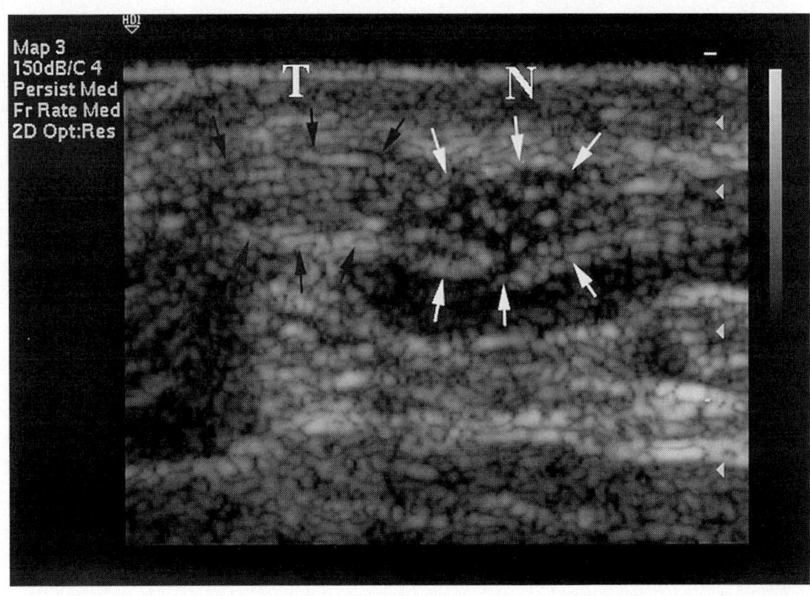

Figure 16–17 ■ Nerve texture: transverse sonogram. A normal median nerve (*white arrows*) adjacent to a normal echogenic tendon (*black arrows*) is identified. The nerve appears slightly less echogenic than the tendon but more echogenic than the muscle lying deep to this structure. A stippled pattern of echos also helps distinguish the nerve from adjacent tendons. Abbreviations: tendon (*T*), nerve (*N*).

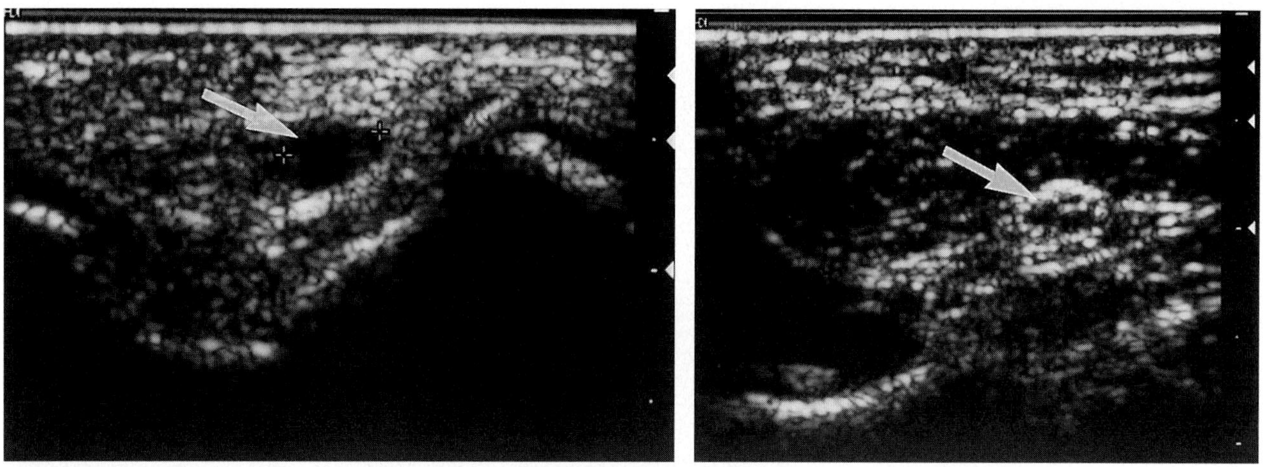

Figure 16–18 ■ Contrast changes of the ulnar nerve: transverse sonograms. The ulnar nerve behind the medial epicondyle (image on the left) has a hypoechoic appearance despite attempts to adjust for anisotropy. It appears much less echogenic than the surrounding fat. In the image on the right, the ulnar nerve is imaged approximately 1 inch distal to the epicondyle, and the nerve appears more echogenic than the surrounding structures. This is probably attributable to differences in attenuation of the sound beam in the more superficial structures. Ulnar nerve (*white arrows*).

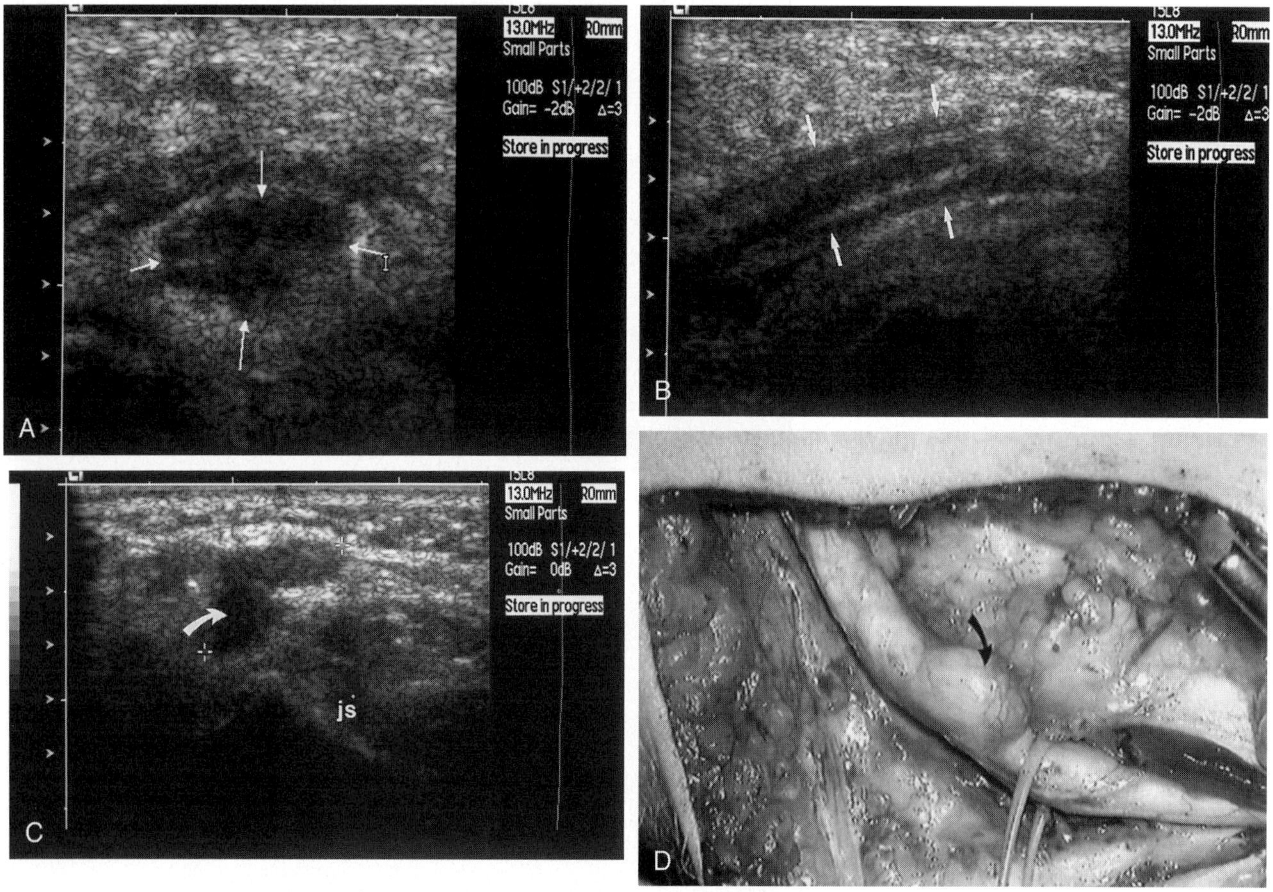

Figure 16–19 ■ **A**, Traumatic neuroma of the ulnar nerve: transverse sonogram. This 24-year-old male suffered a fracture of the elbow several years ago and now presents with paresthesias involving the medial aspect of the palm of the hand. The ulnar nerve (*arrows*) is enlarged (1 cm diameter) and hypoechoic distal to the medial epicondyle. Abbreviation: medial epicondyle (*I*). **B**, Traumatic neuroma of the ulnar nerve: longitudinal sonogram. Same patient as in **A**. In longitudinal images, the nerve (*arrows*) is thickened diffusely and appears hypoechoic. However, the fascicular pattern within the nerve is preserved. **C**, Traumatic neuroma of the ulnar nerve: transverse sonogram. Same patient as in **A**. An exophytic nodule (*curved arrow*) is observed arising from the nerve (+) at the level of the joint space (*js*). **D**, Traumatic neuroma of the ulnar nerve: surgical photograph. Same patient as in **A**. A diffusely swollen nerve with a focal posttraumatic neuroma (*curved arrow*) was demonstrated at the time of surgery and confirmed histologically. (Case courtesy of Drs. Bartel van Holsbeeck, Philippe Lefere, and Luc Fidlers, Stedelijk Ziekenhuis Roeselare.)

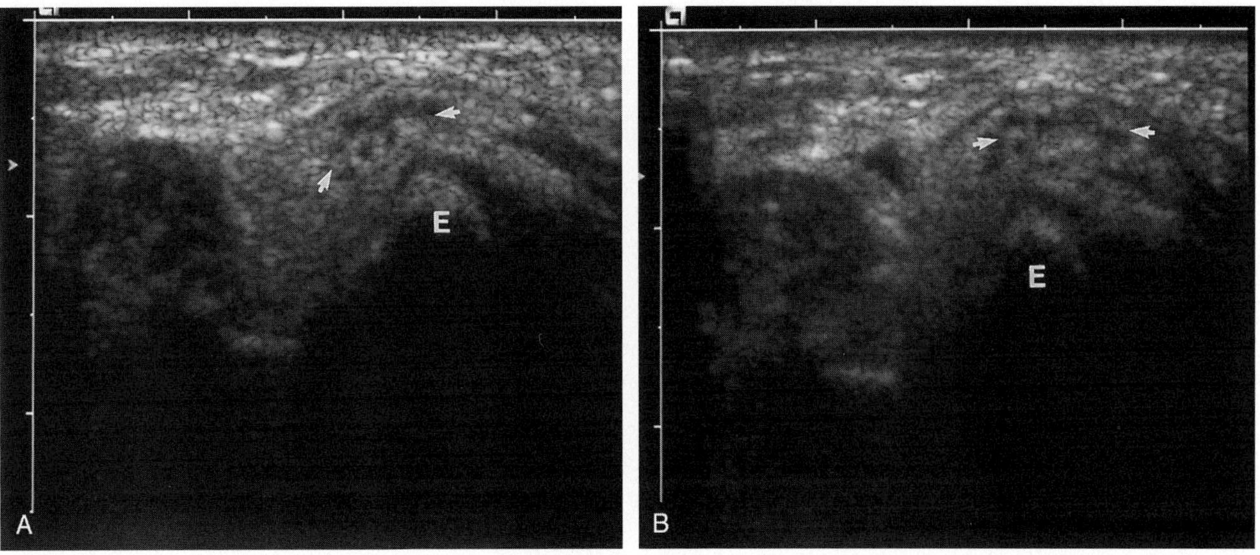

Figure 16-20 ■ **A**, Ulnar nerve subluxation: transverse sonogram. A 40-year-old female presented with pain radiating over the medial forearm and wrist. This transverse sonogram was obtained with the supinated forearm in extension. The ulnar nerve (*arrows*) is slightly displaced anteriorly relative to the medial epicondyle (*E*). **B**, Ulnar nerve subluxation: transverse sonogram. Same patient as in **A**. The forearm was then flexed, revealing further anterior migration of the ulnar nerve. The nerve (*arrows*) now lies directly over the epicondyle (*E*). (Case courtesy of Drs. Bartel van Holsbeeck, Philippe Lefere, and Philippe Gunst, Stedelijk Ziekenhuis Roeselare.)

extended on the examination table. The tendon origins appear as hyperechoic triangles. Right–left comparison is absolutely necessary to detect slight differences in dimension. Tendinitis is characterized by tendon swelling and inhomogeneity, as elsewhere in the extremities (see Fig. 16–1). If a joint effusion is present and loose bodies are not identified, the posterior joint recess should be examined with the arm in 90 degrees of flexion and with the forearm planted perpendicular to the surface of the examination table. The olecranon fossa should be examined very carefully in both longitudinal and transverse planes. Varying degrees of flexion can be used to show mobility of loose bodies. Triceps tendon and muscle cover the posterior elbow, providing a sonographic window to the joint when scanned posteriorly. The transducer is then moved across the cubital tunnel, with the alignment corrected so that the medial aspect touches the medial epicondyle and the lateral aspect contacts the olecranon process. The ulnar nerve is noted as a hypoechoic ovoid structure adjacent to the medial epicondyle. The longitudinal image shows its characteristic fascicular structure. An interesting feature of this structure is that the nerve appears hypoechoic relative to surrounding tissues of the elbow but hyperechoic relative to the musculature of the forearm (see Fig. 16–18). Examination of the elbow is completed by evaluation of the distal biceps tendon. This tendon can be examined longitudinally with the arm extended. Pronation is necessary for visualization of the distal biceps tendon.

A different approach to the elbow can be tried with the patient in the supine position. This is helpful for the posterior recess exam, which is easily performed with the arm at the side and the elbow flexed and lifted 45 degrees off the table, because the fluid then gravitates into the dependent olecranon fossa. The flexor tendon origin and ulnar nerve are then examined with the arm extended and abducted. The upper arm is externally rotated and the forearm supinated. The origin of the extensor tendon can be examined with the arm partially pronated and resting on the lower abdomen.

The Wrist and Hand

Indications for Scanning

The principal indications for ultrasound examination of the wrist and hand are evaluation of tendon pathology and identification of the origin of swelling (Fig. 16–26). Tendon ruptures are easily detected on longitudinal images. Real-time examination of the tendons of the hand is valuable in the diagnosis of tendon dislocation and entrapment. Tenosynovitis of the flexor tendons of the wrist can result in carpal

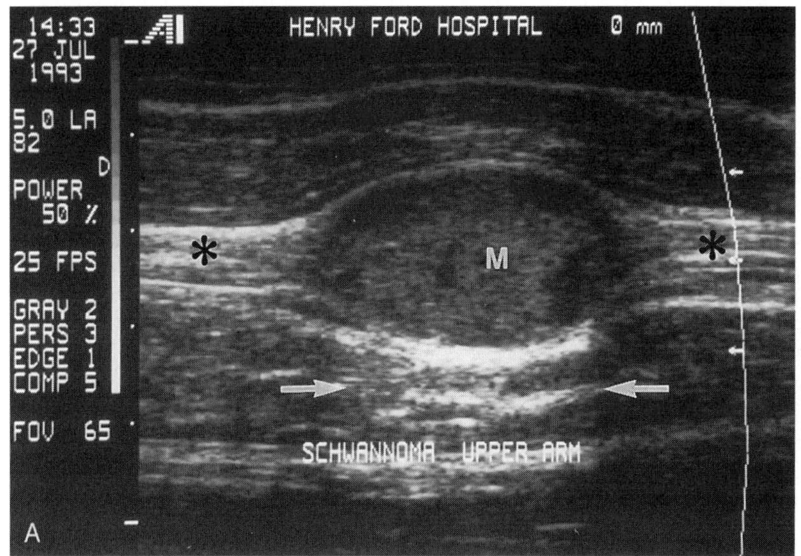

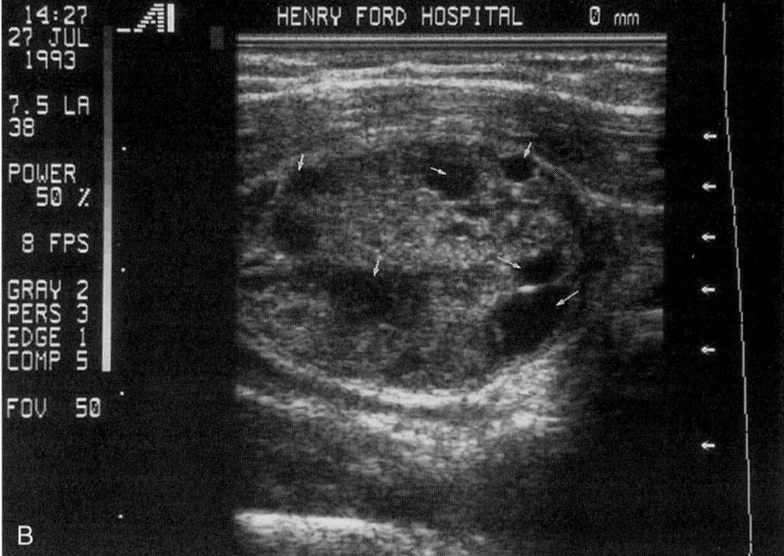

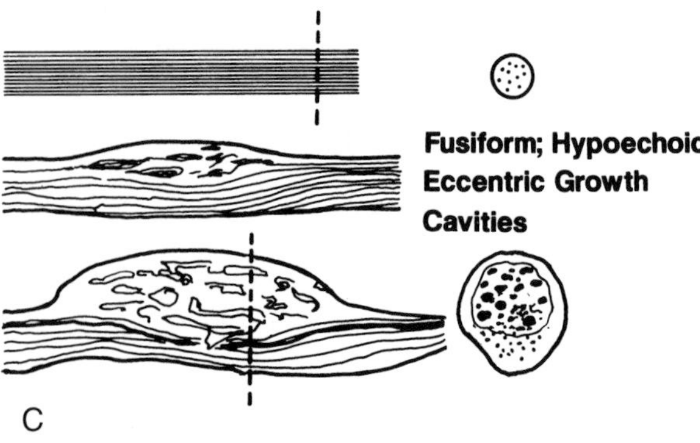

Figure 16–21 ▪ **A**, Median nerve neurilemmoma: longitudinal sonogram. After recently undertaking a weight-lifting regimen, this 36-year-old male experienced paresthesias in the middle and ring fingers. He had a positive Tinel sign but normal forearm strength. A fusiform, hypoechoic soft tissue mass (*M*) is seen in continuity with the median nerve (*) on this image obtained using a 5 MHz. transducer. Acoustic enhancement (*arrows*) deep to the mass is noted. **B**, Median nerve neurilemmoma: longitudinal sonogram. Same patient as in **A**. Greater detail within the mass is demonstrated on this longitudinal image obtained using a 7.5 MHz transducer. Tiny cystic cavities (*small arrows*) are identified within the well-encapsulated mass. **C**, Median nerve neurilemmoma: diagram. This diagram depicts the morphological changes which occur in the development of a schwannoma. A normal nerve and its cross section are shown at the top.

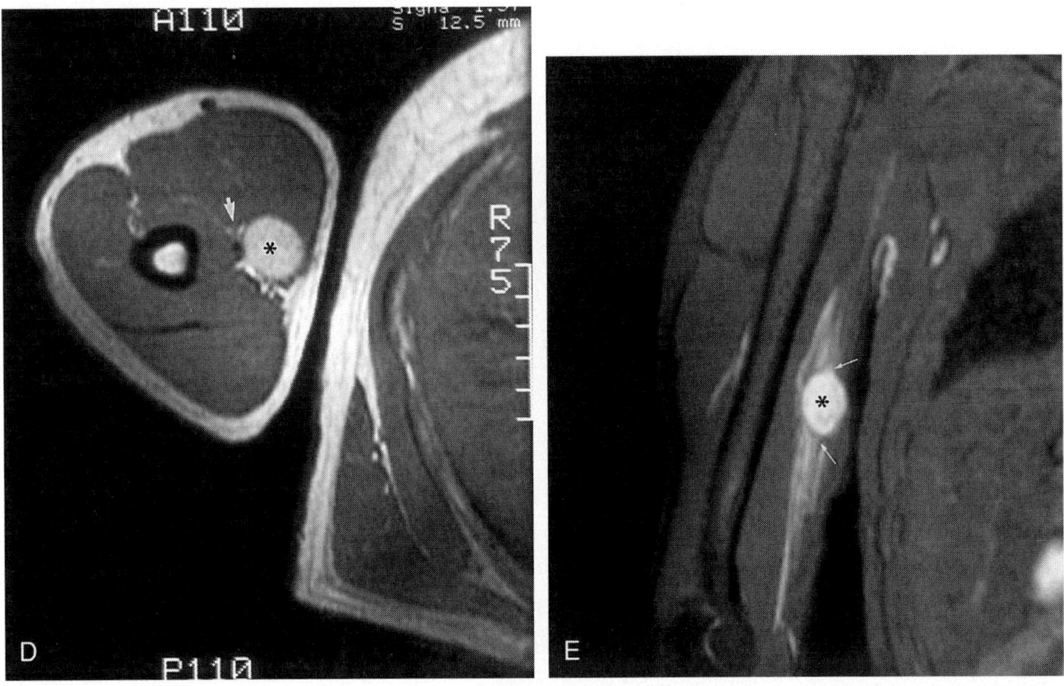

Figure 16–21 *Continued* ▪ **D**, Median nerve neurilemmoma: proton density axial MRI. Same patient as in **A**. A round lesion with a homogeneous high signal (*) is seen in the expected location of the median nerve. The internal architecture demonstrated on ultrasound images is not evident on MRI. Note the proximity to the brachial artery (*small white arrow*). **E**, Median nerve neurilemmoma: sagittal T_2 weighted fat saturation MRI. Same patient as in **A**. The exact relationship of the mass (*) to the nerve (*small arrows*) is not as clear on MRI as on ultrasound images.

tunnel syndrome. Although this is one of the less common causes of carpal tunnel syndrome, it is important to identify the entity due to the greater likelihood of success with conservative therapy. Unusual acute onset of carpal tunnel disease may occur with synovitis in rheumatoid arthritis and gonococcal synovitis. The diagnosis can be confirmed with ultrasound imaging and guided aspiration. Treatment, in the form of carpal tunnel release, must be performed on an emergent basis in those cases (Box 16–2).

Diagnosis of synovial cysts (ganglia) and identification of their origin is possible with ultrasound (Fig. 16–27). Surgical management of a ganglion cyst arising from a tendon sheath differs from that of a ganglion cyst originating from a joint (Fig. 16–28). Wide surgical resection has been recommended in ganglia which recur after treatment with pressure or after aspiration (Crenshaw, 1996). Ideally, the wide resection should include the communication with the adjacent synovium (Crenshaw, 1996). Ultrasound's strength in diagnosis is its ability to find occult ganglia and identify the small communications to the synovium (Figs. 16–29 through 16–33). Often these cysts are very hard and may be mistaken for bony hypertrophy on physical exam. It is noteworthy that ganglia or bursae may form over bony prominences or spurs. Some ganglia may cause nerve compression if they are located within

Box 16–2
Carpal Tunnel Sonography

- Rule out ganglia and tenosynovitis (relatively rare)
- Rule out rheumatoid or amyloid synovitis from the radiocarpal/midcarpal joint (rare)
- Rule out tophi or hydroxyapatite deposition (rare)
- Rule out tumors—fibroma, (very rare)
- If none of the above:

  Nerve cross-sectional area >15 mm^2 (diagnosis established)

  Nerve cross-sectional area <15 mm^2 → EMG

Text continued on page 539

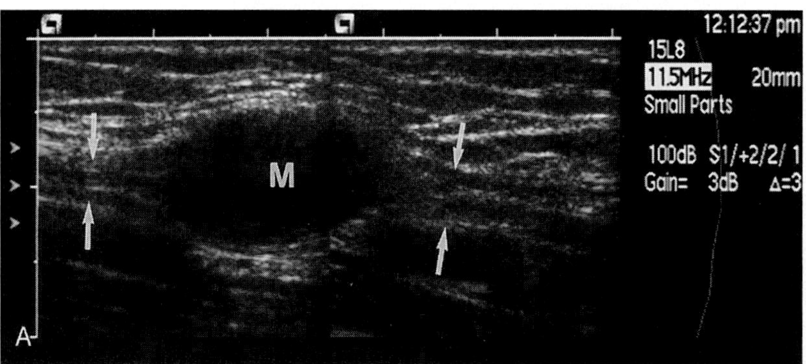

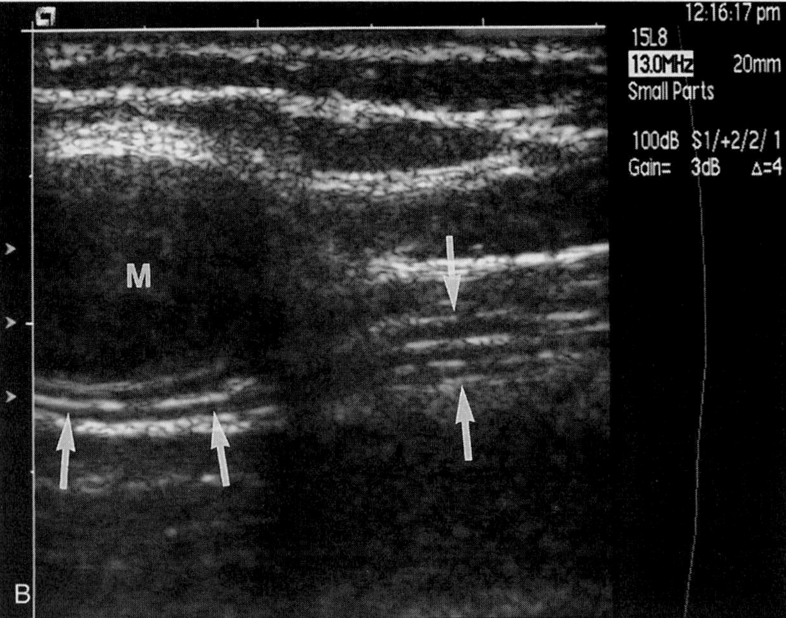

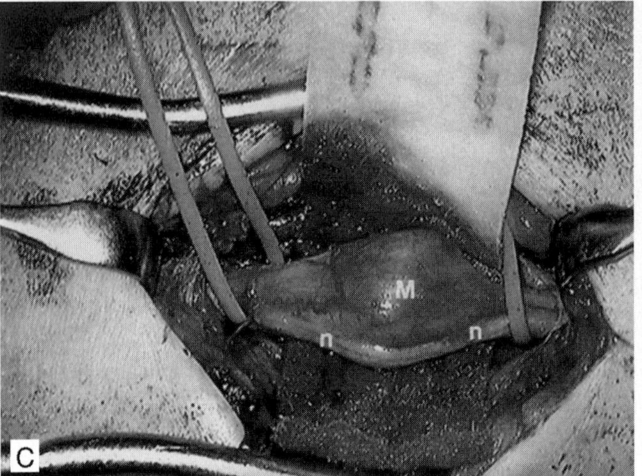

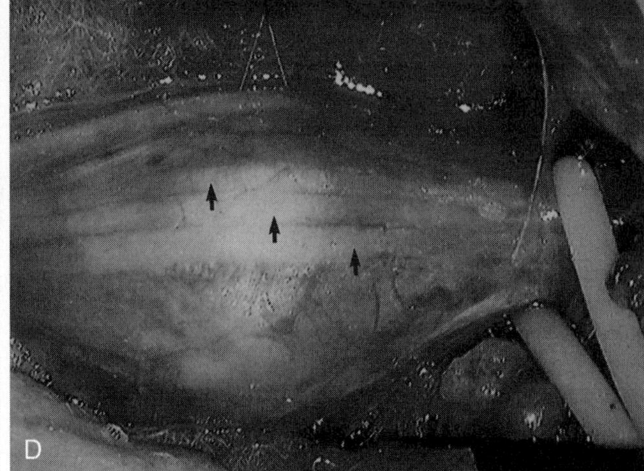

Figure 16–22 ■ **A**, Arm neurilemmoma: longitudinal sonogram. This 31-year-old female presented with swelling over the medial aspect of the upper arm and pain shooting into the hand. In this longitudinal sonogram, the mass (*M*) is seen in continuity with the nerve (*arrows*). **B**, Arm neurilemmoma: longitudinal sonogram. Same patient as in **A**. The mass involving the nerve clearly arises eccentrically from the nerve. Three normal nerve bundles (*arrows*) are identified along the deep margin of the mass and continuing distally on this 13 MHz. image. **C**,**D**, Arm neurilemmoma: surgical photograph. Same patient as in **A**. At surgery, the eccentric relationship of the mass (M) to the remainder of the nerve (*n*) is confirmed. Note the three distinct nerve bundles (*arrows*) seen along the deep aspect of the mass, which is slightly rotated in this close-up photo. (Case courtesy of Drs. Bartel van Holsbeeck, Philippe Gunst, and Luc Fidlers, Stedelijk Ziekenhuis Roeselare.)

Figure 16–23 ■ Normal distal biceps tendon: longitudinal sonogram. In this longitudinal image, a normal distal biceps tendon is seen coursing to its insertion (*curved arrow*) on the radial tuberosity.

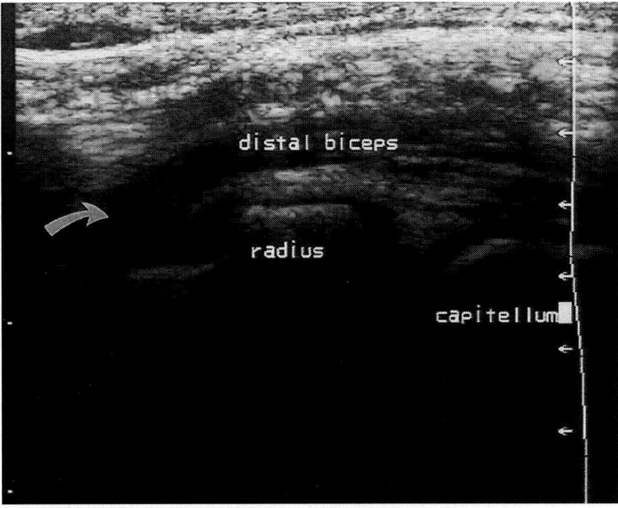

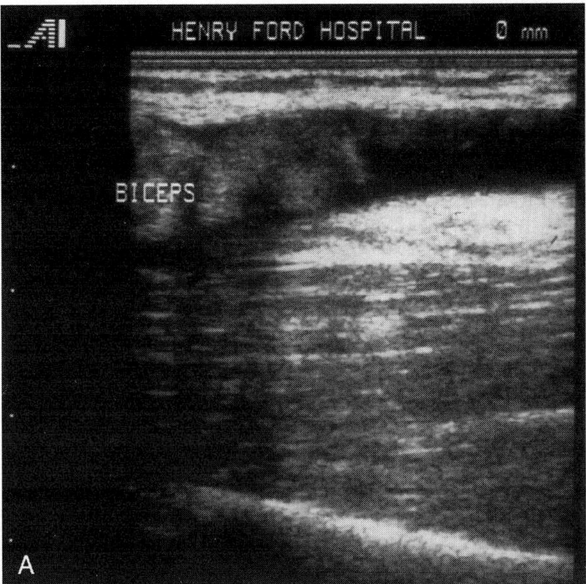

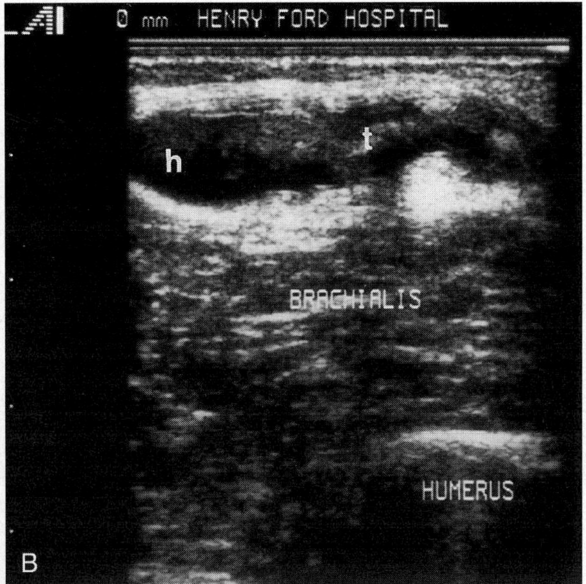

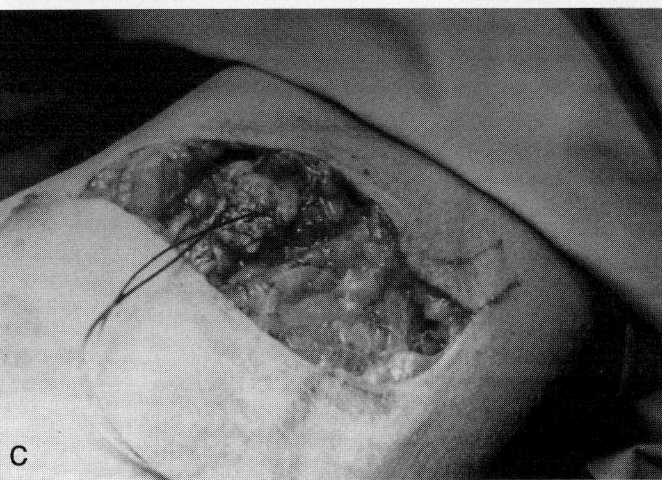

Figure 16–24 ■ **A**, Torn distal biceps tendon: longitudinal sonogram. While trying to climb a wall during a chase, this 36-year-old police officer experienced a sharp, stabbing pain in his lower forearm. He now has little strength in flexion for lifting. An irregular, retracted biceps tendon is identified in the distal aspect of the upper arm. An anechoic fluid collection fills the void created by the retracted tendon. **B**, Torn distal biceps tendon: transverse sonogram. Same patient as in **A**. Ultrasound provides excellent contrast between the frayed torn end of the tendon (*t*), the surrounding hematoma (*h*), and the adjacent brachialis muscle. **C**, Torn distal biceps tendon: surgical photograph. Same patient as in **A**. A suture has been placed through the frayed end of the tendon. (Photograph **C** courtesy of Dr. Patricia Kolowich, Henry Ford Health System.)

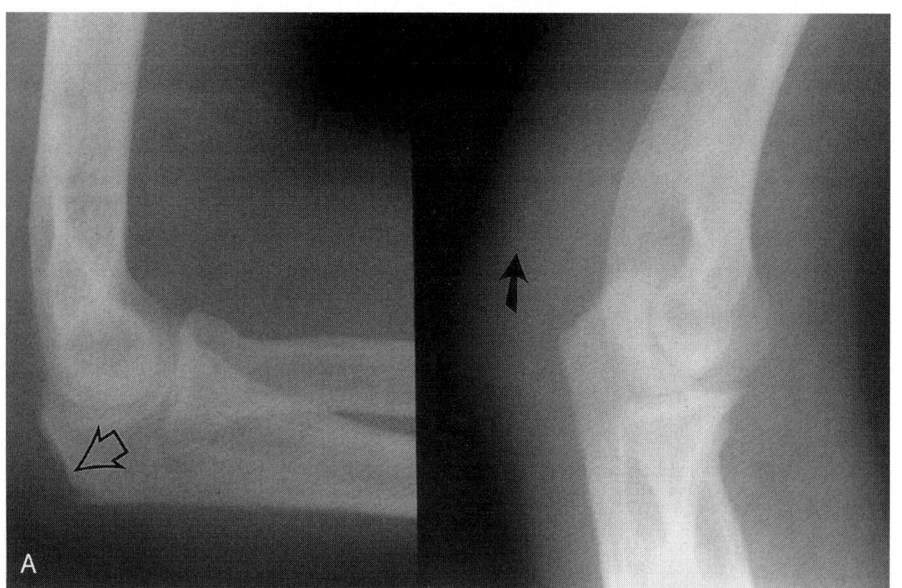

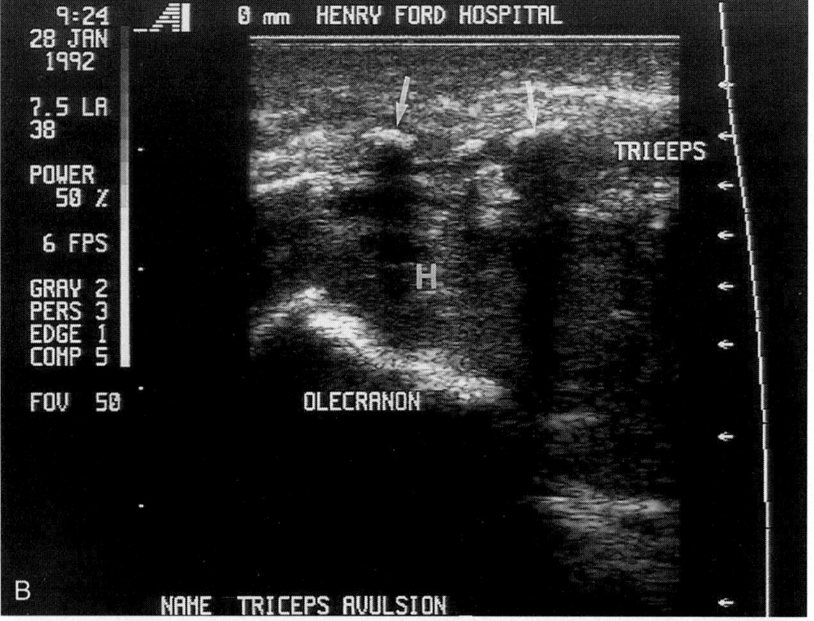

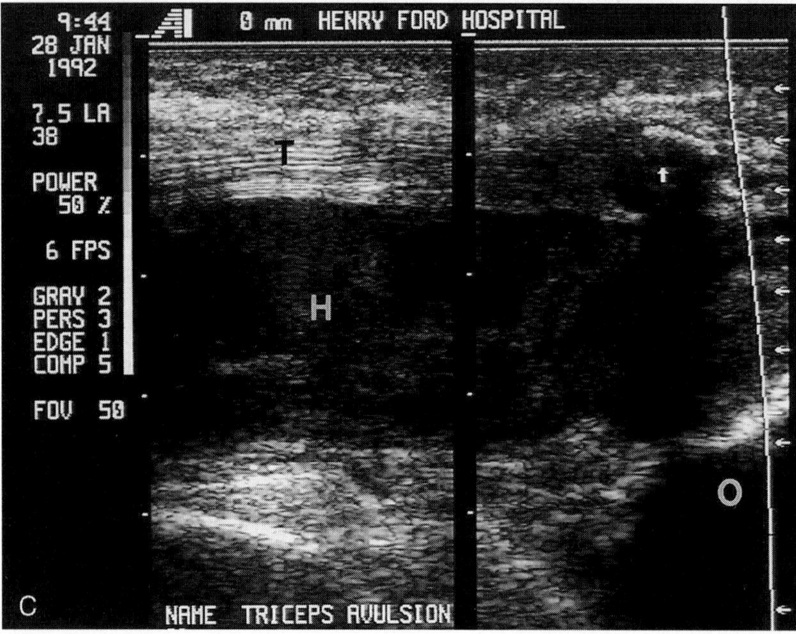

Figure 16–25 ■ **A**, Distal triceps tendon rupture: conventional radiograph. This 40-year-old dialysis patient experienced sudden onset of pain in his right elbow. He now lacks active extension of the forearm. Note the irregularity of the cortical surface of the olecranon (*open arrow*). Small ossific opacities (*solid black arrow*) are seen within the soft tissues posterior to the olecranon fossa on the image with the forearm in extension. **B**, Distal triceps tendon rupture: transverse sonogram. Same patient as in **A**. Several calcified fragments (*arrows*) with acoustic shadowing are separated from the surface of the bone by a hypoechoic hematoma (*H*). **C**, Distal triceps tendon rupture: longitudinal sonogram. Same patient as in **A**. These small, calcified fragments (*small arrow*) are attached to the distal triceps tendon (*T*), which is separated from the olecranon by a hematoma (*H*). Abbreviation: Olecranon (*O*).

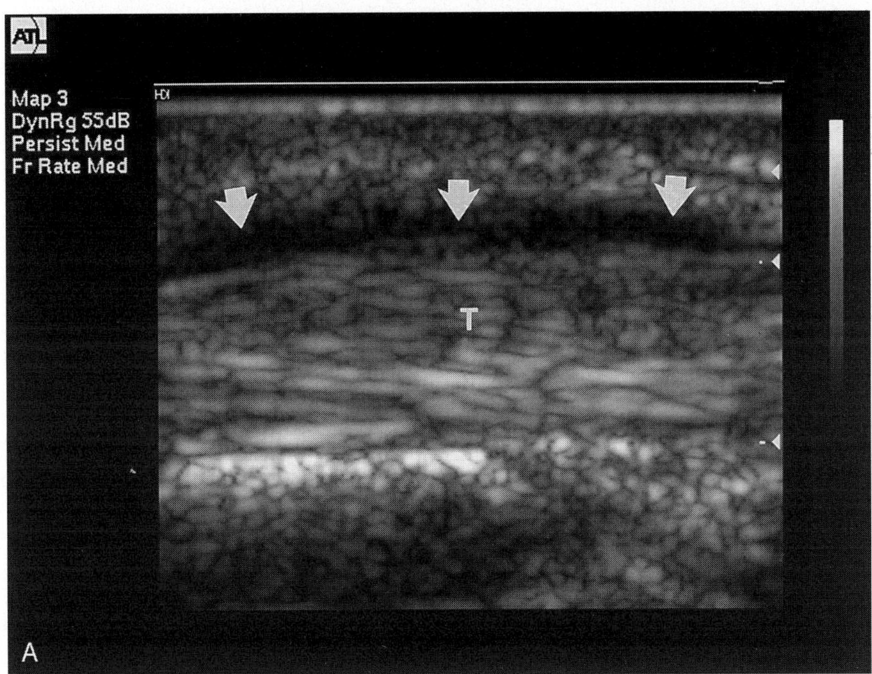

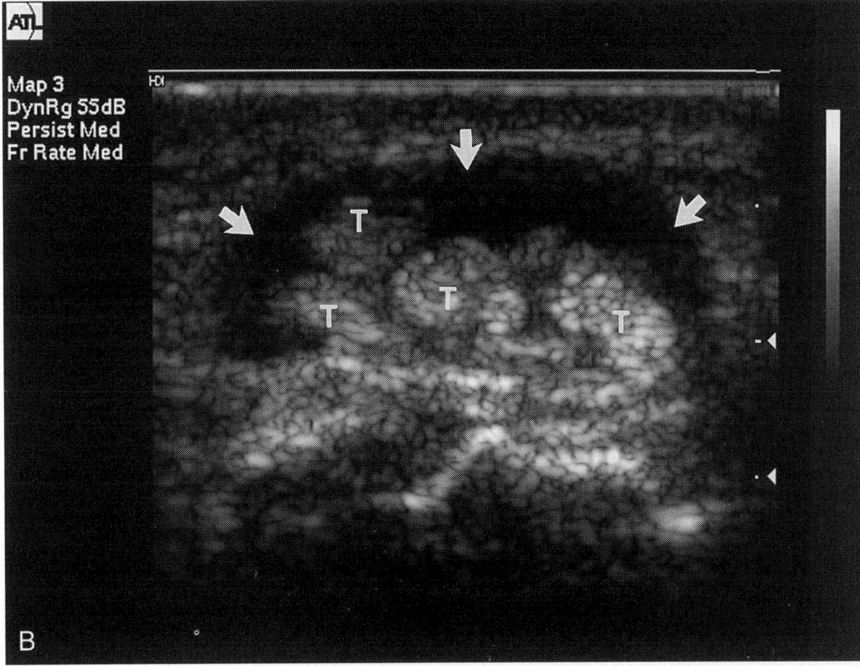

Figure 16-26 ■ **A**, Extensor tenosynovitis: longitudinal sonogram. A 36-year-old male complained of pain over the dorsum of the hand. A thin, uniform layer of fluid (*arrows*) is present along the superficial surface of the extensor tendons (*T*) of the hand within the tendon sheath. **B**, Extensor tenosynovitis: transverse sonogram. Same patient as in **A**. Fluid (*arrows*) within the tendon sheath often accumulates in an eccentric fashion, as seen here. Abbreviation: extensor tendons (*T*).

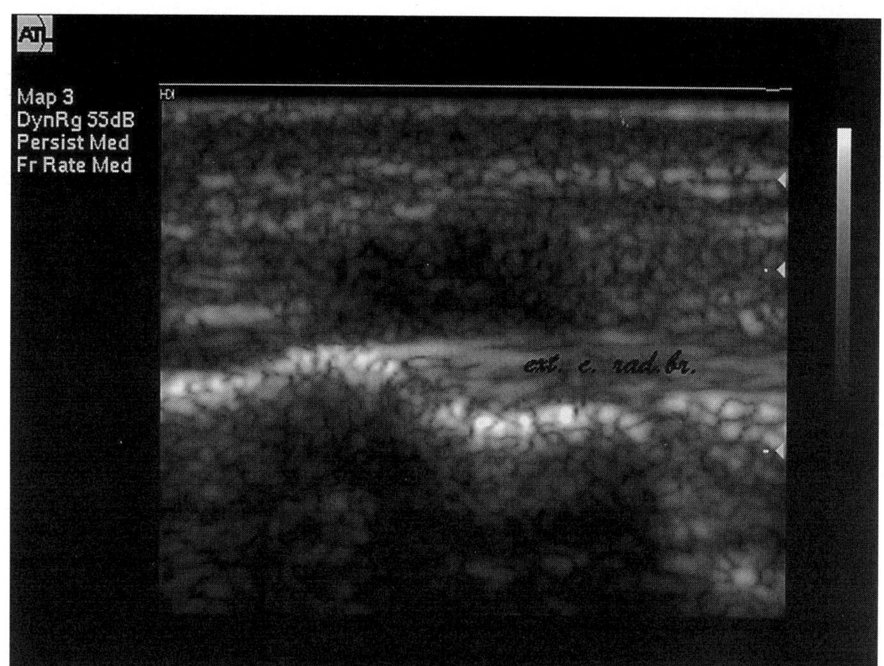

Figure 16–27 ■ Ganglion: longitudinal sonogram. Pain and swelling over the dorsum of the hand prompted this 32-year-old female to seek treatment. A focal mass-like, fluid-filled structure is identified in close association with the extensor carpi radialis brevis tendon. The appearance of this ganglion cyst distinctly differs from that of fluid within the tendon sheath resulting from tenosynovitis.

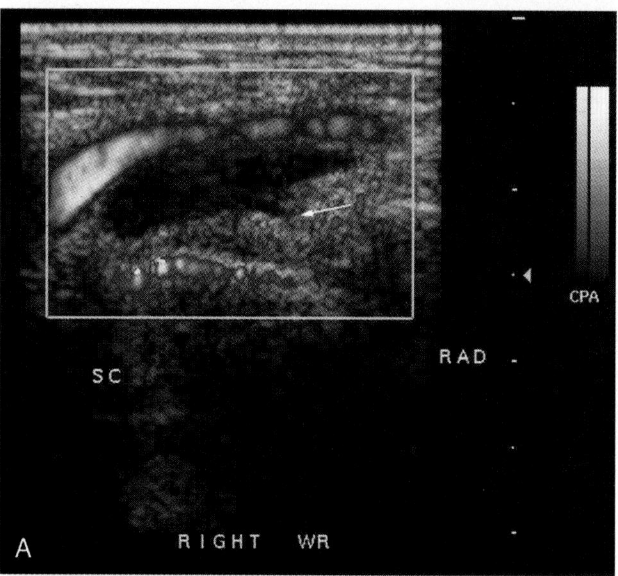

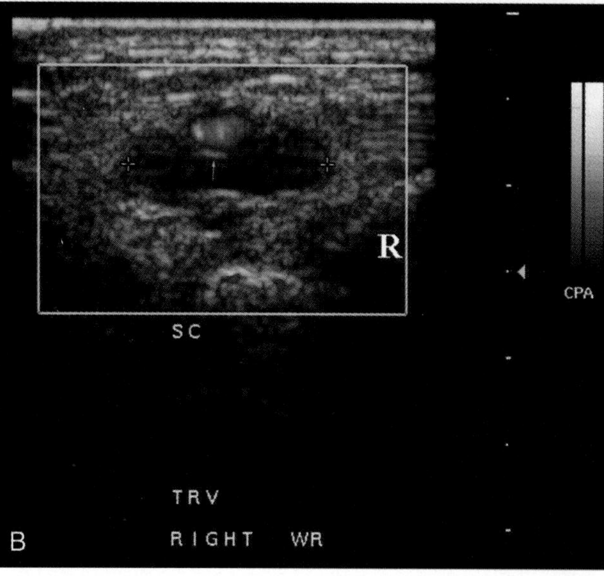

Figure 16–28 ■ **A**, Snuff box ganglion: longitudinal sonogram. The patient, a 28-year-old female, noticed a painful pulsatile mass in the anatomical snuff box. An anechoic mass is identified deep to the radial artery on this longitudinal power Doppler image. A narrow channel is noted extending toward the radiocarpal joint (*arrow*). Abbreviations: scaphoid (*SC*), radius (*RAD*). **B**, Snuff box ganglion: transverse sonogram. Same patient as in **A**. The anechoic mass (+) deep to the radial artery demonstrates a distinct wall (*arrow*) separating it from the artery, excluding the possibility of a thrombosed pseudoaneurysm. Abbreviations: scaphoid (*SC*), radius (*R*).

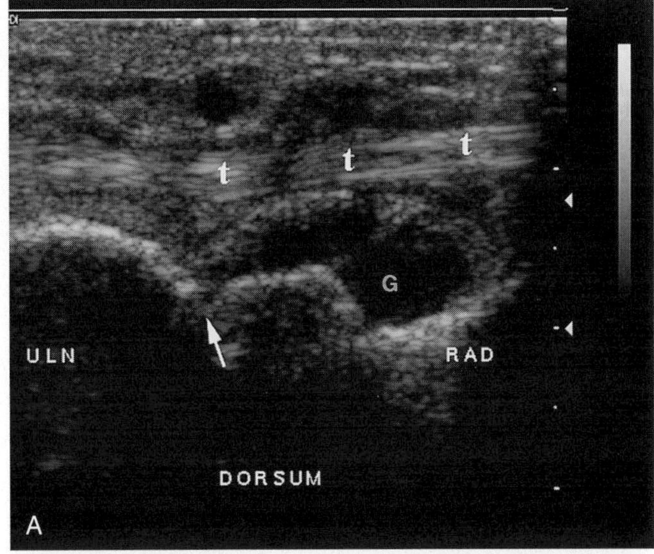

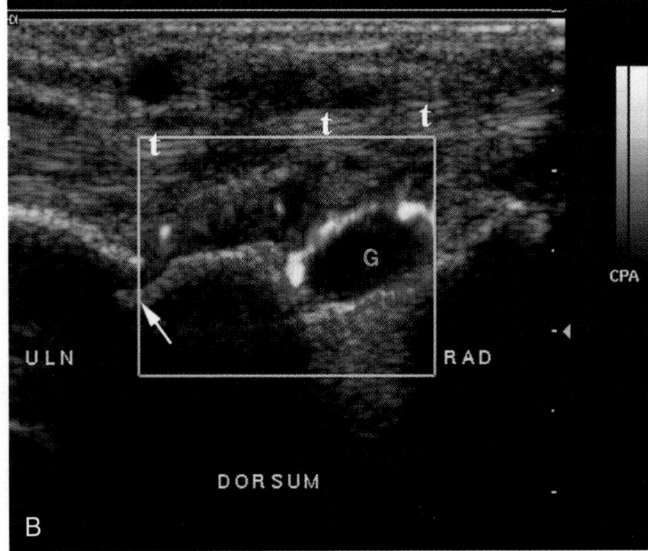

Figure 16–29 ■ **A**, Recurrent dorsal ganglion: transverse sonogram. Six months following surgical resection of a dorsal wrist ganglion, this 29-year-old female returned with recurrent pain and swelling over the distal dorsal radius. A recurrent ganglion (*G*) is noted deep to the extensor tendons (*t*) and lateral to the radioulnar joint (*arrow*). Abbreviations: distal ulna (*ULN*), distal radius (*RAD*). **B**, Recurrent dorsal ganglion: transverse power Doppler sonogram. Same patient as in **A**. Hyperemia is observed in the wall of the recurrent ganglion (*G*). This appearance is not uncommon and should not be interpreted as a sign of infection. Abbreviations: distal ulna (*ULN*), distal radius (*RAD*).

anatomically restricted spaces such as the carpal tunnel and the Guyon canal (see Figs. 16–30 and 16–33). A ganglion that deserves special attention is the scapholunate ganglion. This benign mass lesion is common and has been related to tears of the dorsal scapholunate ligament. The search for occult ganglia should always include the dorsal scapholunate space. Ganglia over the snuff box may present as pulsatile masses. The radial artery is often draped over the mass (see Fig. 16–28). The differential diagnosis includes aneurysm of the radial artery (see Figs. 16–31 and 16–32). Duplex Doppler sonography demonstrates the lack of flow within the ganglion.

The exact role of ultrasound in chronic carpal tunnel disease has not been fully established. Its role in showing the cause of chronic carpal tunnel disease is rather limited because the majority of cases represent idiopathic diseases of the median nerve. However, ultrasound can demonstrate swelling of the median nerve proximal to and at the entrance of the carpal tunnel in cases of idiopathic carpal tunnel disease (Figs. 16–34 through 16–39) (Buchberger et al., 1991, 1992). A recent study emphasized the use of a measurement of the cross-sectional area of the median nerve over the proximal carpal crease. A cross-sectional area above 15 mm^2 corresponds to carpal tunnel disease in all cases (Lee, 1999). It is possible that ultrasound will replace electromyography (EMG) as a noninvasive study of the carpal tunnel. EMG would then be utilized for further evaluation only if the ultrasound

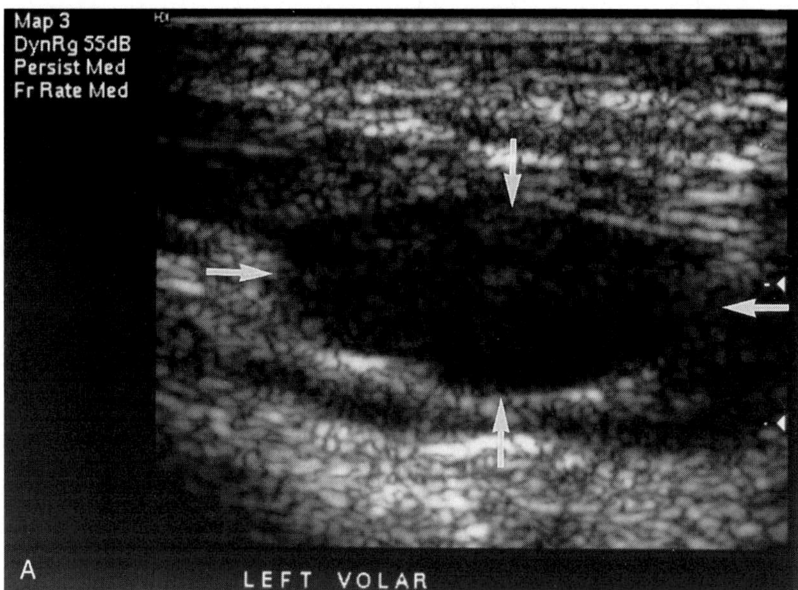

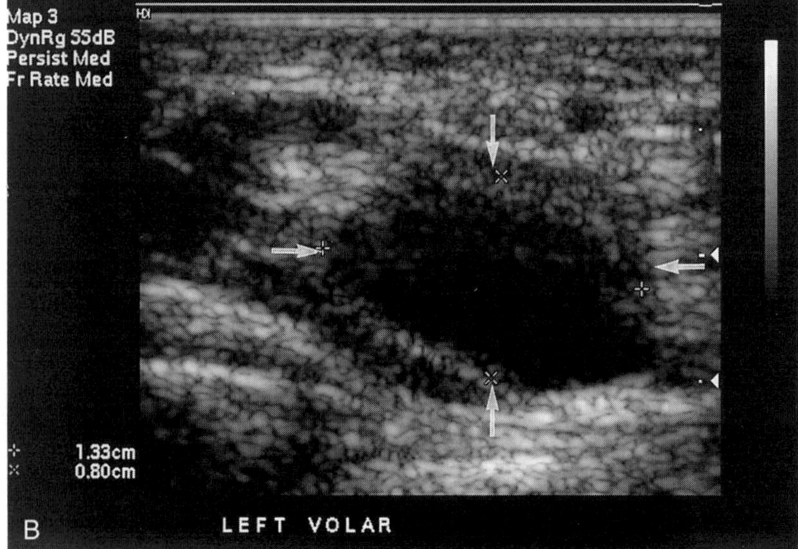

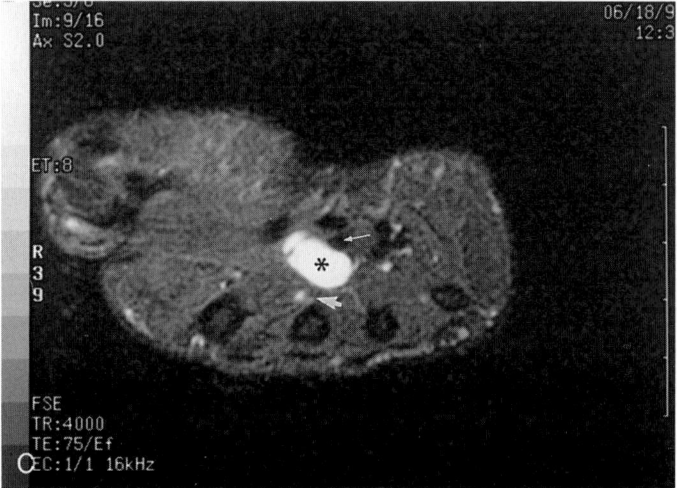

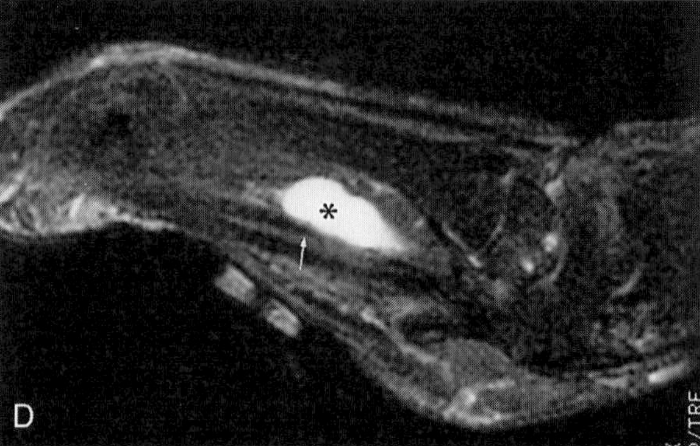

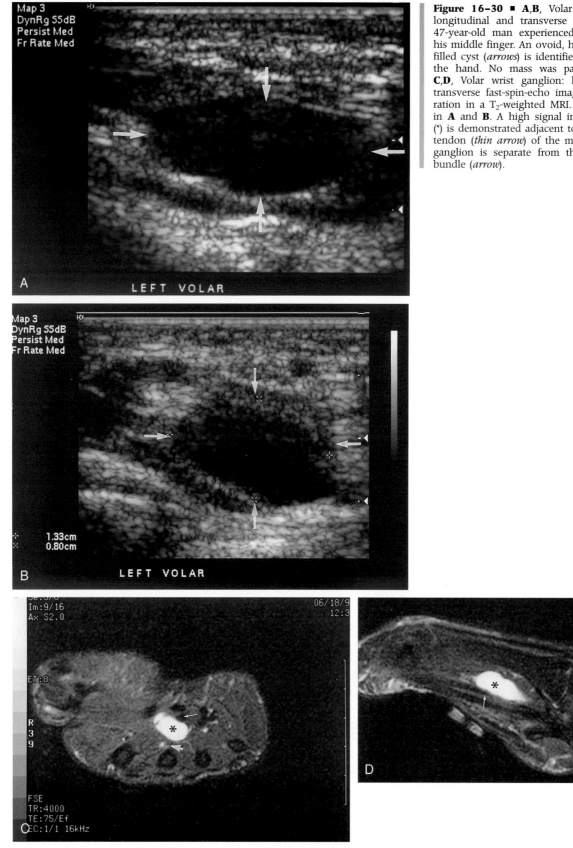

Figure 16–30 ■ **A**,**B**, Volar wrist ganglion: longitudinal and transverse sonograms. This 47-year-old man experienced paresthesias in his middle finger. An ovoid, hypoechoic, fluid-filled cyst (*arrows*) is identified in the palm of the hand. No mass was palpable clinically. **C**,**D**, Volar wrist ganglion: longitudinal and transverse fast-spin-echo image with fat-saturation in a T_2-weighted MRI. Same patient as in **A** and **B**. A high signal intensity ganglion (*) is demonstrated adjacent to the deep flexor tendon (*thin arrow*) of the middle finger. The ganglion is separate from the neurovascular bundle (*arrow*).

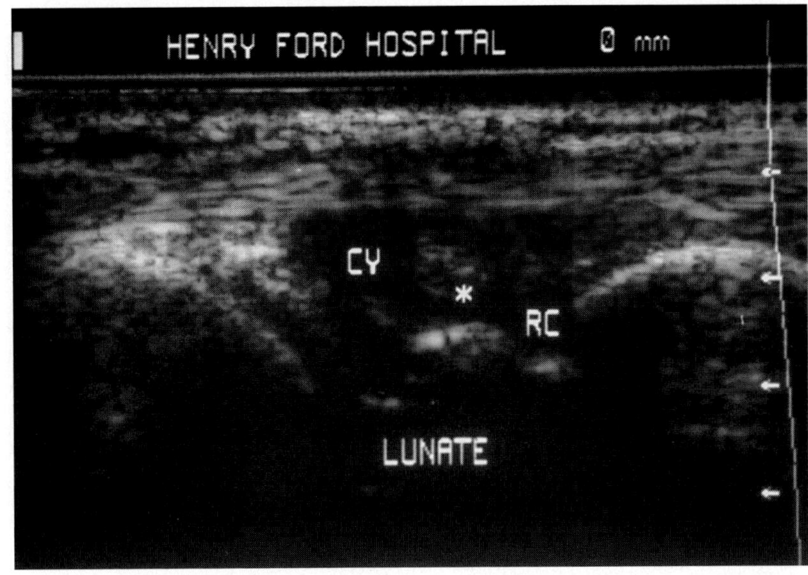

Figure 16–31 ▪ Occult wrist ganglion: longitudinal sonogram. The patient is a 37-year-old female with diffuse wrist pain. An anechoic ganglion (*CY*) is identified deep to the extensor tendons. A clear communication (*) with the radiocarpal joint (*RC*) is seen.

exam is negative in patients with positive clinical findings. There seems to be a difference in the appearance of the median nerve in idiopathic carpal tunnel disease, in which the nerve is almost always swollen proximally, and the appearance of this nerve in cases of chronic compression (Fig. 16–39). In comparison with the large number of patients with idiopathic carpal tunnel disease, only a few patients have median nerve paresthesias because of mass effect from within the tunnel.

Flexor and extensor tendons of the hand and wrist can tear. Flexor tendon tears can occur in the forearm, wrist, palm, or finger. Ruptures occur most frequently in the fingers. Ultrasound has a role in the diagnosis and staging of tears. In addition, ultrasound is invaluable in locating tears accurately prior to surgery. This allows the surgeon to limit the incision and to anticipate the complexity of the reconstructive procedure.

Injuries of flexor tendons (Fig. 16–40) have been divided into five zones (Fig. 16–41). The surgical approach and the success rate depend on the site of the rupture relative to these zones (Figs. 16–42 and 16–43) (Crenshaw, 1996). Zone 1 repre-

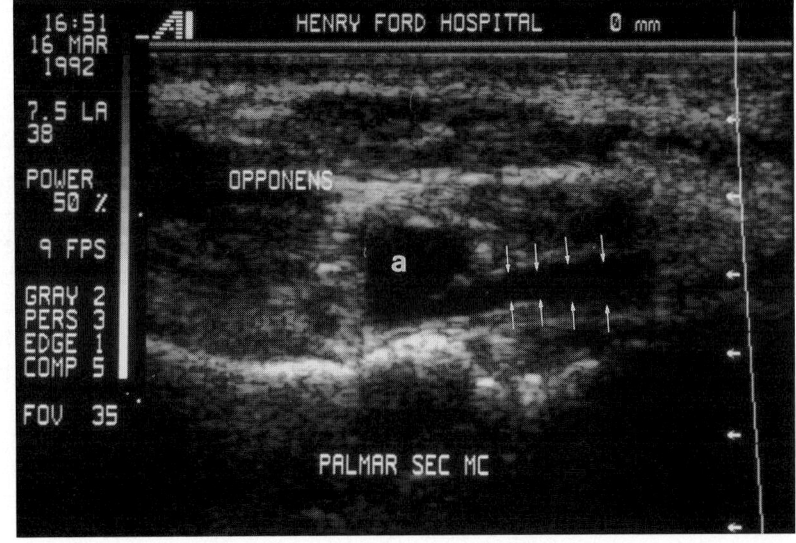

Figure 16–32 ▪ Pseudoaneurysm: longitudinal sonogram. Several years ago, this 42-year-old factory worker sustained a crush injury to the right hand. He now presents with chronic swelling of the right hand. Longitudinal images over the base of the second metacarpal revealed an anechoic mass communicating (*arrows*) with the deep palmar arterial arch. When examining lesions in the hand and wrist, it is important to identify the associated structures definitively. In this case, the lesion communicated with an artery rather than with the nearby joint. Abbreviation: pseudoaneurysm (*a*).

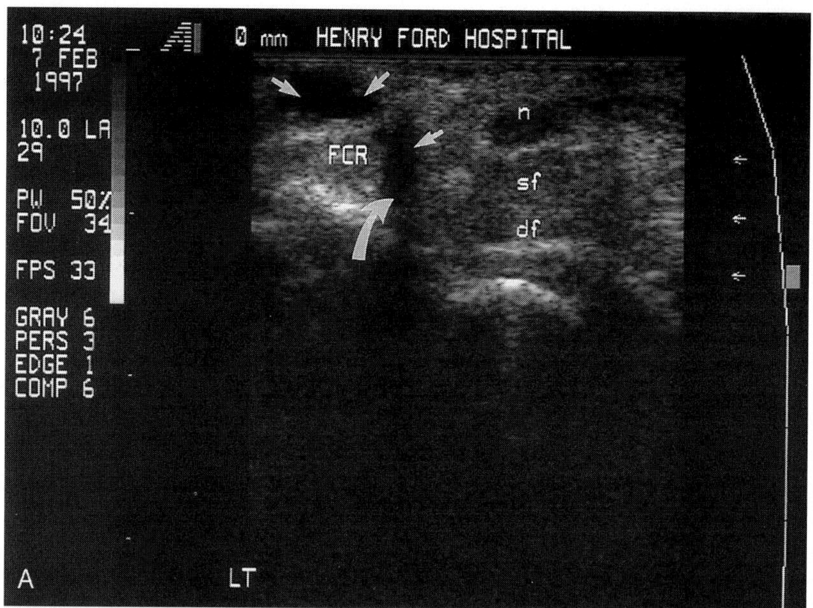

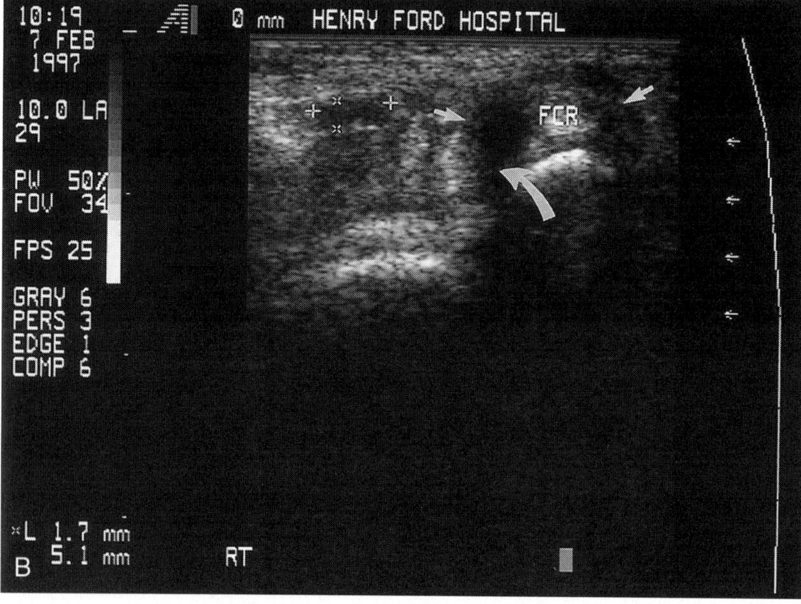

Figure 16–33 ■ **A**, Bilateral carpal tunnel disease caused by mass effect: transverse sonogram. Bilateral carpal tunnel disease resulted in disability in this 33-year-old female postal worker. An anechoic mass (*small arrows*) is demonstrated around the flexor carpi radialis tendon (*FCR*) of the left wrist. This tendon is located outside of the carpal tunnel. However, mass effect (*curved arrow*) on the lateral carpal tunnel is obvious. The median nerve (*n*) is less echogenic than the superficial (*sf*) and deep (*df*) flexor tendons located deep to the nerve. **B**, Bilateral carpal tunnel caused by mass effect: transverse sonogram. Same patient as in **A**. An anechoic mass (*small arrows*), similar to the one identified in the left wrist, is seen around the flexor carpi radialis tendon (*FCR*) of the right wrist. The median nerve (*calipers*) is not swollen, but note the close proximity of the mass to the nerve. The patient underwent carpal tunnel surgery and flexor carpi radialis tendon release. The surgeon removed a ganglion from the flexor carpi radialis tendon sheath. Ultrasound images, however, were more suggestive of a flexor tendon tenosynovitis because of the circumferential rather than focal swelling. Again, note the mass effect (*curved arrow*) on the soft tissue structures of the carpal tunnel.

sents ruptures in the distal finger. Ruptures in zone 2 are lesions in the finger through the flexor tendons in the fibro-osseous tunnel. Zone 3 lesions are located in the palm of the hand. Zone 4 lesions lie within the carpal tunnel, and zone 5 lesions are proximal to the carpal tunnel.

A rupture of the annular ligaments or pulleys will result in separation of the flexor tendons from the proximal phalanx (Fig. 16–44). The A_2 pulley injury occurs most commonly in rock climbers. Complications of tendon rupture and repair may also lead to pulley injury and tendon displacement. These lesions are aggravated by finger flexion against resistance. The typical bowstringing of the tendon then becomes more obvious.

Tenosynovitis of the flexor tendons can also be responsible for tendon dysfunction. Sonography is very helpful in evaluating foreign body penetration as a cause of tendon sheath inflammation (Fig. 16–45). Ultrasound allows detection of radiopaque and nonopaque foreign bodies (Jacobson et al., 1998). The technique is therefore more useful than radiography (Jacobson et al., 1998). Thorns and wood slivers smaller than 1 mm have been detected using sonography (see Fig. 12–12) (Failla et al., 1995).

Figure 16–34 ■ **A**, Normal median nerve: transverse sonogram. The median nerve (*mn*) in this asymptomatic 35-year-old male volunteer is seen as a flattened ovoid structure on top of superficial (*FS*) and deep flexor tendons (*FP*). The tendons appear more rounded and demonstrate more specular echos in their structure compared with the nerve. **B**, Normal median nerve anatomy: transverse section. This frozen cadaver wrist was cut in the axial plane through the carpal tunnel and Guyon's canal. The carpal tunnel is oval-shaped and contains the median nerve (*small arrows*) and flexor tendons. Guyon's canal (*oblique arrow*) is triangular and contains the ulnar nerve and artery. The oval-shaped median nerve is the most superficial structure in the carpal tunnel. The flexor superficialis and profundus tendons deep to the nerve have an anteroposterior diameter twice that of the median nerve. The flexor carpi radialis tendon (*open arrow*) at the lateral aspect of the median nerve is an important landmark which can assist in locating the nerve. This tendon is located outside the carpal tunnel.

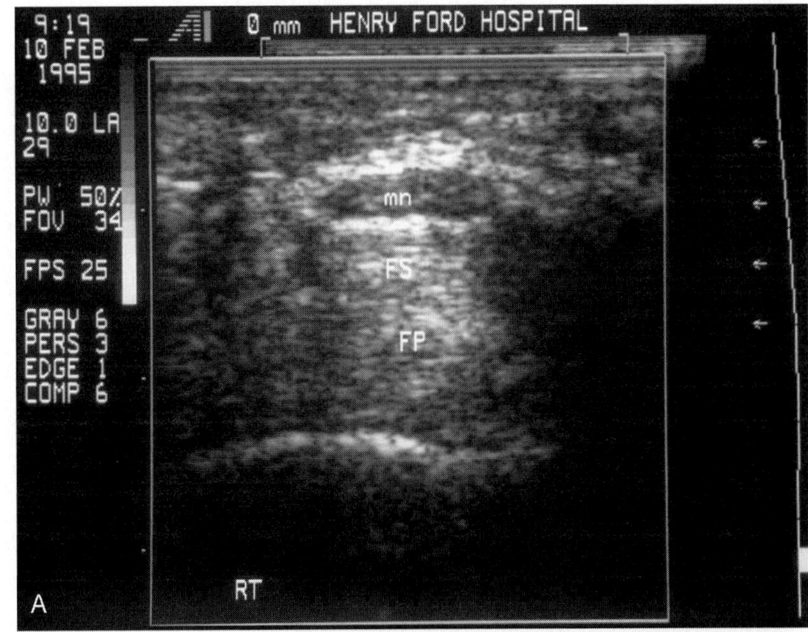

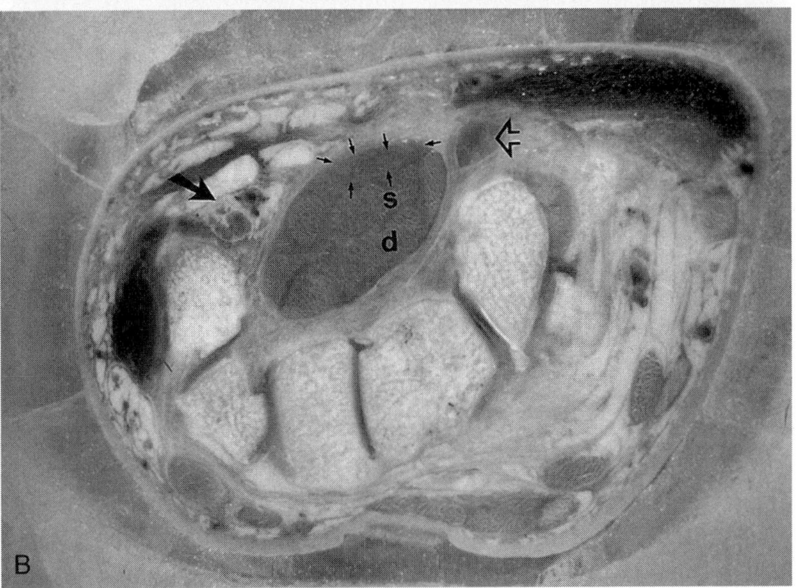

Figure 16–35 ■ Normal tendon and nerve structure: transverse section. Transverse anatomical sections were obtained through the hand. Compare the fine network of septations of the endotendineum in the flexor tendon (*arrow*) with the coarse connective stroma around the nerve fascicles (*curved arrows*). Differences in the connective tissue network of tendons and nerves result in differences in echogenicity observed with ultrasound. (Courtesy of Dr. Donald Ditmars, Henry Ford Health System.)

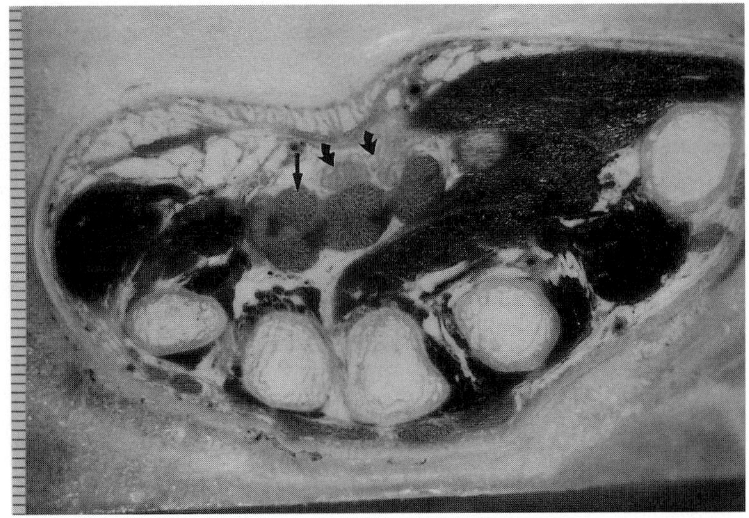

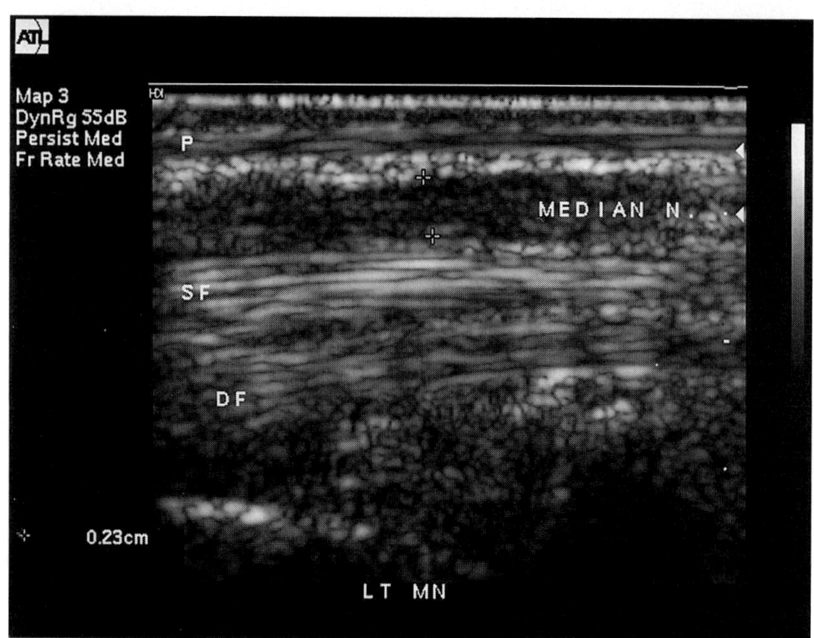

Figure 16–36 ▪ Normal median nerve: longitudinal ultrasound. The median nerve (*calipers*) of this asymptomatic 30-year-old woman courses between the palmaris longus tendon (*P*) on one side and between the superficial (*SF*) and deep (*DF*) flexor tendons of the index finger on the other side. There are fewer bright linear interfaces in tendon than in nerve.

A trigger finger is a diagnostic challenge in some patients. Stenosing tenosynovitis is the most common cause of triggering. Tendon and/or tendon synovium are caught under the A_1 flexor pulley. Sonography may demonstrate tendinitis, synovitis, or associated ganglia. However, locking and catching can relate to other causes. Bony impediments to movement may be due to osteophytosis, loose bodies, hypertrophic sesamoids, or bony irregularity. Soft tissue causes include tears of the volar capsule, tears of collateral ligaments, and torn or displaced volar plate injuries. Ultrasound is valuable in narrowing the differential diagnosis. All these structures are easily visualized sonographically. Thickening of the A_1 pulley is most frequently observed (Fig. 16–46).

Extensor tendon lesions are often posttraumatic and occur quite frequently in the fingers (Fig. 16–47). Lesions of extensors in the wrist can relate to trauma, lacerations, or rheumatoid synovitis

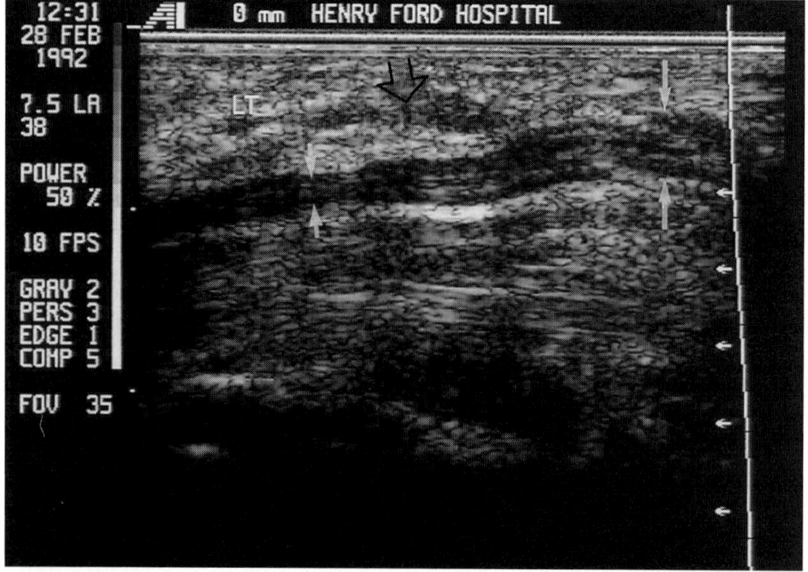

Figure 16–37 ▪ Median nerve changes in carpal tunnel disease: longitudinal ultrasound. Paresthesias in the right wrist resulted in a significant handicap in this 52-year-old transcriptionist. The longitudinal image through the median nerve demonstrates a swollen nerve (*large arrows*) proximal to the transverse carpal ligament (*open arrow*) and constriction of the nerve in the carpal tunnel (*small arrows*). The distal aspect of the extremity is displayed on the left for the examiner's convenience.

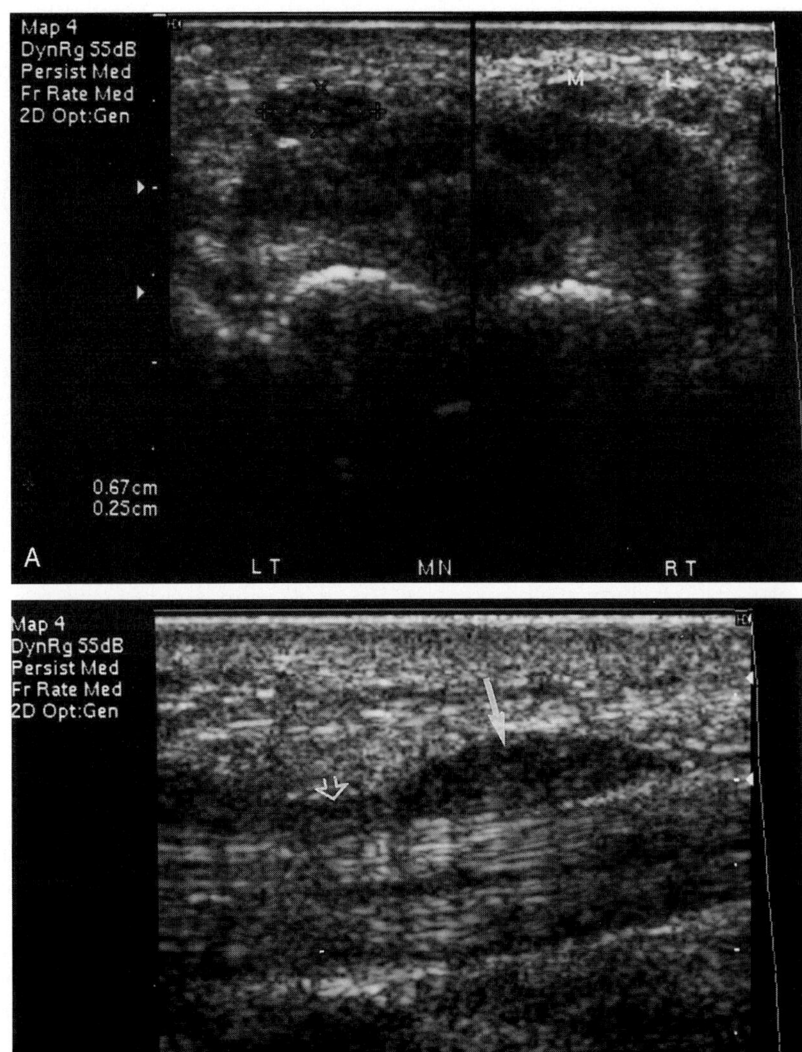

Figure 16–38 ■ **A**, Median nerve changes in carpal tunnel disease: split-screen comparison of symptomatic and asymptomatic wrists. Night pain and paresthesias in the left wrist wake up this 49-year-old man in the middle of the night. The size of the symptomatic left (*LT*) median nerve (*between the calipers*) is almost double that of the asymptomatic right (*RT*) median nerve, which has been marked as *M*. The normal cross-sectional area of the median nerve in men is about 8.3 (SD = 1.9) mm^2; a definitely abnormal cross-section is above 15 mm^2. **B**, Median nerve changes in carpal tunnel disease: longitudinal sonogram through the carpal tunnel. Same patient as in **A**. The symptomatic median nerve is focally swollen (*arrow*). Compare its size with that of the underlying tendons and that of its more normal segment proximally (*open arrow*).

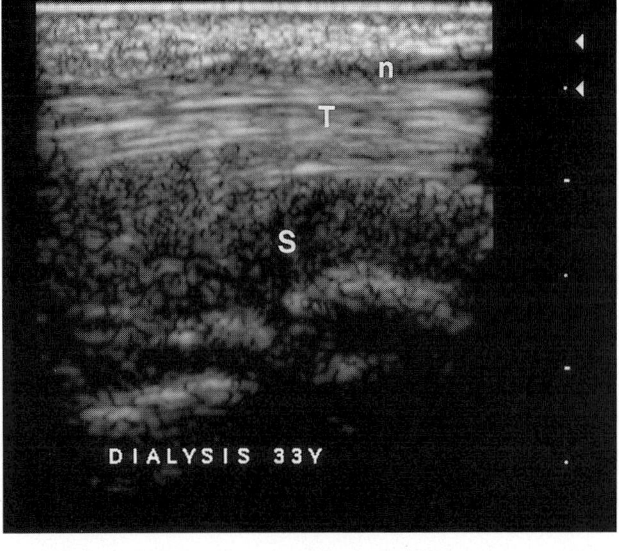

Figure 16–39 ■ Carpal tunnel disease in amyloid arthropathy: longitudinal ultrasound. This 47-year-old woman with chronic renal failure has been treated for 33 years with hemodialysis. Now she is crippled by amyloid arthropathy. In addition to her joint complaints, she experiences paresthesias in the median nerve distribution in both hands. The thenar muscles in the palms of her hands are atrophied. The wrist synovium (*S*), probably infiltrated with amyloid, compresses the flexor tendons (*T*) and the median nerve (*n*). The nerve appears thinned, probably because of the chronic pressure.

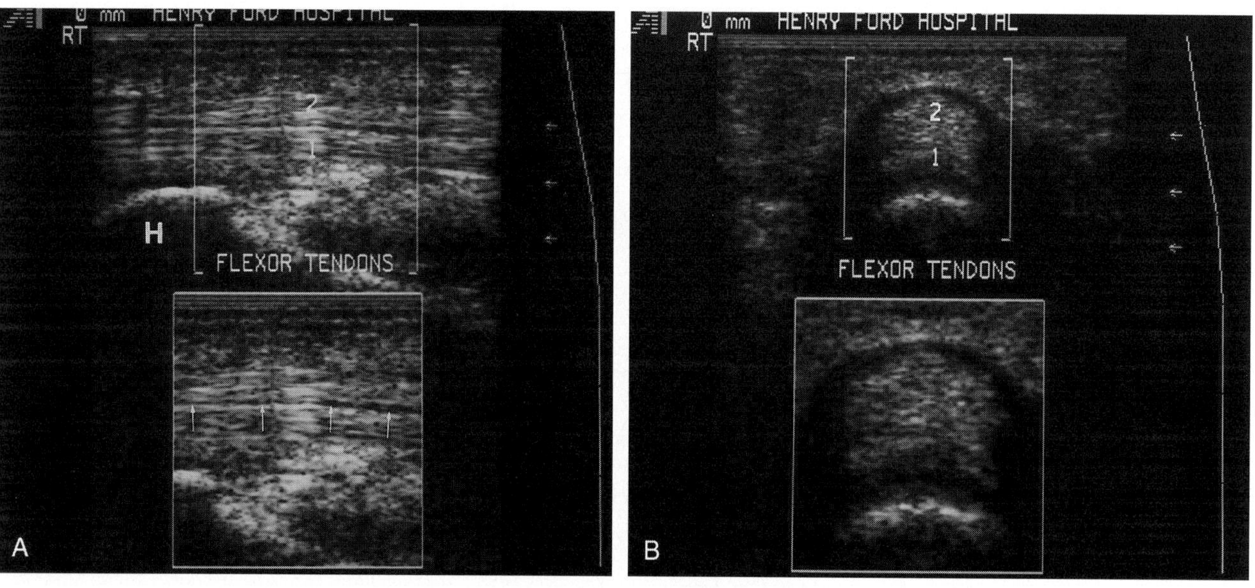

Figure 16-40 ▪ **A**, Normal flexor tendons: longitudinal ultrasound. A 10 MHz transducer, aligned along the flexor tendons of the index finger, shows the deep (*1*) and superficial (*2*) flexor tendons proximal to the metacarpal head (*H*). The insert at the bottom of the image focuses on the interface (*arrows*) between the tendons. **B**, Normal flexor tendons: transverse ultrasound. Same normal volunteer as in **A**. The transverse image of the flexor tendons at the level of the metacarpal head shows a layered architecture. The thick, hypoechoic strap, which surrounds the tendons at this level, corresponds to the A_1 pulley.

(Figs. 16-48 through 16-53). The Mallet finger, a rupture of the distal extensor tendon, is easy to diagnose clinically. Sonographic diagnosis is possible but adds unnecessary cost to the workup. A difficult clinical diagnosis is rupture of the central slip of the extensor digitorum, just distal to the proximal interphalangeal (PIP) joint (Fig. 16-54). This small lesion is very significant because it results in capsular contraction, extension deficit, and boutonniere deformity if not treated in a timely manner. The lesion can be missed at the time of injury because of swelling. Often in the initial clinical examination, the finger lesion can be mistaken for a collateral ligament tear or volar plate injury. Ultrasound examination reveals retraction at the level of the PIP joint or proximal to it. The dorsal hood should be examined if the patient has a traumatic knuckle injury. The clinical diagnosis of rupture of one of the sagittal bands might be impaired because of persistent swelling. Sagittal band rupture follows sudden, forceful extension of the finger against resistance, as in a flicking or thumping motion (Crenshaw, 1996). Discontinuity can be noted in some dorsal hood injuries. Typically, because of delay in diagnosis, the rupture is more often seen as focal swelling of one of the sagittal bands. The ultrasound report should specify whether the ulnar or radial sagittal bands are injured. Traumatic dislocation of the extensor tendon can occur secondarily, most often in the middle finger. Only ruptures of the radial slip of the dorsal hood result in ulnar dislocation of the extensor tendon (Figs. 16-55 through 16-57).

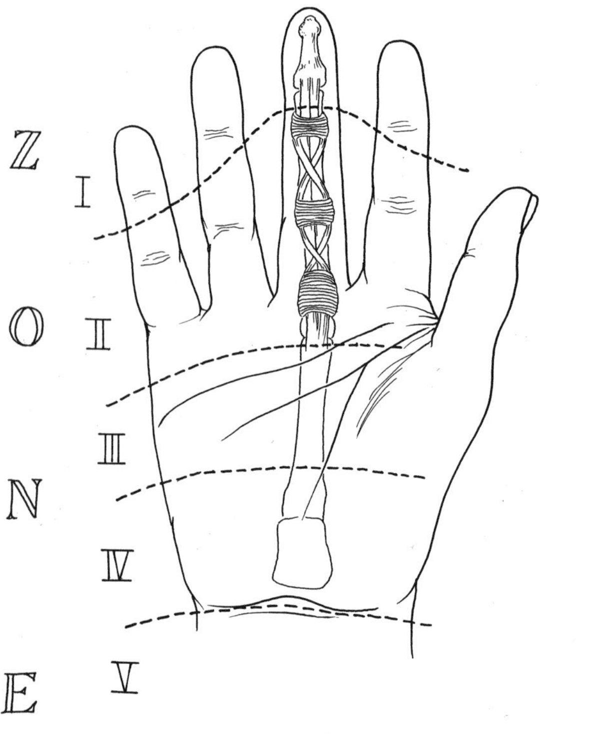

Figure 16-41 ▪ Diagram of different types of flexor tendon injuries by location.

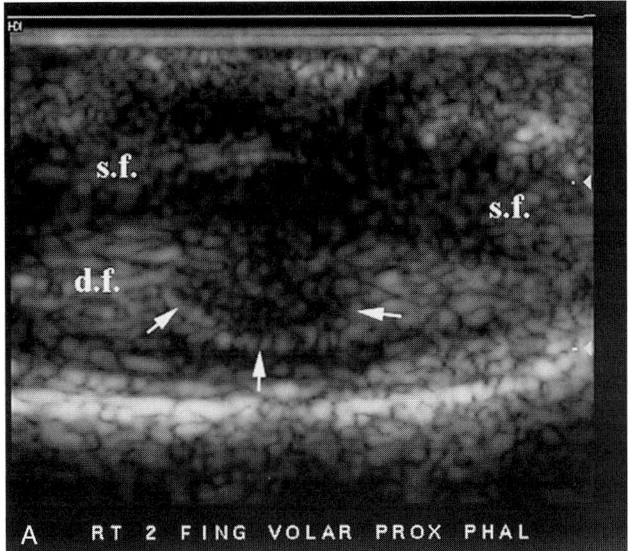

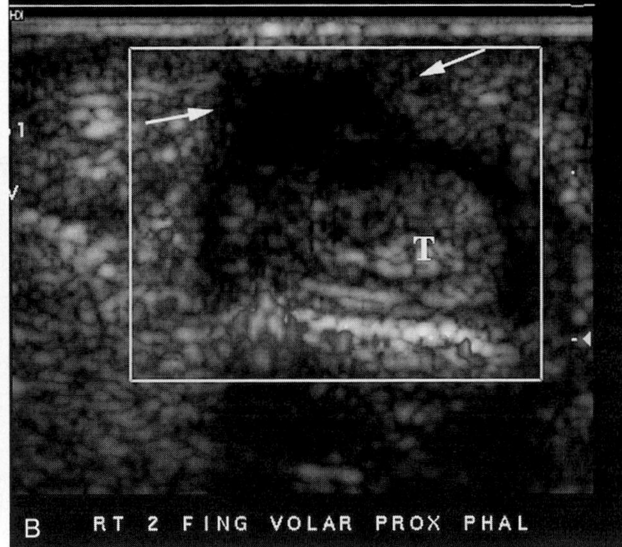

Figure 16–42 ■ **A**, Torn flexor tendons: longitudinal ultrasound. This young man was injured with a knife during a fight. The laceration along the lateral palmar aspect of the hand and at the base of the index finger healed, but he has not been able to flex his index finger. The ultrasound study shows that both the superficial (*s.f.*) and deep (*d.f.*) flexor tendons have been affected. The injury is located precisely at the level of the A_1 pulley. Laceration of the flexor digitorum superficialis (*s.f.*) seems almost complete, and laceration of the flexor digitalis profundus (*d.f.*) is quite deep (*arrows*). However, the tendons are not retracted into the palm. **B**, Torn flexor tendons: transverse ultrasound. Same patient as in **A**. This image obtained with a 12 MHz transducer demonstrates hypoechoic tissue (*arrows*) at the ulnar aspect of the index finger. Almost 50% of the ulnar side of both tendons (*T*) appears affected. The surgeon was surprised upon hearing the results of the ultrasound study because the clinical exam had suggested that the tears were complete. At surgery, the hypoechoic tissue proved to be granulation tissue.

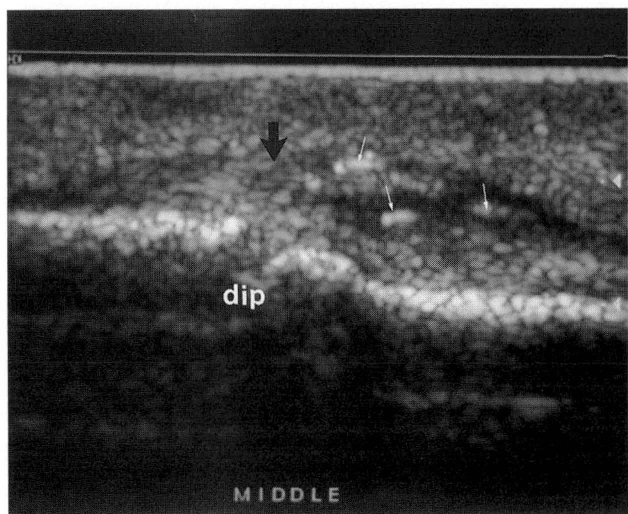

Figure 16–43 ■ Postoperative evaluation of tendon repair: longitudinal ultrasound. Finger flexion is limited in this young woman who underwent flexor digitorum profundus tendon reconstruction several months ago. Flexion of the distal interphalangeal joint (*dip*) was not possible when the proximal interphalangeal joint was fixed in extension. This made the surgeon wonder whether his sutures had come loose. The longitudinal ultrasound image demonstrates continuity (*arrow*) of tendon tissue over the dip joint. Several sutures are visible as hyperechoic structures (*white arrows*) within the tendon. A simple tendon release could now be performed, since the surgeon knew that the reconstruction was intact.

Other causes of swelling of the metacarpophalangeal region (Box 16–3) include volar plate injury, osteochondral fracture, infection, and bursal swelling. The extensor tendon can be lacerated longitudinally (Fig. 16–58). This injury results in swelling and tendon dysfunction as well. Longitudinal tears of the extensor tendon and tears of the dorsal hood often require surgical repair. Longitudinal tears along the tendon axis are not only due to direct injury (hitting,

Box 16–3
"Knuckle Injury" with Persistent Swelling

- Rupture of the dorsal hood
- Bursal synovitis
- Osteochondral injury
- Infection
- Tendon laceration
- Volar plate injury
- Collateral ligament tear

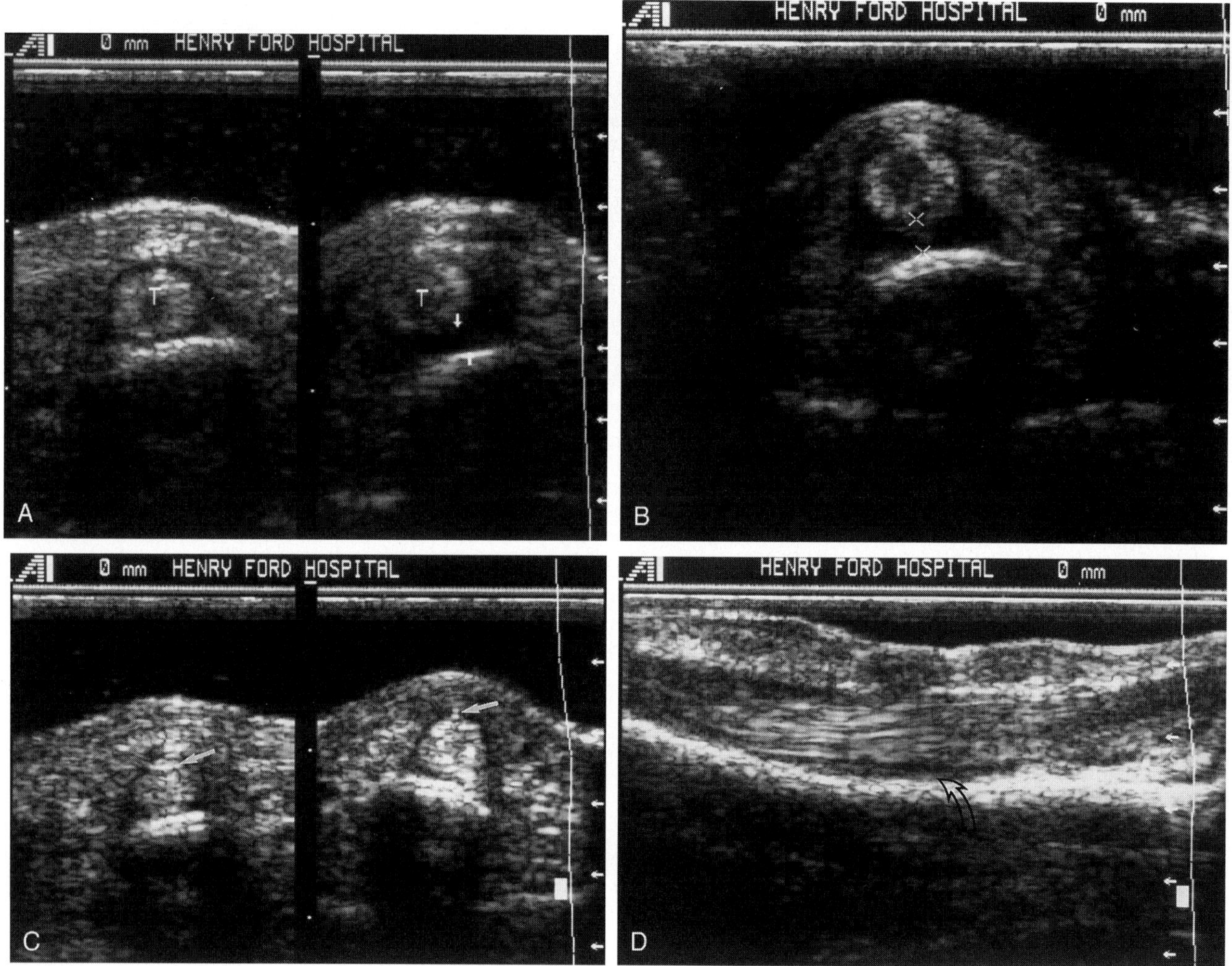

Figure 16-44 ■ **A**, Climber's finger: transverse ultrasound with split-screen technique. A 20-year-old extreme rock climber hurt his middle finger. Weakness of the finger does not allow him to continue in his sport. For the ultrasound study, we applied ample gel over the flexor surface of the tendon. The 7.5 MHz transducer is positioned perpendicularly and transversely over the flexor tendons. Gel is used as standoff, and no pressure is applied to the tissues. The finger is extended on the left side of the split screen. The flexor tendons (*T*) are resting directly on the surface of the proximal phalanx. The image on the right side of the split screen is obtained with the patient's finger trying to flex against the resistance of the examiner's finger. There is abnormal separation of the tendon from the bone surface (*arrows*). Note that when the level of scanning is at the decussation, the flexor digitorum superficialis has a doughnut shape, with the central hypoechogenicity representing the flexor digitorum profundus viewed obliquely. **B**, Climber's finger: transverse ultrasound during active finger flexion. Same patient as in **A**. The separation, which is significant, measures no more than 2 mm (measurement between calipers). **C**, Climber's finger: transverse ultrasound with split-screen technique of the contralateral normal side. Same patient as in **A**. The middle finger on the asymptomatic side depicts the normal relationship of the tendons in extension (left side of the split screen) and active flexion against resistance (right side of the split screen). There is no separation of the tendons. A normal tendon vinculum is noted in the synovium over the volar aspect (*arrow*). **D**, Climber's finger: longitudinal ultrasound of abnormal tendons at rest. Same patient as in **A**. There is slight separation of the tendons from the bone surface (*curved arrow*) on the symptomatic side.

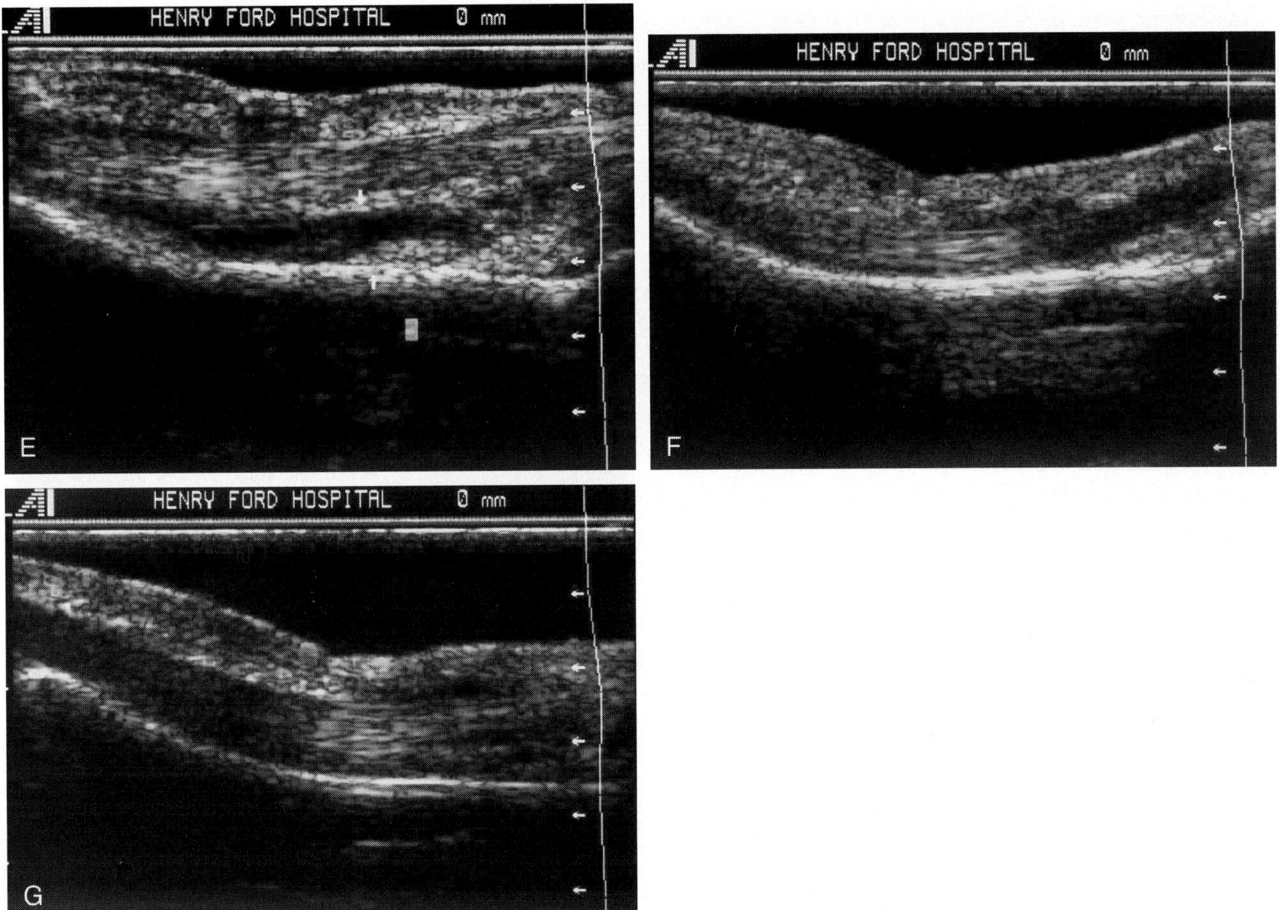

Figure 16–44 *Continued* ■ **E**, Climber's finger: longitudinal ultrasound of abnormal tendons in flexion against resistance. Same patient as in **A**. The transducer is now aligned along the tendons of the symptomatic climber's finger. The gap (*arrows*) between the bone and the tendons widens significantly. A rupture of the pulley system causes the climber's finger. Usually, the A_2 pulley ligament ruptures and allows the bowstringing of deep and superficial flexor tendons away from the cortex of the proximal phalanx. **F**, Climber's finger: longitudinal ultrasound of normal tendons at Rest. Same patient and transducer alignment as in **E**. The normal tendons of the asymptomatic contralateral middle finger at rest seem strongly affixed to the cortex of the phalanx. Note the anisotropic reflection with high-level echogenicity of tendon tissue when visualized perpendicularly and hypoechogenicity when visualized obliquely. The tendon curves with the bone toward the metacarpophalangeal joint at the observer's right and toward the proximal interphalangeal joint at the observer's left. **G**, Climber's finger: longitudinal ultrasound of normal tendons in flexion against resistance. Same patient (asymptomatic side) and transducer alignment as in Figure **F**. The middle finger contracts, and the patient's finger tries to move the observer's finger against strong resistance. Flexion in a normal finger does not cause the tendon to pull away from the bone. The pulleys fix the tendons very tightly to the bone surface.

boxing) over the metacarpal heads. The extensor carpi ulnaris (ECU), which is closely related to the bone surface of the distal ulna, may rupture longitudinally secondary to chronic stress (Figs. 16–59 and 16–60).

Collateral ligament tears of the hand are common injuries. Ultrasound examination can be valuable in acute cases, which cannot be evaluated clinically because of pain. Other indications for sonographic examination are cases in which the clinical examination suggests a more complex differential diagnosis. A small avulsion can occur at the site of ligament injury, or a small impaction fracture can occur at the opposite side. Lesions at the base of the thumb pose a more complex diagnostic challenge. The ligaments of the first metacarpophalangeal joint are often injured when a violent force suddenly abducts the thumb. A tear of the ulnar collateral ligament (UCL) happens in a fall when the thumb is caught in the strap of a ski pole or behind an obstacle. In the acute phase, ultrasound will show disruption of the layered ligamentous structure and swelling (O'Callaghan et al., 1994; Hergan et al., 1995). Ultrasound diagnosis is a considerable improvement over the earlier methods of diagnosis, which included repeated

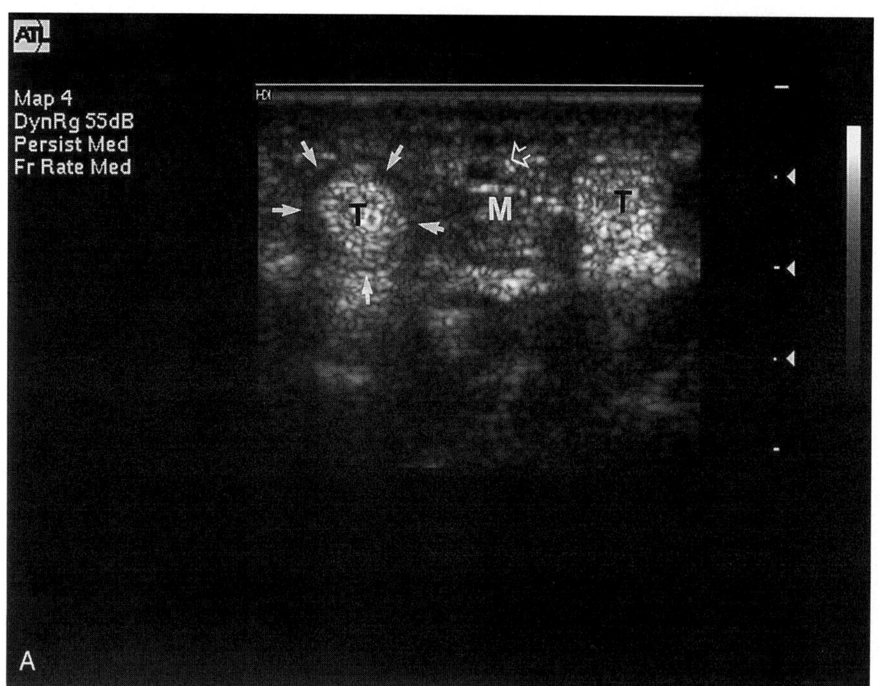

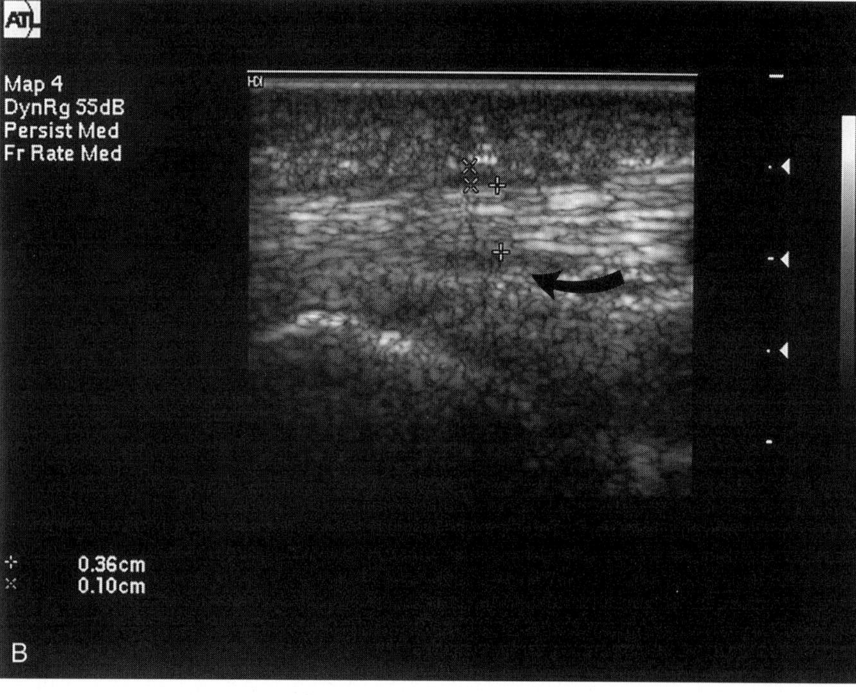

Figure 16–45 ▪ **A**, Flexor tendon tenosynovitis: transverse ultrasound. Increasing swelling and pain of the index finger of this 45-year-old radiological technologist followed a paper cut injury a few days ago. This transverse ultrasound scan over the distal palmar crease reveals a hypoechoic halo (*arrows*) surrounding the abnormal tendon, consistent with infection within the tendon sheath. The neurovascular bundle (*open arrow*) rests on the lumbrical muscles (*M*) between the flexor tendons (*T*). The septic tenosynovitis was treated urgently with surgical debridement and IV antibiotic therapy. **B**, Flexor tendon tenosynovitis: longitudinal ultrasound. Same patient as in **A**. This longitudinal image of the tendon sheath obtained with a 12 MHz transducer demonstrates hypoechoic thickening (×–×) of the tendon sheath of the flexor tendons. The volar aspect of the tendon sheath measures 1 mm. It is important to note that tendon synovium surrounds the tendon circumferentially, and swollen synovium (*curved arrow*) is present between the tendon and the metacarpophalangeal joint.

stress tests, stress radiographs, and arthrography (Figs. 16–61 and 16–62). None of these tests was efficacious, and the stress tests could displace an undisplaced ligament tear (Bronstein et al., 1994). The diagnostic challenge in tears of the UCL of the thumb is to select patients who will require surgery. A displaced ligament tear or a Stener lesion of the first metacarpophalangeal joint represents herniation of the proximal UCL dorsal to the adductor fascia (Figs. 16–62 through 16–64). A Stener lesion at the first metacarpophalangeal joint will not heal spontaneously and will require surgical repair. MRI of the UCL has been attempted, and this technique seems helpful as well. However, it is less dynamic and more expensive than ultrasound.

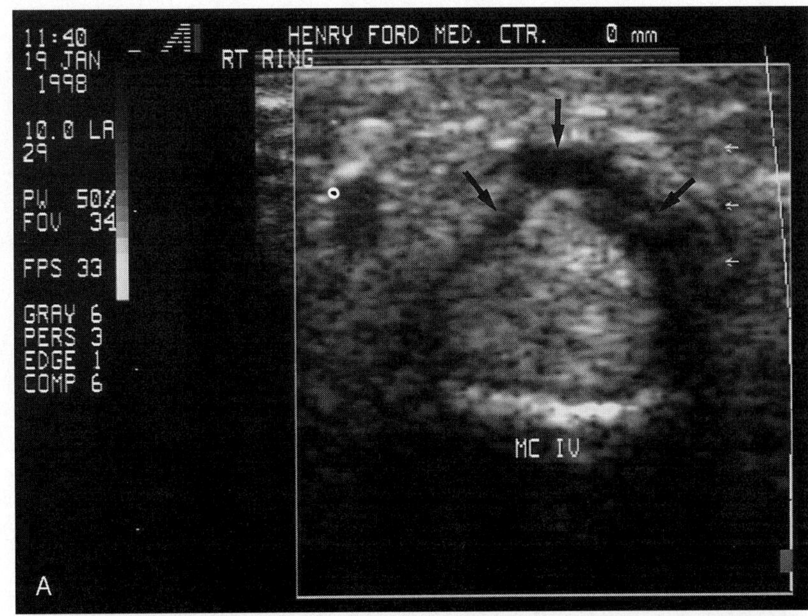

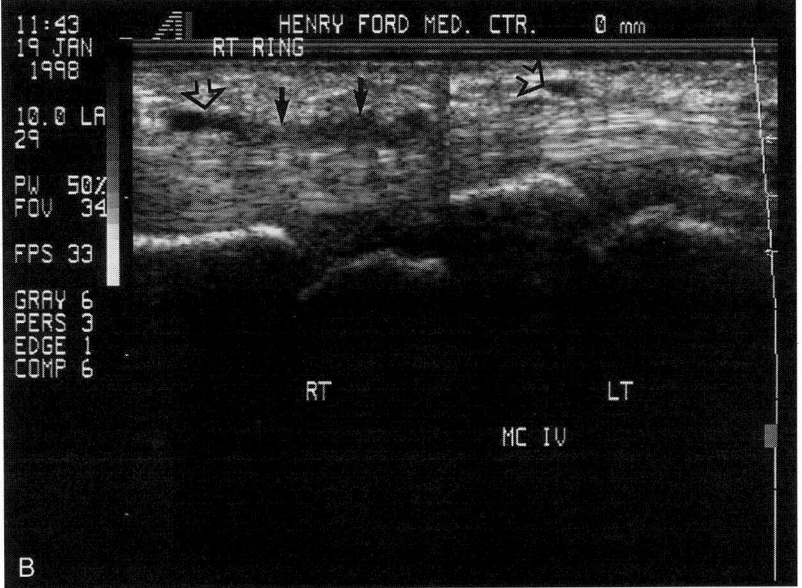

Figure 16-46 ■ **A**, Trigger finger: transverse ultrasound. Extension of the right ring finger of this 40-year-old man is impaired, painful, and discontinuous. The transverse image obtained with a 10 MHz transducer over the fourth metacarpal head depicts hypoechoic swelling (*arrows*) around the flexor tendons. The swelling is eccentric, predominantly over the volar aspect of the tendons. There is no change deep to the tendon, as in Figure 16–45. The A_1 pulley is thickened in patients with trigger fingers. This pulley does not surround the tendon in a circular fashion, as the tendon sheath does, but it surrounds the tendon in a hoof shape. Abbreviation: fourth metacarpal (*MC IV*). **B**, Trigger finger: longitudinal ultrasound. Same patient as in **A**. The A_1 pulley extends over the distal palm, proximal to and at the metacarpophalangeal joint. The thickened pulley appears as hypoechoic tissue (*arrows*). Sometimes one can observe slight thickening of the tendon sheath just distal to the pulley. In this patient it is seen both on the asymptomatic left side and on the symptomatic right side (*open arrows*).

Diagnosis of traumatic disruption of the intercarpal and capsular ligaments of the wrist is rarely based on sonographic findings. The only exception might be the diagnosis of acute ligamentous injury. Ultrasound is capable of diagnosing acute avulsion of the dorsal scapholunate ligament, for example (Fig. 16–65). It is not unusual to find a small, avulsed fragment at the dorsal aspect of the carpal bones, with associated hematoma (Fig. 16–65). This significant lesion can be repaired if it is detected quickly and assessed accurately (Crenshaw, 1996). The triangular fibrocartilage (TFC) of the wrist may also be examined sonographically (Chiou et al., 1997). Tears of the TFC result from rotational trauma during pronation and supination. Arthrography can detect smaller TFC tears than ultrasound. However, ultrasound adds value because it is able to detect subluxability of the radioulnar joint and can show irritation of the ECU tendon by identification of tenosynovitis and partial tears (see Figs. 16–59 and 16–60). Tenosynovitis and radioulnar subluxation can occur as a complication of TFC injury. Subluxation and dislocation of the ECU can occur in combination with TFC tears or as an isolated finding. This lesion is secondary to rupture of supporting ligaments of this extensor tendon. A

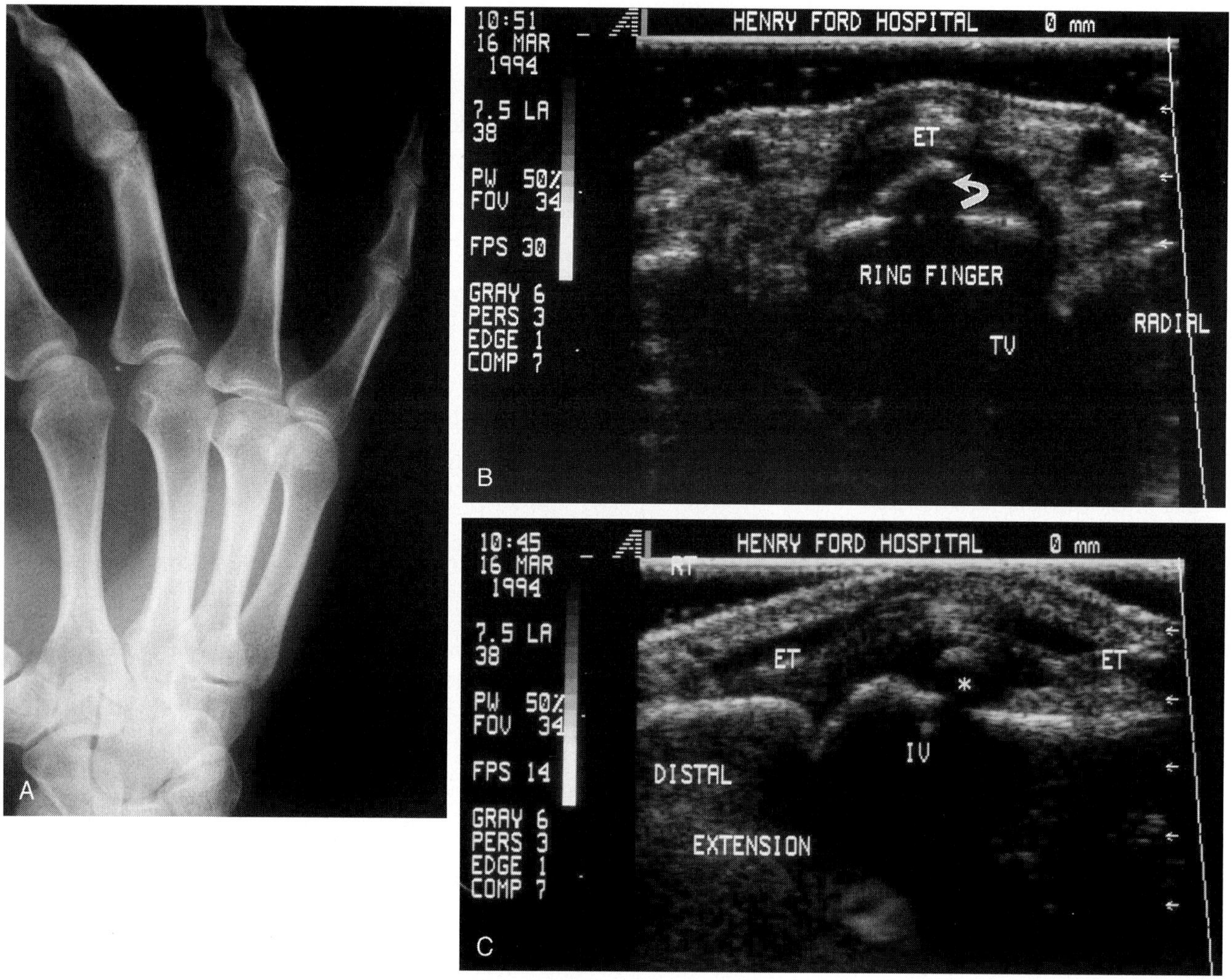

Figure 16–47 ■ **A**, Extensor tendon dysfunction: oblique hand radiograph. A middle-aged woman has difficulty extending the ring finger of her right hand. Radiographs had been interpreted as showing posttraumatic and arthritic change at the fourth metacarpophalangeal joint. **B**, Extensor tendon dysfunction: transverse ultrasound of the ring finger. Same patient as in Figure **A**. The extensor tendon (*ET*) appears displaced by a curvilinear, hyperechoic structure (*curved arrow*). Abbreviation: transverse (*TV*). **C**, Extensor tendon dysfunction: longitudinal ultrasound of the ring finger. Same patient as in **B**. An intra-articular loose body (*) is noted in the fourth metacarpophalangeal joint between the extensor tendon (*ET*) and the bone surface of the distal fourth metacarpal (*IV*). The overstretched extensor mechanism cannot function properly.

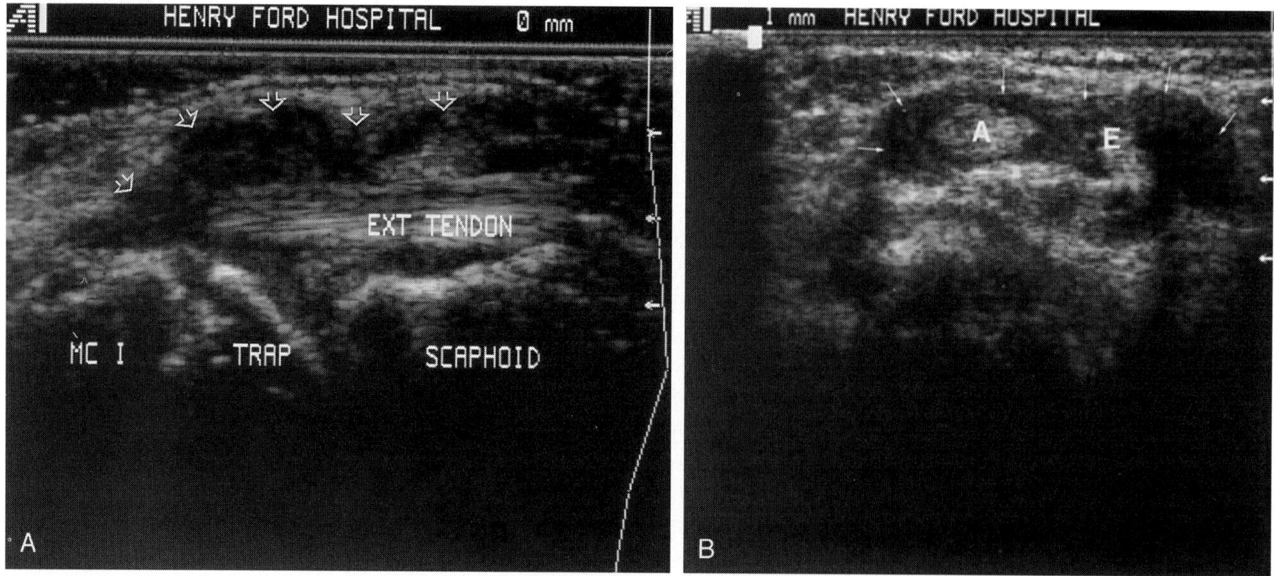

Figure 16–48 ■ *See legend on opposite page*

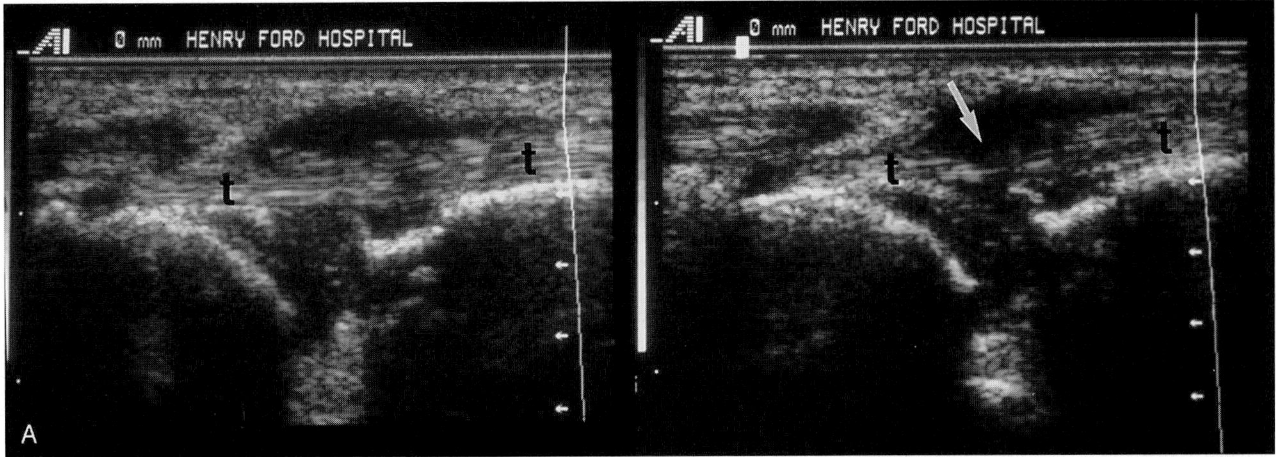

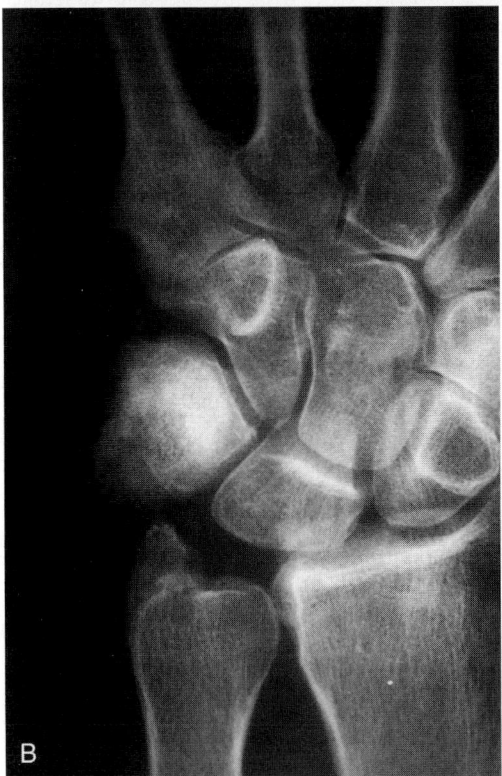

Figure 16–49 ■ **A**, Follow-up of psoriatic tenosynovitis: longitudinal ultrasound with split-screen technique. Afflicted by active psoriatic arthritis and tenosynovitis, this middle-aged woman continued to have a swollen wrist while under treatment. The extensor carpi ulnaris (*t*) appears irregular on the longitudinal image at the right side of the split screen. Irregular synovium surrounds the diseased tendon. The right side of the split screen demonstrates the tendon abnormality 6 months later. The tendon has thinned to a thread (*arrow*). **B**, Follow-up of psoriatic tenosynovitis: anteroposterior wrist radiograph. Same patient as in **A**. Characteristic proliferative bone changes are seen around the pisiform, triquetrum, and ulnar styloid in this patient with psoriatic tenosynovitis.

Figure 16–48 ■ **A**, Rheumatoid synovitis of extensor tendons: longitudinal ultrasound. This 50-year-old woman complains of pain and swelling over the lateral wrist. Her thumb extension is limited on the affected side. With a 7.5 MHz transducer aligned along the extensor pollicis brevis tendon, one detects a tendon sheath that exceeds the thickness of the tendon. The inhomogeneous, hypoechoic character of the swelling probably reflects a mixture of fluid, fibrinous debris, synovial edema, and cell proliferation. Abbreviations: first metacarpal (*MCI*), trapezium (*TRAP*). **B**, Rheumatoid synovitis of extensor tendons: transverse ultrasound. Same patient as in **A**. This transverse sonogram over the first extensor compartment reveals hypoechoic distention (*arrows*) of the tendon sheath surrounding the extensor pollicis brevis and abductor pollicis longus (*A*).

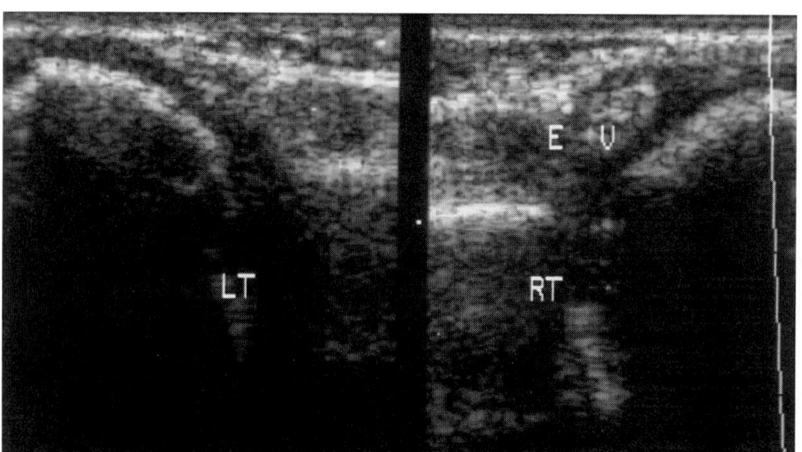

Figure 16–50 ■ Tear of the extensor of the fifth finger: transverse ultrasound. An acute drop of her fifth finger brings this 44-year-old patient to her rheumatologist for an emergency visit. The patient had been treated with Ridaura for rheumatoid arthritis, which was diagnosed 8 years ago. The split-screen transverse images over the ulnar aspect of both wrists demonstrate a normal extensor tendon of the fifth finger (*EV*) on the right and an absent torn tendon on the left. Abbreviation: fifth (*V*) extensor tendon (*E*).

palpable click in the wrist or pain over the ulnar styloid suggests the diagnosis. Sonographic evaluation of the joints of the carpus is limited due to the very tightly adherent joint capsule. These joints are best evaluated by radiographic examination and arthrography.

Soft tissue masses involving the fingers and wrist are relatively common findings. The sonographic appearance of tumors and their location are often pathognomonic for their respective diseases. Small, very vascular tumors located beneath the nail plate typically represent glomus tumors (Fig. 16–66). These lesions are very painful and can erode the surface of bone, resulting in punched-out lytic defects that are visible on radiographs and ultrasound scans. Some glomus tumors are located

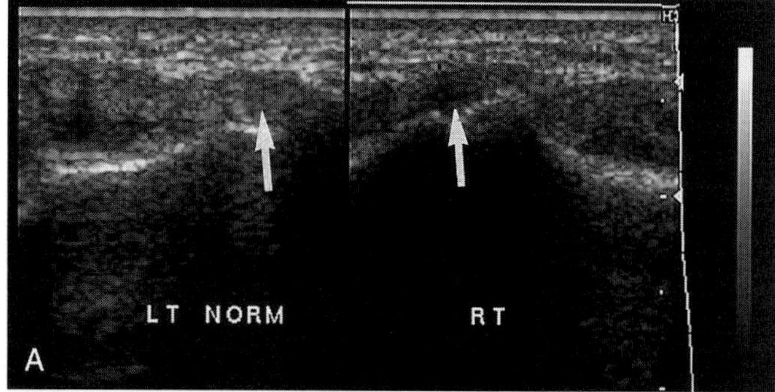

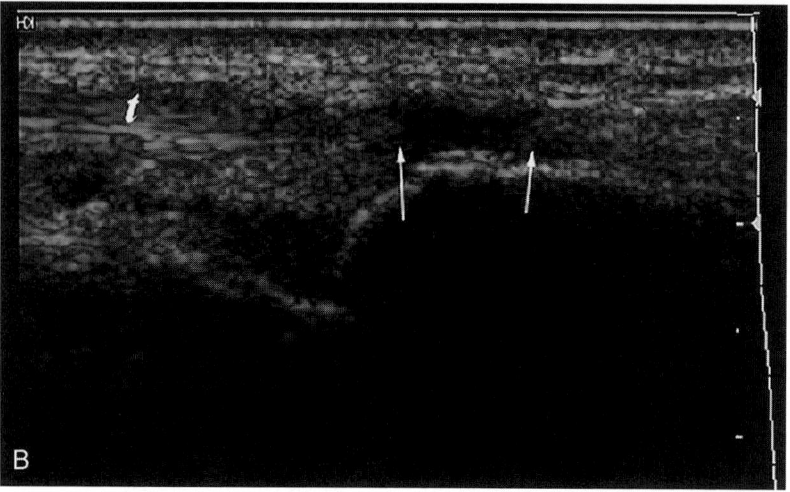

Figure 16–51 ■ **A**, Extensor pollicis longus tear: transverse ultrasound. Three months after jamming his wrist at work, this 51-year-old man noticed loss of extension of the interphalangeal joint of the right thumb. It took 1 month for the swelling of the wrist to subside after the injury, and he observed a "knot" developing over his thumb. This split-screen image compares the normal left (*LT*) transverse image of the wrist and the abnormal right image (*RT*). The groove for the extensor pollicis longus (*arrow*) appears empty on the right, and a normal tendon is identified on the left. The ultrasound examination confirms that the rupture is present at the wrist rather than in the thumb. A more proximal rupture necessitates an extensor indicis proprius transfer rather than a Mallet finger type of operation. **B**, Extensor pollicis longus tear: longitudinal ultrasound. Same patient as in **A**. Complete disruption (*arrows*) of the fibrillar pattern of the tendon (*t*) in the bony groove at the distal radius.

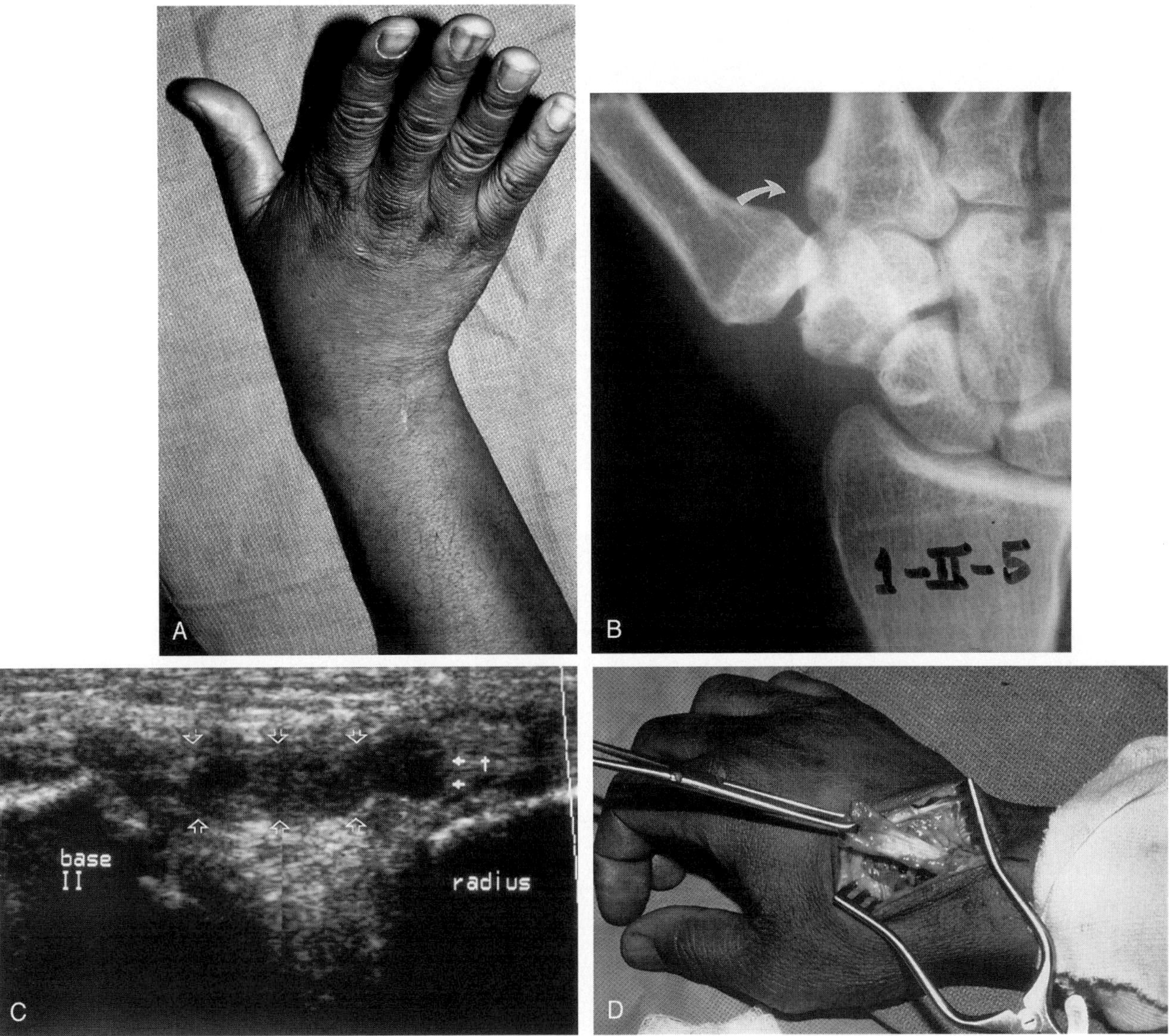

Figure 16–52 ■ **A**, Tear of the extensor carpi radialis longus: clinical photograph. A middle-aged man injured his hand at work. He experiences difficulty extending his wrist when he tries to grasp objects from a shelf. The clinician notices spontaneous ulnar deviation of the hand on full extension of the wrist. **B**, Tear of the extensor carpi radialis longus: conventional radiograph. Same patient as in **A**. Soft tissue swelling is noted at the lateral aspect of the wrist. A small defect and calcification (*curved arrow*) are noted at the base of the second metacarpal. **C**, Tear of the extensor carpi radialis longus: longitudinal ultrasound. Same patient as in **A**. The transducer is aligned along the long axis of the forearm and over the radial aspect of the wrist. There is retraction of the extensor radialis longus (*t*) proximal to the level of the distal radius (*small arrows*). A hypoechoic, probably blood-filled space (*open arrows*) extends from the distal radius to the proximal second metacarpal (*base II*), on which the extensor carpi radialis should insert. **D**, Tear of the extensor carpi radialis brevis and longus: surgical exploration. Same patient as in **A**. The surgeon grabs the end of the retracted tendon. The tendon can be restored to its original length by pulling on it. Subsequently, the tendon was reinserted on the second metacarpal. (Clinical and surgical photographs courtesy of Dr. J. Failla, Henry Ford Health System.)

within the pulp of the distal-most soft tissue of the fingers (Fornage and Rifkin, 1988). Mucoid cysts are frequently found in the region of the nail and around the distal interphalangeal joints. These cysts are part of the differential diagnosis of glomus tumors because of their hypoechoic appearance and their overlap in typical locations (Fornage and Rifkin, 1988). However, these lesions do not cause

Text continued on page 561

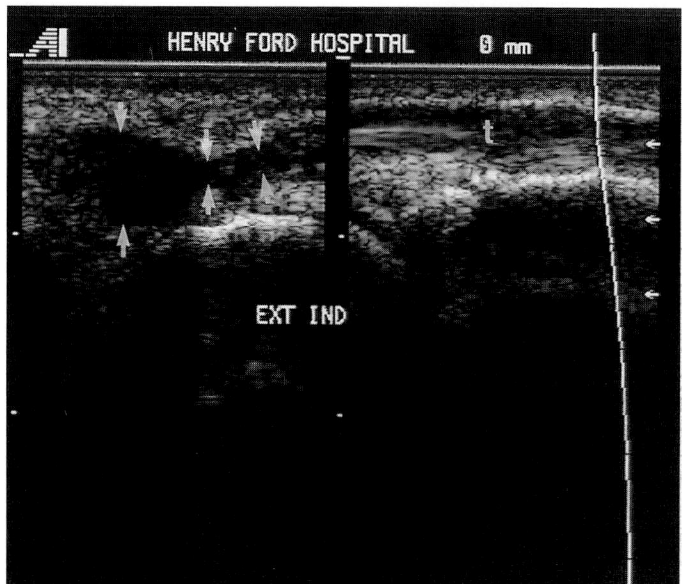

Figure 16–53 ■ Tear of the extensor tendon of the index finger: split-screen comparison of normal and abnormal wrists. A sudden drop of the index finger developed several months after a distal radius fracture in this 58-year-old woman. This longitudinal sonogram through the extensor compartment over the distal radius reveals that the tear is located in the wrist, not in the hand or finger. The empty synovium (*arrows*) filled with fluid is noted on the affected side and at the left side of the split screen. The normal tendon (*t*) of the opposite wrist is depicted on the right. Because of the significant retraction, the patient needed grafting for repair.

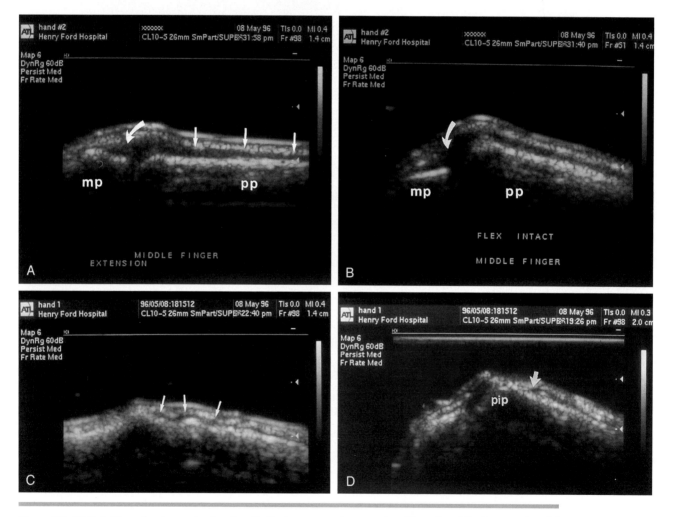

Figure 16–54 ■ **A**, Normal extensor tendon: longitudinal sonogram in extension. Normal middle finger with solid attachment of the central slip (*curved arrow*) of the extensor tendon (*arrows*) at the base of the middle phalanx (*mp*). Abbreviation: proximal phalanx (*pp*). **B**, Normal extensor tendon: longitudinal sonogram in flexion. Same normal finger as in **A**. With the proximal interphalangeal joint flexed, the central slip (*curved arrow*) is still visible with its attachment on the base of the middle phalanx (*mp*). Abbreviation: proximal phalanx (*pp*). **C**, Tear of the extensor tendon: longitudinal sonogram in extension. The middle finger of the contralateral hand of the same patient as in **A** exhibits a mild extension deficit of the proximal interphalangeal joint. The distal extensor tendon seems thin, wavy, and retracted (*arrows*). **D**, Tear of the extensor tendon: longitudinal sonogram in flexion. Same finger as in **C**. With the proximal interphalangeal joint (*pip*) flexed, the tendon retraction becomes more obvious. No tendon tissue is visible between the distal torn tendon (*solid arrow*) and the pip joint.

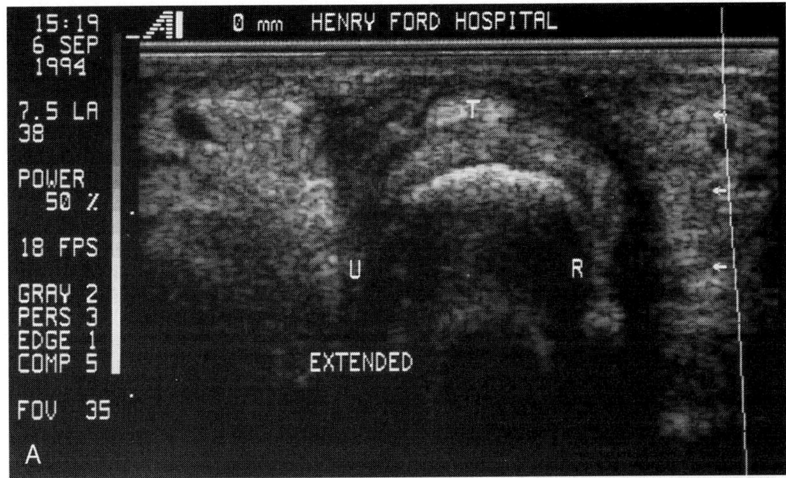

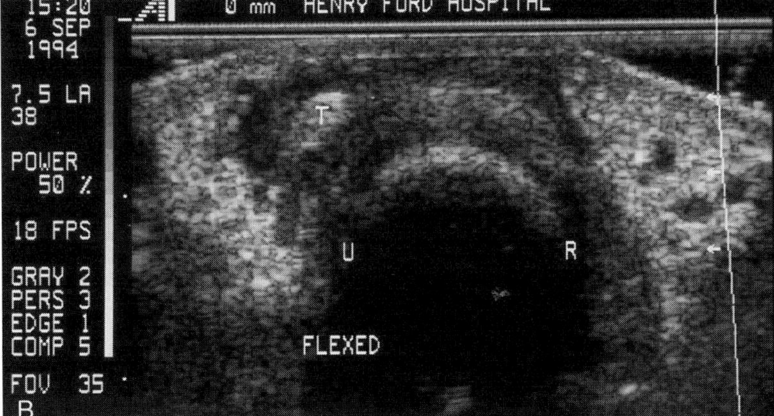

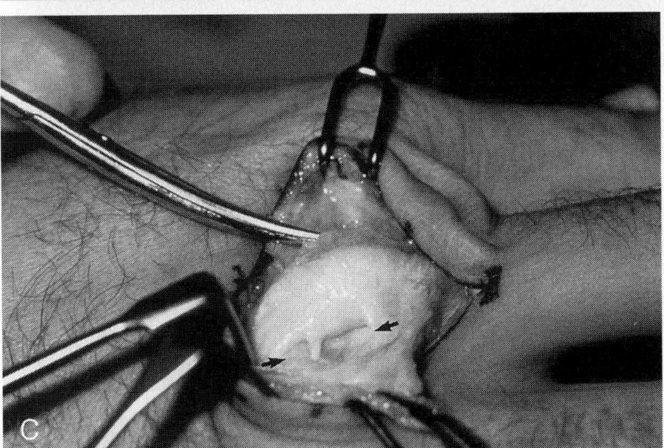

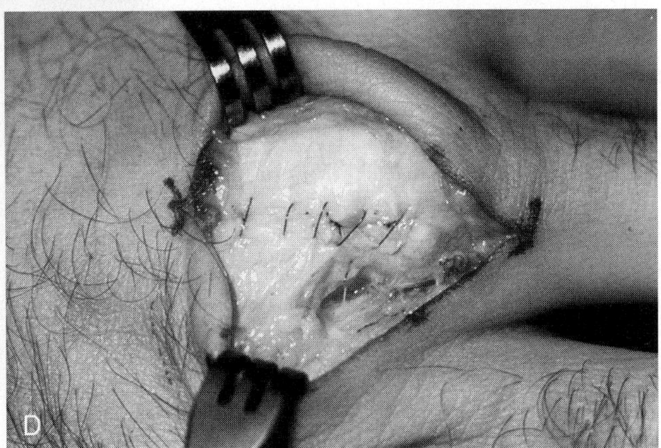

Figure 16-55 ■ **A**, Tear of the dorsal hood: transverse sonogram of the extended finger. While bowling, this 46-year-old barber twisted his left middle finger, with subsequent onset of swelling and pain. Now, 3 weeks later, he has difficulty gripping and a feeling of something popping over the knuckle. A 7.5 MHz transducer is placed over the dorsal aspect of the patient's third metacarpophalangeal joint. Very light pressure is applied on the instrument. Significant edema is noted over the third metacarpal head. The extensor tendon (*T*) with associated hypoechoic swelling is noted. The ulnar (*U*) and radial (*R*) sides of the middle finger have been indicated. **B**, Tear of the dorsal hood: transverse sonogram of the flexed finger. Same patient as in **A**. With the fist clenched, one observes the extensor tendon (*T*) sliding toward the ulnar side of the middle finger. Hypoechoic edema or granulation tissue surrounds the tendon. This lesion is due to rupture of the sagittal band on the radial side of the finger (*R*). **C**, Tear of the dorsal hood: surgical exploration. Same patient as in **A**. A defect (*arrows*) is seen in the sagittal band on the radial side of the dorsal hood. **D**, Tear of the dorsal hood: surgical repair. Same patient as in **A**. The dorsal hood defect is closed with sutures. The patient was asymptomatic 5 weeks after surgery, and he returned to work 1 month later.

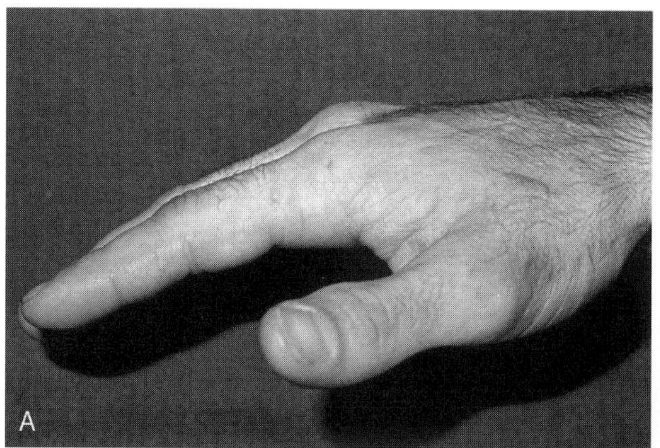

Figure 16–56 ■ **A**, Acute tear of the dorsal hood: clinical picture. A professional hockey player took a hit across the knuckles of his right hand. Swelling of the soft tissues over the metacarpals III, IV, and V makes a good clinical examination impossible. **B**, Acute tear of the dorsal hood: transverse ultrasound of the dorsum of the hand. Same patient as in **A**. With the ultrasound transducer over the metacarpal heads and the wrist clenched, one can see that the extensor tendon slipped (*curved arrows*) toward the ulnar side of the hand. **C**, Acute tear of the dorsal hood: split-screen ultrasound comparison of the dorsum of both hands. Same patient as in **A**. A 7.5 MHz transducer is positioned transversely over the left and right fourth metacarpals with the hand in the clenched fist position. The right extensor tendon (*RT*) has slipped toward the ulnar side of the fourth metacarpal condyle, while the left (*LT*) extensor tendon stays centered over the middle of the condyle. Abbreviation: fourth extensor tendon (*T*).

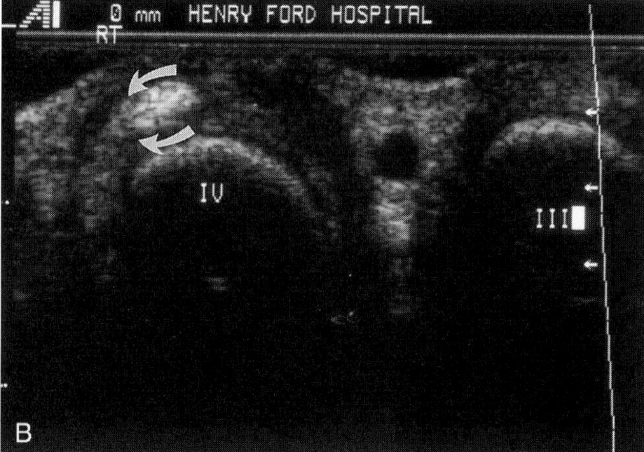

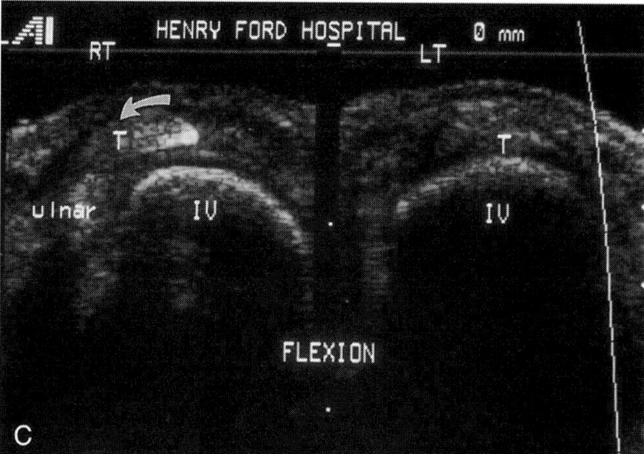

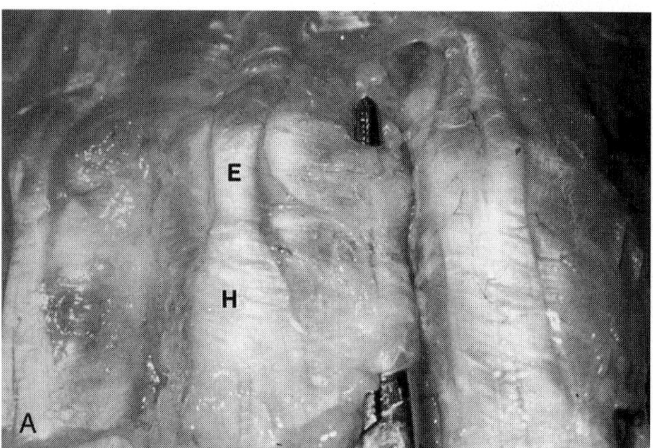

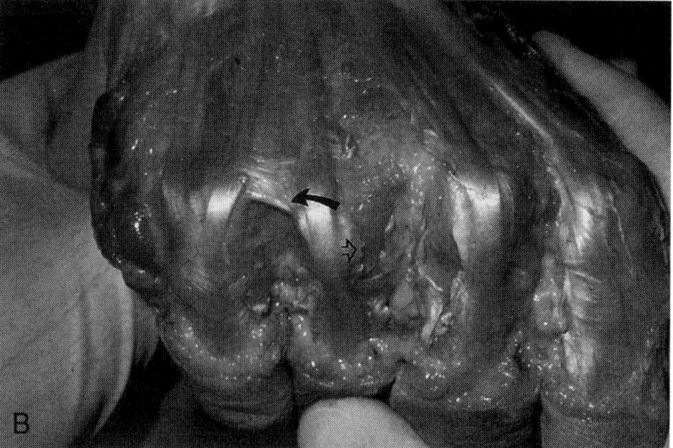

Figure 16–57 ■ **A**, Cadaver model of the dorsal hood injury: dorsal view of the dorsal hood. A hemostat has been placed under the sagittal band of the dorsal hood (*H*) on the radial side of the extensor tendon (*E*). **B**, Cadaver model of the dorsal hood injury: dorsal view of the dorsal hood. The extensor tendon of the fourth finger subluxes (*curved arrow*) toward the ulnar side of the hand after the radial slip of the dorsal hood has been severed (*open arrow*). (Courtesy of Dr. Mark Koniuch, Beaumont Hospital.)

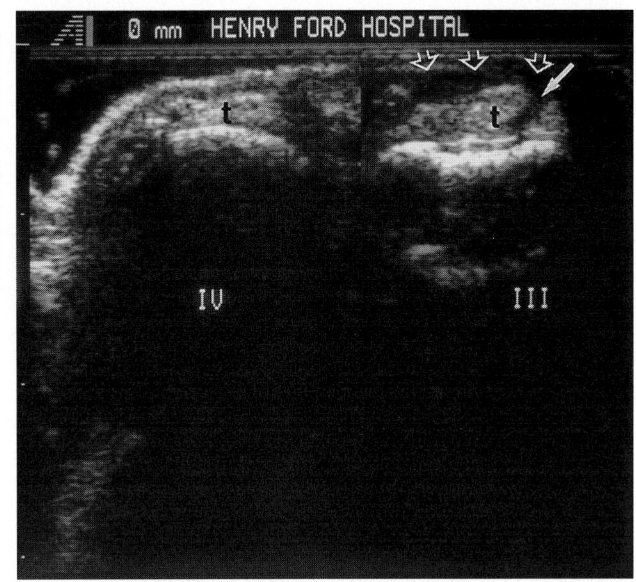

Figure 16–58 ■ Extensor tendon laceration: transverse sonogram. Chronic pain and swelling of the knuckle over the dorsum of the left hand was the chief complaint of this patient. A penetrating injury to the hand had occurred at work months ago. Transverse images obtained with a 10 MHz transducer over the dorsal aspect of the metacarpophalangeal joints demonstrate a significant difference between the extensor tendon (*t*) of the affected middle finger (*III*) and the extensor tendon (*t*) of the normal ring finger (*IV*) of the same hand. Soft tissue swelling (*open arrows*) appears around the abnormal tendon. A deep cut (*arrow*) is noted along the radial aspect of the tendon. This longitudinal tear needed surgical repair.

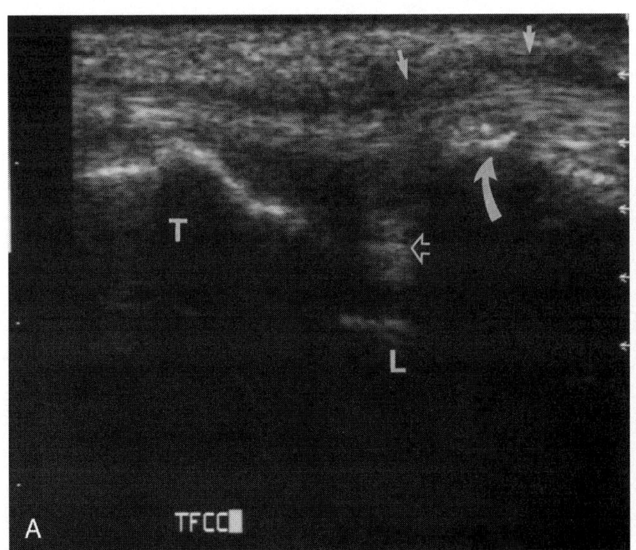

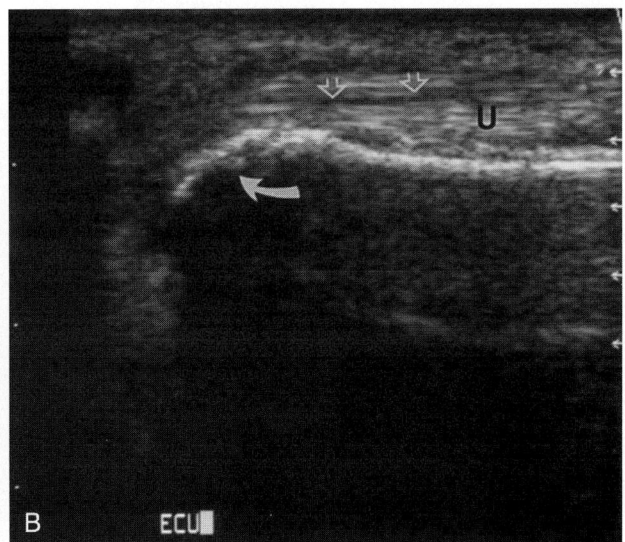

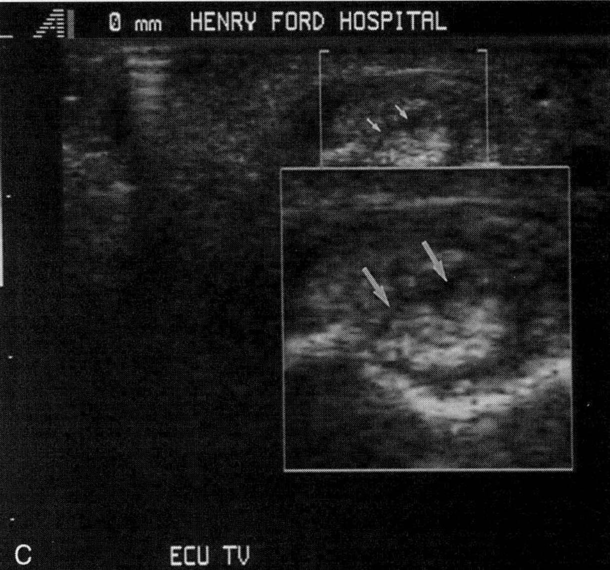

Figure 16–59 ■ **A**, Longitudinal tear of the extensor carpi ulnaris: longitudinal sonogram. This 57-year-old female presents with pain at the ulnar aspect of the wrist. A single-contrast wrist arthrogram was performed and revealed no abnormality. Bony irregularity (*curved arrow*) involving the styloid process of the ulna is noted. The tendon and sheath of the extensor carpi ulnaris (*arrows*) are irregular and inhomogeneous. The visualized peripheral portion of the triangular fibrocartilage (*open arrow*) is normal. Abbreviations: lunate (*L*), triquetrum (*T*). **B**, Longitudinal tear of the extensor carpi ulnaris: longitudinal sonogram. Same patient as in **A**. The transducer is positioned more proximally over the extensor carpi ulnaris (*U*). A longitudinal tear (*open arrows*) is demonstrated extending along the length of the tendon. Again noted is bony irregularity (*curved arrow*) of the styloid process. **C**, Longitudinal tear of the extensor carpi ulnaris: transverse sonogram. Same patient as in **A**. This image with magnification demonstrates the extensor carpi ulnaris tendon in transverse section. A hypoechoic cleft (*arrows*) is identified running obliquely through the tendon, consistent with a longitudinal tear.

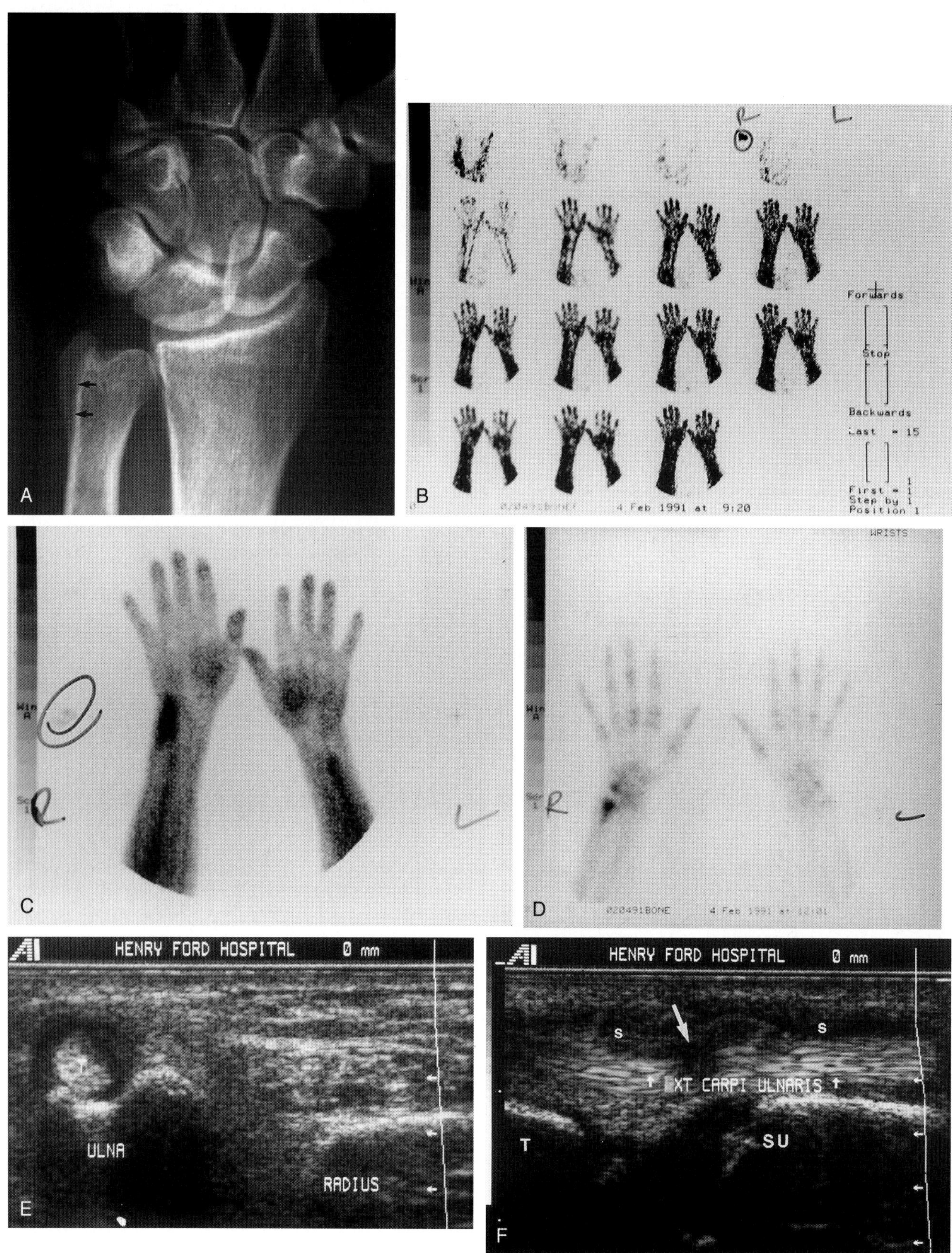

Figure 16–60 ▪ *See legend on opposite page*

Figure 16-60 ■ **A**, Extensor carpi ulnaris (ECU) tenosynovitis: anteroposterior radiograph. A 65-year-old female patient presented with a 3-month history of pain over the ulnar aspect of the wrist. This radiographic examination is normal. Note the bony groove (*arrows*) over the medial aspect of the distal ulna for the ECU tendon. **B**,**C**,**D**, ECU tenosynovitis: triple phase bone scan. Same patient as in **A**. Arterial phase and blood pool images from a triple phase bone scan demonstrate increased activity at the distal aspect of the ulna and surrounding soft tissues. Delayed images demonstrate increased activity within the bone despite a normal radiograph. **E**, ECU tenosynovitis: transverse sonogram. Same patient as in **A**. The ECU tendon (*T*) is seen within the shallow groove along the dorsal aspect of the distal ulna. A hypoechoic halo surrounding the tendon represents an inflamed tendon sheath. **F**, ECU tenosynovitis: longitudinal sonogram. Same patient as in **A**. A focused image on the tendon between the styloid process of the ulna (*SU*) and the triquetrum (*T*) shows changes in addition to synovitis (*s*). With the 7.5 MHz transducer placed along the long axis of the extensor carpi ulnaris tendon, one observes subtle damage (*arrow*) of the synovial surface and of the substance of the tendon.

bone erosion and are typically avascular. Another lesion found in the finger tip is the epidermoid inclusion cyst. This cyst is also hypoechoic but often contain keratin, which appears as hyperechoic foci within the lesion (Fornage and Rifkin, 1988). Of course, the differential diagnosis of these lesions also includes foreign body granuloma. Differentiation of the above-mentioned lesions from a foreign body granuloma is often challenging, but is possible by careful examination for the foreign body. A single hyperechoic focus surrounded by hypoechoic fluid or granulation tissue on all sides usually represents a foreign body (Fig. 16-67). Foreign bodies detected by ultrasound may be so small that they must be removed with magnifying lenses.

Ganglia are anechoic or markedly hypoechoic, with a very homogeneous appearance. Fibrous sep-

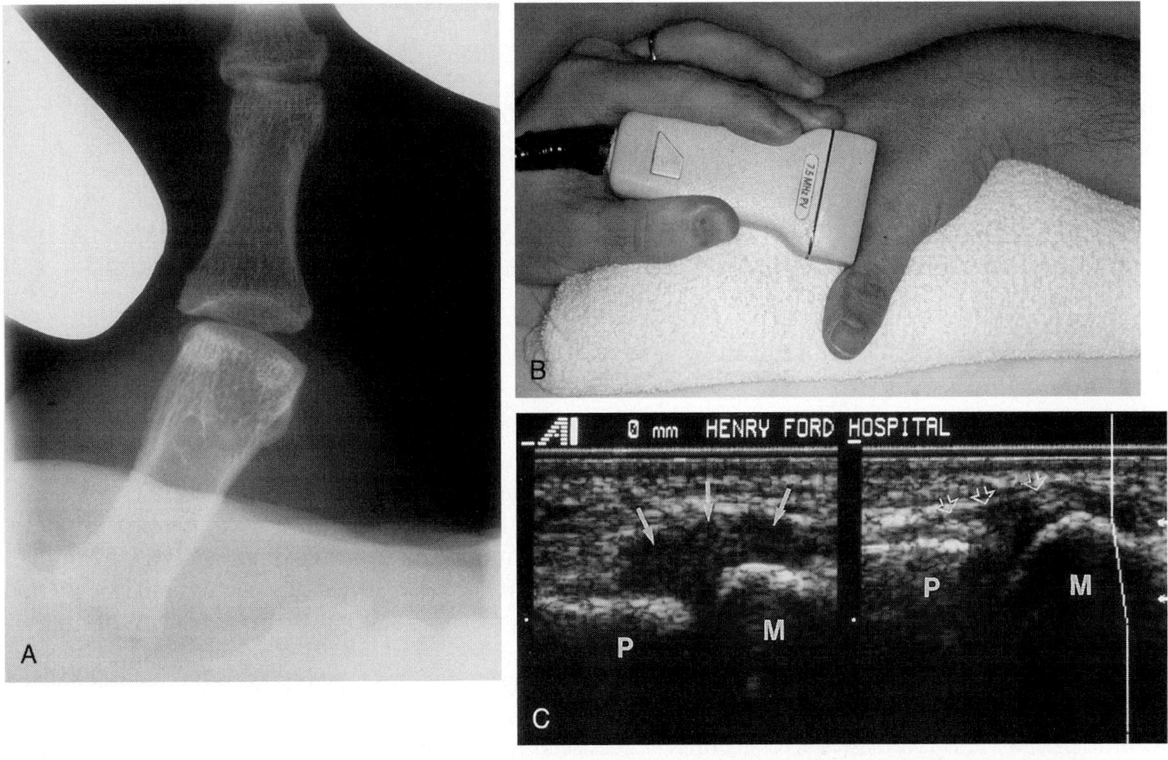

Figure 16-61 ■ **A**, Ulnar collateral ligament tear: stress radiograph. While skiing 2 weeks ago, this patient caught a thumb in the strap of a ski pole. In this radiograph, radial stress is applied with a gloved hand. Widening of the medial joint space is observed, indicative of ulnar collateral ligament injury. This technique is no longer utilized, because it does not allow us to distinguish displaced from nondisplaced tears. Furthermore, in some cases, a nondisplaced tear would be converted into a displaced tear. **B**, Ulnar collateral ligament tear: clinical photograph. Same patient as in **A**. The transducer is positioned along the long axis of the abducted thumb at the medial aspect of the metacarpophalangeal joint. **C**, Ulnar collateral ligament tear: longitudinal sonograms, split screen. Same patient as in **A**. The normal collateral ligament of the contralateral ulnar side is seen on the right. A finely layered, smoothly contoured ligament (*open arrows*) is identified bridging the joint space. The symptomatic torn ligament (*arrows*) on the left demonstrates disruption of the normal architecture and associated swelling. Abbreviations: metacarpal (*M*), proximal phalanx (*P*).

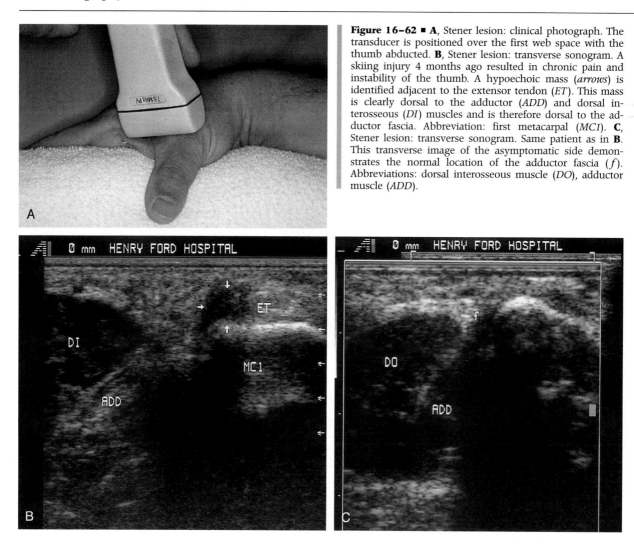

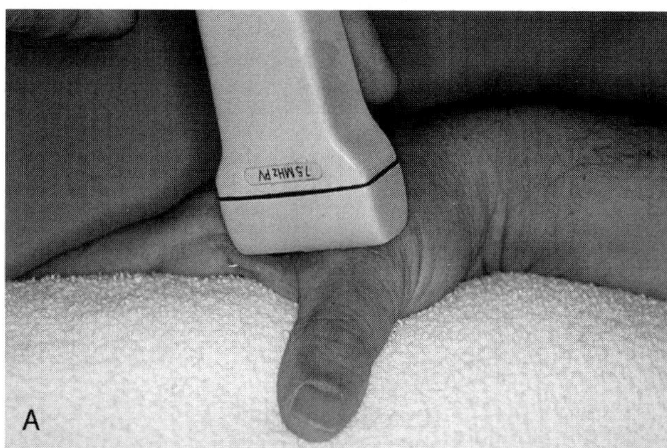

Figure 16–62 ■ **A**, Stener lesion: clinical photograph. The transducer is positioned over the first web space with the thumb abducted. **B**, Stener lesion: transverse sonogram. A skiing injury 4 months ago resulted in chronic pain and instability of the thumb. A hypoechoic mass (*arrows*) is identified adjacent to the extensor tendon (*ET*). This mass is clearly dorsal to the adductor (*ADD*) and dorsal interosseous (*DI*) muscles and is therefore dorsal to the adductor fascia. Abbreviation: first metacarpal (*MC1*). **C**, Stener lesion: transverse sonogram. Same patient as in **B**. This transverse image of the asymptomatic side demonstrates the normal location of the adductor fascia (*f*). Abbreviations: dorsal interosseous muscle (*DO*), adductor muscle (*ADD*).

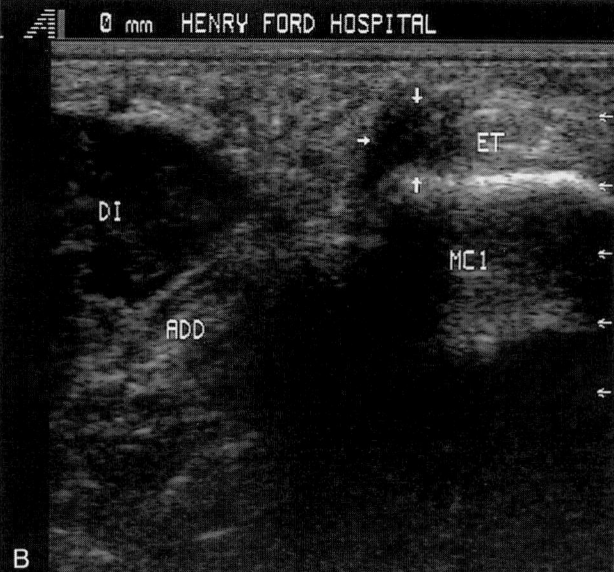

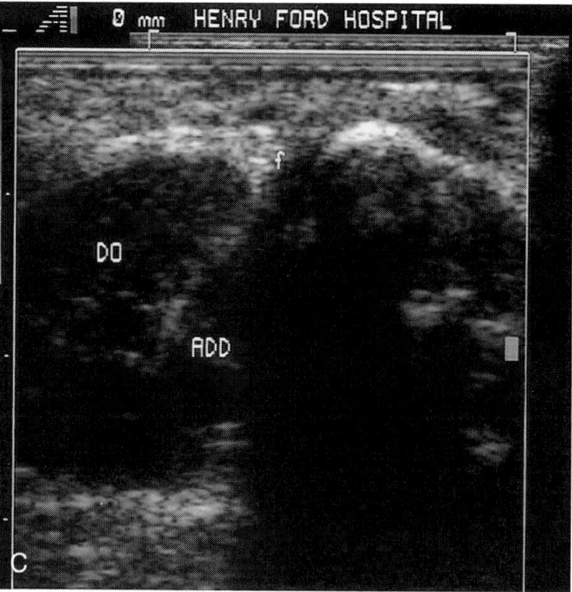

tations may be the only inhomogeneity in their internal architecture. A more inhomogeneous and vascular lesion with a broad base along the tendon sheath is the giant cell tumor (Fig. 16–68). Rare tumors of the tendon sheath include synovial fibromas (Fig. 16–69) and synovial chondromatosis (Fig. 16–70). Subcutaneous lesions of the palm of the hand include nodular fasciitis and Dupuytren's palmar fibrosis. The latter lesion is characteristically located over the palmar aponeurosis. Early lesions are identified on the ulnar side of the palm of the hand. Trauma is often an inciting factor. A genetic predisposition, alcohol abuse, and barbiturate treatment appear to be significant contributory factors (Mattson et al., 1989). The disease is also more common in diabetics. Associated fibromatoses include Ledderhose syndrome or plantar fibromatosis, Peyronie's disease, knuckle pads, and, more rarely, retroperitoneal fibromatosis. Trigger fingers are often observed at the onset of palmar fibrosis. The nodules in palmar fibromatosis appear hypoechoic and are often inhomogeneous in texture. Power Doppler sonography shows little or no vascularity. More advanced disease results in contracture of digits, flexion of joints, and nodules adhering to the flexor tendons. Diabetics and other immune-compromised patients may also be affected by infection. Hand infections invade a variety of compartments in the hand. Ultrasound allows us to diagnose and locate infections with great precision (Figs. 16–71 through 16–73).

Examinations of the wrist and hand performed for diffuse pain are generally low-yield studies. This is in marked contrast to sonographic examination of the shoulder, where investigation of nonspecific complaints will usually establish the cause.

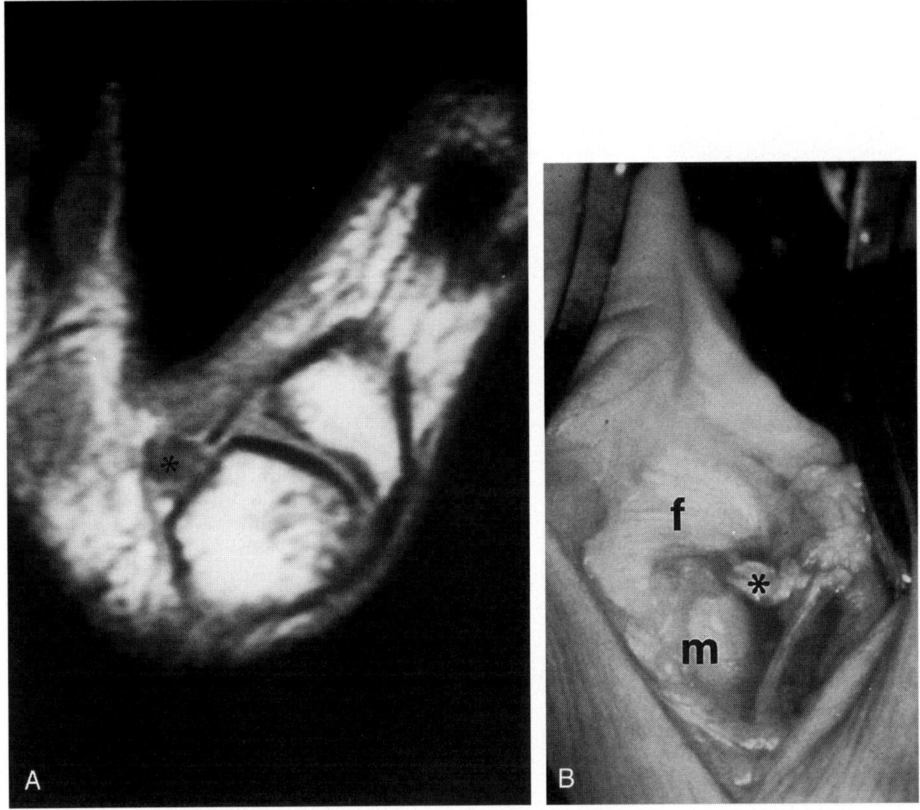

Figure 16-63 ▪ **A**, Stener lesion: coronal T_1-weighted MRI. This coronal T_1-weighted MRI scan of the thumb in a patient with a Stener lesion demonstrates a round low-signal mass in the dorsal aspect of the first web space over the metacarpal head. This is the classic location of a Stener lesion (asterisk). **B**, Stener lesion: cadaver dissection. This dissection of a cadaver specimen demonstrates a Stener lesion (*) with the ulnar collateral ligament retracted and folded over the adductor fascia (*f*). Abbreviation: metacarpal head (*m*).

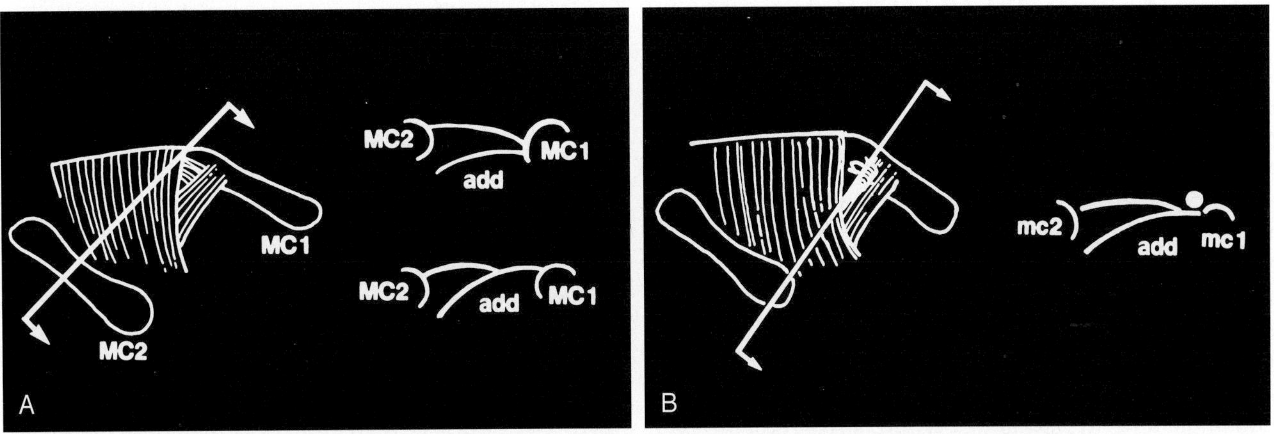

Figure 16-64 ▪ **A**, Normal first web space anatomy: scanning technique diagram. The diagram on the left indicates the orientation of the transducer, with *arrows* showing the direction of transducer movement. The top diagram on the right demonstrates the initial image in this scan sweep, and the lower image is at a level distal to the first metacarpophalangeal joint. Abbreviations: first metacarpal (*MC1*), second metacarpal (*MC2*), adductor muscle (*add*). **B**, Stener lesion: scanning technique diagram. Again, the diagram on the left depicts the transducer's position and motion relative to the torn ligament. The diagram on the right depicts the torn, retracted ligament dorsal to the adductor muscle. Abbreviations: first metacarpal (*MC1*), second metacarpal (*MC2*), adductor muscle (*add*). (Reprinted with permission from O'Callaghan BI, Kohut G, Hoogewoud HM: Gamekeeper thumb: Identification of the Stener lesion with US. *Radiology* 192:477–480, 1994.)

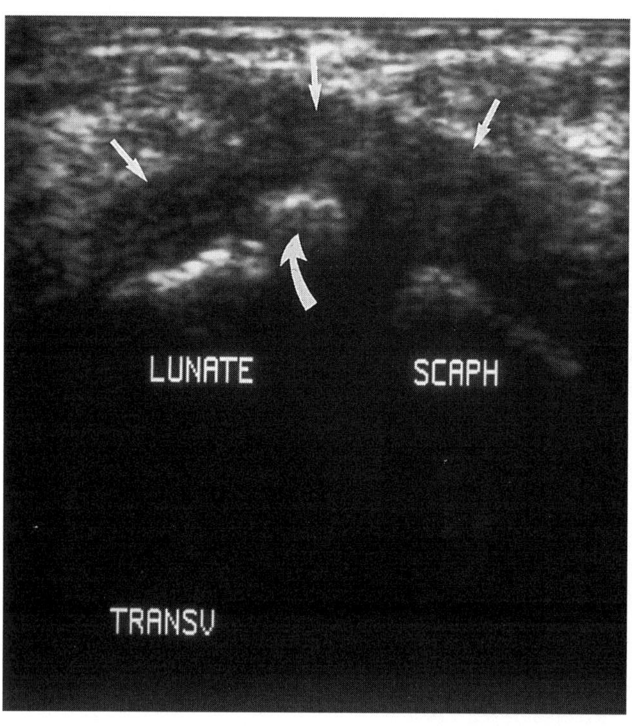

Figure 16-65 ▪ Scapho-lunate ligament avulsion: transverse sonogram. A 23-year-old radiological technologist fell onto his wrist while snowboarding. Radiographs were normal. This transverse image demonstrates significant hypoechoic swelling adjacent to the dorsal scapho-lunate joint (*arrows*). An avulsion fragment (*curved arrow*) is noted arising from the lunate. He was then treated with percutaneous pinning of the fracture. Five years after the injury, the patient remains asymptomatic.

Sonographic examination of the wrist and hand is most beneficial in investigation of a specific clinical question.

Technical Guidelines and Scanning Technique

Ideally, examination of the hand and wrist is performed using 10-, 12-, 15-, or 20-MHz linear array transducers. These are currently available only on state-of-the-art machines. A 7.5-MHz linear array will provide adequate visualization of hand and wrist anatomy. Often a standoff pad must be utilized to visualize these superficial structures. Lavish use of sonographic gel facilitates transverse imaging of the tendons of the fingers as a group. Transverse imaging of the tendons is performed first. This is essential for the identification of swelling of the tendons and tendon sheaths. Measurement of the transverse diameters of tendons allows easy identification of tendon swelling. When involvement of multiple adjacent tendons is suspected, comparison with the asymptomatic side is diagnostic. Evaluation of the echogenicity of tendons of the wrist, as elsewhere, must be performed with the beam perpendicular to the tendon surface. The anisotropic properties of tendons are most noticeable in the wrist. On a transverse image through the carpal tunnel, the flexor retinaculum is seen as a hyperechoic line. Two rows of superficial flexor tendons and one row of deep tendons are identified within the carpal tunnel.

The median nerve is an ovoid structure on the radial side of the carpal tunnel immediately beneath the flexor retinaculum. It is slightly less echogenic than the surrounding tendons and flatter in appearance. The median nerve rests on the deep flexor tendon of the index finger. Flexion and extension of the fingers during real-time examination will clearly demonstrate which structure is the median nerve. Punctate echogenic foci, noted on transverse images, are evenly distributed throughout the structure of the normal median nerve. The contour of the nerve may be slightly concave along one surface. Longitudinal images clearly demonstrate the fascicular architecture of the nerve with long, parallel fibers within its substance. The distal end of the nerve is tapered at the site of its distal divisions for the hand. Normal dimensions of the median nerve have been studied with the transducer just distal to the proximal carpal crease. The cross-sectional area of the median nerve is approximately 8–10 mm^2. Inflamed nerves in carpal tunnel disease are over 15 mm^2 in cases with significant impairment on EMG. Buchberger worked out a more complex ratio using internal landmarks. He also found that the pathological median nerve swells proximal to and at the entrance of the carpal tunnel. In addition, the nerve

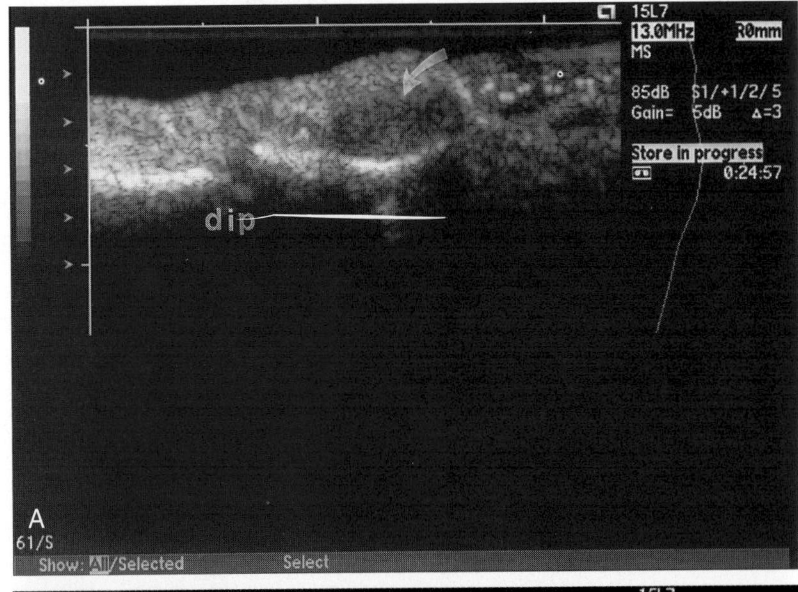

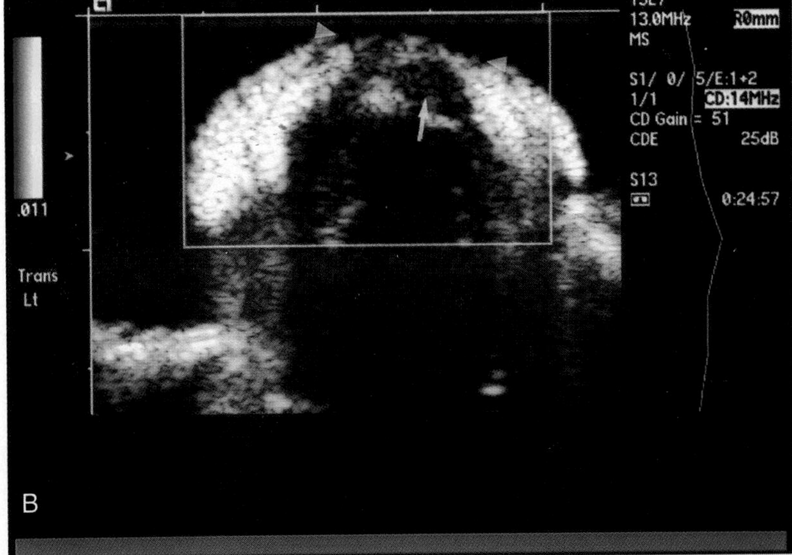

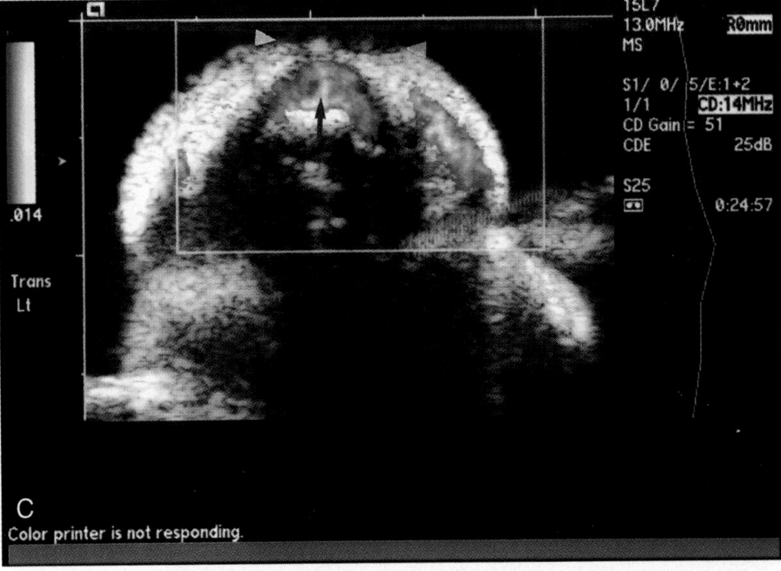

Figure 16-66 ■ **A**, Glomus tumor of the fingernail bed: longitudinal sonogram. Pain and focal swelling at the base of the nail of the left index finger of this 31-year-old female resulted in progressive limitation of function. Clinically, there was discoloration of the nail bed proximally. A small focal, firm, hypoechoic mass (*curved arrow*) is identified at the proximal aspect of the fingernail. Abbreviation: distal interphalangeal joint (*dip*). **B**, Glomus tumor of the fingernail bed: transverse sonogram. Same patient as in **A**. The mass (*arrow*) is well defined on this transverse image adjacent to the cortex of the phalanx. Note the irregular contour of the fingernail (*arrowheads*). **C**, Glomus tumor of the fingernail bed: transverse sonogram, power Doppler. Same patient as in **A**. Marked hypervascularity is noted within the mass (*arrow*), with prominent adjacent digital vessels. This appearance is pathognomonic for a glomus tumor, which was confirmed surgically.

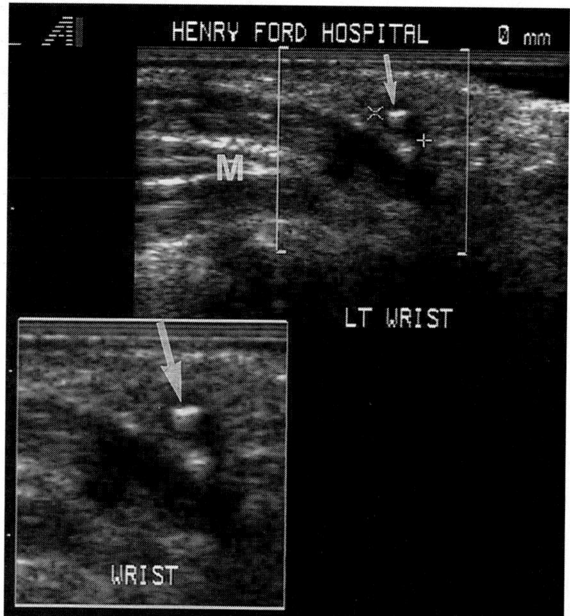

Figure 16–67 ■ Subcutaneous foreign body: transverse sonogram. Several years ago, this woman sustained a penetrating injury to the base of the thumb and continues to have significant pain. This transverse image identifies a hyperechoic foreign body (*arrow*) superficial to the thenar musculature (*M*) surrounded by hypoechoic granulation tissue (× –+). A 1-mm thorn fragment was surgically removed.

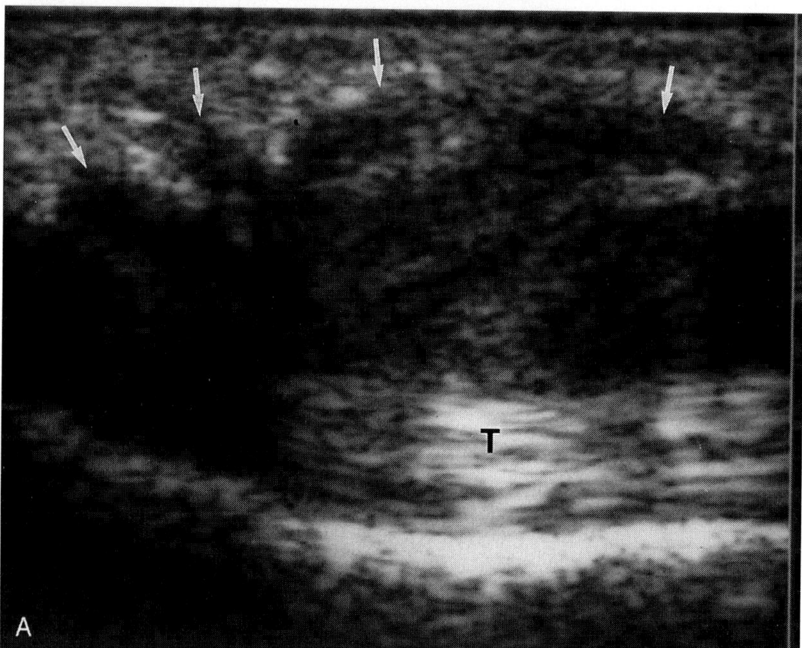

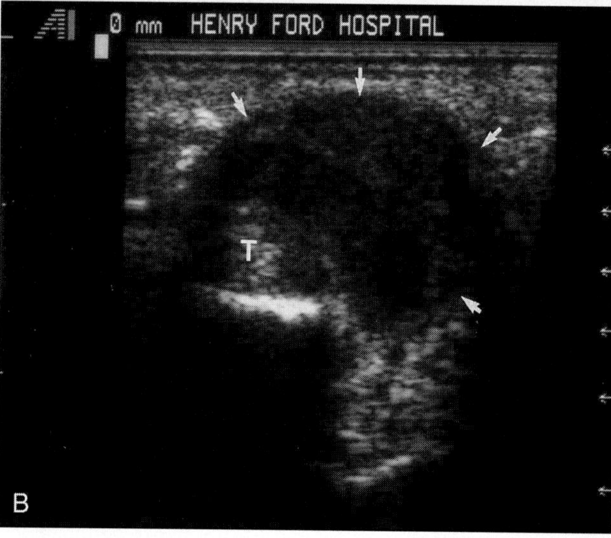

Figure 16–68 ■ **A**, Giant cell tumor of the tendon sheath: longitudinal sonogram. Soft tissue swelling of the middle finger of this 29-year-old man was present for 1 year. Irregular hypoechoic swelling (*arrows*) within the tendon sheath is noted on this longitudinal image. This appearance is very atypical of tenosynovitis because of its thickness and irregularity. Abbreviation: flexor tendons (*T*). **B**, Giant cell tumor of the tendon sheath: transverse sonogram. Same patient as in **A**. This transverse image demonstrates the mass (*arrows*) around the tendon (*T*) to be eccentric and inhomogeneous. The diagnosis of a tendon sheath tumor was suggested, and surgical excision was performed. Histological examination demonstrated a giant cell tumor of the synovial sheath.

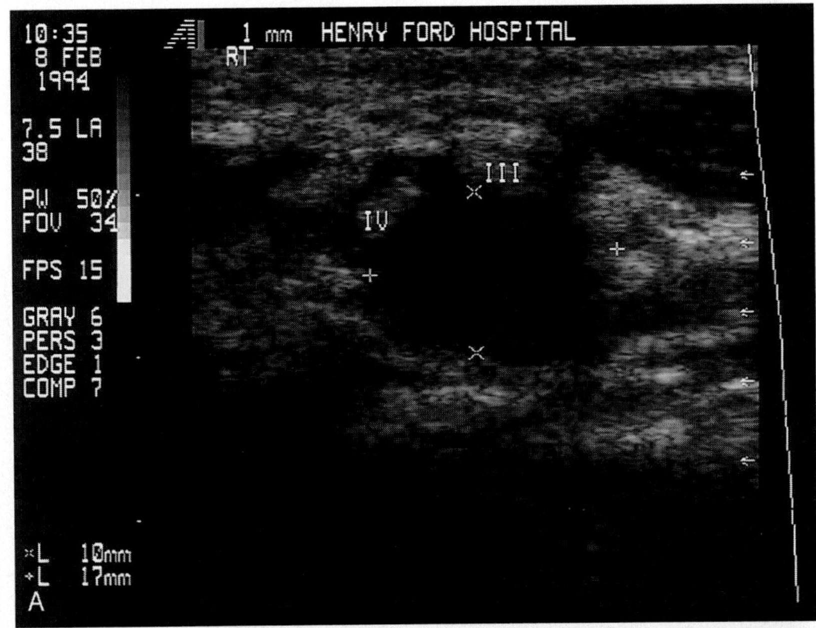

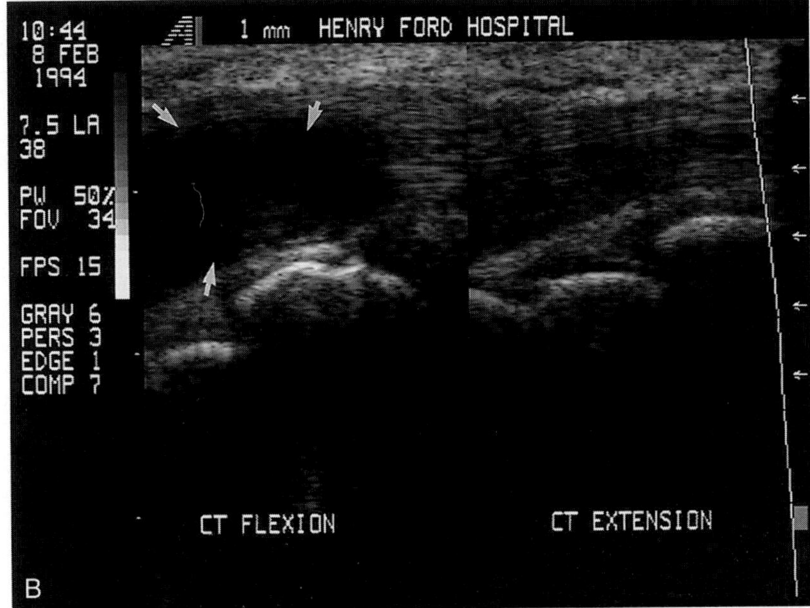

Figure 16-69 ■ **A**, Fibroma of the tendon sheath: transverse sonogram. This 19-year-old male presented with median nerve paresthesias only when he clenched his fist. A hypoechoic mass (*x-X*) displacing the flexor tendons is identified. The first impression of the sonographic findings was that this mass represented a ganglion. However, upon closer examination, no increased through-transmission was found to be present, definite internal echos were identified, and the mass was very firm. The flexor tendon of the middle finger (*III*) and the flexor tendon of the ring finger (*IV*) could be identified by flexion of the tendons under real-time observation. **B**, Fibroma of the tendon sheath: longitudinal sonogram, split screen. Same patient as in **A**. These two images demonstrate the location of the mass with finger flexion and extension. The mass (*arrows*) moves into the carpal tunnel in flexion and distal to the carpal tunnel in extension. Compression of the median nerve resulted from movement of the mass into the carpal tunnel. Subsequently, a fibroma arising from the flexor tendon synovium was resected, with resolution of the patient's symptoms.

is flattened within the carpal tunnel (Buchberger et al., 1991, 1992; Lee et al., 1999).

The TFC is then located by placing the index finger of the examiner's free hand over the tip of the ulnar styloid. The transducer is positioned immediately proximal to the examiner's index finger. If the cartilage of the ulnar head is seen, the transducer is slowly moved distally until the TFC is visualized. Dorsal and volar scanning will ensure a more complete examination of the triangular fibrocartilage complex (TFCC), including the radioulnar ligaments, the ECU, and the meniscus homologue. We have found relatively small tears using a coronal approach with the hand in maximal radial deviation. The gain should be increased until the attachment of the TFC to the distal radius is clearly visible. The position of the ECU tendon must be examined with the transducer across the ECU groove in the distal ulna. It is important to perform this examination with the hand in both supination and pronation and with minimal pressure on the transducer. Subluxation of the ECU tendon may be intermittent and may be present only in supination. Too much pressure on the transducer reduces the abnormality. Comparison with the contralateral side is mandatory because there is a normal range of ligamentous

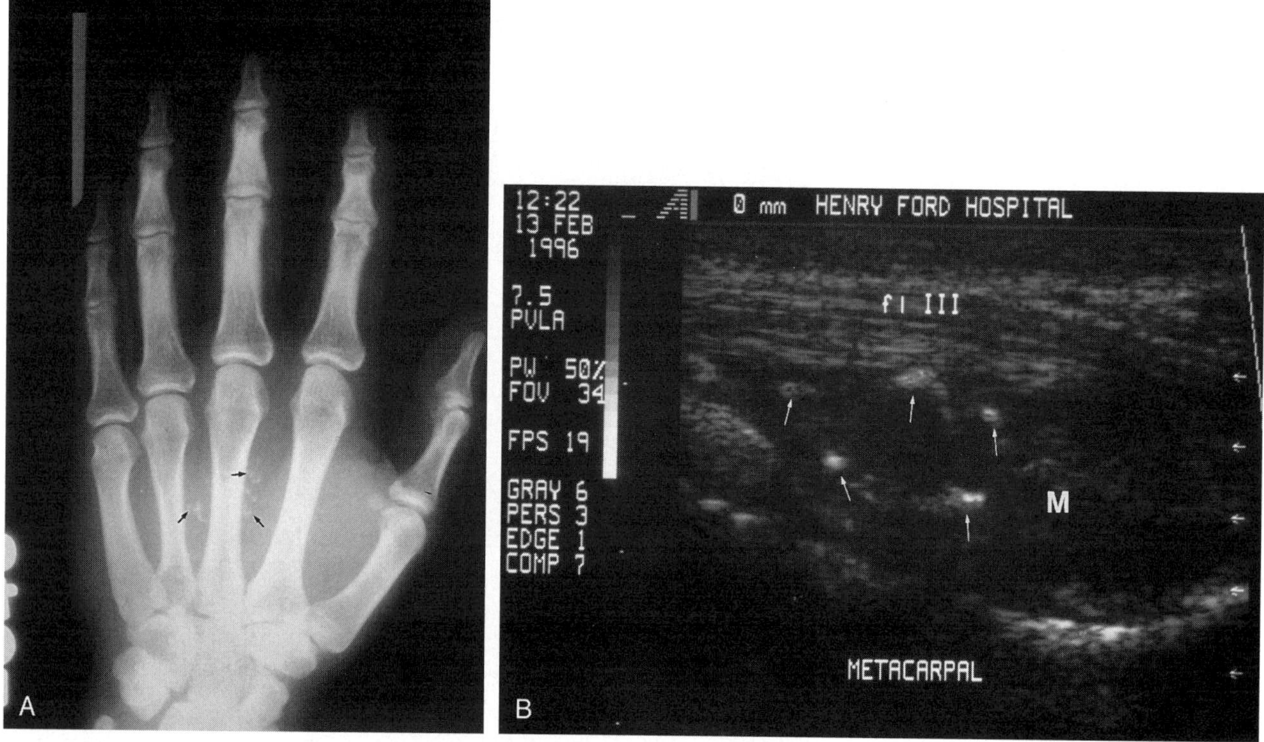

Figure 16–70 ■ **A**, Synovial osteochondromatosis of the tendon sheath: anteroposterior radiograph. Calcifications (*small arrows*) are noted adjacent to the third metacarpal in this 29-year-old male. No osseous abnormality is demonstrated in the metacarpals. **B**, Synovial osteochondromatosis of the tendon sheath: longitudinal sonogram. Same patient as in **A**. A large, heterogeneous mass is noted deep to the flexor tendons of the middle finger (*fl III*). The calcifications seen on the radiograph correspond to the hyperechoic foci (*small arrows*), with incomplete shadowing within the mass. Note the interruption of the cortex of the metacarpal secondary to the acoustic shadowing. Surgical synovectomy was performed, and the diagnosis of synovial osteochondromatosis was confirmed. The hypoechoic mass (*M*) observed between and proximal to the calcifications represented noncalcified cartilage of hyaline origin pathologically.

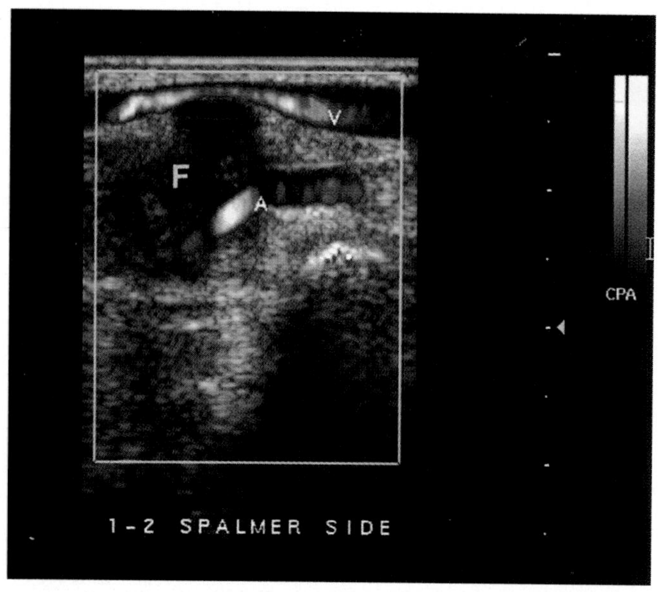

Figure 16–71 ■ Subcutaneous abscess in a diabetic: longitudinal sonogram. This 64-year-old diabetic female presented with fever and swelling distal to the anatomical snuff box. A hypoechoic mass separates two vessels with moderate compression of the superficial vessel. Movement of debris within this fluid collection (*F*) was observed on real-time imaging. Aspiration under ultrasound guidance was performed, and 1 mm of pus obtained. Cultures yielded *Staphylococcus aureus.* Abbreviations: vessel with arterial pulsations (*A*), vessel with venous flow (*V*).

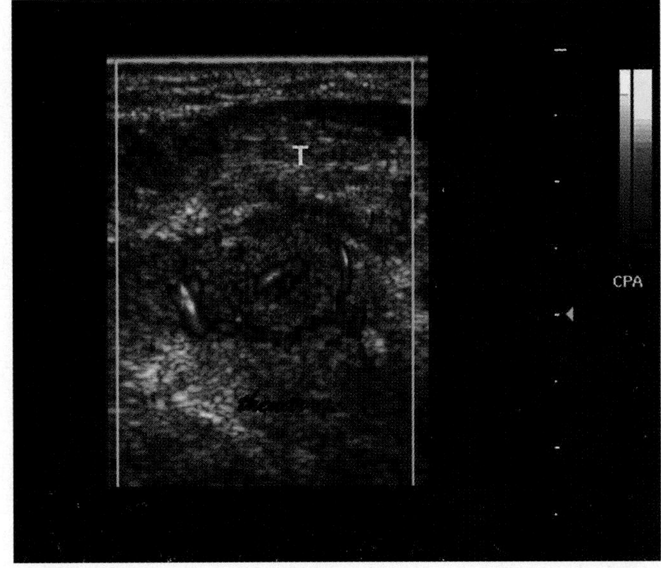

Figure 16–72 ■ Pyomyositis in a diabetic: transverse sonogram. A solid mass within the thenar musculature (*T*) is identified on this transverse sonogram of a 58-year-old diabetic woman. Power Doppler imaging demonstrates hypervascularity within this solid mass. Given the clinical presentation of fever and an elevated white cell count, an aspiration was performed. Since this was not a fluid collection, nonbacteriostatic saline was injected and reaspirated. *Staphylococcus aureus* was cultured from the aspirate.

laxity which should not be confused with tendon instability.

After evaluation of the tendons and TFC on transverse images, continuity of the tendons is examined with longitudinal images. Again, dynamic real-time examination easily differentiates tendons from nerves. The longitudinal axis of the median nerve appears slightly flatter and more hypoechoic than the flexor tendons within the carpal tunnel. Tendons are tubular, but the nerve has a tapered end distal to the carpal tunnel as it divides. Flexor tendon movement can be assessed with the help of color Doppler sonography (Buyruk et al., 1996). Tendon motion has to be smooth, continuous, and constant in velocity. In the examination for tendon injury, we follow tendons from the myotendinous junction to the point of tendinous insertion. In trigger fingers, controlled extension against resistance should be used, with the transducer placed longitudinally over the tendon and pulley system. Changes in the trigger tendon may be revealed on longitudinal images approximately at the level of the distal metacarpals (Serafini, 1996). The position of the transducer should be past the distal palmar crease and over the proximal digital creases. The abnormal side should always be compared with the normal side. In suspected tear of the A_2 pulley, controlled flexion against resistance is necessary, with the transducer positioned longitudinally and transversely over the proximal phalanx and the PIP joint. Bowstringing of the tendon is then clearly visible. All other flexor tears should be assessed longitudinally with respect to the five possible zones of injury.

Extensor tendons are examined in a fashion similar to that utilized for the flexor tendons. More gel should be applied over the extensor surface because the extensor mechanism is very superficial in location. Improvements in imaging are expected with new transducers that have a center frequency higher than 10 MHz and a design which allows the focal zones to be brought up to skin level. The distal insertions of the extensor tendons should be checked carefully to assess for rupture. The central slip of the extensor tendon inserts past the PIP joint. This insertion should be checked routinely in finger injuries.

The dorsal hood, a ligamentous support structure of the extensor tendons over the knuckles, can be identified on transverse images over the metacarpophalangeal joints and proximal web spaces. In some cases, it is possible to identify the paper-thin radial and ulnar sagittal slips of the dorsal hood. Transverse examination of the dorsal hood should be performed in flexion and extension. Finger flexion aggravates subluxation of the extensor tendon, which accompanies dorsal hood injury in some patients.

In evaluation of collateral ligaments, the transducer must be aligned along medial and lateral joint capsules. The lesions are diagnosed easily with varus and valgus stress. The UCL of the thumb can be assessed longitudinally by pressing the transducer into the soft tissue of the medial first web space. A small, bony crest can be used as an internal landmark. This crest over the medial distal first metacarpal is located at the origin of the ligament. A small, bony avulsion may accompany ligament rupture. This avulsion may occur at the base of the proximal phalanx or at the distal end of the first metacarpal. The displaced ligament can be detected sonographically with the transducer oriented transversely over the first web space. Two muscle layers will be noted when a 10-MHz transducer is

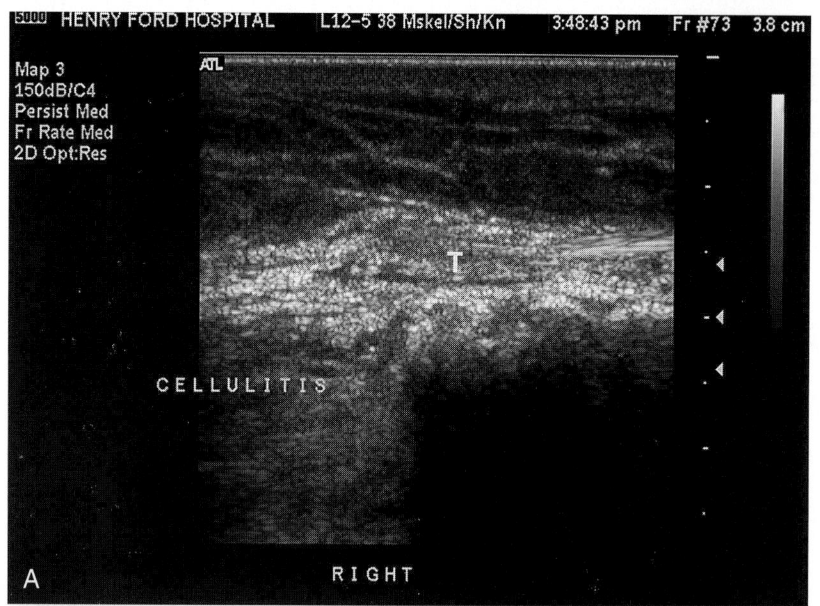

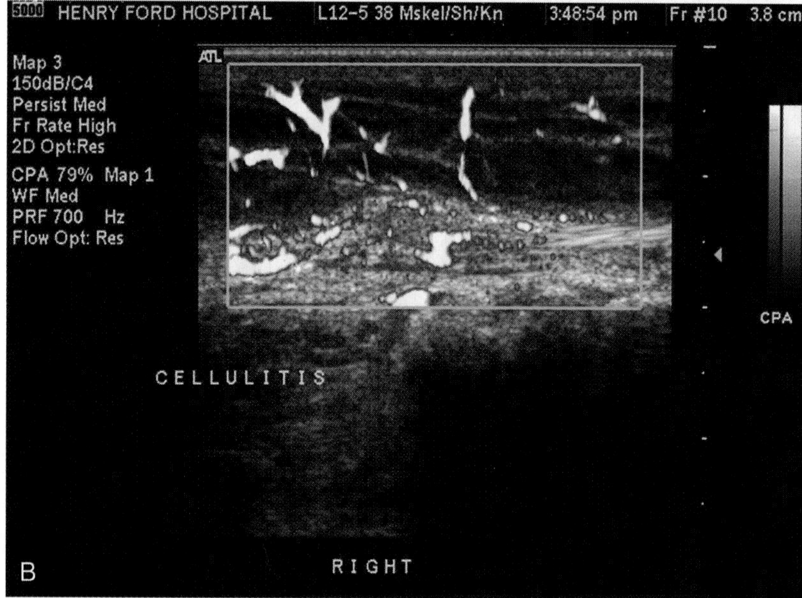

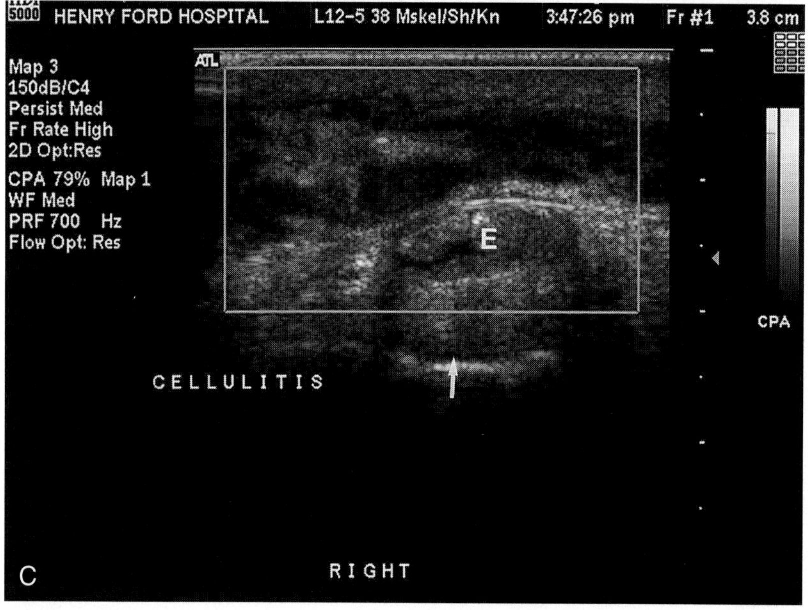

Figure 16–73 ■ **A**, Cellulitis of the dorsum of the wrist: longitudinal sonogram. Fever, chills, and diffuse swelling of the right wrist in this 44-year-old patient were attributed clinically to septic arthritis. A splinter had penetrated the wrist 1 week ago while he was pruning a pine tree. The ultrasound scan shows the swelling to be superficial to the wrist extensor tendons (*T*). The reticular architecture of the swollen tissues is consistent with subcutaneous swelling and is probably likely due to lymphangitis. A saline washout cultured many colonies of group A *Streptococcus pyogenes*. **B**, Cellulitis: longitudinal sonogram with power Doppler sonography. Same patient as in **A**. The transducer position is unchanged from **A**. Diffuse flow is noted in the septations of the subcutaneous fat. **C**, Cellulitis: transverse sonogram. Same patient as in **A**. The 12 MHz transducer is now positioned transversely over the distal radius. This scan shows clearly that the swelling is contained to the tissues superficial to the extensor digitorum compartment (*E*). The synovial compartment of the dorsal aspect of the radiocarpal joint (*arrow*) appears unaffected. The amount of fluid in the extensor synovium and within the radiocarpal joint is within the normal range.

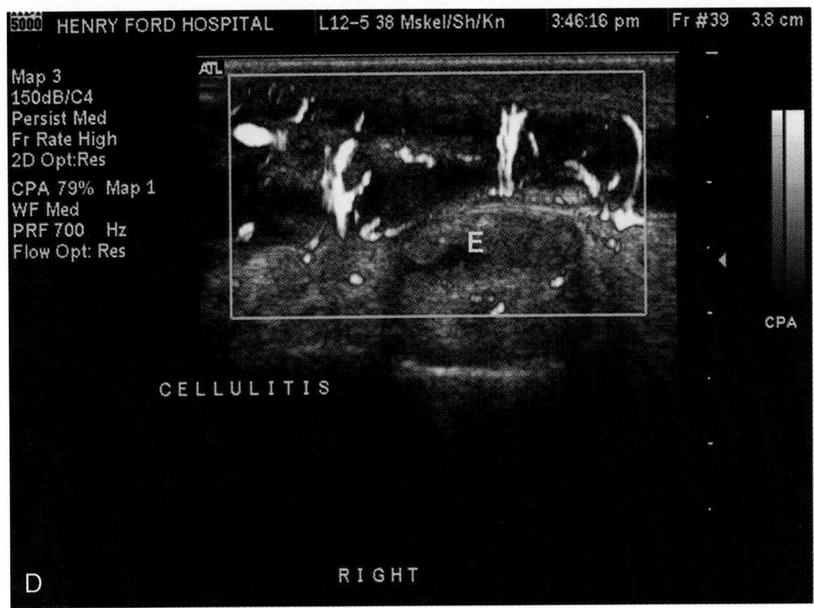

Figure 16–73 *Continued* ■ **D**, Cellulitis: transverse sonogram with power Doppler sonography. Same patient and transducer position as in **C**. The increased vascular and/or lymphatic flow predominates in the hypodermis deep to the dermis and superficial to the extensor digitorum communis tendon sheath (*E*).

applied over the dorsal aspect of the space. The most superficial layer is the dorsal interosseous muscle, and the layer deep to this is the adductor muscle. The adductor ends laterally in the adductor aponeurosis. The normal UCL and the torn but nondisplaced UCL remain deep to the aponeurosis. Stener lesions, however, are demonstrated over the adductor fascia. Transverse ultrasound images will reveal the displaced and retracted ligament as a small, round structure adjacent to the medial side of the extensor pollicis longus tendon. The adductor fascia will be identified deep to the displaced ligament. In typical cases, longitudinal images will have a characteristic notched appearance because of indentation of the adductor aponeurosis.

References

Bronstein AJ, Koniuch MP, van Holsbeeck M: Ultrasonographic detection of thumb ulnar collateral ligament injuries: A cadaveric study. *J Hand Surg* 19A (2): 304–312, 1994.

Buchberger W, et al: High resolution ultrasonography of the carpal tunnel. *J Ultrasound Med* 10:531–537, 1991.

Buchberger W, et al: Carpal tunnel syndrome: Diagnosis with high-resolution sonography. *AJR* 159:793–798, 1992.

Buyruk HM, et al: Colour Doppler ultrasound examination of hand tendon pathologies. *J Hand Surg* 21B(4): 469–473, 1996.

Chiou HJ, et al: Triangular fibrocartilage of wrist: The presentation of high resolution ultrasound. *J Ultrasound Med* 16S:46–47, 1997.

Crenshaw AH: *Campbell's Operative Orthopaedics*, CD-ROM ed. Philadelphia, Mosby–Year Book, 1996.

Failla JM, van Holsbeeck M, Vanderschueren G: Detection of a 0.5-mm-thick thorn using ultrasound: A case report. *J Hand Surg* 20A(3):456–457, 1995.

Fornage BD, Rifkin MD: Ultrasound examination of the hand and foot. *Radiol Clin North Am* 26(1):109–129, 1988.

Frankel DA, et al: Synovial joints: Evaluation of intraarticular bodies with US. *Radiology* 206:41–44, 1998.

Hergan K, Mittler C, Oser W: Ulnar collateral ligament: Differentiation of displaced and nondisplaced tears with US and MRI imaging. *Radiology* 194:65, 1995.

Jacobson JA, et al: Wooden foreign bodies in soft tissue: Detection at US. *Radiology* 206:45–48, 1998.

Lee D, et al: Diagnosis of carpal tunnel syndrome: Ultrasound versus electromyography. *Radiol Clin North Am* 37(4):859–872, 1999.

Mattson RH, Cramer JA, McCutchen CB: Barbiturate-related connective tissue disorders. *Arch of Intern Med* 149(4):911–914, 1989.

O'Callaghan BI, Kohut G, Hoogewoud HM: Gamekeeper thumb: Identification of the Stener lesion with US. *Radiology* 192:477–480, 1994.

Serafini G, et al: High-resolution sonography of the flexor tendons in trigger fingers. *J Ultrasound Med* 15: 213–219, 1996.

Silvestri E, et al: Echotexture of peripheral nerves: Correlation between US and histologic findings and criteria to differentiate tendons. *Radiology* 197:291, 1995.

Chapter 17
Sonography of the Hip

David P. Fessell, M.D., and Marnix T. van Holsbeeck, M.D.

Hip Pain: Imaging Options and the Role of Ultrasound

Hip pain can be due to bone, joint, or soft tissue pathology. A variety of imaging modalities are available (Table 17–1). Conventional radiography is the initial assessment for all types of pathology. For assessment of occult fractures, bone marrow pathology, and tumors, MRI is the modality of choice (Hayes and Balkissoon, 1997). When cortical bone or complex acetabular fractures are to be imaged, CT is superior (Berquist, 1997). The role of ultrasound in the patient with hip pain is multifaceted: assessment of intra- and extra-articular fluid collections, including bursal and synovial pathology; guiding aspiration and biopsy; assessment of muscle and tendon pathology; and assessment of the snapping, locking, or clicking hip (Table 17–2). The advantages of ultrasound include its wide availability, relatively low cost, portability, and rapidity of examination. It can also be used in patients in whom metal is present and would create artifacts with CT or MRI. This section reviews the scanning technique and specific indications for ultrasound of the symptomatic adult hip.

Scanning Technique

For evaluation of the hip, a 2–5 MHz transducer is used. The dynamic capabilities of ultrasound allow the hip to be examined in multiple positions, with easy comparison to the contralateral hip. For evaluation of the joint, the patient is examined in the supine position. The joint is evaluated in longitudinal and transverse orientations by scanning anteriorly, approximately at the level of the inguinal crease. For sagittal (longitudinal) scanning, the transducer is angled slightly toward the axis of the femoral neck (Zieger et al., 1987). Both the symptomatic and asymptomatic hips are routinely scanned (Shiv et al., 1990; Berman et al., 1995), and comparison with the asymptomatic side can aid evaluation when a small effusion may be present.

Scanning is also performed over the lateral hip to evaluate the greater trochanteric bursae, and it is extended into the proximal thigh to exclude a fluid collection such as a hematoma or an abscess. Assessment of the anterior labrum is performed with the transducer perpendicular to the labrum. For assessment of the proximal hamstrings, the patient is examined in the prone position. Scanning transversely over the proximal thigh identifies the hamstring muscles, and scanning is extended cranially to the origin of these muscles on the ischial tuberosity. Both transverse and longitudinal evaluation is performed. The adductors and anterior superior iliac crest are evaluated with the patient supine (Marcelis et al., 1996).

If there is concern about the possibility of an inguinal hernia, scanning is extended over the ostium of the inguinal canal. This structure is found at the origin of the inferior epigastric artery, a branch of the external iliac. Scanning during the Valsalva maneuver or with the patient standing aids evaluation.

Hip Pain

Joint Effusion

A joint effusion is a common finding in the patient with hip pain. The etiology of a joint effusion includes infection, inflammatory and noninflammatory arthritis, avascular necrosis, trauma, and neoplastic conditions. History, plain radiographs, ultrasounds, CT, and MRI can help differentiate these conditions, as listed in Table 17–3. In the patient with joint pain and an effusion, a septic joint must be excluded.

Table 17–1
Hip Pathology: Imaging Options

Modality	Advantages	Disadvantages	Primary Use
Radiographs	Inexpensive Widely available Familiar	Overlapping structures Poor soft tissue contrast Relative insensitivity for early marrow or cortical pathology	Initial assessment for essentially all pathology
MRI	Superior soft tissue contrast Bone marrow evaluation Multiplanar imaging	Expense Limited availability Contraindicated with certain electric/metal implants	Occult fractures AVN/bone marrow tumors MR arthrography
CT	Superior detail of cortex and calcification	Limited soft tissue contrast Expense	Acetabular fractures Metastatic disease
Ultrasound	Inexpensive Widely available Rapid Can be used at the bedside Can be used when metal is present	Operator dependent Limited to joint and soft tissue pathology	R/O intra- or extra-articular fluid Guide aspiration or biopsy
Arthrography	Allows aspiration and injection	Invasive Assesses only the joint	R/O infection or loosening of hip prosthesis
Nuclear study	Sensitive Assesses perfusion	Nonspecific Relatively poor spatial resolution	Occult fractures AVN Osteomyelitis

Source: Berquist, 1997; Hayes and Balkissoon, 1997.

Ultrasound provides a rapid and efficient method of assessing for joint fluid and guiding aspiration.

Joint infections are most commonly due to a bacterial etiology, but they can also be due to fungal, mycobacterial, viral, or parasitic causes. Gram-positive cocci are the most common species. *Staphylococcus aureus* is the most frequent organism, found in approximately 70% of cases of adult pyarthrosis (Middleton, 1993; Cimmino, 1997). Streptococci and gram-negative organisms, especially *Neisseria gonorrhoeae*, are also common (Middleton, 1993). The usual route of joint infection is hematogenous dissemination due to the absence of a basement membrane protecting the highly vascular synovium. Conditions which predispose to joint infection include immune suppression; systemic disease, especially diabetes, sickle cell anemia, and drug abuse; preexisting joint damage; and iatrogenic causes such as joint replacement (Middleton, 1993; Cimmino, 1997). The diagnosis may be suspected on clinical grounds, but definitive diagnosis and treatment require culture of the synovial fluid. Amplification of DNA by the polymerase chain reaction (PCR) is gaining widespread use and will probably aid in providing a rapid, accurate diagnosis of joint infections (Cimmino, 1997). Successful treatment of joint infections is based on early diagnosis, joint drainage, and antibiotics.

When evaluating for an effusion, the hip is best examined in extension and slight abduction (Chan

Table 17–2
Clinical Indications for Ultrasound of the Adult Hip

1. Hip pain in the native and prosthetic hip
   a. Evaluate for effusion or synovitis and guide aspiration or biopsy
   b. Evaluate for bursal and periarticular fluid collections and guide aspiration
2. Hip pain in the athlete
   a. Evaluate for muscle, tendon, bursal pathology, and hernia
3. The snapping, locking, or clicking hip
   a. Evaluate for snapping of the iliopsoas tendon
   b. Evaluate for loose bodies
   c. Evaluate for anterior labral pathology

Table 17–3
Differential Diagnosis of Hip Joint Effusion in the Adult

1. Septic arthritis: Ultrasound-guided aspiration and culture
2. Avascular necrosis: correlate with conventional radiographs and MRI
3. Inflammatory and noninflammatory arthritis: correlate with history and conventional radiographs
4. Hemorrhage: correlate with a history of trauma or bleeding disorder
5. Tumors such as PVNS and synovial osteochondromatosis: correlate with conventional radiographs and MRI

Source: Zieger et al., 1987; Koski, 1989.

et al., 1997). Effusions are best detected along the femoral neck, seen as fluid causing the capsule and iliofemoral ligament to bulge away from the neck (Fig. 17–1) (Shiv et al., 1990; Berman et al., 1995). Effusions as small as 1–2 mL are detectable by US (Zieger et al., 1987). A difference in joint distention of ≥2 mm between the symptomatic and asymptomatic hips has been reported as significant (Koski et al., 1989; Shiv et al., 1990; Nimityongskul et al., 1996). Capsular thickening (≥2 mm) and bony changes along the femur have also been reported with septic arthritis (Shiv et al., 1990).

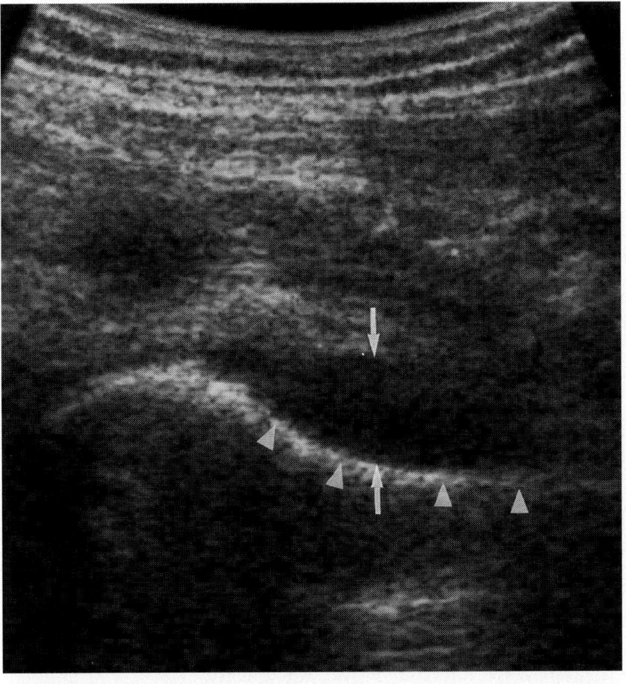

Figure 17–1 ■ Hip effusion: longitudinal ultrasound. This pregnant woman with right hip pain is suspected of having an infected hip. The leg-roll test is positive, and her sedimentation rate is elevated. A hypoechoic effusion (*arrows*) distends the capsule. *Arrowheads* mark the echogenic cortex of the femur. Aspiration showed inflammatory fluid, with no signs of intra-articular pus and negative cultures.

The size and gray scale appearance of the effusion (anechoic, hypoechoic, complex) do not predict an infectious or inflammatory etiology (Shiv et al., 1990; Zawin et al., 1993; Breidahl et al., 1996). Increased power Doppler flow around a fluid collection has been shown to correlate with an infectious/inflammatory versus a noninflammatory etiology. Increased power Doppler flow does not, however, distinguish between inflammatory collections of infectious versus noninfectious etiologies, and flow is not always increased in the presence of a septic joint effusion (Breidahl et al., 1996; Strouse et al., 1998).

Traditionally, the evaluation of a suspected septic joint has included joint aspiration by the orthopedic surgeon utilizing only external anatomical landmarks or by the radiologist utilizing fluoroscopically guided aspiration. Evaluation and aspiration utilizing ultrasound offers several advantages over the traditional approach (Table 17–4). Most importantly, the use of ultrasound can avoid a dry tap, detect extra-articular fluid collections, and guide aspiration to avoid contamination of the joint from an extra-articular fluid collection.

Table 17–4
Advantages of Ultrasound in the Diagnosis and Aspiration of Joint Effusions and Periarticular Fluid Collections

1. Avoidance of a painful "dry tap." If no joint fluid is detected by ultrasound, no aspiration is required.
2. Detection of fluid collections outside of the joint (e.g., in bursa), with ultrasound guidance of the optimal aspiration approach to avoid contamination of an unaffected joint.
3. The aspiration needle can be visualized within the fluid collection. Postaspiration ultrasound can document complete removal of fluid and assess for loculated collections.
4. Solid masses such as synovitis and amyloid can be identified and biopsied under ultrasound guidance.
5. Increased power Doppler flow surrounding a fluid collection can help distinguish inflammatory/infectious fluid collections from noninflammatory collections.
6. Ultrasound is widely available, rapid, and inexpensive, and can be performed at the bedside if necessary.

Source: Shiv et al., 1990; Zawin et al., 1993; Breidahl et al., 1996; Nimityongskul et al., 1996.

Synovitis

Utilizing ultrasound, aseptic synovitis may appear as an anechoic or hypoechoic collection or mass. Aspiration yields increased WBCs without other evidence of infection. Such effusions may be seen in patients with rheumatoid arthritis, osteoarthritis, and avascular necrosis, and they have been detected in asymptomatic hips of patients with rheumatoid arthritis in other joints (Koski, 1989; Koski and Isomaki, 1990). The presence of flow on power Doppler can be seen within thickened synovium. This can aid in distinguishing synovitis from a small or complex effusion which does not demonstrate internal flow. Power Doppler may also aid in the detection and follow-up of hyperemia associated with inflammatory arthritis (Newman et al., 1996). When synovial biopsy is desired, ultrasound with real-time imaging of the needle tip can be used to ensure a safe and successful biopsy.

Hip Bursae

Periarticular or extra-articular fluid collections can be a source of hip pain, including those contained in bursae. The greater trochanteric bursae and the iliopsoas bursa are the major bursae of the hip evaluated by ultrasound. The greater trochanteric bursae are composed of three separate bursae. The gluteus minimus and medius bursae are located anterior to the greater trochanter. The gluteus maximus bursa is the largest of the three and is located posterior to the greater trochanter (Gray, 1985; Varma et al., 1993). Ultrasound evaluation is performed by scanning transversely and longitudinally over the trochanteric eminence. Isolated greater trochanteric septic bursitis has been observed in patients without a joint effusion (Steinbach et al., 1985). Therefore, the greater trochanter should always be assessed whenever the hip is evaluated. Ultrasound also allows evaluation of bursae in

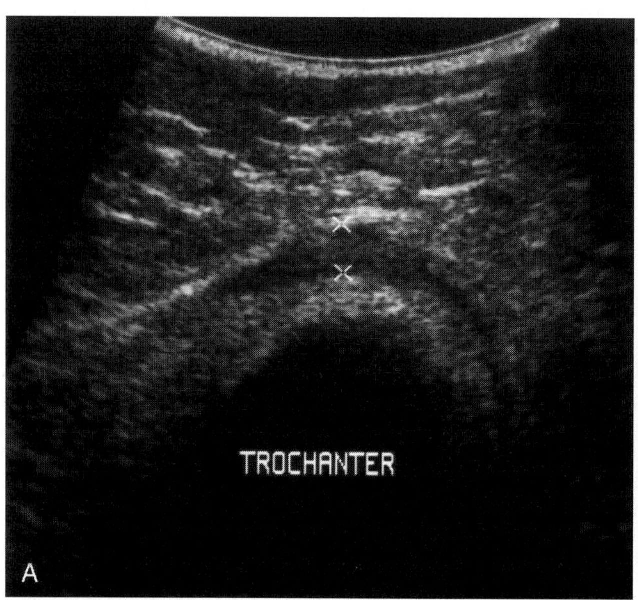

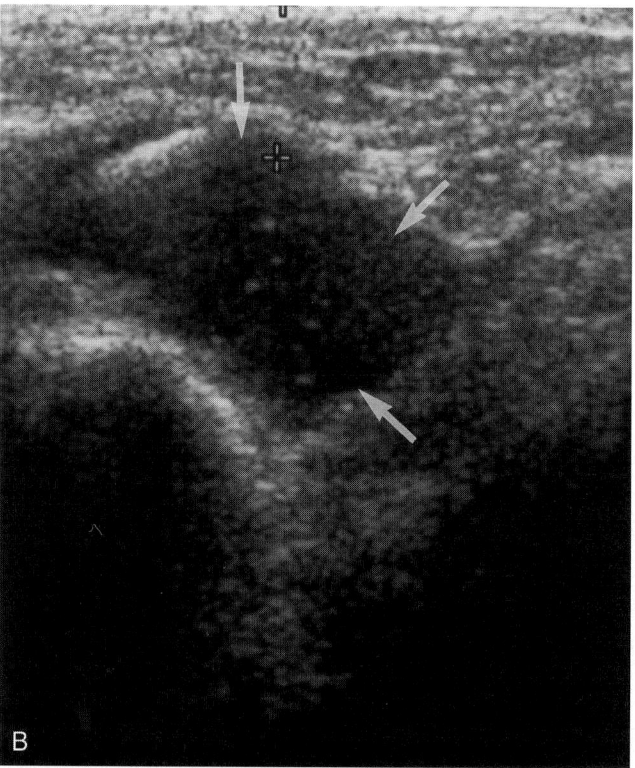

Figure 17–2 ■ **A**, Bursitis: transverse ultrasound. This 69-year-old woman underwent left total hip replacement 16 months ago. She claims that she was never without pain after surgery. Transverse ultrasound over the greater trochanter demonstrates a small amount of fluid within the bursa (5.4 mm between the × cursors). Aspiration for infection was negative. The diagnosis, based on the clinical exam, radiographs and ultrasound was frictional bursitis. **B**, Bursitis: transverse ultrasound. Transverse ultrasound over the right greater trochanter in a 69-year-old man demonstrates a markedly distended bursa (*arrows*) adjacent to the greater trochanter. This patient recently had surgery, with placement of a right hemiarthroplasty. The clinician was worried because of recent increases in the sedimentation rate and a high C-reactive protein level. The bursa is located 0.84 cm deep to the skin surface (between the + cursors). Culture of the aspirate demonstrated no growth consistent with aseptic bursitis.

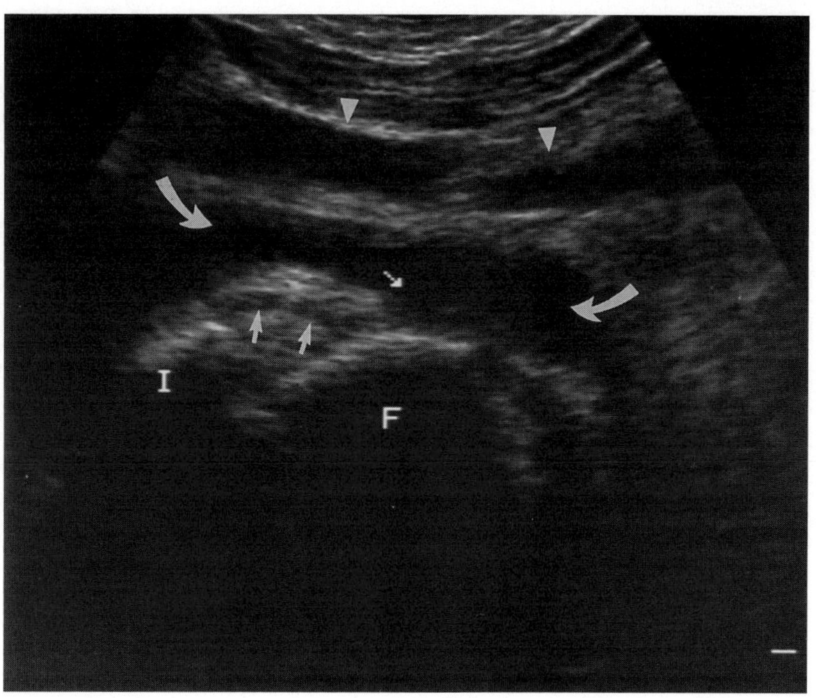

Figure 17–3 ■ Distended iliopsoas bursa: longitudinal ultrasound. A pulsatile groin mass was palpated in this 60-year-old woman. The longitudinal ultrasound scan shows an anechoic mass (*curved arrows*) deep to the femoral vessels (*arrowheads*) and superficial to the femur (*F*). A *small white arrow* marks the communication with the hip joint. The location and appearance are consistent with an iliopsoas bursa. A hypoechoic cleft within the labrum is consistent with a labral tear (*small arrows*). Abbreviation: ileum (*I*).

patients with a prosthetic hip or other metallic hardware that would produce artifacts when imaged by MRI or CT (Steiner et al., 1996).

Bursitis is demonstrated as an enlarged, anechoic or hypoechoic bursa when compared to the contralateral, asymptomatic hip (Fig. 17–2). Posttraumatic, infectious, and inflammatory etiologies are most frequent. Predisposing factors include gait abnormalities, obesity, and prior surgery (Varma et al., 1993; Laorr and Helms, 1997). Fluid distention of the bursae may be asymptomatic (Varma et al., 1993). In such cases, the bursa is nontender when pressure is applied on the transducer. In symptomatic cases, ultrasound can be used to guide aspiration and injection of steroids.

The iliopsoas bursa is located between the hip capsule and the iliacus and psoas major muscles. It normally measures 5–7 cm in length by 2–4 cm in width, making it the largest bursa in the human body (Flanagan et al., 1995; Chandler, 1934). The bursa is normally collapsed and is not visualized by US unless it is pathologically enlarged. Communication with the joint in 15% of cases explains the close association between iliopsoas bursitis and pathology of the hip joint (Chandler, 1934; Flanagan et al., 1995). The communication is probably due to friction produced by the iliopsoas tendon on the joint capsule (Chandler, 1934). When enlarged, the bursa can produce pain, a palpable mass, and pressure symptoms on the femoral nerve and vein, leading to neuropathy and peripheral edema. The enlarged bursa can even extend into the retroperitoneum and compress the bladder and bowel. Rupture or soft tissue dissection is also possible. The etiologies of iliopsoas bursitis include rheumatoid arthritis, osteoarthritis, gout and pseudogout, pigmented villonodular synovitis, synovial osteochondromatosis, trauma, and infection (Steinbach et al., 1985; Flanagan et al., 1995; Laorr and Helms, 1997; Steiner et al., 1996).

In the patient with hip pain, and especially in association with a palpable mass, the diagnosis of iliopsoas bursitis must be considered and its ultrasound appearance recognized to avoid misdiagnosis. An enlarged bursa appears anechoic/hypoechoic (Fig. 17–3) and may contain echogenic foci of synovial proliferation as well as septa. Ultrasound allows differentiation from other masses in this region, including solid neoplasms, inguinal hernias, undescended testes, and lymphadenopathy. Doppler evaluation can help distinguish a femoral artery aneurysm or varices from an enlarged bursa (Steinbach et al., 1985). Ultrasound-guided aspiration and steroid injection can aid the treatment (Flanagan et al., 1995).

Abscesses, Hematomas, and Seromas

Extra-articular fluid collections unrelated to the bursa can also be a source of hip pain. Such fluid

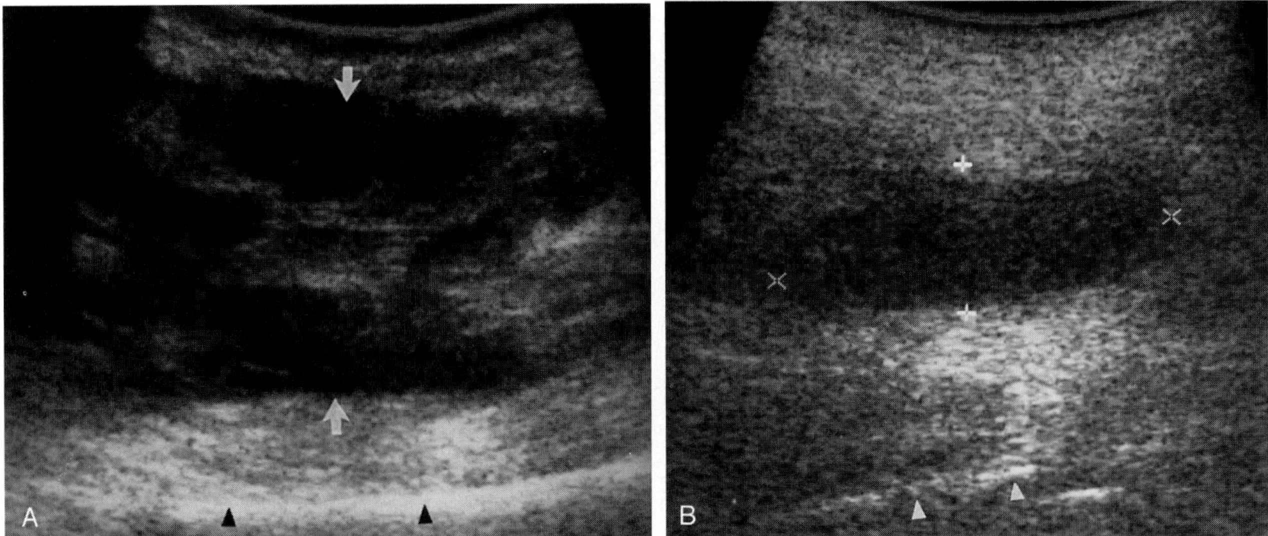

Figure 17–4 ■ **A**, Postoperative hematoma: longitudinal ultrasound. An 87-year-old woman fractured her hip, and a hemiarthroplasty was inserted. Two weeks later, she returns to the hospital with a painful, swollen thigh. The longitudinal ultrasound scan shows a mixed echogenicity fluid collection (*arrows*) superficial to the femur (*arrowheads*). The differential diagnosis includes abscess and hematoma. Aspiration yielded 500 mL of bloody fluid with visible clot. Cultures demonstrated no growth, consistent with a hematoma. **B**, Abscess: longitudinal ultrasound. Pain in the hip started about 2 weeks ago in this 57-year-old woman on renal dialysis. She was admitted to the hospital with bacteremia. Longitudinal ultrasound scan of a uniformly hypoechoic collection superficial to the lateral femur (*arrowheads*). Purulent fluid was aspirated and grew *Staphylococcus aureus*. Dimensions of the abscess: 45 mm between the × cursors and 16 mm between the + cursors.

collections include abscesses, hematomas, and seromas. Pyomyositis, while relatively unusual, has been reported in the adductors and iliacus. Clinically it can mimic a septic hip and can cause a sterile sympathetic hip effusion (Chen and Wan, 1996; Howell and Guly, 1997). MRI with gadolinium also can aid evaluation. Hematomas and abscesses can have a similar ultrasound appearance of mixed hyper-, hypo-, and anechoic areas (Fig. 17–4). Long-standing hematomas become hypoechoic or anechoic. Clinical history and aspiration can aid in differentiating these processes.

Large subcutaneous seromas can occur after soft tissue injury or contusion, especially in the thigh and buttocks, and can be a source of pain. In these cases, the etiology is probably shear forces acting on the subcutaneous tissues and causing rupture of the lymphatic and venous drainage along the fascial interface. The mixture of subcutaneous fat and fluid can interfere with the normal healing process. These collections can easily go undetected on physical exam, especially in the obese patient. We have observed anechoic or hypoechoic fluid collections up to 1–2 L in volume. Such collections can persist years after an injury. On an ultrasound scan, a seroma appears anechoic or hypoechoic (Fig. 17–5). Ultrasound-guided aspiration can relieve pain and, assess for infection and may promote more rapid healing.

Assessment of Muscle and Tendon Pathology

Muscle and tendon pathology around the hip can also be a source of pain. The proximal hamstring tendons are frequently injured in athletes. The typical injury is a partial tear due to tension while lengthening (eccentric exercise). The diagnosis is usually made clinically, with loss of function and localized pain noted and treated conservatively (Kujala et al., 1997). Imaging has a role if pain is persistent or if there is an unclear history of injury, confusing symptoms, or the need to define the severity of injury in the high-performance athlete (Brandser et al., 1995). Ultrasound or MRI can differentiate a partial tear from a complete tear; the latter is often treated surgically. Both modalities can also diagnose avulsion from the ischial tuberosity. This condition requires longer immobilization than with a partial tear, or it may be treated surgically (Brandser et al., 1995; Kujala et al., 1997).

Since the normal tendons are stronger than the musculotendinous junction or the bony insertion into the ischium, the site of hamstring injury is usually at the conjoined tendon or ischial apophysis. Fusion of the ischial apophysis does not occur until late adolescence or 20–29 years of age, and this site is the weakest link in the muscle-tendon-bone unit. Avulsion of the apophysis can demonstrate mixed

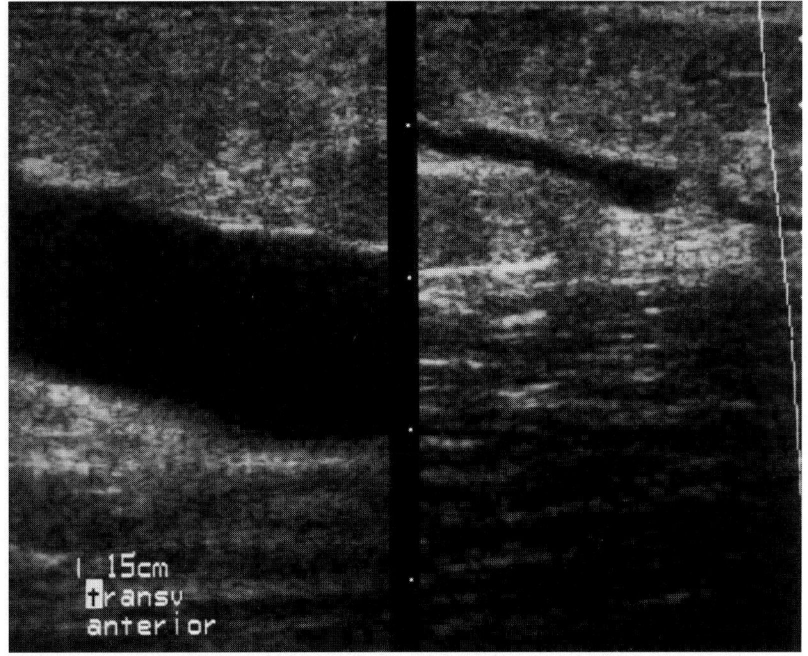

Figure 17–5 ■ Seroma of the lateral thigh: transverse ultrasound. This 25-year-old man had his upper thigh crushed in a side impact collision. Split-screen transverse ultrasound scan of an anechoic fluid collection imaged without (*left image*) and with compression (*right image*). The fluid appeared straw-colored, and culture of the aspirate yielded no growth. Those findings are characteristic of a seroma.

areas of lucency and sclerosis on conventional radiographs. With an appropriate history, this should not be mistaken for an aggressive process such as a tumor. Follow-up radiographs or ultrasound can ensure healing and callus formation. CT can best demonstrate the oblique course of the ischial apophysis, as well as a fracture or callus formation (Brandser et al., 1995).

A partial hamstring tear is demonstrated by ultrasound as an anechoic or hypoechoic gap in the tendon. Complete tears demonstrate tendon retraction and can present as a palpable mass, which can be confused with a tumor. If a rupture is chronic, atrophy may be present. Apophyseal avulsion may be demonstrated as an enlarged, irregular apophysis when compared to the asymptomatic side (Brandser et al., 1995). Muscle strain may show hypoechogenicity of the muscle with indistinctness of the muscle fibers. MRI may be more sensitive to subtle edema and muscle strain. An enlarged, hypoechoic insertion on the ischial tuberosity is consistent with tendinitis/tendinosis (Fig. 17–6).

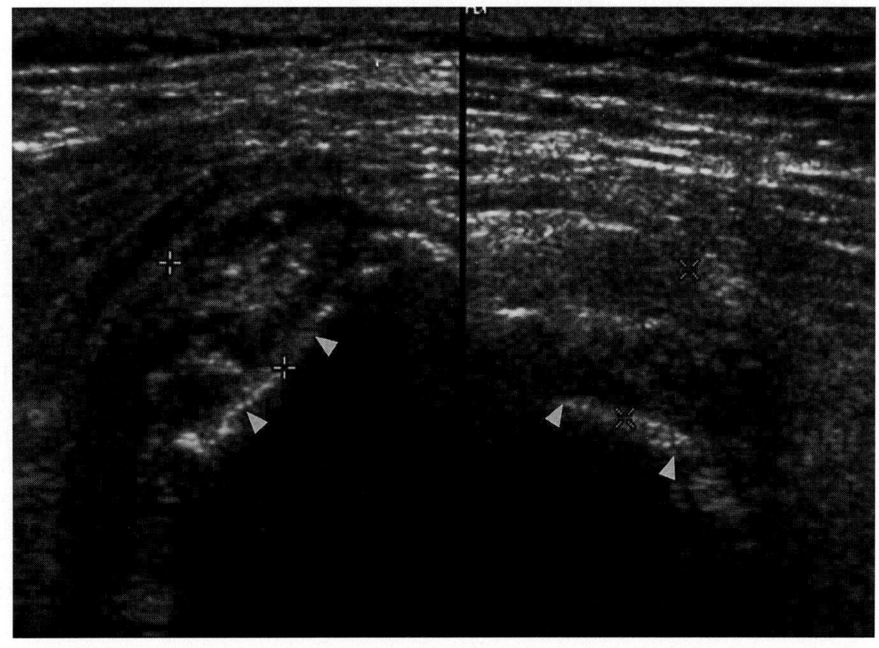

Figure 17–6 ■ Hamstrings tendinitis: transverse ultrasound. At the age of 60, this former gold medal oarsman is still engaged in competitive rowing. Three years ago, he noticed pain developing in his buttocks while rowing. The pain intensified and is now so severe that he cannot sit on his ischial tuberosities for very long. Split-screen transverse image of the right and left proximal hamstrings (*between the cursors*) at the level of the ischial tuberosity (*arrowheads*). The patient is placed in the procubitus position for this study. Thickening, hypoechogenicity, and inhomogeneity of the hamstrings are consistent with tendinitis/tendinosis. The left hamstring origin is more severely affected sonographically, corresponding to the more severe pain felt by the patient.

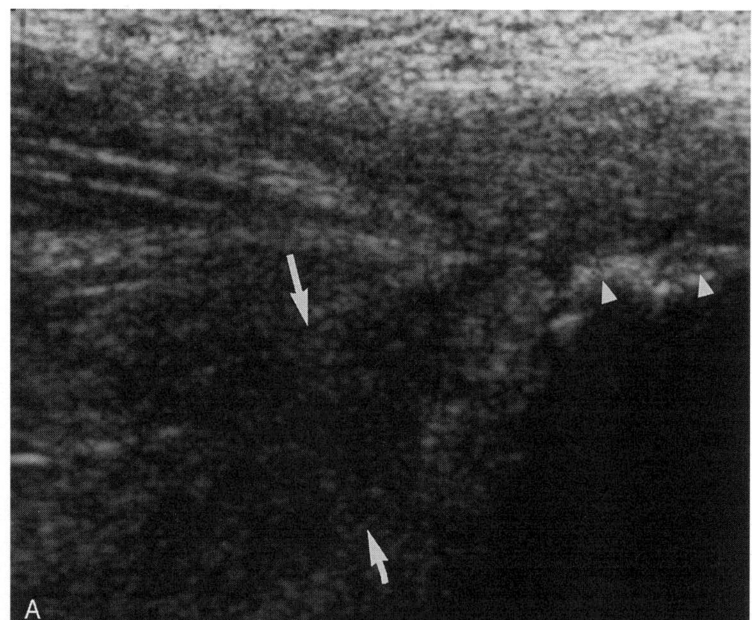

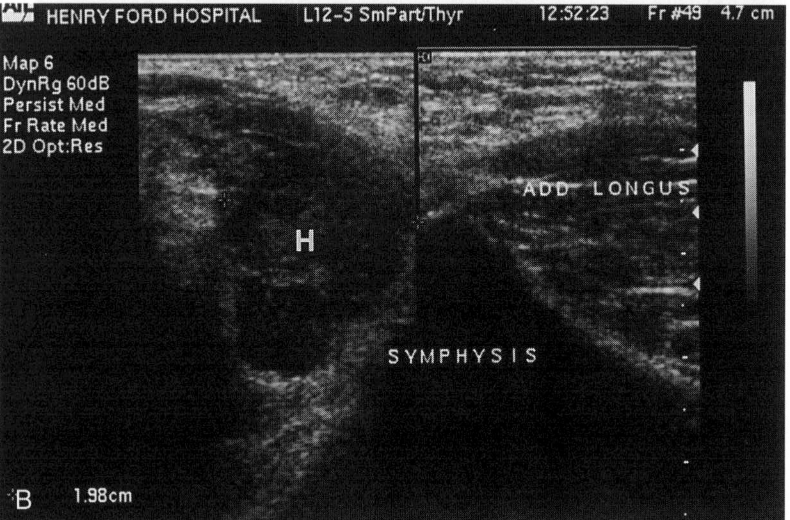

Figure 17-7 ▪ **A**, Adductor strain: transverse ultrasound. A National Hockey League player with groin pain of recent onset. Ultrasound exam along the length of the adductor longus. The adductor origin over the pubic symphysis (*arrowheads*) appears irregular. Hypoechogenicity and posterior ill definition (*arrows*) are demonstrated, consistent with a partial tear. **B**, Adductor strain: transverse ultrasound. Same patient as in **A**. Three months after the initial scan and during the 1998 Stanley cup finals, this player feels a sudden stabbing pain in his right groin. The split screen demonstrates complete separation of the right adductor longus from the pubis (*distance between the calipers*). A large hematoma (*H*) is noted on the patient's right. The retracted muscle is noted on the lateral aspect of the affected side. The normal, nonaffected side is noted on the right side of the split screen (patient's left).

Ultrasound localization of the site of injury can aid injection of steroids or analgesics.

Injury to the adductor muscles, iliopsoas, anterior superior iliac crest, and anterior inferior iliac crest, and their associated tendinous insertions, can also be a source of pain around the hip. These structures can also be evaluated with ultrasound, (Figs. 17-7 and 17-8). Radiographic diagnosis of apophyseal injuries requires the presence of an ossification center. Ultrasound does not, and it can therefore be more sensitive than radiography. Ultrasound can also diagnose instability at the site of an apophyseal avulsion (Lazovic et al., 1996).

Ultrasound of the Prosthetic Hip

Intra- and Extra-articular Fluid

Ultrasound has also been used to detect joint effusions and guide aspiration in patients with hip prostheses (Fig. 17-9) (Komppa et al., 1985; Foldes et al., 1992; van Holsbeeck et al., 1994). Extra-articular fluid collections (Fig. 17-10) may go undetected or may be misdiagnosed as joint effusions using fluoroscopic aspiration or a blind approach (Brandser et al., 1997). Bursal communication of the greater trochanter bursae, iliopsoas bursa, and

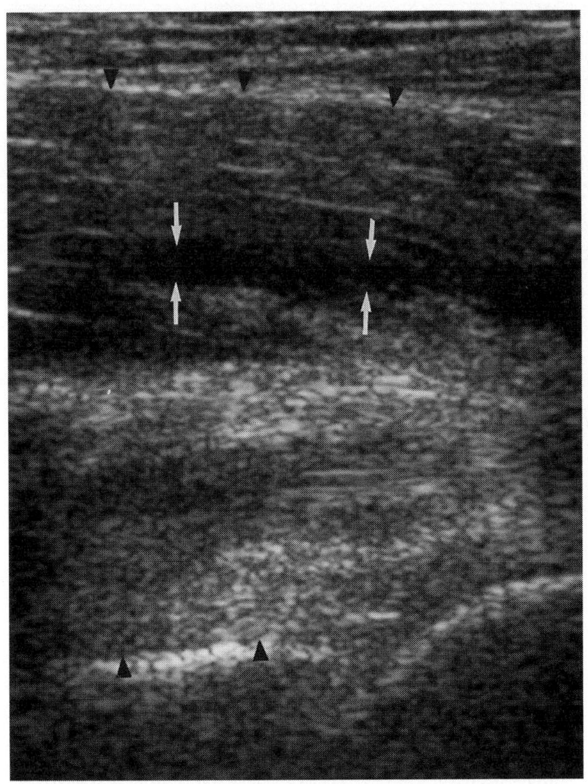

Figure 17–8 ■ Iliopsoas strain: longitudinal ultrasound. A 30-year-old National Hockey League defenseman played in the same final against the player represented in Figure 17–7. He felt a snap in his hip when leaving the bench and while speeding up to join the game. Longitudinal ultrasound scan of a hypoechoic defect (*arrows*) in the iliopsoas muscle (*arrowheads*). The findings are consistent with a longitudinal tear. The edema noted on the MRI scan far overestimated the degree of retraction. The player was able to return to play three games later.

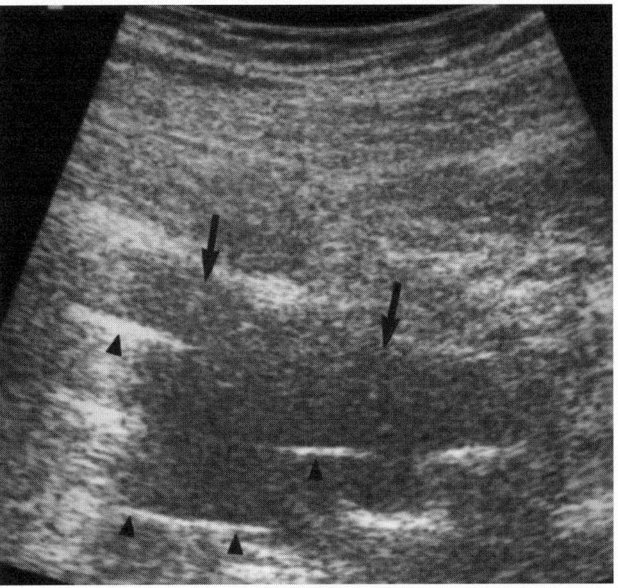

Figure 17–9 ■ Loosening of a prosthetic hip: longitudinal ultrasound. Sixteen years after the placement of left hemiarthroplasty, this 74-year-old lady complains of new groin pain. The pain started 3 months ago; the discomfort interferes with her daily activities. Longitudinal ultrasound scan of a hypoechoic hip effusion (*arrows*) within the pseudocapsule. The echogenic metal prosthesis is noted (*arrowheads*). The aspirate obtained under ultrasound showed no growth on culture but contained wear debris.

supra-acetabular region is common in the patient with a painful hip arthroplasty (Berquist et al., 1987). Such fluid collections can be assessed with ultrasound. An intra- or extra-articular fluid collection may not be visualized utilizing CT or MRI secondary to artifacts caused by a metallic prosthesis. An intra-articular effusion $\geq$3.2 mm measured at the prosthesis–bone junction with an associated extra-articular fluid collection has been reported to have high specificity for infection (van Holsbeeck et al., 1994).

Incisional Drainage in the Postoperative Patient

In patients who have undergone total hip arthroplasty or pelvic reconstruction surgery, persistent serous or bloody drainage from the skin wound is a common occurrence. Ultrasound can be used to assess for a hematoma or seroma and identify its location as superficial or adjacent to the prosthesis. Such fluid collections, especially when large and adjacent to the prosthesis, may contribute to infection and delay wound healing (Magnussen et al., 1988; Parrini et al., 1988). US-guided aspiration can assess for infection and may promote more rapid healing.

Hip Snaps, Locks, and Clicks

Hip snapping, locking, and clicking can be due to external and internal etiologies (Cardinal et al., 1996; Janzen et al., 1996) (Table 17–5). Clinical discrimination between internal and external causes can be difficult. External etiologies include friction of the gluteus maximus muscle or tensor fascia lata over the greater trochanter (Vaccaro et al., 1995). Rarely, snapping can be due to movement of the iliofemoral ligaments over the femoral head or snapping of the biceps femoris over the ischial tuberosity (Paletta and Andrish, 1995). Internal causes include intra-articular bodies, synovial osteochondromatosis, labral tears, articular surface abnormalities, intermittent subluxation of the femoral head, and snapping of the iliopsoas tendon as it moves

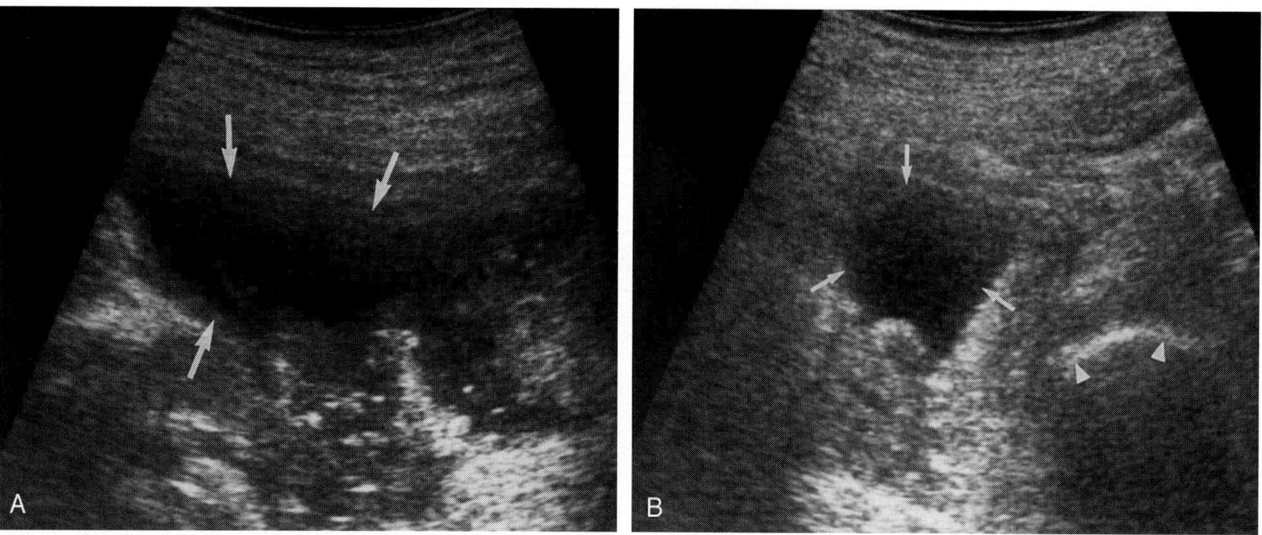

Figure 17-10 ■ **A**, Mass around a prosthetic hip: longitudinal ultrasound. Thigh swelling was first noticed on a 3-month postoperative follow-up study after total hip replacement. This middle-aged man had constantly complained of hip pain after surgery. The longitudinal ultrasound scan demonstrates a hypoechoic extra-articular fluid collection (*arrows*) anterior and lateral to the prosthesis. The differential diagnosis includes abscess and hematoma. **B**, Mass around a prosthetic hip: longitudinal ultrasound. Transverse ultrasound scan shows fluid (*arrows*) lateral to the femur (*arrowheads*). Culture of the aspirate demonstrated no growth. Findings are consistent with a late-stage hematoma.

over the iliopectineal eminence (Schaberg et al., 1984; Cardinal et al., 1996; Janzen et al., 1996).

The snapping hip syndrome produces a painful and audible snap during hip motion. MRI or CT frequently does not detect the tendon pathology since tendon thickening and abnormal fluid in the iliopsoas bursa are usually absent (Schaberg et al., 1984; Cardinal et al., 1996; Janzen et al., 1996). Iliopsoas bursography or hip tenography demonstrates the abnormal movement of the iliopsoas tendon, but these procedures are invasive, not widely performed, and technically difficult (Cardinal et al., 1996; Janzen et al., 1996).

Table 17-5
Differential Diagnosis and Imaging of the Snapping, Locking, or Clicking Hip

1. External etiologies
   a. Iliotibial band syndrome—MRI and ultrasound
2. Internal etiologies
   a. Intra-articular bodies—arthrography, ultrasound
   b. Synovial osteochondromatosis—radiographs, CT, MRI, ultrasound
   c. Labral tears—MR arthrography, ultrasound
   d. Articular surface abnormalities—radiographs, MRI
   e. Intermittent subluxation of the femoral head
   f. Snapping iliopsoas syndrome—ultrasound, bursography

Source: Schaberg et al., 1984; Cardinal et al., 1996; Janzen et al., 1996.

Ultrasound has proved valuable as a noninvasive method of diagnosing the snapping iliopsoas tendon. A linear 5–7 MHz transducer is utilized. Transverse imaging is performed at the approximate level of the femoral head (Janzen et al., 1996). The dynamic scanning capabilities of ultrasound provide an advantage over static techniques such as MRI. With the hip flexed and externally rotated, scanning is performed in the transverse plane as the hip is rotated internally and extended. The dynamic capability of ultrasound allows direct visualization of the abnormal lateral to medial movement of the tendon as the patient extends and internally rotates the hip (Fig. 17-11). The abnormal tendon motion can be directly correlated with the palpable click felt through the transducer and with the audible click heard secondary to abnormal tendon movement. Mediolateral movement of the iliopsoas tendon is not present in the normal patient, and comparison with the contralateral hip can aid in assessing normal tendon motion and thickness (Janzen et al., 1996). Rubbing of the tendon over the iliopubic eminence can cause pain and discomfort. Additional cross-sectional imaging may be required to assess for intra-articular pathology, but ultrasound can accurately diagnose the snapping tendon when it otherwise would not be imaged (Cardinal et al., 1996; Janzen et al., 1996).

It is also possible that ultrasound may aid the diagnosis of snapping tendons in other locations, such as over the greater trochanter. Ultrasound has also been used to diagnose iliopsoas tendinitis, seen

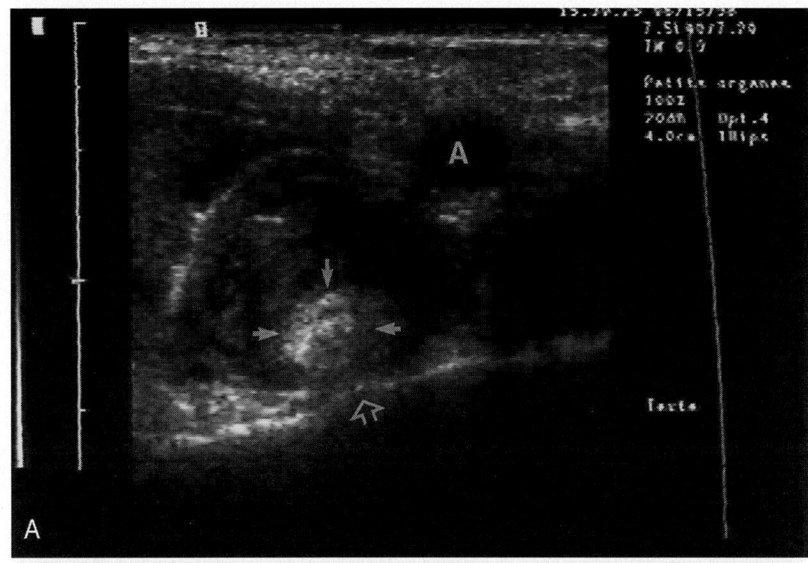

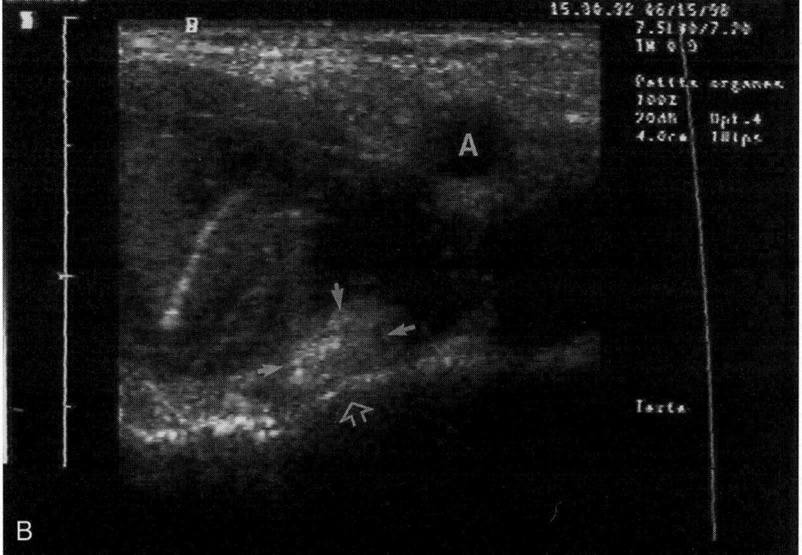

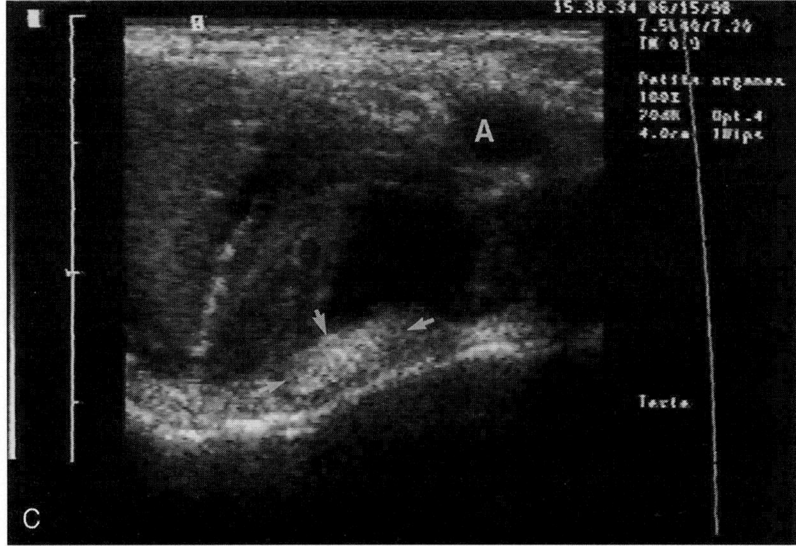

Figure 17–11 ■ **A**, Snapping iliopsoas tendon: transverse sonogram of the hip in the neutral position. This video frame of a dynamic hip study shows the iliopsoas (*arrows*) tendon in neutral position. The ileopubic eminence presents as an osseous protuberance (*open arrow*) deep to the tendon. Abbreviation: external iliac artery (*A*). **B**, Snapping iliopsoas tendon: transverse sonogram with the hip in flexion and external rotation. The tendon (*arrows*) jerks over the iliopubic eminence (*open arrow*). The dynamic study (video) documents this unusual tendon mobility. Ultrasound, so far, is the only modality that has been able to document an abnormal snapping of the iliopsoas tendon. Abbreviation: artery (*A*). **C**, Snapping iliopsoas tendon: transverse sonogram of the hip in neutral position. The hypermobile iliopsoas tendon (*arrows*), flattens considerably at the endpoint of the jerk. Abbreviation: external iliac artery (*A*). (Photos courtesy of Etienne Cardinal, M.D., Montreal, Canada.)

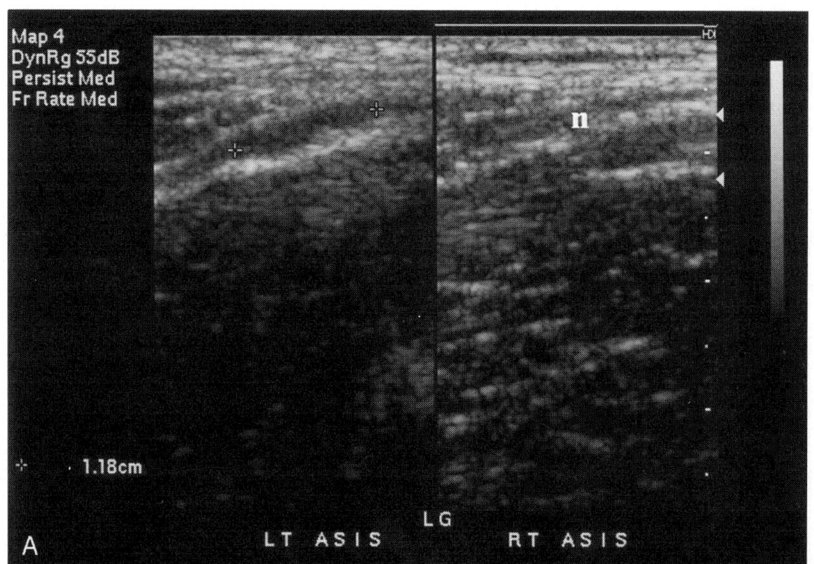

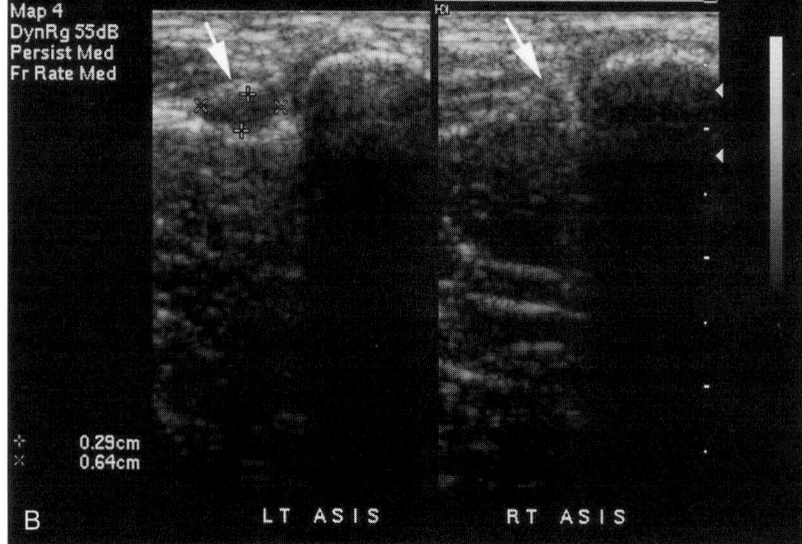

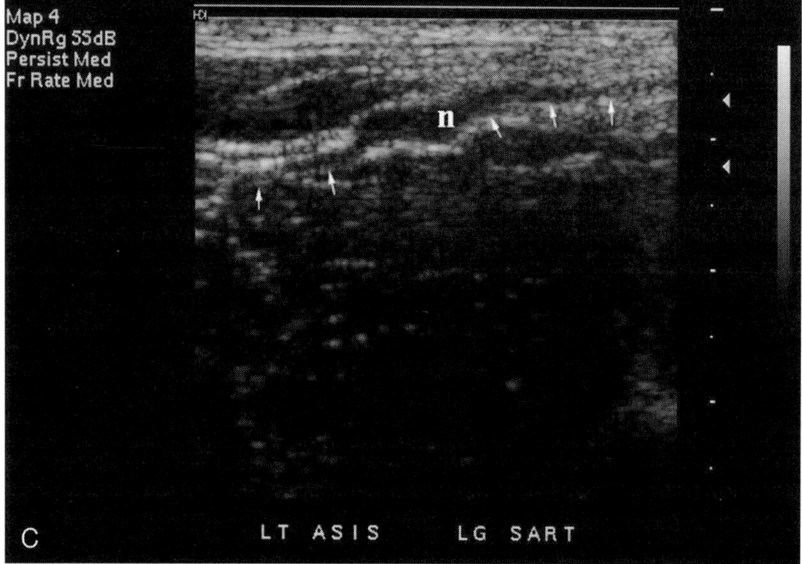

Figure 17-12 ■ **A**, Meralgia paresthetica: Split-screen longitudinal ultrasound. A 20-year-old college student developed pain and numbness over the left lateral aspect of his thigh. Swinging a baseball bat aggravates the pain. With the transducer medial to the anterior superior iliac spine and aligned with the long axis of the thigh, we can observe the swelling of the lateral femoral cutaneous nerve (*between the calipers*) on the symptomatic left side in comparison with the normal nerve (*n*) on the right. **B**, Meralgia paresthetica: transverse ultrasound. Same patient as in **A**. Comparison of the normal right nerve (*arrow*) and the abnormal left (*calipers*) nerve (*arrow*) visualized with a transverse transducer position. Note the more hypoechoic edematous left femoral cutaneous nerve. **C**, Meralgia paresthetica: longitudinal ultrasound. Same patient as in **A**. Detail of the affected lateral femoral cutaneous nerve. The nerve swells fusiformly (*n*) at the level of the anterior superior iliac spine. Entrapment of the nerve and abnormal friction have been blamed for this pathology, which occurs at the site where the nerve exits the pelvis. The ultrasound detail is exquisite. The nerve tissue (*small arrows*) proximal and distal to the site of swelling is no more than 2 mm in diameter.

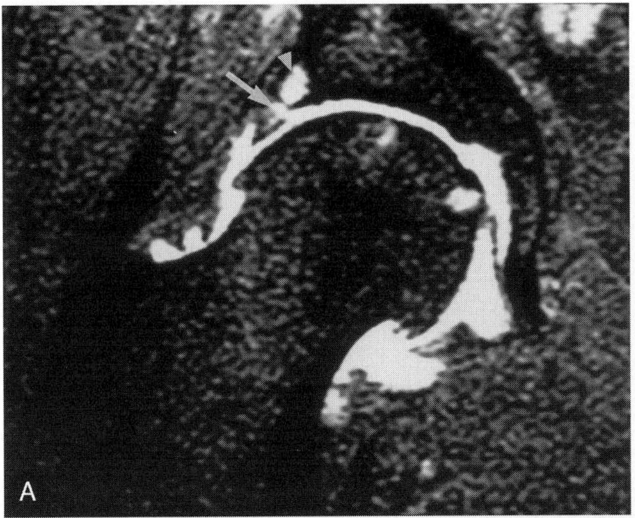

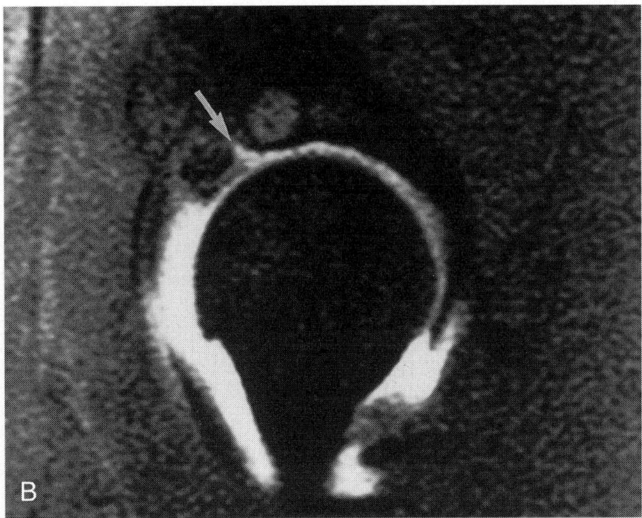

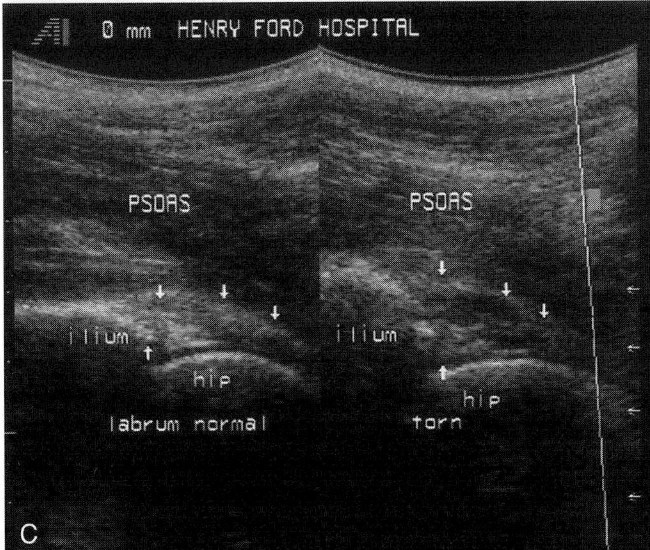

Figure 17–13 ■ **A,** Labral tear: coronal T_1-weighted gadolinium arthrogram. Persistent hip pain and hip click interfere with the athletic endeavors of this 53-year-old patient. Coronal T_1-weighted image of the hip after an intra-articular gadolinium arthrogram shows a labral tear (*arrow*) and a communicating acetabular cyst (*arrowhead*). Osteophytes, subchondral cysts, and joint space narrowing are present. **B,** Labral tear: sagittal T_1-weighted gadolinium arthrogram. Same patient as in **A**. Sagittal T_1-weighted image after an intra-articular gadolinium arthrogram demonstrates the anterior labral tear (*arrow*). **C,** Labral tear: ultrasound with split-screen comparison sagittal images. Similar pathology as in **A** and **B**. This 32-year-old man feels groin pain and a click while preparing for a marathon. He is an experienced marathon runner, but this recent injury slows him down considerably. The left side of the split screen shows a normal anterior labrum appearing triangular and hyperechoic. The right side of the split screen shows hypoechoic damage due to tear of the anterior hip labrum. The normal and abnormal labrums are both outlined by *small arrows.* Note that ultrasound can be done without the injection of intra-articular contrast material; this is considered a major advantage over MRI.

as enlargement of the tendon when compared to the asymptomatic side, and to guide local injection of corticosteroids (Fredberg and Hansen, 1995). Constant rubbing of nerve tissue over the anterior iliac crest can cause lateral thigh pain called *meralgia paresthetica.* Split-screen imaging of the lateral femoral cutaneous nerve may show the unilateral swelling on the affected side (Fig. 17–12).

Tears of the acetabular labrum can be a source of pain and cause clicking of the hip (Byrd, 1996). The acetabular labrum is a fibrocartilaginous structure similar to the glenoid labrum and meniscus in the knee, with similar pathology seen in each of these structures. MR arthrography can be used to assess the acetabular labrum, (Fig. 17–13) (Czerny et al., 1996). However, this technique is invasive and expensive, and can cause scheduling difficulties in coordinating fluoroscopy and MRI. In some cases, ultrasound can detect labral tears. The normal labrum appears as a hyperechoic triangle along the acetabulum. A labral tear appears anechoic or hypoechoic (Fig. 17–3), and can be associated with fluid-filled cysts within the labrum or acetabulum (Fig. 17–13).

Additional intra-articular and bony pathology including articular surface abnormalities, occult or complex acetabular fractures, avascular necrosis (AVN), and bone marrow abnormalities are best assessed with CT or MRI. In some cases, intra-articular loose bodies can be detected by ultrasound, especially when an effusion is present (Frankel et al., 1998).

References

Berman L, et al: Technical note: Identifying and aspirating hip effusions. *Br J Radiol* 68:306–310, 1995.

Berquist TH: Imaging of articular pathology: MRI, CT, arthrograpy. *Clin Anat.* 10:1–13, 1997.

Berquist TH, et al: Pseudobursae: A useful finding in patients with painful hip arthroplasty. *AJR* 148: 103–106, 1987.

Brandser EA, El-Khoury GY, FitzRandolph RL: Modified technique for fluid aspiration in patients with prosthetic hips. *Radiology* 204:580–582, 1997.

Brandser EA, et al: Hamstring injuries: Radiographic, conventional tomographic, CT, and MR imaging characteristics. *Radiology* 197:257–262, 1995.

Breidahl WH, et al: Power Doppler sonography in the assessment of musculoskeletal fluid collections. *AJR* 166: 1443–1446, 1996.

Byrd, JW: Labral lesions: An elusive source of hip pain. Case reports and literature review. *Arthroscopy* 12: 603–612, 1996.

Cardinal E, et al: US of the snapping iliopsoas tendon. *Radiology* 198:521–522, 1996.

Chan YL, Cheng JC, Metreweli C: Sonographic evaluation of hip effusion in children. Improved visualization with the hip in extension and abduction. *Acta Radiol* 38:867–869, 1997.

Chandler SB: The iliopsoas bursa in man. *Anat Rec* 58:235–240, 1934.

Chen WS, Wan YL: Iliacus pyomyositis mimicking septic arthritis of the hip joint. *Arch Orthop Trauma Surg* 115:233–235, 1996.

Cimmino MA: Recognition and management of bacterial arthritis. *Drugs* 54:50–60, 1997.

Czerny C, et al: Lesions of the acetabular labrum: Accuracy of MR imaging and MR arthrography in detection and staging. *Radiology* 200:225–230, 1996.

Flanagan FL, et al: Symptomatic enlarged iliopsoas bursa in the presence of a normal plain hip radiograph. *Br J Rheumatol* 34:365–369, 1995.

Foldes K, et al: Ultrasonography after hip arthroplasty. *Skeletal Radiol* 21:297–299, 1992.

Frankel DA, et al: Synovial joints: Evaluation of intraarticular bodies with US. *Radiology* 206:41–44, 1998.

Fredberg U, Hansen LB: Ultrasound in the diagnosis and treatment of iliopsoas tendonitis: A case report. *Scand J Med Sci Sports* 5:369–370, 1995.

Gray H, Clemente CD (eds): *Anatomy of the Human Body*, ed 13. Philadelphia, Lea & Febiger, 1985, pp 566–568.

Hayes CW, Balkissoon AR: Current concepts in imaging of the pelvis and hip. *Orthop Clin North Am* 28: 617–642, 1997.

Howell MA, Guly HR: A case of muscle abscess presenting to an accident and emergency department. *J Accid Emerg Med* 14:180–182, 1997.

Janzen DL, et al: The snapping hip: Clinical and imaging findings in transient subluxation of the iliopsoas tendon. *Can Assoc Radiol J* 47:202–208, 1996.

Komppa GH, et al: Ultrasound guidance for needle aspiration of the hip in patients with painful hip prosthesis. *J Clin Ultrasound* 13:433, 1985.

Koski JM: Ultrasonographic evidence of hip synovitis in patients with rheumatoid arthritis. *Scand J Rheumatol* 18:127–131, 1989.

Koski JM, Anttila PJ, Isomaki HA: Ultrasonography of the adult hip joint. *Scand J Rheumatol* 18:113–117, 1989.

Koski JM, Isomaki H: Ultrasonography may reveal synovitis in a clinically silent hip joint. *Clin Rheumatol* 9:539–541, 1990.

Kujala UM, Orava S, Jarvinen M: Hamstring injuries. Current trends in treatment and prevention. *Sports Med* 23:397–404, 1997.

Laorr A, Helms CA: *MRI of Musculoskeletal Masses.* New York, Igaku-Shoin, 1997, pp 73–76.

Lazovic D, et al: Ultrasound for diagnosis of apophyseal injuries. *Knee Surg Sports Traumatol Arthrosc* 3: 234–237, 1996.

Magnussen PA, Crozier AE, Gregg PJ: Detecting haematomas by ultrasound: Brief report. *J Bone Joint Surg [Br]* 70:150, 1988.

Marcelis S, Daenen B, Ferrara MA: Dondelinger RF: *Peripheral Musculoskeletal Ultrasound Atlas.* New York, Thieme, 1996.

Middleton DB: Infectious arthritis. *Primary Care* 20: 943–953, 1993.

Newman JS, et al: Power Doppler sonography of synovitis: Assessment of therapeutic response, preliminary observations. *Radiology* 198:582, 1996.

Nimityongskul P, et al: Ultrasonography in the management of painful hips in children. *Am J Orthop* 25:411–414, 1996.

Paletta GA, Andrish JT: Injuries about the hip and pelvis in the young athlete. *Clin Sports Med* 14:591–628, 1995.

Parrini L, Baratelli M, Parrini M: Ultrasound examination of haematomas after total hip replacement. *Int Orthop* 12:79–82, 1988.

Schaberg JE, Harper MC, Allen WC: The snapping hip syndrome. *Am J Sports Med* 12:361–365, 1984.

Shiv VK, et al: Sonography of hip joint in infective arthritis. *Can Assoc Radiol J* 41:76–78, 1990.

Steinbach LS, et al: Bursa and abscess cavities communicating with the hip. Diagnosing using arthrography and CT. *Radiology* 156:303, 1985.

Steiner E, et al: Ganglia and cysts around joints. *Radiol Clin North Am* 34:395–425, 1996.

Strouse PJ, DiPietro MA, Adler RS: Pediatric hip effusions: Evaluation with power Doppler sonography. *Radiology* 206;731–735, 1998.

Vaccarro JP, Sauser DD, Beals RK: Iliopsoas bursa imaging: Efficacy in depicting abnormal iliopsoas tendon motion in patients with internal snapping hip syndrome. *Radiology* 197:853–856, 1995.

van Holsbeeck MT, et al: Detection of infection in loosened hip prostheses: Efficacy of sonography. *AJR* 163: 381–384, 1994.

Varma DGK, Parihar A, Richli WR: CT appearance of the distended trochanteric bursa. *J Comput Assist Tomogr* 17:141–143, 1993.

Zawin JK, et al: Joint effusion in children with an irritable hip: US diagnosis and aspiration. *Radiology* 187: 459–463, 1993.

Zieger MM, Dorr U, Schulz RD: Ultrasonography of hip joint effusions. *Skeletal Radiol* 16:607–611, 1987.

Chapter 18
Sonography of the Knee

Ruth Y. Ceulemans, M.D., and Marnix T. van Holsbeeck, M.D.

MRI and ultrasound are the modalities of choice for evaluation of soft tissue pathology of the knee. MRI is typically preferred for evaluation of chronic symptoms of internal derangement. Ultrasound is a better choice as the initial study when clinical features suggest tendon disease, bursal inflammation, synovial abnormality, or capsular disease. Unique advantages of ultrasound in the examination of the knee include dynamic testing of ligaments and tendons, high-resolution imaging of internal tendon structure, and the capacity to distinguish collections of fluid accurately from soft tissue edema.

Technical Guidelines and Scanning Technique

Ultrasound examination of the knee is first directed to the anterior aspect of the joint, followed by the medial and lateral aspects, and concludes with the study of the popliteal fossa. A 7.5 MHz linear array transducer is used for the adult patient of average body habitus. The structures in the posterior knee joint space, seated deep in the popliteal fossa, may be best examined with a 5 MHz linear array transducer. Rarely, a 5 MHz curved array transducer may be of value in examining the popliteal fossa. The longitudinal view offers the best imaging plane for the anatomical structures shown at the anterior, medial, and lateral aspects of the knee; a few specific exceptions are noted in the text. In the popliteal fossa, the transverse view is best for an initial survey. The entire routine examination of the knee can be completed in 20 minutes.

Examination is initiated with the patient supine and the knee in full extension. Imaging of the anterior aspect of the knee allows identification and evaluation of the suprapatellar pouch, the medial and lateral patellar recesses of the joint (transverse view), the quadriceps tendon, the distal muscle components of the quadriceps, and the anterior horns of the medial and lateral menisci. The knee is then placed in moderate flexion (30–45 degrees) and the patellar tendon, Hoffa's fat pad, the deep infrapatellar bursa, and the subcutaneous soft tissue, including the site of the prepatellar and superficial infrapatellar bursae, are studied. Complete flexion of the knee is utilized to examine the middle and distal portions of the anterior cruciate ligament, the articular cartilage covering the intercondylar notch (femoral trochlea), and the weight-bearing aspects of both femoral condyles.

When the transducer is positioned anteriorly in the midline of the distal thigh with the leg straight and scanning along the long axis, both the quadriceps tendon and the suprapatellar bursa are examined. Moderate knee flexion is required for optimal filling of the bursa. The base of the patella is the inferior landmark of this image. Maintaining this longitudinal imaging plane, the transducer should be moved gently from medial to lateral, encompassing the entire width of the suprapatellar bursa and the quadriceps tendon. Only a thin layer of fluid, no more than 2 mm thick, should be present in the normal suprapatellar bursa. As the suprapatellar bursa is not the dependent portion of the knee joint space in a supine patient, care should be taken to image both the medial and lateral patellar recesses for additional fluid or to move any fluid into the anterior suprapatellar bursa using manual compression. The latter can be done by an assistant or with the free hand of the examiner. Any increase in suprapatellar fluid by this maneuver is considered abnormal. The medial and lateral patellar recesses are imaged on either side of the patella with the transducer held transversely, perpendicular to the long axis of the leg. Firm transducer compression of the suprapatellar pouch displaces any fluid into the adjacent joint space and allows accurate measurement of the thickness of the synovium. The ability to displace fluid confirms its nature. This is especially valuable in the setting of hyperechoic blood or pus. It also demonstrates the communication between the suprapatellar bursa and the adjacent knee joint space. Since in the fetus the suprapatellar bursa is initially sequestered by a suprapatellar septum, which should perforate by the fifth month in utero, confirmation of the communication is often desirable.

The anterior infrapatellar soft tissues are imaged with the knee in moderate flexion (30–45 degrees). A longitudinal midline transducer position at the apex of the patella enables imaging of the proximal and middle portions of the patellar tendon. Sliding the transducer distally, the inferior portion of the tendon is followed to its insertion on the tibial tuberosity. Medial to lateral translation of the transducer will ensure coverage of the full width of the tendon. Transverse imaging is performed by rotating the transducer 90 degrees from the longitudinal plane. The ultrasound beam should be perpendicular to the tendon surface to avoid anisotropy, which causes falsely decreased tendon echogenicity. The correct transducer angulation can be selected by gentle craniocaudal angulation of the transverse transducer. Images in this region also reveal Hoffa's fat pad deep to the patellar tendon, the prepatellar bursa, the superficial infrapatellar bursa in the subcutis, and the deep infrapatellar bursa interposed between the proximal anterior tibia and the patellar tendon insertion.

Articular cartilage of the weight-bearing surfaces of the femoral condyles and the femoral trochlea can be displayed by using a 7.5 MHz linear transducer positioned transversely, proximal to the patella (Aisen et al., 1984). Complete flexion of the knee is required so that the weight-bearing portions of the femoral condyles are no longer in apposition to the tibial plateau. Normal hyaline cartilage appears as a well-defined hypoechoic band with sharp anterior and posterior margins. The cartilage is thickest over the intercondylar area and thinner over the femoral condyles. Because of the wide range of normal thickness, the opposite knee is routinely imaged for comparison. Arthritic patients often have limitation of flexion, in which case the contralateral knee is examined in the same position (Harcke et al., 1988).

Examination of the anterior cruciate ligament also requires flexion of the knee joint to open up the anterior aspect of the intercondylar fossa and limit superimposition of bony structures. The optimal degree of flexion varies from 45 to 60 degrees (Laine et al., 1987) to maximum flexion (Suzuki et al., 1991). In flexion, the middle and distal thirds of the anterior cruciate ligament can be examined. When evaluating patients in the acute posttraumatic setting with ligamentous injury or hemarthrosis, flexion may be very limited. A 5 MHz linear or curved array transducer should be used. Align the transducer along the longitudinal course of the anterior cruciate ligament. The transducer should be positioned anteriorly below the patella and medial to the midline along the longitudinal axis of the tibia, followed by a 30 degree counterclockwise rotation of the transducer for the right knee and similar clockwise rotation for the left knee. A transverse section through the anterior cruciate ligament can then be obtained by rotating the transducer 90 degrees. Another method is to image the patellar tendon transversely at the level of the joint space, followed by a 30 degree counterclockwise (for right) or clockwise rotation (for left). The transducer should sweep from superior lateral to inferior medial along the expected course of the ligament.

The medial aspect of the knee is examined with the patient turned to a lateral decubitus position or supine with external rotation of the leg. The lateral decubitus position is preferred, as it permits full extension of the leg and easier application of stress. Examination of the medial aspect of the knee allows identification and analysis of the medial (tibial) collateral ligament, the body of the medial meniscus, the medial femorotibial joint space, and the pes anserine tendon insertion. Centering the linear 7.5 MHz transducer to the medial joint line with a longitudinal orientation images the medial collateral ligament. In this plane, craniocaudal movement of the transducer from the proximal aspect of the medial femoral condyle down to the proximal tibial metaphysis, as well as anteroposterior movement of the transducer, is necessary to visualize the entire medial collateral ligament. In order to study the internal margin of the meniscus, the gain setting should be increased. Mild valgus stress will open the joint space and allow better delineation of the meniscus. Placing the knee at the edge of the examination table or over a triangular cushion will provide sufficient stress. The meniscus is normally hyperechoic, and its configuration in a longitudinal view is triangular, with its apex pointing toward the center of the joint. Its base is anchored to the linear hyperechoic knee joint capsule without any intervening tissue. Subsequent examination of the meniscus in the transverse plane facilitates the detection of radial tears. In this plane, the normal meniscus is hyperechoic and ribbon-like, with a smooth, continuous inner margin.

The *lateral aspect of the knee* may be studied with the patient in one of three positions: (1) internally rotating the leg, maintaining full extension, (2) assuming a lateral decubitus position, or (3) for the lateroposterior structures, prone. This portion of the examination identifies ligaments and tendons from anterior to posterior: the iliotibial band, popliteal tendon origin, lateral (fibular) collateral ligament, and distal biceps femoris tendon. The body of the lateral meniscus and the lateral femorotibial joint space are imaged deep to these structures. The iliotibial band, the origin of the popliteal tendon, the body of the lateral meniscus, and the lateral joint space can be visualized in a longitudinal plane, parallel to the long axis of the leg. The origin of the popliteal tendon is easily localized in relation to the popliteal groove on the lateral femoral condyle, just anterior to the origin of the lateral collateral ligament. The lateral collateral ligament and distal biceps tendon have a conjoint V-shaped insertion on the fibular head, which serves as a bony landmark. Mild angulation of the longitudinally positioned transducer to a paracoronal plane, oriented from posterosuperior to anteroinferior, can depict the tendon in its entire extent. When the transducer is oriented from anterosuperior to posteroinferior, the lateral collateral ligament is imaged. The normal lateral collateral ligament appears as a thin, band-like, hypoechoic structure. The common peroneal nerve may be identified in its course posteromedial to the distal biceps femoris muscle and its tendon.

The *posterior aspect of the knee*, the popliteal fossa, is examined with the patient prone. Most anatomical structures in the popliteal fossa are initially imaged in the transverse plane. The following structures of the posterior aspect of the knee can be identified: the popliteal artery, vein and nerve; medial and lateral heads of the gastrocnemius muscle; distal tendon of the semimembranosus muscle; pes anserine tendons; and the crural fascia. The popliteal artery, vein, and nerve can be identified in that order from deep to superficial and from medial to lateral. The diameter of the popliteal artery should not exceed 1.5 cm. The patency of the popliteal artery and vein is assessed by the anechogenicity and compressibility of these structures with gray scale technique and by the application of duplex, color flow, or power Doppler mode. The patency of the popliteal vein and the subcutaneous lesser saphenous vein can be ensured when there is complete venous collapse under transducer compression at multiple levels. The neck of a Baker's cyst is found between the semimembranosus tendon and the medial head of the gastrocnemius muscle. The cyst may have an inverted Y shape, with one limb deep and the other superficial to the medial head of the gastrocnemius. The inferior pole of the cyst usually exhibits a smooth convex contour. If the contour is irregular, the calf distal to the most inferior extent of the cyst should be examined to look for fluid tracking down either beneath the fascia or between the soleus and gastrocnemius muscles, indicative of cyst rupture. Inflammation of the overlying subcutaneous tissues is a good secondary indicator of pseudothrombophlebitis.

A longitudinal view, using a linear or curved linear array 5 MHz transducer, displays the posterior cruciate ligament, the posterior joint space, the joint capsule, and the posterior horn of the medial and lateral menisci. In the popliteal fossa, the posterior cruciate ligament is easily examined with the transducer positioned in the midline and oriented along the long axis of the leg. The posterior aspect of the distal femoral and the proximal tibial epiphysis serve as landmarks for positioning the transducer over the posterior joint space. The transducer is then rotated 30 degrees counterclockwise for the right leg or 30 degrees clockwise for the left leg. From this position, the transducer is gently moved from medially to laterally to find the correct imaging plane that will display the ligament over its entire length (Suzuki et al., 1991). On the longitudinal view, the normal posterior cruciate ligament appears as a taut, posteriorly convex, hypoechoic band in the posterior aspect of the intercondylar fossa. It is nicely outlined by contrast with the surrounding normal intra-articular hyperechoic fat. Its tibial insertion is better delineated than its femoral origin on the longitudinal view.

For the transverse view, the transducer is rotated 90 degrees from the longitudinal imaging plane described above and moved from the superior medial to the inferior lateral aspect of the surface along the expected course of the posterior cruciate ligament. The ligament runs from the intercondylar aspect of the medial femoral condyle toward the posterior aspect of the lateral tibial condyle. Another method of obtaining the transverse imaging plane is to position the transducer at 90 degrees to the long axis of the leg, followed by a 30 degree counterclockwise rotation for the right leg or a 30 degree clockwise rotation for the left leg (Suzuki et al., 1991). In the transverse view, the posterior cruciate ligament is visualized as a hypoechoic, well-defined ovoid structure. The posterior horn of the medial meniscus is tightly anchored to the linear hyperechoic knee joint capsule without any intervening tissue. The posterior horn of the lateral meniscus differs in that the popliteus canal intervenes between the capsule and the meniscus at the middle and posterior portions of the lateral meniscus (Selby et al., 1986; Richardson et al., 1988). The canal is

Table 18–1
Anterior, Medial, Lateral, and Posterior Examination of the Knee

Extension	Flexion
Anterior	
Suprapatellar pouch	Patellar tendon
Medial and lateral patellar recess	Hoffa's fat pad
Quadriceps tendon	Deep infrapatellar bursa
Medial	**Lateral**
Medial collateral ligament	Iliotibial band
Body of the medial meniscus	Popliteal tendon
Medial femorotibial joint space	Lateral collateral ligament
	Distal biceps femoris tendon
	Body of the lateral meniscus
	Lateral femorotibial joint space
Posterior	
7.5 MHz	5 MHz
Popliteal a, v [and n]	Posterior cruciate ligament
Gastrocnemius muscle	Posterior joint space
Baker's cyst (+/− calf distally)	Posterior horn of menisci

identified as a hypoechoic region interposed between the periphery of the lateral meniscus and the capsule; superiorly and inferiorly, it is delineated by hyperechoic struts, which allow passage of the popliteus tendon. The posterior horn is the largest part of either meniscus.

The anterior cruciate ligament, the articular cartilage, the anterior horns of both the lateral and medial menisci, and the pes anserine insertion are not routinely used in our standard ultrasound examination of the knee. Their examination is done at the clinician's request or when indicated by the chief complaint of the patient.

Summary of the Routine Examination

The routine examination of the knee is summarized in Table 18–1. Additional studies include the anterior cruciate ligament, articular cartilage, and anterior horn of the menisci.

Swelling

A swelling or palpable mass, which fills the popliteal space, is a common clinical presentation in both children and adults. Transillumination has been used to distinguish an uncomplicated Baker's cyst from a vascular or neoplastic process. A large number of cysts are complicated by hemorrhage or chronic inflammation and as a result will not transilluminate. On ultrasound, a Baker's cyst should originate from the posteromedial aspect of the knee and should have a distinct neck situated between the medial head of the gastrocnemius muscle and the semimembranosus tendon. Popliteal aneurysm (Fig. 18–1) and popliteal venous thrombosis (Fig. 18–2) are easily diagnosed by gray scale and/or Doppler sonography. Aneurysms are then referred to a vascular surgeon for evaluation. Soft tissue masses that are not cysts and do not appear to originate from the popliteal vessels require biopsy for definitive diagnosis (Pathria et al., 1988). Ultrasound is very helpful in targeting smaller, nonpalpable lesions and avoiding major vessels.

Painful swelling of the calf may result from a Baker's cyst dissecting into the calf (Rudikoff et al., 1976), rupture of the cyst (Gompels and Darlington, 1979; Harper et al., 1982), thrombophlebitis, muscle tear, or occasionally Achilles tendon rupture. Muscle tears most often involve the medial head of the gastrocnemius (Bianchi et al., 1998). If the muscle or tendon injury is acute posttraumatic or sports-related, the clinical findings and history will in-

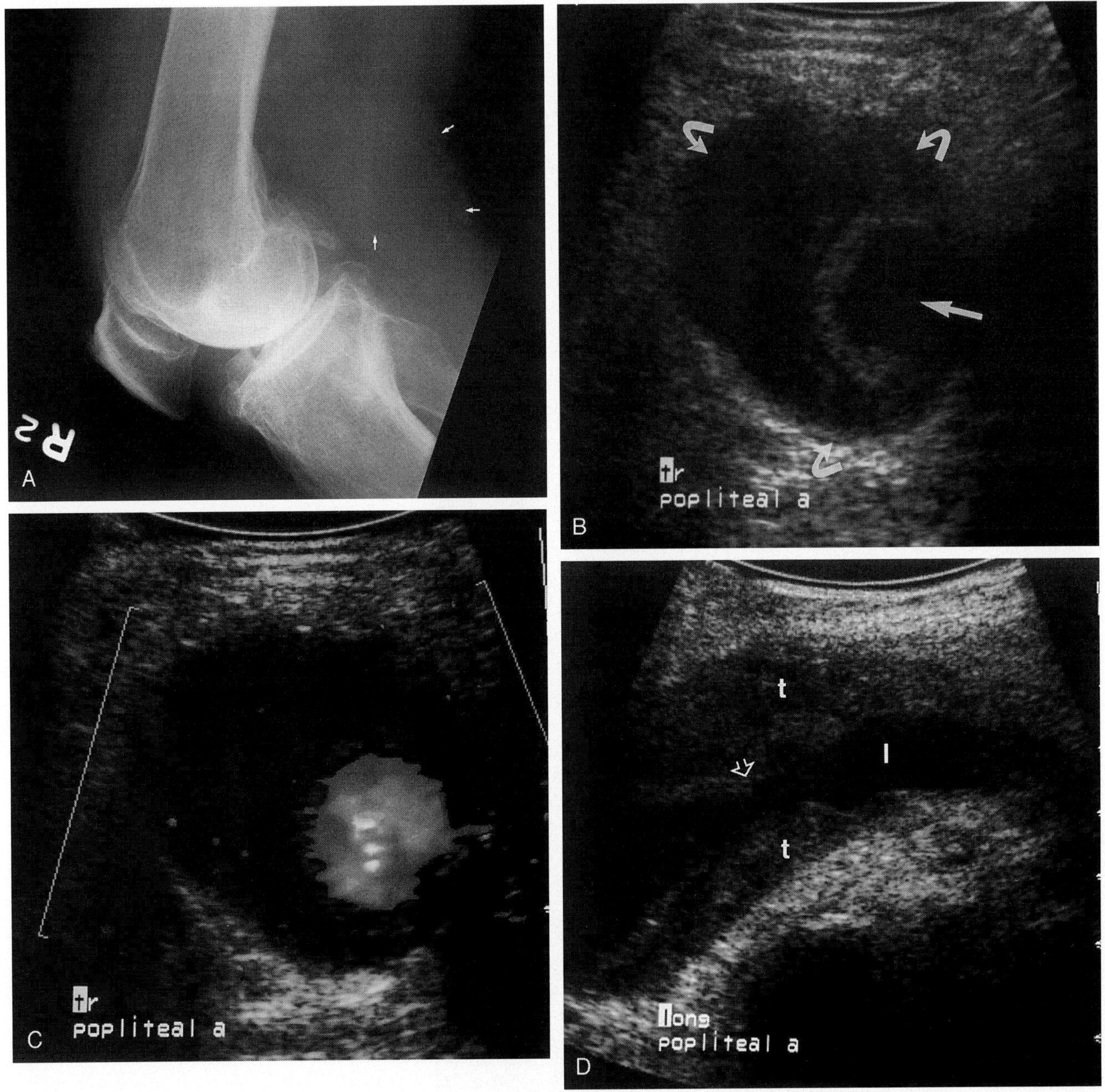

Figure 18–1 ■ **A**, Popliteal artery aneurysm: lateral radiograph of the right knee. In the preoperative workup prior to total knee replacement, this 77-year-old male was referred for a nonpulsatile popliteal fossa mass. The clinical exam suggested a Baker's cyst. The lateral radiograph of the right knee shows osteoarthritis and a large soft tissue mass with a thin rim of peripheral calcification (*arrows*). **B**, Popliteal artery aneurysm: transverse sonogram. Same patient as in **A**. A 5 MHz transverse ultrasound image shows marked enlargement of the popliteal artery. There are two components within the arterial mass. Hypoechoic thrombus (*curved arrows*) is identified superficial to and around the smaller patent lumen (*arrow*). This patient had a popliteal artery aneurysm due to atherosclerotic disease. An anechoic mass associated with an arterial lesion can also represent adventitial cystic disease in the younger patient population. **C**, Popliteal artery aneurysm: transverse color Doppler sonogram. Same patient as in **A**. Color Doppler flow clearly identifies the smaller component to be the true arterial lumen. The eccentric peripheral echos without blood flow represent the thrombosis. **D**, Popliteal artery aneurysm: longitudinal sonogram. Aneurysmal dilatation, peripheral thrombus (*t*) and stenosis (*open arrow*) of the patent lumen (*l*) are demonstrated. After the results of the ultrasound examination, the planned joint replacement surgery was postponed and the patient was scheduled for surgical repair of this popliteal artery aneurysm.

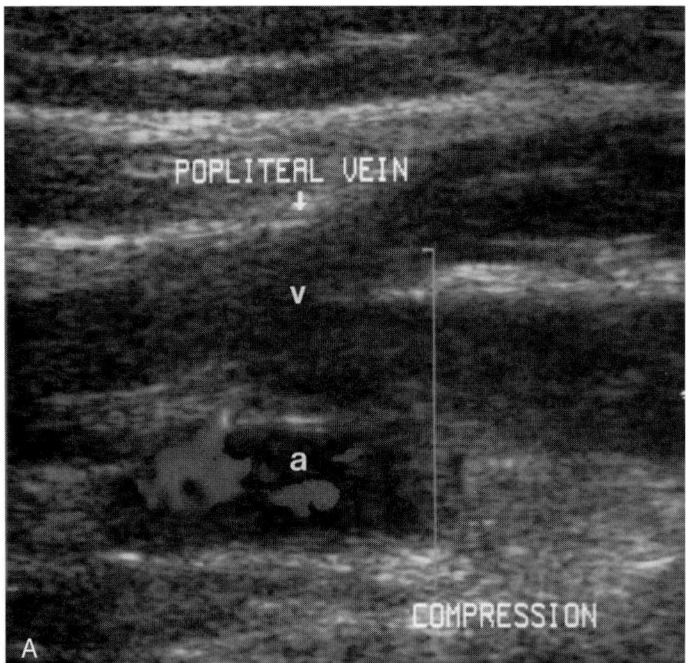

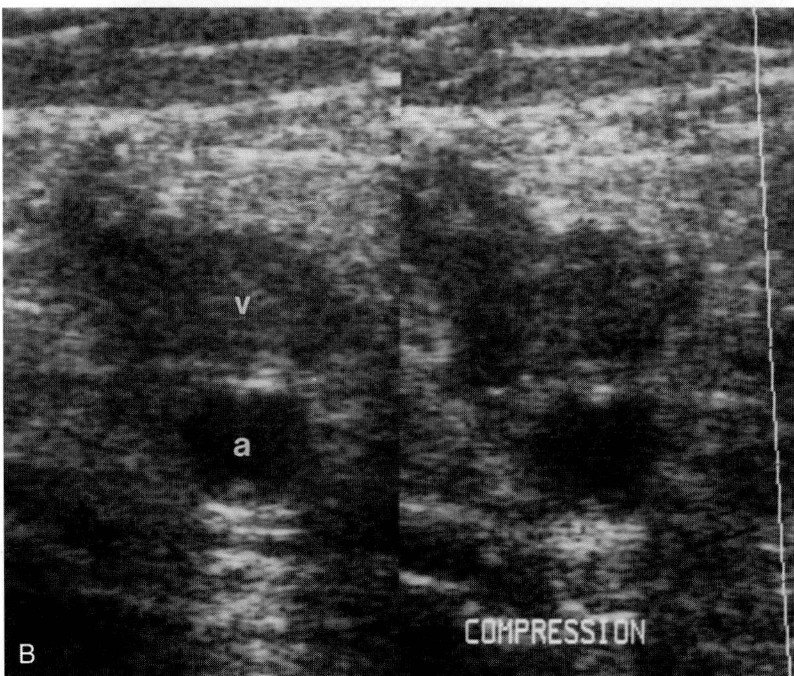

Figure 18–2 ■ **A**, Popliteal vein thrombosis: longitudinal sonogram through the midline of the popliteal fossa. The marked increase in caliber, hypoechoic vessel lumen, lack of compressibility, and lack of color Doppler flow of the popliteal vein (*v*) and its branches are diagnostic of deep vein thrombosis. Abbreviation: popliteal artery (*a*). **B**, Popliteal vein thrombosis: transverse sonogram of the popliteal fossa. This split-screen image depicts the confluence of the lower leg veins into the popliteal vein (*v*). The popliteal vein is located superficially in the popliteal fossa, and the popliteal artery (*a*) is positioned deep to the vein. No change in the caliber of the vein occurs with transducer compression. Abnormal vessel distention and hypoechogenicity within the lumen of the vein are again identified.

dicate the correct diagnosis. In some instances, the injury may be trivial and the diagnosis may not be suspected. These clinical scenarios are routinely encountered in daily practice, and ultrasound should be the first imaging modality used in the diagnostic evaluation.

Any soft tissue swelling around the medial, lateral, or anterior aspect of the knee can be initially assessed by ultrasound. Ultrasound is valuable in the diagnosis of hematoma, abscess, acute bursitis, meniscal cyst, intra- and extra-articular ganglia, synovial cyst (Steiner et al., 1996), and subcutaneous lipoma (Fornage and Tassin, 1991). A solid soft tissue mass may be a benign process such as chronic traumatic bursitis, inflammatory or benign tumoral synovial diseases affecting a bursa (Present et al., 1986; Katz and Levinsohn, 1994; Schofield et al., 1995), hemangioma, posttraumatic neuroma, or be-

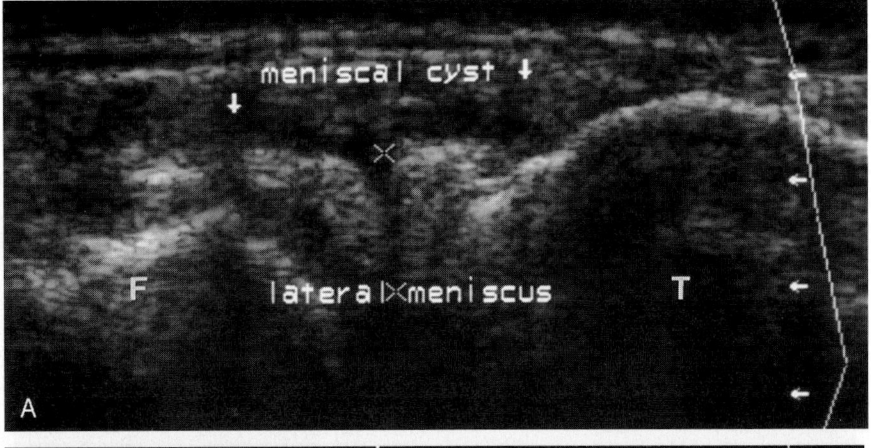

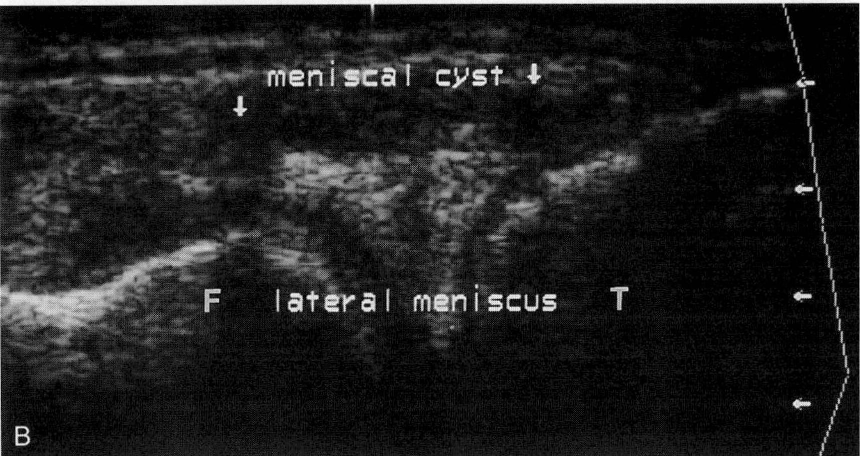

Figure 18–3 ■ **A**, Lateral meniscal cyst: longitudinal sonogram. A horizontal hypoechoic band extends from the periphery of the meniscus to its inner margin (*between the x cursors*). This represents a nondisplaced meniscal tear. A nonpalpable, well-defined hypoechoic soft tissue mass (*arrows*) is consistent with a small meniscal cyst. Abbreviations: distal femur (*F*), proximal tibia (*T*). **B**, Lateral meniscal cyst: longitudinal sonogram. Same patient as in **A**. This image visualizes the extent of the lateral meniscal cyst (*arrows*) more clearly.

nign neurogenic tumor. Malignant tumors including synovial sarcoma and malignant fibrous histiocytoma are also among the considerations. Most tumors are hypoechoic, and their appearance on ultrasound examination will not distinguish benign from malignant tumors. A specific diagnosis can occasionally be made when an anatomical connection can be established between the mass and a landmark soft tissue structure. Examples of such characteristic lesions are masses arising from bursae, cysts arising from menisci, and a variety of lesions originating from the neurovascular bundle. In other tumors, biopsy will often be required.

The knee harbors the largest number of anatomical bursae surrounding a single joint in the body (Brantigan and Voshell, 1943; Lee and Yao, 1991; Hennigan et al., 1994; Forbes et al., 1995; Rothstein et al., 1996; Steiner et al., 1996; Bonaldi et al., 1998). Acute or chronic repetitive trauma and deposition of chemical agents like urate crystals may cause bursal inflammation. Bursal infection may occur, usually following penetrating injury. Extra-articular ganglia and synovial cysts are common around the knee and the proximal tibiofibular joint (Bianchi et al., 1995). If these cysts arise from the proximal tibiofibular joint, they may dissect either laterally into the peroneal compartment or anteriorly into the anterior tibial compartment. A stalk-like connection with the joint cannot always be demonstrated; a ganglion may arise from a nerve sheath, typically from the common peroneal nerve or one of its branches.

Intra-articular ganglia of the knee are less common. They arise from the alar folds that cover Hoffa's fat pad or, more often, from the cruciate ligaments. Intra-articular ganglia usually present with retropatellar, medial, or lateral joint pain (Bui-Mansfield and Youngberg, 1997). Only when they are large and not confined to the intercondylar notch can they present as a palpable mass or interfere with full range of motion (Yasuda and Majima, 1988). Ultrasound-guided aspiration can restore full motion in some patients.

A meniscal cyst may present as a palpable soft tissue swelling centered over the joint line. The cyst may change size, depending on the position of the knee, being largest when the knee is extended. Meniscal cysts are most often seen in association

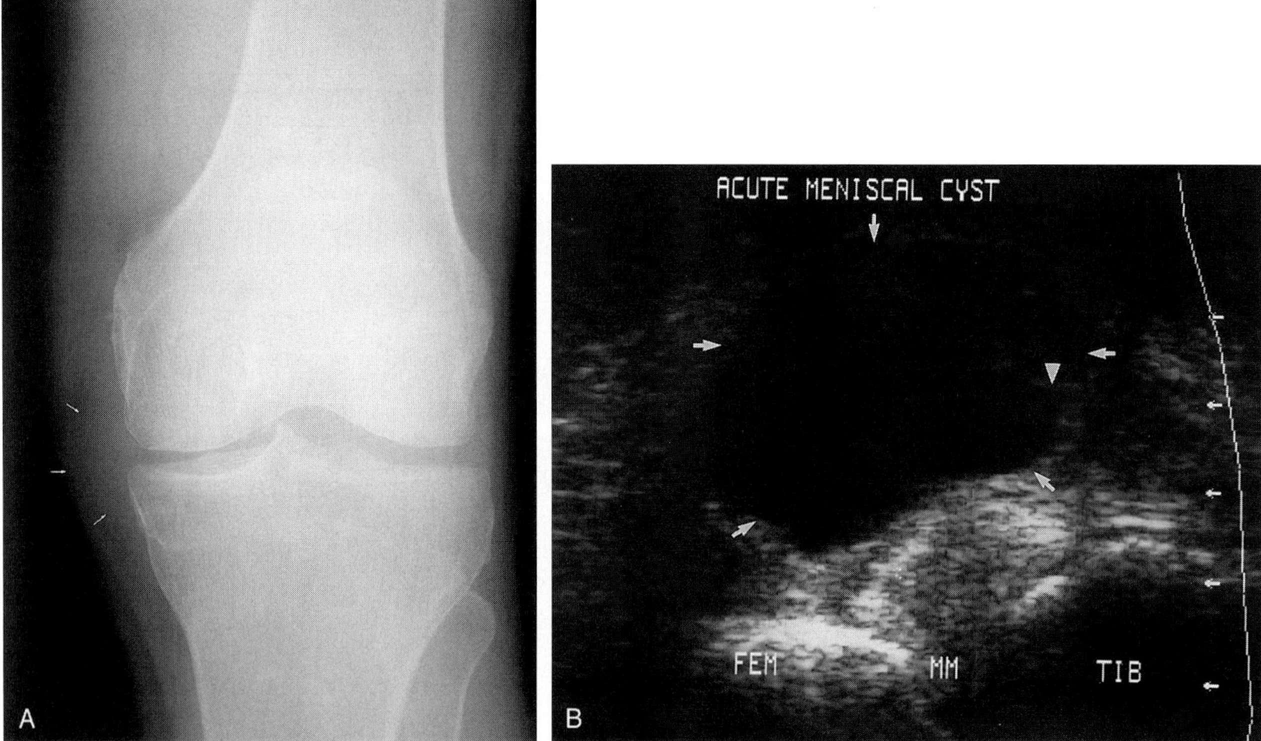

Figure 18–4 ■ **A**, Medial meniscal cyst: low-kilovoltage conventional radiograph of the left knee. Following a fall, this 55-year-old man developed a palpable, hard mass on the medial aspect of his left knee. This low-kilovoltage anteroposterior conventional radiograph displays the soft tissue mass (*arrows*) centered over the medial knee joint line. **B**, Medial meniscal cyst: longitudinal sonogram. Same patient as in **A**. Protrusion of the medial meniscus beyond the bony margins of the joint space is noted. A large, well-defined mass abuts the periphery of the meniscus. The mass is predominantly anechoic, demonstrating increased through-transmission (*arrows*). It contains a few septations in its inferior aspect (*arrowhead*). The meniscal cyst functions as an acoustic window and assists in the evaluation of the medial meniscus (*MM*) beneath it. Abbreviations: medial femoral condyle (*FEM*), medial tibial plateau (*TIB*).

with horizontal and complex tears of the lateral meniscus (Fig. 18–3). Less commonly, they are associated with tears involving the medial meniscus (Fig. 18–4). Controversy exists about whether they are invariably associated with a meniscal tear. Given the tight attachment of the medial meniscus to the medial collateral ligament, medial meniscal cysts have a greater tendency to migrate away from their site of origin. They track anteriorly into Hoffa's fat pad or posteriorly toward the popliteal fossa, deep to the ligament. When small to medium-sized and located medially, they are also less likely to present clinically as a palpable mass.

Swelling may result from an inflammatory arthropathy. The suprapatellar bursa, medial and lateral patellar recesses, knee joint space posterior to the posterior cruciate ligament (an arthroscopic blind spot), or Baker's cyst are frequently involved (Cooperberg et al., 1978; Tiliakos et al., 1985; Spiegel et al., 1987; van Holsbeeck et al., 1988; Sureda et al., 1994; Leeb et al., 1995; Fiocco et al., 1996; Rutten et al., 1998). Ultrasound has proven its value in evaluating the extent of synovial edema and pannus, monitoring the therapeutic response of the synovium and cartilage, and timing synovectomy. Other synovial diseases such as chronic infection, hemophilia (Hermann et al., 1992), pigmented villonodular synovitis (Kaufman et al., 1982), osteochondromatosis, lipoma arborescens, synovial hemangioma and amyloidosis can affect the joint and its surrounding bursae. With the exception of synovial (osteo)chondromatosis, these processes are nonspecific sonographically, but ultrasound can easily guide percutaneous biopsy in selected cases.

Acute Knee Injury

Swelling that occurs in the first 12 hours after an injury usually represents hemarthrosis. This may be secondary to a complete quadriceps tendon tear, capsular injury, osteochondral fracture, peripheral meniscal tear, or acute intra-articular injury, usually to the anterior cruciate ligament. A good clinical examination is difficult when there is acute swelling because of pain and poor muscle relaxation. Arthroscopy is almost impossible with intra-articular hemorrhage. In addition, an MRI study can rarely be obtained on the spur of the moment. Patients with hyperacute knee swelling are good candidates for ultrasound evaluation to identify the cause of the hemorrhage. Ultrasound can detect anterior cruciate ligament disruption cost-effectively. In these cases, the anterior cruciate ligament itself is not visualized. Instead, a hypoechoic hematoma at the femoral attachment of the anterior cruciate ligament, along the posterior aspect of the lateral wall of the intercondylar notch, indicates an acute tear. This site corresponds to the femoral attachment of the anterior cruciate ligament. A transverse posterior approach with a 5 MHz curved transducer is utilized. In 1995, Ptasznik et al. achieved sensitivity of 91%, specificity of 100%, a positive predictive value (PPV) of 100%, and a negative predictive value (NPV) of 63% in ultrasound examinations performed within 10 weeks of the acute injury. The hemorrhagic collection has an average size of 7.7 mm and a convex medial border, which obscures the underlying hypoechoic synovium and displaces the intercondylar fat medially. Since the hematoma resolves over approximately 10 weeks, there is a finite sonographic window of opportunity. In Ptasznik et al.'s study, patients with a prior history of knee injury associated with knee swelling were excluded from the study group. The authors assumed that an acute anterior cruciate ligament injury superimposed on a chronic anterior cruciate ligament injury would not result in significant hematoma.

Lateral and medial collateral ligaments (Lee et al., 1996) are readily evaluated. Collateral and cruciate ligaments can rupture in isolation or in

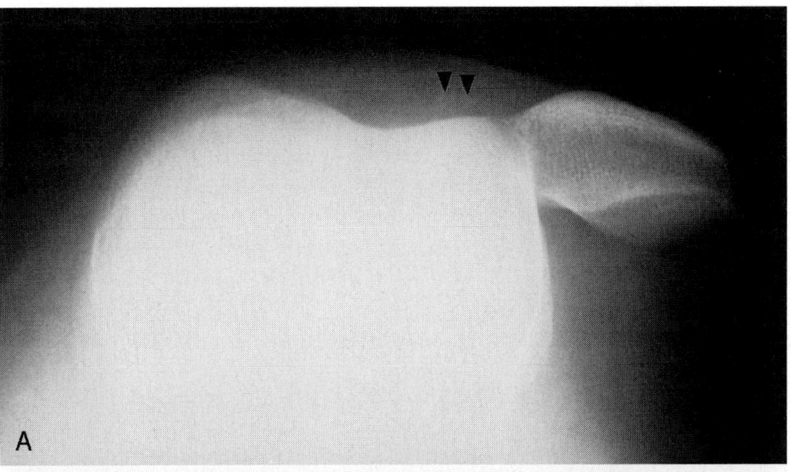

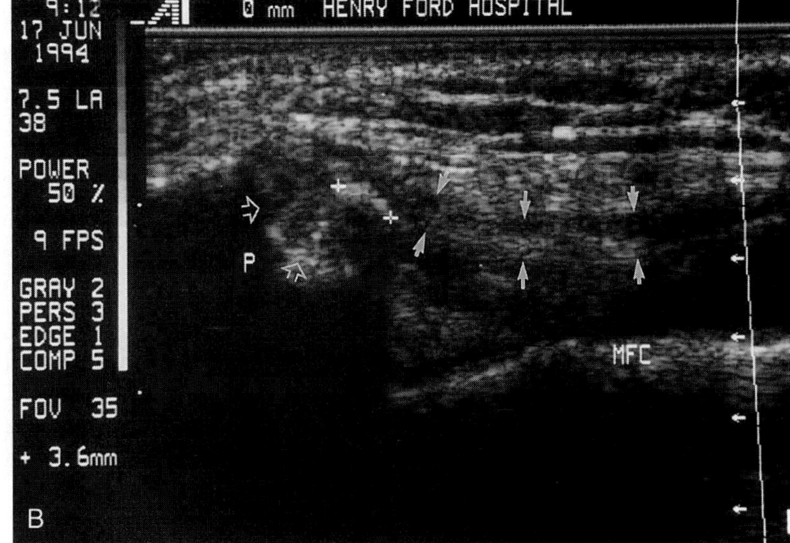

Figure 18–5 ■ **A**, Medial retinacular avulsion fracture: sunrise view of the left patella. This 19-year-old woman experienced several spontaneous bilateral patellar dislocations. Her knee problems first began 7 years ago. Now, during a twisting movement 5 days ago, she dislocated her left patella. For the first time, a physician had to relocate the patella. The radiograph shows the patella in a dislocated position over the lateral femoral condyle. Small avulsions (*arrowheads*) are noted anterior to the lateral femoral trochlea. **B**, Medial retinacular avulsion fracture: transverse sonogram. Same patient as in **A**. The transducer is positioned transversely, centered over the medial edge of the patella. A minimally displaced 4 mm bony fragment (*outlined by + cursors*), which is avulsed from the medial aspect of the patella and attached to the medial retinaculum (*outlined by arrows*), is identified. The fragment's site of origin is clearly shown (*open arrows*). Abbreviations: patella (*p*), medial femoral condyle (*MFC*).

combination with other soft tissue injuries. Only extensive injury results in hemarthrosis.

Osteochondral and chondral fractures are other causes of intra-articular hemorrhage. Fractures of cartilage frequently involve the medial patella and lateral femoral condyle due to subluxation and impaction of the patella against the lateral femoral condyle. Patellar dislocations often reduce spontaneously, making the diagnosis difficult to establish. Edema, disruption, or avulsion of the medial retinaculum and/or medial capsule (Fig. 18–5) (Spritzer et al., 1997; Starok et al., 1997) and hemarthrosis are all well displayed sonographically. Fractures of cartilage most frequently involve the medial femoral condyle and result from a rotational injury or a direct blow. Ultrasound can be used to evaluate transchondral injuries if the articular surface can be projected free of overlying bone by knee flexion or by using medial or lateral patellar subluxation. A transchondral fracture may be seen as a hyperechoic fissure traversing the hypoechoic cartilage. In intra-articular fracture extension, fluid may insinuate and undermine the articular surface, displacing the fracture fragment from its bed. The dynamic characteristics of the ultrasound examination allow manual palpation and direct visualization of the movement of loose fragments. If a fragment has been dislodged, only a cartilaginous defect remains. In cases of unstable fracture, arthroscopic removal, curettage, subchondral drilling, or anchoring with internal fixation devices may be indicated. Intra-articular loose bodies resulting from chondral or osteochondral fractures can be detected sonographically, especially in the presence of joint effusion.

Meniscal abnormalities are evaluated with MRI more often than with ultrasound. Diagnostic errors in MRI evaluation of the menisci may occur in instances of meniscocapsular separation (Rubin et al., 1996) and in subtle tears of the posterior horn, particularly of the lateral meniscus (De Smet et al., 1994; De Smet and Graf, 1994; Justice and Quinn, 1995). Meniscocapsular separation is an uncommon injury. Because it involves the peripheral, vascularized fibrous tissue at the meniscosynovial interface,

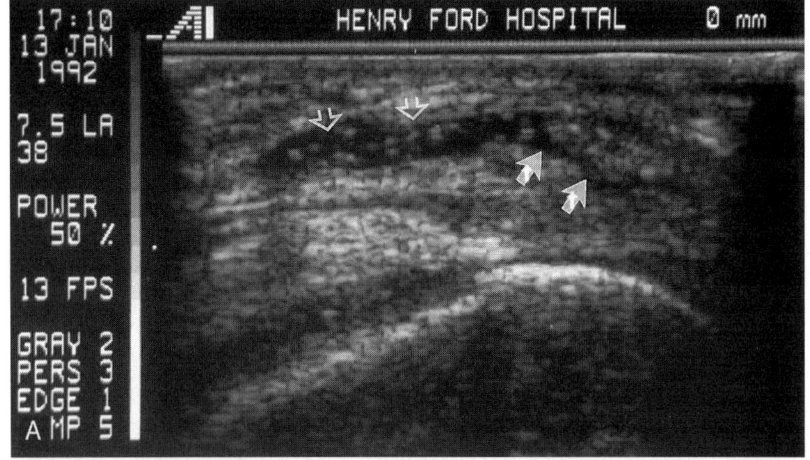

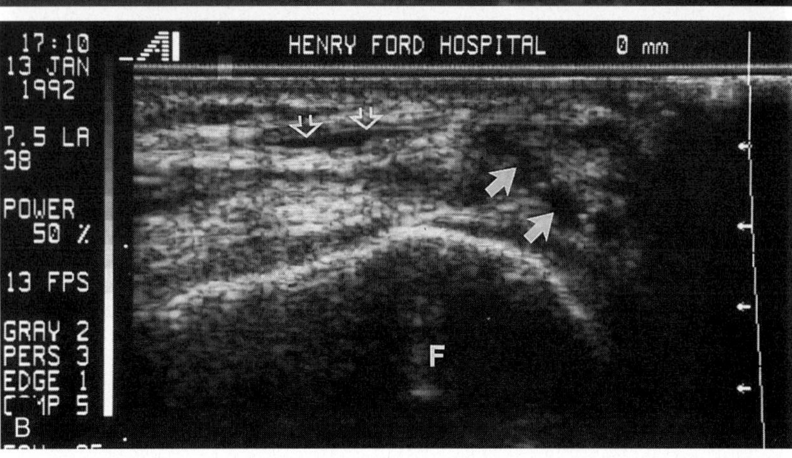

Figure 18–6 ■ **A**, Capsular tear: longitudinal sonogram. This 17-year-old male recalled an old penetrating injury to his knee with glass fragments. He presented with focal pain and intermittent swelling along the lateral aspect of his knee. Extracapsular fluid is noted in a pocket over the lateral knee (*open arrows*). The fluid is of mixed echogenicity. *Solid arrows* outline a hypoechoic cleft extending through the swollen lateral retinaculum. **B**, Capsular tear: longitudinal sonogram. Same patient as in **A**. While the extra-articular pouch is compressed, real-time ultrasound examination demonstrates return of fluid through the capsular rent (*solid arrows*) and the collapse of the extracapsular mass (*open arrows*). In the process, the patient's presenting complaint was elicited. Abbreviation: femur (*F*).

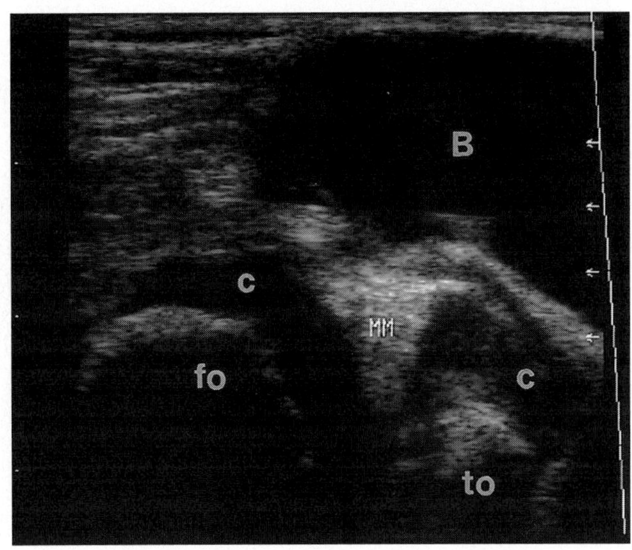

Figure 18–7 ▪ Baker's cyst and normal medial meniscus: longitudinal sonogram. On clinical examination, this 5-year-old girl was found to have a medial popliteal fossa mass. An ultrasound examination was requested to confirm the presence of a Baker's cyst. The normal posterior horn of the medial meniscus (*MM*) is clearly visualized as a hyperechoic triangular structure. The meniscus is outlined nicely, sharply contrasting with the hypoechoic epiphyseal cartilage of the abutting femur and tibia. In addition, the large Baker's cyst serves as an excellent acoustic window. A communication of the cyst with the joint could not be demonstrated. Abbreviations: Baker's cyst (*B*), femoral epiphyseal ossification center (*fo*), tibial epiphyseal ossification center (*to*), articular and growth cartilage (*c*).

there is a good chance of healing. If it is an isolated injury, it can be treated conservatively. When it is associated with ligamentous injury, arthroscopic repair by suturing the meniscus back to the capsule is preferred to meniscectomy. MRI has poor sensitivity and poor positive predictive value in diagnosing meniscocapsular separation. In our hands, ultrasound is more reliable.

Tendon injuries range from strains followed by tendinitis to partial or complete tendon tear. The extensor mechanism is most frequently injured in acute sports-related or other trauma. Focal tendinitis is almost always caused by chronic repetitive trauma, but occasionally acute blunt trauma may produce the same effect. Complete tears are the result of excessive loading of a tendon, as in a fall or a motor vehicle accident. If there is no history of trauma, tendon degeneration should be suspected as the predisposing factor. Degeneration may result from repetitive athletic trauma, hyperparathyroidism, gout, diabetes, rheumatoid arthritis, systemic lupus erythematosus, chronic steroid use, or

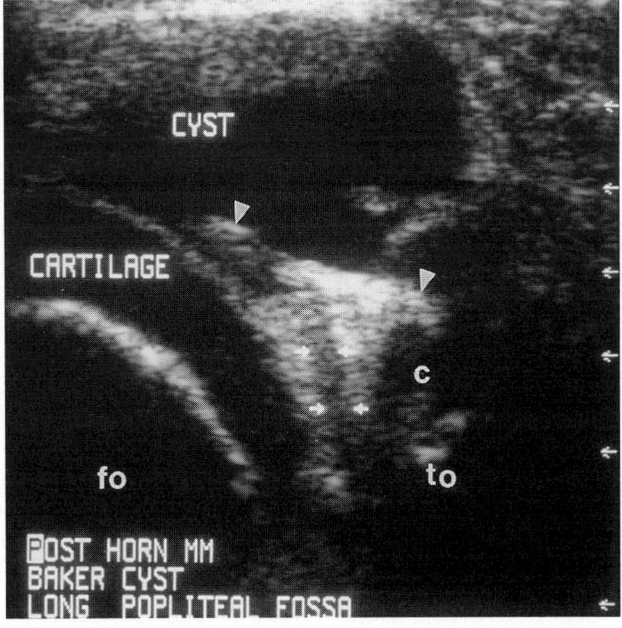

Figure 18–8 ▪ Baker's cyst and oblique tear of the posterior medial meniscus: longitudinal sonogram. This 9-year-old girl developed a medial popliteal fossa mass after a fall. An ultrasound examination was requested to confirm the presence of a Baker's cyst. A hypoechoic tear (*arrows*) traverses the hyperechoic posterior horn of the medial meniscus. It extends to its blunted inner margin and inferior articular surface. Both the meniscofemoral and meniscotibial ligaments are identified (*arrowheads*). Abbreviations: Baker's cyst (*CYST*); femoral epiphyseal ossification center (*fo*), tibial epiphyseal ossification center (*to*), articular and growth cartilage of distal femur (*CARTILAGE*), articular and growth cartilage of proximal tibia (*c*.)

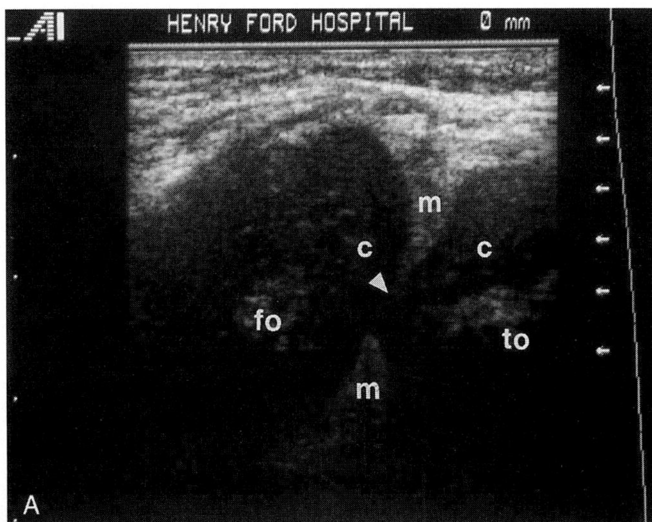

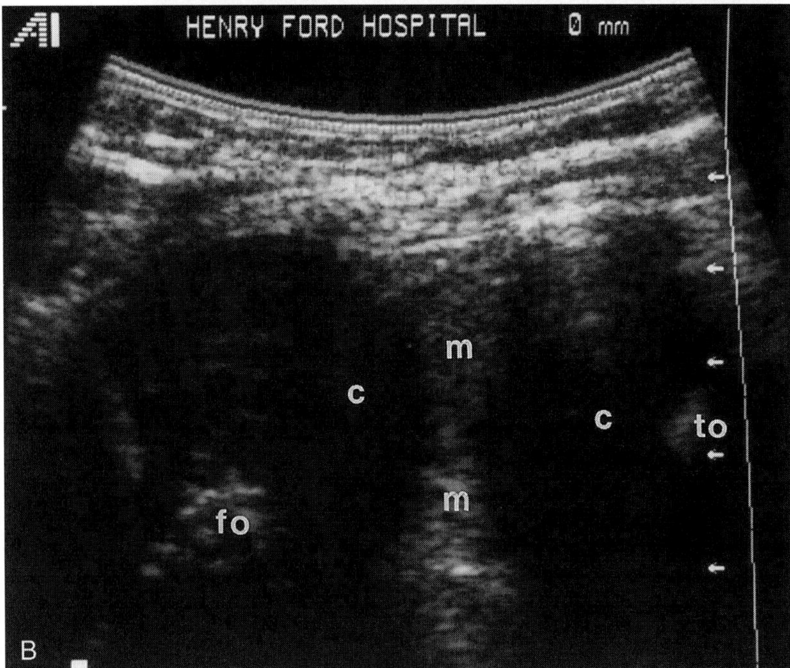

Figure 18–9 ■ **A**, Discoid lateral meniscus: longitudinal sonogram. Asymptomatic 16-month-old boy. His mother had noticed an audible click with knee motion from the age of 3 months. Both the anterior and posterior horns of the medial meniscus (*m*) are visualized in this single scan plane. The normal meniscus has a triangular configuration, with its apex corresponding to the free inner margin. The anterior and posterior horns are separated by intervening joint space (*arrowhead*). Abbreviations: articular and growth cartilage (*c*), femoral epiphyseal ossification center (*fo*), tibial epiphyseal ossification center (*to*). **B**, Discoid lateral meniscus: longitudinal sonogram. Same patient as in **A**. The lateral meniscus has a bulky bow tie appearance, with meniscal substance filling the entire lateral joint space. This is indicative of a discoid meniscus.

postoperative degeneration following total knee replacement.

Chronic Localized Knee Pain

Anterior knee pain may be caused by chondromalacia patellae, pre- and infrapatellar bursal disease, lesions affecting Hoffa's infrapatellar fat pad (Jacobson et al., 1997), inflammation from any cause, partial rupture, insertion tendinopathy, or unrecognized partial avulsion fracture involving the extensor tendons. If avulsion is complete, it will be apparent clinically when the swelling subsides. Anterolateral pain may follow injury to the capsule (Fig. 18–6) or retinaculum. Medial and lateral joint line tenderness may be due to a wide variety of conditions including meniscal tear, meniscal cyst (Coral et al., 1989; De Flaviis et al., 1990; Peetrons et al., 1990), intra-articular ganglion, and other problems relating to tendons, ligaments (Bonaldi et al., 1998), capsule, fascia, or bursae. Following arthroscopy, the capsular portal may persist, a neuroma may form, or a metallic fragment from the arthroscope may remain.

When examining structures which are anisotropic, such as tendons, capsular ligaments, and

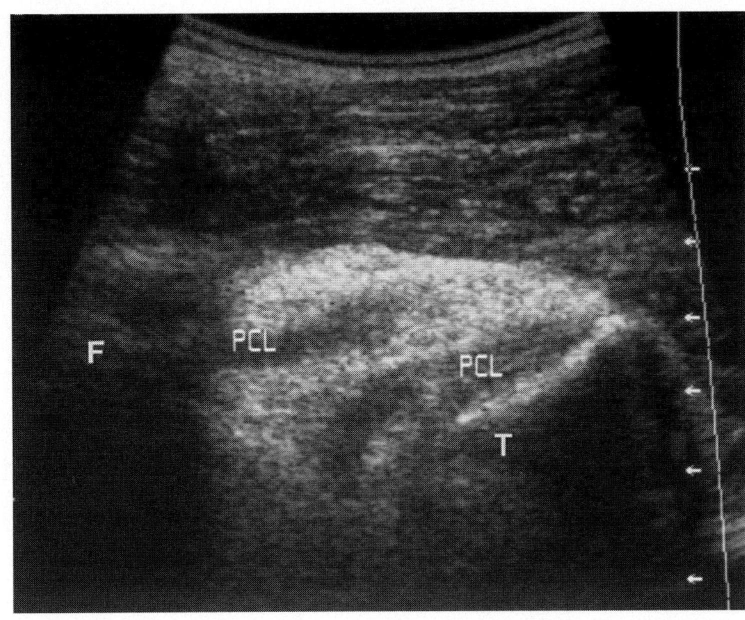

Figure 18–10 ▪ Chronic full-thickness posterior cruciate ligament tear: longitudinal sonogram. A football player presents with knee pain 5 years after a significant knee-to-knee collision. The individual suffers from claustrophobia and is unwilling to undergo MRI. This scan was performed with a 5 MHz curved array transducer placed over the midline of the popliteal space. A complete posterior cruciate ligament rupture has resulted in two elongated, discontinuous ligamentous stumps (*PCL*). The distal portion of the ligament curves down over the tibial condyle (*T*). Abbreviation: femur (*F*).

fascia, the spatial resolution of ultrasound is superior to that of MRI (Erickson, 1997). Sonography is also targeted to the patient's complaints through the technique of sonographic palpation using the transducer during the examination. In cases of minimal abnormality, meticulous comparison between the symptomatic and asymptomatic sides is useful.

Limited Use in Internal Derangement

While indications for the use of ultrasound in examination of the knee are limited, young children and adults who cannot undergo MRI may be well served. Young children usually require deep sedation or general anesthesia for MRI, but none is required for ultrasound examination. The large amount of hypoechoic, nonossified epiphyseal cartilage, in addition to the articular cartilage, provides excellent contrast for visualization of the menisci (Figs. 18–7 and 18–8), including detection of a discoid meniscus (Fig. 18–9). Sonographic imaging of the cartilaginous structures of a child's knee can be used in Osgood-Schlatter disease (Lanning and Heikkinen, 1991), congenital patellar abnormalities (Walker et al., 1991; Baron et al., 1995; Miller et al., 1998) and suspected traumatic fracture or dislocation of the unossified skeleton (Davidson et al., 1994). Intra-articular fracture extension can be identified and alignment of fracture fragments at an articular surface assessed. For adults with suspected internal knee derangement who cannot undergo the MRI exam because of claustrophobia, very large size, an incompatible implant, or an intra-orbital foreign body, ultrasound can be useful (Fig. 18–10).

Peripheral meniscal tears, meniscal cysts, and intra-articular ganglia are readily demonstrated sonographically. Above the age of 50, the menisci become more accessible to ultrasound examination, as they are positioned somewhat more peripherally. Increased laxity of capsular tissues, increased stiffness of the subchondral bone, repetitive microtrauma, and mucoid degeneration of the menisci may be responsible for this peripheral migration. The improvement in visibility using ultrasound coincides with another change, which increases the difficulty of the diagnostic interpretation of the aging meniscus using MRI. Increased intrasubstance signal intensity in all MRI sequences caused by mucoid degeneration makes diagnosis of meniscal lesions much more difficult using MRI (Fig. 18–11). Small tears become progressively more difficult to detect.

Intra-articular loose bodies may cause locking, restriction of range of motion, or recurrent effusions or may be clinically asymptomatic. They arise from meniscal or articular cartilage fragments (Fig. 18–11). In rare cases, locking may be due to meniscal cyst or intra-articular ganglion. Loose bodies may continue to grow by diffusion of ions from the surrounding synovial fluid. Only if calcified or ossified can they be completely assessed by conventional radiography, resulting in underestimation of their presence, true size, and number. MRI will

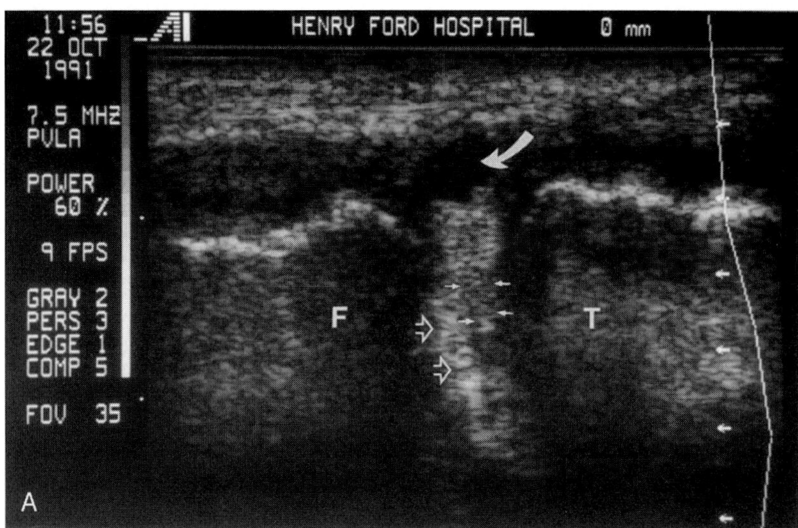

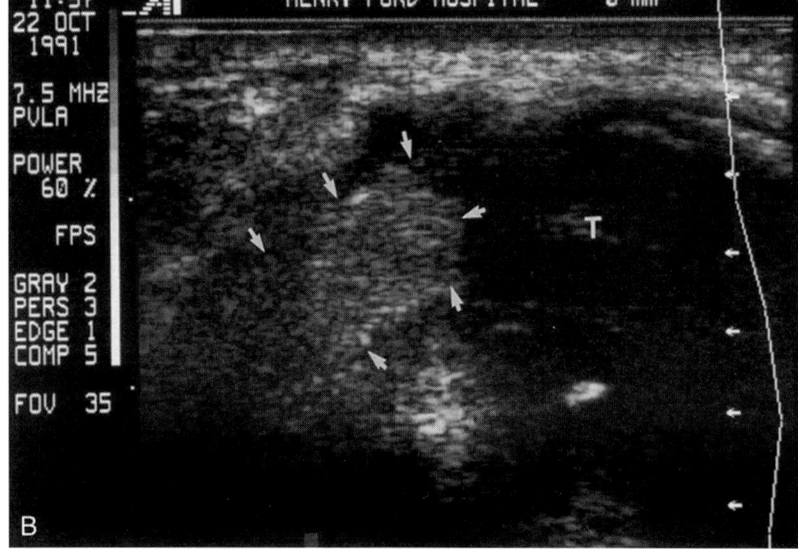

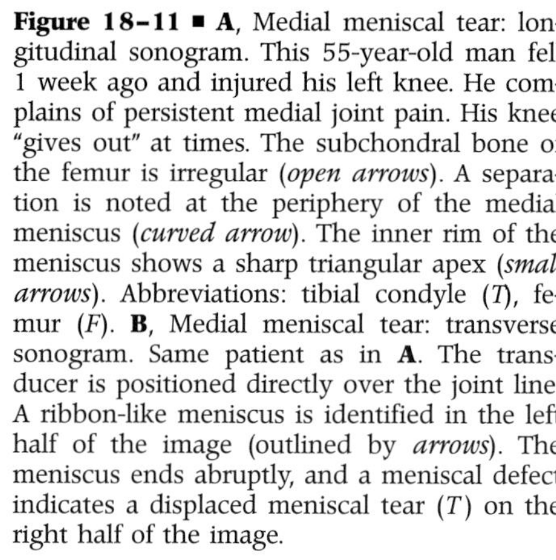

Figure 18–11 ■ **A**, Medial meniscal tear: longitudinal sonogram. This 55-year-old man fell 1 week ago and injured his left knee. He complains of persistent medial joint pain. His knee "gives out" at times. The subchondral bone of the femur is irregular (*open arrows*). A separation is noted at the periphery of the medial meniscus (*curved arrow*). The inner rim of the meniscus shows a sharp triangular apex (*small arrows*). Abbreviations: tibial condyle (*T*), femur (*F*). **B**, Medial meniscal tear: transverse sonogram. Same patient as in **A**. The transducer is positioned directly over the joint line. A ribbon-like meniscus is identified in the left half of the image (outlined by *arrows*). The meniscus ends abruptly, and a meniscal defect indicates a displaced meniscal tear (*T*) on the right half of the image.

detect loose bodies if they are large enough; comparison to the corresponding radiographs is helpful. When small, loose bodies may easily be overlooked by MRI due to volume averaging. The hypointense signal of meniscal loose bodies, calcified or not, may be difficult to separate from adjacent hypointense cortical bone. The advantage of ultrasound is that it identifies purely cartilaginous loose bodies, in addition to ossified and calcified intra-articular loose bodies demonstrated radiographically. Ultrasound is particularly useful in the presence of joint fluid or Baker's cyst (Moss and Dishuk, 1984; Frankel et al., 1998) (Fig. 18–12).

Sonographically, loose bodies present as hyperechoic foci, which are discontinuous with the skeletal structures and may be surrounded by joint fluid. This appearance can be mimicked by punctate, hyperechoic foci within fluid of an infected joint. If apposed to the bony surface, intra-articular loose bodies present as focal cortical irregularities with mobility in relation to the skeletal surface during real-time dynamic scanning. Rarely is saline injection required to distend the joint and thereby distinguish an apposed intra-articular loose body from a degenerative osteophyte.

Postoperative Knee

Postoperatively, joints are often screened for infection or a ruptured extensor tendon. Ultrasound can detect particles of bone, cement, metal, or polyethylene due to intra-articular wear or may reveal loosening of hardware and staples. Ultrasound has

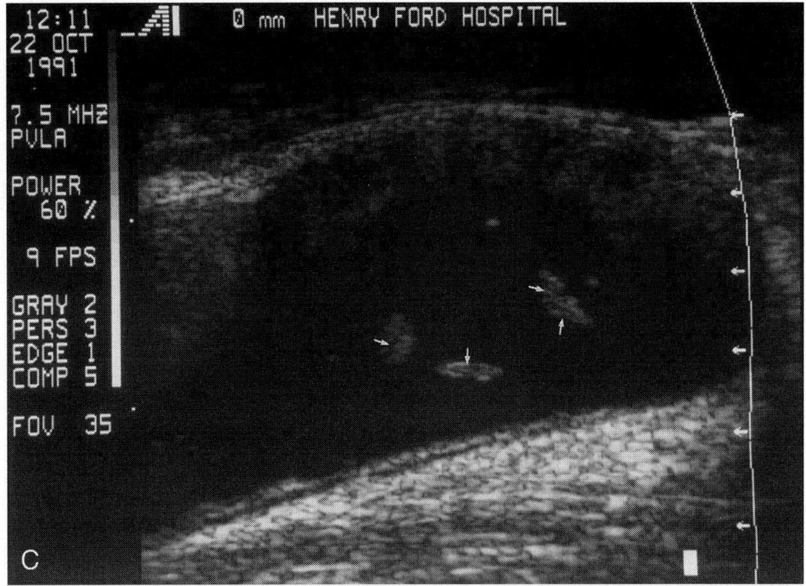

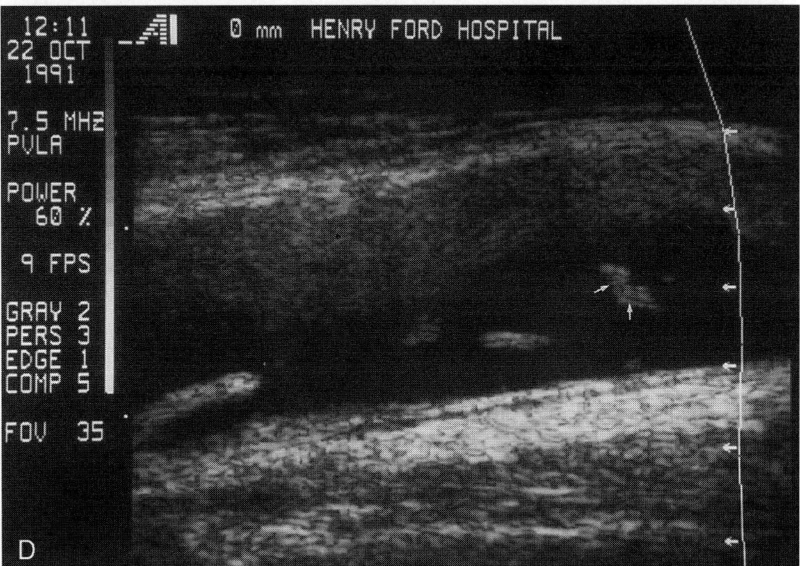

Figure 18-11 *Continued* ■ **C**, Baker's cyst: longitudinal sonogram. Same patient as in **A**. A large Baker's cyst is filled with anechoic fluid. Hyperechoic debris (*arrows*) within the cyst represents small cartilage fragments. **D**, Baker's cyst: longitudinal sonogram with compression. Same patient as in **A**. Compression on the Baker's cyst moves the loose bodies around. The configuration of the fragments does not change, but note the change of orientation of the triangular piece of cartilage in comparison with **C** (*arrows*).

revealed wear of the polyethylene component of total knee arthroplasty prostheses (Yashar et al., 1996). The metallic retropatellar and tibial plateau surfaces of a total knee prosthesis are coated with an ultra-high molecular weight polyethylene. The polyethylene lining is radiolucent, and with the exception of ultrasound, arthroscopy is the only way to document its failure. Arthroscopy carries the risk of general anesthesia and possible introduction of infection. By scanning the entire circumference of the tibial component in the longitudinal plane with a 10 MHz linear array transducer, an ultrasound examination visualizes the bone-cement-metal-polyethylene surfaces and interfaces and permits assessment of the integrity and thickness of the tibial polyethylene spacer. Sonographically, the metal backing of the prosthesis is recognized by its comet tail artifact. The normal polyethylene liner appears as a regular reflecting surface with no posterior echos. Irregularity or partial or complete loss of its specular reflecting surface is indicative of structural failure of the plastic. Abnormal movement of the surfaces may be observed in cases of dislodged polyethylene components (Fig. 18-13). Chronic wear will result in effusion. The fluid may appear echogenic because of the presence of fragmented polyethylene debris.

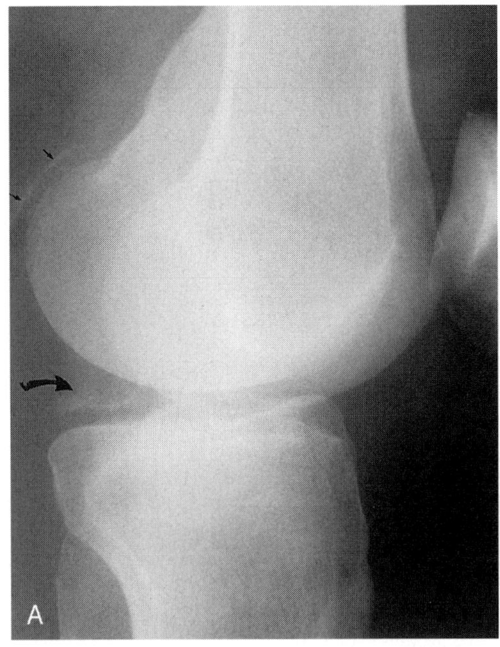

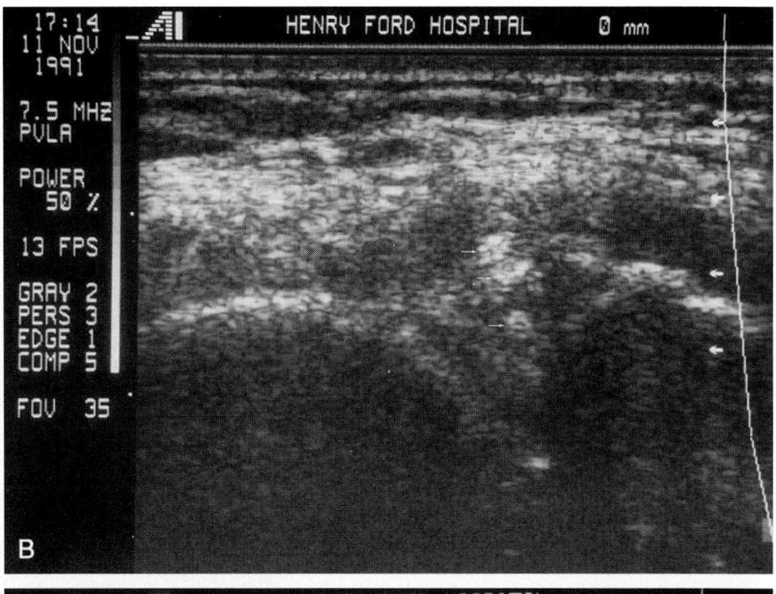

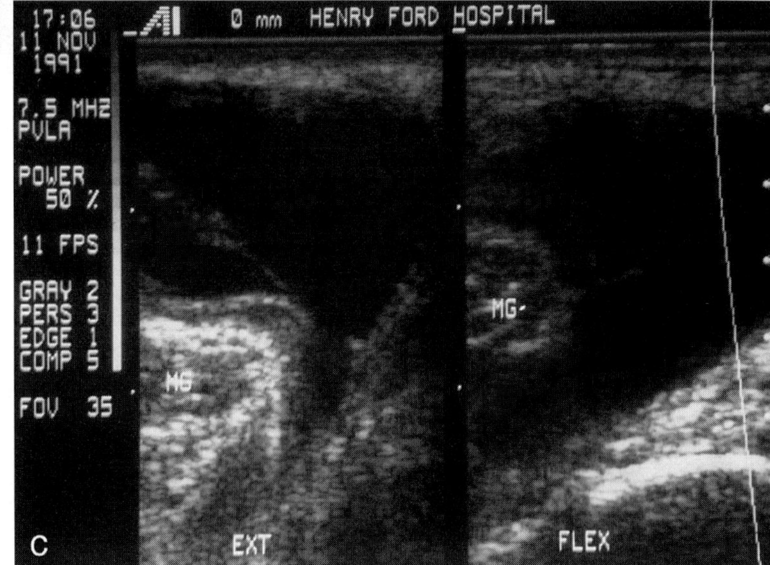

Figure 18–12 ■ **A**, Meniscal chondrocalcinosis: lateral radiograph of the left knee. Both chondral (*arrows*) and meniscal (*curved arrow*) calcifications are visualized in the posterior knee joint capsule. **B**, Meniscal chondrocalcinosis: longitudinal sonogram. Same patient as in **A**. Hyperechoic foci without acoustic shadowing (*white arrows*) are identified within the lateral meniscal substance. The meniscus has a heterogeneous echotexture, indicating degeneration. **C**, Neck of Baker's cyst: transverse sonogram documenting the valve mechanism. Same patient as in **A**. The joint communication of the Baker's cyst is noted to close and open during extension (*EXT*) and flexion (*FLEX*), respectively. Abbreviation: medial head of gastrocnemius (*MG*).

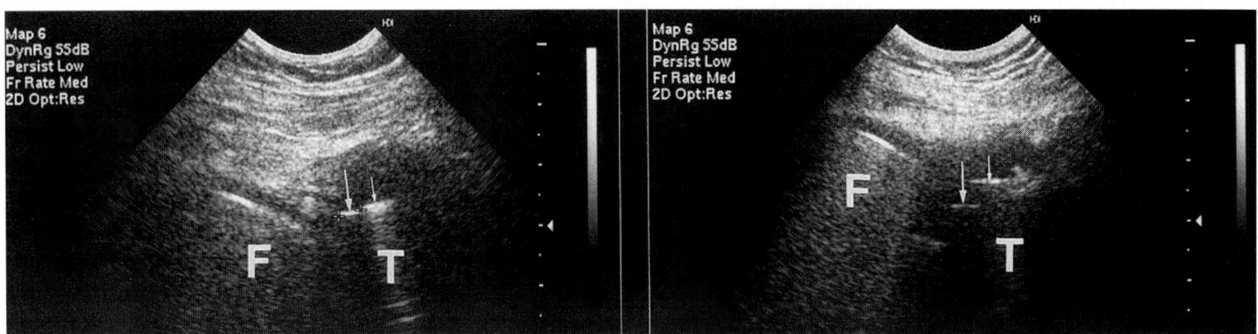

Figure 18–13 ■ Dislodged tibial component in total knee arthroplasty: longitudinal sonogram. A patient with intermittent locking of his knee 2 years after total knee replacement. This split-screen image was obtained using a 5 MHz curved array transducer. The left image was obtained with the knee in extension, and the right image shows the knee in flexion. The metallic femoral (*F*) and tibial (*T*) components are identified by their strong ring down artifacts. The polyethylene tibial spacer (*long arrow*) is the strong specular reflector aligned along and immediately proximal to the metallic tibial component (*short arrow*). It is outlined by the + cursors. In knee flexion, the two components of the prosthesis are subluxed relative to each other. The surgeon removed the cracked polyethylene liner after the sonographic demonstration of its abnormal intra-articular mobility during knee flexion and extension.

References

Aisen AM, et al: Sonographic evaluation of the cartilage of the knee. *Radiology* 153:781–784, 1984.

Baron E, Howard CB, Porat S: The use of ultrasound in the diagnosis of atypical pathology in the unossified skeleton. *J Pediatr Orthop* 15:817–820, 1995.

Bianchi S, et al: Sonographic evaluation of intramuscular ganglia. *Clin Radiol* 50:235–236, 1995a.

Bianchi S, et al: Sonographic evaluation of lipohemarthrosis: Clinical and in vitro study. *J Ultrasound Med* 14:279–282, 1995b.

Bianchi S, et al: Sonographic evaluation of tears of the gastrocnemius medial head ("Tennis leg"). *J Ultrasound Med* 17:157–162, 1998.

Bonaldi VM, et al: Iliotibial band friction syndrome: Sonographic findings. *J Ultrasound Med* 17:257–260, 1998.

Brantigan OC, Voshell AF: Tibial collateral ligament: Its function, its bursae and its relation to the medial meniscus. *J Bone Joint Surg* 25:121–131, 1943.

Bui-Mansfield LT, Youngberg RA: Intraarticular ganglia of the knee: Prevalence, presentation, etiology and management. *AJR* 168:123–127, 1997.

Cooperberg PL, et al: Gray scale ultrasound in the evaluation of rheumatoid arthritis of the knee. *Radiology* 126:759–763, 1978.

Coral A, van Holsbeeck M, Adler RS: Imaging of meniscal cyst of the knee in three cases. *Skeletal Radiol* 18: 451–455, 1989.

Davidson RS, et al: Ultrasonographic evaluation of the elbow in infants and young children after suspected trauma. *J Bone Joint Surg* 76A:1804–1813, 1994.

De Flaviis L, et al: Ultrasound in degenerative cystic meniscal disease. *Skeletal Radiol* 19:441–445, 1990.

De Smet AA, et al: MR diagnosis of meniscal tears: Analysis of causes of errors. *AJR* 163:1419–1423, 1994.

De Smet AA, Graf B: Meniscal tears missed on MR imaging: Relationship to meniscal tear patterns and anterior cruciate ligament tears. *AJR* 162:905–911, 1994.

Erickson SJ: High-resolution imaging of the musculoskeletal system. *Radiology* 205:593–618, 1997.

Fiocco U, et al: Long-term sonographic follow-up of rheumatoid and psoriatic proliferative knee joint synovitis. *Br J Rheumatol* 35:155–163, 1996.

Forbes JR, Helms CA, Janzen DL: Acute pes anserine bursitis: MR imaging. *Radiology* 194:525–527, 1995.

Fornage BD, Tassin GB: Sonographic appearances of superficial soft tissue lipomas. *J Clin Ultrasound* 19: 215–220, 1991.

Frankel DA, et al: Synovial joints: Evaluation of intraarticular bodies with US. *Radiology* 206:41–44, 1998.

Gompels BM, Darlington LG: Grey scale ultrasonography and arthrography in evaluation of popliteal cysts. *Clin Radiol* 30:539–545, 1979.

Harcke TH, Grissom LE, Finkelstein MS: Evaluation of the musculoskeletal system with sonography. *AJR* 150: 1253–1261, 1988.

Harper J, et al: Ultrasound and arthrography in the detection of ruptured Baker's cysts. *Australas Radiol* 26: 281–283, 1982.

Hennigan SP, et al: The semimembranosus-tibial collateral ligament bursa. *J Bone Joint Surg* 76A:1322–1327, 1994.

Hermann G, Gilbert MS, Abdelwahab IF: Hemophilia: Evaluation of musculoskeletal involvement with CT, sonography and MR imaging. *AJR* 158:119–123, 1992.

Jacobson JA, et al: MR imaging of the infrapatellar fat pad of Hoffa. *Radiographics* 17:675–691, 1997.

Justice WW, Quin SF: Error patterns in MR imaging evaluation of menisci of the knee. *Radiology* 196:617–621, 1995.

Katz DS, Levinsohn EM: Pigmented villonodular synovitis of the sequestered suprapatellar bursa. *Clin Orthop Relat Res* 306:204–208, 1994.

Kaufman RA, et al: Arthrosonography in the diagnosis of pigmented villonodular synovitis. *AJR* 139:396–398, 1982.

Laine HR, Harjula A, Peltokallio P: Ultrasound in the evaluation of the knee and patellar regions. *J Ultrasound Med* 6:33–36, 1987.

Lanning P, Heikkinen E: Ultrasonic features of the Osgood-Schlatter lesion. *J Pediatr Orthop* 11:538–540, 1991.

Lee JI, et al: Medial collateral ligament injuries of the knee: Ultrasonographic findings. *J Ultrasound Med* 15: 621–625, 1996.

Lee JK, Yao L: Tibial collateral ligament bursa: MR imaging. *Radiology* 178:855–857, 1991.

Leeb BF, et al: Diagnostic use of office-based ultrasound. *Arthritis Rheum* 38:859–861, 1995.

Miller TT, et al: Sonography of patellar abnormalities in children. *AJR* 171:739–744, 1998.

Moss GD, Dishuk W: Ultrasound diagnosis of osteochondromatosis of the popliteal fossa. *J Clin Ultrasound* 12: 232–233, 1984.

Pathria MN, et al: Ultrasonography of the popliteal fossa and lower extremities. *Radiol Clin North Am* 26:77–85, 1988.

Peetrons P, Allaer D, Jeanmart L: Cysts of the semilunar cartilages of the knee: A new approach by ultrasound imaging. A study of six cases and review of the literature. *J Ultrasound Med* 9:333–337, 1990.

Present DA, Bertoni F, Enneking WF: Case report 348: Pigmented villonodular synovitis arising from bursa of the pes anserinus muscle with secondary involvement of the tibia. *Skeletal Radiol* 15:236–240, 1986.

Ptasznik R, et al: The value of sonography in the diagnosis of traumatic rupture of the anterior cruciate ligament of the knee. *AJR* 164:1461–1463, 1995.

Richardson ML, et al: Ultrasonography of the knee. *Radiol Clin North Am* 26:63–75, 1988.

Rothstein CP, et al: Semimembranosus-tibial collateral ligament bursitis: MR imaging findings. *AJR* 166:875–877, 1996.

Rubin DA, et al: Are MR imaging signs of meniscocapsular separation valid? *Radiology* 201:829–836, 1996.

Rudikoff JC, et al: Ultrasound diagnosis of Baker cyst. *JAMA* 235(10):1054–1055, 1976.

Rutten MJCM, et al: Meniscal cysts: Detection with high-resolution sonography. *AJR* 171:491–496, 1998.

Schofield TD, Pitcher JD, Youngberg R: Synovial chondromatosis simulating neoplastic degeneration of osteochondroma: Findings on MRI and CT. *Skeletal Radiol* 23:199–203, 1995.

Selby B, et al: High-resolution sonography of the menisci of the knee. *Invest Radiol* 21:332–335, 1986.

Selby B, Richardson ML, Nelson BD: Value of sonography in the detection of meniscal injuries of the knees: Evaluation in cadavers. *AJR* 149:549–553, 1987.

Spiegel TM, et al: Measuring disease activity: Comparison of joint tenderness, swelling and ultrasonography in rheumatoid arthritis: Evaluation with US. *Arthritis Rheum* 30(11):1283–1288, 1987.

Spritzer CE, et al: Medial retinacular complex injury in acute patellar dislocation: MR findings and surgical implications. *AJR* 168:117–122, 1997.

Starok M, et al: Normal patellar retinaculum: MR and sonographic imaging with cadaveric correlation. *AJR* 168:1493–1499, 1997.

Steiner E, et al: Ganglia and cysts around joints. *Radiol Clin North Am* 34:395–425, 1996.

Sureda D, et al: Juvenile rheumatoid arthritis of the knee: Evaluation with US. *Radiology* 190:403–406, 1994.

Suzuki S, et al: Ultrasound diagnosis of pathology of the anterior and posterior cruciate ligaments of the knee joint. *Arch Orthop Trauma Surg* 110:200–203, 1991.

Tiliakos N, Morales R, Wilson CH Jr: Use of ultrasound in identifying tophaceous versus rheumatoid nodules. *Arthritis Rheum* 25:478–479, 1985.

van Holsbeeck M, et al: Staging and follow-up of rheumatoid arthritis of the knee. Comparison of sonography, thermography and clinical assessment. *J Ultrasound Med* 7:561–566, 1988.

Walker J, Rang M, Daneman A: Ultrasonography of the unossified patella in young children. *J Pediatr Orthop* 11:100–102, 1991.

Yashar AA, et al: An ultrasound method to evaluate polyethylene component wear in total knee replacement arthroplasty. *Am J Orthop* 25:702–704, 1996.

Yasuda K, Majima J: Intraarticular ganglion blocking extension of the knee: Brief report. *J Bone Joint Surg* 70B:837, 1988.

Chapter 19
Sonography of the Ankle and Foot

David P. Fessell, M.D., and Marnix T. van Holsbeeck, M.D.

Ultrasound is an efficient, inexpensive, and widely available modality for evaluation of the ankle and foot. Tendon, joint, and soft tissue pathology can be diagnosed by ultrasound. Rapid comparison with the asymptomatic ankle and direct correlation of sonographic findings with the patient's symptoms are advantages of ultrasound. A focused foot or ankle ultrasound study can usually be performed more efficiently than with MRI. Demand for ultrasound of the ankle will probably increase given its significantly lower cost compared to that of MRI. This chapter reviews the scanning technique and role of ultrasound in evaluation of traumatic injuries and chronic ankle pain. Knowledge of the location of the pain and the acuity of the injury usually narrows the differential diagnosis; this clinically oriented approach will be utilized in this chapter.

Technical Guidelines and Scanning Technique

Ankle ultrasound requires a high-frequency (7.5 MHz or higher) linear array transducer. Table 19–1 describes patient positioning for evaluation of the ankle and foot. Details of patient positioning and scanning technique have been described previously and are summarized below (Fessell et al., 1998; Vanderscheuren et al., 1998). For an experienced sonographer, examination of the ankle usually requires 10–15 minutes. A tailored examination of a specific tendon can be performed in even less time. The dynamic capabilities of ultrasound allow examination in multiple planes including stress views.

Anterior Joint

Examination of the ankle begins with the patient in the supine position, with the knee flexed and the foot flush with the examination table. The anterior joint is first examined in the longitudinal orientation to assess for synovitis or a joint effusion. The normal anterior joint capsule is hyperechoic and is seen adjacent to the anterior tibia and hypoechoic cartilage of the talar dome (van Holsbeeck and Introcaso, 1991; Chhem et al., 1993). In normal volunteers, up to 3 mm of anechoic fluid has been demonstrated in the anterior joint (Table 19–2) (Nazarian et al., 1995).

Extensor Tendons

Evaluation of the extensor tendons is performed with the patient in the same position used for evaluation of the anterior joint. The anterior tibial tendon is the most medial of the three extensor tendons, and is approximately twice the diameter of the extensor hallucis longus and extensor digitorum longus. The anterior tibial tendon is evaluated in both longitudinal and transverse orientations from its superior extent to its insertion on the first cuneiform. The extensor hallucis longus is similarly evaluated and can be followed to its insertion on the great toe. Scanning transversely from superior to inferior demonstrates the extensor digitorum longus as a single tendon proximally which extends into four individual tendons which insert on the second through fifth toes.

Lateral Ankle Tendons

The peroneal tendons are examined from their supramalleolar musculotendinous junction through their inframalleolar course in both longitudinal and transverse planes. Only a "trace" amount of fluid is visualized in the peroneal tendon sheath. The only exception is within the sheath just distal to the fibula, where up to 3 mm of fluid can usually be observed in normal volunteers (Nazarian et al.,

Table 19–1
Positioning for Ankle and Foot Ultrasound

Structure	Patient Position	Foot Position
1. Extensor tendons and anterior joint	Seated or supine	Plantar foot flush with examination table
2. Peroneal tendons	Seated or supine	Plantar foot flush with table and slightly inverted
3. Flexor tendons	Seated or supine	Plantar foot flush with table or frog leg
4. Achilles tendon, retrocalcaneal bursa, plantar fascia	Prone	Foot hanging over table or dorsiflexed
5. Morton neuroma	Supine	Heel on table, foot dorsi- or plantarflexed

Source: Fessell et al., 1998; Vanderscheuren et al., 1998.

1995). The peroneus brevis is examined to its insertion at the base of the fifth metatarsal. The longus can be examined to the cuboid groove, where it turns medial to course along the plantar foot. Examination of the plantar foot can follow the longus to its insertion at the medial cuneiform/first metatarsal.

Medial Ankle Tendons

The supra- and inframalleolar posterior tibial tendons, flexor digitorum longus, and flexor hallucis longus are examined in both longitudinal and transverse planes. To aid orientation, the posterior tibial tendon is first evaluated transversely in a supramalleolar location where the tendon is easily demonstrated within its shallow, bony groove. In the inframalleolar location, the posterior tibial tendon is evaluated first in the longitudinal orientation just proximal to its navicular insertion. The tendon is more difficult to evaluate, as it fans out to insert on the navicular, tarsals, and proximal metatarsals. In this zone, it is difficult to diagnose tendinitis or a partial tendon tear unless a high-frequency transducers (12 MHz or higher) is used or the patient is symptomatic. A complete tear with retraction of the torn tendon is, however, readily diagnosed even with 7.5 or 10 MHz transducers. Comparison with the asymptomatic ankle aides assessment of this region.

In normal subjects, up to 4 mm of anechoic fluid has been demonstrated around the posterior tibial tendon (Fig. 19–1). The fluid is usually located posterior to the inframalleolar tendon (Table 19–2). (Nazarian et al., 1995). The posterior tibial tendon is the largest of the three medial tendons, usually measuring 4–6 mm in diameter (Miller et al., 1996). When scanning from anterior to posterior, the posterior tibial tendon is anterior to the flexor digitorum longus, followed by the tibial nerve and adjacent vessels (two veins, one artery) and the flexor hallucis longus. In the longitudinal orientation, the talonavicular joint is used as a landmark in evaluating the inframalleolar posterior tibial tendon and the flexor digitorum longus. Due to its depth, evaluation of the flexor hallucis longus is more difficult. A posterior approach, just medial to the Achilles tendon, can aid evaluation.

Table 19–2
Distribution and Amount of Fluid in the Asymptomatic Ankle

Site	Dimensions
1. Posterior tibial tendon	≤4 mm*
2. Common peroneal tendon sheath	≤3 mm†
3. Flexor digitorum, anterior tibial tendon, Achilles tendon, posterior ankle joint	No detectable fluid
4. Anterior joint	≤3 mm
5. Retrocalcaneal bursa	<2.5 mm
6. Flexor hallucis longus	Undefined; trace fluid in our experience

*Usually posterior to the tendon and inferior to the medial malleous; no extension to the navicular insertion.
†Up to 3 mm just distal to the lateral malleolus; trace fluid elsewhere.
Source: Nazarian et al., 1995. Data are from a normal population and do not define the upper limits of normal by strict definition. Physiological fluid can be unilateral or asymmetric in amount when bilateral.

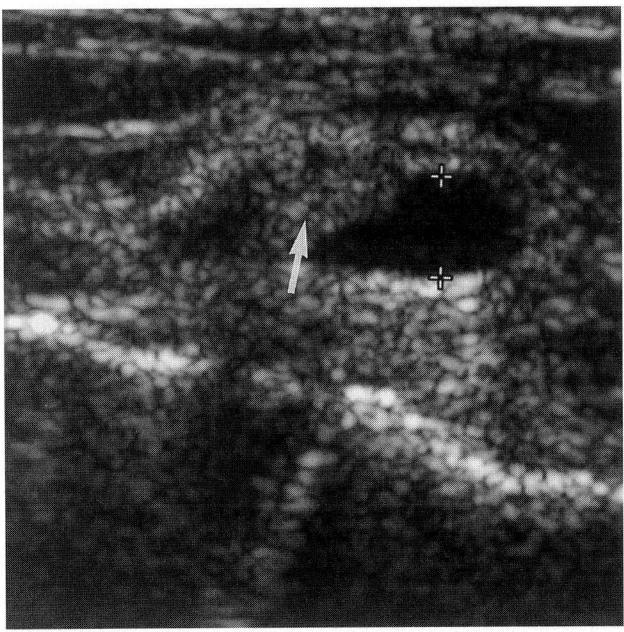

Figure 19–1 ■ Normal posterior tibial tendon sheath: transverse sonogram. A 30-year-old woman with distal plantar fasciitis. The patient's tarsal tunnels and the posterior tibial tendons appear symmetric and normal. The transducer is positioned transversely over the inframalleolar portion of the posterior tibial tendon (*arrow*). A normal amount of fluid (3 mm between the + cursors) is demonstrated inferior to the tendon.

Achilles Tendon and Retrocalcaneal Bursa

For examination of the Achilles tendon and retrocalcaneal bursa the patient is supine, with the foot hanging over the examination table or resting on the toes. The tendon is examined from its origin from the gastrocnemius and soleus muscles to its insertion on the calcaneus in both transverse and longitudinal orientations. The anteroposterior diameter of the normal Achilles tendon is dependent upon the habitus and gender of the patient and usually measures 5–6 mm when measured on a transverse scan (van Holsbeeck and Introcaso, 1991). Measurements of the tendon diameter in the longitudinal plane should be avoided since they can overestimate the tendon thickness due to the oblique course of the tendon (Fornage, 1986). Dynamic evaluation by actively plantarflexing and dorsiflexing the ankle aids evaluation of suspected tendon tears. The plantaris tendon may also be visualized along the medial Achilles tendon as it courses from the posterolateral knee to insert on the posteromedial calcaneus.

The retrocalcaneal bursa is evaluated with the Achilles tendon. The bursa is located between the Achilles tendon and the superior calcaneus. The normal bursa is shaped like a comma, with the tail of the comma extending between the Achilles and calcaneus. The normal bursa can measure up to 3 mm in diameter (Table 19–2) (Fornage and Rifkin, 1988a; Nazarian et al., 1995). The posterior ankle joint and deeper structures, such as the flexor hallucis, can also be evaluated with the Achilles tendon and retrocalcaneal bursa utilizing a 5 MHz transducer.

Plantar Fascia

With the patient prone and the foot hanging freely over the examination table or resting on the toes, the plantar fascia can also be examined (Cardinal et al., 1996). For longitudinal evaluation, the transducer is oriented with the long axis of the plantar fascia. The normal plantar fascia is uniformly fibrillar. The only exception is where the fascia curves slightly to insert on the calcaneal tuberosity. In this region, the fascia may normally appear hypoechoic due to anisotropy; however, there is no thickening. The thickness of the plantar fascia is measured in the longitudinal orientation near its insertion onto the calcaneal tuberosity. The normal fascia measures 3–4 mm in thickness when measured perpendicular to the long axis of the calcaneus (Cardinal et al., 1996).

Interdigital Web Spaces

The web spaces of the foot can be evaluated from the plantar (Shapiro and Shapiro, 1995) or dorsal foot (Redd et al., 1989; Pollak et al., 1992; Sobiesk et al., 1997). The patient is examined supine, with the heel resting on or hanging over the examination table. As each interspace is examined sonographically from the dorsal approach, the sonographer applies finger pressure to each plantar interspace. If ultrasound is used to evaluate from the plantar approach, finger pressure is applied to each dorsal interspace. The dorsal approach is more widely used in the literature, probably because the convex soft tissues of the plantar foot can make the plantar examination somewhat more difficult (Redd et al., 1989; Pollak et al., 1992). However, we routinely evaluate from the plantar approach since there is no intervening intermetatarsal bursa and the interdigital nerve is closer to the plantar surface of the foot. Both approaches can be used to optimize visualization of pathology (Pollak et al., 1992). The interspace is composed of echogenic fat and is bounded by the echogenic cortex of the metatarsals, which demonstrates posterior acoustic shadowing.

Acute Injuries of the Ankle

Acute injury of the ankle can involve the bones, joints, tendons, or ligaments. Frequently more than

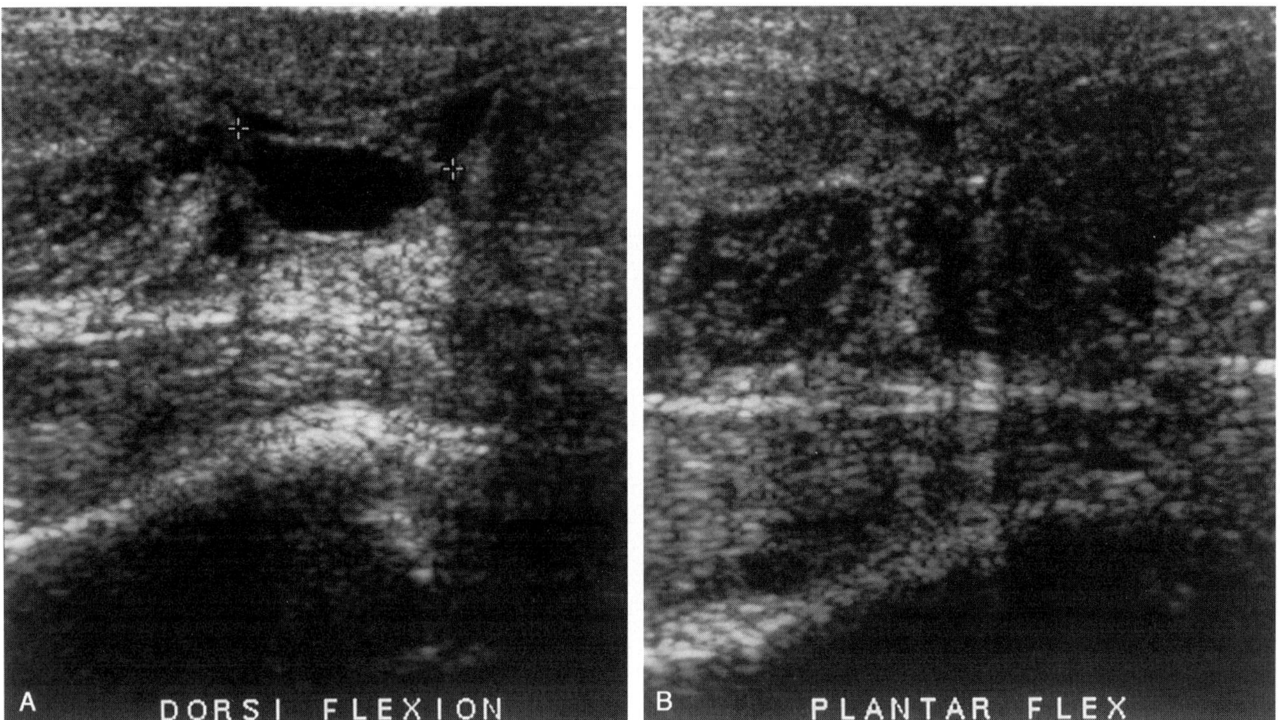

Figure 19–2 ■ **A**, Full-thickness tear of the Achilles tendon: longitudinal sonogram. This 42-year-old man felt a sudden sharp pain and a popping sensation in his heel during aerobic exercises. The scan along the long axis of the Achilles tendon shows a hypoechoic gap in the tendon. With the foot in dorsiflexion, 1.2 cm of distraction is shown between the + cursors. **B**, Full-thickness tear of the Achilles tendon: longitudinal sonogram. Same patient and same technique as in **A**. The foot is now brought in plantar flexion with gentle assistance of the examiner's hand. Due to the absence of distraction between the torn tendon ends in plantarflexion, the patient was treated nonoperatively.

one of these structures is injured. Evaluation begins with conventional radiographs to detect fractures and bony pathology. Conventional radiographs also provide clues to suggest ligamentous or tendonous injury. MRI can reveal occult fractures, bone bruises, and osteochondral injuries. Both MRI and ultrasound can diagnose tendon, ligament, joint, and soft tissue pathology. In the acute setting, ultrasound can often be performed more efficiently and rapidly.

Acute Achilles Tendon Injuries

The Achilles tendon is the most frequently injured ankle tendon (Reinherz et al., 1986). A zone of relative avascularity 2–6 cm proximal to the calcaneal insertion is the most frequent site of a tear (Scheller et al., 1980). Clinical examination including a positive Thompson test (failure of plantar flexion with squeezing of the calf) is often sufficient to make the diagnosis. Opacity in Kager's fat (normally a lucent triangle between the Achilles tendon and the posterior tibia) on a lateral ankle radiograph suggests pathology involving the Achilles tendon. When an acute Achilles tendon injury is suspected, the role of ultrasound is twofold. First, ultrasound can confirm a full- or partial-thickness tear. When there is complete tendon rupture, the magnitude of the tendon gap, measured with the foot in dorsiflexion and plantarflexion (Fig. 19–2) is useful in planning surgical versus conservative treatment (Thermann et al., 1992). Second, ultrasound can evaluate the plantaris tendon. A false-negative Thompson test can be elicited with a complete Achilles tendon tear if the plantaris tendon is intact. Assessment of the condition of the plantaris tendon (Fig. 19–3) is also important since it can be used as a graft for repair of the Achilles tendon.

Distention of the retrocalcaneal bursa can mimic Achilles tendon pathology clinically. Bursal distention >3 mm is frequently due to inflammation or hemorrhagic bursitis and is easily separated from Achilles tendon pathology by ultrasound (Fig. 19–4). A ruptured Baker's cyst can track to the level of the Achilles tendon and mimic tendon pathology. Therefore, if the Achilles tendon and retrocalcaneal bursa are normal, ultrasound examination of the popliteal space may be warranted.

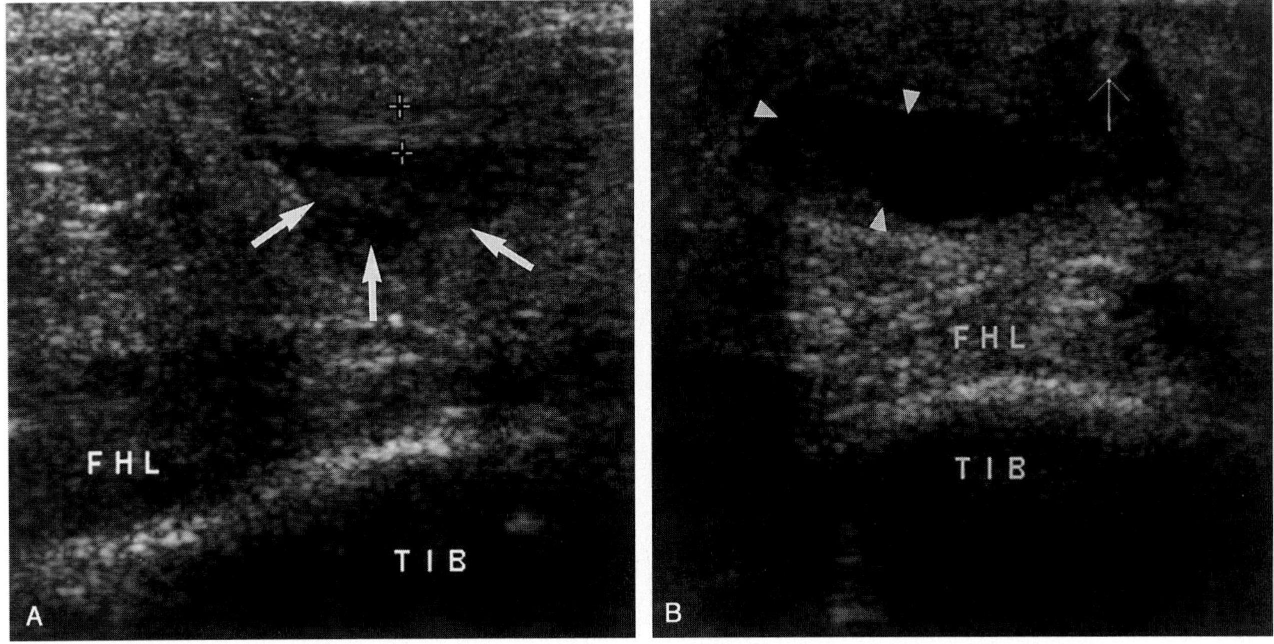

Figure 19–3 ■ **A**, Full-thickness tear of the Achilles tendon: longitudinal sonogram. Same patient as in Figure 19–2. The longitudinal exam is now extended over the medial aspect of the torn Achilles tendon (*arrows*). The plantaris tendon (*between the cursors*) is intact. **B**, Full-thickness tear of the Achilles tendon: transverse sonogram. Same patient as in Figure 19–2 and 19–3**A**. Transverse ultrasound identifies the intact plantaris tendon (*arrow*). The normal Achilles tendon is absent, and fluid fills the empty paratenon (*arrowheads*). Abbrevations: flexor hallucis longus (*FHL*), tibia (*TIB*).

Medial gastrocnemius tears can present with the same symptoms as Achilles tendon tears at the musculo-tendinous junction. Ultrasound can easily distinguish these entities.

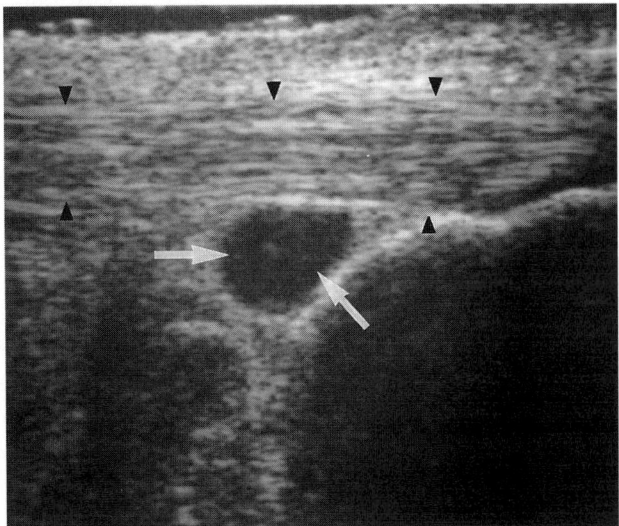

Figure 19–4 ■ Traumatic retrocalcaneal bursitis: longitudinal sonogram. A professional hockey player, age 23, was hit against his heel during recreational sport. Clinical assessment suggested an Achilles tear. The ultrasound exam showed a normal Achilles tendon (*arrowheads*). A distended retrocalcaneal bursa (*arrows*) measuring 6 mm in diameter surrounds the distal end of the tendon.

Acute Ligamentous Injuries

The diagnosis of ligamentous injury is usually made clinically or by radiographs showing an avulsed bony fragment. Diagnosis of a single torn ligament usually does not change the clinical management. The most frequently injured ankle ligament is the anterior talofibular ligament (Reinherz et al., 1986). Communication of a joint effusion with the peroneal tendon sheaths indicates injury to the calcaneofibular ligament (Frieberger and Kaye, 1979). A tear of the calcaneofibular ligament implies a disruption of the anterior talofibular ligament. Stress radiographs which reveal a tilt of 10 degrees or more may prompt operative repair. Injury to all three of the lateral ligaments (anterior talofibular, calcaneofibular, posterior talofibular) is usually an indication for surgery (Leach and Schepsis, 1990).

Ligamentous injury is diagnosed by ultrasound as thickening and hypoechogenicity of the ligament compared with the contralateral asymptomatic side. If the region is tender when scanning, an acute injury is suggested. A complete tear can be diagnosed when a hypoechoic gap or cleft is demonstrated through the substance of a ligament. Bony avulsion or calcification from an old injury is demonstrated as an echogenic focus within the ligament (see also Chapter 6).

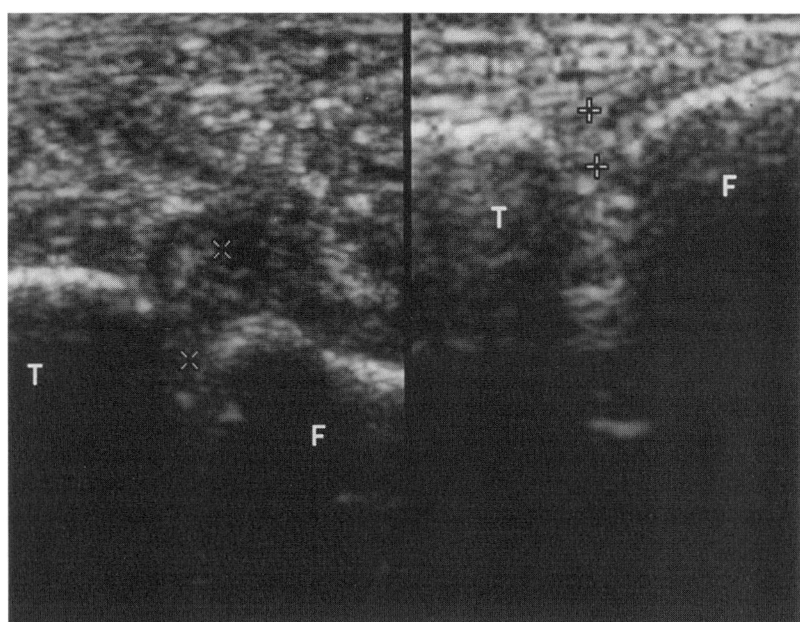

Figure 19–5 ■ Ankle ligament tear: transverse sonogram. A 67-year-old woman slipped going down steps; her ankle twisted and was swollen for 2 weeks. She was seen in the orthopedic clinic because of persistent pain. Split-screen transverse ultrasound of a torn anterior tibiofibular ligament (*image on the left*) with comparison to the contralateral normal ligament (*image on the right*). The torn ligament is bulbous and retracted, measuring 4.8 mm (*between the x cursors*) versus 1.8 mm for the normal ligament (*between the + cursors*). Abbreviations: tibia (*T*), fibula (*F*).

Widening of the medial joint space >4 mm indicates injury to the deltoid ligament. Such injuries are associated with fractures of the proximal fibula (Maisonneuve fracture), distal fibula, and anterior tibiofibular ligament (Leach and Schepsis, 1990). Stress radiographs, MRI, and ultrasound can aid in the diagnosis of deltoid ligament pathology.

Ligament injury can also be caused by an external rotation force on the tibiofibular syndesmosis. These injuries occur in football players, usually when the foot is pronated and twisted or suffers blunt trauma to the posterior aspect of the tibia. Ultrasound of the anterior tibiofibular space shows slight widening with an associated tibiotalar effusion when compared to the asymptomatic ankle. The disrupted tibiofibular ligament appears hyperechoic, with a surrounding hypoechoic collection which can extend into the cleft within the ligament (Fig. 19–5) (see also Chapter 6).

Acute Joint Pathology

Acute pathology of the anterior tibiotalar joint can be due to a number of etiologies. Anechoic fluid causes the capsule to bulge from the joint with a simple joint effusion. A complex effusion is demonstrated as a heterogeneous fluid collection with hypoechoic and hyperechoic regions. The etiology of a complex effusion includes infection, inflammatory conditions, hemorrhage, intra-articular air, pigmented villonodular synovitis, and synovial osteochondromatosis (Fig. 19–6). Conventional radiographs, clinical history, laboratory values, and joint aspiration usually can provide a specific diagnosis. Ultrasound can aid joint aspiration by assessing for fluid, confirming the intra-articular location of the needle, and guiding aspiration with real-time scanning.

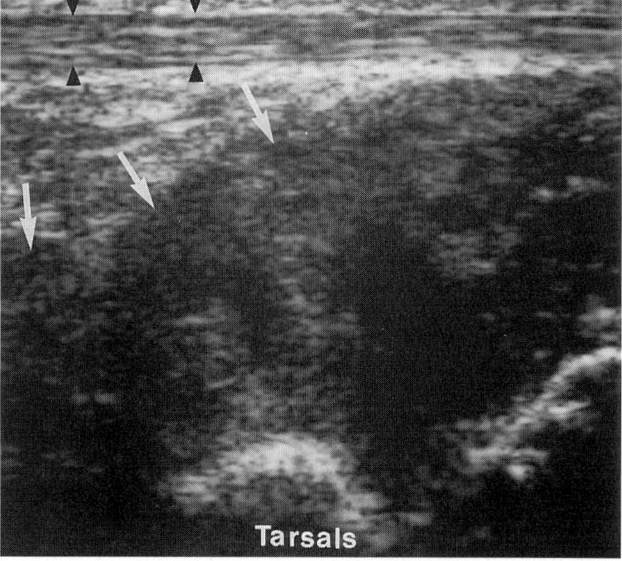

Figure 19–6 ■ Pigmented villonodular synovitis: longitudinal sonogram. Ankle swelling and pain brought this 47-year-old man to the clinic. He was first treated with a presumptive diagnosis of gout. The ultrasound study was obtained 3 months after the start of the failing hyperuricemic treatment. It shows a complex mass over the dorsum of the foot. A mixed echogenicity joint distention (*arrows*) is seen anterior to the tarsal bones and posterior to the extensor tendon (*arrowheads*). The peripheral joint thickening suggests a synovial mass. Biopsy-proved pigmented villonodular synovitis in the tarsus.

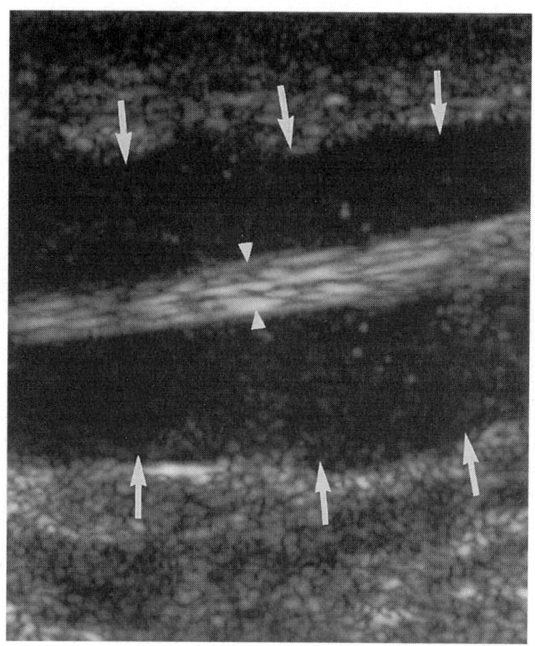

Figure 19–7 ■ Septic tenosynovitis: longitudinal sonogram. An 82-year-old diabetic female has had pain, swelling, and redness over the dorsal aspect of her foot for 1 week. Longitudinal ultrasound of the extensor digitorum tendon (*arrowheads*) was performed in this patient, who was referred for suspicion of a septic joint. Extensive hypoechoic tenosynovitis (*arrows*) surrounds the tendon. Needle aspiration and culture grew *Nocardia asteroides*. Blind aspiration, without prior imaging, could have infected normal joint spaces.

Septic tenosynovitis (Fig. 19–7) can mimic a septic joint clinically. A blind joint aspiration in such cases could infect an aseptic joint, and imaging prior to aspiration should always be considered. Ultrasound may be especially helpful in guiding aspiration of joints with deformity, and can assess for synovial hypertrophy and guide synovial biopsy.

Foreign Bodies

Evaluating for a radiolucent foreign body following a penetrating injury is common in the emergency room. Conventional radiographs should be obtained and correlated with ultrasound scans. Prompt diagnosis and removal is imperative to avoid complications including infection and malpractice litigation (Jacobson et al., 1998). A focused ultrasound examination can be performed if the area of clinical concern is first marked by the referring service (Rockett et al., 1995). A 10 MHz or higher frequency transducer is utilized, with evaluation in both longitudinal and transverse orientations.

Foreign bodies appear uniformly hyperechoic by ultrasound (Jacobson et al., 1998). A hypoechoic reaction develops around the hyperechoic foreign body in subacute and chronic settings, aiding detection (Fig. 19–8) (Jacobson et al., 1998). The sensitivity, specificity, and accuracy of ultrasound detection of foreign bodies have been reported to be 90–100% (Rockett et al., 1995; Jacobson et al., 1998). A foreign body as small as 1 × 0.5 mm has been localized using ultrasound (Failla et al., 1995). Ultrasound has been shown to be superior to both CT and MRI, especially for metallic foreign bodies, which can create artifacts that hinder precise localization (Fig. 19–9) (Oikarinen et al., 1993). When the foreign body is located near bone, ultrasound may not be able to differentiate the echogenic bony cortex from the echogenic foreign body (Mizel et al., 1994), but newer 12 MHz and higher frequency transducers will probably improve detection in such cases (J. A. Jacobson, personal communication). Air from a puncture wound can potentially be mistaken for a small foreign body by ultrasound. However, the absence of posterior acoustic shadowing associated with most wooden foreign bodies helps prevent this error (see also Chapter 12).

Chronic Ankle Pain

The etiology of chronic ankle pain can involve pathology of the bones, joints, tendons, or soft

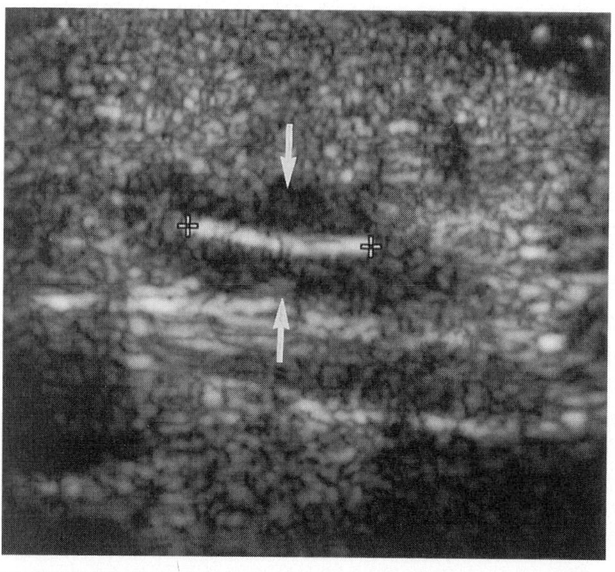

Figure 19–8 ■ Radiolucent foreign body: longitudinal sonogram. A 7-year-old boy stepped on a splinter 1 month ago. His mother thought she had removed the entire piece at the time of the injury, but the child kept complaining and a large, painful callous had formed over the medial aspect of the child's left foot sole. Conventional radiographs were normal. Longitudinal ultrasound scan of the plantar foot demonstrating a linear echogenic foreign body measuring 0.7 cm between the + cursors. A hypoechoic reaction (*arrow*) is noted. A wooden splinter was found at surgery.

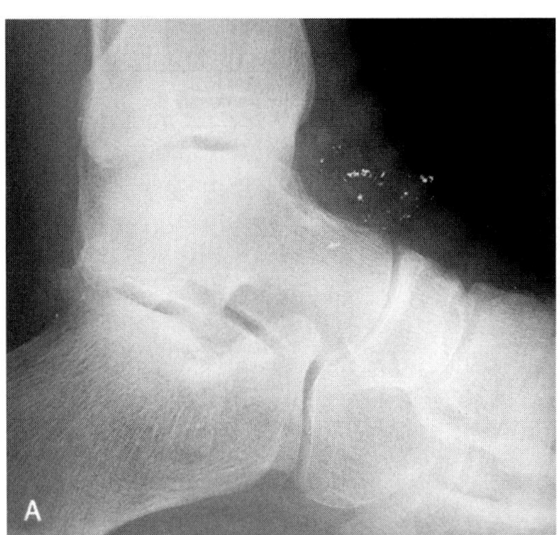

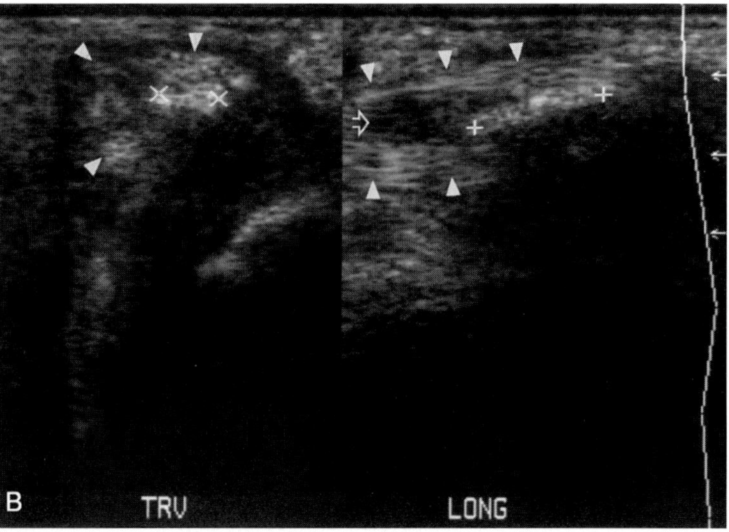

Figure 19–9 ■ **A**, Foreign body in tendon: lateral foot radiograph. Lateral radiograph shows evidence of a prior gunshot wound to the ankle in this 66-year-old male who had ankle pain and denied having had prior trauma. Multiple metallic fragments are present in the soft tissues. **B**, Foreign body in tendon: tendon sonography. Same patient as in **A**. Split-screen transverse (*left image*) and longitudinal (*right image*) ultrasound images demonstrate an echogenic foreign body (*between the cursors*) within the posterior tibial tendon (*arrowheads*) with surrounding tenosynovitis. A partial tear in the distal tendon was caused by the shrapnel impact (*open arrow*). Artifact from the multiple metallic fragments would severely limit imaging by MRI or CT.

tissues. Evaluation begins with conventional radiographs, which can reveal fractures, subluxation/dislocation, and arthritic and degenerative disease and grossly can suggest soft tissue abnormality. Conventional radiographs, including stress views, also provide clues suggesting ligamentous or tendonous injury. CT is useful for evaluation of complex fractures, osteoid osteoma, and tarsal coalition. MRI is superior for the detection of occult fractures, osteochondral or cartilage injuries, bone marrow pathology, and osteomyelitis. In the setting of chronic ankle pain, ultrasound can rapidly evaluate the ankle tendons and assess for pathology, including tenosynovitis (Fig. 19–10), tendinosis, and tendon tears. Orthopedic hardware can be a source of mechanical impingement and pain and complications can be diagnosed with ultrasound (Fig. 19–11). Such hardware often produces artifacts which preclude adequate imaging by CT or MRI. Knowledge of the site of chronic pain narrows the differential diagnosis and allows for a more focused exam.

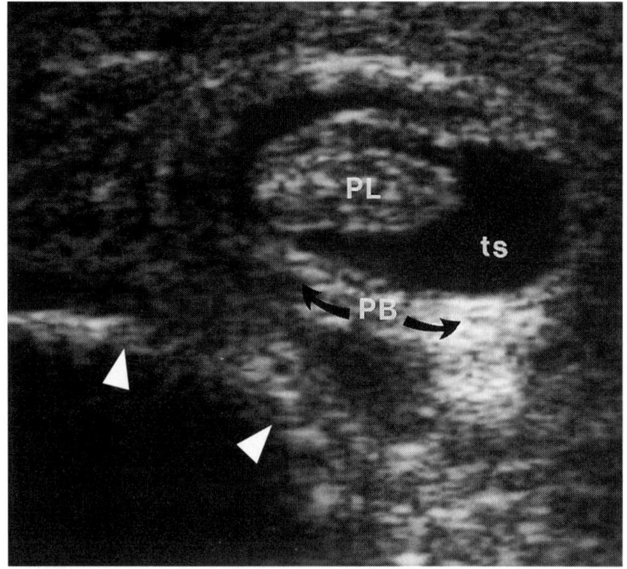

Figure 19–10 ■ Peroneal tendon subluxation: transverse sonography. This 40-year-old man sustained an ankle injury 6 months ago. Pain and swelling around the ankle persisted after the injury. An excruciating lateral ankle pain often accompanied an audible popping and clicking in the ankle. Abnormal alignment could be induced during the study in passive dorsiflexion and eversion of the foot. The transducer is applied transversely over the lateral malleolus, with almost no pressure on the skin surface. The tendons are subluxed anterior to the lateral malleolus (*arrowheads*). Marked tenosynovitis (*ts*) is present. The peroneus brevis (*PB*, *curved arrows*) is markedly flattened adjacent to the peroneus longus (*PL*).

Chronic Lateral Pain

Injury to the superior peroneal retinaculum allows subluxation/dislocation of the peroneal tendons, causing tendinosis/tendinitis, tenosynovitis, and pain

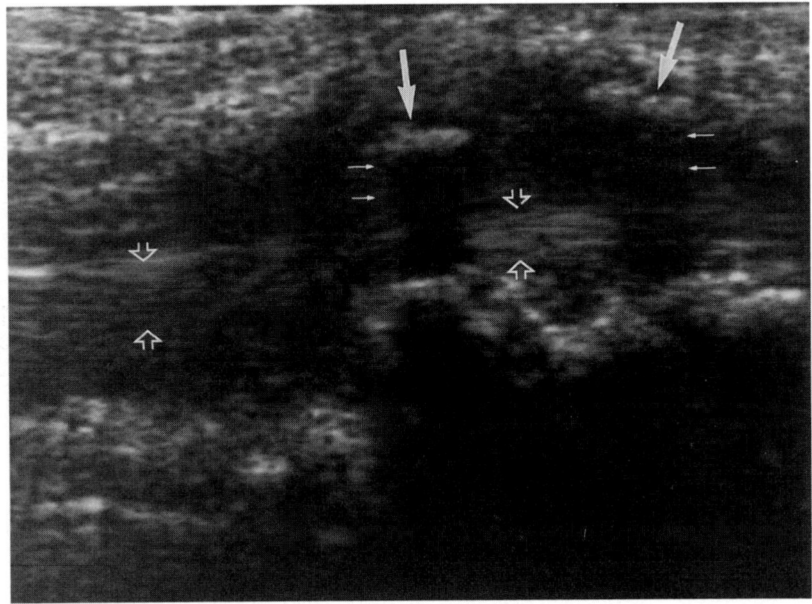

Figure 19–11 ■ Postsurgical tenosynovitis of the posterior tibial tendon: longitudinal sonogram. A 65-year-old woman underwent ankle arthrodesis after posttraumatic degenerative disease of the tibiotalar joint. She developed focal pain at the medial aspect of the ankle over the 6 months following surgery. The posterior tibial tendon (*open arrows*) is intact, but anechoic tenosynovitis surrounds the tendon. The irritation is secondary to impinging screw threads (*large arrows*) from prior surgical fixation. Posterior shadowing from the hardware is noted (*small arrows*).

(Sammarco, 1994). Rupture of the superior peroneal retinaculum often occurs with a calcaneal fracture or avulsion fracture of the lateral malleolus (Fig. 19–12) (Church, 1977; McConkey and Favero, 1987; Cheung et al., 1992). Ski injuries causing a dorsiflexion, eversion ankle injury are also a common etiology of retinacular and peroneal tendon injuries (Church, 1977; McConkey and Favero, 1987). Congenital abnormalities including a congenitally flat or convex fibular groove can predispose to peroneal tendon dislocation (McConkey and Favero, 1987; Cheung et al., 1992). The depth of the fibular groove can be assessed on transverse scans and is normally slightly concave. Transient dislocation or

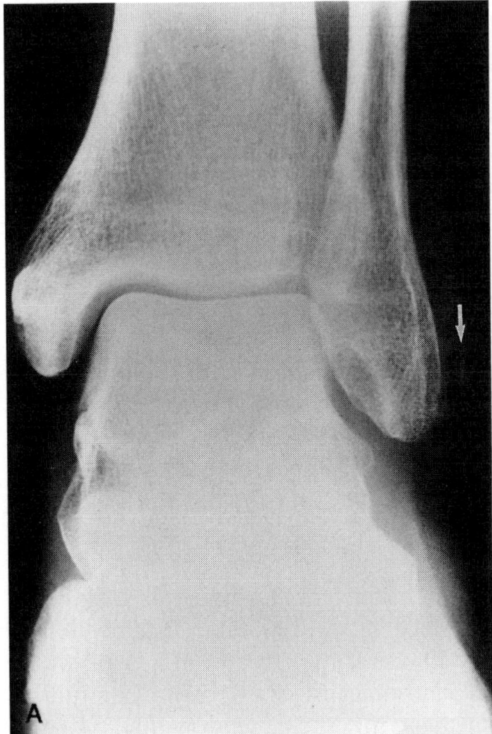

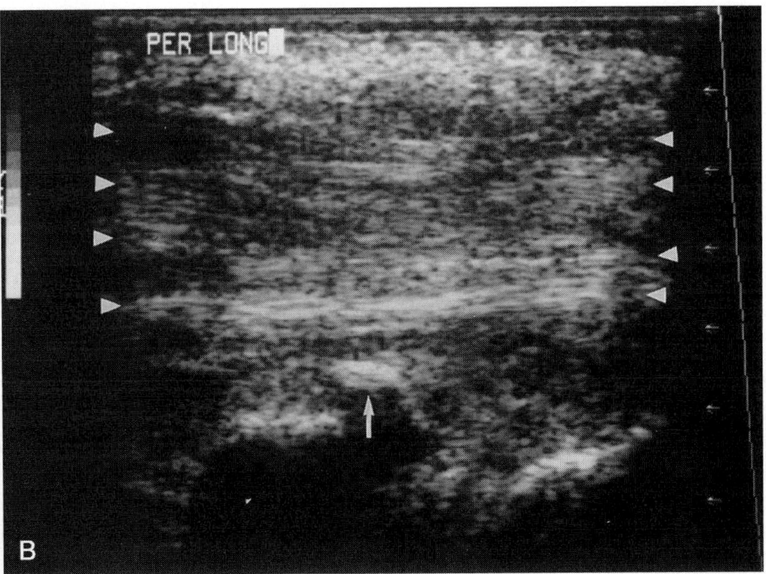

Figure 19–12 ■ **A**, Avulsion of superior peroneal retinaculum: anteroposterior radiograph of the ankle. Radiograph demonstrating an avulsion fracture of the lateral malleolus (*arrow*). **B**, Longitudinal ultrasound scan shows the lateral malleolus avulsion fracture (*arrow*) and a markedly swollen, hypoechoic peroneus longus with duplicated tubular structure (*arrowheads*). (Reproduced with permission from Diaz GC, van Holsbeeck M, et al: Longitudinal split of the peroneus longus and peroneus brevis tendons with disruption of the superior peroneal retinaculum. *J Ultrasound Med* 17:525–529, 1998.)

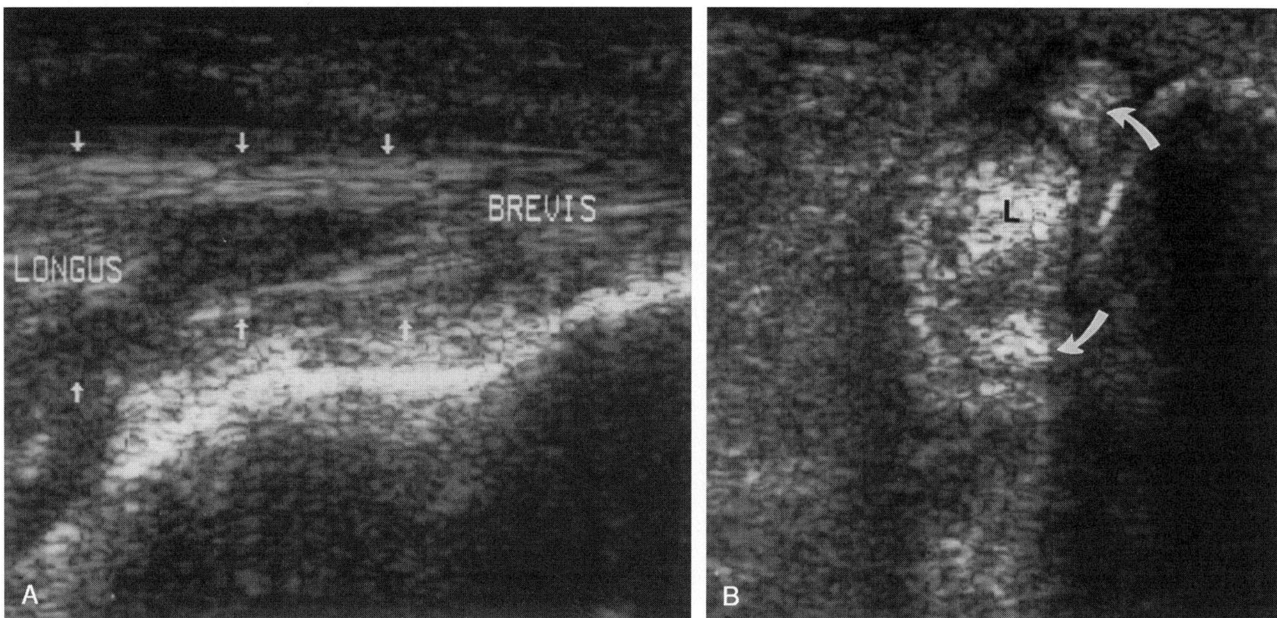

Figure 19–13 ■ **A**, Partial-thickness tear of the peroneus brevis: longitudinal sonogram. This woman, who is now 45 years old, was diagnosed with poliomyelitis 25 years ago. Her foot has been swollen and tender for weeks. Local tenderness over the lateral maleolus is noted. The ultrasound scan shows a longitudinal split in the peroneus brevis (*arrows*), with the longus insinuated into the split in the brevis. **B**, Partial-thickness tear of the peroneus brevis: transverse sonogram. Same patient as in **A**. The transverse ultrasound scan demonstrates the longus (*L*) within the split in the brevis (*curved arrows*).

subluxation can be demonstrated by scanning while simultaneously dorsiflexing and everting the ankle.

A longitudinal split in the peroneus brevis can also cause chronic lateral ankle pain. Longitudinal splits usually begin just distal to the fibula (Sammarco, 1994). Peroneal splits are most often seen in athletes due to repetitive trauma and in the elderly due to degeneration (Sammarco, 1994; Khoury et al., 1996; Rosenberg et al., 1997). The etiology of peroneal splits includes peroneal subluxation, a bony spur at the lateral fibula, and accessory peroneal tendons (Sammarco, 1994; Rosenberg et al., 1997; Schweitzer et al., 1997). The peroneus quartus is the most common accessory peroneal tendon. When present, it can stretch the retinaculum and compress the peroneus brevis against the fibula, leading to a peroneal split (Sammarco, 1994; Rosenberg et al., 1997). When a longitudinal split of the peroneus brevis occurs (Fig. 19–13), the peroneus longus often insinuates within the tendon cleft of the brevis. A complete transverse tear of the peroneus brevis is much less common than a longitudinal split (see also Chapter 4).

Chronic Medial Pain

Chronic spontaneous rupture of the posterior tibial tendon is a common cause of chronic medial ankle pain. A chronic rupture is more common than an acute tear and is often overlooked clinically. A chronic rupture occurs more commonly in females and is associated with seronegative arthropathies; less commonly, a chronic rupture is associated with rheumatoid arthritis (approximately 13% and 5%, respectively). Bilateral chronic ruptures occur in approximately 5% of cases (Cheung et al., 1992). When a complete rupture is chronic, a flat foot deformity develops. Posterior tibial tendon tears most commonly occur just distal to the medial malleolus; the second most common location is at its insertion on the navicular (Johnson, 1983).

Partial tears of the posterior tibial tendon (Fig. 19–14) can also be a source of chronic medial pain. The etiology of partial tears includes overuse, trauma, and mechanical impingement by a bony osteophyte from the adjacent tibial surface (Cheung et al., 1992; Fessell et al., 1998). Ultrasound can demonstrate a bony spur or osteophyte (Fig. 19–15) along with the tendon tear. An osteophyte may be difficult to identify by MRI if fatty marrow is not present within the spur (Cheung et al., 1992; Miller et al., 1996; Schweitzer et al., 1997). Longitudinal tears in the posterior tibial tendon (Fig. 19–16) are not uncommon and are best imaged in the transverse orientation. Longitudinal scanning is also performed but may not demonstrate the tear as

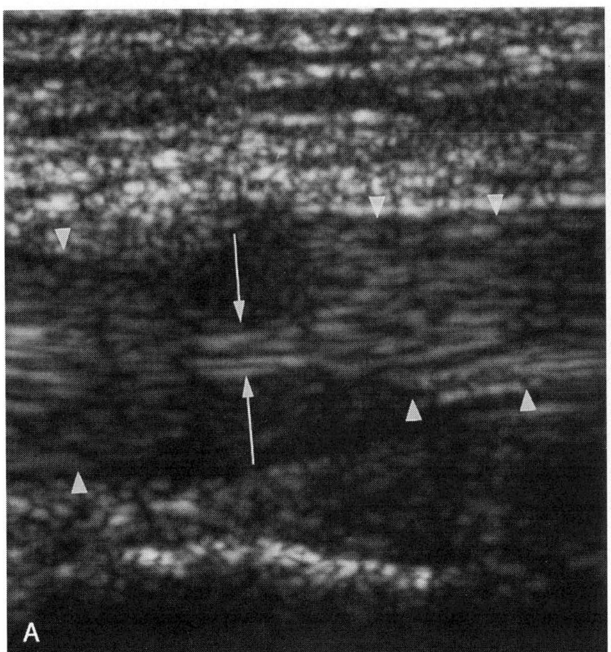

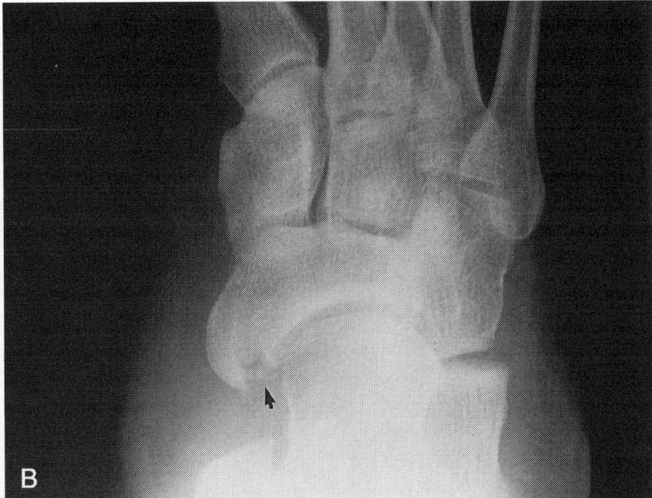

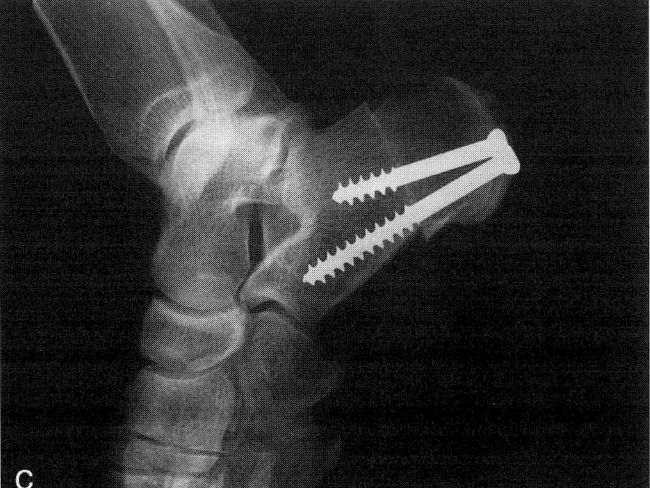

Figure 19-14 ■ **A**, Significant partial-thickness tear of the posterior tibial tendon: longitudinal sonogram. Extensive damage to the posterior tibial tendon is noted in this overweight 46-year-old nurse. She experienced gradual onset medial ankle pain. The pain became very noticeable during a 16-hour drive. A hypoechoic gap is noted in the tendon fibers. A small strand of normal tendon tissue (*arrows*) remains intact; it is less than half the thickness of the original tendon (*arrowheads*). Surgery confirmed a 75% tear of the tendon. The patient was treated with a flexor digitorum longus tendon graft and calcaneal osteotomy to correct the valgus heel deformity. **B**, Significant partial-thickness tear of the posterior tibial tendon: anteroposterior radiograph. Same patient as in **A**. Anterior-posterior radiograph of the foot following surgery demonstrates the insertion of the flexor digitarum longus tendon graft (*arrow*) on the navicular. **C**, Significant partial-thickness tear of the posterior tibial tendon: lateral radiograph. Same patient as in **A** and **B**. Lateral radiograph of the foot following surgery demonstrates osteotomy as treatment of the valgus heel deformity.

effectively, since the imaging plane is parallel to the tendon tear. In a study involving predominantly the posterior tibial tendon, Waitches et al. (1998) reported sensitivity of 100%, accuracy of 93%, and specificity of 88% for ultrasound in detecting ankle tendon tear. Tendon thickening, as seen with rheumatoid arthritis and tendinosis, can have an appearance similar to that of a longitudinal tear. Detection of a hypoechoic cleft in the tendon favors the diagnosis of a tear (Waitches et al., 1998). Ultrasound has been shown to be effective in diagnosing tendinitis/tendinosis, tenosynovitis, and complete and partial tears of the posterior tibial tendon (Miller et al., 1996; Chen and Liang, 1997).

Injury or degeneration of the cartilaginous synchondrosis of an os naviculare type II can also be a source of chronic medial ankle pain. Clinically this injury can mimic rupture or degeneration of the posterior tibial tendon. Ultrasound evaluation can visualize the defect in the synchondrosis and assess the posterior tibial tendon to exclude injury to this structure (Chen et al., 1997). The normal synchondrosis appears echogenic and homogeneous. Injury to the synchondrosis (Fig. 19-17) is seen as heterogeneity or diastasis of the synchondrosis or as fluid around the synchondrosis (Chen et al., 1997). The dynamic capability of ultrasound, allowing imaging in multiple planes and direct correlation with the site of pain, is helpful in differentiating an asymptomatic type I accessory navicular (os tibiale externum) from a symptomatic type II os naviculare.

Tarsal tunnel syndrome can also be a source of chronic medial ankle pain. Compression on the posterior tibial nerve causes pain, altered sensation, and

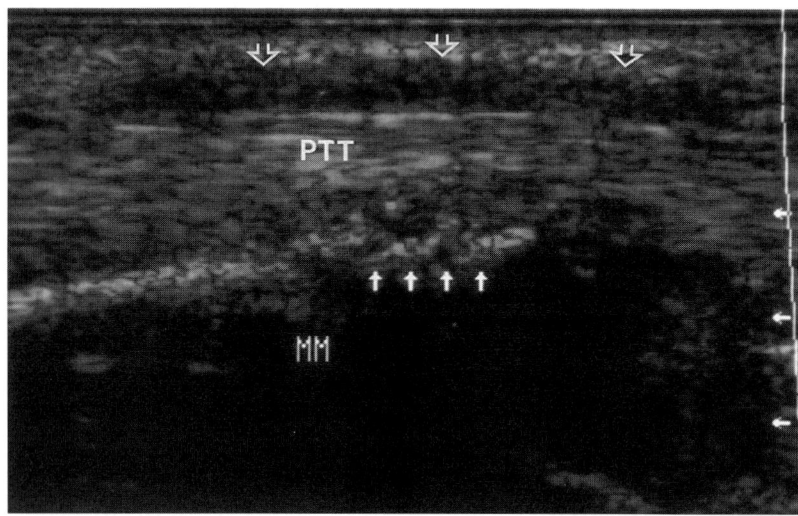

Figure 19-15 ■ Posterior tibial tendinosis and bone spur: longitudinal sonogram. This 40-year-old woman sprained her ankle and needed a syndesmotic screw to restore the ankle mortise. She kept complaining of medial ankle pain for months after the injury until an ultrasound study discovered posterior tibial tendon thinning and a large, irregular bone spur (*arrows*) in the posterior tibial tendon groove. The thinner tendon (*PTT*) over the spur contrasts sharply with the more normal tendon proximal to the abnormality. Associated tenosynovitis surrounds the posterior tibial tendon (*open arrows*). The bone spur was surgically removed and the tendon repaired. Abbreviation: medial malleolus (*MM*). (Reprinted with permission from Fessell DP et al., Ankle ultrasound: Technique, anatomy and pathology. *Radiographics* 18:325–340, 1998.)

muscle function deficit. Such impingement can be due to a soft tissue mass including a ganglion, neuroma, lipoma, posttraumatic fibrosis, or tendinous pathology (Stoller, 1997). Swelling of the plantar fascia can compress branches of the tibial nerve, also resulting in tarsal tunnel-type symptoms. In some cases, ultrasound can demonstrate the etiology of tarsal tunnel syndrome and its relationship to the tendon and surrounding structures.

Pathology of the flexor digitorum longus and flexor hallucis longus is less common but can also be evaluated with ultrasound. Tendinitis of the flexor hallucis longus is seen in ballet dancers (Fornage & Rifkin, 1988a; Cheung et al., 1992) and soccer players. Longitudinal splits of the flexor hallucis longus have been reported at the knot of Henry, the crossing point of the flexor digitorum and flexor hallucis. The etiology in these cases is repetitive hyperextension of the metatarsophalangeal joint of the great toe. Focal pain at the knot of Henry is noted, as well as pain with prolonged walking or running (Boruta and Beauperthuy, 1997).

Chronic Posterior Pain

Chronic Achilles tendon pathology is a common cause of posterior ankle pain. In chronic rupture of the Achilles tendon, physical examination may be limited. In chronic rupture, ultrasound can demonstrate the tendon discontinuity filled by echogenic

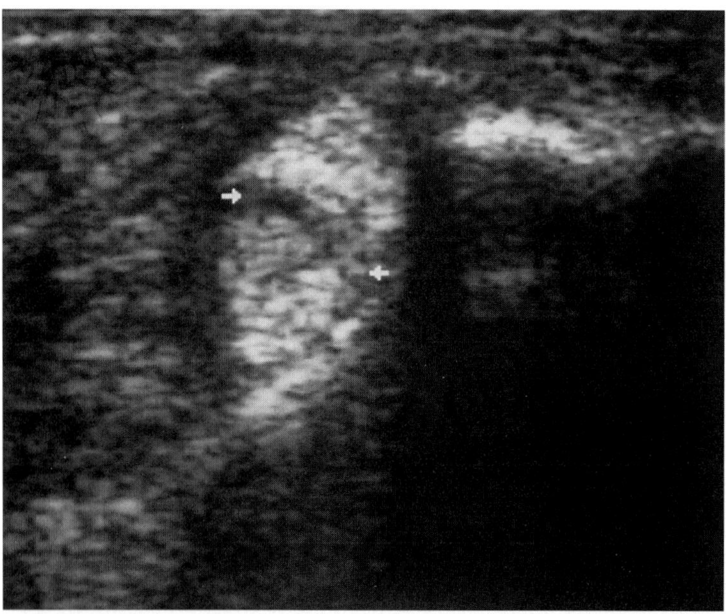

Figure 19-16 ■ Longitudinal tear of the posterior tibial tendon: transverse ultrasound. A 28-year-old woman sprained her ankle stepping down from a curb. The tendon appears bisected when scanned with the transducer transversely over the shallow posterior tibial tendon groove. This longitudinal split of the tendon communicates (*arrows*) with the synovial sheath on either side of the tendon. Transverse ultrasound image of a longitudinal split in the posterior tibial tendon (*arrows*).

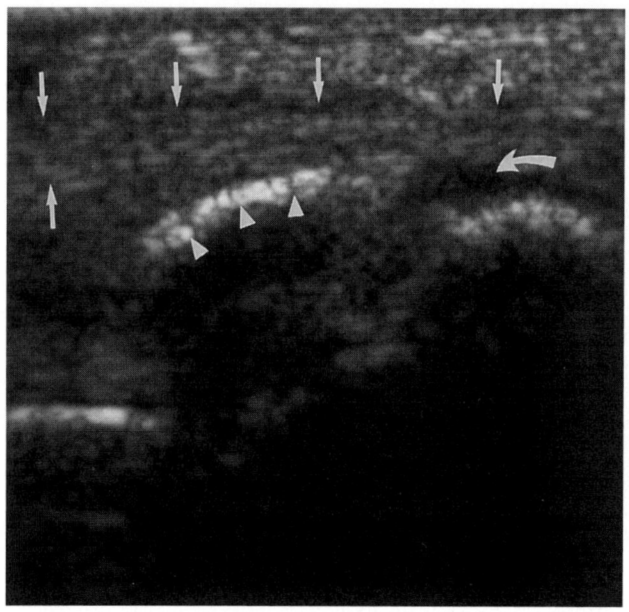

Figure 19–17 ■ Ruptured synchondrosis of the navicular: longitudinal sonogram. This podiatrist has chronic medial foot pain. He does not remember a specific injury. Scanning along the distal posterior tibial tendon (*arrows*) shows a normal tendon and tendon sheath. An os naviculare type II (*arrowheads*) is present, with separation and hypoechoic fluid between the navicular and the accessory ossification center (*curved arrow*). It was possible to move the os naviculare accessorium relative to the navicular under sonographic observation. In normal feet, these two bones are fixed to each other through a synchondrosis.

fluid or granulation tissue which is distinguishable from the echogenic tendon by the absence of a fibrillar echotexture (Fornage, 1986). Chronic Achilles tendon thickening can be due to chronic tendinosis and may have echogenic areas of calcification at the calcaneal insertion (Fig. 19–18). Partial tears usually have an appearance similar to that of tendinosis. Currently there are no definitive discriminators that distinguish tendinosis from a partial tear by ultrasound or MRI. However, a sagittal diameter greater than 10 mm and severe abnormality within the tendon favor the diagnosis of a partial tear (Astrom et al., 1996). Chronic Achilles tendon thickening can also be due to tendon tophi in patients with gout and to tendon xanthomas in patients with hypercholesterolemia (Blei et al., 1986; Fornage and Rifkin, 1988a). Ultrasound can also be used to detect subclinical xanthomatous deposition in patients with primary hypercholesterolemia (Bude et al., 1998).

In some patients, chronic posterior pain may be secondary to bursal pathology. Clinically retrocalcaneal bursal pathology can mimic Achilles tendon pathology. Ultrasound can assess both the bursa and the tendon. A thickened Achilles tendon, distended bursa, and soft tissue bump ("pump bump") are present with Haglund's syndrome. This syndrome is thought to be due to compression of the Achilles tendon and soft tissues between the calcaneus and the shoe (Resnick, 1995).

Chronic Joint and Anterior Ankle Pain

A cartilaginous or bony intra-articular loose body can be a source of chronic joint pain. Intra-articular bodies (Fig. 19–19) can be accurately imaged with ultrasound and are demonstrated as echogenic nodules which move within the joint capsule during

Figure 19–18 ■ Achilles tendinosis: longitudinal sonogram. A 50-year-old marathon runner with heel pain. Areas of hypoechogenicity (*arrowheads*) surround an enthesophyte (*arrow*) at the calcaneal insertion.

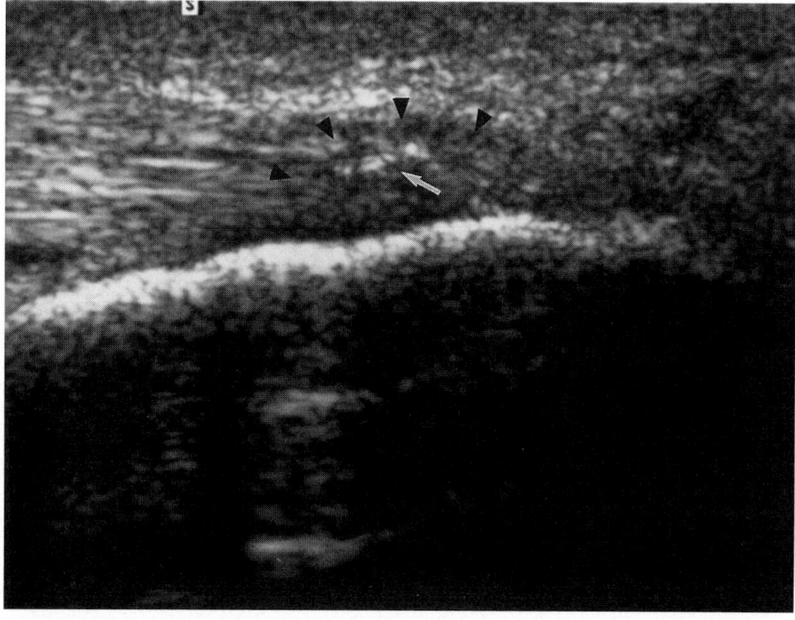

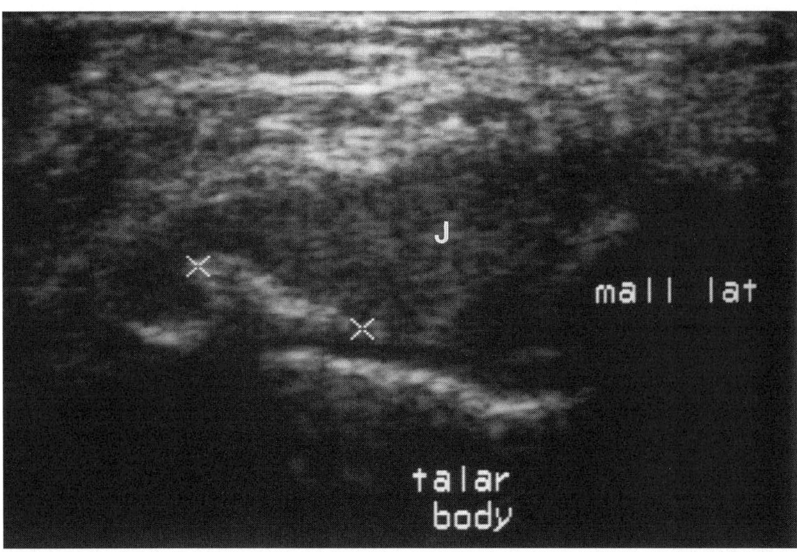

Figure 19–19 ■ Loose body: coronal sonogram. Persistent lateral ankle pain and swelling was a constant nuisance in this 40-year-old man. Coronal sonographic images showed capsular swelling at the lateral joint space. An intra-articular loose body (*between the x cursors*) with surrounding joint effusion (*J*) is demonstrated. The body was surgically removed. Abbreviation: lateral malleolus (*mall lat*).

dynamic scanning (Frankel et al., 1998). When 12 or 15 MHz transducers are used, intra-articular bodies may demonstrate a hyperechoic bony center surrounded by a hypoechoic rim of cartilage (Bianchi, 1997). Detection of a loose body usually requires the presence of a joint effusion. Sterile saline can be injected to aid detection of loose bodies in joints without an effusion (Frankel et al., 1998). Loose bodies can also be a source of pain when they occur in the synovial recesses around tendons or in a tendon sheath. Synovitis can be present with both inflammatory and noninflammatory arthridities and can be a source of an aseptic joint effusion. Synovitis is seen as thickening and increased echogenicity of the synovium of the anterior joint capsule. A bone spur at the insertion of the tibiotalar capsule can also be a source of pain secondary to impingement on the extensor tendons and can be visualized with ultrasound.

Chronic anterior pain in a number of patients may be due to pathology of the extensor tendons. Extensor tendon pathology is the least common of all ankle tendon pathologies. This is probably due to the absence of a bony fulcrum and a strong vascular supply of the anterior tibial tendon (Scheller et al., 1980). Rupture of the anterior tibial tendon does occur, however, and is usually due to blunt or penetrating trauma. Bulbous retraction of the proximal tendon is usually seen with complete rupture. Tendinosis of the anterior tibial tendon (Fig. 19–20) is unusual but can be a source of anterior pain, especially with dorsiflexion.

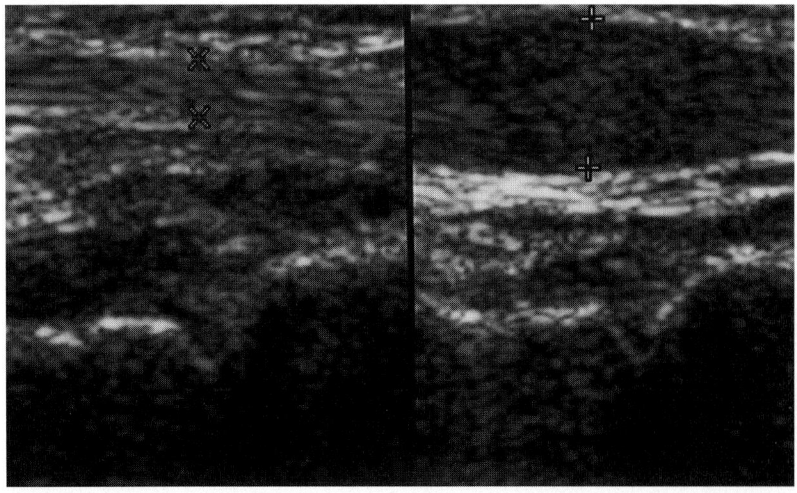

Figure 19–20 ■ Tibialis anterior tendinitis longitudinal sonograms. This 81-year-old woman was involved in a car accident 4 years ago. At that time, she needed pelvic surgery because of extensive retroperitoneal bleeding. Sciatic nerve injury complicated the postoperative period and the patient's gait altered, resulting in persistent ankle complaints. Longitudinal scanning with split-screen comparison shows an enlarged, hypoechoic, symptomatic anterior tibial tendon measuring 57 mm (*right image*) compared with the asymptomatic tendon (*left image*), which measures 22 mm. The anteroposterior dimension of the tendons is noted between callipers. Findings are consistent with tendinosis. Clinically, the patient had difficulty with dorsiflexion, and Achilles pathology was suspected. The study showing anterior tibial tendon pathology allowed more effective treatment by precise local injection.

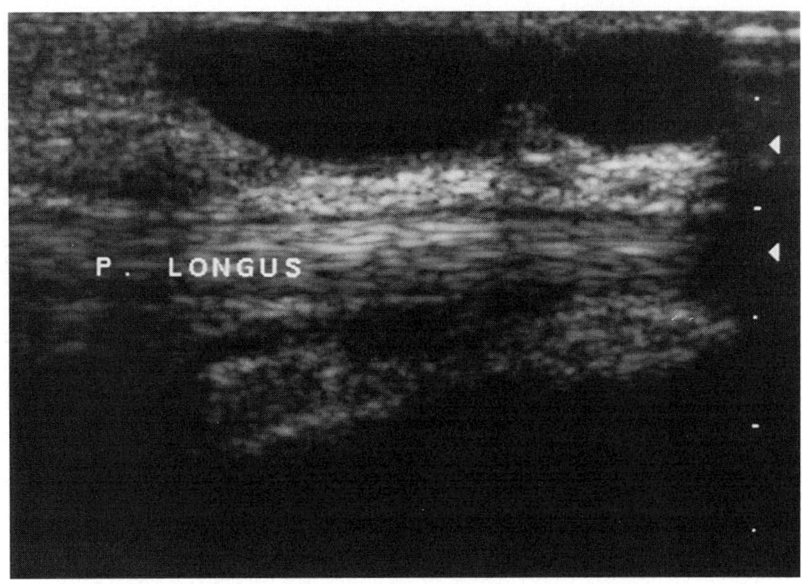

Figure 19–21 ▪ Ganglion of the peroneal tendon sheath: longitudinal sonogram. This 53-year-old man developed a swelling over his lateral ankle. The mass grew within a few months. The patient was worried because the mass felt hard and bone-like. The ultrasound image shows a cystic mass superficial to the peroneus longus (*P. LONGUS*). The sharp edge, the septated structure, and the anechoic character are all consistent with a ganglion.

Soft Tissue Masses

Ultrasound is utilized primarily to determine if a soft tissue mass is cystic or solid (Fig. 19–21) and to aid biopsy by localization and real-time imaging of the needle during biopsy (Ceulemans and van Holsbeeck, 1997; Jacobson and van Holsbeeck, 1998). Ultrasound can also determine the size of the mass and its relationship to surrounding structures (e.g., intra- vs. extra-articular) (Ceulemans and van Holsbeeck, 1997). If the mass is not completely anechoic, compressibility of the mass by the transducer and absence of blood flow with Doppler imaging support a cystic etiology (Jacobson and van Holsbeeck, 1998). In most cases, MRI provides superior imaging of soft tissue masses of the foot and ankle. Advantages of MRI include superior soft tissue resolution, bone marrow evaluation, and information regarding perfusion when gadolinum is utilized.

While ultrasound is generally not able to provide a high degree of specificity regarding the benign versus malignant nature of soft tissue masses, some common benign masses do have typical imaging features. A cystic and completely anechoic fluid collection about the ankle commonly represents a ganglion or synovial cyst (Reinherz et al., 1986; Fornage and Rifkin, 1988a, 1988b; Chhem et al., 1993). Ultrasound can be used to demonstrate the cystic nature of the mass, define its extent, and in some cases reveal its origin from a specific tendon sheath or joint. A subcutaneous mass is frequently due to a lipoma (Fig. 19–22). The typical lipoma is parallel to the skin surface, with an elongated shape (Ceulemans and van Holsbeeck, 1997). The echogenicity and internal architecture of lipomas are highly variable. Considerable overlap exists with other benign and malignant masses. MRI can provide further specificity in some cases. A plantar fibroma can appear as a hypoechoic mass along the medial aspect of the plantar fascia. A soft tissue abscess generally has areas of both hypo- and hyperechogenicity. The hypoechoic areas may be due to fluid or necrosis. Doppler evaluation should be included with evaluation of all ankle masses. Doppler assessment especially aids evaluation of vascular masses such as hemangiomas and arteriovenous malformations. The presence of echogenic foci within a mass which correspond to phleboliths on a conventional radiograph confirms the presence of a hemangioma.

Heel Pain

The differential diagnosis of heel pain includes bony and soft tissue pathology. Conventional radiographs, CT, and MRI can be used to assess for bony pathology including fractures, bone spurs, tumors, and bone dysplasia. Ultrasound can assess for foreign bodies (see above), as well as the most common cause of inferior heel pain, plantar fasciitis (Cardinal et al., 1996).

Plantar Fasciitis

Plantar fasciitis is due to inflammation of the fascia and surrounding structures and is seen in athletes,

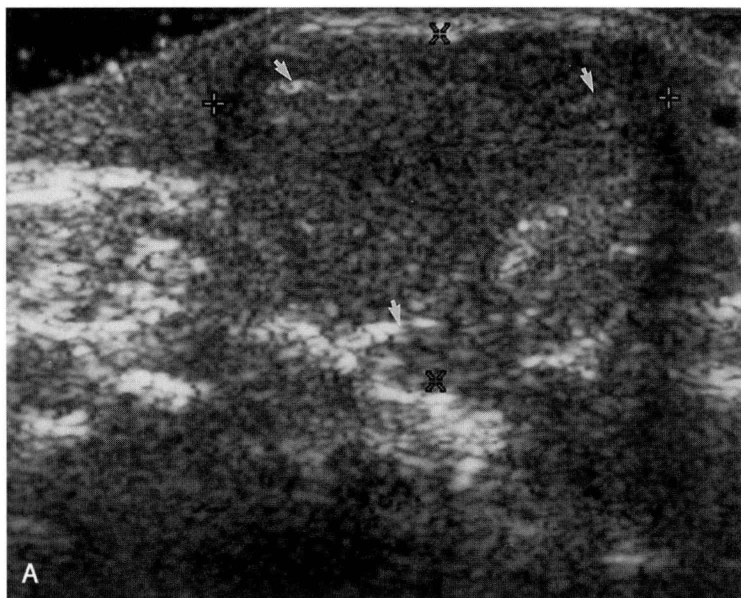

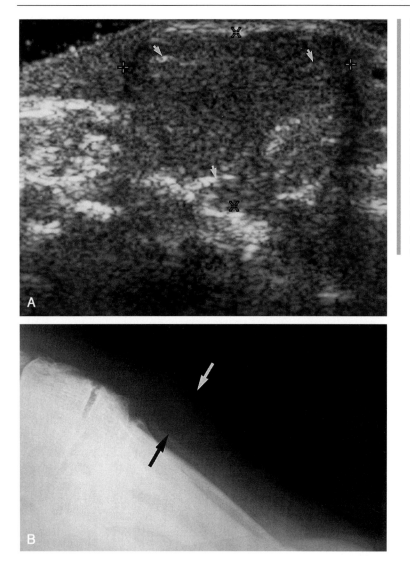

Figure 19–22 ■ **A**, Lipoma of the dorsum of the foot: transverse sonogram. This 36-year-old woman presents with a foot mass that she wants removed as quickly as possible. The mass feels soft, and the surgeon believes it to be a ganglion. An ultrasound scan is performed, with gel cupped over the dorsum of the foot and the transducer positioned across the proximal metatarsals. The mass appears solid and slightly hypoechoic relative to surrounding tissues. It measures 2 × 1.4 cm between the + and × cursors. Linear echogenic foci (*arrows*) are noted within the lipoma. Lipomas can be easily removed, with little scar and nerve damage. Ganglia are more difficult to remove surgically. The ultrasound scan facilitated presurgical planning in this case. **B**, Lipoma of the dorsum of the foot: lateral magnification radiograph. Same patient as in **A**. Lateral magnification radiograph of the foot demonstrating a lucent soft tissue mass (*arrows*) with soft tissue density similar to that of subcutaneous fat. The findings suggest a lipoma.

commonly runners. In addition to trauma, etiologies include mechanical and systemic factors (Resnick, 1995; Jacobson and van Holsbeeck, 1998). Hypoechoic thickening of the fascia greater than 4 mm in the symptomatic patient is consistent with fasciitis, especially when it is asymmetric with the asymptomatic foot (Fig. 19–23) (Cardinal et al., 1996; Gibbon and Long, 1997).

Metatarsalgia

Evaluation of metatarsalgia includes imaging with conventional radiographs to detect bony pathology including fractures and osteochondral injury, avascular necrosis, subluxation/dislocation, osteomyelitis, and arthritis. When conventional radiographs are unrevealing or show widening of a web space, an interdigital neuroma commonly known as *Morton's neuroma* may be considered. Additional causes of metatarsalgia which can be imaged by ultrasound include foreign bodies, ganglion cysts, synovitis, loose bodies, and extensor and flexor tendon pathology.

Morton's Neuroma

Clinical examination is usually sufficient to diagnose Morton's neuroma, defined as a benign mass of perineural fibrosis affecting a plantar interdigital nerve. However, clinical examination may not indicate a specific web space or may suggest more than one etiology for metatarsalgia (Mendicino and Rockett, 1997; Zanetti et al., 1997a). Ultrasound imaging can enhance the likelihood of successful

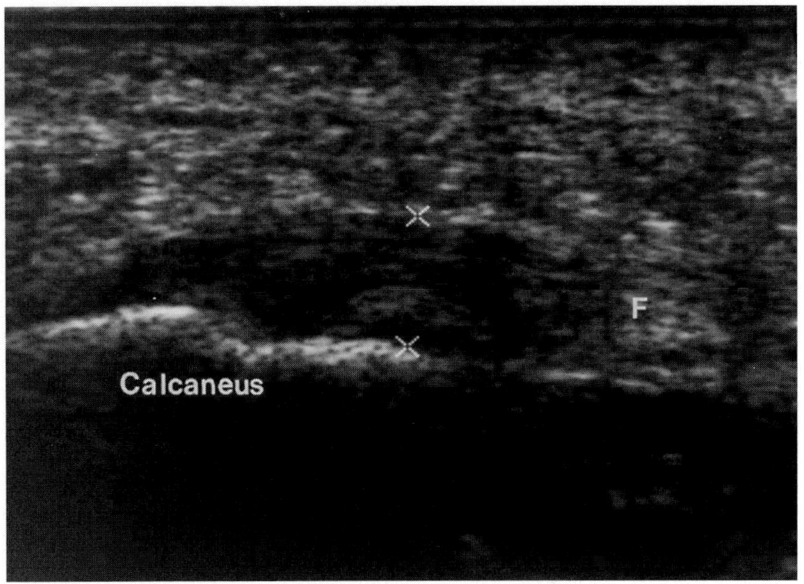

Figure 19–23 ■ Plantar fasciitis: longitudinal ultrasound. Persistent heel pain continued to plague this 36-year-old woman for months. The proximal plantar fascia appears hypoechoic and thickened and measures 5.2 mm. Compare it with the more normal fascia on the right of the image (*F*). After conservative treatment failed, the patient was treated with surgery. The swollen segment of the fascia is identified with callipers.

surgery by confirmation and localization of the neuroma and prevention of a delay in definitive surgical treatment (Redd et al., 1989). Numerous etiologies for Morton's neuroma have been proposed. The most common etiology involves mechanical compression or repetitive trauma which may be due to the use of high-heeled shoes (Sobiesk et al., 1997; Zanetti et al., 1997b). Presenting symptoms are pain and paresthesias with walking. Manual compression of the affected web space elicits exquisite tenderness (Sobiesk et al., 1997; Zanetti et al., 1997b).

The interdigital nerve, formed by branches of the medial and lateral plantar nerves, courses in the intermetatarsal space deep to the transverse intermetatarsal ligament. The normal interdigital nerve is approximately 2 mm in diameter. It has not typically been imaged with ultrasound (Redd et al., 1989; Kaminsky et al., 1997; Sobiesk et al., 1997). Higher-frequency transducers may allow imaging of the normal nerve. The pulsations of the adjacent artery can often be visualized on gray scale imaging, and the artery and adjacent vein can be visualized with Doppler imaging (Redd et al., 1989; Kaminsky et al., 1997; Sobiesk et al., 1997). In some cases the intermetatarsal bursa, demonstrated as a cystic fluid collection, may be visualized along the dorsal aspect of a neuroma (Shapiro and Shapiro, 1995). Compressibility of the bursa can aid in diagnosis; a neuroma, in contrast, is not compressible. Pressure applied by the transducer is used to elicit the patient's symptoms when Morton's neuroma is suspected. The adjacent and contralateral interspaces can be used as a control when pathology is suspected (Mendicino and Rockett, 1997).

The ultrasound appearance of Morton's neuroma (Fig. 19–24) is typically that of an ovoid, well-defined, hypoechoic mass located in the interspace at or just proximal to the metatarsal heads (Sobiesk et al., 1997). The mass may be hourglass shaped due to compression by the transverse intermetatarsal ligament. The neuroma is usually located at the bifurcation point of the interdigital nerve. In advanced cases, the neuroma grows adherent to the adjacent bursa and the hypoechoic mass appears even larger (Enzinger and Weiss, 1995). Visualization of the nerve entering or exiting the neuroma increases diagnostic confidence. The characteristics of Morton's neuroma are listed in Table 19–3.

Table 19–3
Characteristics of Morton Neuromas

1. Third web space is most common location
2. Bilateral in approximately 10%
3. Multiple in up to 28%
4. When symptomatic: usually middle-aged; approximately 80% female
5. Ultrasound appearance: hypoechoic, well-defined, ovoid mass, usually 5–7 mm in diameter

Source: Pollak et al., 1992; Sobiesk et al., 1997; Redd et al., 1989; Kaminsky et al., 1997.

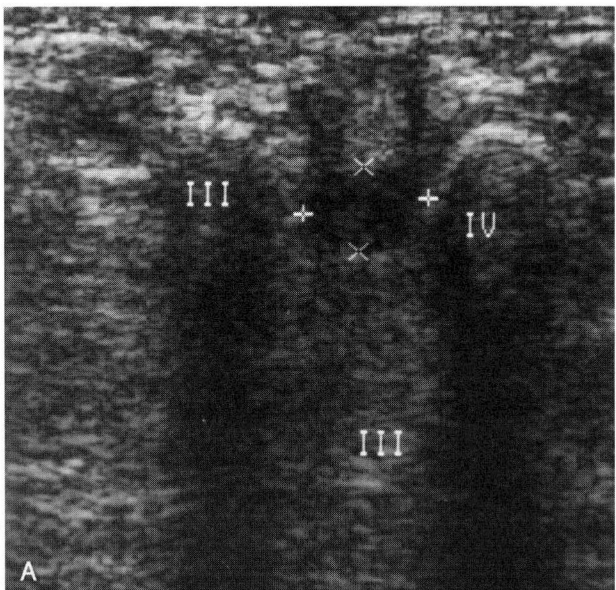

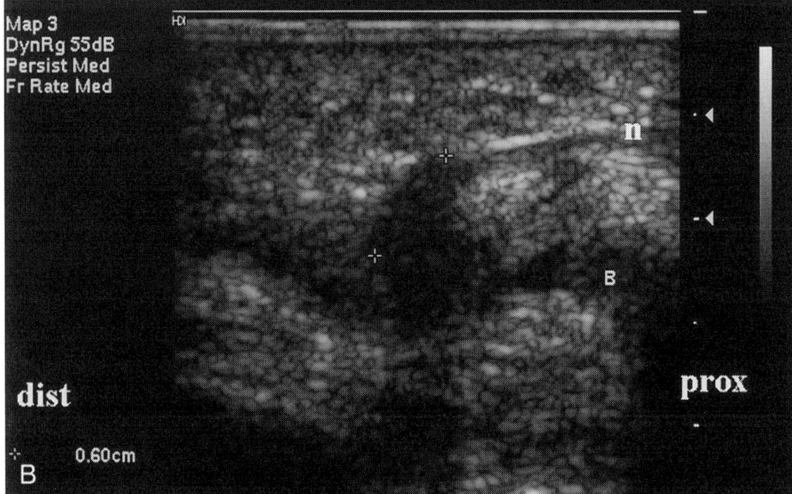

Figure 19-24 ■ **A**, Morton's neuroma: transverse sonogram. A 52-year-old woman complains of persistent pain in her forefoot. The focal pain is accompanied by numbness in her third and fourth toes. While scanning with the transducer positioned transversely over the metatarsal heads, a hypoechoic mass was found. This small mass measuring 5.5 × 3.6 mm was located between the third (*III*) and fourth (*IV*) metatarsals. Surgical resection confirmed a Morton neuroma. (Reprinted with permission from Fessell DP, van Holsbeeck M, *Seminars in Musculoskeletal Radiology* 2:271–281, 1998.) **B**, Morton's neuroma: longitudinal sonogram. Same patient as in **A**. With the transducer aligned along the plantar aspect of the web space and with finger pressure applied along the dorsal aspect of this space, one can observe the normal nerve (*n*) feeding the Morton's neuroma (*between the calipers*). Adjacent hypoechoic tissue dorsal to the nerve represents associated bursal inflammation (*B*). With the palpating finger one can compress the bursal tissue.

Morton's neuromas detected by ultrasound average 5–7 mm in diameter (Redd et al., 1989; Pollak et al., 1992; Kaminsky et al., 1997).

The sensitivity of ultrasound in detecting Morton's neuromas has been reported to be 96–100% (Redd et al., 1989; Sobiesk et al., 1997), with specificity of 83% and accuracy of 95% (Sobiesk et al., 1997). Additional studies have shown that ultrasound has predicted the presence and location of the neuroma in 95–98% of cases (Pollak et al., 1992; Shapiro and Shapiro, 1995). The most accurate data reported by MRI are comparable: sensitivity 87%, specificity 100%, accuracy 89% (Zanetti et al., 1997a). Both MRI and ultrasound studies suggest the diagnosis of Morton's neuroma only when the transverse diameter of the hypoechoic mass equals or exceeds 5 mm in the presence of appropriate clinical findings.

References

Astrom M, et al: Imaging chronic Achilles tendinopathy: A comparison of ultrasonography, magnetic resonance imaging and surgical findings in 27 histologically verified cases. *Skeletal Radiol* 25:615–620, 1996.

Bianchi S: Intraarticular free bodies. Presented at the Seventh Annual Conference on Musculoskeletal Ultrasound, Portofino, Italy, September 1–14, 1997.

Blei CL, Nirschl RP, Grannt EG: Achilles tendon: Ultrasound diagnosis of pathologic conditions. *Radiology* 159:765–767, 1986.

Boruta PM, Beauperthuy GD: Partial tear of the flexor hallucis longus at the knot of Henry: Presentation of three cases. *Foot Ankle Int* 18:243–246, 1997.

Bude RO, et al: Sonographic detection of xanthomas in normal-sized Achilles tendons of individuals with heterozygous familial hypercholesterolemia. *AJR* 170: 621–625, 1998.

Cardinal E, et al: Plantar fasciitis: Sonographic evaluation. *Radiology* 201:257–259, 1996.

Ceulemans R, van Holsbeeck MT: Ultrasonography. In Schepper AM (ed): *Imaging of Soft Tissue Tumors.* Berlin, Heidelberg, Springer-Verlag, 1997, pp 3–18.

Chen YJ, Hsu RW, Liang SC: Degeneration of the accessory navicular synchondrosis presenting as rupture of the posterior tibial tendon. *J Bone Joint Surg* 79A:1791–1798, 1997.

Chen YJ, Liang SC: Diagnostic efficacy of ultrasound in stage I posterior tibial tendon dysfunction: Sonographic–surgical correlation. *J Ultrasound Med* 16: 417–423, 1997.

Cheung Y, et al: Normal anatomy and pathologic conditions of ankle tendons: Current imaging techniques. *Radiographics* 12(3):429–444, 1992.

Chhem RK, et al: Ultrasonography of the ankle and hindfoot. *Can Assoc Radiol J* 44:337–341, 1993.

Church CC: Radiographic diagnosis of acute peroneal tendon dislocation. *AJR* 129:1065–1068, 1977.

Enzinger FM, Weiss SW: *Soft Tissue Tumors,* ed 3. St. Louis, Mosby–Year Book, 1995.

Failla JM, van Holsbeeck MT, Vanderschueren G: Detection of a 0.5 mm-thick thorn using US: A case report. *J Hand Surg [Am]* 20:456–457, 1995.

Fessell DP, et al: Ankle ultrasound: Technique, anatomy and pathology. *Radiographics* 18:325–340, 1998.

Fornage BD: Achilles tendon: Ultrasound examination. *Radiology* 159:759–764, 1986.

Fornage BD, Rifkin MD: Ultrasound examination of tendons. *Radiol Clin North Am* 26:87–107, 1988a.

Fornage BD, Rifkin MD: Ultrasound examination of the hand and foot. *Radiol Clin North Am* 26:109–129, 1988b.

Frankel DA, et al: Synovial joints: Evaluation of intraarticular bodies with US. *Radiology* 206:41–44, 1998.

Freiberger RH, Kaye JJ (eds): *Arthrography.* New York, Appleton-Century-Crofts, 1979, p 239.

Gibbon W, Long G: Plantar fasciitis: Ultrasound evaluation. *Radiology* 203:290, 1997.

Gray H, Clemente CD (eds): *Anatomy of the Human Body,* ed 13. Philadelphia, Lea & Febiger, 1985, pp 577–584.

Jacobson JA, et al: Wooden foreign bodies in soft tissue: Detection at US. *Radiology* 206:45–48, 1998.

Jacobson JA, van Holsbeeck, MT: Musculoskeletal ultrasound. *Orthop Clin North Am* 29:135–167, 1998.

Johnson K: Tibialis posterior tendon rupture. *Clin Orthop* 177:140–147, 1983.

Kaminsky S, Griffin L, Milsap J, et al: Is ultrasonography a reliable way to confirm the diagnosis of Morton's neuroma? *Orthopedics* 20:37–39, 1997.

Khoury NJ, et al: Peroneus longus and brevis tendon tears: MR imaging evaluation. *Radiology* 200:833–841, 1996.

McConkey JP, Favero KJ: Subluxation of the peroneal tendons within the peroneal tendon sheath: A case report. *Am J Sports Med* 15:511–513, 1987.

Mendicino SS, Rockett MS: Morton's neuroma. Update on diagnosis and imaging. *Clin Podiatr Med Surg* 145: 303–311, 1997.

Miller SD, et al: Ultrasound in the diagnosis of posterior tibial tendon pathology. *Foot Ankle Int* 17:555–558, 1996.

Mizel MS, Steinmetz M, Trepman E: Detection of wooden foreign bodies in muscle tissue: Experimental comparison of computed tomography, magnetic resonance imaging and ultrasonography. *Foot Ankle Int* 15: 437–443, 1994.

Nazarian LN, et al: Synovial fluid in the hindfoot and ankle: Detection of amount and distribution with US. *Radiology* 197:275–278, 1995.

Oikarinen KS, et al: Visibility of foreign bodies in soft tissue in plain radiographs, computed tomography, magnetic resonance imaging and US. *Int J Oral Maxillofac Surg* 22:119–124, 1993.

Pollak RA, et al: Sonographic analysis of Morton's neuroma. *J Foot Ankle Surg* 31:534–537, 1992.

Redd RA, et al: Morton neuroma: Sonographic evaluation. *Radiology* 171:415–417, 1989.

Reinherz RP, Zawada SJ, Sheldon DP: Recognizing unusual tendon pathology at the ankle. *J Foot Ankle Surg* 25: 278–283, 1986.

Resch S, et al: The diagnostic efficacy of magnetic resonance imaging in Morton's neuroma. A radiological–surgical correlation. *Foot Ankle Surg* 15:88, 1994.

Resnick D: Internal derangement of joints. In Resnick D (ed): *Diagnosis of Bone and Joint Disorders,* ed 3. Philadelphia, WB Saunders Co, 1995, p 3205.

Rockett MS, et al: The use of ultrasonography for the detection of retained wooden foreign bodies in the foot. *J Foot Ankle Surg* 34:478–484, 1995.

Rosenberg ZS, et al: MR features of longitudinal tears of the peroneus brevis tendon. *AJR* 168:141–147, 1997.

Saltzman CL, Bonar SK: Tendon problems of the foot and ankle. In Lutter LD, Mizel MS, Pfeffer GB (eds): *Orthopaedic Knowledge Update: Foot and Ankle.* Chicago, American Academy of Orthopaedic Surgeons, 1994, pp 269–282.

Sammarco GJ: Peroneal tendon injuries. *Orthop Clin North Am* 25:135–145, 1994.

Scheller AD, Kasser JR, Quigley TB: Tendon injuries about the ankle. *Orthop Clin North Am* 11:801–811, 1980.

Schweitzer ME, et al: Using MR imaging to differentiate peroneal splits from other peroneal disorders. *AJR* 168:129–133, 1997.

Shapiro PP, Shapiro SL: Sonographic evaluation of interdigital neuromas. *Foot Ankle Int* 16:604–606, 1995.

Sobiesk GA, et al: Sonographic evaluation of interdigital neuromas. *J Foot Ankle Surg* 36:364–366, 1997.

Stoller DW: *Magnetic Resonance Imaging in Orthopaedics and Sports Medicine*, ed 2. Philadelphia and New York, Lippincott & Raven, 1997, pp 578–579.

Thermann H, et al: The use of ultrasound in the foot and ankle. *Foot Ankle Surg* 13:386–390, 1992.

van Holsbeeck MT, Introcaso JH: *Musculoskeletal Ultrasound.* St Louis, Mosby–Year Book, 1991, pp 1–327.

van Holsbeeck MT, Powell A: Ankle and foot. In Fornage BD (ed): *Musculoskeletal Ultrasound.* New York, Churchill Livingstone, 1995, pp 221–237.

Vanderschueren G, Fessell DP, van Holsbeeck MT: Ankle ultrasound. In Chhem RK, Cardinal E (eds): *Guidelines and Gamuts in Musculoskeletal Ultrasound.* New York, Wiley, 1998, pp 213–245.

Waitches GM, et al: Ultrasonographic-surgical correlation of ankle tendon tears. *J Ultrasound Med* 17:249–256, 1998.

Zanetti M, et al: Efficacy of MR imaging in patients suspected of having Morton's neuroma. *AJR* 168: 529–532, 1997a.

Zanetti M, et al: Morton neuroma and fluid in the intermetatarsal bursa on MR images of 70 asymptomatic volunteers. *Radiology* 203:516–520, 1997b.

Appendix
Table of Normal Values

Achilles Tendon Measurements

Transverse Image

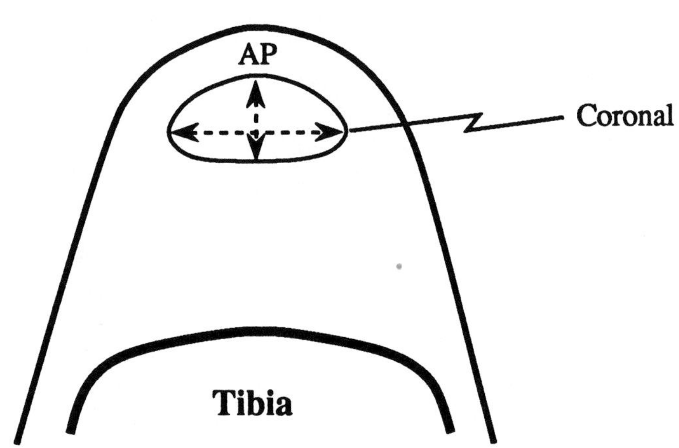

	Sedentary Males (n = 24)	Sedentary Females (n = 21)	Male Athletes (n = 52)	Female Athletes (n = 43)
AP right tendon	6.2 mm (SD ± 0.8)	5.5 mm (SD ± 0.7)	5.7 mm (SD ± 0.8)	5.4 mm (SD ± 0.7)
AP left tendon	6.1 mm (SD ± 0.8)	5.7 mm (SD ± 1.1)	5.9 mm (SD ± 1.0)	5.5 mm (SD ± 0.7)
Coronal right tendon	9.0 mm (SD ± 1.0)	9.2 mm (SD ± 0.9)	13.0 mm (SD ± 2.8)	12.3 mm (SD ± 1.4)
Coronal left tendon	8.8 mm (SD ± 0.8)	8.7 mm (SD ± 1.0)	12.8 mm (SD ± 2.4)	12.3 mm (SD ± 1.5)

Biceps Tendon Measurements

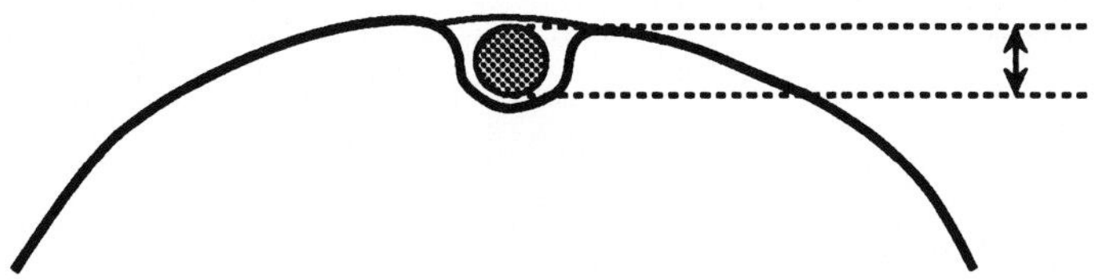

	Sedentary Males (n = 22)	Sedentary Females (n = 21)	Male Athletes (n = 24)	Female Athletes (n = 29)
Biceps, right shoulder	3.2 mm (SD ± 0.5)	2.7 mm (SD ± 0.3)	3.5 mm (SD ± 0.4)	3.0 mm (SD ± 0.3)
Biceps, left shoulder	3.3 mm (SD ± 0.4)	3.0 mm (SD ± 0.3)	3.7 mm (SD ± 0.5)	3.2 mm (SD ± 0.3)

MCL Measurements

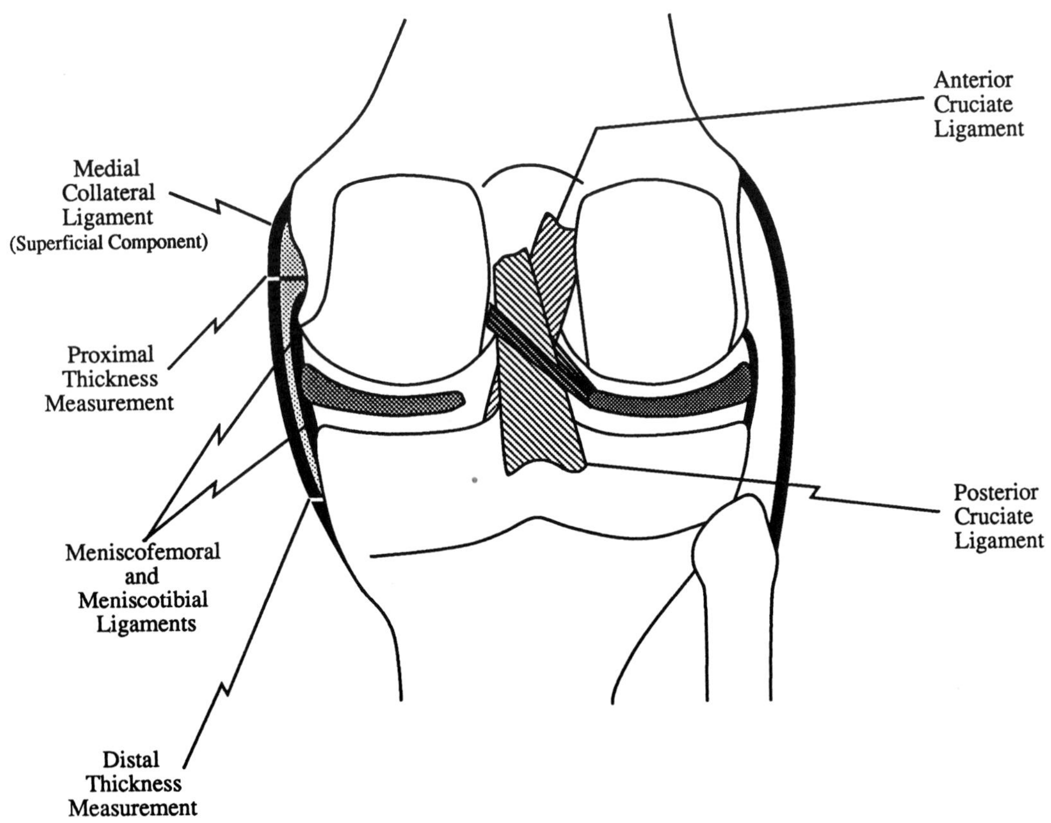

	Sedentary Males (n = 24)	Sedentary Females (n = 21)	Male Athletes (n = 52)	Female Athletes (n = 43)
Right proximal MCL	3.8 mm (SD ± 0.5)	3.6 mm (SD ± 0.7)	3.8 mm (SD ± 0.5)	3.8 mm (SD ± 0.5)
Left proximal MCL	3.7 mm (SD ± 0.6)	3.3 mm (SD ± 0.7)	3.8 mm (SD ± 0.5)	3.6 mm (SD ± 0.5)
Right distal MCL	2.3 mm (SD ± 0.3)	2.3 mm (SD ± 0.4)	2.0 mm (SD ± 0.4)	2.1 mm (SD ± 0.3)
Left distal MCL	2.3 mm (SD ± 0.4)	2.3 mm (SD ± 0.3)	2.0 mm (SD ± 0.4)	2.1 mm (SD ± 0.3)

Quadriceps and Patellar Tendon Measurements

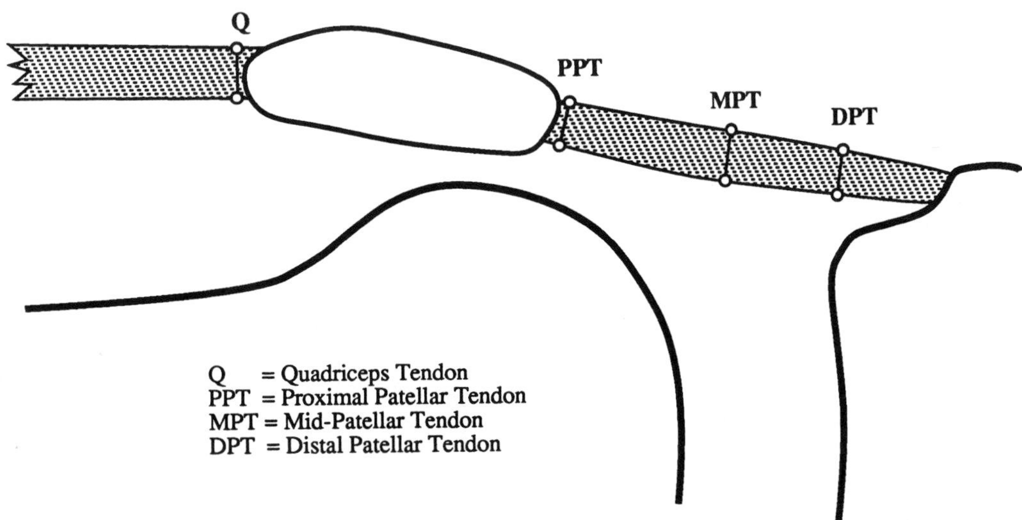

	Sedentary Males (n = 24)	Sedentary Females (n = 21)	Male Athletes (n = 52)	Female Athletes (n = 43)
Right Q	5.1 mm (SD ± 0.6)	4.9 mm (SD ± 0.6)	4.9 mm (SD ± 0.8)	5.1 mm (SD ± 0.7)
Left Q	5.2 mm (SD ± 0.8)	4.8 mm (SD ± 0.5)	5.2 mm (SD ± 0.9)	5.1 mm (SD ± 0.6)
Right PPT	3.0 mm (SD ± 0.4)	2.6 mm (SD ± 0.4)	3.4 mm (SD ± 0.9)	3.3 mm (SD ± 0.8)
Left PPT	3.1 mm (SD ± 0.3)	2.7 mm (SD ± 0.4)	3.5 mm (SD ± 0.7)	3.1 mm (SD ± 0.4)
Right MPT	3.1 mm (SD ± 0.4)	2.9 mm (SD ± 0.5)	3.6 mm (SD ± 0.7)	3.3 mm (SD ± 0.8)
Left MPT	3.2 mm (SD ± 0.4)	2.9 mm (SD ± 0.3)	3.5 mm (SD ± 0.6)	3.1 mm (SD ± 0.4)
Right DPT	3.1 mm (SD ± 0.4)	2.6 mm (SD ± 0.4)	3.4 mm (SD ± 0.9)	3.3 mm (SD ± 0.8)
Left DPT	3.1 mm (SD ± 0.4)	2.7 mm (SD ± 0.4)	3.5 mm (SD ± 0.7)	3.1 mm (SD ± 0.4)

Suprapatellar Bursa Measurements

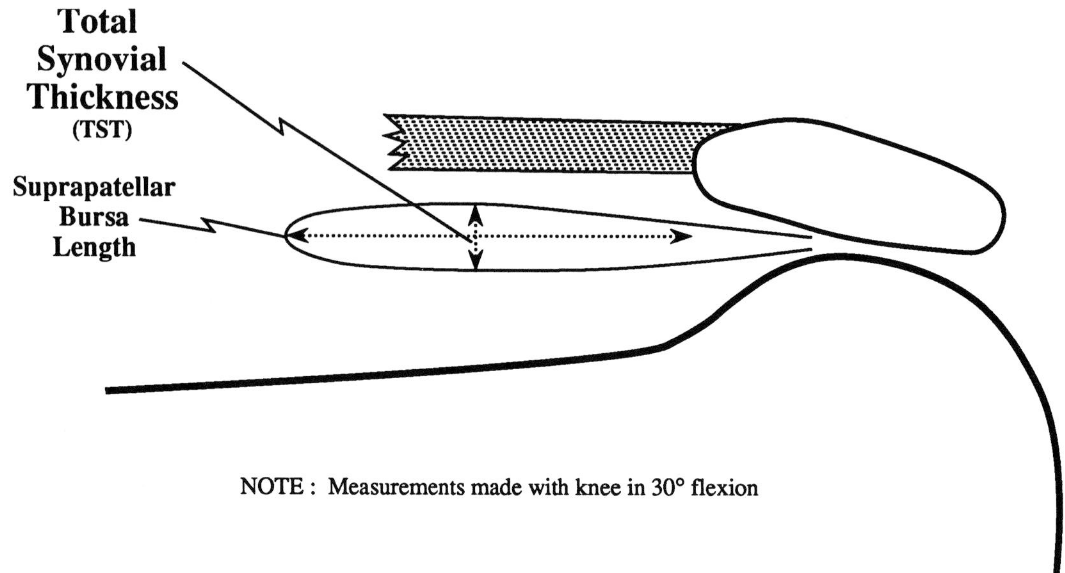

	Sedentary Males (n = 24)	Sedentary Females (n = 21)	Male Athletes (n = 52)	Female Athletes (n = 43)
TST, right knee	2.5 mm (SD ± 0.5)	2.3 mm (SD ± 0.5)	2.5 mm (SD ± 0.7)	2.3 mm (SD ± 0.6)
TST, left knee	2.5 mm (SD ± 0.4)	2.3 mm (SD ± 0.5)	2.6 mm (SD ± 0.6)	2.2 mm (SD ± 0.6)
Bursa length, right	22.3 mm (SD ± 3.8)	21.2 mm (SD ± 4.3)	21.2 mm (SD ± 4.2)	19.5 mm (SD ± 5.0)
Bursa length, left	21.8 mm (SD ± 4.2)	20.6 mm (SD ± 5.3)	23.9 mm (SD ± 4.8)	20.8 mm (SD ± 4.9)

Index

Note: Page numbers in *italics* indicate figures; those followed by t indicate tables; those followed by b indicate boxed material.

Abdominal musculature, rupture of, *36, 37*
Abscess, aspiration of, 431–432
  due to pyogenic myositis, 47–52
  hardware-related, 409, *411–412*
  of hip, 577–578
  periosteal, 333–336, *335*
  subcutaneous, 329–330
    in diabetic, *568*
Absorption, 5
Acetabular labrum, tears of, 585, *585*
Acetabulum, development of, 282–285, *284,* 284t, *285*
Achilles tendon, frictional bursitis of, *139, 140*
  insertion of, 81, *82*
  insertion tendinopathy of, 113
  refractile shadowing of, *11*
  rupture of, 117–126, *120–126*
    acute, 608
    chronic, 122–126, *125, 126,* 616–617
    complete, *121–123, 227,* 608, *608*
    differential diagnosis of, 608–609
    healing, 122, *124*
    musculotendinous, 198, *198*
    partial, *226*
    plantaris tendon in, 608, *609*
    re-, *125*
  sonographic anatomy of, *81,* 607
  tendinitis of, *101,* 112–113, *223*
    calcifying, *105*
    differential diagnosis of, 112–113, *113–115*
    distal, *110,* 112
    peri-, *111,* 112, *112*
    proximal, *108, 109,* 112
  tendinosis of, *101,* 221–223, *223,* 617, *617*
    distal, *110,* 112
    proximal, *108, 109,* 112
    with hypercholesterolemia, 112, *113–114*
ACL (anterior cruciate ligament), *178*
  disruption of, 595
  sonographic examination of, 588
Acoustic impedance, 1, 2t
Acromioclavicular joint, degenerative changes within, 490
  inflammation of, 467–468, *468,* 490
  pseudoganglion of, 488, *489*
  septic arthritis of, 490–491, *491*
  sonography of, 467–468, *468,* 490–491
  sprains of, 490
Acromioplasty, 496
Adductor magnus muscle, pyomyositis of, *52*
Adductor muscles, strain of, 580, *580*
Adhesive capsulitis, 155, *160,* 504–505, *505*
  brisement procedure for, 446
  joint fluid in, 473, *474*
Adolescent(s), knee of, *238*
  tendon injuries in, 200
Aliasing, 5
Alpha angle, 283, *284,* 284t, *285*
Amyloid arthropathy/amyloidosis, Baker's cyst in, *386*
  carpal tunnel disease in, *545*
  hemodialysis-related, 508–511, *511, 512*
  in rheumatoid arthritis, *390,* 390–391
  of shoulder, *250, 390,* 508–511, *511, 512*
    osteoarticular, *364,* 364–365, *365*
  synovial, *452*
  vs. rheumatoid arthritis, 380
Anesthesia, for core biopsy of bone, 454–459
  for interventional ultrasound, 428
  for synovial biopsy, 449
Aneurysm(s), periarticular, 268–271, 268b, *269, 270*
  popliteal, 268b, *269, 270,* 590, *591*
  poststenotic, 268
Aneurysm(s) (*Continued*)
  pseudo-, arterial, after arthroscopy, 424
    of hand, *541*
Angiomatosis, intramuscular, *368*
Angle of incidence, 1–2, *2*
Anisotropic reflectors, *16–19,* 17–18
Anisotropy, of rotator cuff, 202–203, *207*
Ankle, 605–622
  acute injuries of, 607–611
  anterior joint of, 605
  chronic pain of, 611–618
    joint and anterior, 617–618, *618*
    lateral, 612–614, *613, 614*
    medial, 614–616, *615–617*
    posterior, 616–617, *617*
  effusion of, *445*
    in children, *298*
  fluid in, 605, 606, 606t, *607*
  foreign bodies in, 611, *612*
  ganglion of, 619, *619*
    mirror image artifact of, *16*
  joint pathology of, *610,* 610–611, *611*
  ligamentous injuries of, 177–180, *179–181,* 180b, 609–610, *610*
  loose bodies in, 617–618, *618*
  retrocalcaneal bursa of, 607
  septic arthritis of, *443*
  soft tissue masses of, 619, *619*
  synovitis of, 618
    pigmented villonodular, *610*
  technical guidelines and scanning technique for, 605–607, 606t
  tendons of, Achilles. See *Achilles tendon.*
    extensor, 605, 618
    lateral, 605–606
    medial, 606, *607*

Ankle (*Continued*)
tenosynovitis of, *388, 612*
postsurgical, *612*
septic, 611, *611*
Ankle sprain, high, 179
of deltoid ligament, 180
of fibulocalcaneal ligament, 177
of fibulotalar ligament, 177, *179*
of tibiofibular ligament, 177–179, *180, 181*
Annular arrays, *3,* 3–4
Anterior cruciate ligament (ACL), *178*
disruption of, 595
sonographic examination of, 588
Anterior fibulotalar ligament, normal, *179*
rupture of, 177, *179*
Anterior tibial compartment syndrome, 55–56, *55–57*
Anterior tibial muscle, hernia of, *64, 66*
Anterior tibial tendon, anisotropy of, *18*
Anterior tibiofibular ligament, sprain of, 177–179, *180, 181*
Anterior tibiotalar impingement, *181*
Anus, imperforate, *312,* 315
Aponeurosis, *27*
Apophyseal avulsion, of hamstring, 578–579
Arterial pseudoaneurysm, after arthroscopy, 424
Arteriovenous fistulas, 271
Arthritis, gonococcal, *442*
Lyme, *436*
psoriatic, 380
reactive, *447*
rheumatoid. See *Rheumatoid arthritis.*
septic. See *Septic arthritis.*
synovial biopsy for, 446–453, *447–452*
thorn-induced, 402, *402*
Arthrography, of shoulder, 513
Arthropathy, amyloid, Baker's cyst in, *386*
carpal tunnel disease in, *545*
hemodialysis-related, 508–511, *511, 512*
in rheumatoid arthritis, *390,* 390–391
of shoulder, *250, 390*
osteoarticular, *364,* 364–365, *365*
synovial, *452*
vs. rheumatoid arthritis, 380
inflammatory, Baker's cysts due to, 162–165, *163–165*
of knee, 594
sonographic aspiration for, *441*
rotator cuff, 487–488, *488, 489,* 506
Arthroscopy, complication rate for, 419, *420*
diagnostic, pain syndromes after, 425–426
instrument breakage during, *394,* 424
pain syndromes after, 419–426
Arthroscopy (*Continued*)
sites of, 419, 420t
therapeutic, pain syndromes after, 419–425, *421–425*
portals for, 419, *420*
Articular cartilage. See *Cartilage.*
Articular masses, *363–365,* 363–367
Articular recesses, in rheumatoid arthritis, 378, 379t
Artifact(s), 9–21
anisotropic reflectors as, *16–19,* 17–18
beam width, 20, *20*
comet tail, 12–14, *14, 15,* 395, *397, 399*
electrical noise, 21, *21*
enhanced through-transmission as, 10–12, *13, 14*
frame buffer dropout as, 21
mirror image, *16,* 17
motion, 21
refraction, 15, *15*
reverberation, 15–17, *16*
shadowing as, 9–10, *10–13*
speed of sound, 18–20, *20*
vs. rotator cuff tear, 203, *208*
Aspiration, double-needle, 434, *435*
of hip, *445, 446,* 575, *575,* 575t
of joints, *381,* 381–382, *408,* 409, 434–442, *436–446*
of soft tissue, 428–438, *429*
with abscess and phlegmon, 431–432
with calcium deposits, *429,* 432, *433–434,* 490
with cellulitis, 434, *435*
with hematoma, 428–431, *430, 431*
with seroma, 431, *432*
Attenuation, 5
Avulsion. See also *Rupture.*
muscle-aponeurosis, 61–64, *62, 63*
of scapholunate ligament, 551, *564*
Avulsion fractures, of greater tuberosity, 490, 491, *492*
of lateral malleolus, 613, *613*
of medial retinaculum, *595,* 596
Axial resolution, 5

Baker's cyst(s), 160–167, *161–168,* 589, 590
anatomical parts of, *161,* 162
aspiration of, *437*
benign synovioma within, *165,* 167
differential diagnosis of, 165–167
due to increased intra-articular fluid, *161,* 162
due to inflammatory arthropathy, 162–165, *163–165*
formation of, 153, 159, 160–162, *161, 162*
in amyloid arthropathy, *386*
in child, *166, 597*
infected, *152*
loose body entrapment in, 167, *167, 168,* 254, *256, 257, 266*
Baker's cyst(s) (*Continued*)
pseudothrombophlebitis due to, 162–165, *164, 165*
refractile shadowing with, *13*
rheumatoid, 162–165, *163–165, 266, 379,* 385, *385, 386*
ruptured, *330, 385*
valve mechanism of, 159, *161*
with medial meniscal tear, *600–601*
with meniscal chondrocalcinosis, *602*
Bankart lesion, 505–506, *508*
Bare area, in rotator cuff tear, *215*
Beam width, 5
Beam width artifact, 20, *20*
Bell clapper sign, 33, *34, 36*
Beta angle, 283, *284,* 284t, *285*
Biceps femoris tendon, superficial, partial rupture of, *33*
Biceps muscle, contusion of, *37*
Biceps tendon, 498–504
anatomy of, 498
bony spurs of, 502, *503*
displacement (dislocation) of, 498–499, 502–504, *503*
function of, 498
longitudinal view of, 465–466, *466*
luxation of, 91–95
normal, *79, 466,* 499
pathology of, 498–504
rupture of, 85–88, *89,* 499–500
distal, 194, *194, 195,* 526–528, *535*
full-thickness, *195, 499, 500,* 502
partial-thickness, *118,* 502, *502*
scanning technique for, *79,* 499
soft tissue restraint of, 498
subluxation of, 498–499, 502
tendonitis of, *501*
tenosynovitis of, 498
transverse imaging of, 465, *466*
Biceps tendon sheath, fluid within, 473, *474,* 500–501, *501*
in amyloid arthropathy, 509–510, *511*
inflammatory distention of, *253*
osteochondral loose bodies in, 501, *501*
Bicipital groove, 498
shallow, 84, *86*
Bicipital tenosynovitis, 498, 500, *501*
Biopsy, core, 453–459
needles for, 428, *429*
of bone lesion, 454–459, *455–457*
of soft tissue mass, 453–454, *454*
synovial, 446–453, *447–452*
Bipennate structure, *26,* 27
Blood flow, to muscles, 29
Bone(s), 337–354
abnormal development of, 354, *354–358,* 355–359
contour defects of, 337–340
core biopsy of, 454–459, *455–457*
needles for, 428, *429*
distraction callus formation on, 348, *348–350*

Bone(s) (*Continued*)
fractures of. See *Fracture(s).*
heterotopic formation of, *vs.* myositis ossificans, 44
Hill-Sachs lesions of, 337–340, 469, *469,* 473, 506, *507*
in children, 348–354, *351–354*
abnormal development of, 354, *354–358,* 355–359
fractures of, *352–354,* 354
in Legg-Calvé-Perthes disease, 349–352, *351*
in rheumatoid arthritis, 337
sonographic examination of, 337
subluxations of, 340, *341, 342*
tumors of, 367
core biopsy of, 454–459, *455–457*
Bony spurs, at long head of biceps tendon, 502, *503*
at tibialis posterior tendon, 614, *616*
Borrelia burgdorferi, in joint fluid, 440
Brisement procedure, 446
Burns, 325, *326*
Bursa(e), 131–168
Achilles tendon, frictional bursitis of, *139, 140*
adventitious, 141, *141, 142*
Baker's cyst of. See *Baker's cyst(s).*
communicating, 153–167, 153b
deep, 131, 133t
examination techniques for, 131, *133*
gastrocnemius-semimembranosus, fluid in. See *Baker's cyst(s).*
iliopsoas, 577, *577*
fluid in, 153, *154, 155*
infrapatellar, bursitis of, *134*
acute, *137*
chronic, *145*
loose body entrapment in, 167, *167, 168*
noncommunicating, 136–153
normal sonographic structure of, 131–136, *132–134*
of hip, *576,* 576–577, *577*
of knee, 593
frictional bursitis of, *140*
olecranon, bursitis of, acute, *138*
chronic, *145*
septic, *152*
prepatellar, 131–134, *133, 134*
bursitis of, *134*
chronic, *143*
hemorrhagic, *146, 147*
septic, *440*
retrocalcaneal, bursitis of, *82, 133*
frictional, *139, 140*
rheumatoid, *151*
vs. Achilles tendinitis, 112–113
with Achilles tendinosis, *110,* 112
distention of, 608
Bursa(e) (*Continued*)
normal, *82*
sonographic examination of, 607
tendinobursitis of, *133*
subacromial-subdeltoid, *132*
arthropathies of, 494–495, *495*
bursitis of, calcific, 146, *148–151*
hemorrhagic, 494
in impingement syndrome, 474–475, *475*
septic, *153*
traumatic, *141*
communicating abnormalities of, 493–494
fluid in, 153, *156–160, 210, 483,* 492–493, *494*
herniation of, 483
impingement in, 155, *159*
in amyloid arthropathy, 510, *512*
infiltrative disorders of, 494–495, *495*
noncommunicating distention of, 494–495, *495*
normal, *472*
pannus in, 155, *158*
sonographic views of, 471–472, *472*
thickening of, 203, *211, 218, 221*
subcutaneous, 131, 133t
suprapatellar, loose bodies in, *256*
sonographic anatomy of, *133, 237, 239,* 587–588
trochanteric, bursitis of, *576,* 576–577
acute frictional, *138, 139*
hemorrhagic, *148*
Bursal calcifications, 490
Bursal fluid, and intra-articular disease, 153–160, *154–157*
gastrocnemius-semimembranosus. See *Baker's cyst(s).*
iliopsoas, 153, *154, 155*
subacromial-subdeltoid, 153, *156–160, 210,* 492–493, *493, 494*
with rotator cuff tear, 203, *209, 493,* 493–494, *494*
Bursitis, 136–153
calcific, 146–152, *148,* 432, *433–434*
chemical, 144–152, *148–151,* 151b
frictional, 136–139, *137–141*
hemorrhagic, 142–144, *146–148, 249,* 494
iliopsoas, 577, *577*
infrapatellar, *134*
acute, *137*
chronic, *145*
of Achilles tendon, frictional, *139, 140*
of distal patellar tendon, *146*
of hip, *576,* 576–577, *577*
of knee, frictional, *140*
of medial collateral ligament, *184,* 185
of medial malleolus, *144*
of olecranon, acute, *138*
Bursitis (*Continued*)
chronic, *145*
septic, *152*
prepatellar, *134*
chronic, *143*
hemorrhagic, *146, 147*
retrocalcaneal, *82, 133*
frictional, *139, 140*
rheumatoid, *151*
vs. Achilles tendinitis, 112–113
with Achilles tendinosis, *110,* 112
rheumatoid, *151,* 152–153, 379, 386
septic, *152,* 152–153, *153,* 495
sites of, 133t
subacromial-subdeltoid, calcific, 146, *148–151*
hemorrhagic, 494
in impingement syndrome, 474–475, *475*
septic, *153*
traumatic, *141*
traumatic, acute, 136–139, *137–141*
chronic, *139,* 139–142, *141–146*
of communicating bursa, 167
trochanteric, *576,* 576–577
acute frictional, *138, 139*
hemorrhagic, *148*

Calcific bursitis, 146–152, *148,* 432, *433–434*
Calcific tendinitis, *97,* 488–490
aspiration of, 432, *433–434,* 490
clinical presentation of, 488–489
natural history of, 488–489
of Achilles tendon, *105*
of elbow, *519*
of supraspinatus tendon, *489*
"slurry," 489, 490
stages of, 489, 490
types of, 489–490
vs. rotator cuff tear, 486, 488
Calcification(s), bursal, 490
in medial collateral ligament, 189–191, *189–191*
in myositis ossificans, 43–44, *49–51*
in rotator cuff tear, 203, *208*
venous thrombus with, *429*
Calcified loose bodies, in Baker's cyst, 167, *168*
Calcium deposits, aspiration of, *429,* 432, *433–434*
Calf, claudication of, 271
painful swelling of, 590–592
Calf muscles, contusion of, *39*
cyst of, *45*
hematoma of, *40*
muscle-aponeurosis avulsion of, 61–64, *62, 63*
rupture of, *40*
healing of, *41, 42*
Callus, distraction, 348, *348–350*
in fracture healing, *344–347,* 344–348

Candida parapsilosis synovitis, 447
Capillary hemangiomas, *367*
Capital femoral epiphysis, slipped, 294–295
Capitellum, osteochondral injury of, 232, *233*
  Panner's disease of, *527–528*
Capsular rupture, 185, *185,* 504–505, *505*
  after arthroscopy, 425, *425*
  of knee, *596,* 598
Capsulitis, adhesive, 155, *160,* 504–505, *505*
    brisement procedure for, 446
    joint fluid in, 473, *474*
Carpal tunnel syndrome (CTS), *387,* 390–391, 531, 533b, 539–541, *542–545*
Cartilage, costal, abnormalities of, 354, *354*
    bifid, *354*
    fracture of, 354, *355*
  diseases of, 252–265, *254–265*
  edema of, 252, *254*
    in rheumatoid arthritis, 376, 379, 380
  fibro-, 251–252
    triangular, sonographic examination of, 567
      tear of, *176,* 551–554
  fractures of, costal, 354, *355*
    of knee, 596
  hyaline, 352
  loose bodies of, 252–254, *255–257*
    in elbow, 517, *523–526*
  of knee, fractures of, 596
  of large synovial joints, diseases of, 252–265, *254–265*
    edema of, 252, *254*
  structure of, 251–252
  triradiate, 282, *284, 286*
Cartilage sign, 207, *221, 222, 485*
Cartilaginous callus, 344
Cauda equina, in child, 306, *309*
  in infant, *302–304,* 303, *306*
CDH (congenital dislocation of the hip). See *Developmental dysplasia of the hip (DDH).*
Cellulitis, 329
  aspiration of, 434, *435*
  of wrist, *570–571*
Central echo complex, 303, *305,* 315–317, *316*
Chemical bursitis, 144–152, *148–151,* 151b
Child(ren), 277–320
  Baker's cyst in, *166, 597*
  bones in, 348–354, *351–354*
    abnormal development of, 354, *354–358,* 355–359
    fractures of, *352–354,* 354
    in Legg-Calvé-Perthes disease, 349–352, *351*
  effusions in, 295–296, *297, 298*
    of hip, 238–243, *241, 242*
Child(ren) (*Continued*)
  epiphyseal alignment in, 292–295, *292–295*
  extremities in, abnormal development of, *354–358,* 355–359
    deformities of, 295, *296*
  fibromatosis colli in, 299, *300*
  fractures in, *352–354*
    occult, 298–299, *299*
  hip in, developmental dysplasia of, 277–292
      background of, 277–279
      coronal view of, *280,* 282–288, *283, 284, 286, 287, 290*
      defined, 278
      diagnosis, 289–291
      etiology of, 277–278
      Graf's classification of, 283, 284t, *285*
      incidence of, 278
      management of, 278–279, 291–292
      neonatal *vs.* true, 290
      screening for, 290, 291
      sonographic examination of, 279–282, *279–283*
      transverse view of, *283, 288,* 288–289, *289*
    effusions of, 238–243, *241, 242*
    normal, *240*
  inflammation in, 295–299, *297–299*
  joint infection in, 295–299, *297–299,* 441, *445*
  knees of, *597, 598,* 599
  Legg-Calvé-Perthes disease in, 349–352, *351*
  osteomyelitis in, 298, *299,* 333
  septic arthritis in, 296, *298*
  spinal canal in, 299–320
    filum terminale of, *317,* 318, *318*
    hydromyelia of, *317,* 318
    masses of, 300, *300, 301*
    meningocele and myelomeningocele of, 318–320, *319, 320*
    normal anatomy of, 301–310, *302–311*
    normal variants of, 315–318, *316, 317*
    sonographic technique for, 301–310, *302–311*
    tethered spinal cord in, 310–315, *312–315*
    use of sonography of, 299–301, *300, 301*
    vertebral anomaly of, 301, *301*
  tendon injuries in, 200
  transient synovitis in, 238–243, *241*
Chlamydia infection, *246*
Chondral defects, 252
Chondrocalcinosis, meniscal, *602*
Chondromalacia, knee effusion in, *379*
Chondromatosis, synovial, 562, *568*
Circumpennate structure, *26,* 27, *27*
Claudication, calf, 271
Clicking, of hip, 581–585, 582t, *583–585*
Climber's finger, 542, *548–549*
Coccyx, neonatal, 309–310, *310*
Collateral ligament(s), lateral, normal, *172*
    rupture of, *172*
  medial, bursitis in, *184,* 185
    calcification of, 189–191, *189–191*
    normal, 172–173, *173*
    rupture of, acute, *173,* 181–185, *182–184*
      after arthroscopy, *425*
      chronic, 187–191, *187–191*
      mechanism of, 227
    sonographic examination of, 588
    thickness of, 184
  of hand, rupture of, 548–551, *561–563*
    sonographic examination of, 569–571
  ulnar, rupture of, 185–187, 227, 549–551, *561*
      acute, *185*
      chronic, 185, *186*
      with Panner's lesion, 521, *529*
      with Stener lesion, 550, *562, 563*
    sonographic evaluation of, 569–571
Color flow Doppler images, 5, 344
Comet tail artifact, 12–14, *14, 15,* 395, *397, 399*
Compartment syndrome, 52–56
  acute, 52–54, *53, 54, 430*
  after arthroscopy, 423
  anterior tibial, 55–56, *55–57*
  chronic, 54–56, *55–57*
Composite image, 24, *24*
Compression injury, intramuscular hematoma after, *40*
  muscle rupture due to, 30, *31*
Congenital dislocation of the hip (CDH). See *Developmental dysplasia of the hip (DDH).*
Congenital myositis ossificans, 44–46
Contusion, muscle, 36–39, *37–40*
Conus medullaris, in child, 306, *309*
  in infant, *302,* 304, *304,* 306, *308*
Coracoacromial arch, 474
Core biopsy, 453–459
  of bone lesion, 454–459, *455–457*
    needles for, 428, *429*
  of soft tissue mass, 453–454, *454*
Corium, 325
Cortical changes, with rotator cuff tear, *216, 217, 220*
Cortical irregularity, of greater tuberosity, 484, *484*

Corticosteroid therapy, intra-articular, destructive changes due to, 391
  loose bodies due to, 266, *268,* 391
  septic arthritis due to, 391
Costal cartilage, abnormalities of, 354, *354*
  bifid, *354*
  fracture of, 354, *355*
Craig bone biopsy set, 459
Cramps, 30
Creeping tendon ruptures, 201
Critical angle shadowing, 9, *10–13*
Critical zone, in rotator cuff tears, *201,* 202–203, *208,* 464, 475
Cruciate ligament(s), anterior, *178*
  disruption of, 595
  sonographic examination of, 588
  posterior, normal, *176, 177, 237*
  sonographic examination of, 589
  tear of, *177, 178, 599*
  reconstruction of, infection after, *410*
Crystal-related synovitis, *155*
CTS (carpal tunnel syndrome), *387,* 390–391, 531, 533b, 539–541, *542–545*
Currarino triad, 315
Curved object, imaging of, 2, *2, 3*
Cyst(s), Baker's (popliteal). See *Baker's cyst(s).*
  epidermoid inclusion, of finger, 561
  filar, *316, 317,* 317–318
  labral, 254–255
  meniscal, 258, 263–264, *264, 593,* 593–594, *594*
  mucoid, of fingers, 555
  muscle, after muscle rupture, 42, *45*
  enhanced through-transmission with, *13*
  of large synovial joints, 254–255, *258–260,* 263–264, *264*
  pilonidal, 310, *310*
  synovial, *385,* 385–386, 385t, *386*
  after arthroscopy, *420,* 421–423, *422, 423*
  of wrist and hand, 537–539, *538, 539–541*

DDH. See *Developmental dysplasia of the hip (DDH).*
De Quervain's tendinitis, 84–85, *86*
Deep venous thrombosis, 271, *272*
  after arthroscopy, 423–424
Degenerative changes, of acromioclavicular joint, 490
  of menisci, 264–265, *265*
  with rotator cuff tear, 203–207, *212–218, 220*
Delamination, in rotator cuff tear, *202,* 202–203, *203*
Delayed muscle soreness, 30
Deltoid ligament, rupture of, 180
Deltoid muscle, herniation of, *482,* 483
Demerol, for soft tissue core biopsy, *449*
Dermal sinus, 310, *311*
Dermis, 325, *326*
Developmental dysplasia of the hip (DDH), 277–292
  background of, 277–279
  coronal view of, *280,* 282–288, *283, 284, 286, 287, 290*
  defined, 278
  diagnosis, 289–291
  etiology of, 277–278
  Graf's classification of, 283, 284t, *285*
  incidence of, 278
  management of, 278–279, 291–292
  neonatal *vs.* true, 290
  screening for, 290, 291
  sonographic examination of, 279–282, *279–283*
  transverse view of, *283, 288,* 288–289, *289*
Diabetic, hand infections in, *568, 569*
  muscle infarct in, *58–59,* 59–60, *61*
  myonecrosis in, *58–59,* 59–60, *61*
  pyomyositis in, *58–59*
Diaphragm, speed of sound artifact of, 18, *20*
Diastematomyelia, *306,* 315
Dimple, sacral cutaneous, 311
Dirty shadowing, 9
Discoid meniscus, *598*
Dislocation, fracture-, of elbow, 293, *293*
  of hip, 294–295
  of shoulder, *292,* 293
  of elbow, 293, *294*
  of extensor tendons, 546–547
  of knee, 294, *294, 295*
  of long head of biceps tendon, 498–499, 502–504, *503*
  of patella, *595,* 596
  of peroneus tendons, 95, 97b, *99, 100*
  of shoulder, 506
  of tendon, 91–95, 97b, *99, 100*
  sternoclavicular, *341*
Distraction callus, 348, *348–350*
Distraction injury, muscle rupture due to, 30–35, *31*
Divergence, of sound beam, 5
Doppler flow imaging, 5–6
  color, 5, 344
Dorsal hood, injuries of, 546–547, *557, 558*
  sonographic examination of, 569
Double-needle aspiration, 434, *435*
Dupuytren fracture, 179
Dupuytren's palmar fibrosis, 562
Dynamic examination, 279
  of shoulder, 472–473
  of wrist and hand, 569

Echo index, *351,* 351–352
ECU. See *Extensor carpi ulnaris (ECU).*
Edema, cartilage, 252, *254*
  in rheumatoid arthritis, 376, 379–380
  muscle, 52, *53*
  of hypodermis, 325–329, *329, 330*
  rotator cuff, 116–117, *119*
  synovial, 248, *250,* 251, *251*
Effusion(s), around prostheses, 407–409, *407–409,* 414
  differential diagnosis of, 380–382
  follow-up of, 243
  in children, 295–296, *297, 298*
  in chondromalacia, *379*
  in Legg-Calvé-Perthes disease, *241,* 243
  in rheumatoid arthritis, 376, *376–378*
  in septic arthritis, 243–248, *244–247*
  in transient synovitis, 238–243, *241*
  in trauma, 248, *248–250*
  of ankle, *445*
  in children, *298*
  of elbow, 517, *520, 522,* 531
  of hip, 238–243, *241, 242,* 573–575
  aspiration of, *445, 446,* 575, *575,* 575t
  differential diagnosis of, 574t
  due to infection, 242–243, 573–575, *575*
  examination technique for, 575
  in children, 295–296, *297*
  in Legg-Calvé-Perthes disease, *242,* 243
  in transient synovitis, 238–243, *241*
  subchondral fracture with, *340*
  with prostheses, 580–581, *581, 582*
  of knee, *239, 240*
  in chondromalacia, *379*
  of shoulder, 507
  reactive, of elbow, *522*
Elbow, 517–531
  dislocation of, 293, *294*
  effusion of, 517, *520, 522,* 531
  epicondylitis of, 517, *518*
  flexor tendons of, *186*
  fracture-dislocation of, 293, *293*
  golfer's, 517
  indications for scanning of, 517–528
  loose bodies in, *257,* 517, *523–526,* 531
  nerves of, 521, *529, 530*
  normal, *519*
  Panner's disease of, 517, *527–528*
  pannus of, *252–253*
  periarticular ganglion of, *520,* 526
  periarticular swelling of, 526
  peripheral nerve tumors of, 521–526, 524b, *532–534*
  reactive inflammatory arthropathy of, *441*
  rheumatoid arthritis of, *378, 521*

Elbow (*Continued*)
synovitis of, *521*
technical guidelines and scanning technique for, 528–531
tendinitis of, 531
calcific, *519*
tendinosis of, 115, 225–227
tennis, 115, 225–227, 517
traumatic neuroma of, 521, *530–531*
ulnar nerve subluxation of, 521, *531*
Electrical noise artifact, 21, *21*
Electrocautery equipment, electrical noise artifact due to, *21*
Elongation injury, of muscle, *31*, 31–32, *32*
"Empty groove" sign, 499–500, *500*
Endometrioma, 325, *328*
Endomysium, 26
Enhanced through-transmission, 10–12, *13, 14*
Epicondylitis, 517, *518*
Epidermis, 325, *326*
Epidermoid inclusion cyst, of finger, 561
Epigastric hernia, *66*
Epimysium, 27
Epiphyseal alignment, 292–295, *292–295*
Epiphyseal fractures, *353–354*, 354
Epiphysis, slipped capital femoral, 294–295
Epitendineum, 81
Epitrochlear lymph node, *360*
Equipment, *3*, 3–4, *4*
Exostoses, hereditary multiple, popliteal aneurysm with, *269*
Extended field of view (FOV) imaging, 6, *24*, 24–25, *25*
Extensor carpi radialis brevis tendon, ganglion of, *538*
Extensor carpi radialis longus tendon, tear of, *555*
Extensor carpi radialis tendon, tendinitis of, 115
Extensor carpi ulnaris (ECU), rupture of, 547–548, *559*
sonographic examination of, 567
tenosynovitis of, *560–561*
Extensor pollicis longus tendon, tear of, *554*
tenosynovitis of, *386, 387*
Extensor tendons, of ankle and foot, 605, 618
of fingers, dislocation of, 546–547
laceration of, 547, *559*
tears of, 546, 547, *554, 556–557*
of wrist, dysfunction of, 544–547, *552–557*
rheumatoid synovitis of, *552–553*
tenosynovitis of, *83, 84, 537, 553*
Extremities, abnormal development of, *355–358*, 355–359
deformities of, 295, *296*
Feet. See *Foot.*
Femoral condyle, osteochondritis dissecans of, *254*
sonographic anatomy of, *237*, 588
Femoral epiphysis, slipped capital, 294–295
Femoral head, displacement of, coronal view of, 285–288, *286, 287*
transverse view of, *288*, 288–289, *289*
Femoral neck, fracture of, *341*
Femur, anteversion of, *356*, 356–357, *357*
osteomyelitis of, *335*
Fibroadipose septa, 26, *27, 28*
contusion of, 36, *37–39*
Fibrocartilage, 251–252
triangular, sonographic examination of, 567
tear of, *176*, 551–554
Fibroma, of tendon sheath, 562, *567*
Fibromatosis, plantar, 73, *73, 359*
Fibromatosis colli, 299, *300*
Fibro-osseous junction, 27
Fibrosarcoma, *362*
Fibrosis, after muscle rupture, 40–42, *43–45*
Fibrous callus, 344
Fibrous histiocytoma, malignant, *369*
Fibula, fracture of, *342*
Fibulocalcaneal ligament, rupture of, 177
Fibulotalar ligament, normal, *179*
rupture of, 177, *179*
Field of view (FOV), 24
extended, 6, *24*, 24–25, *25*
Filar cyst, *316, 317*, 317–318
Filum terminale, *316–318*, 318
Finger(s), climber's, 542, *548–549*
epidermoid inclusion cyst of, 561
extensor tendons of, dislocation of, 546–547
tears of, 546, *554, 556–557*
foreign bodies in, 561, *566*
glomus tumors of, 554–555, *565*
mallet, 546
mucoid cysts of, 555
rheumatoid nodule of, *390*
trigger, 544, *551*
First metatarsal head, adventitious bursa over, 141, *142*
Flexor carpi radialis tendon, anisotropy of, *16*
ganglion of, *542*
tendinosis of, *101*
Flexor digitorum longus tendon, pathology of, 616
Flexor hallucis longus tendon, longitudinal split of, 616
muscle-aponeurosis avulsion of, *62*
tendinitis of, 616
Flexor tendons, of elbow, tear of, *186*
of wrist, anisotropy of, *16*
normal, *546*
tear of, 541–542, *546, 547*
tenosynovitis of, 531, 542, *550*
Fluid collection. See *Effusion(s).*
Foot, 605–622
extensor tendons of, 605, 618
foreign bodies in, 611, *611*
interdigital web spaces of, 607
lipoma of, 620, *620*
plantar fascia of, 607
rheumatoid arthritis of, *377*
soft tissue masses of, 619, *620*
technical guidelines and scanning technique for, 605–607, 606t
vertical talus of, 295, *296*
Foreign body(ies), 393–417
acoustic shadowing with, *10*
diagnostic approach to, *405*, 405–407, *406*
due to instrument breakage, *394*
examination technique for, 393–395, *394*
glass as, 395, *397, 399*
in ankle and foot, 611, *611, 612*
in fingers, 561, *566*
metal, *394*, 395, *398, 400*, 402–405, *404*, 611, *612*
migration of, *404*, 414, *416*
Norplant contraceptive devices as, *405*, 406–407
orthopedic implants as, 407–414
acute complications of, *406–409*, 407–409
chronic complications of, 409–414, *410–416*
infection due to, 409–412, *410–413*, 414
loosening of, 412–414, *414, 415*
soft tissue erosion due to, 414, *416*
plastic, 395, *398, 401*
removal of, 460
secondary signs of, 395
thorns as, 395, *398*, 402, *402, 403*
ultrasound *vs.* radiography of, 395–405, *396–404*
wooden, 395, *396, 399*, 399–402, *403, 611*
Foreign body granulomas, 412–414
Foreign body phantom, *398*
FOV (field of view), 24
extended, 6, *24*, 24–25, *25*
Fracture(s), *340–343*, 340–344
avulsion, of greater tuberosity, 490, 491, *492*
of lateral malleolus, 613, *613*
of medial retinaculum, *595*, 596
cartilage, costal, 354, *355*
of knee, 596
Dupuytren, 179
epiphyseal, *353–354*, 354
femoral neck, *341*
hairline, 336, *336*
healing of, *344–347*, 344–348
in children, *343, 352–354*
occult, 298–299, *299*
metaphyseal corner, of tibia, 299, *299*
neonatal, *343*

Fracture(s) (*Continued*)
occult, 340–344, *342, 343*
in children, 298–299, *299*
of fibula, *342*
of greater tuberosity, 340–342, 491
avulsion, 490, 491, *492*
of lateral malleolus, avulsion, 613, *613*
of medial retinaculum, avulsion, *595,* 596
osteochondral, 232, *233*
Salter-Harris 2, 299, *299*
stress, 336, *337*
subchondral, *340*
tibial, healing of, 344, *344–347*
metaphyseal corner, 299, *299*
stress, *337*
Fracture-dislocation, of elbow, 293, *293*
of hip, 294–295
of shoulder, *292,* 293
Frame buffer dropout, 21
Fraunhofer zone, 4, *4*
Freiberg infraction, of metatarsal head, *343*
Fresnel zone, 4, *4*
Frictional bursitis, 136–139, *137–141*
Frozen shoulder disease, brisement procedure for, 446

Gamekeeper's injury, 227, 229
Ganglion(ia), after arthroscopy, *420,* 421–423, *422, 423*
of acromioclavicular joint, pseudo-, 488, *489*
of ankle, 619, *619*
of elbow, periarticular, *520,* 526
of knee, 593
of peroneal tendon sheath, *619*
of wrist and hand, 537–539, *538, 539–542*
periarticular, of elbow, *520,* 526
pseudo-, of acromioclavicular joint, 488, *489*
scapholunate, 539
snuff box, *437, 538,* 539
suprascapular, 255, *258–260*
Gastrocnemius, cyst of, *45*
hematoma of, *40*
hernia of, *65*
muscle-aponeurosis avulsion of, 61–63, *62*
rupture of, *40, 194*
healing of, *41, 42*
vs. Achilles tendon tears, 609
Gastrocnemius-semimembranosus bursa, fluid in. See *Baker's cyst(s).*
Gelosis, in myositis ossificans, 43, *47, 48*
Geremia needle, 459
Geyser sign, 488, *489*
Giant cell tumor, of tendon sheath, 562, *566*
Glass, as foreign body, 395, *397, 399*
comet tail artifact due to, 12–14, *14*
Glenohumeral joint, joint fluid in, 473–474
translation of, 506
Glenoid labrum, anterior, Bankart lesion of, 506, *508*
detached, 506, *509*
sonography of, 473, *473*
posterior, sonography of, *468,* 468–469, *469*
superior, sonography of, 473
Glomus tumors, 325, 554–555, *565*
Gluteus muscle, healing of rupture of, *44*
Golfer's elbow, 517
Gonococcal arthritis, *442*
Gonococcal synovitis, *244–245*
Gout, aspiration of, *438*
uric acid-related synovitis in, 495
Graf's classification, of developmental dysplasia of the hip, 283, 284t, *285*
Granulomas, foreign body, 412–414
reparative, of synovium, *448–449*
Gray scale images, 4–5, 344
Greater trochanteric bursae, bursitis of, *576,* 576–577
acute frictional, *138, 139*
hemorrhagic, *148*
Greater tuberosity, cortical irregularity of, 484, *484*
fractures of, 340–342, 491
avulsion, 490, 491, *492*
in rotator cuff tear, 203, *212–215, 218*

Haglund's disease, 112, *115*
Hairline fracture, 336, *336*
Hamartoma, *368*
Hamstring tendon, 578–580
apophyseal avulsion of, 578–579
rupture of, full-thickness, 579
healing of, *43*
partial-thickness, *33, 34,* 579
site of injury of, 578–579
strain of, 579
tendinitis/tendinosis of, *579,* 579–580
Hand, 531–571
collateral ligaments of, tears of, 548–551, *561–563*
dynamic imaging of, 569
ganglia of, 537–539, *538, 539–542*
indications for scanning of, 531–564
infections of, 562, *568–571*
pseudoaneurysm of, *541*
technical guidelines and scanning techniques for, 564–571
tenosynovitis of, 531, *537*
Heel pain, 619–620, *621*
Hemangiomas, 367, *367, 368*
Hemangiopericytoma, *300*
Hemarthrosis, after arthroscopy, *424,* 424–425
of knee, *248,* 594–596
Hematoma(s), aspiration of, 428–431, *430, 431*
of hip, 577–578, *578*
of muscle, 35–39, *37–40*
postoperative, *406,* 407–409
subcutaneous, 330, *330*
subperiosteal, *332–333, 338–339*
superficial *vs.* deep, 409
Hemodialysis-related amyloid arthropathy, 508–511, *511, 512*
Hemorrhage, subcutaneous, *330*
subperiosteal, *332–333, 338–339*
Hemorrhagic bursitis, 142–144, *146–148, 249,* 494
Hereditary multiple exostoses, popliteal aneurysm with, *269*
Herniation, muscle, 64–67, *64–68*
anterior tibial, *64, 66*
deltoid, *482,* 483
epigastric, *66*
gastrocnemius, *65*
tibialis anterior, *64, 66*
of subacromial-subdeltoid bursa, 483
Spigelian, 66, *67, 68*
Heterotopic bone formation, *vs.* myositis ossificans, 44
Hill-Sachs deformity, 337–340, 469, *469,* 473, 506, *507*
Hip, 573–585
abscesses of, 577–578
adductor strain of, 580, *580*
bursitis of, *576,* 576–577, *577*
coronal view of, 279, *279–281,* 282–288, *283–287,* 284t
developmental dysplasia of, 277–292
background of, 277–279
coronal view of, *280,* 282–288, *283, 284, 286, 287, 290*
defined, 278
diagnosis, 289–291
etiology of, 277–278
Graf's classification of, 283, 284t, *285*
incidence of, 278
management of, 278–279, 291–292
neonatal *vs.* true, 290
screening for, 290, 291
sonographic examination of, 279–282, *279–283*
transverse view of, *283, 288,* 288–289, *289*
effusions of, 573–575
aspiration of, *445, 446,* 575, *575,* 575t
differential diagnosis of, 575t
due to infection, 242–243, 573–575, *575*
examination technique for, 575
in children, 295–296, *297*
in Legg-Calvé-Perthes disease, *242,* 243
in transient synovitis, 238–243, *241*

Hip (*Continued*)
subchondral fracture with, *340*
with prostheses, 580–581, *581, 582*
examination technique for, 235–236, *236,* 573
hamstring injury of, 578–580, *579*
hematomas of, 577–578, *578*
iliopsoas strain of, 580, *581*
imaging options for, 574t
in Legg-Calvé-Perthes disease, 349–352, *351*
indications for ultrasound of, 574t
meralgia paresthetica of, *584,* 585
of child, *240*
pain in, 573–580
due to abscesses, hematomas, and seromas, 577–578, *578, 579*
due to bursitis, *576,* 576–577, *577*
due to joint effusion, 573–575, 574t, *575,* 575t
due to muscle and tendon pathology, 578–580, *579–581*
due to synovitis, 576
pyomyositis of, 577–578
rheumatoid arthritis of, *377*
septic arthritis of, 243, *247*
seromas of, 578, *579*
slipped capital femoral epiphysis of, 294–295
snaps, locks, and clicks of, 581–585, 582t, *583–585*
sonographic anatomy of, 236–238, *240–242*
synovitis of, 576
transverse view of, 279, *280–283, 288,* 288–289, *289*
Hip prostheses, 580–581
hyperemia with, 414, *415*
incisional drainage with, 581
infected, 409, *412, 413, 443*
joint effusions with, 580–581, *581, 582*
loosening of, *581*
normal, *442*
Histiocytoma, malignant fibrous, *369*
Histological examination, of synovial fluid, 453
Hoffa's fat pad, after arthroscopy, 419–421, *421,* 423, *423*
Hookwire localization, presurgical, *458–459,* 459–460
Horizontal resolution, 5
Humeral head, erosion of, *377*
retroversion of, *355,* 355–356, *356*
subluxation of, 480, *480,* 488
Humerus, fracture-dislocation of, *292,* 293, *293*
neonatal fracture of, *343*
osteomyelitis of, *334*
Hyaline cartilage, 352
Hydromyelia, *316, 317,* 318
Hydroxyapatite synovitis, *149–151,* 151
Hypercholesterolemia, tendinosis with, 112, *113–114*
Hyperemia, in prosthetic hip replacement, 414, *415*
synovial, 135–136, *135–136*
Hypervascularity, with rotator cuff tear, 206, *216*
Hypodermis, edema of, 325–329, *329, 330*
melanoma in, 325, *327*
normal, 325, *326*
pathology of, 325–333, *327–331*

Iliac line, 282, *284, 285*
Iliofemoral ligament, *240*
Iliopsoas bursa, 577, *577*
fluid in, 153, *154, 155*
Iliopsoas muscle, contusion of, *38*
strain of, 580, *581*
Iliopsoas tendon, snapping, 582, *583*
tendinitis of, 585
Iliotibial band friction syndrome, *69–71, 71, 72*
frictional bursitis in, *142*
Ilizarov external fixation, distraction callus with, 348, *348–350*
Image(s), color flow Doppler, 5–6, 344
gray scale, 4–5, 344
Imaging, 4–5
Doppler flow, 5–6, 344
extended field of view, *6, 24,* 24–25, *25*
of curved object, 2, *2, 3*
pulse-echo, 1
Siescape, *24,* 24–25, *25*
tissue harmonic, 6, *6*
transmission, 6–7
Imperforate anus, *312,* 315
Impingement, 474–476
by osteophyte, *503*
defined, 464
conventional radiography of, *464*
stages of, 116–117, 465, 474–476
subacromial, 155, *159,* 476, 494
subacromial-subdeltoid bursitis in, 474–475, *475*
with rotator cuff edema, 116, *119*
Incisional drainage, with hip prostheses, 581
Increased through-transmission, 10–12, *13, 14*
Infants. See *Child(ren).*
Infarction, muscle, 54, *54*
diabetic, *58–59,* 59–60, *61*
Infection(s), of hand, 562, *568–571*
of hip, 242–243, 573–575, *575*
of joint, 243–248, 243b, *244–247*
due to intra-articular steroid injections, 391
due to orthopedic implants, 409–412, *410–413,* 414
in children, 295–299, *297–299,* 441, *445*
in rheumatoid arthritis, 382–385, *384*
vs. rheumatoid arthritis, 380–381
of vascular graft, *401*
Inflammation, in children, 295–299, *297–299*
of acromioclavicular joint, 467–468, *468,* 490
Inflammatory arthropathy, Baker's cysts due to, 162–165, *163–165*
of knee, 594
sonographic aspiration for, *441*
Infrapatellar bursa, bursitis of, *134*
acute, *137*
chronic, *145*
Infraspinatus fossa, suprascapular ganglion of, *258, 260*
Infraspinatus muscle, sonography of, *468,* 468–469, *469*
Infraspinatus tendon, sonography of, 469
tears of, 465
Injection, intra-articular steroid, destructive changes due to, 391
loose bodies due to, 266, *268,* 391
septic arthritis due to, 391
of joints and soft tissue, 442–446
Insertion tendinopathy, Achilles, 113
of patellar tendon, *108,* 111–112
Instability, of shoulder, 473, *473,* 505–506, *507–509*
Instrument breakage, during arthroscopy, *394,* 424
Interdigital nerve, 621
Interdigital web spaces, sonographic examination of, 607
Internal oblique muscle, rupture of, *36*
Interventional ultrasound, 427–460
examination technique for, 427–428, *429*
for aspiration of joint, 434–442, *436–446*
for aspiration of soft tissue, 428–438, *429*
with abscess and phlegmon, 431–432
with calcium deposits, *429,* 432, *433–434*
with cellulitis, 434, *435*
with hematoma, 428–431, *430, 431*
with seroma, 431, *432*
for core biopsy, 453–459
of bone lesion, 454–459, *455–457*
of soft tissue mass, 453–454, *454*
for image guided surgery, 460
for injection of joints and soft tissue, 442–446
for presurgical hookwire localization, *458–459,* 459–460
for synovial biopsy, 446–453, *447–452*
Intra-articular debris. See *Loose bodies.*
Intra-articular disease, 238
bursal fluid and, 153–160, *154–157*
ultrasound evaluation of, 235

Intra-articular steroid therapy, destructive changes due to, 391
loose bodies due to, 266, *268,* 391
septic arthritis due to, 391
Ischemia, muscle, 52, 55

Joint(s), aspiration of, *381,* 381–382, *408,* 409, 434–442, *436–446*
effusions of. See *Effusion(s).*
injection of, 442–446
large synovial. See *Large synovial joints.*
Joint fluid, aspirated, 438–439
in adhesive capsulitis, 473, *474*
in ankle, 605, 606, 606t, *607*
in shoulder, 473–474, *474,* 500–501, *501*
infectious organisms in, 439, 440, *442*
Jumper's knee, 97–112
differential diagnosis of, *108,* 110–112
focal thickening in, *106,* 107, *107*
global thickening in, *107,* 107–110
pathologic changes in, 97–110, *100, 102–104*
Juvenile rheumatoid arthritis, *446*

Knee, 587–602
acute injury of, 594–598, *595*
anterior aspect of, 587–588
arthroscopy of, pain syndromes after, *420–425*
Baker's cyst of. See *Baker's cyst(s).*
bursae of, 593
bursitis of, frictional, *140*
hemorrhagic, *249*
capsular tear of, *596,* 598
cartilage edema of, *254*
cartilage fractures of, 596
chronic localized pain of, *596,* 598–599
dislocation of, 294, *294, 295*
effusion of, *239, 240*
in chondromalacia, *379*
examination technique for, 235–236, *236*
ganglia of, 593
hemarthrosis of, *248,* 594–596
inflammatory arthropathy of, 594
internal derangement of, *597–602,* 599–601
jumper's, 97–112
differential diagnosis of, *108,* 110–112
focal thickening in, *106,* 107, *107*
global thickening in, *107,* 107–110
pathologic changes in, 97–110, *100, 102–104*
lateral aspect of, 588–589
ligaments of, *184*
collateral. See *Collateral ligament(s).*
Knee (*Continued*)
meniscofemoral, 172
meniscotibial, 172
longitudinal view of, 589
loose bodies in, *255–257,* 599–601
medial aspect of, 588
medial retinaculum of, tear of, 185, *185*
of adolescent, *238*
of child, *597, 598,* 599
osteochondritis dissecans of, *254*
posterior aspect of, 589
postoperative, 600, *602*
rheumatoid arthritis of, *251, 379, 380, 383*
runner's, 69–71, *71, 72*
septic arthritis of, 243
sonographic anatomy of, 236–238, *237–240*
summary of routine examination of, 590, 590t
swelling of, 590–594, *591–594*
technical guidelines and scanning technique for, 587–590
tendon injuries of, 597–598
transverse view of, 589–590
tumors of, 593
Knee prostheses, 601, *602*
"Knuckle injury," 547–548, 547b

Labral cysts, 254–255
Labral tear, 255, *260*
Labrum, acetabular, tears of, 585, *585*
glenoid, anterior, Bankart lesion of, 506, *508*
detached, 506, *509*
sonography of, 473, *473*
posterior, sonography of, *468,* 468–469, *469*
superior, sonography of, 473
Laceration, of extensor tendons, 547, *559*
Laminae, in infant, 304, *308*
Large synovial joints, 235–275
aneurysms of, 268–271, 268b, *269, 270*
cartilage of, diseases of, 252–265, *254–265*
edema of, 252, *254*
structure of, 251–252
cysts of, 254–255, *258–260,* 263–264, *264*
degenerative changes of, 264–265, *265*
development of, 354
edema of, 248, *250,* 251, *251*
effusions of, follow-up, 243
in trauma, 248, *248–250*
entrapment syndrome of, 271
examination techniques for, 235–236, *236*
intra-articular disease of, 238
loose bodies in, 252–254, *255–257,* 265–266, *266–268*
Large synovial joints (*Continued*)
nerve lesions of, 271–275, 271b, *273, 274*
pannus of, 248–249, *251–253*
periarticular disease of, 266–275
septic arthritis of, 243–248, 243b, *244–247*
sonographic anatomy of, 236–238, *237–242*
tears of, 255–258, *260–263*
transient synovitis of, 238–243, *241*
venous pathology of, 271, *272*
Larsen syndrome, 293, *294, 295*
Larsen-Johansson syndrome, 200
Lateral collateral ligament, injury to, *172*
normal, *172*
Lateral malleolus, avulsion fracture of, 613, *613*
Ledderhose's disease, 73, *73, 359*
Leg lengthening, distraction callus with, 348, *348–350*
Legg-Calvé-Perthes disease, 349–352, *351*
hip effusion in, *241,* 243
vs. slipped capital femoral epiphysis, 295
Leptomyelolipoma, 311, 314
LHB. See *Long head of biceps tendon (LHB).*
Lidocaine, for soft tissue core biopsy, 449
Ligament(s), 171–191
anterior cruciate, *178*
disruption of, 595
sonographic examination of, 588
deltoid, rupture of, 180
examination technique for, 171
extra-articular, acute injury of, 175–187, *179–186,* 180b, 185b
chronic injury of, 187–191, *187–191*
fibulocalcaneal, rupture of, 177
fibulotalar, normal, *179*
rupture of, 177, *179*
healing of, 180–181
iliofemoral, *240*
intra-articular, pathology of, 175, *176–178*
lateral collateral, normal, *172*
rupture of, *172*
medial (tibial) collateral, bursitis in, *184,* 185
calcification of, 189–191, *189–191*
normal, 172–173, *173*
rupture of, *529*
acute, *173,* 181–185, *182–184*
after arthroscopy, *425*
chronic, 187–191, *187–191*
mechanism of, 227
sonographic examination of, 588
thickness of, 184
meniscofemoral, 172
meniscotibial, 172
nonunion of, 187–191, *187–191*

Ligament(s) (*Continued*)
normal sonographic structure of, 171–173, *172–175*
of ankle, 177–180, *179–181,* 180b, 609–610, *610*
of hand, collateral, sonographic examination of, 569–571
tears of, 548–551, *561–563*
of knee, *184*
posterior cruciate, normal, *176, 177, 237*
rupture of, *177, 178, 599*
sonographic examination of, 589
rupture of, acute, 175–187, *179–186,* 180b, 185b
anterior cruciate, 595
chronic, 187–191, *187–191*
deltoid, 180
fibulocalcaneal, 177
fibulotalar, 177, *179*
lateral collateral, *172*
medial (tibial) collateral, *529*
acute, *173,* 181–185, *182–184*
after arthroscopy, *425*
chronic, 187–191, *187–191*
mechanism of, 227
of hand, collateral, 548–551, *561–563*
pathophysiology of, 227–233, *233*
posterior cruciate, *177, 178, 599*
tibiofibular, 177–179, *180, 181, 610*
ulnar collateral, 185–187, 227, 549–551, *561*
acute, *185*
chronic, 185, *186*
with Panner's lesion, 521, *529*
with Stener lesion, 550, *562, 563*
scapholunate, avulsion of, 551, *564*
tibiofibular, rupture of, 177–179, *180, 181, 610*
sprain of, 177–179, *180, 181*
ulnar collateral, rupture of, 185–187, 227, 549–551, *561*
acute, *185*
chronic, 185, *186*
with Panner's lesion, 521, *529*
with Stener lesion, 550, *562, 563*
sonographic evaluation of, 569–571
Linear array(s), 3, *3*
Linear array transducers, 79
Lipohemarthrosis, 428, *430*
Lipoma(s), atypical, *366*
biopsy of, 453
intramuscular, *365*
intraspinal, 311–314, *312–315,* 315
of foot, 620, *620*
of subcutaneous tissues, *365, 366,* 367
Lipoma arborescens, *363,* 364
Lipomatosis, synovial, *450–451*
Lipomyelocele, 311
Lipomyelomeningocele, 311, *315*
Lipomyeloschisis, 311–314
Liposarcoma, myxoid, 364
Locking, of hip, 581–585, 582t, *583–585*
Long head of biceps tendon (LHB), 498–504
anatomy of, 498
bony spurs at, 502, *503*
displacement (dislocation) of, 498–499, 502–504, *503*
function of, 498
longitudinal view of, 465–466, *466*
luxation of, 91–95
normal, *79, 466,* 499
pathology of, 498–504
rupture of, 85–88, *89,* 499–500
distal, 194, *194, 195,* 526–528, *535*
full-thickness, *195, 499, 500,* 502
partial-thickness, *118,* 502, *502*
scanning technique for, *79,* 499
soft tissue restraint of, 498
subluxation of, 498–499, 502
tendonitis of, *501*
tenosynovitis of, 498
transverse imaging of, 465, *466*
Loose bodies, after meniscal surgery, *267*
cartilaginous, 252–254, *255–257*
in elbow, 517, *523–526*
classification of, 265–266
in ankle, 617–618, *618*
in Baker's cysts, 167, *167, 168,* 254, *256, 257, 266*
in biceps tendon sheath, 501, *501*
in bursae, 167, *167, 168*
in elbow, 517, *523–526,* 531
in knee, 599–601
in olecranon fossa, *257, 524*
in rheumatoid arthritis, 265, *266, 267*
osteochondral, in biceps tendon sheath, 501, *501*
steroid-related, 266, *268*
Luxation. See *Dislocation.*
Lyme arthritis, *436*
Lymph node, epitrochlear, *360*
Lymphedema, 329
Lymphoma, core biopsy of, *456–457*

Magic angle phenomenon, *95*
Magnetic resonance imaging (MRI), of shoulder, 512–513
Maisonneuve injury, 179
Malignant fibrous histiocytoma, *369*
Malignant melanoma, 325, *327*
Malleolus, medial, chronic bursitis over, *144*
Mallet finger, 546
Marginal erosions, in rheumatoid arthritis, 373–375, 376, *376–378,* 380
Medial collateral ligament (MCL), bursitis in, *184,* 185
calcification in, 189–191, *189–191*
Medial collateral ligament (*Continued*)
rupture of, *529*
acute, *173,* 181–185, *182–184*
after arthroscopy, *425*
chronic, 187–191, *187–191*
mechanism of, 227
sonographic examination of, 588
thickness of, 184
Medial malleolus, chronic bursitis over, *144*
Medial meniscectomy, pain syndromes after, *421, 424*
Medial retinaculum, avulsion fracture of, *595,* 596
tear of, 185, *185*
Median nerve, in carpal tunnel disease, *544, 545*
neurilemmoma of, *532–533*
normal, *529, 543, 544*
sonographic examination of, 564–567
Melanoma, malignant, 325, *327*
Meningocele, *318,* 318–320, *319*
Meniscal cyst, *593,* 593–594, *594*
Meniscal surgery, meniscal fragment after, *267*
Meniscectomy, medial, pain syndromes after, *421, 424*
Meniscocapsular separation, 596–597
Meniscofemoral ligament, 172
Meniscotibial ligament, 172
Meniscus(i), chondrocalcinosis of, *602*
cysts of, 258, 263–264, *264*
degenerative changes of, 264–265, *265*
discoid, *598*
normal, *237, 261*
sonographic examination of, 256–258, 588, 599
tears of, 255–258, *261–263, 600–601*
bucket handle, 258, *262*
horizontal, 258
longitudinal, 258, *262*
radial, 258, *263*
Meralgia paresthetica, *584,* 585
Mesenchymal syndrome, 226
Mesothelioma, core biopsy of, *455*
Metal, as foreign body, *394,* 395, *398, 400,* 402–405, *404,* 611, *612*
comet tail artifact due to, 12–14, *14, 15, 400*
Metaphyseal corner fracture, of tibia, 299, *299*
Metatarsal head, Freiberg infraction of, *343*
Metatarsalgia, 620–622, 621t, *622*
Mirror image artifact, *16,* 17
Monopty biopsy system, 449
Morton's neuromas, 274–275, 620–622, 621t, *622*
Motion artifact, 21
MRI (magnetic resonance imaging), of shoulder, 512–513
Mucoid cysts, of fingers, 555
Muscle(s), 23–73
abdominal, rupture of, *36, 37*

Muscle(s) (*Continued*)
adductor, strain of, 580, *580*
adductor magnus, pyomyositis of, *52*
anisotropy of, *19*
anterior tibial, hernia of, *64, 66*
biceps, contusion of, *37*
boundary lesions of, 30, 61–73
calf, contusion of, *39*
cyst of, *45*
hematoma of, *40*
muscle-aponeurosis avulsion of, 61–64, *62, 63*
rupture of, *40*
healing of, *41, 42*
contusion of, 36–39, *37–40*
cramps of, 30
cyst of, after muscle rupture, 42, *45*
enhanced through-transmission with, *13*
delayed soreness of, 30
deltoid, herniation of, *482,* 483
edema of, 52, *53*
examination techniques for, 23–26, *24, 25*
gastrocnemius, cyst of, *45*
hematoma of, *40*
hernia of, *65*
muscle-aponeurosis avulsion of, 61–63, *62*
rupture of, *40, 194*
healing of, *41, 42*
vs. Achilles tendon rupture, 609
gluteus, healing of rupture of, *44*
herniation of, 64–67, *64–68*
anterior tibial, *64, 66*
deltoid, *482,* 483
epigastric, *66*
gastrocnemius, *65*
tibialis anterior, *64, 66*
iliopsoas, contusion of, *38*
strain of, 580, *581*
in compartment syndrome, 52–56, *53–57*
in runner's knee, 69–71, *71, 72*
in shin splints, 67, *68–70*
infarction of, 54, *54*
diabetic, *58–59,* 59–60, *61*
infraspinatus, sonography of, *468,* 468–469, *469*
internal oblique, rupture of, *36*
ischemia of, 52, *54,* 55
myositis of, 46–52, *51, 52*
myositis ossificans of, *25,* 43–46, *46–51,* 46b
acoustic shadowing with, *10*
necrosis of, 57–61, 57b, *58–61,* 59b
diabetic, *58–59,* 59–60, *61*
normal sonographic anatomy of, 26–29, *26–29*
pathology of, 29–73
intramuscular, 29–61
value of ultrasound for, 23, 23b
pectoral, pyogenic myositis of, *51*
pectoralis major, elongation injury of, *32*
Muscle(s) (*Continued*)
pseudomasses of, 27–29, *29*
quadriceps, hematoma of, *39*
rectus, gelosis of, *47, 48*
myositis ossificans of, *48*
rupture of, complete, *35*
healing of, *42–45*
partial, *34*
volume loss after, *44*
rhabdomyolysis of, 57–61, 57b, *58–61,* 59b
rupture of, 30–35, *31–37*
abdominal, *36, 37*
calf, *40*
healing of, *41, 42*
common sites of, 30, *34*
complete, *31,* 34–35, *35–37*
compression, 30, *31*
distraction, 30–35, *31*
elongation type of, *31,* 31–32, *32*
etiology of, 193
gastrocnemius, *40, 194*
healing of, *41, 42*
vs. Achilles tendon rupture, 609
gluteus, *44*
hamstring, healing of, *43*
partial-thickness, *33, 34*
healing of, 40–42, *41–45*
hematoma with, 35–36, 37, *39*
internal oblique, *36*
partial, *31,* 32–34, *33–34*
pathophysiology of, 193
rectus, complete, *35*
healing of, *42–45*
partial, *34*
volume loss after, *44*
signs and symptoms of, 31
soleus, *40*
healing of, *41*
transverse abdominis, *36*
vastus intermedius, *35, 36*
vastus lateralis, *31*
semitendinosus, muscle-aponeurosis avulsion of, *63*
soleus, contusion of, *39*
cyst of, *45*
hematoma of, *40*
muscle-aponeurosis avulsion of, 61–64, *62, 63*
rupture of, *40*
healing of, *41*
strain of, adductor, 580, *580*
iliopsoas, 580, *581*
tibialis anterior, hernia of, *64, 66*
transverse abdominis, rupture of, *36*
vastus intermedius, complete rupture of, *35, 36*
myositis ossificans of, *46, 49–51*
vastus lateralis, compressive rupture of, *31*
Muscle cramps, 30
Muscle tissue, accessory, 27–29, *29*
Muscle-aponeurosis avulsion, 61–64, *62, 63*
Musculotendinous tear, 198, *198*
Mycobacterium, in joint fluid, 440
Mycotic aneurysms, 271
Myelomeningocele, 311, *316,* 318–320, *320*
Myeloschisis, 311, 318
Myonecrosis, diabetic, *58–59,* 59–60, *61*
Myositis, 46–52, *51, 52*
bacterial (pyogenic), 47–52, *51, 52*
core biopsy of, *454*
diabetic, *58–59, 569*
of hip, 577–578
vs. rhabdomyolysis, 61
defined, 46
subcutaneous and fascial changes in, 60, *60*
viral, 46–47
Myositis ossificans, 43–46, 367, *369*
acoustic shadowing with, *10*
calcification in, 43–44, *49–51*
congenital, 44–46
defined, 43
extended field of view imaging of, *25*
gelosis in, 43, *47, 48*
signs and symptoms of, 43, 46b
stages of, 43–44, *46–51*
vs. heterotopic bone formation, 44
vs. parosteal sarcoma, 44
zonal phenomenon in, *46, 49*
Myositis ossificans progressiva, 44–46

Navicular, synchondrosis of, ruptured, 615, *617*
Necrosis, muscle, 57–61, 57b, *58–61,* 59b
diabetic, *58–59,* 59–60, *61*
Needles, as foreign bodies, *394,* 395, *398, 400*
for biopsy, 428, *429*
of bone, 459
synovial, 449–453
Neisseria gonorrhoeae, hip infection due to, 574
in joint fluid, 439, *442*
Neonates. See *Child(ren).*
Neoplasia. See *Tumor(s).*
Neovascularity, with rotator cuff tear, 206, *216*
Nerve(s), of elbow, 521, *529, 530*
Nerve entrapment, 273–274
Nerve lesions, 271–275, 271b, *273, 274*
Neurilemmoma, median nerve, *532–533*
of elbow, 524, 524b, *532–534*
Neurofibroma(s), 360–363, *362*
in popliteal fossa, 271, *274*
of elbow, 521, 524–525, 524b
plexiform, 525
Neurofibrosarcomas, of elbow, 525
Neuroma(s), after arthroscopy, 421, *422*
Morton's, 274–275, 620–622, 621t, *622*
traumatic, of ulnar nerve, 521, *530–531*
Newborns. See *Child(ren).*

Nodules, rheumatoid, 388, *390*
Nonunion, of ligaments, 187–191, *187–191*
Norplant contraceptive devices, ultrasound-guided removal of, *405,* 406–407

Obese patients, seroma in, 431, *432*
Occult fractures, in children, 298–299, *299*
Olecranon bursa, bursitis of, acute, *138*
chronic, *145*
septic, *152*
Olecranon fossa, loose body in, *257, 524*
sonographic examination of, 531
Orthographic transmission ultrasound, 344
Orthopedic implants, 407–414
acute complications of, *406–409,* 407–409
chronic complications of, 409–414, *410–416*
hyperemia with, 414, *415*
infection due to, 409–412, *410–413,* 414, *443*
loosening of, 412–414, *414, 415*
soft tissue erosion due to, 414, *416*
Os naviculare, 615, *617*
Osgood-Schlatter disease, 200, *200*
Osseous callus, 344
Osteoarticular amyloidosis, *364,* 364–365, *365*
Osteochondral defects, 252
Osteochondral fractures, 232, *233*
Osteochondral loose bodies, in biceps tendon sheath, 501, *501*
Osteochondritis dissecans, 252, *254*
Osteochondromatosis, synovial, 562, *568*
OSTEOCUT needle, 459
Osteomyelitis, 333–336
acute, *331,* 333, *334*
chronic, 333–336, *335*
in children, 298, *299,* 333
Osteophytes, impingement by, *503*
of tibialis posterior tendon, 614, *616*
Oxymorphone, for core biopsy, of bone, 454
of soft tissue, 449

Paget's disease, periosteal thickening in, 336–337, *339*
Pain, after arthroscopy, 419–426
diagnostic, 425–426
therapeutic, 419–425, *421–425*
ankle, 611–618
joint and anterior, 617–618, *618*
lateral, 612–614, *613, 614*
medial, 614–616, *615–617*
posterior, 616–617, *617*
heel, 619–620, *621*
Pain (*Continued*)
hip, 573–580
due to abscesses, hematomas, and seromas, 577–578, *578, 579*
due to bursitis, *576,* 576–577, *577*
due to joint effusion, 573–575, 574t, *575,* 575t
due to muscle and tendon pathology, 578–580, *579–581*
due to synovitis, 576
knee, chronic localized, *596,* 598–599
Palmar fibrosis, 562
Palpation, sonographic, 26, 342
Panner's disease, 517, *527–528*
Pannus, 248–249, 379
defined, 373
in subacromial-subdeltoid bursa, 155, *158*
of elbow, *252–253, 378*
of hip, *377*
of knee, *251*
of shoulder, *374, 377*
synovial, *375, 378, 388*
Paratenon, 77
Parker-Pearson needle, 453
Parosteal mass, wire localization of, *458–459*
Parosteal processes, 367
Parosteal sarcoma, *vs.* myositis ossificans, 44
Patella, dislocation of, *595,* 596
Patellar tendon, anisotropy of, *17*
chronic bursitis around, *146*
insertion tendinopathy of, *108,* 111–112
normal, *102*
rupture of, 127–128, 194, *197, 228*
after arthroscopy, 419, *421, 422*
refractile shadowing with, *12, 13*
sonographic examination of, 588
tendinitis of, 97–112
after arthroscopy, 419, *421*
differential diagnosis of, *108,* 110–112
focal thickening in, *106,* 107, *107*
global thickening in, *107,* 107–110
pathologic changes in, 97–110, *100, 102–104*
tendinosis of, *224, 225*
Pavlik harness, 291
PCL. See *Posterior cruciate ligament (PCL).*
Pectoral muscle, pyogenic myositis of, *51*
Pectoralis major, elongation injury of, *32*
Pectoralis tendon, tear of, 117, *120*
Pediatric patients. See *Child(ren).*
Pennate structure, *26–28,* 27
Periarticular complications, of rheumatoid disease, *385–390,* 385–391, 385t
Periarticular disease, 266–275
aneurysms as, 268–271, 268b, *269, 270*
nerve lesions as, 271–275, 271b, *273, 274*
popliteal entrapment syndrome as, 271
venous thrombosis as, 271, 271b
Periarticular ganglion, of elbow, *520,* 526
Periarticular swelling, of elbow, 526
Perimysium, 26
Periosteum, *331–339,* 333–337
in stress and hairline fractures, 336, *336, 337*
osteomyelitis of, *331,* 333–336, *334, 335*
thickening of, 333
in Paget's disease, 336–337, *339*
Periostitis, of tibia, *70*
Peripheral nerve lesions, 359–363, *361, 362*
Peripheral nerve tumors, of elbow, 521–526, 524b, *532–534*
Peritendinitis, Achilles, *111,* 112, *112*
Peritenon, *81*
Peroneal tendon sheath, ganglion of, *619*
Peroneus tendons, instability of, *198*
luxation of, 95, 97b, *99, 100*
normal, *199*
rupture of, 91, *98, 99,* 198–200, *199,* 614, *614*
sonographic examination of, 605–606
subluxation of, *612*
Phantom echoes, 17
Phleboliths, 367, *368*
Phlegmon, aspiration of, 432
Piezoelectric crystal, 4
Pigmented villonodular synovitis (PVNS), *363,* 364, 380, *610*
Pilonidal cyst, 310, *310*
Pixels, 5
Plantar fascia, rupture of, 71–73, *72, 73*
sonographic examination of, 607
Plantar fasciitis, 619–620, *620*
Plantar fibromatosis, 73, *73, 359*
Plantaris tendon, 608, *609*
Plastic foreign bodies, 395, *398, 401*
Plicae, normal, 238, *239*
thickened, *240*
Polyester vascular graft, *401*
Polyp, synovial, *380*
Popliteal aneurysms, 268b, *269, 270,* 590, *591*
Popliteal artery, 589
Popliteal cysts. See *Baker's cyst(s).*
Popliteal entrapment syndrome, 271
Popliteal fossa, hernia of, *65*
nerve lesions in, 271, *273, 274*
sonographic anatomy of, *237,* 589
Popliteal vein, 589
Popliteal venous thrombosis, 590, *592*
Popliteus canal, 589

Posterior cruciate ligament (PCL), normal, *176, 177, 237*
sonographic examination of, 589
tear of, *177, 178, 599*
Posterior tibial tendon (PTT). See *Tibialis posterior tendon.*
Poststenotic aneurysms, 268
Power Doppler, 5–6
Pregnancy, joint aspiration during, 441, *446*
Prepatellar bursa, 131–134, *133, 134*
bursitis of, *134*
chronic, *143*
hemorrhagic, *146, 147*
septic, *440*
Presurgical hookwire localization, *458–459,* 459–460
Prostheses, hip, 580–581
hyperemia with, 414, *415*
incisional drainage with, 581
infected, 409, *412, 413, 443*
joint effusions with, 580–581, *581, 582*
loosening of, *581*
normal, *442*
hyperemia with, 414, *415*
infection of, 409–412, *410–413,* 414, *443*
knee, 601, *602*
loosening of, 412–414, *414, 415*
soft tissue erosion due to, 414, *416*
Pseudoaneurysm(s), 268–270, *269*
arterial, after arthroscopy, 424
of hand, *541*
Pseudoganglion, of acromioclavicular joint, 488, *489*
Pseudomasses, of muscle, 27–29, *29*
Pseudothrombophlebitis, 162–165, *164, 165*
Pseudotumor, of upper arm, *358*
Psoriatic arthritis, 380
Psoriatic tenosynovitis, *553*
PTT (posterior tibial tendon). See *Tibialis posterior tendon.*
Pubic symphysis, instability of, 340, *342*
Pulse-echo imaging, 1
Purity, of sound, 4
PVNS (pigmented villonodular synovitis), *363,* 364, 380, *610*
Pyogenic myositis. See *Pyomyositis.*
Pyomyositis, 47–52, *51, 52*
core biopsy of, *454*
diabetic, *58–59, 569*
of hip, 577–578
vs. rhabdomyolysis, 61

Q factor, 4
Quadriceps muscle, hematoma of, *39*
Quadriceps tendon, rupture of, 126–127, *127, 128,* 194, *196*
sonographic anatomy of, *237,* 587

Radial arrays, 3, *3*
Reactive arthritis, *447*
Reactive inflammatory arthropathy, *447*
Reactive joint effusion, of elbow, *522*
Rectus muscle, gelosis of, *47, 48*
myositis ossificans of, *48*
rupture of, complete, *35*
healing of, *42–45*
partial, *34*
volume loss after, *44*
Reflection, of sound, 1–2, *2,* 2t
Reflectors, anisotropic, *16–19,* 17–18
Refractile shadowing, *9, 10–13*
Refraction, 2
Refraction artifact, 15, *15*
Regeneration, in healing of muscle rupture, 40
Reiter's disease, 380
Reparative granuloma, of synovium, *448–449*
Resolution, 5
Resonant frequency, 4
Retrocalcaneal bursa, bursitis of, *82*
frictional, *139, 140*
rheumatoid, *151*
vs. Achilles tendinitis, 112–113
with Achilles tendinosis, *110,* 112
distention of, 608
normal, *82*
sonographic examination of, 607
tendinobursitis of, *133*
Reverberation artifact, 15–17, *16*
comet tail, 12–14, *14, 15*
Rhabdomyolysis, 57–61, *58–61*
defined, 57
etiology of, 57, 57b, 59b
vs. pyomyositis, 61
Rheumatoid arthritis, 373–391
advanced, *378*
amyloid arthropathy in, *390,* 390–391
articular recesses in, 378, 379t
Baker's cysts in, 162–165, *163–165, 266, 379,* 385, *385, 386*
bony contours in, 337
bursitis in, *151,* 152–153, 379, 386
cartilage edema in, 376, 379, 380
complications of, 382–391
periarticular, *385–390,* 385–391, 385t
diagnosis of, 373–380, *375–380*
differential, 380–382, 380t, *381*
early, *374, 375–376, 376, 378*
effusion in, 376, *376–378*
follow-up of, 382, *383*
infection in, 382–385, *384*
intra-articular steroid therapy for, complications of, 391
joints affected by, 375, 376t
juvenile, *446*
loose bodies in, 265, *266, 267*
marginal erosions in, 373–375, 376, *376–378,* 380
of ankle, *388*
of elbow, *378, 521*
of foot, *377*
of hip, *377*
Rheumatoid arthritis (*Continued*)
of knee, *251, 379, 380, 383*
of posterior tibial tendon, 225
of shoulder, *374, 376, 377, 384, 389,* 506–508, *510*
of wrist, *386, 387*
pannus in. See *Pannus.*
rheumatoid nodules in, 388, *390*
rotator cuff tear with, 155
septic arthritis in, *381, 384*
sonography *vs.* arthrography of, 373, *374*
synechiae in, 379, *379*
synovial cysts in, *385,* 385–386, 385t, *386*
synovial proliferation in, 373, *374,* 375, *375, 379*
synovitis in. See *Rheumatoid synovitis.*
tendon ruptures in, 386–388, *389*
tenosynovitis in, 386–388, *386–388*
Rheumatoid nodules, 388, *390*
Rheumatoid synovitis, 378–379
follow-up of, *383*
of ankle, *388*
of foot, *87–88*
of knee, *379, 380*
of wrist, *387, 552–553*
Rib cage, abnormalities of, 354, *354, 355*
Rib cartilage, abnormalities of, 354, *354*
bifid, *354*
fracture of, 354, *355*
Ring down time, 4
Rotator cuff, absence of, 480, *480, 481*
adhesive capsulitis of, 155, *160*
anisotropy of, 202–203, *207*
clinical pathology of, 463–464
compression of, *483,* 483–484
edema of, 116–117, *119*
focal nonvisualization of, 481, *481*
herniation of deltoid muscle or subacromial-subdeltoid bursa in, *482,* 483
hypoechoic or anechoic cleft in, 481, *482*
in amyloid arthropathy, 509, *511*
limitations in sonography of, 486–487
tendinopathy of, 200–212, 201b
thickening of, 494–495, *495*
Rotator cuff arthropathy, 487–488, *488, 489,* 506
Rotator cuff interval, 485, *486*
Rotator cuff tear(s), 115–117, 477–488
arthropathy with, 487–488, *488, 489*
articular surface, 202, 477, *477, 478,* 479
artifacts *vs.*, 203, *208*
asymptomatic, 201, 209–210
bare area in, *215*
bony abnormalities *vs.*, 486

Rotator cuff tear(s) (*Continued*)
bursal fluid in, 153–155, *156–160, 493,* 493–494, *494*
bursal surface, 202, *205, 206,* 479
bursal thickening with, 203, *211, 218, 221*
calcific tendinitis *vs.*, 486
calcifications in, 203, *208*
cartilage sign in, 207, *221, 222, 485*
chronic, 116, 207–209, 495
classification of, 479
cortical changes in, *216*
critical zone in, *201,* 202–203, *208,* 464, 475
degenerative bony changes with, 203–207, *212–218, 220*
delamination in, *202,* 202–203, *203*
differential diagnosis of, 116–117, 210–211
earliest signs of, 202, *202*
epidemiology of, 116, 463–464
errors in sonographic interpretation of, 484–487, *486*
factors contributing to, 200–201, 212
full-thickness, 116, *118,* 207, 479
absence of rotator cuff in, 480, *480, 481*
bursal thickening in, *218, 221*
cartilage interface sign in, *221, 222*
compression of tendon in, *483,* 483–484
cortical irregularity of greater tuberosity in, 484
focal nonvisualization of rotator cuff in, 481, *481*
herniation of deltoid muscle or subacromial-subdeltoid bursa in, *482,* 483
horizontal, 207, *220, 221*
hypoechoic or anechoic cleft in cuff in, 481, *482*
longitudinal (vertical), 207, *221, 222*
osseous changes with, *213, 214, 217, 220*
primary signs of, 479–484, *480–483*
secondary signs of, 484, *484, 485*
tendon retraction in, *219*
hypervascularity with, 206, *216*
hypoechoic or anechoic, 202, *205, 206*
in men *vs.* women, 201
intrasubstance (intratendinous), *115–117,* 116, 479
mirror bone change in, *204*
normal anatomy mimicking, 485–486, *486*
partial-thickness, *201,* 202, 477–479
articular surface, 202, *203, 204,* 477, *477, 478,* 479
bursal surface, 202, *205, 206,* 479
criteria for, *477,* 477–478, *478*
intratendinous, *115–117,* 116, 479

Rotator cuff tear(s) (*Continued*)
pathophysiology of, 200–212, 463–464
plain films of, 487
postoperative assessment of, 495–498, *496, 497*
primary signs of, 479–484, *480–483*
pseudomasses *vs.*, 28–29, *29*
recurrent, 495–498, *497*
refractile shadowing *vs.*, *11*
repair of, 495–498, *496*
secondary signs of, 203–207, *209–218,* 484, *484, 485*
sensitivity/specificity of ultrasound for, 487
soft tissue abnormalities *vs.*, 486
"stub" in, *204*
symptomatic, 201, 211–212
synovial thickening in, 203, *211*
synovitis with, 203, *209–211*
tendon retraction in, *219,* 480
with mixed echogenicity, 202, *203, 204*
with rheumatoid arthritis, 155
Runner's knee, *69–71, 71, 72*
Rupture, capsular, 185, *185*
after arthroscopy, 425, *425*
of knee, *596,* 598
dorsal hood, 546–547, *557, 558*
infraspinatus, 465
labral, 255, *260*
acetabular, 585, *585*
ligament, acute, 175–187, *179–186,* 180b, 185b
anterior cruciate, 595
chronic, 187–191, *187–191*
deltoid, 180
fibulocalcaneal, 177
fibulotalar, 177, *179*
healing of, 180–181
lateral collateral, *172*
medial (tibial) collateral, *529*
acute, 181–185, *182–184*
after arthroscopy, *425*
chronic, 187–191, *187–191*
mechanism of, 227
of hand, 548–551, *561–563*
pathophysiology of, 227–233, *233*
posterior cruciate, *177, 178, 599*
tibiofibular, 177–179, *180, 181, 610*
ulnar collateral, 185–187, 227, 549–551, *561*
acute, *185*
chronic, 185, *186*
with Panner's lesion, 521, *529*
with Stener lesion, 550, *562, 563*
medial retinaculum, 185, *185*
meniscal, 255–258, *261–263, 600–601*
muscle, 30–35, *31–37*
abdominal, *36, 37*
calf, *40*
healing of, *41, 42*

Rupture (*Continued*)
causes of, 30
common sites of, 30, *34*
complete, *31,* 34–35, *35–37*
compression, 30, *31*
distraction, 30–35, *31*
elongation type of, *31,* 31–32, *32*
etiology of, 193
gastrocnemius, *40, 194*
healing of, *41, 42*
vs. Achilles tendon rupture, 609
gluteus, *44*
hamstring, healing of, *43*
partial-thickness, *33, 34*
healing of, 40–42, *41–45*
hematoma with, 35–36, *37, 39*
internal oblique, *36*
partial, *31,* 32–34, *33–34*
pathophysiology of, 193
rectus, complete, *35*
healing of, *42–45*
partial, *34*
volume loss after, *44*
signs and symptoms of, 31
soleus, *40*
healing of, *41*
transverse abdominis, *36*
vastus intermedius, *35, 36*
vastus lateralis, *31*
navicular synchondrosis, 615, *617*
plantar fascia, 71–73, *72, 73*
sagittal band, 546
superior peroneal retinaculum, *100, 613*
tendon, Achilles, 117–126, *120–126*
acute, 608
chronic, 122–126, *125, 126,* 616–617
complete, *121–123, 227,* 608, *608*
differential diagnosis of, 608–609
healing, 122, *124*
musculotendinous, 198, *198*
partial, *226*
plantaris tendon in, 608, *609*
re-, *125*
biceps, 85–88, *89,* 499–500
distal, 194, *194, 195*
full-thickness, *195, 499, 500,* 502
partial-thickness, *118,* 502, *502*
creeping, 201
due to chronic overuse, 224–227, *229–232*
due to degeneration, 200–212
due to tendinosis, 221–224
etiology of, 194–198
extensor, of fingers, 546, 547, *554, 556–557*
extensor carpi radialis longus, *555*
extensor carpi ulnaris, 547–548, *559*
extensor pollicis longus, *554*
factors predisposing to, 198

Rupture (*Continued*)
flexor, of elbow, *186*
of wrist, 541–542, *546, 547*
flexor hallucis longus, 616
hamstring, full-thickness, 579
healing of, *43*
partial-thickness, *33, 34,* 579
in children and adolescents, 200
in rheumatoid arthritis, 386–388, *389*
infraspinatus, 465
musculotendinous, 198
patellar, 127–128, 194, *197*
after arthroscopy, 419, *421, 422*
refractile shadowing with, *12, 13*
pathophysiology of, 194–200
pectoralis, 117, *120*
peroneal, 91, *98, 99,* 198–200, *199,* 614, *614*
quadriceps, 126–127, *127, 128,* 194, *196*
rotator cuff. See *Rotator cuff tear(s).*
sites of, 198–200
subscapularis, 465, *483,* 484
superficial biceps femoris, *33*
supraspinatus, *115–118*
bursal fluid in, *157*
full-thickness, *213, 220*
horizontal, *220*
partial-thickness, *218, 477*
re-, *497*
tibialis anterior, 618
tibialis posterior, 88–91
acute, 90–91
chronic, 614
complete, 88–91, *90, 92, 228, 231,* 614
late-stage, 91, *92*
longitudinal, *231, 232,* 614–615, *616*
partial, 91, *93–97, 230,* 614, *615*
presentation of, 88, 89b
transverse, *229*
with bony spur or osteophyte, 614, *616*
triceps, 528, *536*
with synovial sheath, 85–91, *89–99,* 89b
without synovial sheath, 115–128, *115–128*

Sacral cutaneous dimple, 311
Sagittal band rupture, 546
Salter-Harris 1 fracture-dislocation, of hip, 294–295
of humerus, *292, 293*
Salter-Harris 2 fracture, 299, *299*
Sarcoma(s), fibro-, *362*
lipo-, myxoid, 364
neurofibro-, of elbow, 525
of elbow, 526
neurofibro-, 525
parosteal, *vs.* myositis ossificans, 44
synovial, 364, 367
Scapholunate ganglion, 539
Scapholunate ligament, avulsion of, 551, *564*
Scar formation, after muscle rupture, 40–42, *43–45*
Scattering, 5
SCFE (slipped capital femoral epiphysis), 294–295
Schwannoma(s), 360, *361*
in popliteal fossa, 271, *273*
of elbow, 521–525, 524b, *532–534*
Second harmonic, 6
Sector scanners, 3, *3*
Semitendinosus muscle, muscle-aponeurosis avulsion of, *63*
Septic arthritis, 243–248, 243b, *244–247*
aspiration of, *443*
due to intra-articular steroid therapy, 391
in children, 296, *298*
in rheumatoid arthritis, *381, 384*
of ankle, *443*
of hip, *444*
of shoulder, 243, *247, 381, 384,* 490–491, *491*
vs. transient synovitis, 242–243
Septic bursitis, *152,* 152–153, *153,* 495
Septic tenosynovitis, *85, 404, 444, 550, 611*
Seroma(s), 333
aspiration of, 431, *432*
of hip, 578, *579*
post-traumatic, enhanced through-transmission with, *14*
Shadowing, 9–10, *10–13*
Sharpey's fibers, 27, 194
Shin splints, 67, *68–70*
Shoulder, 463–513
acromioclavicular joint inflammation of, 490–491, *491*
adhesive capsulitis of, 155, *160,* 504–505, *505*
brisement procedure for, 446
joint fluid in, 473, *474*
amyloidosis of, *250,* 508–511, *511, 512*
osteoarticular, *364,* 364–365, *365*
anatomical variations in, 511–512
arthropathy of, 506
clinical pathology of, 463–465
dislocation of, 506
dynamic scanning of, 472–473
effusion of, 507
fracture-dislocation of, *292,* 293
fractures of, greater tuberosity, 491, *492*U
occult, 340–342
impingement of, 474–476
by osteophyte, *503*
defined, 464
plain radiography of, *464*
stages of, 116–117, 465, 474–476
subacromial, 155, *159,* 476, 494
Shoulder (*Continued*)
subacromial-subdeltoid bursitis in, 474–475, *475*
with rotator cuff edema, 116, *119*
infection of, *384*
instability of, 473, *473,* 505–506, *507–509*
joint fluid in, 473–474, *474,* 500–501, *501*
labral tear of, 255, *260*
plain radiography of, 463, *464*
postoperative assessment of, 495–498, *496, 497*
rheumatoid arthritis of, *374, 376, 377, 384, 389,* 506–508, *510*
rotator cuff tears of. See *Rotator cuff tear(s).*
septic arthritis of, 243, *247, 381, 384*
sonographic anatomy of, 236–238
subacromial-subdeltoid bursa of. See *Subacromial-subdeltoid bursa.*
suprascapular ganglia of, 255, *258–260*
suprascapular nerve compression of, 491
tendinitis of, *476,* 476–477
calcific, 488–490, *489*
tendinopathy of, 477
ultrasound examination of, examination technique for, 235–236, *236*
instrumentation for, 465
patient position for, 465–473, *466–473*
reporting of, 512
technique of, 465–473
vs. arthrography, 513
vs. MRI, 512–513
Shrug position, 472
Siescape imaging, *24,* 24–25, *25*
Sinus, dermal, 310, *311*
Skin, 325, *326*
Slipped capital femoral epiphysis (SCFE), 294–295
Snapping, of hip, 581–585, 582t, *583–585*
Snuff box ganglion, *538,* 539
aspiration of, *437*
Soft tissue, aspiration of, 428–438, *429*
with abscess and phlegmon, 431–432
with calcium deposits, *429,* 432, *433–434*
with cellulitis, 434, *435*
with hematoma, 428–431, *430, 431*
with seroma, 431, *432*
erosion of, due to orthopedic implants, 414, *416*
injection of, 442–446
masses of, core biopsy of, 453–454, *454*
of ankle and foot, 619, *619, 620*

Soleus, contusion of, *39*
cyst of, *45*
hematoma of, *40*
muscle-aponeurosis avulsion of, 61–63, *62, 63*
rupture of, *40*
healing of, *41*
Sonographic palpation, 26, 342
Sonography. See *Ultrasound imaging.*
Soreness, delayed muscle, 30
Sound, purity of, 4
reflection of, 1–2, *2,* 2t
speed of, through various substances, 2t
Sound beam, divergence of, 5
zones of, 4, *4*
Speed of sound artifact, 18–20, *20*
Spigelian hernias, *66, 67, 68*
Spina bifida, 311
Spinal canal, in children, 299–320
filum terminale of, *317,* 318, *318*
hydromyelia of, *317,* 318
masses of, 300, *300, 301*
meningocele and myelomeningocele of, 318–320, *319, 320*
normal anatomy of, 301–310, *302–311*
normal variants of, 315–318, *316, 317*
sonographic technique for, 301–310, *302–311*
tethered spinal cord in, 310–315, *312–315*
use of sonography of, 299–301, *300, 301*
vertebral anomaly of, 301, *301*
Spinal cord, oscillation of, 314–315
tethered, 310–315, *312–315*
Spinous processes, in infant, 303–304, *308*
Splinters, 395, *396, 399,* 399–402, *403, 611*
Sprain(s), ankle. See *Ankle sprain.*
of acromioclavicular joint, 490
Spurs, of long head of biceps tendon, 502, *503*
of tibialis posterior tendon, 614, *616*
Standoff cushion, 26
Staphylococcus aureus, hip infection due to, 574
Staple, surgical, intra-articular migration of, *406*
Stener lesion, 550, *562, 563*
Sternoclavicular joint, dislocation of, *341*
infected, *439*
Steroid therapy, intra-articular, destructive changes due to, 391
loose bodies due to, 266, *268,* 391
septic arthritis due to, 391
Strain, adductor, 580, *580*
hamstring, 579
iliopsoas, 580, *581*
Stress fracture, 336, *337*
Subacromial-subdeltoid bursa, *132,* 492–495
arthropathies of, 494–495, *495*
bursitis of, calcific, 146, *148–151*
hemorrhagic, 494
in impingement syndrome, 474–475, *475*
septic, *153*
traumatic, *141*
communicating abnormalities of, 493–494
fluid in, 153, *156–160, 210,* 492–493, *493, 494*
herniation of, 483
impingement in, 155, *159,* 476, 494
in amyloid arthropathy, 510, *512*
infiltrative disorders of, 494–495, *495*
noncommunicating distention of, 494–495, *495*
normal, *472*
pannus in, 155, *158*
sonographic views of, 471–472, *472*
thickening of, 203, *211,* 494–495, *495*
Subchondral fracture, *340*
Subcutaneous abscess, 329–330
in diabetic, *568*
Subcutaneous hemorrhage, *330*
Subcutaneous tissue, lipomas of, *365, 366,* 367
measurement of, 325
normal, 325, *326*
pathology of, 325–333, *327–331*
Subdeltoid bursa. See *Subacromial-subdeltoid bursa.*
Subluxation, 340
of humeral head, 480, *480,* 488
of long head of biceps tendon, 498–499, 502
of peroneus tendon, *612*
of posterior tibial tendon, 225, *232*
of ulnar nerve, 521, *531*
Subperiosteal hemorrhage, *332–333, 338–339*
Subscapularis tendon, longitudinal view of, 467
tears of, 465, *483,* 484
transverse view of, 466–467, *467*
Superficial biceps femoris tendon, partial rupture of, *33*
Superior peroneal retinaculum, rupture of, *100, 613*
Suprapatellar bursa, loose bodies in, *256*
sonographic anatomy of, *133, 237, 239,* 587–588
Suprapatellar plica, normal, 238, *239*
thickened, *240*
Suprascapular ganglia, 255, *258–260*
Suprascapular nerve, compression (entrapment) of, 491
Supraspinatus fossa, suprascapular ganglion of, *259, 260*
Supraspinatus tendon, clinical pathology of, 464
comparison views of, 474
critical zone of, *201,* 202–203, *208,* 464, 475
edema of, 116–117, *119*
longitudinal hyperextended internal rotation view of, 474, *474*
longitudinal partial internal rotation (shrug position) view of, 472
normal, *470, 471*
retraction of, *219*
rupture of, *115–118*
bursal fluid in, *157*
full-thickness, *213, 220*
horizontal, *220*
partial-thickness, *218, 477*
re-, *497*
tendinitis of, *476,* 476–477
calcific, 488, *489*
transverse hyperextended, internal rotation view of, 469–471, *470*
transverse partial internal rotation (shrug position) view of, 472
Surgery, hookwire localization prior to, *458–459,* 459–460
image guided, 460
meniscal, loose bodies after, *267*
tenosynovitis after, *612, 613*
Surgical staple, intra-articular migration of, *406*
Sutures, synovitis due to, 414, *416*
Swelling, of knee, 590–594, *591–594*
Synchondrosis, of navicular, ruptured, 615, *617*
Synechiae, in rheumatoid arthritis, *379, 379*
Synovial amyloidosis, *452*
Synovial biopsy, 446–453, *447–452*
Synovial chondromatosis, 562, *568*
Synovial cysts, *385,* 385–386, 385t, *386*
after arthroscopy, *420,* 421–423, *422, 423*
of wrist and hand, 537–539, *538, 539–541*
Synovial edema, 248, *250,* 251, *251*
Synovial fibroma, 562, *567*
Synovial fluid, *80*
extravasation of, after arthroscopy, *420*
Synovial hyperemia, 135–136, *135–136*
Synovial hypertrophy, *375*
Synovial joints, large. See *Large synovial joints.*
Synovial lipomatosis, *450–451*
Synovial pannus, *375, 378, 388*
Synovial polyp, *380*
Synovial proliferation, differential diagnosis of, 380, 380t
in rheumatoid arthritis, 373, *374,* 375, *375, 379*
Synovial sarcoma, 364, 367

Synovial sheath, 77, *80,* 81
tendons with, *80,* 82–95
tendons without, *81,* 95–128
Synovial thickening, in rheumatoid arthritis, 378
in rotator cuff tear, 203, *211*
Synovial thickness, total, *251*
Synovianalysis, 453
Synovioma, benign, within Baker's cyst, *165,* 167
Synovitis, *Candida parapsilosis,* 447
crystal-related, *155*
due to sutures, 414, *416*
gonococcal, *244–245*
hydroxyapatite, *149–151,* 151
iliopsoas bursa in, 153, *154, 155*
metal-induced, 405
of ankle, 618
of elbow, *521*
of hip, 576
pigmented villonodular, *363,* 364, 380, *610*
proliferative, differential diagnosis of, 380, 380t
in rheumatoid arthritis, 373, *374,* 375, *375, 379*
rheumatoid, 378–379
follow-up of, *383*
of ankle, *388*
of foot, *87–88*
of knee, *379, 380*
of wrist, *387, 552–553*
thorn-induced, 402, *403*
transient (toxic), 238–243, *241*
uric acid-related, *495*
with rotator cuff tear, 203, *209–211*
wood-induced, 402, *403*
Synovium, hyperechoic foci within, 151b
reparative granuloma of, *448–449*
Syringohydromyelia, *316,* 318

Talus, vertical, 295, *296*
Tarsal tunnel syndrome, 615–616
Tear. See *Rupture.*
Tendinitis. See also *Tendinopathy; Tendinosis.*
Achilles, 112–113
calcifying, *105*
differential diagnosis of, 112–113, *113–115*
distal, *110,* 112
peri-, *111,* 112, *112*
proximal, *108, 109,* 112
acute, *80,* 82–84, *83–85*
calcific, *97,* 488–490
aspiration of, 432, *433–434,* 490
clinical presentation of, 488–489
natural history of, 488–489
of Achilles tendon, *105*
of elbow, *519*
of supraspinatus tendon, *489*
"slurry," 489, 490
stages of, 489, 490
types of, 489–490
vs. rotator cuff tear, 486, 488
Tendinitis (*Continued*)
chronic, 85
De Quervain's, 84–85, *86*
differential diagnosis of, 85, *87–88*
extensor carpi radialis, 115
flexor hallucis longus, *616*
iliopsoas, 585
of elbow, 531
calcific, *519*
of hamstring, *579,* 579–580
of shoulder, *476,* 476–477
calcific, 488–490, *489*
patellar, 97–112
after arthroscopy, 419, *421*
differential diagnosis of, *108,* 110–112
focal thickening in, *106,* 107, *107*
global thickening in, *107,* 107–110
pathologic changes in, 97–110, *100, 102–104*
peri-, Achilles, *111,* 112, *112*
subacute, 84–85, *86*
supraspinatus, *476,* 476–477
calcific, 488, *489*
tibialis anterior, 618, *618*
tibialis posterior, *80*
vs. rheumatoid synovitis, 85, *87–88*
with synovial sheath, 82–85, *83–88*
without synovial sheath, 95–115, *100–115*
Tendinobursitis, retrocalcaneal, *133*
Tendinopathy. See also *Tendinitis; Tendinosis.*
insertion, Achilles, 113
of patellar tendon, *108,* 111–112
rotator cuff, 200–212, 201b, 477
Tendinosis. See also *Tendinitis; Tendinopathy.*
Achilles, *101,* 221–223, *223,* 617, *617*
distal, *110,* 112
proximal, *108, 109,* 112
with hypercholesterolemia, 112, *113–114*
flexor carpi radialis, *101*
of elbow, 115, 225–227
of hamstring, *579,* 579–580
patellar, *224, 225*
pathophysiology of, 221–224
tibialis anterior, 618, *618*
tibialis posterior, 225, *229–232*
with hypercholesterolemia, 112, *113–114*
Tendon(s), 77–128
Achilles, frictional bursitis of, *139, 140*
insertion of, 81, *82*
insertion tendinopathy of, 113
refractile shadowing of, *11*
rupture of, 117–126, *120–126*
acute, 608
chronic, 122–126, *125, 126,* 616–617
complete, *121–123, 227,* 608, *608*
Tendon(s) (*Continued*)
differential diagnosis of, 608–609
healing, 122, *124*
musculotendinous, 198, *198*
partial, *226*
plantaris tendon in, 608, *609*
re-, *125*
sonographic anatomy of, *81,* 607
tendinitis of, 112–113
calcifying, *105*
differential diagnosis of, 112–113, *113–115*
distal, *110,* 112
peri-, *111,* 112, *112*
proximal, *108, 109,* 112
tendinosis of, *101,* 221–223, *223,* 617, *617*
distal, *110,* 112
proximal, *108, 109,* 112
with hypercholesterolemia, 112, *113–114*
anterior tibial, anisotropy of, *18*
biceps, anatomy of, 498
bony spurs of, 502, *503*
displacement of, 502–504, *503*
function of, 498
longitudinal view of, 465–466, *466*
luxation of, 91–95
normal, *79, 466,* 499
pathology of, 498–504
rupture of, 85–88, *89,* 499–500
distal, 194, *194, 195,* 526–528, *535*
full-thickness, *195, 499, 500,* 502
partial-thickness, *118,* 502, *502*
scanning technique for, *79*
soft tissue restraint of, 498
tendonitis of, *501*
tenosynovitis of, 498
transverse imaging of, 465, *466*
chronic overuse of, 224–227, *229–232*
degeneration of, 200–212
erosion of, by orthopedic devices, 414, *416*
extensor, of ankle and foot, 605, 618
of fingers, dislocation of, 546–547
laceration of, 547, *559*
tears of, 546, 547, *554, 556–557*
of wrist, dysfunction of, 544–547, *552–557*
rheumatoid synovitis of, *552–553*
tendinitis of, 115
tenosynovitis of, *83, 84*
extensor carpi radialis, tendinitis of, 115
extensor carpi radialis brevis, ganglion of, *538*
extensor carpi radialis longus, rupture of, *555*

Tendon(s) (*Continued*)
extensor carpi ulnaris, rupture of, 547–548, *559*
sonographic examination of, 567
tenosynovitis of, *560–561*
extensor pollicis longus, rupture of, *554*
tenosynovitis of, *386, 387*
flexor, of elbow, rupture of, *186*
of wrist, anisotropy of, *16*
normal, *546*
rupture of, 541–542, *546, 547*
tenosynovitis of, 531, 542, *550*
flexor carpi radialis, anisotropy of, *16*
ganglion of, *542*
tendinosis of, *101*
flexor digitorum longus, pathology of, *616*
flexor hallucis longus, longitudinal split of, *616*
muscle-aponeurosis avulsion of, *62*
tendinitis of, 616
hamstring, 578–580
apophyseal avulsion of, 578–579
rupture of, full-thickness, 579
healing of, *43*
partial-thickness, *33, 34,* 579
site of injury of, 578–579
strain of, 579
tendinitis/tendinosis of, *579,* 579–580
iliopsoas, snapping of, 582, *583*
tendinitis of, 585
infraspinatus, rupture of, 465
sonography of, 469
luxation of, 91–95, 97b, *99, 100*
of ankle, Achilles. See *Tendon(s), Achilles.*
extensor, 605
lateral, 605–606
medial, 606, *607*
patellar, anisotropy of, *17*
chronic bursitis around, *146*
insertion tendinopathy of, *108,* 111–112
normal, *102*
rupture of, 127–128, 194, *197, 228*
after arthroscopy, 419, *421, 422*
refractile shadowing with, *12, 13*
sonographic examination of, 588
tendinitis of, 97–112
after arthroscopy, 419, *421*
differential diagnosis of, *108,* 110–112
focal thickening in, *106,* 107, *107*
global thickening in, *107,* 107–110
pathologic changes in, 97–110, *100, 102–104*
tendinosis of, *224, 225*
pectoralis, rupture of, 117, *120*

Tendon(s) (*Continued*)
peroneus, instability of, *198*
luxation of, 95, 97b, *99, 100*
normal, *199*
rupture of, 91, *98, 99,* 198, *199,* 614, *614*
sonographic examination of, 605–606
subluxation of, *612*
plantaris, 608, *609*
quadriceps, rupture of, 126–127, *127, 128,* 194, *196*
sonographic anatomy of, *237,* 587
rotator cuff. See *Rotator cuff.*
rupture of, Achilles, 117–126, *120–126*
acute, 608
chronic, 122–126, *125, 126,* 616–617
complete, *121–123, 227,* 608, *608*
differential diagnosis of, 608–609
healing, 122, *124*
musculotendinous, 198, *198*
partial, *226*
plantaris tendon in, 608, *609*
re-, *125*
biceps, 85–88, *89,* 499–500
distal, 194, *194, 195,* 526–528, *535*
full-thickness, *195, 499, 500,* 502
partial-thickness, *118,* 502, *502*
creeping, 201
due to chronic overuse, 224–227, *229–232*
due to degeneration, 200–212
due to tendinosis, 221–224
etiology of, 194–198
extensor, of fingers, 546, 547, *554, 556–557*
extensor carpi radialis longus, *555*
extensor carpi ulnaris, 547–548, *559*
extensor pollicis longus, *554*
factors predisposing to, 198
flexor, of elbow, *186*
of wrist, 541–542, *546, 547*
flexor hallucis longus, 616
hamstring, full-thickness, 579
healing of, *43*
partial-thickness, *33, 34,* 579
in children and adolescents, 200
in rheumatoid arthritis, 386–388, *389*
infraspinatus, 465
musculotendinous, 198
patellar, 127–128, 194, *197, 228*
after arthroscopy, 419, *421, 422*
refractile shadowing with, *12, 13*
pathophysiology of, 194–200
pectoralis, 117, *120*

Tendon(s) (*Continued*)
peroneus, 91, *98, 99,* 198, *199,* 614, *614*
quadriceps, 126–127, *127, 128,* 194, *196*
rotator cuff. See *Rotator cuff tear.*
sites of, 198–200
subscapularis, 465, *483,* 484
superficial biceps femoris, *33*
supraspinatus, *115–118*
bursal fluid in, *157*
full-thickness, *213, 220*
horizontal, *220*
partial-thickness, *218, 477*
re-, *497*
tibialis anterior, 618
tibialis posterior, 88–91
acute, 90–91
chronic, 614
complete, 88–91, *90, 92, 228, 231,* 614
late-stage, 91, *92*
longitudinal, *231, 232,* 614–615, *616*
partial, 91, *93–97, 230,* 614, *615*
presentation of, 88, 89b
transverse, *229*
with bony spur or osteophyte, 614, *616*
triceps, 528, *536*
with synovial sheath, 85–91, *89–99,* 89b
without synovial sheath, 115–128, *115–128*
sonographic anatomy of, 79–81, *80–82*
sonographic examination of, advantages of, *77, 78*
equipment for, 77–79, 79b
scanning technique for, *79, 79*
subscapularis, longitudinal view of, *467*
rupture of, 465, *483,* 484
transverse view of, 466–467, *467*
superficial biceps femoris, partial rupture of, *33*
supraspinatus, clinical pathology of, 464
comparison views of, 474
critical zone of, *201,* 202–203, *208,* 464, 475
edema of, 116–117, *119*
longitudinal hyperextended internal rotation view of, 474, *474*
longitudinal partial internal rotation (shrug position) view of, 472
normal, *470, 471*
retraction of, *219*
rupture of, *115–118*
bursal fluid in, *157*
full-thickness, *213, 220*
horizontal, *220*
partial-thickness, *218, 477*
re-, *497*

Tendon(s) (*Continued*)
tendinitis of, *476,* 476–477
calcific, 488, *489*
transverse hyperextended, internal rotation view of, 469–471, *470*
transverse partial internal rotation (shrug position) view of, 472
tendinitis of. See *Tendinitis.*
tibialis anterior, anisotropy of, *18*
pathology of, 618, *618*
tibialis posterior, *79*
normal, *80,* 606, *607*
overuse of, 225, *229–232*
rheumatoid arthritis of, 225
rupture of, 88–91
acute, *90–91*
chronic, 614
complete, 88–91, *90, 92, 228, 231,* 614
late-stage, 91, *92*
longitudinal, *231, 232,* 614–615, *616*
partial, 91, *93–97, 230,* 614, *615*
presentation of, 88, 89b
transverse, *229*
with bony spur or osteophyte, 614, *616*
sonographic examination of, 79, 606
subluxation of, 225, *232*
surface erosion of, *96*
tendinitis of, *80*
tendinosis of, 225, *229–232*
tenosynovitis of, *78, 83, 85, 90, 388, 613*
triceps, rupture of, 528, *536*
sonographic examination of, 531
with synovial sheath, *80,* 82–95
luxation of, 91–95, 97b, *99, 100*
rupture of, 85–91, *89–99,* 89b
tendinitis of, 82–85, *83–88*
without synovial sheath, *81,* 95–128
rupture of, 115–128, *115–128*
tendinitis of, 95–115, *100–115*
Tendon insertion, 81, *82*
Tendon sheath, fibroma of, 562, *567*
giant cell tumor of, 562, *566*
synovial chondromatosis of, 562, *568*
Tennis elbow, 115, 225–227, 517
Tennis leg, 63
Tenosynovitis, acute, *80,* 82–84, *83–85*
bicipital, 498, 500, *501*
chronic, *84,* 85
differential diagnosis of, 85, *87–88*
in rheumatoid arthritis, 386–388, *386–388*
of ankle, *388, 612*
postsurgical, *612*
septic, 611, *611*
of extensor carpi ulnaris, *560–561*
Tenosynovitis (*Continued*)
of extensor tendons of wrist, *83, 84, 386, 387, 537, 553*
of flexor tendons of wrist, 531, 542, *550*
of foot, *611*
of posterior tibial tendon, *78, 83, 85, 90, 388*
postsurgical, *613*
of wrist and hand, extensor, *83, 84, 386, 387, 537, 553*
flexor, 531, 542, *550*
psoriatic, *553*
septic, *85, 404, 444, 550, 611*
subacute, 84–85, *86*
vs. rheumatoid synovitis, 85, *87–88*
Tethered spinal cord, 310–315, *312–315*
Tethering, secondary, 319
TFC (triangular fibrocartilage), sonographic examination of, 567
tear of, *176,* 551–554
TFCC (triangular fibrocartilage complex), 567
Thompson test, 608
Thorns, as foreign bodies, 395, *398,* 402, *402, 403*
Three-dimension (3-D) sonography, 24
Thrombophlebitis, edema in, 329
pseudo-, 162–165, *164, 165*
Thrombosis, venous, 271, 271b
deep, 271, *272*
after arthroscopy, 423–424
popliteal, 590, *592*
with calcification, *429*
Thrombus, in tibiotalar joint, *250*
Through-transmission, enhanced, 10–12, *13, 14*
Thumb, gamekeeper's, 227, 229
Tibia, fracture of, healing of, 344, *344–347*
metaphyseal corner, 299, *299*
stress, *337*
osteomyelitis of, *331, 334*
periostitis of, *70*
subperiosteal hematoma of, *332–333*
Tibial collateral ligament. See *Medial collateral ligament (MCL).*
Tibial nerve, schwannoma of, *361*
Tibial torsion, 357–359, *358*
Tibialis anterior muscle, hernia of, *64, 66*
Tibialis anterior tendon, anisotropy of, *18*
pathology of, 618, *618*
Tibialis posterior tendon, normal, *80,* 606, *607*
overuse of, 225, *229–232*
rheumatoid arthritis of, 225
rupture of, 88–91
acute, 90–91
chronic, 614
complete, 88–91, *90, 92, 228, 231,* 614
late-stage, 91, *92*
Tibialis posterior tendon (*Continued*)
longitudinal, *231, 232,* 614–615, *616*
partial, 91, *93–97, 230,* 614, *615*
presentation of, 88, 89b
transverse, *229*
with bony spur or osteophyte, 614, *616*
sonographic examination of, 79, 606
subluxation of, 225, *232*
surface erosion of, *96*
tendinitis of, *80*
tendinosis of, 225, *229–232*
tenosynovitis of, *78, 83, 85, 90, 388*
postsurgical, *613*
Tibiofibular ligament, rupture of, 177–179, *180, 181, 610*
sprain of, 177–179, *180, 181*
Tibiotalar joint, acute pathology of, *610,* 610–611, *611*
impingement of, *181*
thrombus in, *250*
Time gain compensation, 5
Time of flight, 18
Tissue harmonic imaging, 6, *6*
Tissue sparing, 453
Total hip arthroplasty, 580–581
hyperemia with, 414, *415*
incisional drainage with, 581
infection with, 409, *412, 413, 443*
joint effusions with, 580–581, *581, 582*
loosening of, *581*
normal, *442*
Total knee arthroplasty, 601, *602*
Total synovial thickness (TST), *251, 383*
Toxic synovitis, 238–243, *241*
Transducer(s), for interventional ultrasound, 427
frequency of, 2–3
operating characteristics of, 4, *4*
types of, *3,* 3–4
Transient synovitis, 238–243, *241*
Transmission ultrasound, *6–7,* 344
Transverse abdominis muscle, rupture of, *36*
Trauma, effusions in, 248, *248–250*
Traumatic bursitis, acute, 136–139, *137–141*
chronic, *139,* 139–142, *141–146*
of communicating bursa, 167
Traumatic neuroma, of ulnar nerve, 521, *530–531*
Triangular fibrocartilage (TFC), sonographic examination of, 567
tear of, *176,* 551–554
Triangular fibrocartilage complex (TFCC), 567
Triceps tendon, sonographic examination of, 531
tear of, 528, *536*
Trigger finger, 544, *551*
Triradiate cartilage, 282, *284, 286*

Trochanteric bursa, bursitis of, *576,* 576–577
acute frictional, *138, 139*
hemorrhagic, *148*
Tru-Cut system, 449
TST (total synovial thickness), *251, 383*
Tumor(s), bone, *358–369,* 359–367
core biopsy of, 454–459, *455–457*
giant cell, of tendon sheath, 562, *566*
glomus, 325, 554–555, *565*
image guided ablation of, 460
of elbow, peripheral nerve, 521–526, 524b, *532–534*
of knee, 593
peripheral nerve, of elbow, 521–526, 524b, *532–534*
presurgical hookwire localization of, *458–459,* 459–460
pseudo-, *358*
soft tissue, *358–369,* 359–367
core biopsy of, 453–454, *454*

Ulna, hairline fracture of, *336*
Ulnar collateral ligament (UCL), rupture of, 185–187, 227, 549–551, *561*
acute, *185*
chronic, 185, *186*
with Panner's lesion, 521, *529*
with Stener lesion, 550, *562, 563*
sonographic evaluation of, 569–571
Ulnar nerve, *530*
sonographic examination of, 531
subluxation of, 521, *531*
traumatic neuroma of, 521, *530–531*
Ultrasonic geyser sign, 488, *489*
Ultrasonic volume imaging, 24
Ultrasound, frequency range of, 1
Ultrasound imaging, Doppler flow, 5–6
color, 5, 344
equipment for, *3,* 3–4, *4*
extended field of view, 6, *24,* 24–25, *25*
fundamental principles of, 1–3, *2,* 2t, *3*
gray scale, 4–5, 344
historical development of, 1
images in, 4–5
three-dimension (3-D), 24
tissue harmonic, 6, *6*
transmission, 6–7, 344
Unipennate structure, *26,* 27
Uric acid-related synovitis, *495*

Valium, for core biopsy, of bone, 454
of soft tissue, 449
Varices, refractile shadowing with, *10*
Vascular dissections, 270–271
Vascular grafts, infection due to, 330, *331*
infections due to, *401*
Vastus intermedius, complete rupture of, *35, 36*
myositis ossificans of, *46, 49–51*
Vastus lateralis, compressive rupture of, *31*
Venous thrombosis, 271, 271b
deep, 271, *272*
after arthroscopy, 423–424
popliteal, 590, *592*
with calcification, *429*
Vertebral anomaly, 301, *301*
Vertebral levels, estimation of, 306–309, *309*
Vertical talus, 295, *296*
Volume averaging, 20

Web spaces, of foot, 607
Wire localization, presurgical, *458–459,* 459–460
Wood, as foreign body, 395, *396, 399,* 399–402, *403, 611*
Wrist, 531–571
carpal tunnel syndrome of, *387,* 390–391, 531, 533b, 539–541, *542–545*
cellulitis of, *570–571*
chlamydia infection of, *246*
De Quervain's tendinitis of, 84–85, *86*
dynamic imaging of, 569
extensor tendons of, dysfunction of, 544–547, *552–557*
ganglion of, *538*
tendinitis of, 115
tenosynovitis of, *83, 84, 386, 387, 537*
flexor tendons of, anisotropy of, *16*
normal, *546*
tear of, 541–542, *546, 547*
tenosynovitis of, 531
ganglia of, 537–539, *538, 539–542*
gonococcal synovitis of, *244–245*
indications for scanning of, 531–564
rheumatoid arthritis of, *386, 387*
scapholunate ligament of, avulsion of, 551, *564*
technical guidelines and scanning techniques for, 564–571
tenosynovitis of, extensor, *83, 84, 386, 387, 537, 553*
flexor, 531, 542, *550*
triangular fibrocartilage tear in, *176,* 551–554

Zonal phenomenon, in myositis ossificans, *46, 49*

ISBN 0-323-00018-5